DEDICATION

To my children, Lauren, Kathryn, and Keith: May your future be increasingly bright with promise.

Barbara Hodgson

To all health care professionals who, in the expectation of little glory or material reward, dedicated themselves to the art and science of healing.

Robert Kizior

To my grandchildren and their future: Steven, Cheyenne, Dan, Tyler, and Nicholas.

Ruth Kingdon

NURSE'S DRUG HANDBOOK 1996

BARBARA B. HODGSON, RN

Drug Research Coordinator
Diabetes Center
University of South Florida
Tampa, Florida

ROBERT J. KIZIOR, BS, RPh

Education Coordinator
Department of Pharmacy
Alexian Brothers Medical Center
Elk Grove Village, Illinois;
Formerly, Adjunct Faculty
William Rainey Harper College
Palatine, Illinois

RUTH T. KINGDON, MSN, RN

Assistant Hospital Administrator
Kaiser Foundation Hospital
Fontana, California

W.B. SAUNDERS COMPANY

A Division of Harcourt Brace & Company

Philadelphia / London / Toronto / Montreal / Sydney / Tokyo

W.B. SAUNDERS COMPANY
A Division of Harcourt Brace & Company

The Curtis Center
Independence Square West
Philadelphia, Pennsylvania 19106

Library of Congress Cataloging-in-Publication Data

Hodgson, Barbara B.
Nurse's drug handbook 1996 / Barbara B. Hodgson, Robert J. Kizior, Ruth T. Kingdon.
p. cm.
Includes bibliographical references and index.
ISBN 0-7216-6377-X
1. Clinical pharmacology—Handbooks, manuals, etc. 2. Nursing——Handbooks, manuals, etc. I. Kizior, Robert J. II. Kingdon, Ruth T. III. Title.
[DNLM: 1. Drugs—handbooks. 2. Drugs—nurses' instruction. QV 39 H688n 1996]
RM125.H57 1995
615'.1—dc20
DNLM/DLC
for Library of Congress 95-21835
CIP

NURSE'S DRUG HANDBOOK 1996 ISBN 0-7216-6377-X

Printed in the United States of America.

Last digit is the print number: 9 8 7 6 5 4 3 2 1

ACKNOWLEDGMENTS

I offer a heartfelt thank you to my co-authors, Robert Kizior, RPh, and Ruth Kingdon, MSN, RN, for their superb work and incredible tenacity in this major endeavor; our nursing editor, Daniel Ruth, for his patience and friendship; and especially to Karl Schumann, Carolyn Steele, Anne Caplan, Deborah Kline, Jane and Mike Sperry, Greg Boyd, and Sherry and Tony Zemaitis for their unflagging support of me and my family when it was needed the most.

Barbara Hodgson

TO THE READER

Nurses and other health care practitioners face many challenges in today's environment, not the least of which is familiarity with a large volume of complex drugs. And drugs, like everything else in health care, keep changing! New applications of current drugs, new drugs to replace current drugs entirely, new routes—all this knowledge must be integrated into patient care in the limited time available. So this book was designed not just as a quick reference, but as a quick reference geared to the specific information needed in the clinical setting. Instructions on administration are detailed for each route. Side effects are given by *frequency* so the practitioner can focus on patient care without wading through a myriad of signs and symptoms. Nursing implications are organized as care is organized, that is, "What needs to be assessed/done before the first dose?" "What interventions and evaluations are needed during therapy?" and 'What explicit teaching is needed by patient/family?" These and other features are written for ease in understanding and application.

The authors of *Nurse's Drug Handbook* have carefully verified the dosages, administration, contraindications, and pregnancy category with officially accepted standards at the time of this publication. However, we recommend that the reader always check product information for such changes before administering any drug.

What separates this drug book from others is that it guides the user through patient care, from beginning to end. To better practice, to better care . . .

Barb, Bob, and Ruth

PREFACE

We are very pleased to present the 1996 edition of *NURSE'S DRUG HANDBOOK,* the most current and practical source of drug information for nurses available.

In this edition we have included 25 new drugs approved by the Food and Drug Administration to those previously listed in the Latest Drug Supplement (in the very back of the book), bringing the total number of drugs listed in the Supplement to 37. The Latest Drug Supplement offers the user a quick review and reference for the very latest medications available.

All drug entries in this edition have been reviewed and updated as appropriate to include new uses and dosages. As in the previous edition, dosages for the elderly are included in the entries where applicable, and the introductory pharmacokinetics section now comprises protein binding and half-life as well as absorption, distribution, metabolism, and elimination.

The classification section overviews 45 drug classifications, including opiate equi-analgesic equivalents. Additionally, the tables and grids of the classifications have been updated, reflecting new medications in the category (for example, anticonvulsants, antidepressants, and angiotensin-converting enzyme inhibitors).

The Appendix of the previous edition introduced the rate of administration of intravenous intermittent medications (piggybacks). This entry has been retained, along with those for commonly used abbreviations, the bibliography, calculation of drug dosages, explanations of controlled drug categories for Canada and the United States, normal laboratory values, FDA pregnancy categories, and signs and symptoms of toxic effects/adverse reactions.

PREFACE
to the First Edition

Every book has its own characteristics, and the following remarks are intended to familiarize the reader with this writing.

Classifications: Drugs are categorized by classification to help the reader organize drugs and quickly retrieve information on an entire group of drugs. Classifications are not intended to substitute for the more specific information available on individual drug monographs.

Pediatric usage: Dosage and recommendations for pediatric use are included. However, it should be noted that the content is generally directed toward the adult patient, and the practitioner needs to adapt some material for pediatric usage. For example, injection sites and amounts/rates of IV infusions are stated for adults and must be appropriately modified for the very young.

Elderly patients: There are cautions about specific drugs that may cause paradoxical reaction or require dosage reduction in elderly patients. In all cases, dosage in the older patient should be carefully evaluated, particularly if any known renal or hepatic limitations are superimposed.

Side effects/adverse reactions: For purposes of clarity, the authors have defined side effects as those responses that are more predictable with the drug, are generally not life threatening, and that may or may not require discontinuation of the drug. Adverse reactions/toxic effects, on the other hand, are very serious, often life threatening, undesirable responses that require prompt intervention.

Occasionally, when a drug produces no known side effects or major adverse reactions, "None significant" will appear.

Pregnancy/lactation: Additional information on drug use during pregnancy or lactation is given, expanding on the FDA Pregnancy Category. It is of the utmost importance that patients be asked about the possibility of pregnancy before any drug therapy is initiated. Ideally, no drugs would be administered during pregnancy, but there are situations that may demand a risk/benefit decision by the physician and patient.

Antineoplastic agents: Some general guidelines are provided for spills, extravasation, and other aspects of antineoplastic agents because of their toxic properties. These guidelines are not intended to supersede the organizational procedures required for therapy with highly toxic substances.

Allergies: Not enough can be said about obtaining an accurate history from the patient or family. Allergy, also referred to as hypersensitivity, to a drug is vital information to avoid preventable and potentially life-threatening reactions. Since the stress of the present illness may make people forget about previous drug reactions, it is recommended that the patient be asked about hypersensitivity every time a drug is being given.

Narcotic analgesics: While the practitioner should be alert to patients who present with drug abuse, it is important to note that narcotics given for short-term pain are not usually addicting. Unrelieved pain may require higher dosage or more frequent administration, and the practitioner should not hesitate to seek appropriate comfort measures. Medicating the patient for pain on a regular, uninterrupted schedule breaks the pain cycle and assists in better analgesia.

Because the patient with intractable pain of terminal cancer or other illness may develop an extremely high tolerance for a narcotic, it is still essential that pain relief be sought to the greatest degree possible, even though dosages may far exceed the "normal" range.

Each patient is an individual and, as such, may vary in needs and response to any medication. This book is intended to support the practitioner in assessment and intervention to achieve optimal care for each patient.

CONTENTS

NOTICE

Medicine is an ever-changing field. Standard safety precautions must be followed, but as new research and clinical experience broaden our knowledge, changes in treatment and drug therapy become necessary or appropriate. The editors of this work have carefully checked the generic and trade drug names and verified drug dosages to ensure that the dosage information in this work is accurate and in accord with the standards accepted at the time of publication. Readers are advised, however, to check the product information currently provided by the manufacturer of each drug to be administered to be certain that changes have not been made in the recommended dose or in the contraindications for administration. This is of particular importance in regard to new or infrequently used drugs. It is the responsibility of the treating physician, relying on experience and knowledge of the patient, to determine dosages and the best treatment for the patient. The editors cannot be responsible for misuse or misapplication of the material in this work.

THE PUBLISHER

acebutolol

ah-see-beaut´oh-lol
(Sectral)

CANADIAN AVAILABILITY:
Monitan, Sectral

CLASSIFICATION

Beta$_1$-adrenergic blocker

PHARMACOKINETICS

	ONSET	PEAK	DURATION
PO (hypotensive)	1-1.5 hrs	2-8 hrs	24 hrs
PO (antiarrhythmic)	1 hr	4-6 hrs	10 hrs

Well absorbed from GI tract. Protein binding: 25%. Undergoes extensive first-pass liver metabolism to active metabolite. Eliminated via bile, secreted into GI tract via intestine, excreted in urine. Removed by hemodialysis. Half-life: 3-4 hrs; metabolite: 8-13 hrs.

ACTION

Selectively blocks beta$_1$-adrenergic receptors, slowing sinus heart rate, decreasing cardiac output, decreasing B/P (exact mechanism unknown but may block peripheral adrenergic receptors, decrease sympathetic outflow from CNS or decrease renin release from kidney). Large dose may block beta$_2$-adrenergic receptors, increasing airway resistance. Exhibits antiarrhythmic activity, slowing AV conduction, increasing refractory period in AV node.

USES

Management of mild to moderate hypertension. Used alone or in combination w/diuretics, especially thiazide-type. Management of cardiac arrhythmias (primarily PVCs).

PO ADMINISTRATION

1. May be given w/o regard to meals.

INDICATIONS/DOSAGE/ROUTES

Mild to moderate hypertension:
PO: Adults: Initially, 400 mg/day in 1-2 divided doses. **Maintenance:** 200-800 mg/day.

Severe hypertension:
PO: Adults: Up to 1,200 mg/day given in 2 divided doses.

Ventricular arrhythmias:
PO: Adults: Initially, 200 mg q12h. Increase gradually up to 600-1,200 mg/day in 2 divided doses.

Usual elderly dosage:
PO: Elderly: Initially, 200-400 mg/day. **Maximum:** 800 mg/day.

Dosage in renal impairment:

CREATININE CLEARANCE	% OF NORMAL DOSAGE
<50 ml/min	50
<25 ml/min	25

PRECAUTIONS

CONTRAINDICATIONS: Overt cardiac failure, cardiogenic shock, heart block greater than first degree, severe bradycardia. **CAUTIONS:** Impaired renal or hepatic function, peripheral vascular disease, hyperthyroidism, diabetes, inadequate cardiac function, bronchospastic disease. **PREGNANCY/LACTATION:** Readily crosses placenta; distributed in breast milk. May produce bradycardia, apnea, hypoglycemia, hypothermia during delivery, small birth weight infants. **Pregnancy Category B.**

INTERACTIONS

DRUG INTERACTIONS: Diuretics, other hypotensives may increase hypotensive effect; sympathomimetics, xanthines may mutually inhibit effects; may mask symptoms of hypoglycemia, prolong hypoglycemic effect of insulin, oral hypoglycemics; NSAIDs may decrease antihypertensive effect; Cimetidine may increase concentration. **ALTERED LAB VALUES:** May increase ANA titer, SGOT (AST), SGPT (ALT), alkaline phosphatase, LDH, bilirubin, BUN, creatinine, K, uric acid, lipoproteins, triglycerides.

SIDE EFFECTS

Generally well tolerated, w/mild and transient side effects. **FREQUENT:** Hypotension manifested as dizziness, nausea, diaphoresis, headache, fatigue; constipation/ diarrhea, shortness of breath. **OCCASIONAL:** Insomnia, flatulence, urinary frequency. **RARE:** Ocular effects (dry eye, conjunctivitis, eye pain), unusual dreams, arthralgia, myalgia, rhinitis, rash, depression edema, chest pain, cough, wheezing.

ADVERSE REACTIONS/TOXIC EFFECTS

Excessive dosage may produce profound bradycardia, hypotension. Abrupt withdrawal may result in sweating, palpitations, headache, tremulousness, arrhythmias. May precipitate CHF, myocardial infarction in those w/cardiac disease, thyroid storm in those w/thyrotoxicosis, peripheral ischemia in those w/existing peripheral vascular disease. Hypoglycemia may occur in previously controlled diabetics.

NURSING IMPLICATIONS

BASELINE ASSESSMENT:

Assess baseline renal/liver function tests. Assess B/P, apical pulse immediately before drug is administered (if pulse is 60/min or below, or systolic B/P is below 90 mm Hg, withhold medication, contact physician).

INTERVENTION/EVALUATION:

Monitor B/P for hypotension, respiration for shortness of breath. Assess pulse for strength/weakness, irregular rate, bradycardia. Monitor EKG for cardiac arrhythmias, particularly shortening of QT interval, prolongation of PR interval. Assess frequency and consistency of stools. Assist w/ambulation if dizziness occurs. Assess for evidence of CHF: dyspnea (particularly on exertion or lying down), night cough, peripheral edema, distended neck veins, decreased urine output, weight gain. Monitor I&O, daily weight. Assess for nausea, diaphoresis, headache, fatigue.

PATIENT/FAMILY TEACHING:

Do not abruptly discontinue medication. Compliance w/therapy regimen is essential to control hypertension, arrhythmias. To avoid hypotensive effect, rise slowly from lying to sitting position, wait momentarily before standing. Avoid tasks that require alertness, motor skills until response to drug is established. Report shortness of breath, excessive fatigue, weight gain, prolonged dizziness or headache. Do not use nasal decongestants, over-the-counter cold preparations (stimulants) w/o physician approval. Take B/P, pulse before taking medication (instruct on proper technique, when to contact physician). Avoid smoking; follow physician's instructions for weight loss, exercise. Restrict salt, alcohol intake.

acetaminophen

ah-see-tah-min′oh-fen
(Datril, Tempra, Tylenol)

FIXED-COMBINATION(S): W/codeine, a narcotic analgesic (Tylenol w/codeine); w/hydrocodone, a narcotic analgesic (Vicodin); w/oxycodone, a narcotic analgesic (Percocet, Tylox); w/propoxyphene, an analgesic (Darvocet).

CANADIAN AVAILABILITY: Apo-Acetaminophen, Tempra, Tylenol

CLASSIFICATION

Nonnarcotic analgesic, antipyretic

PHARMACOKINETICS

	ONSET	PEAK	DURATION
PO	15-30 min	1-1.5 hrs	4-6 hrs

Rapid, completely absorbed from GI tract; rectal absorption variable. Widely distributed to most body tissues. Protein binding: 20-50%. Metabolized in liver; excreted in urine. Half-life: 1-4 hrs (increased in hepatic disease, elderly, neonates; decreased in children).

ACTION

Exact mechanism of analgesia unknown (may be related to inhibition of prostaglandin synthesis). Antipyresis produced by direct effect on hypothalamic heat regulating center.

USES

Relief of mild to moderate pain, fever.

PO/RECTAL ADMINISTRATION

PO:

1. Give w/o regard to meals.
2. Tablets may be crushed.

RECTAL:

1. Moisten suppository w/cold water before inserting well up into rectum.

INDICATIONS/DOSAGE/ROUTES

Analgesia, antipyresis:
NOTE: Children may repeat doses 4-5 times/day; maximum of 5 doses/24 hrs.
PO: Adults, elderly: 325-650 mg q4-6h. **Maximum:** 4 Gm/day. **Children (11 yrs):** 480 mg/dose; **(9-10 yrs):** 400 mg/dose; **(6-8 yrs):** 320 mg/dose; **(4-5 yrs):** 240 mg/dose; **(2-3 yrs):** 160 mg/dose; **(1-2 yrs):** 120 mg/dose; **(4-11 months):** 80 mg/dose; **(0-3 months):** 40 mg/dose.
RECTAL: Adults: 650 mg q4-6h. **Maximum:** 6 doses/24 hrs. **Children (6-12 yrs):** 325 mg q4-6h. **Maximum:** 2.6 Gm/24 hrs. **Children (3-6 yrs):** 120 mg q4-6 h. **Maximum:** 720 mg/24 hrs. **Children (<3 months):** Consult physician.

PRECAUTIONS

CONTRAINDICATIONS: Hypersensitivity to acetaminophen. **CAUTIONS:** Impaired hepatic function, anemia. **PREGNANCY/LACTATION:** Crosses placenta; distributed in breast milk. Routinely used in all stages of pregnancy, appears safe for short term use. **Pregnancy Category C.**

INTERACTIONS

DRUG INTERACTIONS: Alcohol (chronic use), liver enzymes inducers (e.g., cimetidine), hepatotoxic medications (e.g., phenytoin) may increase risk of hepatotoxicity w/prolonged high dose or single toxic dose. **ALTERED LAB VALUES:** May increase SGOT (AST), SGPT (ALT), bilirubin, prothrombin levels (may indicate hepatotoxicity).

SIDE EFFECTS

Well tolerated. **RARE:** Hypersensitivity reaction.

ADVERSE REACTIONS/TOXIC EFFECTS

Early signs of acetaminophen toxicity: anorexia, nausea, diaphoresis, generalized weakness within first 12-24 hrs. Later signs of toxicity: vomiting, right upper quadrant tenderness, elevated liver function tests within 48 to 72 hrs after ingestion. Antidote: Acetylcysteine.

NURSING IMPLICATIONS

BASELINE ASSESSMENT:

Question for sensitivity to acetaminophen. Assess onset, type, location, and duration of pain. Effect of medication is reduced if full pain recurs before next dose. *Fixed-combination:* Obtain vital signs before giving medication. If respirations are 12/min or lower (20/min or lower in children), withhold medication, contact physician.

INTERVENTION/EVALUATION:

Assess for clinical improvement and relief of pain, fever.

PATIENT/FAMILY TEACHING:

Do not exceed dosage. Consult physician for use in children <3 yrs, oral use >5 days (children), >10 days (adults), or fever >3 day duration. Severe/recurrent pain or high/continuous fever may indicate serious illness. *Fixed-combination:* Avoid tasks that require alertness, motor skills until response to drug is established. Tolerance/dependence may occur w/prolonged use.

acetazolamide

ah-seat-ah-zole´ah-myd

(Dazamide, Diamox, AK-Zol)

acetazolamide sodium

(Diamox) [injection]

CANADIAN AVAILABILITY:
Acetazolam, Apo-Acetazolamide, Diamox

CLASSIFICATION

Carbonic anhydrase inhibitor

PHARMACOKINETICS

	ONSET	PEAK	DURATION
PO	60-90		
(tablets)	min	2-4 hrs	8-12 hrs
(capsules)	2 hrs	8-18 hrs	18-24 hrs
IV	2 min	15 min	4-5 hrs

Well absorbed from GI tract. Protein binding: 90%. Primarily excreted unchanged in urine. Half-life: 10-15 hrs.

ACTION

Reduces formation of hydrogen and bicarbonate ions from carbon dioxide and water by inhibiting, in proximal renal tubule, the enzyme carbonic anhydrase, thereby promoting renal excretion along w/ potassium, bicarbonate, water. *Ocular effects:* reduces rate of aqueous humor formation, lowers intraocular pressure. *Renal, metabolic effects:* increases excretion of bicarbonate, sodium, potassium, water-producing alkaline diuresis. *Diamox only:* anticonvulsant; exact mechanism unknown.

USES

Treatment of open-angle (noncongestive, chronic simple) glaucoma. Used prior to surgery in correction of acute angle-closure (obstructive, narrow-angle) glaucoma. Used for prevention, treatment of high-altitude sickness. Adjunctive treatment of edema associated w/ CHF, drug-induced edema, management of petit mal, or unlocalized seizures.

STORAGE/HANDLING

Store tablets, capsules, parenteral form at room temperature. Syrup suspension mixed w/acetazolamide is stable for 1 week at room temperature. After reconstitution, IV solution stable for 24 hrs.

PO/IV ADMINISTRATION

PO:

1. When oral liquid is needed, tablet may be crushed and mixed w/5 ml cherry, chocolate, raspberry, or other highly flavored carbohydrate syrup. Each tablet may be softened in 2 tsp hot water, then added to 2 tsp honey or syrup (mix just prior to administration). Drug will not dissolve in fruit juice.
2. Scored tablets may be crushed; do not crush or break extended-release capsules.
3. May give w/food if GI upset occurs.

IV:

NOTE: IM injection painful due to alkaline pH. IV preferred.

1. Reconstitute 500 mg vial w/5 ml sterile water for injection to provide solution containing 100 mg/ml.

INDICATIONS/DOSAGE/ROUTES

Glaucoma:
PO: Adults: 250 mg 1-4 times/day.
EXTENDED-RELEASE: 500 mg 1-2 times/day usually given in morning and evening.

Secondary glaucoma, preop treatment of acute congestive glaucoma:
PO/IV: Adults: 250 mg q4h, 250 mg q12h; or 500 mg, then 125-250 mg q4h.
PO: Children: 10-15 mg/kg/day in divided doses.
IV: Children: 5-10 mg/kg q6h.

Edema secondary to CHF, drug therapy:
PO: Adults: Initially, 250-375 mg/day. (If pt fails to diurese, hold drug 1-2 days allowing kidneys to recover, then give drug intermittently.)
PO/IV: Children: 5 mg/kg/dose daily in morning.

Epilepsy:
PO: Adults, children: 375-1,000 mg/day in 1-4 divided doses.

Acute mountain sickness:
PO: Adults: 500-1,000 mg/day in divided doses. If possible, begin 24-48 hrs before ascent, continue at least 48 hrs at high altitude.

Usual elderly dosage:
PO: Elderly: Initially, 250 mg 2 times/day; use lowest effective dose.

PRECAUTIONS

CONTRAINDICATIONS: Hypersensitivity to sulfonamides, severe renal disease, adrenal insufficiency, hypochloremic acidosis. **CAUTIONS:** History of hypercalcemia, diabetes mellitus, gout, digitalized patients, obstructive pulmonary disease. **PREGNANCY/LACTATION:** Drug crosses placenta, unknown if distributed in breast milk. May produce skeletal anomalies, embryocidal effects at high doses. **Pregnancy Category C.**

INTERACTIONS

DRUG INTERACTIONS: May increase excretion of lithium; decrease excretion of quinidine, procainamide, methenamine. May increase digoxin toxicity (due to hypokalemia). **ALTERED LAB VALUES:** May increase ammonia, bilirubin, glucose, chloride, uric acid, calcium; may decrease bicarbonate, potassium.

SIDE EFFECTS

OCCASIONAL: Paresthesia in extremities/lips/mouth/anus; anorexia, polyuria, drowsiness, confusion. **RARE:** Nausea, vomiting, diarrhea, altered taste or smell, excessive thirst, headache, malaise, irritability, sedation, dizziness.

ADVERSE REACTIONS/TOXIC EFFECTS

Long-term therapy may result in acidotic state. Bone marrow depression may be manifested as aplastic anemia, thrombocytopenia, thrombocytopenic purpura, leukopenia, agranulocytosis, hemolytic anemia. Renal effects may include dysuria, crystalluria, renal colic/calculi.

NURSING IMPLICATIONS

BASELINE ASSESSMENT:

Glaucoma: Assess peripheral vision, acuity. Assess affected pupil for dilation, response to light. *Epilepsy:* Take history of seizure disorders (length, intensity, duration of seizures, presence of auras, LOC).

INTERVENTION/EVALUATION:

Monitor I&O, BUN, electrolytes (particularly serum potassium). Monitor pattern of daily bowel activity and stool consistency. Observe for signs of infection (fever, sore throat, unusual bleeding/bruising, fatigue) due to bone marrow depression. Monitor for acidosis (headache, lethargy progressing to drowsiness, CNS depression, Kussmaul's respiration).

PATIENT/FAMILY TEACHING:

Report presence of tingling or tremor in hands or feet, unusual bleeding/bruising, unexplained fever, sore throat, flank pain. Avoid tasks that require alertness, motor skills until response to drug is established.

acetohexamide

a-seet-oh-hex´a-mide
(Dymelor)

CANADIAN AVAILABILITY:
Dimelor

CLASSIFICATION

Hypoglycemics: Oral

PHARMACOKINETICS

	ONSET	PEAK	DURATION
PO	—	1-2 hrs	12-24 hrs

Rapid absorption from GI tract. Protein binding: 90%. Metabolized in liver to active metabolite. Primarily excreted in urine. Half-life: 1.3-1.5 hrs; metabolite: 5-6 hrs.

ACTION

Promotes release of insulin from beta cells of pancreas, decreases hepatic glycogenolysis and gluconeogenesis, increases insulin sensitivity at peripheral sites.

USES

As adjunct to diet/exercise in management of stable, mild to moderately severe non–insulin-dependent diabetes mellitus (type II, NIDDM). May be used to supplement insulin in patients w/type I diabetes mellitus.

PO ADMINISTRATION

May take w/food. Responses better if taken 15-30 min before meals.

INDICATIONS/DOSAGE/ROUTES

Diabetes mellitus:
PO: Adults: Initially, 250 mg up to 1,500 mg/day in 2 divided doses. **Maintenance:** 1,000 mg/day. Patients on 1,000 mg/day or less usually receive 1 dose/day.

Usual elderly dosage:
PO: Elderly: Initially, 125-250 mg/day; gradually increased to optimal control of diabetes.

PRECAUTIONS

CONTRAINDICATIONS: Sole therapy for: type I diabetes mellitus, diabetic complications (ketosis, acidosis, diabetic coma), stress situations (severe infection, trauma, surgery); hypersensitivity to drug, severe renal or hepatic impairment. **CAUTIONS:** Elderly, malnourished or debilitated, those w/renal or hepatic dysfunction, cardiac disease, adrenal or pituitary insufficiency, history of hepatic porphyria. Cardiovascular risks may be increased. **PREGNANCY/LACTATION:** Insulin is drug of choice during pregnancy; acetohexamide given within 2 weeks of delivery may cause neonatal hypoglycemia. Drug crosses placenta; excreted in breast milk. **Pregnancy Category C.**

INTERACTIONS

DRUG INTERACTIONS: May have disulfiram reaction w/ alcohol; may increase effect of oral anticoagulants; chloramphenicol, MAOI, salicylates, sulfonamides may increase effect; beta-blockers may impair hyperglycemic response; may increase effects of insulin; mask signs of hypoglycemia. **ALTERED LAB VALUES:** May increase alkaline phosphatase, SGOT (AST), LDH, creatinine, BUN; may decrease uric acid.

SIDE EFFECTS

FREQUENT: Nausea, heartburn, epigastric fullness. **OCCASIONAL:** Anorexia, vomiting, diarrhea, pruritus. **INFREQUENT:** Skin reactions, headache, photosensitivity.

ADVERSE REACTIONS/TOXIC EFFECTS

Hypoglycemia may occur due to overdosage, insufficient food intake esp. w/increased glucose demands. Hepatic porphyria, cholestatic or mixed hepatic jaundice, leukopenia, thrombocytopenia, pancytopenia, agranulocytosis, aplastic or hemolytic anemia occur rarely.

NURSING IMPLICATIONS

Baseline Assessment:

Question for hypersensitivity to acetohexamide. Check blood glucose level. Discuss lifestyle to determine extent of learning, emotional needs.

Intervention/Evaluation:

Monitor blood glucose and food intake. Assess for hypoglycemia (cool/wet skin, tremors, dizziness, headache, anxiety, tachycardia, numbness in mouth, hunger, diplopia) or hyperglycemia (polyuria, polydipsia, polyphagia, nausea and vomiting, dim vision, fatigue, deep rapid breathing). Check for adverse skin reactions, jaundice. Monitor hematology reports. Assess for bleeding or bruising. Be alert to conditions altering medication requirements: fever, increased activity or stress, surgical procedure.

Patient/Family Teaching:

Prescribed diet is a principal part of treatment; do not skip or delay meals. Diabetes mellitus requires life-long control. Check blood glucose/urine as ordered. Signs and symptoms, treatment of hypo/hyperglycemia. Carry candy, sugar packets, or other sugar supplements for immediate response to hypoglycemia. Wear, carry medical alert identification. Check w/physician in event of fever, infection, trauma, stress, heavy physical activity. Avoid alcoholic beverages. Do not take other medication w/o consulting physician. Weight control, exercise, hygiene (including foot care), nonsmoking are essential part of therapy. Protect skin, limit sun exposure. Avoid exposure to infections. Select clothing, positions that do not restrict blood flow. Notify physician promptly of skin eruptions, itching, bleeding, yellow skin, dark urine. Inform dentist, physician, or surgeon of this medication before any treatment. (Assure follow-up instruction if patient/family does not thoroughly understand diabetes management, glucose testing techniques.)

acetylcysteine (*N*-acetylcysteine)

ah-sea-tyl-sis´teen

(Mucomyst, Mucosil)

CANADIAN AVAILABILITY:
Airbron, Mucomyst, Parvolex

CLASSIFICATION

Antidote, mucolytic

PHARMACOKINETICS

	ONSET	PEAK	DURATION
Inhalant	1 min	5 min	—

After oral inhalation/intratracheal instillation, most of drug involved in sulfhydryl-disulfide reaction. Remainder absorbed from pulmonary epithelium. After oral administration, readily absorbed from GI tract. Metabolized in liver.

ACTION

Sulfhydryl group in acetylcysteine directly splits disulfide linkage of mucoproteins. Reduces viscosity of pulmonary secretions, facilitates removal by coughing, postural drainage, mechanical means. Maintains/restores hepatic concentration of glutathione (necessary for inactivation of hepatotoxic acetaminophen metabolite).

USES

Adjunctive treatment for abnormally viscid mucous secretions present in acute and chronic bronchopulmonary disease and pulmonary complication of cystic fibrosis, tracheostomy care, treatment of acetaminophen overdose.

STORAGE/HANDLING

A light purple color may occur in opened bottle (does not impair safety or effectiveness of medication). After exposure to air, refrigerate solution and use within 96 hrs.

PO/NEBULIZATION ADMINISTRATION

NOTE: A slight, disagreeable odor from solution may be noticed during initial administration but disappears quickly.

NEBULIZATION:

1. 20% solution may be diluted w/0.9% NaCl or sterile water for injection; 10% solution may be used undiluted.
2. Avoid contact w/iron, copper, rubber (reacts w/acetylcysteine).
3. Use parts made of glass, plastic, aluminum, chromed metal, sterling silver, or stainless steel.

ORAL SOLUTION:

1. Give as 5% solution; dilute 1:3 w/cola soft drink or juice.
2. Prepare fresh; use within 1 hr.
3. May give via duodenal tube.

INDICATIONS/DOSAGE/ROUTES

NOTE: Use 20% solution for oral inhalation or intratracheal instillation.

NEBULIZATION: Adults, elderly: (20% solution): 3-5 ml 3-4 times daily. **Range:** 1-10 ml q2-6h. **Adults, elderly: (10% solution):** 6-10 ml 3-4 times daily. **Range:** 2-20 ml q2-6hr.

INTRATRACHEAL INSTILLATION: Adults: 1-2 ml of 10-20% solution instilled into tracheostomy q1-4h.

Acetaminophen overdose:
ORAL SOLUTION (5%): Adults, elderly: Loading dose of 140 mg/kg, followed in 4 hrs by maintenance dose of 70 mg/kg q4h for 17 additional doses (unless acetaminophen assay reveals nontoxic level).

PRECAUTIONS

CONTRAINDICATIONS: None significant. **CAUTIONS:** Bronchial asthma, elderly, debilitated w/severe respiratory insufficiency. **PREGNANCY/LACTATION:** Unknown if drug crosses placenta or is distributed in breast milk. **Pregnancy Category B.**

INTERACTIONS

DRUG INTERACTIONS: None significant. **ALTERED LAB VALUES:** None significant.

SIDE EFFECTS

RARE: Bronchospasm (relieved quickly by bronchodilator), rhinorrhea.

ADVERSE REACTIONS/TOXIC EFFECTS

Large dosage may produce severe nausea, vomiting. Stomatitis occurs rarely.

NURSING IMPLICATIONS

BASELINE ASSESSMENT:

Mucolytic: Assess pretreatment respirations for rate, depth, rhythm. Place tissue within easy reach of patient. *Antidote:* Assess acetominophen plasma level. Determine baselines for AST, ALT, bilirubin, PT, creatinine, BUN, blood sugar, and electrolytes. Assure that the stomach is empty by lavaging or inducing emesis. If activated charcoal has been administered, lavage before administering acetylcysteine.

INTERVENTION/EVALUATION:

Mucolytic: Have suction equipment available in case pt cannot clear airway. If bronchospasm occurs, treatment should be discontinued and physician notified; bronchodilator may be added to therapy. Monitor rate, depth, rhythm, type of respiration (abdominal, thoracic). Assess for evidence of stomatitis (erythema of mucous membranes, dry mouth, burning of oral mucosa). Check sputum for color, consistency, amount. Assess lung sounds for rhonchi, wheezing, rales. *Antidote:* Continue to monitor lab test results (see Baseline Assessment) daily. Monitor I&O. Assess pt for vomiting (potential is increased due to vomiting from acetaminophen). Treat hypoglycemia as necessary. Avoid diuretics. Vitamin K_1 may be administered if PT ratio exceeds 1.5, fresh frozen plasma if ratio exceeds 3. Monitor vital signs.

PATIENT/FAMILY TEACHING:

Mucolytic: A slight, disagreeable odor from solution may be noticed during initial administration but disappears quickly. Explain importance of adequate hydration. Teach proper coughing and deep breathing. *Antidote:* Explain purpose of therapy. Report any bleeding at once.

acitretin (Soriatine)
See supplement

acyclovir

aye-sigh´klo-veer
(Zovirax)

CANADIAN AVAILABILITY:
Zovirax

CLASSIFICATION

Antiviral

PHARMACOKINETICS

Poorly absorbed from GI tract; minimal absorption following topical application. Widely distributed. Protein binding: 10-30%. Partially metabolized by cellular enzymes. Excreted primarily in urine. Removed by hemodialysis. Half-life: 2.5 hrs (increased in decreased renal function).

ACTION

Converted to acyclovir triphosphate, becoming part of DNA chain, interfering w/DNA synthesis and viral replication. Virustatic.

USES

Parenteral: Initial and recurrent mucosal and cutaneous herpes infections (HSV-1, HSV-2) and varicella-zoster (shingles) infection in immunocompromised patients. Herpes simplex encephalitis in pts >6 months and severe first clinical occurrence of genital herpes. *Oral:* Initial and recurrent genital herpes in select pts, localized herpes zoster and chickenpox (varicella). *Topical:* Initial episodes of genital herpes, immunocompromised pts w/limited nonthreatening herpes simplex infections.

STORAGE/HANDLING

Store capsules at room temperature. Solutions of 50 mg/ml stable for 12 hrs at room temperature; may form precipitate when refrigerated. Potency not affected by precipitate and redissolution. IV infusion (piggyback) stable for 24 hrs at room temperature. Yellow discoloration does not affect potency.

PO/IV ADMINISTRATION

NOTE: Space doses evenly around the clock.

PO:

1. Give w/o regard to food.
2. Do not crush or break capsules.

IV:

NOTE: Do not administer by IM, SubQ, or rapid IV infusion or rapid IV injection.

1. For IV infusion (piggyback), reconstitute each 500 mg vial w/10 ml sterile water for injection or bacteriostatic water for injection containing benzyl alcohol. Shake well to assure complete dissolution.
2. Further dilute w/50-125 ml 5% dextrose, 0.9% NaCl, or other compatible IV fluid. Infuse over at least 1 hr.
3. Maintain adequate hydration, especially during urine concentration that occurs 2 hrs following IV administration.
4. Alternating IV sites, use large veins to reduce risk of phlebitis.

INDICATIONS/DOSAGE/ROUTES

Initial genital herpes infections, intermittent treatment of recurrent episodes:
PO: Adults, elderly: 200 mg q4h while awake (5 times/day).

Prophylaxis of recurrent episodes:
PO: Adults, elderly: 400 mg 2 times/day up to 12 months.

Chickenpox:
PO: Adults, elderly, Children (2-12 yrs): 20 mg/kg (maximum 800 mg) 4 times/day for 5 days.

Mucosal or cutaneous herpes simplex, severe genital herpes:
IV: Adults, elderly: 5 mg/kg q8h. **Children <12 yrs:** 250 mg/m² q8h. Continue for 7 days for herpes simplex; 5 days for genital herpes.

Herpes simplex encephalitis:
IV: Adults, elderly: 10 mg/kg q8h for 10 days. **Children, 6 months-12 yrs:** 500 mg/m² q8h for 10 days.

Varicella zoster infections:
IV: Adults, elderly: 10/mg/kg q8h. **Children:** 500 mg/m² q8h. Continue for 7 days.

Herpes zoster (acute):
PO: Adults, elderly: 800 mg q4h (5 times/day) for 7-10 days.

Usual topical dosage:
TOPICAL: Adults, elderly: 3-6 times/day for 7 days.

Dosage in renal impairment:

Dose/frequency is modified based on severity of infection, degree of renal impairment.

Oral: Creatinine clearance of 10 ml/1.73m² or less: 200 mg q12h.
IV:

CREATININE CLEARANCE	DOSAGE (ADULTS)	DOSAGE (CHILDREN)
>50 ml/min	5 mg/kg q8h	250 mg/m² q8h
25-50 ml/min	5 mg/kg q12h	250 mg/m² q12h
10-25 ml/min	5 mg/kg q24h	250 mg/m² q24h
0-10 ml/min	2.5 mg/kg q24h	125 mg/m² q24h

PRECAUTIONS

CONTRAINDICATIONS: Hypersensitivity to acyclovir or components of preparation. Acyclovir reconstituted w/bacteriostatic water containing benzyl alcohol should not be used in neonates. **CAUTIONS:** Renal or hepatic impairment, dehydration, fluid/electrolyte imbalance, concurrent use of nephrotoxic agents, neurologic abnormalities. **PREGNANCY/LACTATION:** Crosses placenta; distributed in breast milk. **Pregnancy Category C.**

INTERACTIONS

DRUG INTERACTIONS: Probenecid may increase half-life. Nephrotoxic medications (e.g., aminoglycosides) may increase nephrotoxicity. **ALTERED LAB VALUES:** May increase BUN, serum creatinine concentrations.

SIDE EFFECTS

FREQUENT: *Parenteral:* Phlebitis at IV site, rash or hives. *Oral:* Nausea, vomiting. *Topical:* Burning, stinging, pruritus. **OCCASIONAL:** Headache. *Parenteral:* Hypotension, hematuria, diaphoresis, nausea. **RARE:** Lethargy, confusion, agitation, tremors, hallucinations, seizures w/IV.

ADVERSE REACTIONS/TOXIC EFFECTS

Rapid parenteral administration, excessively high doses, or fluid/electrolyte imbalance may produce renal failure w/parenteral use. Toxicity not reported w/oral or topical use.

NURSING IMPLICATIONS

BASELINE ASSESSMENT:

Question history of allergies, particularly to acyclovir. Avoid nephrotoxic drugs if possible. Tissue cultures for HSV should be done before giving first dose (therapy may proceed before results are known).

INTERVENTION/EVALUATION:

Monitor I&O, renal function tests if ordered, electrolyte levels. Check food tolerance, vomiting. Assess IV site for phlebitis (heat, pain, red streaking over vein). Evaluate cutaneous lesions. Be alert to neurologic effects: headache, lethargy, confusion, agitation, hallucinations, seizures. Assure adequate ventilation. Manage chicken pox and disseminated herpes zoster with strict isolation. Provide analgesics and comfort measures; esp. exhausting to elderly. Encourage fluids. Keep pt's fingernails short, hands clean.

PATIENT/FAMILY TEACHING:

Drink adequate fluids. Notify physician if side effects develop. Do not touch lesions with fingers to avoid spreading infection to new site. *Genital herpes:* Continue therapy for full length of treatment. Space doses evenly. Use finger cot or rubber glove to apply topical ointment. Avoid sexual intercourse during duration of lesions to prevent infecting partner. Acyclovir does not cure herpes. Notify physician if lesions do not improve or recur. Avoid driving or operating machinery if dizziness is present. Pap smears should be done at least annually due to increased risk of cancer of cervix in women w/genital herpes. *Chicken pox:* Unknown whether treatment of childhood chickenpox will have effect on long-term immunity.

adenosine

ah-den´oh-seen
(Adenocard)

CLASSIFICATION

Antiarrhythmic

PHARMACOKINETICS

Immediate onset of action. Rapidly metabolized by enzymes in erythrocytes and vascular endothelial cells to inosine and adenosine monophosphate.

ACTION

Decreases conduction through SA, AV nodes; may interrupt reentry pathway through AV node. Depresses left ventricular function.

USES

Treatment of paroxysmal supraventricular tachycardia, including those associated w/accessory bypass tracts (WPW syndrome).

STORAGE/HANDLING

Store at room temperature. Solution appears clear. Crystallization occurs if refrigerated; if crystallization occurs, dissolve crystals by warming to room temperature. Discard unused portion.

IV ADMINISTRATION

1. Administer directly into vein, or if using IV line, as proximal as possible. Follow by rapid saline flush.
2. Administer rapidly (>1-2 sec period).

INDICATIONS/DOSAGE/ROUTES

Usual adult dosage:

IV: Adults, elderly: Initially, 6 mg (over 1-2 sec). If 1st dose does not convert within 1-2 min, give 12 mg; may repeat 12 mg dose in 1-2 min if no response has occurred.

PRECAUTIONS

CONTRAINDICATIONS: Second- or third-degree AV block or sick sinus syndrome (w/functioning pacemaker), atrial flutter or fibrillation, ventricular tachycardia. **CAUTIONS:** Heart block, arrhythmias at time of conversion, mutagenesis, asthma, hepatic/renal failure. **PREGNANCY/LACTATION:** Unknown if drug crosses placenta or is excreted in breast milk. **Pregnancy Category C.**

INTERACTIONS

DRUG INTERACTIONS: Methylxanthines (e.g., caffeine, theophylline) may decrease effect. Dipyridamole may increase effect. Carbamazepine may increase degree of heart block caused by adenosine. **ALTERED LAB VALUES:** None significant.

SIDE EFFECTS

FREQUENT: Facial flushing, shortness of breath/dyspnea. **OCCASIONAL:** Chest pressure, nausea, headache, lightheadedness. **RARE:** Blurred vision, hypotension, sweating, metallic taste.

ADVERSE REACTIONS/TOXIC EFFECTS

May produce short lasting heart block.

NURSING IMPLICATIONS

BASELINE ASSESSMENT:

Identify arrhythmia per cardiac monitor and apical pulse

INTERVENTION/EVALUATION:

Assess cardiac performance per continuous EKG. Monitor B/P, apical pulse (rate, rhythm, and strength), and respirations. Monitor I&O; assess for fluid retention. Check electrolytes.

albumin, human

al-byew′min

(Albuminar, Albutein, Buminate, Plasbumin)

CANADIAN AVAILABILITY:
Plasbumin

CLASSIFICATION

Blood derivative

ACTION

Regulates circulating blood volume, tissue fluid balance, and maintains plasma colloid osmotic pressure. Binds and functions as carrier of intermediate metabolites (hormones, enzymes, drugs) in transport and exchange of tissue products.

USES

Symptomatic/supportive treatment of shock due to burns, trauma, surgery, infections. Prevents hemoconcentration and combats water, protein, electrolyte losses in severely burned or hemorrhaging pt, hypoproteinemia, ARDS, cardiopulmonary bypass surgery (preop blood dilution), acute nephrosis, renal dialysis (treat shock or hypotension), hyperbilirubinemia and erythroblastosis fetalis.

STORAGE/HANDLING

Store at room temperature. Clear, brownish, odorless, moderate viscous fluid. Do not use if solution has been frozen, solution appears turbid, or contains sediment, or if not used within 4 hrs of opening vial.

IV ADMINISTRATION

1. Give by IV infusion.
2. 5% administered undiluted; 25% may be administered undiluted or diluted w/0.9% NaCl or 5% dextrose.
3. May give w/o regard to pt blood group or Rh factor.

INDICATIONS/DOSAGE/ROUTES

NOTE: Dosage based on pt's condition; duration of administration based on pt's response.

Usual dosage:
IV: Adults, elderly: 25 Gm by infusion. May be repeated in 15-30 min. Maximum: 125 Gm/24 hrs or 250 Gm/48 hrs.

Shock (greatly reduced blood volume):
IV: Adults, elderly: Administer 5% or 25% fluid as rapidly as possible to improve condition and restore normal blood volume. May be repeated in 15-30 min. **Infants, neonates:** 10-20 ml/kg of 5% solution.

Shock (slightly reduced blood volume):
IV: Adults, elderly: 5%: Give 2-4 ml/min. **Children:** Give 0.5-2 ml/min.
IV: Adults, elderly: 25%: Give 1 ml/min.

Burns (5% or 25%):
IV: Adults, elderly, children: Maintain plasma albumin concentration of 2.5 ± 0.5 Gm/100 ml (or plasma protein level of 5.2 Gm/100 ml).

Hypoproteinemia:
IV: Adults, elderly: 50-75 Gm/day. **Children:** 25 Gm/day. Give at rate not to exceed 5-10 ml/min

(5%) or 2-3 ml/min (25%). (Minimizes circulatory overload, pulmonary edema.)

Acute nephrosis:
IV: Adults, elderly: 25%: 100-200 ml (25-50 Gm) daily for 7-10 days.

Renal dialysis:
IV: Adults, elderly: 25%: 100 ml (25 Gm).

Hyperbilirubinemia, erythroblastosis fetalis:
IV: Infants: 1 Gm/kg 1-2 hrs before transfusion.

PRECAUTIONS

CONTRAINDICATIONS: Severe anemia, cardiac failure, history of allergic reaction to albumin, renal insufficiency, no albumin deficiency. **CAUTIONS:** Low cardiac reserve, pulmonary disease, hepatic or renal failure. **PREGNANCY/LACTATION:** Unknown if drug crosses placenta or is distributed in breast milk. **Pregnancy Category C.**

INTERACTIONS

DRUG INTERACTIONS: None significant. **ALTERED LAB VALUES:** May increase serum alkaline phosphatase concentrations.

SIDE EFFECTS

OCCASIONAL: Hypotension. High dosage, repeated therapy may result in allergy or protein overload (chills, fever, flushing, low back pain, nausea, urticaria, vital sign changes).

ADVERSE REACTIONS/TOXIC EFFECTS

Fluid overload (headache, weakness, blurred vision, behavioral changes, incoordination, isolated muscle twitching) and pulmonary edema (rapid breathing, rales, wheezing, coughing, increased B/P, distended neck veins) may occur.

NURSING IMPLICATIONS

BASELINE ASSESSMENT:

Obtain B/P, pulse, respirations immediately before administration. There should be adequate hydration before albumin is administered.

INTERVENTION/EVALUATION:

Monitor B/P for hypo/hypertension. Assess frequently for evidence of fluid overload, pulmonary edema (see Adverse Reactions/Toxic Effects). Check skin for flushing, urticaria. Monitor hemoglobin, hematocrit. Monitor I&O ratio (watch for decreased output). Assess for therapeutic response (increased B/P, decreased edema).

albuterol

ale-beut´er-all
(Proventil, Ventolin [inhalation])

albuterol sulfate

(Proventil, Ventolin [syrup, tablets, nebulization])

FIXED-COMBINATION(S):
W/ipratropium, a bronchodilator (Combivent)

CANADIAN AVAILABILITY:
Novosalmol, Ventolin

CLASSIFICATION

Bronchodilator

PHARMACOKINETICS

	ONSET	PEAK	DURATION
Inhalation	5-15 min	0.5-2 hrs	3-6 hrs
Oral	<30 min	2-3 hrs	4-8 hrs

Rapid, well absorbed from GI

tract; gradual absorption from bronchi following inhalation. Metabolized in liver. Primarily excreted in urine. Half-life: 3-8 hrs oral; 3.7-5 hrs inhalation.

ACTION

Stimulates $beta_2$-adrenergic receptors in lungs (relaxes bronchial smooth muscle by increasing cAMP. Relieves bronchospasm, reduces airway resistance).

USES

Relief of bronchospasm due to reversible obstructive airway disease, exercise-induced bronchospasm.

PO/INHALATION ADMINISTRATION

1. Do not crush or break extended-release tablets.

INHALATION:

1. Shake container well, exhale completely, then holding mouthpiece 1 inch away from lips, inhale and hold breath as long as possible before exhaling.
2. Wait 1-10 min before inhaling second dose (allows for deeper bronchial penetration).
3. Rinse mouth w/water immediately after inhalation (prevents mouth/throat dryness).

NEBULIZATION:

1. Dilute 0.5 ml of 0.5% solution to final volume of 3 ml w/0.9% NaCl to provide 2.5 mg.
2. Administer over 5-15 min.
3. Nebulizer should be used w/ compressed air or oxygen at rate of 6-10 liters/min.

INDICATIONS/DOSAGE/ROUTES

Bronchospasm:
INHALATION (AEROSOL): Adults, elderly, children >12 yrs: 2 inhalations q4-6h. One inhalation q4h may be sufficient in some pts. Wait 1-10 min before administering second inhalation.
INHALATION (CAPSULES): Adults, elderly, children >4 yrs: 200-400 mcg q4-6h.
INHALATION (SOLUTION): Adults, elderly: 2.5 mg 3-4 times/day by nebulization.
TABLETS: Adults, children >12 yrs: 2 or 4 mg 3-4 times/day. Gradually increased to maximum dose of 8 mg 4 times/day (32 mg/day). **Elderly:** 2 mg 3-4 times/day. Gradually increased to maximum 8 mg 3-4 times/day.
SYRUP: Adults, children >14 yrs: 2-4 mg 3-4 times/day. Maximum: 32 mg/day. **Children 6-14 yrs:** 2 mg 3-4 times/day. Dosage may be gradually increased to 24 mg/day in divided doses. **Children 2-6 yrs:** Initially, 0.1 mg/kg 3 times/day (do not exceed 2 mg 3 times/day). Gradually increased to 0.2 mg/kg 3 times/day (do not exceed 4 mg 3 times/day).
EXTENDED-RELEASE: Adults, children >12 yrs: 4 or 8 mg q12h. May be gradually increased to 16 mg daily.

Exercise-induced bronchospasm:
INHALATION: Adults, elderly, children >12 yrs: 2 inhalations 15 min before exercise.

PRECAUTIONS

CONTRAINDICATIONS: History of hypersensitivity to sympathomimetics. **CAUTIONS:** Hypertension, cardiovascular disease, hyperthyroidism, diabetes mellitus. **PREGNANCY/LACTATION:** Appears to cross placenta; unknown if distributed in breast milk. May inhibit uterine contractility. **Pregnancy Category C.**

INTERACTIONS

DRUG INTERACTIONS: Increased risk of cardiovascular effects if used w/other sympathomimetics. Do not use other orally inhaled beta-adrenergic agonists concurrently. Beta-adrenergic blocking agents (beta blockers) antagonize albuterol effects. MAO inhibitors, tricyclic antidepressants may potentiate cardiovascular effects. **ALTERED LAB VALUES:** May decrease serum potassium levels.

SIDE EFFECTS

OCCASIONAL: Tremor, nausea, nervousness, palpitations, tachycardia, peripheral vasodilation, dryness of mouth and throat.

ADVERSE REACTIONS/TOXIC EFFECTS

Excessive sympathomimetic stimulation may produce palpitations, extrasystoles, tachycardia, chest pain, slight increase in B/P followed by substantial decrease, chills, sweating, blanching of skin. Too-frequent or excessive use may lead to loss of bronchodilating effectiveness and/or severe, paradoxical bronchoconstriction.

NURSING IMPLICATIONS

BASELINE ASSESSMENT:

Offer emotional support (high incidence of anxiety due to difficulty in breathing and sympathomimetic response to drug).

INTERVENTION/EVALUATION:

Monitor rate, depth, rhythm, type of respiration; quality and rate of pulse. Assess lung sounds for wheezing (bronchoconstriction) and rales.

PATIENT/FAMILY TEACHING:

Instruct on proper use of inhaler. Increase fluid intake (decreases lung secretion viscosity). Do not take more than 2 inhalations at any one time (excessive use may produce paradoxical bronchoconstriction or a decreased bronchodilating effect). Rinsing mouth with water immediately after inhalation may prevent mouth/throat dryness. Avoid excessive use of caffeine derivatives (chocolate, coffee, tea, cola, cocoa). Do not take over-the-counter medications w/o physician approval: may increase sympathetic stimulation. Avoid smoking, smoke-filled areas.

alclometasone

(Aclovate)

(See Classifications section under Corticosteroid: topical)

aldesleukin

all-des-lyew'kin

(Proleukin, Interleukin-2, IL-2)

CLASSIFICATION

Antineoplastic

PHARMACOKINETICS

Distributed to extravascular, extracellular space. Metabolized in kidney (to amino acids in cells lining proximal convoluted tubule). Excreted in urine. Half-life: 30-120 min.

ACTION

Promotes proliferation, differentiation, and recruitment of T and B cells, natural killer cells, and thymocytes. Enhances lymphocyte mitogenesis and cytotoxicity, stimulates growth of interleukin-2 dependent cell lines, induces natural killer cells and interferon gamma production. Produces many immunologic effects: Activates cellular immunity, inhibits tumor growth.

USES

Treatment of metastatic renal cell carcinoma.

STORAGE/HANDLING

Refrigerate vial before and after reconstitution. Reconstituted solutions stable for 48 hrs. Discard solution that does not appear clear, colorless to slightly yellow. Discard unused portion.

IV ADMINISTRATION

NOTE: Hold administration in those who develop moderate to severe lethargy or somnolence (continued administration may result in coma).

1. Reconstitute 22 million unit vial w/1.2 ml sterile water for injection to provide concentration of 18 million U/ml.
2. During reconstitution, direct the sterile water for injection at the side of vial. Swirl contents gently to avoid foaming. Do not shake.
3. Further dilute dose in 50 ml 5% dextrose and infuse over 15 min. Do not use an in-line filter.
4. Solution should be warmed to room temperature before pt infusion.
5. Monitor diligently for drop in mean arterial B/P (sign of capillary leak syndrome [CLS]). Continued treatment may result in significant hypotension (<90 mm Hg or a 20 mm Hg drop from baseline systolic pressure), edema, pleural effusion, mental status changes.

INDICATIONS/DOSAGE/ROUTES

NOTE: Restrict therapy to those w/ normal cardiac and pulmonary functions as defined by thallium stress testing, pulmonary function testing. Dosage individualized based on clinical response, tolerance to adverse effects.

Metastatic renal cell carcinoma:
IV: Adults >18: 600,000 IU/kg q8h for 14 doses; rest 9 days, repeat 14 doses. Total: 28 doses. May repeat treatment no sooner than 7 wks from date of hospital discharge.

PRECAUTIONS

CONTRAINDICATIONS: Abnormal thallium stress test or pulmonary function tests, organ allografts, retreatment in those who experience the following toxicities: Sustained ventricular tachycardia, cardiac rhythm disturbances uncontrolled or unresponsive, recurrent chest pain w/EKG changes, angina, MI; intubation >72 hrs, pericardial tamponade, renal dysfunction requiring dialysis >72 hrs, coma or toxic psychosis >48 hrs, repetitive or difficult to control seizures, bowel ischemia/perforation, GI bleeding requiring surgery. **EXTREME CAUTION:** Those w/normal thallium stress tests and pulmonary function tests who have history of prior cardiac or pulmonary disease. **CAUTIONS:** Those w/fixed requirements for large volumes of fluid (e.g., those w/hypercalcemia), history of seizures. **PREGNANCY/LACTATION:** Avoid use in those of either sex not practicing effective contraception. **Pregnancy Category C.**

INTERACTIONS

DRUG INTERACTIONS: Antihypertensives may increase hypotensive effect. Glucocorticoids may decrease effects. Cardiotoxic, hepatotoxic, nephrotoxic, myelotoxic producing medications may increase toxicity. **ALTERED LAB VALUES:** May increase bilirubin, BUN, serum creatinine, transaminase, alkaline phosphatase. May decrease magnesium, calcium, phosphorus, potassium.

SIDE EFFECTS

NOTE: Side effects generally self-limiting and reversible within 2-3 days after discontinuation of therapy.

FREQUENT: Fever, chills, nausea, vomiting, hypotension, diarrhea, oliguria/anuria, mental status changes, sinus tachycardia, pain (abdomen, chest, back), fatigue, dyspnea, pruritus. **OCCASIONAL:** Erythema, rash, edema, anorexia, headache, weight gain, infection (urinary tract, injection site, catheter tip), dizziness. **RARE:** Dry skin, sensory disorders (vision, speech, taste), dermatitis, arthralgia, myalgia, weight loss, conjunctivitis, hematuria, proteinuria.

ADVERSE REACTIONS/TOXIC EFFECTS

Anemia, thrombocytopenia, leukopenia occur commonly. GI bleeding, pulmonary edema occur occasionally. CLS results in hypotension (<90 mm Hg or a 20 mm Hg drop from baseline systolic pressure) and extravasation of plasma proteins and fluid into extravascular space and loss of vascular tone. May result in cardiac arrhythmias, angina, MI, respiratory insufficiency, deficiency in mental status. Fatal malignant hyperthermia, cardiac arrest or stroke, pulmonary emboli as well as bowel perforation/gangrene, severe depression leading to suicide have occurred in less than 1% of pts.

NURSING IMPLICATIONS

BASELINE ASSESSMENT:

Preexisting bacterial infections and those w/indwelling central lines should be treated w/antibiotic therapy (oxacillin, nafcillin, ciprofloxacin, vancomycin) before treatment begins. All pts should be neurologically stable with a negative CT scan before treatment begins. CBC, differential and platelet counts, blood chemistries including electrolytes, renal and hepatic function tests, chest x-ray should be performed before therapy begins and daily thereafter. Obtain baseline B/P, temperature, pulse, weight.

INTERVENTION/EVALUATION:

Determine serum amylase concentration frequently during therapy. Discontinue medication at first sign of hypotension and hold for moderate to severe lethargy (physician must decide whether therapy should continue). Assess B/P and pulse, temperature, mental status changes (irritability, confusion, depression), weight gain or loss. Maintain strict I&O. Check hypovolemia by catheterization and central pressure monitoring (correction may require IV fluid management). Assess for extravascular fluid accumulation: Rales in lungs, edema in dependent areas.

PATIENT/FAMILY TEACHING:

Nausea may decrease during therapy. Evaluation 4 wks after therapy and before each course of therapy to determine additional courses (given only if some tumor shrinkage). At home, increase fluid intake (protects against renal impairment). Do not have immunizations; avoid those who have recently taken live virus vaccine.

alendronate (Fosamax)
See supplement

alfentanil

(Alfenta)

(See Classifications section under Opioid analgesics)

allopurinol

al-low-pure´ih-nawl
(Lopurin, Zyloprim)

CANADIAN AVAILABILITY:
Alloprin, Apo-Allopurinol, Novopurol, Purinol, Zyloprim

CLASSIFICATION

Antigout

PHARMACOKINETICS

Well absorbed from GI tract. Widely distributed. Metabolized in liver to active metabolite. Excreted primarily in urine. Removed by hemodialysis. Half-life: 1-3 hrs; metabolite: 12-30 hrs.

ACTION

Decreases uric acid production by inhibition of xanthine oxidase. Decreases serum, urine uric acid concentrations.

USES

Treatment of chronic gouty arthritis, uric acid nephropathy. Prevents or treats hyperuricemia secondary to blood dyscrasias, cancer chemotherapy. Prevents recurrence of uric acid or calcium stone formation.

PO ADMINISTRATION

1. May give w/or immediately after meals or milk.
2. Instruct pt to drink at least 10-12 8 oz glasses of water/day.
3. Doses >300 mg/day to be administered in divided doses.

INDICATIONS/DOSAGE/ROUTES

Gout, hyperuricemia:
PO: Adults: 200-600 mg/day. **Range:** 100-800 mg/day. **Maximum:** 800 mg/day. **Children (6-10 yrs):** 300 mg/day. **Children (<6 yrs):** 150 mg/day.

Prevention uric acid nephropathy during neoplastic disease therapy:
PO: Adults: 600-800 mg/day for 2-3 days (w/high fluid intake).

Reduce acute gouty attacks:
PO: Adults: Initially, 100 mg/day. May increase by 100 mg/day at weekly intervals (up to maximum of 800 mg/day) until serum uric acid ≤6 mg/dl attained.

Recurrent calcium oxalate stones:
PO: Adults: 200-300 mg/day.

Usual elderly dosage:
PO: Elderly: Initially, 100 mg/day, gradually increased to optimal uric acid level.

Dosage in renal impairment:
Based on creatinine clearance using serum uric acid as index.

CREATININE CLEARANCE	DOSAGE
10-20 ml/min	200 mg/day
3-10 ml/min	100 mg/day maximum
<3 ml/min	100 mg at increased intervals

PRECAUTIONS

CONTRAINDICATIONS: Asymptomatic hyperuricemia. **CAUTIONS:** Impaired renal, hepatic function. **PREGNANCY/LACTATION:** Unknown if drug crosses placenta or is distributed in breast milk. **Pregnancy Category C.**

INTERACTIONS

DRUG INTERACTIONS: Thiazide diuretics may decrease effect. May increase effect of oral anticoagulants. May increase effect, toxicity of azathioprine, mercaptopurine. Ampicillin, amoxicillin may increase incidence of skin rash. **ALTERED LAB VALUES:** May increase alkaline phosphatase, SGOT (AST), SGPT (ALT), BUN, creatinine.

SIDE EFFECTS

OCCASIONAL: Drowsiness. **RARE:** Nausea, diarrhea, headache.

ADVERSE REACTIONS/TOXIC EFFECTS

Pruritic maculopapular rash should be considered a toxic reaction. May be accompanied by malaise, fever, chills, joint pain, nausea, vomiting, leukopenia. Severe hypersensitivity may follow appearance of rash. Bone marrow depression occurs rarely.

NURSING IMPLICATIONS

BASELINE ASSESSMENT:

Question pt for hypersensitivity to allopurinol. Instruct pt to drink 10-12 glasses (8 oz) of fluid daily while on medication.

INTERVENTION/EVALUATION:

Discontinue medication immediately if rash or other evidence of allergic reaction appears. Encourage high fluid intake (3,000 ml/day). Monitor I&O (output should be at least 2,000 ml/day). Assess CBC, serum uric acid levels. Assess urine for cloudiness, unusual color, odor. Assess for therapeutic response (reduced joint tenderness, swelling, redness, limitation of motion).

PATIENT/FAMILY TEACHING:

May take 1 or more wks for full therapeutic effect. Encourage low purine food intake, drinking 10-12 glasses (8 oz) of fluid daily while on medication. Avoid tasks that require alertness, motor skills until response to drug is established. Contact physician/nurse if rash, irritation of eyes, swelling of lips/mouth occurs.

alpha$_1$-proteinase inhibitor (human, alpha$_1$-PI)

(Prolastin)

CANADIAN AVAILABILITY:
Prolastin

CLASSIFICATION

Proteinase inhibitor

ACTION

Protects alveolar epithelial lining of lower respiratory tract by alleviating imbalance between elastase (enzyme capable of degrading elastin tissue in lower respiratory tract) and alpha$_1$-proteinase inhibitor (inhibits neutrophil elastase).

USES

Chronic replacement therapy in patients w/clinically demonstrable panacinar emphysema. Do not use in patients w/PiMZ or PiMS phenotypes (small risk of panacinar emphysema).

STORAGE/HANDLING

Store parenteral form in refrigerator. After reconstitution, do not refrigerate. Use within 3 hrs. Discard unused portion.

IV ADMINISTRATION

1. Reconstitute each vial w/20 or 40 ml sterile water (total functional activity stated in mg is noted on label of each vial). 20 ml = about 500 mg; 40 ml = about 1,000 mg activity.
2. May use 0.9% NaCl as diluent.
3. Infuse at rate of at least 0.08 ml/kg.

INDICATIONS/DOSAGE/ROUTES

Replacement therapy:
IV INFUSION: Adults, elderly: 60 mg/kg once weekly at rate of at least 0.08 ml/kg.

PRECAUTIONS

CONTRAINDICATIONS: None significant. **CAUTIONS:** Those at risk for circulatory overload. Safety in children not established. **PREGNANCY/LACTATION:** Unknown if drug crosses placenta or is distributed in breast milk. **Pregnancy Category C.**

INTERACTIONS

DRUG INTERACTIONS: None significant. **ALTERED LAB VALUES:** None significant.

SIDE EFFECTS

RARE: Delayed fever (occurring 12 hrs after administration, resolves spontaneously), lightheadedness, dizziness.

ADVERSE REACTIONS/TOXIC EFFECTS

Mild leukocytosis occurs rarely.

NURSING IMPLICATIONS

BASELINE ASSESSMENT:

All patients should be immunized against hepatitis B before initial dose is given.

INTERVENTION/EVALUATION:

Maintain blood levels of alpha$_1$-PI at 80 mg/dl. Monitor respiratory status throughout therapy.

PATIENT/FAMILY TEACHING:

Explain purpose of medication, importance of hepatitis B vaccine, periodic pulmonary function tests. Avoid smoking. Notify physician of changes in respiratory condition.

alprazolam

ale-praz´oh-lam
(Xanax)

CANADIAN AVAILABILITY:
Apo-Alpraz, Novo-Alprazol, Xanax

CLASSIFICATION

Antianxiety: Benzodiazepine

PHARMACOKINETICS

Well absorbed from GI tract. Protein binding: 80%. Metabolized in liver. Primarily excreted in urine. Minimal removed by hemodialysis. Half-life: 11-16 hrs.

ACTION

Enhances action of inhibitory neurotransmitter gamma-aminobutyric acid (GABA). Depressant effects occur at all levels of CNS.

USES

Management of anxiety disorders associated w/depression, panic disorder.

PO ADMINISTRATION

1. May be given w/o regard to meals.
2. Tablets may be crushed.

INDICATIONS/DOSAGE/ROUTES

Anxiety disorders:
PO: Adults >18 yrs: Initially, 0.25-0.5 mg 3 times daily. Titrate to max-

imum of 4 mg daily in divided doses. **Elderly/debilitated/liver disease/low serum albumin:** Initially, 0.25 mg 2-3 times daily. Gradually increase to optimum therapeutic response.

Panic disorder:
PO: Adults: Initially, 0.5 mg 3 times/day. May increase at 3-4 day intervals at no more than 1 mg/day. **Range:** 1-10 mg/day.

Usual elderly dosage:
PO: Elderly: Initially, 0.125-0.25 mg 2 times/day; may increase in 0.125 mg increments until desired effect attained.

PRECAUTIONS

CONTRAINDICATIONS: Acute narrow-angle glaucoma, acute alcohol intoxication. **CAUTIONS:** Impaired renal/hepatic function. **PREGNANCY / LACTATION:** Crosses placenta; distributed in breast milk. Chronic ingestion during pregnancy may produce withdrawal symptoms, CNS depression in neonates. **Pregnancy Category D.**

INTERACTIONS

DRUG INTERACTIONS: Potentiated effects when used w/other CNS depressants, (including alcohol). **ALTERED LAB VALUES:** May produce abnormal renal function tests, elevate SGOT (AST), SGPT (ALT), LDH, alkaline phosphatase, serum bilirubin.

SIDE EFFECTS

FREQUENT: Drowsiness/lightheadedness (particularly elderly, debilitated), dry mouth, headache, constipation/diarrhea. **OCCASIONAL:** Nausea, confusion, insomnia, tachycardia, palpitations, nasal congestion, blurred vision. **RARE:** Paradoxical CNS excitement/restlessness in elderly/debilitated (generally noted during first 2 wks of therapy, particularly in presence of pain).

ADVERSE REACTIONS/TOXIC EFFECTS

Abrupt or too-rapid withdrawal may result in pronounced restlessness, irritability, insomnia, hand tremors, abdominal/muscle cramps, sweating, vomiting, seizures. Overdosage results in somnolence, confusion, diminished reflexes, coma.

NURSING IMPLICATIONS

BASELINE ASSESSMENT:

Offer emotional support to anxious pt. Assess motor responses (agitation, trembling, tension) and autonomic responses (cold, clammy hands, sweating).

INTERVENTION/EVALUATION:

For those on long-term therapy, liver/renal function tests, blood counts should be performed periodically. Assess for paradoxical reaction, particularly during early therapy. Assist w/ambulation if drowsiness, lightheadedness occur. Evaluate for therapeutic response: calm facial expression, decreased restlessness and/or insomnia.

PATIENT/FAMILY TEACHING:

Drowsiness usually disappears during continued therapy. If dizziness occurs, change positions slowly from recumbent to sitting position before standing. Avoid tasks that require alertness, motor skills until response to drug is established. Smoking reduces drug effectiveness. Sour hard candy, gum, or sips of tepid water may relieve dry mouth. Do not abruptly withdraw medication after long-term therapy. Avoid alcohol. Do not take other medications w/o consulting physician.

alprostadil (prostaglandin E_1; PGE_1)

ale-pros´tah-dill
(Prostin VR Pediatric)

CANADIAN AVAILABILITY:
Prostin VR

CLASSIFICATION

Prostaglandin

PHARMACOKINETICS

After IV administration, rapidly metabolized in lungs (oxidation). Protein binding: 80-99%. Excreted in urine. Half-life: 5-10 min.

ACTION

Vasodilator having direct effect on vascular smooth muscle, ductus arteriosus.

USES

Temporarily maintains patency of ductus arteriosus until surgery is performed in those w/congenital heart defects and dependent on patent ductus for survival (e.g., pulmonary atresia or stenosis).

STORAGE/HANDLING

Store parenteral form in refrigerator. Must dilute before use. Prepare fresh every 24 hrs. Discard unused portions.

IV ADMINISTRATION

1. Infuse for shortest time, lowest dose possible.
2. If significant decrease in arterial pressure is noted via umbilical artery catheter, auscultation, or Doppler transducer, decrease infusion rate immediately.
3. Discontinue infusion immediately if apnea or bradycardia occurs (overdosage).
4. Dilute 500 mcg amp w/5% dextrose or 0.9% NaCl to volume appropriate for available pump delivery system.

INDICATIONS/DOSAGE/ROUTES

NOTE: Give by continuous IV infusion or through umbilical artery catheter placed at ductal opening.

Maintain patency ductus arteriosus:
IV INFUSION: Neonate: Initially, 0.05-0.1 mcg/kg/min. After therapeutic response achieved, use lowest dose to maintain response. **Maximum:** 0.4 mcg/kg/min.

PRECAUTIONS

CONTRAINDICATIONS: Respiratory distress syndrome (hyaline membrane disease). **CAUTIONS:** Those w/bleeding tendencies.

INTERACTIONS

DRUG INTERACTIONS: Anticoagulants, heparin, thrombolytics may increase risk of bleeding. Sympathomimetics may decrease effect. Vasodilators may increase risk of hypotension. **ALTERED LAB VALUES:** May increase bilirubin. May decrease calcium, glucose, potassium.

SIDE EFFECTS

FREQUENT: Fever. **OCCASIONAL:** Seizures, hypotension, tachycardia. **RARE:** Hyperirritability, diarrhea, hypothermia, jitteriness, lethargy, stiffness, edema.

ADVERSE REACTIONS/TOXIC EFFECTS

Overdosage manifested as flushing, bradycardia, apnea. Cardiac arrest, sepsis occur rarely.

NURSING IMPLICATIONS

INTERVENTION/EVALUATION:

Monitor arterial pressure by umbilical artery catheter, auscultation, or Doppler transducer. If significant decrease in arterial pressure occurs, decrease infusion rate immediately. Maintain continuous cardiac monitoring. Assess heart sounds, femoral pulse (circulation to lower extremities), and respiratory status frequently. Monitor B/P, ABGs, temperature. If apnea or bradycardia occur, discontinue infusion and notify physician.

PATIENT/FAMILY TEACHING:

Explain purpose of this palliative therapy to parents.

alteplase, recombinant

all′teh-place
(Activase)

CANADIAN AVAILABILITY:
Activase rt-PA

CLASSIFICATION

Thrombolytic

PHARMACOKINETICS

Rapidly metabolized in liver. Primarily excreted in urine. Half-life: 35 min.

ACTION

Directly acts on plasminogen to produce plasmin (enxyme that degrades fibrin clots). Selectively binds to fibrin-plasminogen complex within a clot.

USES

Management of acute myocardial infarction (AMI) for lysis of thrombi obstructing coronary arteries (decreases infarct size, improves ventricular function and incidence of CHF, mortality rate) and management of acute massive pulmonary embolus for lysis of acute pulmonary emboli.

STORAGE/HANDLING

Store vials at room temperature. After reconstitution, solutions are colorless to pale yellow. Solution is stable for 8 hrs after reconstitution. Discard unused portions.

IV ADMINISTRATION

1. Give by IV infusion via an infusion pump.
2. Reconstitute immediately prior to use w/sterile water for injection.
3. Reconstitute a 50 mg vial w/ 50 ml sterile water for injection without preservative (20 ml for 20 mg vial) to provide a concentration of 1 mg/ml. (May be further diluted w/50 ml 5% dextrose or 0.9% NaCl to provide a concentration of 0.5 mg/ml.)
4. Avoid excessive agitation; gently swirl or slowly invert vial to reconstitute.
5. If minor bleeding occurs at puncture sites, apply pressure for 30 sec.; if unrelieved, apply pressure dressing.
6. If uncontrolled hemorrhage occurs, discontinue infusion immediately (slowing rate of infusion may produce worsening hemorrhage).
7. Avoid undue pressure when

drug is injected into catheter (can rupture catheter or expel clot into circulation).

INDICATIONS/DOSAGE/ROUTES

Acute myocardial infarction:
IV INFUSION: Adults: 100 mg over 90 min. 15 mg bolus given over 1-2 min; then, 50 mg over 30 min; then, 35 mg over 60 min.

Acute pulmonary emboli:
IV INFUSION: Adults: 100 mg over 2 hrs. Institute or reinstitute heparin near end or immediately after infusion (when PTT or thrombin time returns to twice normal or less).

PRECAUTIONS

CONTRAINDICATIONS: Active internal bleeding, recent (within 2 mo) cerebrovascular accident, intracranial or intraspinal surgery or trauma, intracranial neoplasm, arteriovenous malformation or aneurysm, bleeding diathesis, severe uncontrolled hypertension. **CAUTIONS:** Recent (10 days) of major surgery or GI bleeding, OB delivery, organ biopsy, recent trauma (cardiopulmonary resuscitation, left heart thrombus, endocarditis, severe hepatic/renal disease, pregnancy, elderly, cerebrovascular disease, diabetic retinopathy, thrombophlebitis, occluded AV cannula at infected site. **PREGNANCY/LACTATION:** Use only when benefit outweighs potential risk to fetus. Unknown if drug crosses placenta or is distributed in breast milk. **Pregnancy Category C.**

INTERACTIONS

DRUG INTERACTIONS: Anticoagulants, heparin may increase risk of hemorrhage. Platelet aggregation inhibitors (e.g., aspirin) may increase risk of bleeding. **ALTERED LAB VALUES:** Decreases plasminogen and fibrinogen level during infusion, decreasing clotting time (confirms presence of lysis).

SIDE EFFECTS

FREQUENT: Superficial or surface bleeding at puncture sites (venous cutdowns, arterial punctures, site of recent surgical intervention, IM, retroperitoneal, or intracerebral); internal bleeding (GI/GU tract, vaginal). **RARE:** Mild allergic reaction (rash, wheezing).

ADVERSE REACTIONS/TOXIC EFFECTS

Severe internal hemorrhage may occur. Lysis of coronary thrombi may produce atrial or ventricular dysrhythmias.

NURSING IMPLICATIONS

BASELINE ASSESSMENT:

Evaluate 12-lead EKG, CPK, CPK-MB, electrolytes. Obtain baseline B/P, apical pulse. Record weight. Assess hematocrit, platelet count, thrombin (TT), activated thromboplastin (APTT), prothrombin time (PT), fibrinogen level, before therapy is instituted. Type and hold blood.

INTERVENTION/EVALUATION:

Continuous cardiac monitoring for arrhythmias, B/P, pulse and respirations q 15 min until stable, then hourly. Check peripheral pulses, heart and lung sounds. Monitor chest pain relief and notify physician of continuation or recurrence (note location, type and intensity). Assess for bleeding: overt blood, blood in any body substance. Monitor PTT per protocol. Maintain BR; avoid any trauma that might increase risk of bleeding (injections, shaving, etc.). Assess neurologic status.

PATIENT/FAMILY TEACHING:

Explain the reason for therapy and to report any bleeding.

altretamine (hexamethylmelamine)

all-treh´tih-meen
(Hexalen)

CANADIAN AVAILABILITY:
Hexastat

CLASSIFICATION

Antineoplastic

PHARMACOKINETICS

Well absorbed from GI tract. Protein binding: 6% (metabolites 25-50%). Metabolized in liver to active metabolites (necessary for action). Primarily excreted in urine. Half-life: 4.7-10.2 hrs.

ACTION

Exact mechanism unknown. May inhibit DNA, RNA synthesis.

USES

Palliative treatment for persistent or recurrent ovarian cancer following therapy w/a cisplatin or alkylating combination.

PO ADMINISTRATION

Give after meals and at bedtime.

INDICATIONS/DOSAGE/ROUTES

Ovarian cancer:
NOTE: Give total daily dose as 4 equally divided doses after meals and bedtime.

PO: Adults, elderly: 260 mg/m^2/day in 4 divided doses for 14 or 21 consecutive days in 28-day cycle. May be temporarily held or discontinued w/dose decreased to 200 mg/m^2/day if: GI intolerance, WBC $<$2,000/mm^3 or granulocyte $<$1,000/mm^3, platelets $<$75,000/mm^3, progressive neurotoxicity.

PRECAUTIONS

CONTRAINDICATIONS: Severe bone marrow depression, severe neurologic toxicity. **CAUTIONS:** Decreased neurological function. **PREGNANCY/LACTATION:** Unknown if drug crosses placenta or is distributed in breast milk. **Pregnancy Category D.**

INTERACTIONS

DRUG INTERACTIONS: Bone marrow depressants may increase bone marrow depression. MAOIs may cause severe orthostatic hypotension. Live virus vaccines may potentiate virus replication, increase vaccine side effects, decrease pt's antibody response to vaccine. **ALTERED LAB VALUES:** May increase alkaline phosphatase, BUN, serum creatinine; reduce platelet, WBC count.

SIDE EFFECTS

FREQUENT: Mild to moderate nausea and vomiting, mild sensory peripheral neuropathy, mild anemia. **OCCASIONAL:** Moderate to severe sensory peripheral neuropathy, moderate to severe anemia. **RARE:** Severe nausea and vomiting, anorexia, fatigue, rash, alopecia.

ADVERSE REACTIONS/TOXIC EFFECTS

Mild to moderate myelosuppression expected. Neurologic toxicity generally disappears when drug is discontinued.

NURSING IMPLICATIONS

BASELINE ASSESSMENT:

Give emotional support to patient and family. Perform neurologic function tests prior to chemotherapy. Check blood counts prior to each course of therapy, monthly or as clinically indicated.

INTERVENTION/EVALUATION:

Monitor for hematologic toxicity (fever, sore throat, signs of local infection, easy bruising, unusual bleeding), symptoms of anemia (excessive tiredness, weakness). Measure all vomitus (general guideline requiring immediate notification of physician: 750 ml/8 hrs, urinary output less than 100 ml/hr).

PATIENT/FAMILY TEACHING:

Nausea may decrease during therapy. Do not have immunizations w/o physician's approval (drug lowers body's resistance). Avoid contact w/those who have recently taken live virus vaccine.

aluminum acetate

(Burow's Solution)

FIXED-COMBINATION(S): Aluminum sulfate w/calcium acetate (Domboro Powder, Domboro Tablets, Bluboro Powder, Pedi-Boro Soak Paks, Modified Burow's Solution)

CANADIAN AVAILABILITY:
Acid Mantle

CLASSIFICATION

Astringent

ACTION

Precipitates proteins; lowers pH w/increase in skin acidity; inhibits discharge by causing contraction (shrinkage of tissue). Anti-inflammatory, antipruritic, astringent, mild antiseptic properties.

USES

Relief of inflammation, irritation of the skin such as insect bites, poison ivy, diaper rash, acne, allergy, anal pruritis, eczema, bruises.

TOPICAL ADMINISTRATION

1. Mix 1 tablet or packet w/1 pint of water (warm or cool, as ordered).
2. Do not cover dressing w/plastic or other occlusive covering.
3. Keep away from eyes.

INDICATIONS/DOSAGE/ROUTES

Usual topical dosage:
TOPICAL: Adults, elderly: Apply for 15-30 min q4-8h.

PRECAUTIONS

CONTRAINDICATIONS: Sensitivity to aluminum. **CAUTIONS:** For external use only. **PREGNANCY/LACTATION: Pregnancy Category C.**

INTERACTIONS

DRUG INTERACTIONS: None significant. **ALTERED LAB VALUES:** None significant.

SIDE EFFECTS

RARE: Increased irritation, extension of inflammation.

NURSING IMPLICATIONS

BASELINE ASSESSMENT:

Determine extent of skin irritation, inflammation.

INTERVENTION/EVALUATION:

Assess therapeutic response, increased redness, irritation, discomfort.

PATIENT/FAMILY TEACHING:

Discontinue if increased irritation or inflammation occurs. Avoid using near eyes. Do not cover with plastic or other occlusive material.

aluminum carbonate

(Basaljel)

aluminum hydroxide

(Alternagel, Alu-Cap, Alu-Tab, Amphojel, Dialume)

dihydroxyaluminum sodium carbonate

(Rolaids)

FIXED-COMBINATION(S): W/magnesium, an antacid (Aludrox, Delcid, Gaviscon, Maalox); w/magnesium and simethicone, an antiflatulent (DiGel, Gelusil, Maalox Plus, Mylanta, Silain-Gel); w/magnesium and calcium, an antacid (Camalox)

CANADIAN AVAILABILITY: Amphojel, Basaljel

CLASSIFICATION

Antacid

PHARMACOKINETICS

Small amount absorbed from intestine. Onset of action based on solubility in stomach and reaction w/hydrochloric acid. Duration of action based primarily on gastric emptying time (20 min when given before meals, up to 3 hrs when given after meals).

ACTION

Neutralizes or reduces gastric acid by increasing gastric pH, inhibiting pepsin activity. Binds phosphate in intestine, then excreted in feces (reduces phosphates in urine preventing formation of phosphate urinary stones; reduces serum phosphate levels). May increase absorption of calcium (due to decreased serum phosphate levels). Astringent, adsorbent properties (decreases fluidity of stools).

USES

Symptomatic relief of upset stomach associated w/hyperacidity (heartburn, acid indigestion, sour stomach). Hyperacidity associated w/gastric, duodenal ulcers. Symptomatic treatment of gastroesophageal reflux disease. Prophylactic treatment of GI bleeding secondary to gastritis and stress ulceration. In conjunction w/low phosphate diet, prevents formation of phosphate urinary stones, reduces elevated phosphate levels.

PO ADMINISTRATION

1. Usually administered 1-3 hrs after meals.
2. Individualize dose (based on neutralizing capacity of antacids).
3. Chewable tablets: Thoroughly chew tablets before swallowing (follow w/glass of water or milk).
4. If administering suspension, shake well before use.

INDICATIONS/DOSAGE/ROUTES

NOTE: Usual dose is 30-60 ml.

Aluminum Carbonate:

Antacid:
PO: Adults, elderly: 2 capsules or 10 ml q2h up to 12 times/day.

Hyperphosphatemia:
PO: Adults, elderly: 2 capsules or 12.5 ml 3-4 times/day w/meals.

Aluminum Hydroxide:

Antacid:
PO: Adults, elderly: 500-1,800 mg 3-6 times/day between meals and bedtime.

Hyperphosphatemia:
PO: Children: 50-150 mg/kg/24 hrs in divided doses q4-6h.

PRECAUTIONS

CONTRAINDICATIONS: Fecal impaction. **CAUTIONS:** Impaired renal function, gastric outlet obstruction, elderly, dehydration, fluid restriction. **PREGNANCY/LACTATION:** May produce hypercalcemia, hypo/hypermagnesemia, increase tendon reflexes in neonate/fetus whose mother is a chronic, high-dose user. May be distributed in breast milk. **Pregnancy Category C.**

INTERACTIONS

DRUG INTERACTIONS: May decrease excretion of quinidine, anticholinergics. May decrease effects of methenamine. May increase salicylate excretion. May decrease absorption of quinolones, iron preparations, isoniazid, ketoconazole, tetracyclines. **ALTERED LAB VALUES:** May increase gastrin, systemic/urinary pH. May decrease serum phosphate.

SIDE EFFECTS

FREQUENT: Constipation w/repeated dosage.

ADVERSE REACTIONS/TOXIC EFFECTS

Prolonged constipation may result in intestinal obstruction. Excessive or chronic use may produce hypophosphatemia (anorexia, malaise, muscle weakness, bone pain) resulting in osteomalacia, osteoporosis. Prolonged use may produce urinary calculi.

NURSING IMPLICATIONS

Baseline Assessment:

Do not give other oral medication within 1-2 hrs of antacid administration.

Intervention/Evaluation:

Assess pattern of daily bowel activity and stool consistency. Monitor serum phosphate, calcium, uric acid levels. Assess for relief of gastric distress.

Patient/Family Teaching:

Chewable tablets: Chew tablets thoroughly before swallowing (may be followed by water or milk). Tablets may discolor stool. Maintain adequate fluid intake.

amantadine hydrochloride

ah-man´tih-deen
(Symadine, Symmetrel)

CANADIAN AVAILABILITY:
Symmetrel

CLASSIFICATION

Antiviral, antiparkinson.

PHARMACOKINETICS

Rapid, completely absorbed

from GI tract. Widely distributed. Protein binding: 67%. Primarily excreted in urine. Minimal removed by hemodialysis. Half-life: 11-15 hrs (increased in elderly, decreased renal function).

ACTION

Antiviral action against influenza A virus believed to prevent uncoating of virus, penetration of host cells, release of nucleic acid into host cells. Antiparkinsonism due to increased release of dopamine. Virustatic.

USES

Prevention, treatment of respiratory tract infections due to influenza virus, Parkinson's disease, drug-induced extrapyramidal reactions.

PO ADMINISTRATION

Administer nighttime dose several hours before bedtime (prevents insomnia).

INDICATIONS/DOSAGE/ROUTES

Prophylaxis, symptomatic treatment respiratory illness due to influenza A virus:
NOTE: Give as single or in 2 divided doses.
PO: Adults (10-64 yrs): 200 mg daily. **Adults (>64 yrs):** 100 mg daily. **Children (9-12 yrs):** 100 mg 2 times/day. **Children (1-9 yrs):** 4.4-8.8 mg/kg/day (up to 150 mg/day).

Parkinson's disease, extrapyramidol symptoms:
PO: Adults: 100 mg 2 times/day. May increase up to 400 mg/day in divided doses.

Usual elderly dosage:
PO: Elderly: Based on renal function. Ccr 40-50 ml/min: 100 mg/day; Ccr 20 ml/min: 100 mg 3 times/wk.

Dosage in renal impairment:
Dose and/or frequency is modified based on creatinine clearance.

CREATININE CLEARANCE	DOSAGE
30-50 ml/min	200 mg first day; 100 mg/day thereafter
15-29 ml/min	200 mg first day; 100 mg on alternate days
<15 ml/min	200 mg every 7 days

PRECAUTIONS

CONTRAINDICATIONS: None significant. **CAUTIONS:** History of seizures, orthostatic hypotension, CHF, peripheral edema, liver disease, recurrent eczematoid dermatitis, cerebrovascular disease, renal dysfunction, those receiving CNS stimulants. **PREGNANCY/LACTATION:** Unknown if drug crosses placenta; distributed in breast milk. **Pregnancy Category C.**

INTERACTIONS

DRUG INTERACTIONS: Tricyclic antidepressants, antihistamines, phenothiazine, anticholinergics may increase anticholinergic effects. CNS stimulants may increase CNS stimulation. Hydrochlorothiazide, triamterene may increase concentration, toxicity. **ALTERED LAB VALUES:** None significant.

SIDE EFFECTS

FREQUENT: Nausea, dizziness, difficulty concentrating, insomnia. **OCCASIONAL:** Orthostatic hypotension, anorexia, constipation, irritability, headache, peripheral edema, confusion, depression, hallucinations, livedo reticularis (reddish-blue, net-like blotching of skin). **RARE:** Vomiting, dyspnea, skin rash, weakness, fatigue, urinary retention, slurred speech, eczematoid dermatitis.

ADVERSE REACTIONS/TOXIC EFFECTS

CHF, leukopenia, neutropenia occur rarely. Hyperexcitability, convulsions, ventricular arrhythmias may occur.

NURSING IMPLICATIONS

BASELINE ASSESSMENT:

Question history of allergies, especially to amantadine. When treating infections caused by influenza A virus, obtain specimens for viral diagnostic tests before giving first dose (therapy may begin before results are known).

INTERVENTION/EVALUATION:

Monitor I&O, renal function tests if ordered; check for peripheral edema. Evaluate food tolerance, vomiting. Assess skin for rash, blotching. Be alert to neurologic effects: headache, lethargy, confusion, agitation, blurred vision, seizures. Assess B/P at least twice daily. Determine bowel pattern, modify diet, or administer laxative as needed. Assess for dizziness. *Parkinsonism:* Assess for clinical reversal of symptoms (improvement of tremor of head/hands at rest, mask-like facial expression, shuffling gait, muscular rigidity).

PATIENT/FAMILY TEACHING:

Continue therapy for full length of treatment. Doses should be evenly spaced. Do not take any medications w/o consulting physician. Avoid alcoholic beverages. Do not drive, use machinery, or engage in other activities that require mental acuity if experiencing dizziness, confusion, blurred vision. Get up slowly from a sitting or lying position. Advise physician if no improvement in 2-3 days when taking for viral infection. Inform physician of new symptoms, especially blotching, rash, dizziness, blurred vision, nausea/vomiting. Take nighttime dose several hours before bedtime to prevent insomnia.

amcinonide

(Cyclocort)

(See Classifications section under Corticosteroid: topical)

amikacin sulfate

am-ih-kay´sin

(Amikin)

CANADIAN AVAILABILITY:
Amikin

CLASSIFICATION

Antibiotic: Aminoglycoside

PHARMACOKINETICS

Rapid, complete absorption after IM administration. Widely distributed (does not cross blood-brain barrier, low concentrations in CSF). Protein binding: 10%. Excreted unchanged in urine. Removed by hemodialysis. Half-life: 2-4 hrs (increased in decreased renal function, neonates; decreased in cystic fibrosis, burn or febrile pts).

ACTION

Irreversibly binds to protein on 30S subunit of bacterial ribosome, interfering in protein synthesis of susceptible microorganisms.

USES

Treatment of skin/skin structure, bone, joint, respiratory tract, intra-abdominal and complicated urinary tract infections; postop, burns, septicemia, meningitis.

STORAGE/HANDLING

Store vials at room temperature. Solutions appear clear but may become pale yellow (does not affect potency). Intermittent IV infusion (piggyback) stable for 24 hrs at room temperature. Discard if precipitate forms or dark discoloration occurs.

IM/IV ADMINISTRATION

NOTE: Coordinate peak and trough lab draws w/administration times.

IM:

1. To minimize discomfort, give deep IM slowly. Less painful if injected into gluteus maximus rather than lateral aspect of thigh.

IV:

1. Dilute w/50-200 ml 5% dextrose, 0.9% NaCl, or other compatible fluid. Amount of diluent for infants, children depends on individual needs.
2. Infuse over 30-60 min for adults, older children, and over 60-120 min for infants, young children.
3. Alternating IV sites, use large veins to reduce risk of phlebitis.

INDICATIONS/DOSAGE/ROUTES

NOTE: Space doses evenly around the clock. Dosage based on ideal body weight. Peak, trough serum level is determined periodically to maintain desired serum concentrations (minimizes risk of toxicity). *Recommended peak level:* 15-30 mcg/ml; *trough level:* 5-10 mcg/ml.

Uncomplicated urinary tract infections:
IM/IV: Adults, elderly: 250 mg q12h.

Moderate to severe infections:
IM/IV: Adults, elderly, children: 15 mg/kg/day in divided doses q8-12h. Do not exceed 15 mg/kg or 1.5 Gm/day. **Neonates:** *Loading dose:* 10 mg/kg, then 7.5 mg/kg q12h.

Dosage in renal impairment:
Dose and/or frequency is modified based on degree of renal impairment, serum concentration of drug. After loading dose of 5-7.5 mg/kg, maintenance dose/frequency based on serum creatinine or creatinine clearance.

PRECAUTIONS

CONTRAINDICATIONS: Sulfite sensitivity (may result in anaphylaxis, especially in asthmatics). **CAUTIONS:** Possible cross-sensitivity to other aminoglycosides. Elderly, neonates (potential for renal insufficiency or immaturity); neuromuscular disorders (potential for respiratory depression), prior hearing loss, vertigo, renal impairment. **PREGNANCY/LACTATION:** Readily crosses placenta; unknown if distributed in breast milk. May produce fetal nephrotoxicity. **Pregnancy Category C.**

INTERACTIONS

DRUG INTERACTIONS: Other aminoglycosides, nephrotoxic- and ototoxic-producing medications may increase toxicity. May increase effects of neuromuscular blocking agents. **ALTERED LAB VALUES:** May increase BUN, SGPT (ALT), SGOT (AST), bilirubin, creatinine, LDH concentrations; may decrease serum calcium, magnesium, potassium, sodium concentrations.

SIDE EFFECTS

OCCASIONAL: Pain, induration at IM injection site; phlebitis, thrombophlebitis w/IV administration; hypersensitivity reactions: rash, fever, urticaria, pruritus. **RARE:** Hypotension, nausea, vomiting, weakness.

ADVERSE REACTIONS/TOXIC EFFECTS

Nephrotoxicity (evidenced by increased BUN and serum creatinine, decreased creatinine clearance) may be reversible if drug stopped at first sign of symptoms; irreversible ototoxicity (tinnitus, dizziness, ringing/roaring in ears, reduced hearing) and neurotoxicity (headache, dizziness, lethargy, tremors, visual disturbances) occur occasionally. Risk is greater w/higher dosages, prolonged therapy. Superinfections, particularly w/fungi, may result from bacterial imbalance.

NURSING IMPLICATIONS

BASELINE ASSESSMENT:

Dehydration must be treated before aminoglycoside therapy. Establish pt's baseline hearing ...ty before beginning therapy. ...n for history of allergies, es... to aminoglycosides and sulfite. Obtain specimen for culture, sensitivity before giving the first dose (therapy may begin before results are known).

INTERVENTION/EVALUATION:

Monitor I&O (maintain hydration), urinalysis (casts, RBC, WBC, decrease in specific gravity). Monitor results of peak/trough blood tests. Be alert to ototoxic and neurotoxic symptoms (see Adverse Reactions/Toxic Effects). Check IM injection site for pain, induration. Evaluate IV site for phlebitis (heat, pain, red streaking over vein). Assess for skin rash. Assess for superinfection, particularly genital/anal pruritus, changes of oral mucosa, diarrhea. When treating those w/neuromuscular disorders, assess respiratory response carefully.

PATIENT/FAMILY TEACHING:

Continue antibiotic for full length of treatment. Space doses evenly. Discomfort may occur w/IM injection. Notify physician in event of any hearing, visual, balance, urinary problems even after therapy is completed. Do not take other medication w/o consulting physician. Lab tests are essential part of therapy.

amiloride hydrochloride

ah-mill′or-ride
(Midamor)

FIXED-COMBINATION(S):
W/hydrochlorothiazide, a thiazide diuretic (Moduretic)

CANADIAN AVAILABILITY:
Midamor

CLASSIFICATION

Diuretic: Potassium-sparing

PHARMACOKINETICS

	ONSET	PEAK	DURATION
PO	2 hr	6-10 hrs	24 hrs

Incompletely absorbed from GI tract. Protein binding: minimal. Primarily excreted in urine; partially eliminated in feces. Half-life: 6-9 hrs.

ACTION

Directly interferes w/sodium reabsorption in distal tubule, increasing sodium and water excretion and decreasing potassium excretion. Initial decrease in B/P by decreasing plasma and extracellular fluid volume.

USES

Adjunctive therapy in treatment of diuretic-induced hypokalemia in those w/CHF or hypertension. Used when maintenance of serum potassium levels is necessary (digitalized patients, cardiac arrhythmias).

PO ADMINISTRATION

Give w/food to avoid GI distress.

INDICATIONS/DOSAGE/ROUTES

PO: Adults: Initially, 5 mg daily. May be increased to 10 mg daily, as single dose or in divided doses. If hypokalemia persists, dose may be increased to 15 mg, then to 20 mg, w/electrolyte monitoring.

Usual elderly dosage:
PO: Elderly: Initially, 5 mg/day or every other day.

PRECAUTIONS

CONTRAINDICATIONS: Serum potassium >5.5 mEq/L, those on other potassium-sparing diuretics, anuria, acute or chronic renal insufficiency, diabetic nephropathy. **CAUTIONS:** Those w/BUN >30 mg/dl or serum creatinine >1.5 mg/dl, elderly, debilitated, hepatic insufficiency, those w/cardiopulmonary disease, diabetes mellitus. **PREGNANCY/LACTATION:** Unknown if drug crosses placenta or is distributed in breast milk. **Pregnancy Category B.**

INTERACTIONS

DRUG INTERACTIONS: May decrease effect of anticoagulants, heparin. NSAIDs may decrease antihypertensive effect. ACE inhibitors (e.g., captopril), potassium-containing diuretics, potassium supplements may increase potassium. May decrease lithium clearance, increase toxicity. **ALTERED LAB VALUES:** May increase BUN, calcium excretion, creatinine, glucose, magnesium, potassium, uric acid. May decrease sodium.

SIDE EFFECTS

EXPECTED RESPONSE: Frequent urination, polyuria. **OCCASIONAL:** Fatigue, nausea, diarrhea, abdominal distress, leg aches, headache. **RARE:** Anorexia, weakness, rash, dizziness.

ADVERSE REACTIONS/TOXIC EFFECTS

Severe hyperkalemia may produce irritability, anxiety, heaviness of legs, paresthesia, hypotension, bradycardia, tented T waves, widening QRS, ST depression.

NURSING IMPLICATIONS

BASELINE ASSESSMENT:

Assess baseline electrolytes, particularly for low potassium. Assess renal/hepatic functions. Assess edema (note location, extent), skin turgor, mucous membranes for hydration status. Assess muscle strength, mental status. Note skin temperature, moisture. Obtain baseline weight. Initiate strict I&O. Note pulse rate/regularity.

INTERVENTION/EVALUATION:

Monitor B/P, vital signs, electrolytes (particularly potassium), I&O, weight. Note extent of diuresis. Watch for changes from initial assessment; hyperkalemia may result in muscle strength changes, tremor, muscle cramps, change in mental status (orientation, alertness, confusion), cardiac arrhythmias. Monitor potassium level, particularly during initial therapy. Weigh daily. Assess lung sounds for rales, wheezing.

PATIENT/FAMILY TEACHING:

Expect increase in volume and frequency of urination. Therapeutic effect takes several days to begin and can last for several days when drug is discontinued. High potassium diet/potassium supplements can be dangerous, especially if pt has renal/hepatic problems. Avoid foods high in potassium such as whole grains (cereals), legumes, meat, bananas, apricots, orange juice, potatoes (white, sweet), raisins.

aminocaproic acid

ah-meen-oh-kah-pro´ick
(Amicar)

CANADIAN AVAILABILITY:
Amicar

CLASSIFICATION

Fibrinolysis inhibitor

PHARMACOKINETICS

Rapidly absorbed. Protein binding: none. Primarily excreted in urine.

ACTION

Inhibits activation of plasminogen (reducing plasminogen to plasmin-fibrinolysin). Directly inhibits activity of plasmin.

USES

Treatment of excessive bleeding from hyperfibrinolysis or urinary fibrinolysis. Use only in acute life-threatening situations.

PO/IV ADMINISTRATION

PO:

1. Scored tablets may be crushed.
2. May take w/o regard to food.
3. Syrup used by pts unable to take tablets.

IV:

1. Give only by IV infusion.
2. Dilute w/5% dextrose, 0.9% NaCl, or other compatible solution.
3. Monitor for hypotension during infusion. Rapid infusion may produce bradycardia, arrhythmias.

INDICATIONS/DOSAGE/ROUTES

NOTE: Reduce dosage in presence of cardiac, renal, or hepatic impairment.

Acute bleeding:
PO/IV INFUSION: Adults, elderly: Initially, 4-5 Gm, then 1-1.25 Gm/hr. Continue for 8 hrs or until

bleeding controlled. **Maximum:** Up to 30 Gm/24 hrs.

Chronic bleeding:
PO: Adults, elderly: 5-30 Gm/day, in divided doses at 3-6 hr intervals.

PRECAUTIONS

CONTRAINDICATIONS: Evidence of active intravascular clotting process, disseminated intravascular coagulation w/o concurrent heparin therapy, hematuria of upper urinary tract origin (unless benefits outweigh risk). *Parenteral:* Newborns. **EXTREME CAUTION:** Impaired cardiac, hepatic, or renal disease, those w/hyperfibrinolysis. **PREGNANCY/LACTATION:** Unknown if drug crosses placenta or is distributed in breast milk. **Pregnancy Category C.**

INTERACTIONS

DRUG INTERACTIONS: None significant. **ALTERED LAB VALUES:** May elevate serum potassium level.

SIDE EFFECTS

Frequency of effects unknown, but are generally mild and disappear after drug withdrawal: Nausea, cramping, diarrhea, skeletal weakness/fatigue (myopathy), tinnitus, nasal stuffiness, rash, prolonged menstrual period.

ADVERSE REACTIONS/TOXIC EFFECTS

Rarely, grand mal seizure occurs, generally preceded by weakness, dizziness, headache.

NURSING IMPLICATIONS

INTERVENTION/EVALUATION:

Monitor serum creatine kinase in those undergoing long-term therapy. If increase is noted in serum creatine kinase test, drug should be discontinued. Question any change in skeletal strength as noted by pt (consider possibility of cardiac damage as a result). Skeletal myopathy characterized by increase in creatine kinase, aldolase, and SGOT (AST) serum levels. Monitor these lab results frequently. Monitor heart rhythm. Assess for decrease in B/P, increase in pulse rate, abdominal or back pain, severe headache (may be evidence of hemorrhage). Assess peripheral pulses; skin for bruises, petechiae. Question for increase in amount of discharge during menses. Check for excessive bleeding from minor cuts, scratches. Assess gums for erythema, gingival bleeding. Assess urine output for hematuria.

PATIENT/FAMILY TEACHING:

Use electric razor, soft toothbrush to prevent bleeding. Report any sign of red/dark urine, black/red stool, coffee-ground vomitus, red-speckled mucus from cough. Do not use any over the counter medication w/o physician approval (may interfere w/platelet aggregation).

aminophylline (theophylline ethylenediamine)

am-in-oh´phil-lin
(Aminophylline, Phyllocontin)

theophylline

(Immediate-release: Aerolate, Slo-Phyllin, Theolair) (Extended-release: Slo-Bid, Theo-Dur, Theo-24, Uniphyl)

CANADIAN AVAILABILITY:
aminophylline: Palaron, Phyllocontin; **theophylline:** Theo-Dur, Theolair, Uniphyl

CLASSIFICATION

Bronchodilator

PHARMACOKINETICS

Well absorbed from GI tract (absorption may vary w/dosage form used). Protein binding: 60% (decreased in neonates, pts w/hepatic cirrhosis). Metabolized in liver. Excreted in urine. Half-life: dependent on age, liver, cardiac function, lung disease, smoking.

ACTION

Directly relaxes smooth muscle of bronchial airway, pulmonary blood vessels (relieves bronchospasm, increases vital capacity). Respiratory stimulant.

USES

Symptomatic relief, prevention of bronchial asthma, reversible bronchospasm due to chronic bronchitis, emphysema.

STORAGE/HANDLING

Store solution, suppositories at room temperature. Discard if solution contains a precipitate.

PO/IV/RECTAL ADMINISTRATION

PO:

1. Give w/food to avoid GI distress.
2. Do not crush or break extended-release forms.

IV:

1. Give loading dose diluted in 100-200 ml of 5% dextrose or 0.9% NaCl. Maintenance dose in larger volume parenteral infusion.
2. Do not exceed flow rate of 1 ml/min (25 mg/min) for either piggyback or infusion.
3. Administer loading dose over 20-30 min.
4. Use infusion pump or microdrip to regulate IV administration.

RECTAL:

1. Moisten suppository w/cold water before inserting well up into rectum.

INDICATIONS/DOSAGE/ROUTES

NOTE: Dosage calculated on basis of lean body weight. Dosage based on peak serum theophylline concentrations, clinical condition, presence of toxicity.

Chronic bronchospasm:
PO: Adults, elderly, children: Initially, 16 mg/kg or 400 mg/day (whichever is less) in 2-4 divided doses (6-12 hr intervals). May increase by 25% every 2-3 days up to maximum of 24 mg/kg/day **(1-9 yrs);** 20 mg/kg/day **(9-12 yrs);** 18 mg/kg/day **(12-16 yrs);** 13 mg/kg/day **(>16 yrs).** Doses above maximum based on serum theophylline concentrations, clinical condition, presence of toxicity.

Acute bronchospasm in patients not currently on theophylline:
IV LOADING DOSE: Adults, children (>1 yr): Initially, 6 mg/kg (aminophylline), then begin maintenance aminophylline dosage based on patient group.

PATIENT GROUP	MAINTENANCE AMINOPHYLLINE DOSAGE
Neonates	0.2 mg/kg/hr
Children (1-12 mo)	0.2-0.9 mg/kg/hr
Children (1-9 yrs)	1-1.2 mg/kg/hr
Children (9-16 yrs), young adult smokers	0.8-1 mg/kg/hr

Older patients, patients w/cor pulmonale	0.3-0.6 mg/kg/hr
Patients w/CHF, liver disease	0.1-0.5 mg/kg/hr

PO/LOADING DOSE: Adults, children (>1 yr): Initially, 5 mg/kg (theophylline), then begin maintenance theophylline dosage based on patient group.

PATIENT GROUP	MAINTENANCE THEOPHYLLINE DOSAGE
Children (1-9 yrs)	4 mg/kg q6h
Children (9-16 yrs), young adult smokers	3 mg/kg q6h
Healthy, nonsmoking adults	3 mg/kg q8h
Older patients, patients w/cor pulmonale	2 mg/kg q8h
Patients w/CHF, liver disease	1-2 mg/kg q12h

Acute bronchospasm in patients currently on theophylline:
IV/PO: Adults, children >1 yr: Obtain serum theophylline level. If not possible and pt in respiratory distress, not experiencing toxicity, may give 2.5 mg/kg dose. **Maintenance:** Dosage based on peak serum theophylline concentrations, clinical condition, presence of toxicity.

PRECAUTIONS

CONTRAINDICATIONS: History of hypersensitivity to xanthine, caffeine. **CAUTIONS:** Impaired cardiac, renal, or hepatic function, hypertension, hyperthyroidism, diabetes mellitus, peptic ulcer, glaucoma, severe hypoxemia. **PREGNANCY/LACTATION:** Readily crosses placenta; distributed in breast milk. May inhibit uterine contractions; produce irritability in nursing infants. **Pregnancy Category C.**

INTERACTIONS

DRUG INTERACTIONS: Glucocorticoids may produce hypernatremia. Phenytoin, primidone, rifampin may increase metabolism. Beta-blockers may decrease effects. Cimetidine, ciprofloxacin, erythromycin, norfloxacin may increase concentration, toxicity. Smoking may decrease concentration. **ALTERED LAB VALUES:** None significant.

SIDE EFFECTS

FREQUENT: Momentary change in sense of smell during IV administration; shakiness, restlessness, increased heart rate, mild diuresis.

ADVERSE REACTIONS/TOXIC EFFECTS

Too-rapid rate of IV administration may produce marked fall in B/P w/accompanying faintness and lightheadedness, palpitations, tachycardia, hyperventilation, nausea, vomiting, angina-like pain, seizures, ventricular fibrillation, cardiac standstill.

NURSING IMPLICATIONS

BASELINE ASSESSMENT:

Offer emotional support (high incidence of anxiety due to difficulty in breathing and sympathomimetic response to drug). Peak serum concentration should be taken 1 hr after IV, 1-2 hrs following immediate-release dose, 3-8 hrs following extended-release. Take trough level just before next dose.

INTERVENTION/EVALUATION:

Monitor rate, depth, rhythm, type of respiration; quality, and rate of pulse. Assess lung sounds for rhonchi, wheezing, rales. Monitor arterial blood gases. Observe lips, fingernails for blue or dusky color in light-skinned pts; gray in dark-skinned pts. Observe for clavicular retractions, hand tremor. Evaluate for clinical improvement (quieter, slower respirations, relaxed facial expression, cessation of clavicular retractions). Monitor theophylline blood serum levels (therapeutic serum level range: 10-20 mcg/ml).

PATIENT/FAMILY TEACHING:

Increase fluid intake (decreases lung secretion viscosity). Avoid excessive use of caffeine derivatives (chocolate, coffee, tea, cola, cocoa). Smoking, charcoal broiled food, high-protein, low-carbohydrate diet may decrease theophylline level.

amiodarone hydrochloride

ah-me-oh´dah-roan
(Cordarone)

CANADIAN AVAILABILITY: Cordarone

CLASSIFICATION

Antiarrhythmic

PHARMACOKINETICS

Slowly, variably absorbed from GI tract. Protein binding: 96%. Extensively metabolized in liver to active metabolite. Excreted via bile; not removed by hemodialysis. Half-life: 26-107 days; metabolite: 61 days.

ACTION

Prolongs action potential duration, refractory period by direct action on all cardiac tissue. Decreases AV conduction, sinus node function.

USES

Treatment of documented, life-threatening, recurrent ventricular fibrillation, and recurrent, hemodynamically unstable ventricular tachycardia in those who have not responded adequately to other antiarrhythmic agents.

PO ADMINISTRATION

1. Give w/meals to reduce GI distress.
2. Tablets may be crushed.

INDICATIONS/DOSAGE/ROUTES

Life-threatening ventricular arrhythmias:
PO: Adults, elderly: Initially, 800-1,600 mg/day in 1-2 divided doses for 1-3 wks. After arrhythmias controlled or side effects occur, reduce to 600-800 mg/day for about 4 wks. **Maintenance:** 200-600 mg/day.

PRECAUTIONS

CONTRAINDICATIONS: Severe sinus-node dysfunction, second and third degree AV block, bradycardia-induced syncope (except in presence of pacemaker), severe hepatic disease. **CAUTIONS:** Thyroid disease. **PREGNANCY/LACTATION:** Crosses placenta; distributed in breast milk. May adversely affect fetal development. **Pregnancy Category C.**

INTERACTIONS

DRUG INTERACTIONS: May increase cardiac effects w/other antiarrhythmics. May increase effect of oral anticoagulants. May increase concentration, toxicity of digoxin, phenytoin. **ALTERED LAB VALUES:** May increase SGOT (AST), SGPT (ALT), alkaline phosphatase, ANA titer. May cause changes in EKG, thyroid function tests.

SIDE EFFECTS

Corneal microdeposits are noted in almost all pts. **FREQUENT:** Nausea, vomiting, photosensitivity, malaise, fatigue, tremor, peripheral paresthesia, constipation, anorexia, sleep disturbances. **OCCASIONAL:** Proximal muscle weakness, tremors, bluish skin discoloration due to sun exposure, headache, bradycardia, hypo/hyperthyroidism.

ADVERSE REACTIONS/TOXIC EFFECTS

Serious, potentially fatal pulmonary toxicity (alveolitis, pulmonary fibrosis, pneumonitis, adult respiratory distress syndrome) may begin w/progressive dyspnea and cough w/rales, decreased breath sounds, pleurisy. CHF, hepatotoxicity may be noted. May worsen existing arrhythmias or produce new arrhythmias.

NURSING IMPLICATIONS

BASELINE ASSESSMENT:

Obtain baseline pulmonary function tests, chest x-ray, liver enzyme tests SGOT (AST), SGPT (ALT), alkaline phosphatase). Assess B/P, apical pulse immediately before drug is administered (if pulse is 60/min or below, or systolic B/P is below 90 mm Hg, withhold medication, contact physician).

INTERVENTION/EVALUATION:

Monitor for symptoms of pulmonary toxicity (progressively worsening dyspnea, cough). Dosage should be discontinued or reduced if toxicity occurs. Assess pulse for strength/weakness, irregular rate, bradycardia. Monitor EKG for cardiac changes, particularly widening of QRS, prolongation of PR and QT intervals. Notify physician of any significant interval changes. Assess for nausea, fatigue, paresthesia, tremor. Monitor for signs of hypothyroidism (periorbital edema, lethargy, pudgy hands/feet, cool/pale skin, vertigo, night cramps), and hyperthyroidism (hot/dry skin, bulging eyes [exophthalmos], frequent urination, eye lid edema, weight loss, breathlessness). Monitor SGOT (AST), SGPT (ALT), alkaline phosphatase for evidence of liver toxicity. Assess skin, cornea for bluish discoloration in those who have been on drug therapy longer than 2 mos. Monitor liver function tests, thyroid test results. If elevated liver enzymes, dose reduction or discontinuation is evident. Monitor for therapeutic serum level (1.5-2.5 mcg/ml).

PATIENT/FAMILY TEACHING:

Protect against photosensitivity reaction on skin exposed to sunlight. Bluish skin discoloration gradually disappears when drug is discontinued. Report shortness of breath, cough. Outpatients should monitor pulse before taking medication. Do not abruptly discontinue medication. Compliance w/therapy regimen is essential to control arrhythmias. Do not use nasal decongestants, over-the-counter preparations (stimulants) w/o physician approval. Restrict salt, alcohol intake.

amitriptyline hydrochloride

a-me-trip´tih-leen
(Elavil, Endep)

FIXED-COMBINATION(S): W/chlordiazepoxide, an antianxiety (Limbitrol); w/perphenazine, an antipsychotic (Etrafon, Triavil)

CANADIAN AVAILABILITY: Apo-Amitriptyline, Elavil, Levate, Novotriptyn

CLASSIFICATION

Antidepressant: Tricyclic

PHARMACOKINETICS

Rapid, well absorbed from GI tract. Protein binding: 95%. Metabolized in liver, undergoes first pass metabolism. Primariy excreted in urine. Minimal removal by hemodialysis. Half-life: 10-26 hrs.

ACTION

Increases synaptic concentration of norepinephrine and/or serotonin (inhibits re-uptake by presynaptic membrane).

USES

Treatment of various forms of depression, often in conjunction w/ psychotherapy.

STORAGE/HANDLING

Store parenteral form at room temperature. Protect from light (precipitate may form). Store tablets at room temperature. Protect Elavil tablets (10 mg strength only) from light.

PO/IM ADMINISTRATION

PO:

1. Give w/food or milk if GI distress occurs.

IM:

1. Give by IM only if oral administration is not feasible.
2. Crystals may form in injection. Redissolve by immersing ampoule in hot water for 1 min.
3. Give deep IM slowly.

INDICATIONS/DOSAGE/ROUTES

NOTE: May give entire daily oral dose at one time (preferably bedtime).

Inpatient:
PO: Adults: Initially, 75-100 mg daily in 1-4 divided doses. Gradually increase by 25-50 mg increments to maximum of 300 mg daily, then reduce slowly to minimum therapeutic level. **Elderly, adolescents:** Initially, 10 mg 3 times daily, plus 20 mg at bedtime. **Maintenance:** 40-100 mg/day.
IM: Adults: 20-30 mg 4 times daily.

Outpatient:
PO: Adults: Initially, 50-100 mg daily. May be gradually increased to 150 mg daily. **Elderly patients, adolescents:** 10 mg 3 times daily, plus 20 mg at bedtime. Maximum therapeutic effect should be achieved in 2-4 wks. Dosage should be gradually reduced to minimum therapeutic level.

Usual elderly dosage:
PO: Elderly: Initially, 10-25 mg at bedtime; increase at weekly intervals of 10-25 mg. **Range:** 25-150 mg/day.

PRECAUTIONS

CONTRAINDICATIONS: Acute recovery period following MI, within 14 days of MAO inhibitor ingestion. **CAUTIONS:** Prostatic hypertrophy, history of urinary retention or obstruction, glaucoma, diabetes mellitus, history of seizures, hyperthyroidism, cardiac/

hepatic/renal disease, schizophrenia, increased intraocular pressure, hiatal hernia. **PREGNANCY/LACTATION:** Crosses placenta; minimally distributed in breast milk. **Pregnancy Category C.**

INTERACTIONS

DRUG INTERACTIONS: Alcohol, CNS depressants may increase CNS, respiratory depression, hypotensive effects. Antithyroid agents may increase risk of agranulocytosis. Phenothiazines may increase sedative, anticholinergic effects. Cimetidine may increase concentration, toxicity. May decrease effects of clonidine, guanadrel. May increase cardiac effects w/sympathomimetics. May increase risk of hypertensive crisis, hyperpyretic, convulsions w/ MAO inhibitors. **ALTERED LAB VALUES:** May alter EKG readings, glucose.

SIDE EFFECTS

FREQUENT: Drowsiness, fatigue, dry mouth, blurred vision, constipation, delayed micturition, postural hypotension, excessive sweating, disturbed concentration, increased appetite, urinary retention. **OCCASIONAL:** GI disturbances (nausea, GI distress, metallic taste sensation). **RARE:** Paradoxical reaction (agitation, restlessness, nightmares, insomnia), extrapyramidal symptoms (particularly fine hand tremor).

ADVERSE REACTIONS/TOXIC EFFECTS

High dosage may produce cardiovascular effects (severe postural hypotension, dizziness, tachycardia, palpitations, arrhythmias) and seizures. May also result in altered temperature regulation (hyperpyrexia or hypothermia). Abrupt withdrawal from prolonged therapy may produce headache, malaise, nausea, vomiting, vivid dreams.

NURSING IMPLICATIONS

BASELINE ASSESSMENT:

For those on long-term therapy, liver/renal function tests, blood counts should be performed periodically.

INTERVENTION/EVALUATION:

Supervise suicidal-risk patient closely during early therapy (as depression lessens, energy level improves increasing suicide potential). Assess appearance, behavior, speech pattern, level of interest, mood. Monitor pattern of daily bowel activity and stool consistency. Monitor B/P, pulse for hypotension, arrhythmias. Assess for urinary retention by bladder palpation.

PATIENT/FAMILY TEACHING:

Change positions slowly to avoid hypotensive effect. Tolerance to postural hypotension, sedative and anticholinergic effects usually develop during early therapy. Maximum therapeutic effect may be noted in 2-4 wks. Photosensitivity to sun may occur. Dry mouth may be relieved by sugarless gum or sips of tepid water. Report visual disturbances. Do not abruptly discontinue medication. Avoid tasks that require alertness, motor skills until response to drug is established.

amlodipine

am-low'dih-peen

(Norvasc)

CLASSIFICATION

Calcium channel blocker

PHARMACOKINETICS

	ONSET	PEAK	DURATION
PO	—	—	24 hrs

Slowly absorbed from GI tract. Protein binding: 97-99%. Undergoes first-pass metabolism in liver. Excreted primarily in urine. Half-life: 30-50 hrs (increased in elderly, pts w/hepatic cirrhosis).

ACTION

Inhibits calcium movement across cell membranes of cardiac and vascular smooth muscle (may dilate coronary arteries, peripheral arteries/arterioles); may decrease myocardial contractility. Decreases total peripheral vascular resistance by vasodilation.

USES

Management of hypertension, chronic stable angina, vasospastic (Prinzmetal's or variant) angina. May be used alone or w/other antihypertensives or antianginals.

PO ADMINISTRATION

May take w/o regard to food.

INDICATIONS/DOSAGE/ROUTES

NOTE: Dosage should be titrated >7-14 days.

Hypertension:
PO: Adults: Initially, 5 mg/day as single dose. **Maximum:** 10 mg/day.

PO: Small frame, fragile, elderly: Initially, 2.5 mg/day as single dose.

Angina (chronic stable or vasospastic):
PO: Adults: 5-10 mg.

PO: Elderly, hepatic insufficiency: 5 mg.

PRECAUTIONS

CONTRAINDICATIONS: Hypersensitivity to amlodipine. **CAUTIONS:** Impaired hepatic function, CHF. **PREGNANCY/LACTATION:** Unknown if drug crosses placenta or is distributed in breast milk. **Pregnancy Category C.**

INTERACTIONS

DRUG INTERACTIONS: None significant. **ALTERED LAB VALUES:** May decrease LDL, triglycerides; may increase HDL: cholesterol ratio.

SIDE EFFECTS

COMMON: Peripheral edema, headache. **FREQUENT:** Dizziness/lightheadedness (hypotensive effect), asthenia (loss of strength, weakness), facial flushing. **OCCASIONAL:** Dyspepsia, paresthesia, cough, respiratory infection. **RARE:** Palpitations, nausea, diarrhea/constipation, muscle cramps.

ADVERSE REACTIONS/TOXIC EFFECTS

Overdosage may produce excessive peripheral vasodilation, marked hypotension w/reflex tachycardia.

NURSING IMPLICATIONS

BASELINE ASSESSMENT:

Assess baseline renal/liver function tests, B/P, and apical pulse.

INTERVENTION/EVALUATION:

Assess B/P (if systolic B/P is below 90 mm Hg, withhold medication, contact physician). Assist w/ambulation if lightheadedness, dizziness occurs. Assess for peripheral edema behind medial malleolus (sacral area in bedridden pts). Assess skin for flushing. Monitor liver enzyme tests. Question for headache, asthenia.

PATIENT/FAMILY TEACHING:

Do not abruptly discontinue medication. Compliance w/therapy regimen is essential to control hypertension. To avoid hypotensive effect, rise slowly from lying to sitting position, wait momentarily before standing. Avoid tasks that require alertness, motor skills until response to drug is established. Contact physician/nurse if irregular heart beat, shortness of breath, pronounced dizziness, or nausea occurs.

amoxapine

ah-mocks´ah-peen
(Asendin)

CANADIAN AVAILABILITY:
Asendin

CLASSIFICATION

Antidepressant: Tricyclic

PHARMACOKINETICS

Rapid, well absorbed from GI tract. Protein binding: 92%. Metabolized in liver, undergoes first-pass metabolism. Primarily excreted in urine. Minimal removal by hemodialysis. Half-life: 8-30 hrs.

ACTION

Increases synaptic concentration of norepinephrine and/or serotonin (inhibits re-uptake by presynaptic membrane).

USES

Treatment of neurotic, endogenous depresssion, and mixed symptoms of anxiety, depression.

PO ADMINISTRATION

Give w/food or milk if GI distress occurs.

INDICATIONS/DOSAGE/ROUTES

NOTE: May give entire daily dose at one time (preferably bedtime).
PO: Adults: Initially, 50 mg 2-3 times/day. May gradually increase to 200-300 mg/day by end of first wk of therapy. If therapeutic response does not occur by end of 2 wks, may increase dose to maximum 400 mg/day for outpatients. Hospitalized patients w/no history of seizures may receive up to 600 mg daily in divided doses.

Usual elderly dosage:
PO: Elderly: Initially, 25 mg, then increase at 25 mg increments q3days for hospitalized pts; q7days for outpts. **Range:** 50-150 mg/day. **Maximum:** 300 mg/day.

PRECAUTIONS

CONTRAINDICATIONS: Acute recovery period following MI, within 14 days of MAO inhibitor ingestion. **CAUTIONS:** Prostatic hypertrophy, history of urinary retention or obstruction, glaucoma, diabetes mellitus, history of seizures, hyperthyroidism, cardiac/hepatic/renal disease, schizophrenia, increased intraocular pressure, hiatal hernia. **PREGNANCY/LACTATION:** Crosses placenta; is distributed in breast milk. **Pregnancy Category C.**

INTERACTIONS

DRUG INTERACTIONS: Alcohol, CNS depressants may increase CNS, respiratory depression, hypotensive effects. Antithyroid agents may increase risk of agranulocytosis. Phenothiazines may increase sedative, anticholinergic effects. Cimetidine may increase concentration, toxicity. May decrease effects of clonidine, guanadrel. May increase cardiac effects w/sympathomimetics. May increase risk of hypertensive crisis, hyperpyretic, convulsions w/ MAO inhibitors. **ALTERED LAB VALUES:** May alter ECG readings, glucose.

SIDE EFFECTS

FREQUENT: Drowsiness, fatigue, dry mouth, blurred vision, constipation, delayed micturition, postural hypotension, excessive sweating, disturbed concentration, increased appetite, urinary retention. **OCCASIONAL:** GI disturbances (nausea, GI distress, metallic taste sensation). **RARE:** Paradoxical reaction (agitation, restlessness, nightmares, insomnia), extrapyramidal symptoms (particularly fine hand tremor).

ADVERSE REACTIONS/TOXIC EFFECTS

High dosage may produce cardiovascular effects (severe postural hypotension, dizziness, tachycardia, palpitations, arrhythmias) and seizures. May also result in altered temperature regulation (hyperpyrexia or hypothermia). Abrupt withdrawal from prolonged therapy may produce headache, malaise, nausea, vomiting, vivid dreams.

NURSING IMPLICATIONS

BASELINE ASSESSMENT:

For those on long-term therapy, liver/renal function tests, blood counts should be performed periodically.

INTERVENTION/EVALUATION:

Supervise suicidal-risk patient closely during early therapy (as depression lessens, energy level improves increasing suicide potential). Assess appearance, behavior, speech pattern, level of interest, mood. Monitor pattern of daily bowel activity and stool consistency. Monitor B/P, pulse for hypotension, arrhythmias. Assess for urinary retention by bladder palpation.

PATIENT/FAMILY TEACHING:

Change positions slowly to avoid hypotensive effect. Tolerance to postural hypotension, sedative and anticholinergic effects usually develops during early therapy. Therapeutic effect may be noted within 1-2 wks. Photosensitivity to sun may occur. Dry mouth may be relieved by sugarless gum or sips of tepid water. Report visual disturbances. Do not abruptly discontinue medication. Avoid tasks that require alertness, motor skills until response to drug is established.

amoxicillin

ah-mocks´ih-sill-in

(Amoxil, Polymox, Sumox, Trimox, Wymox)

CANADIAN AVAILABILITY:

Amoxil, Apo-Amoxi, Novamoxin

CLASSIFICATION

Antibiotic: Penicillin

PHARMACOKINETICS

Well absorbed from GI tract.

Protein binding: 17-20%. Partially metabolized in liver. Primarily excreted in urine. Removed by hemodialysis. Half-life: 1-1.3 hrs (increased in reduced renal function).

ACTION

Bactericidal. Binds to bacterial membranes. Inhibits cell wall synthesis.

USES

Treatment of skin/skin structure, respiratory, GI, and genitourinary infections, otitis media, gonorrhea.

STORAGE/HANDLING

Store capsules, tablets at room temperature. Oral solution, after reconstitution, is stable for 14 days at either room temperature or refrigeration.

PO ADMINISTRATION

1. Space doses evenly around the clock.
2. Give orally w/o regard to meals.
3. Instruct pt to chew or crush chewable tablets thoroughly before swallowing.

INDICATIONS/DOSAGE/ROUTES

Ear, nose, throat, genitourinary, skin/skin structure infections:
PO: Adults, children >20 kg: 250-500 mg q8h. **Children <20 kg:** 20-40 mg/kg/day in divided doses q8h.

Lower respiratory tract infections:
PO: Adults, children >20 kg: 500 mg q8h. **Children <20 kg:** 40 mg/kg/day in divided doses q8h.

Acute, uncomplicated gonorrhea, epididymo-orchitis:
PO: Adults: 3 Gm one time w/1 Gm probenecid. Follow w/tetracycline or erythromycin therapy.

PRECAUTIONS

CONTRAINDICATIONS: Infectious mononucleosis, hypersensitivity to any penicillin. **CAUTIONS:** History of allergies (especially cephalosporins). **PREGNANCY/LACTATION:** Crosses placenta, appears in cord blood, amniotic fluid. Distributed in breast milk in low concentrations. May lead to allergic sensitization, diarrhea, candidiasis, skin rash in infant. **Pregnancy Category B.**

INTERACTIONS

DRUG INTERACTIONS: Allopurinol may increase incidence of rash. Probenecid may increase concentration, toxicity risk. May decrease effects of oral contraceptives. **ALTERED LAB VALUES:** May increase SGOT (AST), SGPT (ALT). May cause positive Coombs' test.

SIDE EFFECTS

FREQUENT: Generalized rash, diarrhea, urticaria. **OCCASIONAL:** Nausea, vomiting.

ADVERSE REACTIONS/TOXIC EFFECTS

Superinfections, potentially fatal antibiotic-associated colitis may result from altered bacterial balance. Severe hypersensitivity reactions including anaphylaxis, acute interstitial nephritis occur rarely.

NURSING IMPLICATIONS

BASELINE ASSESSMENT:

Question for history of allergies, especially penicillins, cephalosporins. Obtain specimen for culture and sensitivity before giving first dose (therapy may begin before results of test are known).

INTERVENTION/EVALUATION:

Hold medication and promptly report rash (although common w/ amoxicillin, may indicate hypersensitivity) or diarrhea (w/fever, abdominal pain, mucus and blood in stool may indicate antibiotic-associated colitis). Assess food tolerance. Monitor I&O, urinalysis, renal function tests. Be alert for superinfection: increased fever, sore throat onset, vomiting, diarrhea, black/hairy tongue, ulceration or changes of oral mucosa, anal/genital pruritus.

PATIENT/FAMILY TEACHING:

Continue antibiotic for full length of treatment. Space doses evenly. Take w/meals if GI upset occurs. Thoroughly chew the chewable tablets before swallowing. Notify physician in event of rash, diarrhea, or other new symptom.

amoxicillin / clavulanate potassium

a-mocks-ih-sill´in/klah-view-lan´ate

(Augmentin)

CANADIAN AVAILABILITY:
Clavulin

CLASSIFICATION

Antibiotic: Penicillin

PHARMACOKINETICS

Well absorbed from GI tract. Protein binding: 17-20%. Partially metabolized in liver. Primarily excreted in urine. Removed by hemodialysis. Half-life: 1-1.3 hrs (increase in decreased renal function).

ACTION

Bactericidal. Binds to bacterial membranes. Inhibits cell wall synthesis. Clavulanate: Inhibits bacterial beta-lactamase protecting amoxicillin from enzymatic degradation.

USES

Treatment of skin/skin structure, lower respiratory tract and urinary infections, otitis media, sinusitis.

STORAGE/HANDLING

Store tablets at room temperature. Oral suspension, after reconstitution, is stable for 10 days if refrigerated.

PO ADMINISTRATION

1. Space doses evenly around the clock.
2. Give w/o regard to meals.
3. Instruct pt to chew or crush chewable tablets thoroughly before swallowing.

INDICATIONS/DOSAGE/ROUTES

NOTE: Dosage expressed in terms of amoxicillin. Two 250 mg tablets are not equivalent to one 500 mg tablet (both strengths contain 125 mg of clavulanic acid).

Mild to moderate infections:
PO: Adults, elderly, children >40 kg: 250 mg q8h. **Children <40 kg:** 20 mg/kg/day in divided doses q8h.

Respiratory tract infections, severe infections:
PO: Adults, elderly, children >40 kg: 500 mg q8h. **Children <40 kg:**

40 mg/kg/day in divided doses q8h.

Otitis media, sinusitis, lower respiratory tract infections:
PO: Children <40 kg: 40 mg/kg/day in divided doses q8h.

PRECAUTIONS

CONTRAINDICATIONS: Disulfiram therapy, infectious mononucleosis, hypersensitivity to any penicillin. **CAUTIONS:** History of allergies, especially cephalosporins. **PREGNANCY/LACTATION:** Crosses placenta, appears in cord blood, amniotic fluid. Distributed in breast milk in low concentrations. May lead to allergic sensitization, diarrhea, candidiasis, skin rash in infant. **Pregnancy Category B.**

INTERACTIONS

DRUG INTERACTIONS: Allopurinol may increase incidence of rash. Probenecid may increase concentration, toxicity risk. May decrease effects of oral contraceptive. **ALTERED LAB VALUES:** May increase SGOT (AST), SGPT (ALT). May cause positive Coombs test.

SIDE EFFECTS

FREQUENT: Diarrhea, rash, urticaria, vomiting. **OCCASIONAL:** Flatulence, abdominal discomfort, exfoliative dermatitis.

ADVERSE REACTIONS/TOXIC EFFECTS

Superinfections, potentially fatal antibiotic-associated colitis may result from altered bacterial balance. Severe hypersensitivity reactions including anaphylaxis, acute interstitial nephritis, occur rarely.

NURSING IMPLICATIONS

Baseline Assessment:

Question for history of allergies, especially penicillins, cephalosporins. Obtain specimen for culture and sensitivity before giving first dose (therapy may begin before results of test are known).

Intervention/Evaluation:

Hold medication and promptly report rash (hypersensitivity) or diarrhea (w/fever, abdominal pain, blood and mucus in stool may indicate antibiotic-associated colitis). Assess food tolerance. Monitor I&O, urinalysis, renal function tests. Be alert for superinfection: increased fever, sore throat onset, vomiting, diarrhea, black/hairy tongue, ulceration or changes of oral mucosa, anal/genital pruritus.

Patient/Family Teaching:

Space doses evenly. Take antibiotic for full length of treatment. Take w/meals if GI upset occurs. Thoroughly chew the chewable tablets before swallowing. Notify physician in event of rash, diarrhea, or other new symptom.

amphotericin B

am-foe-tear´ih-sin
(Fungizone)

CANADIAN AVAILABILITY:
Fungizone

CLASSIFICATION

Antifungal

PHARMACOKINETICS

Widely distributed. Protein binding: >90%. Metabolic fate unknown. Primarily excreted in urine. Minimal removal by hemodialysis. Half-life: 24 hrs (increased in neonates, children).

ACTION

Binds to sterols in cell membrane, increasing permeability. Permits loss of potassium, other cell components. Generally fungistatic but may be fungicidal w/ high dosage or very susceptible microorganisms.

USES

Parenteral: Treatment of severe systemic infections/meningitis due to susceptible fungi. Disseminated candidiasis, candidal prophylaxis during immunosuppressive therapy, aspergillosis, histoplasmosis, blastomycosis, coccidioidomycosis, cryptomycosis, sporotrichosis. *Topical:* Treatment of cutaneous/mucocutaneous infections caused by *Candidia albicans* (paronychia, oral thrush, perleche, diaper rash, intertriginous candidiasis).

STORAGE/HANDLING

Refrigerate vials. Concentrated solutions (5 mg/ml) stable for 24 hrs at room temperature, 7 days if refrigerated. Potency unaffected if IV infusion is exposed to light for 8 hrs after preparation. Not necessary to protect IV infusion from light under normal administration conditions. Use solution for IV infusion immediately after preparation. Discard if precipitate forms.

IV ADMINISTRATION

IV:

NOTE: Give by slow IV infusion.

1. Reconstitute each 50 mg vial w/10 ml sterile water for injection w/o bacteriostatic agent to provide concentration of 5 mg/ml.
2. Further dilute only w/5% dextrose (prevents precipitation) to provide concentration of 0.1 mg/ml or less.
3. Infuse over 2-6 hrs.
4. Monitor B/P, temperature, pulse, respirations; assess for adverse reactions q15min ×2, then q30min for 4 hrs of initial infusion.
5. Do not use IV line filters unless pores >1.0 micron.
6. Potential for thrombophlebitis may be less w/use of pediatric scalp vein needles or (w/physician order) adding dilute heparin solution.
7. Therapy on alternate days may reduce anorexia, phlebitis.
8. Observe strict aseptic technique, since no bacteriostatic agent or preservative is present in diluent.

INDICATIONS/DOSAGE/ROUTES

Usual parenteral dosage:

IV: Adults, elderly: Dosage based on pt tolerance, severity of infection. Initially, a 1 mg test dose is given over 20-30 min. If test dose is tolerated, 5 mg dose may be given the same day. Subsequently, increases of 5 mg/dose are made q12-24h until desired daily dose is reached. Alternatively, if test dose is tolerated, a dose of 0.25 mg/kg is given same day; increased to 0.5 mg/kg the second day. Dose increased until desired daily dose reached. **Total daily dose:** 1 mg/kg/day up to 1.5 mg/kg every other day. Do not exceed maximum total daily dose of 1.5 mg/kg.

Cutaneous infections:

TOPICAL: Adults, elderly, children: Apply liberally and rub in 2-4 times/day.

PRECAUTIONS

CONTRAINDICATIONS: Hyper-

sensitivity to amphotericin B, sulfite. **CAUTIONS:** Renal impairment, in combination w/antineoplastic therapy. Give only for progressive, potentially fatal fungal infection. **PREGNANCY/LACTATION:** Crosses placenta; unknown if distributed in breast milk. **Pregnancy Category C.**

INTERACTIONS

DRUG INTERACTIONS: Steroids may cause severe hypokalemia. Bone marrow depressants may increase anemia. May increase digoxin toxicity (due to hypokalemia). Nephrotoxic medications may increase nephrotoxicity. **ALTERED LAB VALUES:** May decrease magnesium, potassium; may increase CPK.

SIDE EFFECTS

FREQUENT: Fever, occasionally w/shaking, chills, generally occurs 1-2 hrs after start of IV infusion, subsides 4 hrs after discontinuance; malaise, muscle and joint pain, nausea, vomiting, dyspepsia, abdominal pain, diarrhea, pain at injection site. **OCCASIONAL:** Anemia, hypokalemia, hypomagnesemia. *Topical:* Drying, irritation, itching, or burning, esp. in intertriginous areas. **RARE:** *Topical:* allergic contact dermatitis.

ADVERSE REACTIONS/TOXIC EFFECTS

Nephrotoxicity occurs commonly. Cardiovascular toxicity (hypotension, ventricular fibrillation), anaphylactic reaction occur rarely. Vision and hearing alterations, seizures, hepatic failure, coagulation defects may be noted.

NURSING IMPLICATIONS

BASELINE ASSESSMENT:

Question for history of allergies, especially to amphotericin B, sulfite. Avoid, if possible, other nephrotoxic medications. Confirm that a positive culture or histologic test was performed. Check for/obtain orders to reduce adverse reactions during IV therapy (antipyretics, antihistamines, antiemetics, or small doses of corticosteroids given before or during amphotericin administration may control reactions).

INTERVENTION/EVALUATION:

Monitor B/P, temperature, pulse, respirations; assess for adverse reactions q15min ×2, then q30min for 4 hrs of initial infusion (fever, shaking chills, anorexia, nausea, vomiting, abdominal pain). slow infusion and administer medication for symptomatic relief. For severe reaction or w/o symptomatic relief orders, stop infusion and notify physician immediately. Evaluate IV site for phlebitis (heat, pain, red streaking over vein). Determine pattern of bowel activity and stool consistency. Assess food intake, tolerance. Monitor I&O, renal function tests for nephrotoxicity. Check potassium and magnesium levels, hematologic and hepatic function test results. Assess for bleeding, bruising, soft tissue swelling. *Topical:* Assess for itching, irritation, burning.

PATIENT/FAMILY TEACHING:

Prolonged therapy (weeks or months) is usually necessary. Discomfort may occur at IV site. Notify physician of bleeding, bruising, soft tissue swelling, other new symptom. Fever reaction may decrease w/continued therapy. Muscle weakness may be noted during therapy (due to hypokalemia). *Topical:* Application may cause staining of skin or nails; soap and water or dry cleaning will remove fabric stains. Do not use other preparations or occlusive coverings w/o consulting physician. Keep areas clean, dry; wear light clothing. Separate personal items w/direct contact to area.

ampicillin sodium

amp-ih-sill′in

(Omnipen, Penamp, Polycillin, Principen)

FIXED-COMBINATION(S):

W/probenecid, (Principen w/probenecid, Polycillin PRB, Proambicin)

CANADIAN AVAILABILITY:

Apo-Ampi, Novo-Ampicillin, Nu-Ampi, Penbriton

CLASSIFICATION

Antibiotic: Penicillin

PHARMACOKINETICS

Moderately absorbed from GI tract. Widely distributed. Protein binding: 17-20%. Partially metabolized in liver. Primarily excreted in urine. Removed by hemodialysis. Half-life: 1-1.5 hrs (increase in decreased renal function).

ACTION

Bactericidal. Binds to bacterial membranes. Inhibits cell wall synthesis.

USES

Treatment of respiratory, GI and GU tract, skin/skin structure, bone and joint infections, otitis media, gonorrhea, endocarditis, meningitis, septicemia, mild to moderate typhoid fever, perioperative prophylaxis.

STORAGE/HANDLING

Store capsules at room temperature. Oral suspension, after reconstituted, is stable for 7 days at room temperature, 14 days if refrigerated. The IV solution, diluted w/0.9% NaCl, is stable for 3 days if refrigerated. If diluted w/5% dextrose, use immediately (drug inactivation). Discard if precipitate forms.

PO/IM/IV ADMINISTRATION

NOTE: Space doses evenly around the clock.

PO:

1. Give orally 1 hr before or 2 hrs after meals for maximum absorption.

IM:

1. Reconstitute each vial w/sterile water for injection or bacteriostatic water for injection (consult individual vial for specific volume of diluent).
2. Give deeply in large muscle mass.

IV:

1. For IV injection, dilute each 125 mg, 250 mg, or 500 mg vial w/5 ml sterile water for injection (10 ml for 1 and 2 Gm vials).
2. Give IV injection over 3-5 min (10-15 mins for 1-2 Gm dose).
3. For intermittent IV infusion (piggyback), further dilute w/50-100 ml 0.9% NaCl, 5% dextrose, or other compatible IV fluid. Infuse over 20-30 min.
4. Alternating IV sites, use large veins to reduce phlebitis risk.
5. Due to potential for hypersensitivity/anaphylaxis, start initial dose at few drops per minute, in-

crease slowly to ordered rate; stay w/pt first 10-15 min, then check q10min.

6. Change to oral route as soon as possible.

INDICATIONS/DOSAGE/ROUTES

Respiratory tract, skin/skin structure infections:
PO: Adults, elderly, children >20 kg: 250 mg q6h. **Children <20 kg:** 50 mg/kg/day in divided doses q6h.
IM/IV: Adults, elderly, children >40 kg: 250-500 mg q6h. **Children <40 kg:** 25-50 mg/kg/day in divided doses q6-8h.

Bacterial meningitis, septicemia:
IM/IV: Adults, elderly: 2 Gm q4h or 3 Gm q6h. **Children:** 100-200 mg/kg/day in divided doses q4h.

Gonococcal infections:
PO: Adults: 3.5 Gm one time w/1 Gm probenecid plus tetracycline, erythromycin, or ampicillin.

Perioperative prophylaxis:
IM/IV: Adults, elderly: 2 Gm 30 min prior to procedure. May repeat in 8 hrs. **Children:** 50 mg/kg using same dosage regimen.

Usual dosage (neonates):
IM/IV: Neonates 7-28 days: 75 mg/kg/day in divided doses q8h up to 200 mg/kg/day in divided doses q6h. **Neonates 0-7 days:** 50 mg/kg/day in divided doses q12h up to 150 mg/kg/day in divided doses q8h.
NOTE: Higher doses may be needed for neonatal meningitis.

PRECAUTIONS

CONTRAINDICATIONS: Infectious mononucleosis, hypersensitivity to any penicillin. Do not give Amcill to those w/asthma (contains bisulfite). **CAUTIONS:** History of allergies, particularly cephalosporins. **PREGNANCY/LACTATION:** Readily crosses placenta; appears in cord blood, amniotic fluid. Distributed in breast milk in low concentrations. May lead to allergic sensitization, diarrhea, candidiasis, skin rash in infant. **Pregnancy Category B.**

INTERACTIONS

DRUG INTERACTIONS: Allopurinol may increase incidence of rash. Probenecid may increase concentration, toxicity risk. May decrease effects of oral contraceptive. **ALTERED LAB VALUES:** May increase SGOT (AST), SGPT (ALT). May cause positive Coombs test.

SIDE EFFECTS

FREQUENT: Rash, diarrhea, nausea/vomiting, urticaria, fever due to hypersensitivity. **OCCASIONAL:** Pain at IM injection site, phlebitis, thrombophlebitis w/IV administration; abdominal discomfort, flatulence. **RARE:** Headache, dizziness, seizures esp. w/IV therapy.

ADVERSE REACTIONS/TOXIC EFFECTS

Hypersensitivity reactions, including anaphylaxis, acute interstitial nephritis may be noted. Superinfections, potentially fatal antibiotic-associated colitis may result from altered bacterial balance.

NURSING IMPLICATIONS

BASELINE ASSESSMENT:

Question for history of allergies, esp. penicillins, cephalosporins. Obtain specimen for culture and sensitivity before giving first dose (therapy may begin before results are known).

INTERVENTION/EVALUATION:

Hold medication and promptly report rash (although common w/ ampicillin, may indicate hypersensitivity) or diarrhea (w/fever, abdominal pain, mucus and blood in stool may indicate antibiotic-associated colitis). Assess food tolerance. Evaluate IV site for phlebitis (heat, pain, red streaking over vein). Check IM injection site for pain, induration. Monitor I&O, urinalysis, renal function tests. Assess for signs of superinfection: increased fever, sore throat onset, vomiting, diarrhea, anal/genital pruritus, changes in oral mucosa, black/hairy tongue.

PATIENT/FAMILY TEACHING:

Space doses evenly. Take antibiotic for full length of treatment. More effective if taken 1 hr before or 2 hrs after food/beverages. Discomfort may occur w/IM injection. Notify physician of rash, diarrhea, or other new symptom.

ampicillin/ sulbactam sodium

amp-ih-sill´in/sull-bak´tam

(Unasyn)

CLASSIFICATION

Antibiotic: Penicillin

PHARMACOKINETICS

Moderately absorbed from GI tract. Widely distributed. Protein binding: low. Partially metabolized in liver. Primarily excreted in urine. Removed by hemodialysis. Half-life: 1 hr (increase in decreased renal function).

ACTION

Bactericidal. Binds to bacterial membranes. Inhibits cell wall synthesis. Sulbactam: inhibits bacterial beta-lactamase protecting ampicillin from enzymatic degradation.

USES

Treatment of intra-abdominal, skin/skin structure, gynecologic infections.

STORAGE/HANDLING

When reconstituted w/0.9% NaCl, IV solution is stable for 8 hrs at room temperature, 48 hrs if refrigerated. Stability may be different w/other diluents. Discard if precipitate forms.

IM/IV ADMINISTRATION

NOTE: Space doses evenly around the clock.

IM:

1. Reconstitute each 1.5 Gm vial w/3.2 ml sterile water for injection to provide concentration of 250 mg ampicillin/125 mg sulbactam/ml.
2. Give deeply into large muscle mass within one hr after preparation.

IV:

1. For IV injection, dilute w/10-20 ml sterile water for injection. Give slowly over minimum of 10-15 min.
2. For intermittent IV infusion (piggyback), further dilute w/50-100 ml 5% dextrose, 0.9% NaCl, or other compatible IV fluid. Infuse over 15-30 min.
3. Alternating IV sites, use large veins to reduce risk of phlebitis.
4. Due to potential for hypersensitivity/anaphylaxis, start initial dose at few drops per min, in-

crease slowly to ordered rate; stay w/pt first 10-15 min, then check q10min.

5. Change to oral route as soon as possible.

INDICATIONS/DOSAGE/ROUTES

Skin/skin structure, intra-abdominal, gynecologic infections:

IM/IV: Adults, elderly: 1.5 Gm (1 Gm ampicillin/500 mg sulbactam) to 3 Gm (2 Gm ampicillin/1 Gm sulbactam) q6h.

Dosage in renal impairment:

Modification of dose and/or frequency based on creatinine clearance and/or severity of infection.

CREATININE CLEARANCE	DOSAGE
≥30 ml/min	1.5-3 Gm q6-8h
15-29 ml/min	1.5-3 Gm q12h
5-14 ml/min	1.5-3 Gm q24h
<5 ml/min	Not recommended

PRECAUTIONS

CONTRAINDICATIONS: Infectious mononucleosis, hypersensitivity to any penicillin. **CAUTIONS:** History of allergies, particularly to cephalosporins. **PREGNANCY LACTATION:** Readily crosses placenta, appears in cord blood, amniotic fluid. Distributed in breast milk in low concentrations. May lead to allergic sensitization, diarrhea, candidiasis, skin rash in infant. **Pregnancy Category B.**

INTERACTIONS

DRUG INTERACTIONS: Allopurinol may increase incidence of rash. Probenecid may increase concentration, toxicity risk. May decrease effects of oral contraceptive. **ALTERED LAB VALUES:** May increase SGOT (AST), SGPT (ALT), alkaline phosphatase, LDH, creatinine. May cause positive Coombs test.

SIDE EFFECTS

FREQUENT: Diarrhea and rash (most common), urticaria, fever due to hypersensitivity; pain at IM injection site; phlebitis, thrombophlebitis w/IV administration. **OCCASIONAL:** Nausea, vomiting, headache, malaise, urinary retention.

ADVERSE REACTIONS/TOXIC EFFECTS

Hypersensitivity reactions, including anaphylaxis, acute interstitial nephritis may be noted. Superinfections, potentially fatal antibiotic-associated colitis may result from altered bacterial balance. Overdose may produce seizures.

NURSING IMPLICATIONS

BASELINE ASSESSMENT:

Question for history of allergies, especially, penicillins, cephalosporins. Obtain specimen for culture and sensitivity before giving first dose (therapy may begin before results are known).

INTERVENTION/EVALUATION:

Hold medication and promptly report rash (although common w/ampicillin, may indicate hypersensitivity) or diarrhea (w/fever, mucus and blood in stool, abdominal pain may indicate antibiotic-associated diarrhea). Assess food tolerance. Evaluate IV site for phlebitis (heat, pain, red streaking over vein). Check IM injection site for pain, induration. Monitor I&O, urinalysis, renal function tests. Assess for initial signs of superinfection: increased fever, sore throat onset, vomiting, diarrhea, anal/genital pruritus, ulceration or changes of oral mucosa.

PATIENT/FAMILY TEACHING:

Space dose evenly. Take antibiotic for full length of treatment. Discomfort may occur w/IM injection. Notify physician of rash, diarrhea, or other new symptom.

amrinone lactate

am'rih-known
(Inocor)

CANADIAN AVAILABILITY:
Inocor

CLASSIFICATION

Cardiac inotropic agent

PHARMACOKINETICS

	ONSET	PEAK	DURATION
IV	—	10 min	0.5-2 hrs

Protein binding: 10-49%. Metabolized in liver. Primarily excreted in urine. Half-life: 3.6 hrs (increase in neonates, infants; pts w/CHF).

ACTION

Reduces preload/afterload by direct peripheral vasodilation. Directly stimulates cardiac contractility (positive inotropic effect) by inhibiting phosphodiesterase.

USES

Short-term management of CHF in those who have not responded adequately to cardiac glycosides, diuretics, and vasodilators.

STORAGE/HANDLING

Use only a clear, yellow solution. Discard if precipitate forms or discoloration occurs. Stable for 24 hrs when diluted w/0.9% NaCl.

IV ADMINISTRATION

1. Do not dilute w/dextrose-containing solutions (chemically incompatible), but may be injected into tubing of freely flowing IV dextrose solution.
2. Avoid furosemide injections into tubing of amrinone IV infusion (precipitate forms immediately).
3. For direct IV injection, may be given undiluted and administered slowly over 2-3 min.
4. For IV infusion, dilute w/0.9% NaCl to provide concentration of 1-3 mg/ml.
5. Monitor for arrhythmias, hypotension during IV therapy.

INDICATIONS/DOSAGE/ROUTES

Congestive heart failure:
IV: Adults, elderly: Initially, give 0.75 mg/kg over 2-3 min. Continue w/maintenance infusion rate of 5-10 mcg/kg/min. If necessary, a bolus dose of 0.75 mg/kg may be given 30 min after initial dose. Do not exceed total daily dose of 10 mg/kg.

PRECAUTIONS

CONTRAINDICATIONS: History of hypersensitivity to bisulfites, severe aortic/pulmonic valvular disease w/o surgical intervention during acute phase of MI. **CAUTIONS:** Hypertrophic subaortic stenosis, impaired renal, hepatic function. **PREGNANCY/LACTATION:** Unknown if drug crosses placenta or is distributed in breast milk. **Pregnancy Category C.**

INTERACTIONS

DRUG INTERACTIONS: None significant. **ALTERED LAB VALUES:** May decrease potassium; may increase liver enzymes.

SIDE EFFECTS

OCCASIONAL: Asymptomatic thrombocytopenia (platelet count less than 150,000/mm^3). **RARE:** Nausea, diarrhea.

ADVERSE REACTIONS/TOXIC EFFECTS

Rarely, hepatotoxicity (manifested as enzyme elevation and/or hepatic cell necrosis), hypersensitivity reaction (wheezing, shortness of breath, pruritus, urticaria, clammy skin, flushing) may occur.

NURSING IMPLICATIONS

BASELINE ASSESSMENT:

Offer emotional support (difficulty breathing may produce anxiety).

INTERVENTION/EVALUATION:

Monitor CVP for hypotension, fluid balance management (hydration status), platelet count, SGOT (AST), SGPT (ALT), alkaline phosphatase, serum electrolytes, I&O, renal function studies. Assess lung sounds for rales at base of lungs, wheezing. Monitor for relief of CHF symptoms (reduction in edema, lessening of dyspnea, improvement of orthopnea and fatigue).

anistreplase

an-is´trep-lace

(Eminase)

CLASSIFICATION

Thrombolytic

PHARMACOKINETICS

	ONSET	PEAK	DURATION
IV	—	—	4-6 hrs

Limited information available. Clearance of fibrinolytic activity due to tissue uptake, inactivation by inhibitors, and degradation by circulating antiplasmin. Half-life: 70-120 min.

ACTION

Inactive complex of streptokinase and human plasminogen. Immediately after injection, complex is deacylated at catalytic binding site (converts plasminogen to plasmin). Conversion occurs within thrombus or embolus, on its surface, and in blood.

USES

Management of acute myocardial infarction (AMI) in adults, lysis of thrombi obstructing coronary arteries, reduce infarct size, improve ventricular function following AMI, reduce mortality associated w/ AMI.

STORAGE/HANDLING

Refrigerate powder. Reconstituted solutions are colorless to pale yellow. Once reconstituted, discard solution if not used within 30 min.

IV ADMINISTRATION

1. Reconstitute 30 U vial w/5 ml sterile water for injection (direct fluid against side of vial).
2. Gently roll vial, mixing fluid and powder. Do not shake (minimizes foaming).
3. Give only by IV injection over 2-5 min into IV line or vein.
4. Do not dilute further w/any infusion fluid or add to other medications.
5. If minor bleeding occurs at puncture sites, apply pressure for 30 min, then apply pressure dressing.
6. If uncontrolled hemorrhage

occurs, discontinue infusion immediately (slowing rate of infusion may produce worsening hemorrhage).

7. Avoid undue pressure when drug is injected into catheter (can rupture catheter or expel clot into circulation).

INDICATIONS/DOSAGE/ROUTES

Management of acute myocardial infarction:
IV: Adults, elderly: 30 units over 2-5 min as soon as possible after onset of symptoms.

PRECAUTIONS

CONTRAINDICATIONS: Active internal bleeding, recent (within 2 mos) cerebrovascular accident, intracranial or intraspinal surgery or trauma, intracranial neoplasm, arteriovenous malformation or aneurysm, bleeding diathesis, severe uncontrolled hypertension. **CAUTIONS:** Recent (10 days) of major surgery or GI bleeding, OB delivery, organ biopsy, recent trauma (cardiopulmonary resuscitation), left heart thrombus, endocarditis, severe hepatic or renal disease, pregnancy, elderly, cerebrovascular disease, diabetic retinopathy, thrombophlebitis, occluded AV cannula at infected site. **PREGNANCY/LACTATION:** Use only when benefit outweighs potential risk to fetus. Unknown if drug crosses placenta or is distributed in breast milk. **Pregnancy Category C.**

INTERACTIONS

DRUG INTERACTIONS: Anticoagulants, heparin, NSAIDs, aspirin, other platelet aggregation inhibitors may increase risk of bleeding. Antifibrinolytics (e.g., aminocaproic acid) may decrease effect. Valproic acid may increase risk of hemorrhage. **ALTERED LAB VALUES:** May increase activated partial thromboplastin time (APTT), prothrombin time (PT), thrombin time (TT). May decrease activity of alpha-2 antiplasmin, factor V, VIII, fibrinogen, plasminogen. May decrease hemoglobin, hematocrit.

SIDE EFFECTS

FREQUENT: Superficial or surface bleeding at puncture sites (venous cutdowns, arterial punctures, site of recent surgical intervention, IM, retroperitoneal, or intracerebral sites; internal bleeding (GI/GU tract, vaginal). **RARE:** Mild allergic reaction (rash, wheezing).

ADVERSE REACTIONS/TOXIC EFFECTS

Severe internal hemorrhage may occur. Lysis of coronary thrombi may produce atrial or ventricular arrhythmias.

NURSING IMPLICATIONS

BASELINE ASSESSMENT:

Avoid arterial invasive technique before and during treatment. If arterial puncture is necessary, use upper extremity vessels. Assess hematocrit, platelet count, thrombin (TT), activated thromboplastin (APTT), prothrombin time (PT), fibrinogen level before therapy is instituted.

INTERVENTION/EVALUATION:

Handle pt carefully and infrequently as possible to prevent bleeding. Never give via IM injection route. Monitor clinical response, vital signs q4h. Do not obtain B/P in lower extremities (possible deep vein thrombi). Monitor TT, PT, APTT, fibrinogen level q4h after initiation of therapy, stool culture for occult blood. Assess for decrease in B/P, increase in pulse rate, complaint of abdominal or back pain, severe headache (may be evidence of hemorrhage). Question for increase in amount of discharge during menses. Assess area of thromboembolus for color, temperature. Assess peripheral pulses; skin for bruises, petechiae. Check for excessive bleeding from minor cuts, scratches. Assess urine output for hematuria.

antihemophilic factor (factor VIII, AHF)

(Koate, Monoclate)

CANADIAN AVAILABILITY:
Koate-HP, Kogenate, Kryobulin VH

CLASSIFICATION

Hemostatic

PHARMACOKINETICS

Rapidly cleared from plasma. Half-life: 4-14 hrs.

ACTION

Assists in conversion of prothrombin to thrombin (essential for blood coagulation), accelerating clotting time. Replaces missing clotting factor, correcting or preventing bleeding episodes.

USES

Treatment of classic hemophilia A (factor VIII deficiency). Used during elective or emergency surgery to improve hemostasis.

STORAGE/HANDLING

Refrigerate, avoid freezing. After reconstitution, solution is clear, colorless, or yellow. Stable for 24 hrs at room temperature, but use within 1-3 hrs. Do not refrigerate reconstituted solution.

IV ADMINISTRATION

NOTE: May be given by slow IV injection or infusion.

1. Filter before administration. Use only plastic syringes for IV injection.
2. Warm concentrate and diluent to room temperature.
3. To dissolve, gently agitate or rotate. Do not shake vigorously. Complete dissolution may take 5-10 min.
4. Check pulse rate before and during administration. If pulse rate increases, reduce or stop administration.
5. After administration, apply prolonged pressure on venipuncture site.
6. Monitor IV site for oozing q5-15min for 1-2 hrs after administration.

INDICATIONS/DOSAGE/ROUTES

NOTE: Dosage is highly individualized, based on patient weight, severity of bleeding, coagulation studies.

Prophylaxis of spontaneous hemorrhage:
IV: Adults, elderly, children: 10 AHF/IU/kg as a single infusion.

Moderate hemorrhage, minor surgery:
IV: Adults, elderly, children: Initially, 15-25 AHF/IU/kg. **Maintenance:** 10-15 IU/kg q8-12h.

Severe hemorrhage (near vital organ):
IV: Adults, elderly, children: Initially, 40-50 AHF/IU/kg. **Maintenance:** 20-25 IU/kg q8-12h.

Major surgery:
IV: Adults, elderly, children: 40-50 AHF/IU/kg 1 hr prior to surgery, 20-25 IU/kg 5 hrs later, then 10-15 IU/kg/day for 10-14 days.

PRECAUTIONS

CONTRAINDICATIONS: None significant. **CAUTIONS:** Hepatic disease, those w/blood type A, B, AB. **PREGNANCY/LACTATION:** Unknown if drug crosses placenta or is distributed in breast milk. **Pregnancy Category C.**

INTERACTIONS

DRUG INTERACTIONS: None significant. **ALTERED LAB VALUES:** None significant.

SIDE EFFECTS

OCCASIONAL: Allergic reaction (fever, chills, urticaria [hives], wheezing, hypotension, feeling of chest tightness). Disappears 15-20 min after discontinuation of IV infusion.

ADVERSE REACTIONS/TOXIC EFFECTS

There is a risk of transmitting viral hepatitis and a slight risk of transmitting AIDS. Possibility of intravascular hemolysis is present if large or frequent doses used in those w/blood group A, B, or AB.

NURSING IMPLICATIONS

BASELINE ASSESSMENT:

When monitoring B/P, avoid overinflation of cuff. Remove adhesive tape from any pressure dressing very carefully and slowly.

INTERVENTION/EVALUATION:

After IV administration, apply prolonged pressure on venipuncture site. Monitor IV site for oozing q5-15min for 1-2 hrs after administration. Assess for allergic reaction (see Side Effects). Report any evidence of hematuria or change in vital signs immediately. Monitor hematocrit, direct antiglobulin (Coombs') test, CBC, urinalysis, PTT, thromboplastin/prothrombin, AHF test results. Assess for decrease in B/P, increase in pulse rate, complaint of abdominal or back pain, severe headache (may be evidence of hemorrhage). Question for increase in amount of discharge during menses. Assess peripheral pulses; skin for bruises, petechiae. Check for excessive bleeding from minor cuts, scratches. Assess gums for erythema, gingival bleeding. Assess urine for hematuria. Evaluate for therapeutic relief of pain, reduction of swelling, and restricted joint movement.

PATIENT/FAMILY TEACHING:

Use electric razor, soft toothbrush to prevent bleeding. Report any sign of red or dark urine, black or red stool, coffee-ground vomitus, red-speckled mucous from cough. Do not use any over-the-counter medication w/o physician approval (may interfere w/platelet aggregation).

---

aprotinin (Trasylol) *See supplement*

---

artificial tears

(Isopto Tears, Liquifilm Forte, Hypotears, Neo-Tears, Just Tears, Tears Naturale, Lacril, Murocel, Lyteers, Isopto Plain, Ultra Tears, Moisture Drops)

CANADIAN AVAILABILITY:
Tears Naturale

CLASSIFICATION

Tear-like lubricant

ACTION

Protects and lubricates the eyes.

USES

Relief of dryness and irritation due to deficient tear production; ocular lubricant for artificial eyes; some products may be used w/ hard contact lenses.

STORAGE/HANDLING

Store at room temperature.

INDICATIONS/DOSAGE/ROUTES

Ophthalmic lubricant:
OPHTHALMIC: Adults, elderly: 1-2 drops 3-4 times/day as needed.

PRECAUTIONS

CONTRAINDICATIONS: Hypersensitivity to any component of preparation. **PREGNANCY/LACTATION: Pregnancy Category C.**

INTERACTIONS

DRUG INTERACTIONS: None significant. **ALTERED LAB VALUES:** None significant.

SIDE EFFECTS

OCCASIONAL: Transient mild stinging or blurred vision. **RARE:** Headache, eye pain, vision changes, increased redness or irritation.

NURSING IMPLICATIONS

BASELINE ASSESSMENT:

Determine extent of dryness, irritation.

INTERVENTION/EVALUATION:

Assess therapeutic response, increased irritation or discomfort.

PATIENT/FAMILY TEACHING:

Wash hands thoroughly. Do not touch the tip of the dropper or container to any surface. Cover immediately after administration. Instruct patient on proper instillation. No one else should use the product. Notify physician if condition worsens or redness, irritation are not relieved within 3 days.

ascorbic acid (vitamin C)

(Cecon, Cevalin)

CANADIAN AVAILABILITY:
Apo-C, Ce-Vi-Sol

CLASSIFICATION

Vitamin

PHARMACOKINETICS

Readily absorbed from GI tract. Protein binding: 25%. Metabolized in liver. Excreted in urine. Removed by hemodialysis.

ACTION

Nutritional supplement necessary for collagen formation, tissue repair, oxidation-reduction reactions. Involved in metabolism, carbohydrate utilization, synthesis of lipids, proteins, carnitine. Preserves blood vessel integrity.

USES

Prophylaxis, treatment of vitamin C deficiency. Increased requirement may be needed in GI disease, malignancy, peptic ulcer, tuberculosis, smokers, oral contraceptive users, hyperthyroidism, prolonged stress, burns, infection, chronic fever, parenteral hyperalimentation, hemodialysis.

PO/SubQ/IM/IV ADMINISTRATION

1. Give orally unless infeasible or malabsorption occurs. Incompatible w/potassium penicillin G.
2. Administer IV slowly to avoid dizziness.

INDICATIONS/DOSAGE/ROUTES

Dietary supplement:
PO: Adults, elderly: 45-60 mg/day. **Children >4 yrs:** 30-40 mg/day.

Deficiency:
PO/IM/IV: Adults, elderly: 75-150 mg/day.

Scurvy:
PO: Adults, elderly: 300 mg-1 Gm/day.

Burns:
PO: Adults, elderly: Up to 2 Gm/day.

Enhance wound healing:
PO: Adults, elderly: 300-500 mg/day for 7-10 days.

PRECAUTIONS

CONTRAINDICATIONS: History of gout. **CAUTIONS:** Those on sodium restriction, daily salicylate treatment, warfarin therapy. **PREGNANCY/LACTATION:** Crosses placenta, excreted in breast milk. Large doses during pregnancy may produce scurvy in neonates. **Pregnancy Category C.**

INTERACTIONS

DRUG INTERACTIONS: May increase iron toxicity w/deferoxamine. **ALTERED LAB VALUES:** May decrease bilirubin, urinary pH. May increase uric acid, urine oxalate.

SIDE EFFECTS

RARE: Abdominal cramps, nausea, vomiting, diarrhea, increased urination with doses exceeding 1 Gm. Parenteral treatment may produce flushing, headache, dizziness, sleepiness or insomnia, soreness at injection site.

ADVERSE REACTIONS/TOXIC EFFECTS

May produce urine acidification leading to crystalluria. Large doses given IV may lead to deep-vein thrombosis. Prolonged use of large doses may result in scurvy when dosage is reduced to normal.

NURSING IMPLICATIONS

INTERVENTION/EVALUATION:

Monitor lab values for improvement of megaloblastic anemia, increased serum ascorbic acid (0.4-1.5 mg/dl), urine acidity. Assess for clinical improvement (improved sense of well-being and sleep patterns). Observe for reversal of deficiency symptoms (gingivitis, bleeding gums, poor wound healing, digestive difficulties, joint pain).

PATIENT/FAMILY TEACHING:

Discomfort may occur w/parenteral administration. Report diarrhea (dosage adjustment may be needed). Abrupt vitamin C withdrawal may produce rebound deficiency. Reduce dosage gradually. Foods rich in vitamin C include rose hips, guava, black currant jelly, brussel sprouts, green peppers, spinach, watercress, strawberries, citrus fruits.

asparaginase

ah-spa-raj´in-ace
(Elspar)

CANADIAN AVAILABILITY:
Kidrolase

CLASSIFICATION

Antineoplastic

PHARMACOKINETICS

Protein binding: 30%. Metabolized via slow sequestration by reticuloendothelial system. Half-life: 39-49 hrs IM; 8-30 hrs IV.

ACTION

Interferes w/DNA, RNA, protein synthesis in leukemic cells by breaking down extracellular supplies of amino acid, asparagine (necessary for survival of these cells). Cell cycle-specific for G-1 phase of cell division.

USES

Treatment of acute lymphocytic leukemia (in combination w/other agents).

STORAGE/HANDLING

NOTE: May be carcinogenic, mutagenic, or teratogenic. Handle w/ extreme care during preparation/ administration.

Refrigerate powder for injection. Reconstituted solutions stable for 8 hrs if refrigerated. Discard solutions not clear, colorless. Gelatinous fiber-like particles may develop (remove via 5 micron filter during administration).

IM/IV ADMINISTRATION

NOTE: Powder, solution may irritate skin on contact. Wash area for 15 min if contact occurs.

IM:

1. Add 2 ml 0.9% NaCl injection to 10,000 IU vial to provide a concentration of 5,000 IU/ml.
2. Administer no more than 2 ml at any one site.

IV:

NOTE: Administer intradermal test dose (2 IU) prior to initiating therapy or when more than 1 wk has elapsed between doses. Observe pt for 1 hr for appearance of wheal or erythema. **Test solution:** Reconstitute 10,000 IU vial w/5 ml sterile water for injection or 0.9% NaCl injection. Shake to dissolve. Withdraw 0.1 ml, inject into vial containing 9.9 ml same diluent for concentration of 20 IU/ml.

1. Reconstitute 10,000 IU vial w/ 5 ml sterile water for injection or 0.9% NaCl injection to provide a concentration of 2,000 IU/ml.
2. Shake gently to assure complete dissolution (vigorous shaking produces foam, difficulty withdrawing entire vial contents).
3. For IV injection, administer into tubing of freely running IV solution of 5% dextrose or 0.9% NaCl over at least 30 min.
4. For IV infusion, further dilute w/ up to 1,000 ml 5% dextrose or 0.9% NaCl.

INDICATIONS/DOSAGE/ROUTES

NOTE: Dosage individualized based on clinical response, tolerance to adverse effects. When used in combination therapy, consult specific protocols for optimum dosage, sequence of drug administration.

Acute lymphocytic leukemia:
IV: Adults, elderly, children: Single agent: 200 IU/kg/day for 28 days.
IV: Children: Combination (w/

prednisone, vincristine): 1,000 IU/kg/day for 10 days beginning day 22 of treatment period.
IM: Children: Combination (w/ prednisone, vincristine): 6,000 IU/m^2 on days 4, 7, 10, 13, 16, 19, 22, 25, 28.

PRECAUTIONS

CONTRAINDICATIONS: Previous anaphylactic reaction, pancreatitis, history of pancreatitis. **CAUTIONS:** None significant. **PREGNANCY/LACTATION:** If possible, avoid use during pregnancy, especially first trimester. Breast feeding not recommended. **Pregnancy Category C.**

INTERACTIONS

DRUG INTERACTIONS: Steroids, vincristine may increase hyperglycemia, risk of neuropathy, disturbances of erythropoiesis. May decrease effect of antigout medications. May block effects of methotrexate. Live virus vaccines may potentiate virus replication, increase vaccine side effects, decrease pt's antibody response to vaccine. **ALTERED LAB VALUES:** May increase blood ammonia, BUN, uric acid, glucose, partial thromboplastin time (PTT), platelet count, prothrombin time (PT), thrombin time (TT), SGOT (AST), SGPT (ALT), alkaline phosphatase, bilirubin. May decrease plasma fibrinogen, antithrombin, plasminogen, albumin, calcium, cholesterol.

SIDE EFFECTS

FREQUENT: Nausea, vomiting, anorexia, weight loss, leukopenia, azotemia, impaired pancreatic function. **OCCASIONAL:** Chills, fever, diaphoresis, transient proteinuria, irritability, confusion, agitation, dizziness. **RARE:** Hair loss, diarrhea, oral/intestinal ulcers.

ADVERSE REACTIONS/TOXIC EFFECTS

Increased risk of allergic reaction (rash, urticaria, arthralgia, facial edema, hypotension, respiratory distress, anaphylactic reaction) after repeated therapy. Severe bone marrow depression more severe in adults than children, and when given daily rather than weekly.

NURSING IMPLICATIONS

BASELINE ASSESSMENT:

Before giving medication, agents for adequate airway and allergic reaction (antihistamine, epinephrine, oxygen, IV corticosteroid) should be readily available (an abrupt fall in serum asparaginase generally precedes allergic reaction). Skin testing, hepatic, renal, pancreatic (including blood glucose), CBC, differential, CNS functions should be performed before therapy begins and when a wk or more has elapsed between doses.

INTERVENTION/EVALUATION:

Determine serum amylase concentration frequently during therapy. Discontinue medication at first sign of renal failure, pancreatitis (abdominal pain, nausea, vomiting). Monitor for hematologic toxicity (fever, sore throat, signs of local infection, easy bruising, unusual bleeding), symptoms of anemia (excessive tiredness, weakness).

PATIENT/FAMILY TEACHING:

Increase fluid intake (protects against renal impairment). Nausea may decrease during therapy. Do not have immunizations w/o physician's approval (drug lowers body's resistance). Avoid contact w/those who have recently taken live virus vaccine. Contact physician if nausea/vomiting continues at home.

aspirin (acetylsalicylic acid, ASA)

as´purr-in
(Ascriptin, Bayer, Bufferin, Ecotrin, Halfprin)

FIXED-COMBINATION(S):
W/butabarbital, a barbiturate, and codeine, a narcotic, (Fiorinal); w/oxycodone, a narcotic (Percodan); w/pentazocine, an analgesic (Talwin Cmpd); w/caffeine, a stimulant (Anacin, Midol).

CANADIAN AVAILABILITY:
Coryphen, Ecotrin, Novasen

CLASSIFICATION

Nonsteroidal anti-inflammatory: Salicylate

PHARMACOKINETICS

Rapidly, completely absorbed from GI tract; enteric coated absorption delayed; rectal absorption delayed, incomplete. Widely distributed. Protein binding: high. Rapidly hydrolyzed to salicylate. Half-life: 15-20 min (aspirin); salicylate: 2-3 hrs at low dose; >20 hrs at high dose.

ACTION

Produces analgesic, anti-inflammatory effect by inhibiting prostaglandin synthesis, reducing inflammatory response and intensity of pain stimulus reaching sensory nerve endings. Antipyresis produced by drug's effect on hypothalamus, producing vasodilation, thereby decreasing elevated body temperature. Inhibits platelet aggregation.

USES

Treatment of mild to moderate pain, fever, inflammatory conditions. Reduces risk of recurrent TIA, stroke. Reduces risk of MI in those w/unstable angina or w/previous MI.

STORAGE/HANDLING

Refrigerate suppositories.

PO/RECTAL ADMINISTRATION

PO:

1. Do not crush or break enteric coated or sustained-release form.
2. May give w/water, milk, or meals if GI distress occurs.

RECTAL:

1. If suppository is too soft, chill for 30 min in refrigerator or run cold water over foil wrapper.
2. Moisten suppository w/cold water before inserting well up into rectum.

INDICATIONS/DOSAGE/ROUTES

Pain, fever:
PO/RECTAL: Adults, elderly: 325-650 mg q4h as needed, up to 4 Gm/day.

Rheumatoid arthritis, osteoarthritis, other inflammatory conditions:
PO: Adults, elderly: 3.2-6 Gm/day in divided doses.

Juvenile arthritis:
PO: Children: 60-110 mg/kg/day in divided doses (q 6-8 h). May increase dose at 5-7 day intervals.

Acute rheumatic fever:
PO: Adults, elderly: 5-8 Gm/day.

Children: 100 mg/kg/day, then decrease to 75 mg/kg/day for 4-6 wks.

Thrombosis (decrease TIAs):
PO: Adults, elderly: 1.3 Gm/day in 2-4 divided doses.

Thrombosis (decrease MI):
PO: Adults, elderly: 300-325 mg/day.

Usual pediatric dosage:
PO/RECTAL: Children: 10-15 mg/kg/dose q4h up to 60-80 mg/kg/day.

PRECAUTIONS

CONTRAINDICATIONS: Chickenpox or flu in children/teenagers, GI bleeding or ulceration, bleeding disorders, history of hypersensitivity to aspirin or NSAIDs, allergy to tartrazine dye, impaired hepatic function. **CAUTIONS:** Vitamin K deficiency, chronic renal insufficiency, those w/"aspirin triad" (rhinitis, nasal polyps, asthma). **PREGNANCY/LACTATION:** Readily crosses placenta; distributed in breast milk. May prolong gestation and labor, decrease fetal birth weight, increase incidence of stillbirths, neonatal mortality, hemorrhage. Avoid use during last trimester (may adversely affect fetal cardiovascular system: premature closure of ductus arteriosus). **Pregnancy Category D.**

INTERACTIONS

DRUG INTERACTIONS: Alcohol, NSAIDs may increase risk of GI effects (e.g., ulceration). Urinary alkalinizers, antacids increase excretion. Anticoagulants, heparin, thrombolytics increase risk of bleeding. Large dose may increase effect of insulin, oral hypoglycemics. Valproic acid, platelet aggregation inhibitors may increase risk of bleeding. May increase toxicity of methotrexate, zidovudine. Ototoxic medications, vancomycin may increase ototoxicity. May decrease effect of probenecid, sulfinpyrazone. **ALTERED LAB VALUES:** May alter SGOT (AST), SGPT (ALT), alkaline phosphatase, uric acid; prolong prothrombin time, bleeding time. May decrease cholesterol, potassium, T_3, T_4.

SIDE EFFECTS

OCCASIONAL: GI distress (cramping, heartburn, abdominal distention, mild nausea).

ADVERSE REACTIONS/TOXIC EFFECTS

High doses may produce GI bleeding and/or gastric mucosal lesions. Low-grade toxicity characterized by ringing in ears, generalized pruritus (may be severe), headache, dizziness, flushing, tachycardia, hyperventilation, sweating, thirst. Febrile, dehydrated children can reach toxic levels quickly. Marked intoxication manifested by hyperthermia, restlessness, abnormal breathing pattern, convulsions, respiratory failure, coma.

NURSING IMPLICATIONS

BASELINE ASSESSMENT:

Do not give to children/teenagers who have flu or chickenpox (increases risk of Reye's syndrome). Do not use if vinegar-like odor is noted (indicates chemical breakdown). Assess type, location, duration of pain, inflammation. Inspect appearance of affected joints for immobility, deformities, skin condition. Therapeutic serum level for anti-arthritic effect: 20-30 mg/

dl (toxicity occurs if levels are over 30 mg/dl).

INTERVENTION/EVALUATION:

In long-term therapy, monitor plasma salicylic acid concentration. Monitor urinary pH (sudden acidification, pH from 6.5 to 5.5) may result in toxicity. Assess skin for evidence of bruising. If given as an antipyretic, assess temperature directly before, and 1 hr after giving medication. Evaluate for therapeutic response: relief of pain, stiffness, swelling, increase in joint mobility, reduced joint tenderness, improved grip strength.

PATIENT/FAMILY TEACHING:

Do not crush or chew sustained-release or enteric-coated form. Report auditory disturbances. Therapeutic anti-inflammatory effect noted in 1-3 wks.

astemizole

az-tem´ih-zole

(Hismanal)

CANADIAN AVAILABILITY:
Hismanal

CLASSIFICATION

Antihistamine

PHARMACOKINETICS

	ONSET	PEAK	DURATION
PO	—	—	24 hrs

Well absorbed from GI tract. Protein binding: 96%. Metabolized in liver to active metabolite. Primarily eliminated in feces. Half-life: 0.9-2.3 days; metabolite: 11.6-14.6 days.

ACTION

Prevents, antagonizes most histamine effects (e.g., urticaria, pruritus). Anticholinergic effects cause drying of nasal mucosa.

USES

Treatment of seasonal allergic rhinitis, chronic idiopathic urticaria.

PO ADMINISTRATION

Give on empty stomach (2 hrs after meal, no additional food intake for 1 hr post-dosing).

INDICATIONS/DOSAGE/ROUTES

Allergic rhinitis, urticaria:
PO: Adults, children >12 yrs: 10 mg once/day.

Usual elderly dosage:
PO: Elderly: 10 mg/day.

PRECAUTIONS

CONTRAINDICATIONS: Acute asthma, concomitant erythromycin, ketoconazole, itraconazole, significant liver dysfunction. **CAUTIONS:** Narrow-angle glaucoma, peptic ulcer, prostatic hypertrophy, pyloroduodenal or bladder neck obstruction, asthma, COPD, increased intraocular pressure, cardiovascular disease, hyperthyroidism, hypertension, seizure disorders. **PREGNANCY/LACTATION:** Unknown if drug crosses placenta or is detected in breast milk. Increased risk of seizures in neonates, premature infants if used during third trimester of pregnancy. May inhibit lactation. **Pregnancy Category C.**

INTERACTIONS

DRUG INTERACTIONS: Alcohol, CNS depressants may increase CNS depressant effects. Anticholinergics may increase anticholinergic effects. Ketoconazole, fluconazole, itraconazole, micoconazole, macrolide antibiotics (e.g., erythromycin) may increase concentrations resulting in cardiotoxic effect. MAOIs may increase anticholinergic, CNS depressant effects. **ALTERED LAB VALUES:** May suppress wheal and flare reactions to antigen skin testing unless antihistamines are discontinued 4 days prior to testing.

SIDE EFFECTS

OCCASIONAL: Headache, increase in appetite, nausea, nervousness, dizziness. **RARE:** Diarrhea, pharyngitis, abdominal pain, conjunctivitis, arthralgia, angioedema.

ADVERSE REACTIONS/TOXIC EFFECTS

Children may experience dominant paradoxical reaction (restlessness, insomnia, euphoria, nervousness, tremors). Hypersensitivity reaction (eczema, pruritus, rash, photosensitivity) may occur.

NURSING IMPLICATIONS

BASELINE ASSESSMENT:

If patient is undergoing allergic reaction, obtain history of recently ingested foods, drugs, environmental exposure, recent emotional stress. Monitor rate, depth, rhythm, type of respiration; quality and rate of pulse. Assess lung sounds for rhonchi, wheezing, rales.

INTERVENTION/EVALUATION:

Monitor B/P, especially in elderly (increased risk of hypotension). Monitor children closely for paradoxical reaction. Assess for therapeutic response from allergy: itching, red, watery eyes, relief from rhinorrhea, sneezing.

PATIENT/FAMILY TEACHING:

Tolerance to antihistaminic effect generally does not occur; tolerance to sedative effect may occur. Avoid tasks that require alertness, motor skills until response to drug is established. Dry mouth, drowsiness, dizziness may be an expected response of drug. Avoid alcoholic beverages during antihistamine therapy. Sugarless gum, sips of tepid water may relieve dry mouth. Coffee or tea may help reduce drowsiness.

atenolol

ay-ten´oh-lol

(Tenormin)

FIXED-COMBINATION(S):

W/chlorthalidone, a diuretic (Tenoretic)

CANADIAN AVAILABILITY:

Apo-Atenolol, Tenormin

CLASSIFICATION

Beta$_1$-adrenergic blocker

PHARMACOKINETICS

	ONSET	PEAK	DURATION
PO (heart rate)	1 hr	2-4 hrs	24 hrs
PO (hypotensive)	—	—	24 hrs

Incompletely absorbed from GI tract. Protein binding: 6-16%. Minimal liver metabolism. Primarily excreted unchanged in urine. Removed by hemodialysis. Half-life: 6-7 hrs (increase in decreased renal function).

ACTION

Selectively blocks beta$_1$-adrenergic receptors, slowing sinus heart rate, decreasing cardiac output, decreasing B/P (exact mechanism unknown but may block peripheral adrenergic receptors, decrease sympathetic outflow from CNS or decrease renin release from kidney). Large dose may block beta$_2$-adrenergic receptors, increasing airway resistance. Decreases myocardial ischemia severity by decreasing oxygen requirements.

USES

Management of mild to moderate hypertension, used alone or in combination w/diuretics, especially thiazide-type. Management of chronic stable angina pectoris. Reduces cardiovascular mortality in those w/definite or suspected acute MI.

STORAGE/HANDLING

After reconstitution, parenteral form is stable for 48 hrs at room temperature.

PO/IV ADMINISTRATION

PO:

1. May be given w/o regard to meals.
2. Tablets may be crushed.

IV:

1. Dilutions w/5% dextrose or 0.9% NaCl may be used.

INDICATIONS/DOSAGE/ROUTES

Hypertension:
PO: Adults: Initially, 25-50 mg once daily. May increase up to 100 mg once daily.

Angina pectoris:
PO: Adults: Initially, 50 mg once daily. May increase up to 200 mg once daily.

Usual elderly dosage:
PO: Elderly: Initially, 25 mg/day for angina/hypertension.

Acute myocardial infarction:
IV: Give 5 mg over 5 min, may repeat in 10 min. In those who tolerate full 10 mg IV dose, begin 50 mg tablets 10 min after last IV dose followed by another 50 mg oral dose 12 hrs later. Thereafter, give 100 mg once/day or 50 mg twice/day for 6-9 days. (Alternatively, for those who do not tolerate full IV dose, give 50 mg orally 2 times/day or 100 mg once daily for at least 7 days.)

Dosage in renal impairment:

CREATININE CLEARANCE	DOSAGE
15-35 ml/min	50 mg daily
<15 ml/min	50 mg q other day

PRECAUTIONS

CONTRAINDICATIONS: Overt cardiac failure, cardiogenic shock, heart block greater than first degree, severe bradycardia. **CAUTIONS:** Impaired renal or hepatic function, peripheral vascular disease, hyperthyroidism, diabetes, inadequate cardiac function, bronchospastic disease. **PREGNANCY/LACTATION:** Readily crosses placenta; distributed in breast milk. Avoid use during first trimester. May produce bradycardia, apnea, hypoglycemia, hypothermia during delivery, small birth weight infants. **Pregnancy Category C.**

INTERACTIONS

DRUG INTERACTIONS: Diuretics, other hypotensives may increase hypotensive effect; sympathomimetics, xanthines may mutually inhibit effects; may mask symptoms of hypoglycemia, prolong hypoglycemic effect of insulin, oral hypoglycemics; NSAIDs may decrease anti-hypertensive effect; Cimetidine may increase concentration. **ALTERED LAB VALUES:** May increase ANA titer, BUN, creatinine, potassium, uric acid, lipoproteins, triglycerides.

SIDE EFFECTS

Generally well tolerated, w/ transient and mild side effects. **FREQUENT:** Hypotension (systolic B/P below 90 mm Hg) manifested as dizziness, nausea, diaphoresis, headache, cold extremities, fatigue; diarrhea; depression. **OCCASIONAL:** Lightheadedness, lethargy, peculiar dreams, rash, sore throat, unusual bruising/ bleeding.

ADVERSE REACTIONS/TOXIC EFFECTS

May produce profound bradycardia, hypotension, bronchospasm. Abrupt withdrawal may result in sweating, palpitations, headache, tremulousness. May precipitate CHF, MI in those w/ cardiac disease, thyroid storm in those w/thyrotoxicosis, peripheral ischemia in those w/existing peripheral vascular disease. Hypoglycemia may occur in previously controlled diabetics.

NURSING IMPLICATIONS

BASELINE ASSESSMENT:

Assess B/P, apical pulse immediately before drug is administered (if pulse is 60/min or below, or systolic B/P is below 90 mm Hg, withhold medication, contact physician). *Antianginal:* Record onset, type (sharp, dull, squeezing), radiation, location, intensity and duration of anginal pain, and precipitating factors (exertion, emotional stress). Assess baseline renal/liver function tests.

INTERVENTION/EVALUATION:

Monitor B/P for hypotension, pulse for bradycardia, respiration for shortness of breath. Assess pattern of daily bowel activity and stool consistency. Assess for evidence of CHF: dyspnea (particularly on exertion or lying down), night cough, peripheral edema, distended neck veins). Monitor I&O (increase in weight, decrease in urine output may indicate CHF). Assess extremities for coldness. Assist w/ambulation if dizziness occurs. Assess skin for rash, bruising. Therapeutic antihypertensive effect noted in 1-2 wks.

PATIENT/FAMILY TEACHING:

Do not abruptly discontinue medication. Compliance w/therapy essential to control hypertension, angina. To reduce hypotensive effect, rise slowly from lying to sitting position and permit legs to dangle from bed momentarily before standing. Avoid tasks that require alertness, motor skills until drug reaction is established. Report dizziness, depression, confusion, rash, unusual bruising or bleeding. Do not use nasal decongestants, over-the-counter cold preparations (stimulants) w/o physician approval. Outpatients should monitor B/P, pulse before taking medication (teach correct technique). Restrict salt, alcohol intake.

atovaquone

ah-tow'vah-quon
(Mepron)

CLASSIFICATION

Antiprotozoal

PHARMACOKINETICS

Poorly absorbed from GI tract (increased when given w/food especially high-fat foods). Protein binding: >99%. Primarily eliminated unchanged in feces. Half-life: 50-77 hrs.

ACTION

Inhibits mitochondrial electron-transport system at the cytochrome bc_1 complex. Interrupts pyrimidine synthesis and nucleic and ATP synthesis.

USES

Treatment of mild to moderate *Pneumocystis carinii* pneumonia (PCP) in those intolerant to trimethoprim-sulfamethoxazole (TMP-SMZ).

PO ADMINISTRATION

Give w/food (especially high-fat foods).

INDICATIONS/DOSAGE/ROUTES

Pneumocystis carinii *pneumonia (PCP):*

PO: Adults: 750 mg w/food 3 times/day for 21 days.

PRECAUTIONS

CONTRAINDICATIONS: Development or history of potentially life-threatening allergic reaction to drug. **CAUTIONS:** Elderly, pts w/ severe PCP, chronic diarrhea, malabsorption syndromes. **PREGNANCY/LACTATION:** May produce maternal toxicity; body length and weight of fetus may be decreased. Unknown if distributed in breast milk. **Pregnancy Category C.**

INTERACTIONS

DRUG INTERACTIONS: None significant. **ALTERED LAB VALUES:** May elevate SGOT (AST), SGPT (ALT), alkaline phosphatase, amylase. May decrease sodium.

SIDE EFFECTS

FREQUENT: Rash, nausea, diarrhea. **OCCASIONAL:** Headache, vomiting, fever, insomnia, abdominal discomfort. **RARE:** Weakness, sweating, cough, constipation.

ADVERSE REACTIONS/TOXIC EFFECTS

None significant.

NURSING IMPLICATIONS

INTERVENTION/EVALUATION:

Assess for GI discomfort, nausea, vomiting. Check consistency and frequency of stools. Assess skin for rash. Monitor I&O, renal function tests. Atovaquone has not been fully evaluated in pts >65 years of age; monitor elderly closely because of decreased hepatic, renal and cardiac function.

PATIENT/FAMILY TEACHING:

Continue therapy for full length of treatment. Doses should be evenly spaced. Do not take any other medication unless approved by physician. Notify physician in event of rash, diarrhea or other new symptom.

atracurium

(Tracrium)

(See Classifications section under Neuromuscular blockers)

atropine sulfate

ah´trow-peen
(Atropine Sulfate, Isopto Atropine, Ocu-Tropine)

FIXED-COMBINATION(S):
W/phenobarbital, a sedative-hypnotic (Antrocol); w/diphenoxylate, a constipating meperidine derivative (Lomotil); w/prednisolone, a steroid (Mydropred Ophthalmic)

CANADIAN AVAILABILITY:
Atropine Minims, Atropisol, Isopto-Atropine

CLASSIFICATION

Anticholinergic

PHARMACOKINETICS

Mydriatic effect: Peak 30-40 min; recovery 7-12 days. *Cycloplegic effect:* Peak 60-180 min; recovery 6-12 days. Rapidly absorbed after IM, oral administration. Protein binding: moderate. Metabolized in liver. Primarily excreted in urine. Half-life: 2-3 hrs. After PO/IM administration, inhibits salivation within 30-60 min (peak 1-2 hrs), duration 4 hrs; increases heart rate within 2-4 min (IV), 5-40 min (IM), or 30-120 min (PO), peak in 0.5-1 hr (IM), 1-2 hrs (PO).

ACTION

Inhibits action of acetylcholine on structures innervated by postganglionic sites: smooth, cardiac muscle, SA, AV nodes, exocrine glands. Larger doses may decrease motility, secretory activity of GI system, tone of ureter, urinary bladder. Blocks responses of sphincter muscle and accommodation muscle ciliary body producing mydriasis, cycloplegia.

USES

Adjunct in treatment of peptic ulcer disease. Treatment of functional disturbances of GI motility, hypermotility disorders of lower urinary tract, GI hypermotility, diarrhea. Preop medication to prevent or reduce salivation, excessive secretions of respiratory tract. May also prevent cholinergic effects during surgery: cardiac arrhythmias, hypotension, reflex bradycardia. Blocks adverse muscarinic effects of anticholinesterase agents (i.e., neostigmine). Management of sinus bradycardia in those w/acute MI who have hypotension and increased ventricular irritability. For cycloplegic refraction and to dilate pupil in inflammatory conditions of iris and uveal tract.

PO/IM/IV/OPHTHALMIC ADMINISTRATION

PO:

1. Administer 30 min before meals and at bedtime.

IM:

1. May be given SubQ or IM.

IV:

1. Generally given rapidly (prevents paradoxical slowing of heart rate).

Ophthalmic:

1. Place finger on lower eyelid and pull out until pocket is formed between eye and lower lid. Hold dropper above pocket and place prescribed number of drops (¼-½ inch ointment) in pocket. Close eye gently. *Drops:* Apply digital pressure to lacrimal sac for 1-2 min (minimize drainage into nose and throat, reducing risk of systemic effects). *Ointment:* Close eye for 1-2

min, rolling eyeball (increases contact area of drug to eye). W/ either method, remove excess solution or ointment around eye w/ tissue.

2. Ophthalmic solutions not to be used for injection.

INDICATIONS/DOSAGE/ROUTES

Usual oral dosage:
PO: Adults, elderly: 0.4-0.6 mg q4-6h. **Range:** 0.1-1.2 mg. **Children:** 0.01 mg/kg, not to exceed 0.4 mg q4-6h.

Usual parenteral dose:
SubQ/IM/IV: Adults, elderly: 0.4-0.6 mg q4-6h. **Range:** 0.3-1.2 mg. **Children:** 0.01 mg/kg, not to exceed 0.4 mg q4-6h.

Bradycardia in advanced cardiac life support:
IV: Adults, elderly: 0.4-1 mg. Repeat at 5 min intervals until desired rate achieved. **Maximum:** 2 mg total dose. **Children:** 0.01-0.03 mg/kg (minimum dose: 0.1 mg). Repeat at 5 min intervals. **Maximum:** 1 mg total dose.

Preoperative:
SubQ/IM/IV: Adults, elderly, children >20 kg: 0.4 mg (range: 0.2-0.6 mg) 30-60 min prior to time of induction of anesthesia or other preanesthetic medications. **Children (3 kg):** 0.1 mg; **(7-9 kg):** 0.2 mg; **(12-16 kg):** 0.3 mg.

Usual ophthalmic dose (mydriasis, cycloplegia):
OPHTHALMIC OINTMENT:
Adults, elderly: 0.3-0.5 cm 1-3 times/day. **Children:** 0.3 cm 3 times/day. Administer for 1-3 days prior to procedure.
OPHTHALMIC SOLUTION:
Adults, elderly: 1 drop 1% solution. **Children:** 1-2 drops 0.5% solution 2 times/day. Administer for 1-3 days prior to and 1 hr before procedure.

Treatment of acute inflammatory ophthalmic conditions:
OPHTHALMIC SOLUTION:
Adults, elderly: 1-2 drops of 0.5-1% solution up to 3-4 times/day. **Children:** 1-2 drops of 0.5% solution up to 3-4 times/day.

PRECAUTIONS

CONTRAINDICATIONS: Narrow-angle glaucoma, severe ulcerative colitis, toxic megacolon, obstructive disease of GI tract, paralytic ileus, intestinal atony, bladder neck obstruction due to prostatic hypertrophy, myasthenia gravis in those not treated w/neostigmine, tachycardia secondary to cardiac insufficiency or thyrotoxicosis, cardiospasm, unstable cardiovascular status in acute hemorrhage. **EXTREME CAUTION:** Autonomic neuropathy, known or suspected GI infections, diarrhea, mild to moderate ulcerative colitis. **CAUTIONS:** Hyperthyroidism, hepatic or renal disease, hypertension, tachyarrhythmias, CHF, coronary artery disease, gastric ulcer, esophageal reflux or hiatal hernia associated w/reflux esophagitis, infants, elderly, systemic administration in those w/COPD. **PREGNANCY/LACTATION:** Crosses placenta; unknown if distributed in breast milk. May produce fetal tachycardia. **Pregnancy Category C.**

INTERACTIONS

DRUG INTERACTIONS: Antacids, antidiarrheals may decrease absorption. Anticholinergics may increase effects. May decrease absorption of ketoconazole. May increase severity of GI lesions with

KCl (wax matrix). **ALTERED LAB VALUES:** None significant.

SIDE EFFECTS

FREQUENT: Dry mouth (sometimes severe), decreased sweating, constipation, pupillary dilation, temporary paralysis of accommodation. **OCCASIONAL:** Blurred vision, bloated feeling, urinary hesitancy, drowsiness (w/high dosage), headache, intolerance to light, loss of taste, nervousness, flushing, insomnia, impotence, mental confusion/excitement (particularly in elderly, children). IM may produce temporary lightheadedness, local irritation. **RARE:** Dizziness, faintness.

ADVERSE REACTIONS/TOXIC EFFECTS

Overdosage may produce temporary paralysis of ciliary muscle, pupillary dilation, tachycardia, palpitation; hot/dry/flushed skin; absence of bowel sounds, hyperthermia, increased respiratory rate, EKG abnormalities, nausea, vomiting, rash over face/upper trunk, CNS stimulation, psychosis (agitation, restlessness, rambling speech, visual hallucination, paranoid behavior, delusions), followed by depression.

NURSING IMPLICATIONS

BASELINE ASSESSMENT:

Before giving medication, instruct pt to void (reduces risk of urinary retention).

INTERVENTION/EVALUATION:

Monitor changes in B/P, pulse, temperature. Assess skin turgor, mucous membranes to evaluate hydration status (encourage adequate fluid intake unless NPO for surgery), bowel sounds for peristalsis. Be alert for fever (increased risk of hyperthermia). Monitor I&O, palpate bladder for urinary retention. Assess stool frequency & consistency.

PATIENT/FAMILY TEACHING:

Take oral form 30 min before meals (food decreases absorption of medication). Avoid becoming overheated during exercise in hot weather (may result in heat stroke). Avoid hot baths, saunas. Avoid tasks that require alertness, motor skills until response to drug is established. Sugarless gum, sips of tepid water relieve dry mouth. Do not take antacids or medicine for diarrhea within 1 hr of taking this medication (decreased effectiveness). For preop use, explain that warm, dry, flushing feeling may occur. Remind pt to remain in bed and not eat or drink anything.

auranofin

aur-an-oh´fin

(Ridaura)

CANADIAN AVAILABILITY: Ridaura

CLASSIFICATION

Antirheumatic: Gold compound

PHARMACOKINETICS

Moderately absorbed from GI tract. Protein binding: 60%. Rapidly metabolized. Primarily excreted in urine. Half-life: 21-31 days.

ACTION

Exact mechanism unknown (may alter cellular mechanisms, enzyme systems, immune responses, collagen biosynthesis; may suppress phagocytic activity).

USES

Management of rheumatoid arthritis in those w/insufficient therapeutic response to nonsteroidal anti-inflammatory agents.

PO ADMINISTRATION

Give w/o regard to food.

INDICATIONS/DOSAGE/ROUTES

Rheumatoid arthritis:
PO: Adults, elderly: 6 mg/day in 1 or 2 divided doses. May increase to 9 mg/day (in 3 divided doses) if no response in 6 months. If response still inadequate, discontinue.

PRECAUTIONS

CONTRAINDICATIONS: *Parenteral:* History of gold-induced pathologies (necrotizing enterocolitis, exfoliative dermatitis, pulmonary fibrosis, blood dyscrasias), hepatic dysfunction or history of hepatitis, uncontrolled diabetes or CHF, urticaria, eczema, colitis, hemorrhagic conditions, systemic lupus erythematosus, recent radiation therapy. *Oral:* History of gold-induced pathologies (necrotizing enterocolitis, exfoliative dermatitis, pulmonary fibrosis, blood dyscrasias), bone marrow aplasia, severe blood dyscrasias. **CAUTIONS:** Renal/hepatic disease, inflammatory bowel disease. **PREGNANCY/LACTATION:** Crosses placenta; distributed in breast milk. Use only when benefits outweigh hazard to fetus. **Pregnancy Category C.**

INTERACTIONS

DRUG INTERACTIONS: Bone marrow depressants, hepatotoxic, nephrotoxic medications may increase toxicity. Penicillamine may increase risk of hematologic or renal adverse effects. **ALTERED LAB VALUES:** May decrease hemoglobin, hematocrit, platelets, WBCs. May alter liver function tests. May increase urine protein.

SIDE EFFECTS

FREQUENT: Diarrhea/loose stools, rash, pruritus, abdominal pain, nausea. **OCCASIONAL:** Vomiting, anorexia, flatulence, dyspepsia, conjunctivitis, photosensitivity. **RARE:** Constipation, urticaria, rash.

ADVERSE REACTIONS/TOXIC EFFECTS

Signs of gold toxicity: decreased hemoglobin, leukopenia (WBC below 4,000/mm^3), reduced granulocyte counts (below 150,000/mm^3), proteinuria, hematuria, stomatitis, blood dyscrasias (anemia, leukopenia, thrombocytopenia, eosinophilia), glomerulonephritis, nephrotic syndrome, cholestatic jaundice.

NURSING IMPLICATIONS

BASELINE ASSESSMENT:

Rule out pregnancy before beginning treatment. CBC, urinalysis, platelet and differential, renal and liver function tests should be performed before therapy begins.

INTERVENTION/EVALUATION:

Monitor daily bowel activity and stool consistency. Assess urine tests for proteinuria or hematuria. Monitor WBC, hemoglobin, differential, platelet count, renal and hepatic function studies. Question for pruritus (may be first sign of impending rash). Assess skin daily for rash, purpura or ecchymoses. Assess oral mucous membranes, borders of tongue, palate, pharynx for ulceration, complaint of metallic taste sensation (sign of stomatitis). Evaluate for therapeutic response: relief of pain, stiffness, swelling, increase in joint mobility, reduced joint tenderness, improved grip strength.

PATIENT/FAMILY TEACHING:

Therapeutic response may be expected in 3-6 mos. Avoid exposure to sunlight (grey to blue pigment may appear). Contact physician if pruritus, rash, sore mouth, indigestion, or metallic taste occurs. Maintain diligent oral hygiene.

aurothioglucose

ah-row-thigh-oh-glu´cose
(Solganal)

CLASSIFICATION

Antirheumatic: Gold compound

PHARMACOKINETICS

Slow, erratic absorption after IM administration. Protein binding: 95-99%. Metabolic fate unknown. Primarily excreted in urine. Half-life: 3-27 days (increased w/increased number of doses).

ACTION

Exact mechanism unknown (may alter cellular mechanisms, enzyme systems, immune responses, collagen biosynthesis; may suppress phagocytic activity.)

USES

Management of rheumatoid arthritis in those w/insufficient therapeutic response to nonsteroidal anti-inflammatory agents.

IM ADMINISTRATION

Give in upper outer quadrant of gluteus.

INDICATIONS/DOSAGE/ROUTES

Rheumatoid arthritis:
NOTE: Give as weekly injections.
IM: Adults, elderly: Initially, 10 mg, then 25 mg for 2 doses, then 50 mg weekly thereafter until total dose of 0.8-1 Gm given. If pt improved and no signs of toxicity, give 50 mg at 3-4 wk intervals for many months.

PRECAUTIONS

CONTRAINDICATIONS: *Parenteral:* History of gold-induced pathologies (necrotizing enterocolitis, exfoliative dermatitis, pulmonary fibrosis, blood dyscrasias), hepatic dysfunction or history of hepatitis, uncontrolled diabetes or CHF, urticaria, eczema, colitis, hemorrhagic conditions, systemic lupus erythematosus, recent radiation therapy. *Oral:* History of gold-induced pathologies (necrotizing enterocolitis, exfoliative dermatitis, pulmonary fibrosis, blood dyscrasias), bone marrow aplasia, severe blood dyscrasias. **CAUTIONS:** Renal/hepatic disease, inflammatory bowel disease. **PREGNANCY/LACTATION:** Crosses placenta, distributed in breast milk. Use only when benefits outweigh hazard to fetus. **Pregnancy Category C.**

INTERACTIONS

DRUG INTERACTIONS: Bone marrow depressants, hepatotoxic, nephrotoxic medications may increase toxicity. Penicillamine may increase risk of hematologic or renal adverse effects. **ALTERED LAB VALUES:** May decrease hemoglobin, hematocrit, platelets,

WBCs. May alter liver function tests. May increase urine protein.

SIDE EFFECTS

FREQUENT: Diarrhea/loose stools, rash, pruritus, abdominal pain, nausea. **OCCASIONAL:** Vomiting, anorexia, flatulence, dyspepsia, conjunctivitis, photosensitivity. **RARE:** Constipation, urticaria, rash.

ADVERSE REACTIONS/TOXIC EFFECTS

Signs of gold toxicity: decreased hemoglobin, leukopenia (WBC below 4,000/mm^3), reduced granulocyte counts (below 150,000/mm^3), proteinuria, hematuria, stomatitis, blood dyscrasias (anemia, leukopenia, thrombocytopenia, eosinophilia), glomerulonephritis, nephrotic syndrome, cholestatic jaundice.

NURSING IMPLICATIONS

BASELINE ASSESSMENT:

Rule out pregnancy before beginning treatment. CBC, urinalysis, platelet and differential, renal and liver function tests should be performed before therapy begins.

INTERVENTION/EVALUATION:

Monitor daily bowel activity and stool consistency. Assess urine tests for proteinuria or hematuria. Monitor WBC, hemoglobin, differential, platelet count, renal, and hepatic function studies. Question for pruritus (may be first sign of impending rash). Assess skin daily for rash, purpura, or ecchymoses. Assess oral mucous membranes, borders of tongue, palate, pharynx for ulceration, complaint of metallic taste sensation (signs of stomatitis). Evaluate for therapeutic response: relief of pain, stiffness, swelling, increase in joint mobility, reduced joint tenderness, improved grip strength.

PATIENT/FAMILY TEACHING:

Therapeutic response may take 6 mos or longer. Avoid exposure to sunlight (grey to blue pigment may appear). Contact physician/nurse if pruritus, rash, sore mouth, indigestion, or metallic taste occurs. Maintain diligent oral hygiene.

azathioprine

azha-thigh´oh-preen

(Imuran [oral])

azathioprine sodium

(Imuran [parenteral])

CANADIAN AVAILABILITY:

Imuran

CLASSIFICATION

Immunosuppressant

PHARMACOKINETICS

Well absorbed from GI tract. Protein binding: 30%. Converted to active metabolite. Further metabolized in liver and erythrocytes. Eliminated via biliary system. Minimal removal by hemodialysis. Half-life: 5 hrs.

ACTION

Antagonizes purine metabolism. May inhibit RNA, DNA, protein synthesis, interfere w/cellular metabolism and inhibit mitosis. Effects on rheumatoid arthritis related to immunosuppression.

USES

Adjunct in prevention of rejection in kidney transplantation; treatment of rheumatoid arthritis in those unresponsive to conventional therapy.

STORAGE/HANDLING

Store oral, parenteral form at room temperature. After reconstitution, IV solution stable for 24 hrs.

PO/IV ADMINISTRATION

PO:

1. Give during or after meal to reduce potential for GI disturbances.

IV:

1. Reconstitute 100 mg vial w/10 ml sterile water for injection to provide concentration of 10 mg/ml.
2. Further dilute w/5% dextrose or 0.9% NaCl; infuse over 30-60 min.

INDICATIONS/DOSAGE/ROUTES

NOTE: May give in divided doses if GI disturbance occurs.

Kidney transplantation:
PO/IV: Adults, elderly, children: Initially, 3-5 mg/kg/day as single dose on day of transplant. **Maintenance:** 1-3 mg/kg/day.

Rheumatoid arthritis:
PO/IV: Adults: Initially, 1 mg/kg/day as single or in 2 divided doses. May increase by 0.5 mg/kg/day after 6-8 wks at 4 wk intervals up to maximum dose of 2.5 mg/kg/day. **Maintenance:** Lowest effective dose. May decrease dose by 0.5 mg/kg or 25 mg/day q4wks (other therapy maintained).

Rheumatoid arthritis:
PO: Elderly: Initially, 1 mg/kg/day (50-100 mg); may increase by 25 mg/day until response or toxicity.

PRECAUTIONS

CONTRAINDICATIONS: Pregnant rheumatoid arthritis pts, those previously treated for rheumatoid arthritis w/alkylating agents (cyclophosphamide, chlorambucil, melphalan). **CAUTIONS:** Immunosuppressed pts. **PREGNANCY/LACTATION:** If at all possible, avoid use. **Pregnancy Category D:** Do not give to nursing mother.

INTERACTIONS

DRUG INTERACTIONS: Allopurinol may increase activity, toxicity. Bone marrow depressants may increase bone marrow depression. Other immunosuppressants may increase risk of infection or development of neoplasms. Live virus vaccines may potentiate virus replication, increase vaccine side effects, decrease patients antibody response to vaccine. **ALTERED LAB VALUES:** May decrease hemoglobin, albumin, uric acid. May increase SGPT (ALT), SGOT (AST), alkaline phosphatase, amylase, bilirubin.

SIDE EFFECTS

OCCASIONAL: Nausea, vomiting, diarrhea, particularly during early treatment and w/large doses. **RARE:** Rash, alopecia, hypotension.

ADVERSE REACTIONS/TOXIC EFFECTS

There is an increased risk of neoplasia. Significant leukopenia, thrombocytopenia may occur, particularly in those undergoing kidney rejection. Hepatotoxicity occurs rarely.

NURSING IMPLICATIONS

BASELINE ASSESSMENT:

Arthritis: Assess onset, type, location and duration of pain, fever, or inflammation. Inspect appearance of affected joints for immobility, deformities, and skin condition.

INTERVENTION/EVALUATION:

CBC, platelet count, liver function studies should be performed weekly during first month of therapy, twice monthly during second and third month of treatment, then monthly thereafter. If rapid fall in WBC occurs, dosage should be reduced or discontinued. Assess particularly for delayed bone marrow suppression. Monitor for fungal, viral, bacterial, protozoal infection vigorously. Report any major change in assessment of pt. Routinely watch for any change from normal. *Arthritis:* Evaluate for therapeutic response: relief of pain, stiffness, swelling, increase in joint mobility, reduced joint tenderness, improved grip strength.

PATIENT/FAMILY TEACHING:

Contact physician if unusual bleeding or bruising, sore throat, mouth sores, abdominal pain, or fever occurs. Therapeutic response in rheumatoid arthritis may take up to 12 wks. Women of childbearing age must avoid pregnancy (assure pt has adequate information and resources to comply).

azithromycin

aye-zith´row-my-sin
(Zithromax)

CLASSIFICATION

Antibiotic: Macrolide

PHARMACOKINETICS

Rapidly absorbed from GI tract. Protein binding: 51% (decreases w/increased doses). Widely distributed. Eliminated primarily unchanged via biliary excretion. Half-life: 68 hrs.

ACTION

Inhibits protein synthesis by binding to ribosomal receptor sites.

USES

Treatment of mild to moderate infections of upper respiratory tract (pharyngitis, tonsillitis), lower respiratory tract (acute bacterial exacerbations, COPD, pneumonia), uncomplicated skin/skin structure infections, and sexually transmitted diseases (nongonococcal urethritis, cervicitis due to *Chlamydia trachomatis*).

PO ADMINISTRATION

1. Administer at least 1 hr before or 2 hrs after meals.
2. Give w/8 oz water.

INDICATIONS/DOSAGE/ROUTES

Lower/upper respiratory tract, skin/skin structure infections:
PO: Adults, elderly: Initially, 500 mg on first day, then 250 mg on days 2-5 (total dose 1.5 Gm).

***Nongonococcal urethritis, cervicitis due to* C. trachomatis:**
PO: Adult: 1 Gm as a single dose.

Usual pediatric dosage:
PO: Children: 10 mg/kg on day 1; then 5 mg/kg on days 2-5.

PRECAUTIONS

CONTRAINDICATIONS: Hypersensitivity to azithromycin, erythromycins, any macrolide antibiotic. **CAUTIONS:** Hepatic/renal dysfunction. **PREGNANCY/LACTATION:** Unknown if distributed in breast milk. **Pregnancy Category B.**

INTERACTIONS

DRUG INTERACTIONS: May increase serum concentrations of carbamazepine, cyclosporine, theophylline, warfarin. **ALTERED LAB VALUES:** May increase serum CPK, SGOT (AST), SGPT (ALT), alkaline phosphatase, bilirubin, BUN, creatinine, LDH.

SIDE EFFECTS

OCCASIONAL: Nausea, vomiting, diarrhea, abdominal pain. **RARE:** Angioedema, cholestatic jaundice.

ADVERSE REACTIONS/TOXIC EFFECTS

Superinfections, esp. antibiotic-associated colitis may result from altered bacterial balance.

NURSING IMPLICATIONS

Baseline Assessment:

Question patient for history of allergies to azithromycin, erythromycins, hepatitis. Obtain specimens for culture, sensitivity before giving first dose (therapy may begin before results are known).

Intervention/Evaluation:

Check for GI discomfort, nausea, vomiting. Determine pattern of bowel activity and stool consistency. Assess skin for rash. Monitor hepatic function tests, assess for hepatotoxicity: malaise, fever, abdominal pain, GI disturbances. Evaluate for superinfection: genital/anal pruritus, sore mouth or tongue, moderate to severe diarrhea.

Patient/Family Teaching:

Continue therapy for full length of treatment. Doses should be evenly spaced. Take medication w/8 oz water at least 1 hr before or 2 hrs after food/beverage. Notify physician in event of GI upset, rash, diarrhea, or other new symptom.

aztreonam

az-tree´oh-nam

(Azactam)

CLASSIFICATION

Antibiotic: Monobactam

PHARMACOKINETICS

Completely absorbed following IM administration. Protein binding: 56-60%. Partially metabolized by hydrolysis. Primarily excreted unchanged in urine. Removed by hemodialysis. Half-life: 1.4-2.2 hrs (increase in decreased renal, liver function).

ACTION

Bactericidal. Binds to bacterial cell wall inhibiting bacterial cell wall synthesis causing cell lysis, death.

USES

Lower respiratory tract, skin/skin structure, intra-abdominal, gynecologic, complicated/uncomplicated urinary tract infections; septicemia.

STORAGE/HANDLING

Solution appears colorless to light yellow. Following reconstitution for IM injection or IV use, solution stable for 48 hrs at room temperature, or 7 days if refrigerated. Discard if precipitate forms. Discard unused portions.

IM/IV ADMINISTRATION

NOTE: Give by deep IM injection, IV injection, intermittent IV infusion (piggyback).

IM:

1. Shake immediately, vigorously after adding diluent.
2. Dissolve each Gm w/at least 3 ml sterile water or 0.9% NaCl for injection to provide concentration of 333 mg/ml.
3. Inject deeply into large muscle mass.

IV:

1. For IV injection, reconstitute each Gm w/6-10 ml sterile water for injection. Give over 3-5 min.
2. For intermittent IV infusion, further dilute w/50-100 ml 5% dextrose, 0.9% NaCl, or other compatible IV fluid. Infuse over 20-60 min. Do not exceed final concentration of 20 mg/ml.
3. Alternating IV sites, use large veins to reduce risk of phlebitis.

INDICATIONS/DOSAGE/ROUTES

NOTE: Space doses evenly around clock.

Urinary tract infections:
IM/IV: Adults, elderly: 500 mg to 1 Gm q8-12h.

Moderate to severe systemic infections:
IM/IV: Adults, elderly: 1-2 Gm q8-12h.

Severe or life-threatening infections:
IV: Adults, elderly: 2 Gm q6-8h.

Dosage in renal impairment:
Dose and/or frequency is modified based on creatinine clearance, severity of infection:

CREATININE CLEARANCE	DOSAGE
10-30 ml/min	1-2 Gm initially; then ½ usual dose at usual intervals
<10 ml/min	1-2 Gm initially; then ¼ usual dose at usual intervals

PRECAUTIONS

CONTRAINDICATIONS: Hypersensitivity to aztreonam. **CAUTIONS:** History of allergy, especially antibiotics, hepatic or renal impairment. **PREGNANCY/LACTATION:** Crosses placenta, distributed in amniotic fluid; low concentration in breast milk. **Pregnancy Category B.**

INTERACTIONS

DRUG INTERACTIONS: None significant. **ALTERED LAB VALUES:** Positive Coombs test. May increase SGOT (AST), SGPT (ALT), LDH, alkaline phosphatase, creatinine.

SIDE EFFECTS

FREQUENT: Phlebitis, thrombophlebitis, pain at IM injection site, eosinophilia. **OCCASIONAL:** Nausea, vomiting, diarrhea, rash. **RARE:** Dizziness, confusion, seizures, hypotension, tinnitus, weakness, headache, jaundice/hepatitis, anaphylaxis.

ADVERSE REACTIONS/TOXIC EFFECTS

Superinfection occurs frequently, anaphylaxis rarely.

NURSING IMPLICATIONS

BASELINE ASSESSMENT:

Question patient for history of allergies, especially to aztreonam, other antibiotics. Obtain culture and sensitivity tests prior to giving first dose (therapy may begin before results are known).

INTERVENTION/EVALUATION:

Evaluate for phlebitis (heat, pain, red streaking over vein), pain at IM injection site. Assess for GI discomfort, nausea, vomiting. Monitor stool frequency and consistency. Assess skin for rash. Monitor vital signs. B/P twice daily. Assess mental status; be alert to tremors, possible seizures. Monitor I&O, renal function tests if indicated. Be alert to superinfection: increased temperature, changes in oral mucosa, sore throat, anal/genital pruritus.

PATIENT/FAMILY TEACHING:

Continue therapy for full length of treatment. Doses should be evenly spaced. Notify physician in event of tremors, seizures, rash, diarrhea, other new symptom.

bacampicillin hydrochloride

back-am-pi-sill′in

(Spectrobid)

CANADIAN AVAILABILITY: Penglobe

CLASSIFICATION

Antibiotic: Penicillin

PHARMACOKINETICS

Rapidly absorbed from GI tract. Protein binding: 17-20%. Metabolized in liver. Primarily excreted in urine. Removed by hemodialysis. Half-life: 0.7-1.1 hrs.

ACTION

Bactericidal. Binds to bacterial membranes. Inhibits cell wall synthesis.

USES

Treatment of respiratory, GI and GU tract, skin/skin structure infections; otitis media, gonorrhea.

STORAGE/HANDLING

Store tabs at room temperature. Oral suspension, after reconstitution, is stable for 10 days if refrigerated.

PO ADMINISTRATION

1. Give tablets w/o regard to meals; give oral solution on empty stomach.
2. Space doses evenly around the clock.

INDICATIONS/DOSAGE/ROUTES

Urinary tract, upper respiratory tract, skin/skin structure infections:

PO: Adults, elderly, children >25 kg: 400 mg q12h. **Children <25 kg:** 25 mg/kg/day in divided doses q12h.

Lower respiratory tract, severe infections:

PO: Adults, elderly, children >25 kg: 800 mg q12h. **Children <25 kg:** 50 mg/kg/day in divided doses q12h.

Gonorrhea:

PO: Adults: 1.6 Gm plus 1 Gm probenecid as single dose.

PRECAUTIONS

CONTRAINDICATIONS: Infectious mononucleosis, disulfiram therapy, hypersensitivity to any penicillin. **CAUTIONS:** History of allergies, especially cephalosporins. **PREGNANCY/LACTA-**

TION: Drug crosses placenta, appears in cord blood, amniotic fluid. Distributed in breast milk in low concentrations. May lead to allergic sensitization, diarrhea, candidiasis, skin rash in infant. **Pregnancy Category B.**

INTERACTIONS

DRUG INTERACTIONS: Probenecid may increase concentration, toxicity risk. May decrease effects of oral contraceptive. May have nausea, vomiting, confusion, CV abnormalities w/disulfiram. **ALTERED LAB VALUES:** May increase SGOT (AST), SGPT (ALT). May cause positive Coombs test.

SIDE EFFECTS

FREQUENT: Diarrhea, rash, urticaria, vomiting. **OCCASIONAL:** Flatulence, abdominal discomfort, anemia, exfoliative dermatitis. **RARE:** Headache, dizziness.

ADVERSE REACTIONS/TOXIC EFFECTS

Severe hypersensitivity reactions, including anaphylaxis. Superinfections, potentially fatal antibiotic-associated colitis may result from altered bacterial balance.

NURSING IMPLICATIONS

BASELINE ASSESSMENT:

Question for history of allergies, especially penicillins, cephalosporins. Obtain specimen for culture, sensitivity before giving first dose (therapy may begin before results of test are known).

INTERVENTION/EVALUATION:

Hold medication and promptly report rash (hypersensitivity) or diarrhea (w/fever, abdominal pain, blood, and mucus in stool may indicate antibiotic-associated colitis). Assess food tolerance. Check for dizziness and assure safety. Be alert for superinfection: increased fever, sore throat onset, vomiting, diarrhea, black/hairy tongue, ulceration or changes of oral mucosa, anal/genital pruritus.

PATIENT/FAMILY TEACHING:

Continue antibiotic for full length of treatment. Space doses evenly. Notify physician in event of diarrhea, rash, or other new symptom.

bacitracin

bah-cih-tray′sin

(Baciguent, Bacitracin, Baci-IM)

FIXED-COMBINATION(S): W/polymixin B, an antibiotic (Polysporin); w/polymixin B and neomycin, antibiotics (Mycitracin, Neosporin).

CANADIAN AVAILABILITY: Baciguent, Bacitin

CLASSIFICATION

Anti-infective

ACTION

Inhibits cell wall synthesis, interferes w/plasma membrane permeability. Bacteriostatic.

USES

Ophthalmic: Superficial ocular infections (conjunctivitis, keratitis, corneal ulcers, blepharitis). *Topical:* Minor skin abrasions, superficial infections.

OPHTHALMIC ADMINISTRATION

1. Place finger on lower eyelid and pull out until a pocket is formed between eye and lower lid.

Place ¼-½ inch ointment in pocket.

2. Close eye gently for 1-2 min, rolling eyeball (increases contact area of drug to eye). Remove excess ointment around eye w/tissue.

INDICATIONS/DOSAGE/ROUTES

Usual ophthalmic dosage:
OPHTHALMIC: Adults: ½-inch ribbon in conjunctival sac q3-4h.

Usual topical dosage:
TOPICAL: Adults, Children: Apply 1-5 times/day to affected area.

PRECAUTIONS

CONTRAINDICATIONS: Severe renal dysfunction. **CAUTIONS:** Neuromuscular disorders. **PREGNANCY/LACTATION:** Avoid parenteral use during pregnancy. **Pregnancy Category C.**

INTERACTIONS

DRUG INTERACTIONS: None significant. **ALTERED LAB VALUES:** None significant.

SIDE EFFECTS

NOTE: It is important to know side effects of components when bacitracin is used in fixed-combination. **RARE:** *Topical:* Hypersensitivity reaction (itching, burning, inflammation) allergic contact dermatitis. *Ophthalmic:* Burning, itching, redness, swelling, pain.

ADVERSE REACTIONS/TOXIC EFFECTS

Severe hypersensitivity reaction (hypotension, apnea) occurs rarely.

NURSING IMPLICATIONS

BASELINE ASSESSMENT:

Question pt for history of allergies, particularly to bacitracin, neomycin.

INTERVENTION/EVALUATION:

Topical: Evaluate for hypersensitivity: itching, burning, inflammation. W/preparations containing corticosteroids, consider masking effect on clinical signs. *Ophthalmic:* Assess eye for therapeutic response or increased redness, swelling, burning, itching.

PATIENT/FAMILY TEACHING:

Continue therapy for full length of treatment. Doses should be evenly spaced. Report burning, itching, rash, or increased irritation. Ophthalmic application may cause temporary blurred vision; check w/physician before using eye makeup.

baclofen

back′low-fin
(Lioresal)

CANADIAN AVAILABILITY:
Lioresal

CLASSIFICATION

Skeletal muscle relaxant

PHARMACOKINETICS

Well absorbed from GI tract. Protein binding: 30%. Partially metabolized in liver. Primarily excreted in urine. Half-life: 2.5-4 hrs.

ACTION

Acts at spinal cord level (decreases frequency/amplitude of muscle spasms in patients w/spinal cord lesions.)

USES

Relief of signs and symptoms of spasticity due to spinal cord injuries or diseases and multiple sclerosis, especially flexor spasms, concomitant pain, clonus, and muscular rigidity.

PO ADMINISTRATION

1. Give w/o regard to meals.
2. Tablets may be crushed.

INDICATIONS/DOSAGE/ROUTES

Musculoskeletal spasm:
PO: Adults: Initially, 5 mg 3 times/day. May increase by 15 mg/day at 3 day intervals. **Range:** 40-80 mg/day. Total dose not to exceed 80 mg/day.

Usual elderly dosage:
PO: Elderly: Initially, 5 mg 2-3 times/day. May gradually increase dose.

PRECAUTIONS

CONTRAINDICATIONS: Skeletal muscle spasm due to rheumatic disorders. **CAUTIONS:** Impaired renal function. **PREGNANCY/LACTATION:** Unknown if drug crosses placenta or is distributed in breast milk. **Pregnancy Category C.**

INTERACTIONS

DRUG INTERACTIONS: Potentiated effects when used w/other CNS depressants (including alcohol). **ALTERED LAB VALUES:** May increase SGOT (AST), alkaline phosphatase, blood sugar.

SIDE EFFECTS

FREQUENT: Transient drowsiness, dizziness, weakness, hypotension, nausea. **OCCASIONAL:** Fatigue, confusion, headache, insomnia, constipation, urinary frequency. **RARE:** Paradoxical CNS excitement/restlessness, paresthesia, tinnitus, slurred speech, tremor, blurred vision, dry mouth, diarrhea, nocturia, impotence.

ADVERSE REACTIONS/TOXIC EFFECTS

Abrupt withdrawal may produce hallucinations, seizures. Ovarian cysts tend to occur, then disappear spontaneously in women on long-term therapy. Overdosage results in vomiting, muscular hypotonia, muscle twitching, respiratory depression, seizures.

NURSING IMPLICATIONS

BASELINE ASSESSMENT:

Record onset, type, location, and duration of muscular spasm. Check for immobility, stiffness, swelling.

INTERVENTION/EVALUATION:

Assess for paradoxical reaction. Assist with ambulation at all times. For those on long-term therapy, liver/renal function tests, blood counts should be performed periodically. Evaluate for therapeutic response: decreased intensity of skeletal muscle pain. Be alert to signs of infection. *Intrathecal:* After bolus in screening phase, observe pt closely for decreased muscle spasm (frequency or severity). After implant, monitor carefully for side effects w/resuscitative equipment immediately available. Check pump function and catheter patency.

PATIENT/FAMILY TEACHING:

Drowsiness usually diminishes w/continued therapy. Avoid tasks that require alertness, motor skills until response to drug is established. Do not abruptly withdraw medication after long-term therapy. Avoid alcohol and CNS depressants. *Intrathecal:* Notify physician of frequency or painful urination, constipation, headache, nausea, confusion, or insomnia.

BCG, intravesical

(Tice BCG, TheraCys)

CANADIAN AVAILABILITY:
Immu Cyst

CLASSIFICATION

Antineoplastic

ACTION

Promotes local inflammation reaction w/histiocytic and leukocytic infiltration in urinary bladder. Inflammatory effects associated w/apparent elimination/reduction of superficial cancerous lesions of urinary bladder.

USES

Treatment of carcinoma in situ w/or w/o associated papillary tumors; therapy for pts w/carcinoma in situ of bladder following failure to respond to other treatment regimens. *TheraCys:* Treatment of primary and relapsed carcinoma in situ of urinary bladder (eliminates residual tumor cells, reduces frequency of tumor recurrence). *Tice BCG:* Primary or secondary treatment in absence of invasive cancer in pts w/contraindication to radical surgery.

STORAGE/HANDLING

Store in refrigerator. Use immediately after reconstitution, avoid exposure to sunlight, direct or indirect. Handle as infectious; use aseptic technique.

INTRAVESICAL ADMINISTRATION

TheraCys:

1. Do not remove rubber stopper from vial, prepare immediately prior to use.
2. Use mask, gloves while preparing solution.
3. Reconstitute only w/diluent provided by manufacturer.
4. After reconstitution, further dilute w/50 ml sterile, preservative-free saline to final volume of 53 ml for intravesical instillation.

Tice BCG:

1. Draw 1 ml sterile, preservative-free saline into syringe (3 ml); add to 1 ampoule Tice BCG.
2. Draw mixture into syringe/gently expel back into ampoule 3 times (ensures mixing; decreased clumping).
3. Dispense BCG suspension into top end of catheter-tip syringe containing 49 ml saline.
4. Gently rotate syringe; do not filter.

INDICATIONS/DOSAGE/ROUTES

Intravesical treatment and prophylaxis for carcinoma in situ of urinary bladder:
TheraCys:

INTRAVESICAL: Adults, elderly: vials (in 50 ml saline) once weekly for 6 wks then one treatment at 3, 6, 12, 18, 24 mos after initial treatment. Begin 7-14 days after biopsy or transurethral resection.

Tice BCG:

INTRAVESICAL: Adults, elderly: One amp in 50 ml preservative-free saline/wk for 6 wks. May repeat once. Thereafter, continue monthly for 6-12 mos.

PRECAUTIONS

CONTRAINDICATIONS: Those on immunosuppressive or corticosteroid therapy, those who have compromised immune system, positive HIV virus, undetermined fever or fever due to infection, urinary tract infection, positive Mantoux test, as immunizing agent for tuberculosis prevention, within 1-2 wks following transurethral resection. **CAUTIONS:** None significant. **PREGNANCY/LACTATION:** If possible, avoid use during pregnancy. Breast feeding not recommended. **Pregnancy Category C.**

INTERACTIONS

DRUG INTERACTIONS: Bone marrow depressants, immunosuppressants may decrease immune response, increase risk of osteomyelitis of disseminated BCG infection. Live virus vaccines may potentiate virus replication, increase vaccine side effects, decrease pt's antibody response to vaccine. **ALTERED LAB VALUES:** None significant.

SIDE EFFECTS

FREQUENT: Dysuria, urinary frequency, hematuria; hypersensitivity reaction manifested as malaise, fever, chills. **OCCASIONAL:** Cystitis, urinary urgency, anemia, nausea, vomiting, anorexia, diarrhea, myalgia/arthralgia. **RARE:** Urinary tract infection, urinary incontinence, cramping.

ADVERSE REACTIONS/TOXIC EFFECTS

Systemic BCG infection manifested as fever >103° F or persistent fever >101° F for more than 2 days or severe malaise has produced deaths. Infectious disease specialist should be notified and fast-acting antituberculosis therapy begun immediately.

NURSING IMPLICATIONS

BASELINE ASSESSMENT:

Use aseptic technique when administering drug (handle as infectious) and avoid introducing contaminants into urinary tract. Pt symptoms usually begin 2-4 hrs after instillation and last 24-72 hrs. Hepatic and renal tests should be performed before therapy begins and when a wk or more has elapsed between doses.

INTERVENTION/EVALUATION:

Have pt sit to void after instillation. For 6 hrs post instillation urine should be disinfected w/equal volume 5% hypochlorite solution (undiluted household bleach) before flushing. Diligently monitor renal status (assess for hematuria, urinary frequency, dysuria, urinalysis for bacterial urinary tract infection). Inform physician immediately if any urinary difficulties arise. Monitor closely for BCG systemic infection (see Adverse Reactions/Toxic Effects) and contact physician immediately if such occur.

PATIENT/FAMILY TEACHING:

Notify physician/nurse immediately if cough develops. Check w/physician if symptoms persist or increase or if any of the following occur: blood in urine, fever, chills, a frequent urge to urinate, joint pain, nausea and vomiting, or painful urination. Do not have immunizations w/o physician's approval (drug lowers body's resistance). Avoid contact w/those who have recently taken live virus vaccine.

beclomethasone dipropionate

beck-low-meth´ah-sewn

(Beclovent, Beconase, Vanceril, Vancenase)

CANADIAN AVAILABILITY:
Beclovent, Beconase, Propaderm, Vancenase, Vanceril

CLASSIFICATION

Corticosteroid

PHARMACOKINETICS

Rapidly absorbed from pulmonary, nasal, and GI tissue. Protein binding: 65-90%. Metabolized in liver, undergoes extensive first pass effect. Primarily eliminated in feces. Half-life: 15 hrs.

ACTION

Decreases immediate and late phase allergic reactions. Reduces influx of inflammatory cells.

USES

Inhalation: Control of bronchial asthma in those requiring chronic steroid therapy. *Intranasal:* Relief of seasonal/perennial rhinitis; prevention of nasal polyps from recurring after surgical removal; treatment of nonallergic rhinitis.

INHALATION ADMINISTRATION

Shake container well, exhale completely, then holding mouthpiece 1 inch away from lips, inhale and hold breath as long as possible before exhaling.

INDICATIONS/DOSAGE/ROUTES

Usual inhalation dosage:
INHALATION: Adults, elderly: 2 inhalations 3-4 times/day. **Maximum:** 20 inhalations/day. **Children 6-12 yrs:** 1-2 inhalations 3-4 times/day. **Maximum:** 10 inhalations/day.

Usual intranasal dosage:
INTRANASAL: Adults, elderly, children >12 yrs: 1 inhalation each nostril 2-4 times/day. **Children 6-12 yrs:** 1 inhalation 3 times/day.

PRECAUTIONS

CONTRAINDICATIONS: Hypersensitivity to any corticosteroid or components, primary treatment of status asthmaticus, systemic fungal infections, persistently positive sputum cultures for *Candida albicans.* **CAUTIONS:** Adrenal insufficiency. **PREGNANCY/LACTATION:** Unknown if drug crosses placenta or is distributed in breast milk. **Pregnancy Category C.**

INTERACTIONS

DRUG INTERACTIONS: None significant. **ALTERED LAB VALUES:** None significant.

SIDE EFFECTS

OCCASIONAL: *Inhalation:* Throat irritation, hoarseness, dry mouth, coughing, temporary wheezing, localized fungal infection in mouth, pharynx, larynx (particularly if mouth is not rinsed w/water after each administration). *Intranasal:* Local irritation, burning, stinging, dryness, headache.

ADVERSE REACTIONS/TOXIC EFFECTS

Acute hypersensitivity reaction (urticaria, angioedema, severe bronchospasm) occurs rarely. Transfer from systemic to local steroid therapy may unmask previously suppressed bronchial asthma condition.

NURSING IMPLICATIONS

BASELINE ASSESSMENT:

Question for hypersensitivity to any corticosteroids, components.

INTERVENTION/EVALUATION:

In those receiving bronchodilators by inhalation concomitantly with inhalation of steroid therapy, advise pt to use bronchodilator several minutes before corticosteroid aerosol (enhances penetration of steroid into bronchial tree).

PATIENT/FAMILY TEACHING:

Do not change dose schedule or stop taking drug; must taper off gradually under medical supervision. *Inhalation:* Maintain careful mouth hygiene. Rinse mouth w/ water immediately after inhalation (prevents mouth/throat dryness, fungal infection of mouth). Contact physician/nurse if sore throat or mouth occurs. *Intranasal:* Contact physician if no improvement in symptoms, sneezing or nasal irritation occur. Clear nasal passages prior to use. Improvement seen in several days.

benazepril

ben-ayz′ah-prill
(Lotensin)

FIXED-COMBINATION(S):
W/hydrochlorothiazide, a diuretic (Lotensin-HCT)

CLASSIFICATION

Angiotensin converting enzyme (ACE) inhibitor

PHARMACOKINETICS

	ONSET	PEAK	DURATION
PO	1 hr	2-4 hrs	24 hrs

Partially absorbed from GI tract. Protein binding: 97%. Metabolized in liver to active metabolite. Primarily excreted in urine. Minimal removal by hemodialysis. Half-life: 35 min; metabolite: 10-11 hrs.

ACTION

Suppresses renin-angiotensin-aldosterone system (prevents conversion of angiotensin I to angiotensin II, a potent vasoconstrictor; may also inhibit angiotensin II at local vascular and renal sites). Decreases plasma angiotensin II, increases plasma renin activity, decreases aldosterone secretion. Reduces peripheral arterial resistance.

USES

Treatment of hypertension. Used alone or in combination w/ other antihypertensives.

PO ADMINISTRATION

May give w/o regard to food.

INDICATIONS/DOSAGE/ROUTES

Hypertension (used alone);
PO: Adults: Initially, 10 mg/day. **Maintenance:** 20-40 mg/day as single dose. **Maximum:** 80 mg/day.

Usual elderly dosage:
PO: Elderly: Initially, 10 mg/day. **Range:** 20-40 mg/day.

Hypertension (combination therapy):
NOTE: Discontinue diuretic 2-3 days prior to initiating benazepril therapy.
PO: Adults: Initially, 5 mg/day titrated to pt's needs.

Dosage in renal impairment (Ccr <30 ml/min):
Initially, 5 mg/day titrated up to maximum of 40 mg/day.

PRECAUTIONS

CONTRAINDICATIONS: MI, coronary insufficiency, angina, evidence of coronary artery disease, hypersensitivity to phentolamine, history of angioedema w/previous treatment w/ACE inhibitors. **CAUTIONS:** Renal impairment, those w/sodium depletion or on diuretic therapy, dialysis, hypovolemia, coronary or cerebrovascular insufficiency. **PREGNANCY/LACTATION:** Crosses placenta; unknown if distributed in breast milk. May cause fetal-neonatal mortality/morbidity. **Pregnancy Category D.**

INTERACTIONS

DRUG INTERACTIONS: Alcohol, diuretics, hypotensive agents may increase effects. NSAIDs may decrease effect. Potassium-sparing diuretics, potassium supplements may cause hyperkalemia. May increase lithium concentration, toxicity. **ALTERED LAB VALUES:** May increase potassium, SGOT (AST), SGPT (ALT), alkaline phosphatase, bilirubin, BUN, creatinine. May decrease sodium. May cause positive ANA titer.

SIDE EFFECTS

Frequency of effects unknown: Weakness, dizziness, flushing, postural hypotension, nasal stuffiness, nausea, vomiting, diarrhea.

ADVERSE REACTIONS/TOXIC EFFECTS

Excessive hypotension ("first-dose syncope") may occur in those w/CHF, severe salt/volume depletion. Angioedema (swelling of face/lips), hyperkalemia occur rarely. Agranulocytosis, neutropenia may be noted in those w/impaired renal function or collagen vascular disease (systemic lupus erythematosus, scleroderma). Nephrotic syndrome may be noted in those w/history of renal disease.

NURSING IMPLICATIONS

BASELINE ASSESSMENT:

Obtain B/P immediately before each dose, in addition to regular monitoring (be alert to fluctuations). If excessive reduction in B/P occurs, place pt in supine position w/legs elevated. Renal function tests should be performed before therapy begins. In those w/renal impairment, autoimmune disease, or taking drugs that affect leukocytes or immune response, CBC and differential count should be performed before therapy begins and q2wks for 3 mos, then periodically thereafter.

INTERVENTION/EVALUATION:

Monitor pattern of daily bowel activity and stool consistency. Assist w/ambulation if dizziness occurs.

PATIENT/FAMILY TEACHING:

To reduce hypotensive effect, rise slowly from lying to sitting position and permit legs to dangle from bed momentarily before standing. Cola, unsalted crackers, dry toast may relieve nausea. Full therapeutic effect may take 2-4 wks. Report any sign of infection (sore throat, fever). Skipping doses or voluntarily discontinuing drug may produce severe, rebound hypertension.

benzocaine

ben´zoe-kane

(Americaine; Anbesol; Orajel; Cetacaine; Chloroseptic Lozenges; Dermoplast; Hurricane)

CANADIAN AVAILABILITY:
Auralgan, Bionet, Rectogel

CLASSIFICATION

Topical anesthetic

PHARMACOKINETICS

	ONSET	PEAK	DURATION
TOPICAL	—	1 hr	0.5-1 hr

Poorly absorbed through intact skin, but readily absorbed through mucous membranes or denuded skin. Primarily excreted in urine as metabolite.

ACTION

Inhibits conduction of nerve impulses from sensory nerves due to alteration of the cell membrane permeability to sodium ions.

USES

Temporary relief of pain. *Skin disorders:* Sunburn, minor burns, insect bites, pruritus, diaper rash, prickly heat, eczema, episiotomy. *Mucous membranes:* Pruritus ani, pruritus vulvae, hemorrhoids; on oral mucous membranes for toothache, sore gums, teething, denture irritation, canker sores; as a lubricant and anesthetic for pharyngeal or nasal airways, intratracheal catheters, nasogastric and endoscopic tubes, urinary catheters, vaginal specula, laryngoscopes, proctoscopes, sigmoidoscopes. *Oral:* Lozenges for sore throat. *Otic:* Acute congestive and serous otitis media, swimmer's ear, otitis externa.

ORAL/TOPICAL/OTIC ADMINISTRATION

NOTE: Avoid inhalation of any sprays. Do not get preparations near eyes.

ORAL:

1. Dissolve lozenge slowly in the mouth.

TOPICAL:

1. For skin disorders, apply to affected area only. May apply ointments or creams directly or to gauze or bandage first.
2. When using aerosol, hold can 12 inches from skin; do not puncture can or use near open flame.
3. For oral mucous membranes, apply as directed by manufacturer. Do not eat, drink, or chew gum for 1 hr following use (may impair swallowing and increase risk of biting trauma).
4. For anorectal use, cleanse and dry area thoroughly before application. Maintain normal bowel function by proper diet, adequate fluid intake, and regular exercise. Adjunctive therapy w/stool softeners or bulk laxatives may be used (avoid excessive use).
5. For use as lubricant/anesthetic on specula, tubes, catheters: apply evenly along external surface w/clean or sterile technique according to procedure.

OTIC:

1. Warm preparation to body temperature by holding in hands for several minutes or setting container in warm water.
2. W/pt lying down, pull outer ear up and back to straighten ear canal; for children under 3 years of age, pull outer ear back and downward.
3. Direct drops along side of auditory canal.
4. Have patient lie on unaffected side for 1-2 min; hold child.
5. Avoid touching dropper to ear.
6. Do not rinse dropper after use.

7. Discard preparation 6 mos after dropper is first placed in solution.

INDICATIONS/DOSAGE/ROUTES

Usual otic dosage:
OTIC: Adults, elderly: 4-5 drops; insert cotton pledget, may repeat q1-2h.

Usual topical dosage:
TOPICAL: Adults, elderly: *(Topical):* Apply to area as needed (may apply to gauze/bandage prior to skin application). *(Mucous membrane):* Dose varies based on area to be anesthesized, vascularity, technique, pt tolerance.

PRECAUTIONS

CONTRAINDICATIONS: Hypersensitivity to benzocaine or other PABA derivatives (e.g., sunscreens) or other components of preparation. Sensitivity to aspirin or tartrazine w/Cepacol Anesthetic Lozenges, Vicks Cough Silencers, and Vicks Oracin Cooling Throat Lozenges. Individuals w/phenylketonuria or others w/restricted intake of phenylalanine w/Kank-a use. Perforated eardrum (otic). **CAUTIONS:** Not for application to large areas; use in children only as indicated by manufacturer. **PREGNANCY/LACTATION:** Not known whether excreted in breast milk. **Pregnancy Category C.**

INTERACTIONS

DRUG INTERACTIONS: Cholinesterase inhibitors may inhibit metabolism, increase risk of toxicity. **ALTERED LAB VALUES:** None significant.

SIDE EFFECTS

OCCASIONAL: Allergic reactions: burning, itching, stinging, redness, urticaria, edema, contact dermatitis. **RARE:** Urethritis w/ and w/o bleeding, sloughing, or necrosis of tissue, cyanosis associated w/methemoglobinemia (esp. w/oral use).

ADVERSE REACTIONS/TOXIC EFFECTS

W/increased absorption, systemic reactions may occur including CNS reactions (excitation or depression, confusion, double or blurred vision, lightheadedness, sensation of heat, cold, or numbness, respiratory depression) and cardiovascular reactions (bradycardia, hypotension). Respiratory or cardiac arrest have occurred.

NURSING IMPLICATIONS

BASELINE ASSESSMENT:

Assess skin or mucous membrane condition, evaluate for pain.

INTERVENTION/EVALUATION:

Check skin or mucous membrane for allergic reaction. Monitor pain relief.

PATIENT/FAMILY TEACHING:

Teach proper administration (see Administration). Do not apply to large or denuded areas. Use lowest effective dose to avoid side effects. In event of skin irritation, discontinue use. Not for prolonged use; notify physician if pain relief not obtained or more severe side effects develop (see Side Effects).

benzonatate

ben-zow′nah-tate
(Tessalon Perles)

CLASSIFICATION

Antitussive

PHARMACOKINETICS

	ONSET	PEAK	DURATION
PO	15-20 min	—	3-8 hrs

ACTION

Anesthetizes stretch receptors in respiratory passages, lungs, pleura, thereby reducing cough production.

USES

Symptomatic relief of cough including acute respiratory conditions (e.g., pneumonia) and chronic diseases (e.g., bronchial asthma).

PO ADMINISTRATION

1. Give w/o regard to meals.
2. Swallow whole, do not chew/dissolve in mouth (may produce temporary local anesthesia/choking).

INDICATIONS/DOSAGE/ROUTES

Antitussive:
PO: Adults, elderly, children >10 yrs: 100 mg 3 times/day up to 600 mg/day.

PRECAUTIONS

CONTRAINDICATIONS: None significant. **CAUTIONS:** None significant. **PREGNANCY/LACTATION:** Unknown if drug crosses placenta or is distributed in breast milk. **Pregnancy Category C.**

INTERACTIONS

DRUG INTERACTIONS: CNS depressants may increase effect. **ALTERED LAB VALUES:** None significant.

SIDE EFFECTS

OCCASIONAL: Drowsiness, sense of chilliness, headache, GI upset, constipation, sensation of burning in eyes (more likely noted in elderly). **RARE:** Mild hypersensitivity reaction (pruritus, skin eruption).

ADVERSE REACTIONS/TOXIC EFFECTS

Paradoxical reaction (restlessness, insomnia, euphoria, nervousness, tremors) has been noted.

NURSING IMPLICATIONS

BASELINE ASSESSMENT:

Assess type, severity, frequency of cough, and production.

INTERVENTION/EVALUATION:

Initiate deep breathing and coughing exercises, particularly in those with impaired pulmonary function. Monitor for paradoxical reaction. Increase fluid intake and environmental humidity to lower viscosity of lung secretions. Assess for clinical improvement and record onset of relief of cough.

PATIENT/FAMILY TEACHING:

Avoid tasks that require alertness, motor skills until response to drug is established. Dry mouth, drowsiness, dizziness may be an expected response of drug. Coffee or tea may help reduce drowsiness.

benzquinamide hydrochloride

benz-quin´ah-mied
(Emete-Con)

CLASSIFICATION

Antiemetic

PHARMACOKINETICS

	ONSET	PEAK	DURATION
IM	15 min	—	3-4 hrs
IV	15 min	—	3-4 hrs

Rapidly absorbed following IM administration. Widely distributed (highest concentration in liver, kidneys). Metabolized in liver. Excreted in urine and bile.

ACTION

Depresses the chemoreceptor trigger zone in the CNS for emesis.

USES

Prevention, treatment of nausea and vomiting due to anesthesia and surgery.

STORAGE/HANDLING

Store vials at room temperature. After reconstitution, stable for 14 days at room temperature.

IM/IV ADMINISTRATION

1. Reconstitute each 50 mg vial w/2.2 ml sterile water for injection or bacteriostatic water for injection to provide a concentration of 25 mg/ml. Do not use saline as diluent (may cause precipitate).
2. Inject deep IM using deltoid muscle (if well developed).
3. For IV injection, administer slowly (1 ml over 30-60 sec).

INDICATIONS/DOSAGE/ROUTES

NOTE: IM route preferable to IV administration.

Nausea, vomiting:
NOTE: To prevent nausea/vomiting, give dose 15 min prior to emergence of anesthesia.
IM: Adults, elderly: 50 mg (0.5-1 mg/kg), may repeat first dose in 1 hr, then give q3-4h as needed.
IV: Adults, elderly: 25 mg (0.2-0.4 mg/kg) one time; then administer IM.

PRECAUTIONS

CONTRAINDICATIONS: None significant. **CAUTIONS:** None significant. **PREGNANCY/LACTATION:** Unknown if drug crosses placenta or is distributed in breast milk. **Pregnancy Category C.**

DRUG INTERACTIONS: CNS depressants may increase sedative effect. **ALTERED LAB VALUES:** None significant.

SIDE EFFECTS

FREQUENT: Drowsiness, dry mouth. **OCCASIONAL:** Shivering, diaphoresis, tremor, paradoxical reaction (restlessness, nervousness), blurred vision. **RARE:** Hypersensitivity reaction (rash, hives).

ADVERSE REACTIONS/TOXIC EFFECTS

Overdosage may produce combination of CNS stimulation and depressant effects.

NURSING IMPLICATIONS

BASELINE ASSESSMENT:

Assess for dehydration if excessive vomiting has occurred (poor skin turgor, dry mucous membranes, longitudinal furrows in tongue).

INTERVENTION/EVALUATION:

Monitor B/P during and following IV administration for sudden B/P increase, transient arrhythmias (PVCs and atrial contractions).

B

PATIENT/FAMILY TEACHING:

Report visual disturbances. Dry mouth is expected response to medication. Relief from nausea/vomiting generally occurs within 15 min of drug administration.

benztropine mesylate

benz´row-peen
(Cogentin)

CANADIAN AVAILABILITY:
Apo-Benztropine, Cogentin, PMS Benztropine, Bensylate

CLASSIFICATION

Anticholinergic, Antiparkison

PHARMACOKINETICS

	ONSET	PEAK	DURATION
PO	1 hr	—	24 hrs
IM	15 min	—	24 hrs

Well absorbed from GI tract.

ACTION

Suppresses central cholinergic activity, may inhibit reuptake/storage dopamine, thus prolonging its action.

USES

Treatment of Parkinson's disease, drug-induced extrapyramidal reactions, except tardive dyskinesia.

INDICATIONS/DOSAGE/ROUTES

Idiopathic parkinsonism:
PO/IM: Adults: Initially, 0.5-1 mg/day at bedtime up to 6 mg/day.

Postencephalitic parkinsonism:
PO/IM: Adults: 2 mg/day as single or divided dose.

Drug-induced extrapyramidal symptoms:
PO/IM: Adults: 1-4 mg 1-2 times/day.

Acute dystonic reactions:
IV: Adults: 1-2 mg, then 1-2 mg orally 2 times/day to prevent recurrence.

Usual elderly dosage:
PO: Elderly: Initially, 0.5 mg 1-2 times/day, may increase by 0.5 mg every 5-6 days. **Maximum:** 6 mg/day.

PRECAUTIONS

CONTRAINDICATIONS: Angle-closure glaucoma, GI obstruction, paralytic ileus, intestinal atony, severe ulcerative colitis, prostatic hypertrophy, myasthenia gravis, megacolon, children <3 yrs. **CAUTIONS:** Treated open-angle glaucoma, autonomic neuropathy, pulmonary disease, esophageal reflux, hiatal hernia, heart disease, hyperthyroidism, hypertension. **PREGNANCY/LACTATION:** Unknown if drug crosses placenta; distributed in breast milk. **Pregnancy Category C.**

INTERACTIONS

DRUG INTERACTIONS: Alcohol, CNS depressants may increase sedation. Amantadine, anticholinergics, MAO inhibitors may increase effects. Antacids, antidiarrheals may decrease absorption, effects. **ALTERED LAB VALUES:** None significant.

SIDE EFFECTS

NOTE: Elderly (>60 yrs) tend to develop mental confusion, disorientation, agitation, psychotic-like symptoms. **FREQUENT:** Drowsiness, dizziness, muscular weakness, dry mouth/nose/throat/lips, urinary retention, thickening of bronchial secretions. Sedation, dizziness, hypotension more likely noted in elderly. **OCCASIONAL:** Epigastric distress, flushing, visual disturbances, hearing disturbances, paresthesia, sweating, chills.

ADVERSE REACTIONS/TOXIC EFFECTS

Children may experience dominant paradoxical reaction (restlessness, insomnia, euphoria, nervousness, tremors). Overdosage in children may result in hallucinations, convulsions, death. Hypersensitivity reaction (eczema, pruritus, rash, cardiac disturbances, photosensitivity) may occur. Overdosage may vary from CNS depression (sedation, apnea, cardiovascular collapse, death) to severe paradoxical reaction (hallucinations, tremor, seizures).

NURSING IMPLICATIONS

BASELINE ASSESSMENT:

If pt is undergoing allergic reaction, obtain history of recently ingested foods, drugs, environmental exposure, recent emotional stress. Monitor rate, depth, rhythm, type of respiration; quality and rate of pulse. Assess lung sounds for rhonchi, wheezing, rales.

INTERVENTION/EVALUATION:

Be alert to neurologic effects: headache, lethargy, mental confusion, agitation. Monitor children closely for paradoxical reaction. Assess for clinical reversal of symptoms (improvement of tremor of head/hands at rest, mask-like facial expression, shuffling gait, muscular rigidity).

PATIENT/FAMILY TEACHING:

Avoid tasks that require alertness, motor skills until response to drug is established. Dry mouth, drowsiness, dizziness may be an expected response of drug. Avoid alcoholic beverages during therapy. Sugarless gum, sips of tepid water may relieve dry mouth. Coffee or tea may help reduce drowsiness.

bepridil hydrochloride

beh´prih-dill

(Bepadin, Vascor)

CLASSIFICATION

Calcium channel blocker

PHARMACOKINETICS

Rapid, completely absorbed from GI tract. Undergoes first-pass metabolism in liver. Protein binding: 99%. Metabolized in liver to active metabolite. Primarily excreted in urine. Not removed by hemodialysis. Half-life: <24 hrs.

ACTION

Inhibits calcium ion entry across cell membranes of cardiac and vascular smooth muscle (may dilate coronary arteries, peripheral arteries/arterioles); may decrease heart rate, myocardial contractility, slow SA and AV conduction.

USES

Treatment of chronic stable angina (effort-associated angina) in those who have failed to respond or are intolerant to other antianginal drugs. May be used alone or concurrent w/beta blockers, nitrates.

PO ADMINISTRATION

1. Do not crush or break film-coated tablets.
2. May give w/o regard to food. May give w/meals and at bedtime (decreases nausea).

INDICATIONS/DOSAGE/ROUTES

Chronic stable angina:
PO: Adults, elderly: Initially, 200 mg/day, after 10 days, dosage may be adjusted. **Maintenance:** 200-400 mg/day.

PRECAUTIONS

CONTRAINDICATIONS: Sick sinus syndrome/second- or third-degree AV block (except in presence of pacemaker), severe hypotension (<90 mm Hg, systolic), history of serious ventricular arrhythmias, uncompensated cardiac insufficiency, congenital QT interval prolongation, use w/other drugs prolonging QT interval. **CAUTIONS:** Impaired renal/hepatic function, CHF. **PREGNANCY/LACTATION:** Unknown if drug crosses placenta. Distributed in breast milk. **Pregnancy Category C.**

INTERACTIONS

DRUG INTERACTIONS: Beta-blockers may have additive effect. May increase digoxin concentration. Procainamide, quinidine may increase risk of QT interval prolongation. Hypokalemia producing agents may increase risk of arrhythmias. **ALTERED LAB VALUES:** QT interval may be increased.

SIDE EFFECTS

FREQUENT: Dizziness, lightheadedness, nervousness, headache, drowsiness, asthenia (loss of strength, weakness), nausea, dyspepsia, dry mouth. **OCCASIONAL:** Tinnitus. constipation/diarrhea, dyspnea/wheezing, respiratory infection, anorexia. **RARE:** Peripheral edema, bradycardia, tachycardia, mental depression, psychosis, visual disturbances, paresthesia, insomnia, anxiety, flatulence, dermatitis/rash, nasal congestion, sweating, cough.

ADVERSE REACTIONS/TOXIC EFFECTS

Can induce serious arrhythmias. CHF, second- and third-degree AV block occur rarely. Overdosage produces nausea, drowsiness, confusion, slurred speech, profound bradycardia.

NURSING IMPLICATIONS

BASELINE ASSESSMENT:

Record onset, type (sharp, dull, squeezing), radiation, location, intensity, and duration of anginal pain, and precipitating factors (exertion, emotional stress). Assess baseline renal/liver function tests. Assess pulse rate, EKG for arrhythmias before drug is administered.

INTERVENTION/EVALUATION:

Assist w/ambulation if lightheadedness, dizziness, drowsiness occur. Question for asthenia, headache, ringing/roaring in ears. Monitor liver enzyme tests. Monitor daily bowel activity and stool consistency. Assess EKG for arrhythmias, lung sounds for rales, wheezing.

PATIENT/FAMILY TEACHING:

Do not abruptly discontinue

medication. Compliance w/therapy regimen is essential to control anginal pain. To avoid hypotensive effect, rise slowly from lying to sitting position, wait momentarily before standing. Avoid tasks that require alertness, motor skills until response to drug is established. Contact physician/nurse if irregular heart beat, shortness of breath, pronounced dizziness, nausea, dyspepsia, ringing/roaring in ears, or constipation occurs.

beractant

(Survanta)

CLASSIFICATION

Lung surfactant

ACTION

Lowers surface tension on alveolar surfaces during respiration, stabilizes alveoli vs. collapse that may occur at resting transpulmonary pressures. Replenishes surfactant, restores surface activity to lungs.

USES

Prevention/treatment (rescue) of respiratory distress syndrome (RDS-hyaline membrane disease) in premature infants. Oxygenation improves within minutes of administration.

STORAGE/HANDLING

Refrigerate vials. Warm by standing vial at room temperature for 20 min or warm in hand 8 min. If settling occurs, gently swirl vial (do not shake) to redisperse. After warming, may return to refrigerator within 8 hrs. Each vial should be injected w/a needle only one time; discard unused portions. Color is off-white to light brown.

INTRATRACHEAL ADMINISTRATION

1. Instill through catheter inserted into infant's endotracheal tube. Do not instill into main stem bronchus.

2. Monitor for bradycardia, decreased oxygen saturation during administration. Stop dosing procedure if these effects occur, begin appropriate measures before reinstituting therapy.

INDICATIONS/DOSAGE/ROUTES

Usual dosage:

INTRATRACHEAL: Infants: 100 mg of phospholipids/kg birth weight (4 ml/kg). Give within 15 min of birth if infant <1250 Gm w/evidence of surfactant deficiency; give within 8 hrs when RDS confirmed by x-ray and requiring mechanical ventilation. May repeat no sooner than 6 hrs after preceding dose.

PRECAUTIONS

CONTRAINDICATIONS: None significant. **CAUTIONS:** Those at risk for circulatory overload.

INTERACTIONS

DRUG INTERACTIONS: None significant. **ALTERED LAB VALUES:** None significant.

SIDE EFFECTS

OCCASIONALLY: Transient bradycardia, oxygen desaturation; transient rales, moist breath sounds immediately after drug administration (endotracheal suctioning unnecessary unless signs of airway obstruction are present). **RARE:** Endotracheal tube reflux, pallor, hypo/hypertension, vasoconstriction.

ADVERSE REACTIONS/TOXIC EFFECTS

Nosocomial sepsis may occur (not associated w/increased mortality).

NURSING IMPLICATIONS

BASELINE ASSESSMENT:

Drug must be administered in highly supervised setting. Clinicians in care of neonate must be experienced w/intubation, ventilator management. Give emotional support to parents.

INTERVENTION/EVALUATION:

Monitor infant w/arterial or transcutaneous measurement of systemic O_2 and CO_2. Assess lung sounds for rales and moist breath sounds.

betamethasone

bay-tah-meth´a-sone

(Celestone)

betamethasone benzoate

(Uticort)

betamethasone sodium phosphate

(Cel-U-Jec, Selestoject)

betamethasone dipropionate

(Alphatrex, Diprolene, Diprosone)

betamethasone valerate

(Valisone, Beta-Val, Betatrex)

FIXED-COMBINATION(S): Betamethasone sodium phosphate w/ betamethasone acetate (Celestone Soluspan). Betamethasone dipropionate w/clotrimazole, an antifungal, (Lotrisone)

CANADIAN AVAILABILITY: Beben, Betaderm, Betnesol, Celestone, Diprolene, Diprosone

CLASSIFICATION

Corticosteroid

PHARMACOKINETICS

Rapid, complete absorption after oral, IM administration. Protein binding: 64%. Metabolized in liver, kidneys, tissue. Primarily excreted in urine. Half-life: 3-5 hrs.

ACTION

Decreases/prevents tissue response to inflammatory process. Inhibits accumulation of inflammatory cells at inflammation sites, phagocytosis, lysosomal enzyme release and synthesis and/or release of mediators of inflammation. Prevents/suppresses cell-mediated immune reactions.

USES

Substitution therapy in *deficiency states:* acute/chronic adrenal insufficiency, congenital adrenal hyperplasia, adrenal insufficiency secondary to pituitary insufficiency. *Nonendocrine disorders:* arthritis, rheumatic carditis, allergic, collagen, intestinal tract, liver, ocular, renal, and skin diseases, bronchial asthma, cerebral edema, malignancies. *Topi-*

cal: Relief of inflammatory and pruritic dermatoses.

PO/IM/TOPICAL ADMINISTRATION

PO:

1. Give w/milk or food (decreases GI upset).
2. Single doses given prior to 9 AM; multiple doses at evenly spaced intervals.

TOPICAL:

1. Gently cleanse area prior to application.
2. Use occlusive dressings only as ordered.
3. Apply sparingly and rub into area thoroughly.
4. When using aerosol, spray area 3 sec from 15 cm distance; avoid inhalation.

IM:

Celestone Soluspan should not be mixed w/diluent or anesthetics containing preservatives.

INDICATIONS/DOSAGE/ROUTES

Usual dosage:
PO: Adults, elderly: 0.6-7.2 mg/day.
IM/IV: Adults, elderly: Up to 9 mg/day.

Usual topical dosage:
TOPICAL: Adults, elderly: 2-4 times/day.

PRECAUTIONS

CONTRAINDICATIONS: Hypersensitivity to any corticosteroid or sulfite, systemic fungal infection, peptic ulcers (except life-threatening situations). Avoid live virus vaccine such as smallpox. *Topical:* marked circulation impairment. **CAUTIONS:** Hypothyroidism, cirrhosis, ocular herpes simplex, history of tuberculosis (may reactivate disease), nonspecific ulcerative colitis, CHF, hypertension, psychosis, renal insufficiency. Prolonged therapy should be discontinued slowly. *Topical:* Do not apply to extensive areas. **PREGNANCY/LACTATION:** Drug crosses placenta, distributed in breast milk. May cause cleft palate (chronic use first trimester). Nursing contraindicated. **Pregnancy Category C.**

INTERACTIONS

DRUG INTERACTIONS: Amphotericin may increase hypokalemia. May decrease effect of oral hypoglycemics, insulin, diuretics, potassium supplements. May increase digoxin toxicity (due to hypokalemia). Hepatic enzyme inducers may decrease effect. Live virus vaccines may potentiate virus replication, increase vaccine side effects, decrease pt's antibody response to vaccine. **ALTERED LAB VALUES:** May decrease calcium, potassium, thyroxine. May increase cholesterol, lipids, glucose, sodium, amylase.

SIDE EFFECTS

FREQUENT: Increased appetite, exaggerated sense of well-being, abdominal distension, weight gain, insomnia, mood swings. *High-dose, prolonged therapy:* **FREQUENT:** Increased susceptibility to infection (signs/symptoms masked); delayed wound healing, hypokalemia, hypocalcemia, GI distress, diarrhea or constipation, hypertension. **OCCASIONAL:** Headache, vertigo. **RARE:** Increased blood coagulability, tachycardia, frequency or urgency or urination, psychosis. *Topical:* Allergic contact dermatitis, telangiectasis, purpura. (Systemic absorption more likely w/occlusive dressings or extensive application.)

ADVERSE REACTIONS/TOXIC EFFECTS

Long-term therapy: muscle wasting (esp. arms, legs), osteoporosis, spontaneous fractures, amenorrhea, cataracts, glaucoma, peptic ulcer, CHF. Abrupt withdrawal following long-term therapy: anorexia, nausea, fever, headache, joint pain, rebound inflammation, fatigue, weakness, lethargy, dizziness, orthostatic hypotension.

NURSING IMPLICATIONS

BASELINE ASSESSMENT:

Question for hypersensitivity to any of the corticosteroids, sulfite. Obtain baselines for: height, weight, B/P, glucose, electrolytes. Check results of initial tests, e.g., TB skin test, x-rays, EKG.

INTERVENTION/EVALUATION:

Monitor I&O, daily weight; assess for edema. Check lab results for blood coagulability and clinical evidence of thromboembolism. Evaluate food tolerance and bowel activity; report hyperacidity promptly. Check B/P, temperature, pulse, respiration at least 2 times/day. Be alert to infection: sore throat, fever, or vague symptoms. Monitor electrolytes. Watch for hypocalcemia (muscle twitching, cramps, positive Trousseau's or Chvostek's signs) or hypokalemia (weakness and muscle cramps, numbness/tingling esp. lower extremities, nausea and vomiting, irritability, EKG changes). Assess emotional status, ability to sleep. Provide assistance w/ambulation.

PATIENT/FAMILY TEACHING:

Take w/food or milk. Carry identification of drug and dose, physicians name and phone number. Do not change dose/schedule or stop taking drug; must taper off gradually under medical supervision. Notify physician of fever, sore throat, muscle aches, sudden weight gain/swelling. W/dietician give instructions for prescribed diet (usually sodium restricted w/ high vitamin D, protein, and potassium). Maintain careful personal hygiene, avoid exposure to disease or trauma. Severe stress (serious infection, surgery, or trauma) may require increased dosage. Do not take aspirin or any other medication w/o consulting physician. Follow-up visits, lab tests are necessary; children must be assessed for growth retardation. Inform dentist or other physicians of betamethasone therapy now or within past 12 mos. Caution against overuse of joints injected for symptomatic relief. Topical: Apply after shower or bath for best absorption. Do not cover unless physician orders; do not use tight diapers, plastic pants or coverings. Avoid contact w/eyes. Do not expose treated area to sunlight.

betaxolol

beh-tax´oh´lol

(Kerlone, Betopic)

CANADIAN AVAILABILITY:

Betoptic

CLASSIFICATION

Beta-adrenergic blocker

PHARMACOKINETICS

	ONSET	PEAK	DURATION
Eye drops	30 min	2 hrs	12 hrs

Completely absorbed from GI tract. Protein binding: 50%. Metabolized in liver. Primarily excreted unchanged in urine. Not removed by hemodialysis. Half-life: 14-22 hrs (increase in decreased renal function).

ACTION

Selectively blocks $beta_1$-adrenergic receptors, slowing sinus heart rate, decreasing cardiac output, decreasing B/P (exact mechanism unknown but may block peripheral adrenergic receptors, decrease sympathetic outflow from CNS or decrease renin release from kidney). Large dose may block $beta_2$-adrenergic receptors, increasing airway resistance. Decreases intraocular pressure by reducing aqueous humor production.

USES

Management of mild to moderate hypertension. Used alone or in combination w/diuretics, especially thiazide-type. Reduces intraocular pressure in management of chronic open-angle glaucoma, ocular hypertension.

STORAGE/HANDLING

Store oral form, ophthalmic solution at room temperature.

PO/OPHTHALMIC ADMINISTRATION

PO:

1. May be given w/o regard to meals.

OPHTHALMIC:

1. Place finger on lower eyelid and pull out until pocket is formed between eye and lower lid. Hold dropper above pocket and place prescribed number of drops in pocket. Instruct pt to close eyes gently so medication will not be squeezed out of sac.
2. Apply gentle finger pressure to the lacrimal sac at inner canthus for 1 min following installation (lessens risk of systemic absorption).

INDICATIONS/DOSAGE/ROUTES

Hypertension:
PO: Adults: Initially, 10 mg/day alone or added to diuretic therapy. Dose may be doubled if no response in 7-14 days. If used alone, addition of another antihypertensive to be considered.

Usual elderly dosage:
PO: Elderly: Initally, 5 mg/day.

Glaucoma:
EYE DROPS: Adults, elderly: 1 drop 2 times/day.

Dosage in renal impairment (dialysis):
Initially 5 mg/day, increase by 5 mg/day q2wks. Maximum: 20 mg/day.

PRECAUTIONS

CONTRAINDICATIONS: Sinus bradycardia, overt cardiac failure, cardiogenic shock, heart block greater than first degree. **CAUTIONS:** Impaired renal or hepatic function, peripheral vascular disease, hyperthyroidism, diabetes, inadequate cardiac function. **PREGNANCY/LACTATION:** Unknown if drug crosses placenta or is distributed in breast milk. May produce bradycardia, apnea, hypoglycemia, hypothermia during delivery, small birth weight infants. **Pregnancy Category C.**

INTERACTIONS

DRUG INTERACTIONS: Diuretics, other hypotensives may increase hypotensive effect; sympathomimetics, xanthines may mutually inhibit effect; may mask symptoms of hypoglycemia, prolong hypoglycemic effect of insulin, oral hypoglycemics; NSAIDs may decrease antihypertensive effect; Cimetidine may increase concentration. **ALTERED LAB VALUES:** May increase ANA titer, BUN, creatinine, potassium, uric acid, lipoproteins, triglycerides.

SIDE EFFECTS

Generally well tolerated, w/ mild and transient side effects. **FREQUENT:** *Oral:* Hypotension manifested as dizziness, nausea, diaphoresis, headache, fatigue; constipation/diarrhea; shortness of breath. *Ophthalmic:* Eye irritation, visual disturbances. **OCCASIONAL:** Insomnia, flatulence, urinary frequency. **RARE:** Ocular effects (dry eye, conjunctivitis, eye pain), unusual dreams, arthralgia, myalgia, rhinitis, rash, depression, edema, chest pain, cough, wheezing.

ADVERSE REACTIONS/TOXIC EFFECTS

Oral form may produce profound bradycardia, hypotension, bronchospasm. Abrupt withdrawal may result in sweating, palpitations, headache, tremulousness. May precipitate CHF, MI in those w/cardiac disease, thyroid storm in those w/thyrotoxicosis, peripheral ischemia in those w/existing peripheral vascular disease. Hypoglycemia may occur in previously controlled diabetics. Ophthalmic overdosage may produce bradycardia, hypotension, bronchospasm, acute cardiac failure.

NURSING IMPLICATIONS

BASELINE ASSESSMENT:

Oral: Assess baseline renal/liver function tests. Assess B/P, apical pulse immediately before drug is administered (if pulse is 60/min or below, or systolic B/P is below 90 mm Hg, withhold medication, contact physician).

INTERVENTION/EVALUATION:

Monitor B/P for hypotension, respiration for shortness of breath. Assess pulse for strength/weakness, irregular rate, bradycardia. Monitor EKG for cardiac arrhythmias. Monitor daily bowel activity and stool activity. Assist w/ambulation if dizziness occurs. Assess for evidence of CHF: dyspnea (particularly on exertion or lying down), night cough, peripheral edema, distended neck veins. Monitor I&O (increase in weight, decrease in urine output may indicate CHF). Assess for nausea, diaphoresis, headache, fatigue.

PATIENT/FAMILY TEACHING:

Do not abruptly discontinue medication. Compliance w/therapy regimen is essential to control glaucoma, hypertension, angina, arrhythmias. To avoid hypotensive effect, rise slowly from lying to sitting position, wait momentarily before standing. Avoid tasks that require alertness, motor skills until response to drug is established. Report shortness of breath, excessive fatigue, prolonged dizziness, or headache. Do not use nasal decongestants, over-the-counter cold preparations (stimulants) w/o physician approval. Monitor B/P, pulse before taking medication. Restrict salt, alcohol intake.

bethanechol chloride

beth-an´eh-coal
(Duvoid, Urecholine)

CANADIAN AVAILABILITY:
Duvoid, Urecholine

CLASSIFICATION

Cholinergic

PHARMACOKINETICS

	ONSET	PEAK	DURATION
PO	>30 min	60-90 min	1 hr
SubQ	5-15 min	15-30 min	2 hrs

Large oral doses (300-400 mg) may give up to 6 hrs duration of action. Poorly absorbed from GI tract.

ACTION

Acts directly at cholinergic receptors of smooth muscle of urinary bladder and GI tract. Increases tone of detrusor muscle, may initiate micturition, bladder emptying. Stimulates gastric, intestinal motility.

USES

Treatment of acute postoperative and postpartum nonobstructive urinary retention, neurogenic atony of bladder w/retention.

STORAGE/HANDLING

Store parenteral form at room temperature. Discard if particulate matter, discoloration occurs.

PO/SubQ ADMINISTRATION

PO:

1. Give on an empty stomach (minimizes risk of GI upset).

SubQ:

1. **Note:** Violent cholinergic reaction if given IM or IV (circulatory collapse, severe hypotension, bloody diarrhea, shock, cardiac arrest). Antidote: 0.6-1.2 mg atropine sulfate.
2. Aspirate syringe before injecting (avoid intra-arterial administration).

INDICATIONS/DOSAGE/ROUTES

Postoperative/postpartum urinary retention, atony of bladder:
PO: Adults, elderly: 10-50 mg 3-4 times/day. Minimum effective dose determined by initially giving 5-10 mg, and repeating same amount at 1 hr intervals until desired response achieved, or maximum of 50 mg reached.
SubQ: Adults, elderly: Initially, 2.5-5 mg. Minimum effective dose determined by giving 2.5 mg (0.5 ml), repeating same amount at 15-30 min intervals up to a maximum of 4 doses. Minimum dose repeated 3-4 times/day.

PRECAUTIONS

CONTRAINDICATIONS: Hyperthyroidism, peptic ulcer, latent or active bronchial asthma, mechanical GI and urinary obstruction or recent GI resection, acute inflammatory GI tract conditions, anastomosis, bladder wall instability, pronounced bradycardia, hypotension, hypertension, cardiac disease, coronary artery disease, vasomoter instability, epilepsy, parkinsonism. **CAUTIONS:** None significant. **PREGNANCY/LAC-**

TATION: Unknown if drug crosses placenta or is distributed in breast milk. **Pregnancy Category C.**

INTERACTIONS

DRUG INTERACTIONS: Cholinesterase inhibitors may increase effects/toxicity. Procainamide, quinidine may decrease effect. **ALTERED LAB VALUES:** May increase amylase, lipase, SGOT (AST).

SIDE EFFECTS

COMMON: Miosis, increased GI and skeletal muscle tone, reduced pulse rate, constriction of bronchi and ureters, salivary and sweat gland secretion. **OCCASIONAL:** Slight, temporary decrease in diastolic B/P w/mild reflex tachycardia, short periods of atrial fibrillation in hyperthyroid pts. Hypertensive pts may react w/ marked fall in B/P.

ADVERSE REACTIONS/TOXIC EFFECTS

Overdosage produces cholinergic reaction manifested as abdominal discomfort/cramping, nausea, vomiting, diarrhea, flushing, feeling of warmth/heat about face, excessive salivation and sweating, lacrimation, pallor, bradycardia/tachycardia, hypotension, urinary urgency, blurred vision, bronchospasm, pupillary contraction, involuntary muscular contraction visible under the skin (fasciculation). *Cholinergic crisis* manifested as increasingly severe muscle weakness, (appears first in muscles involving chewing, swallowing, then muscular weakness of shoulder girdle upper extremities), respiratory muscle paralysis, then pelvic girdle, leg muscle paralysis. Requires withdrawal of all anticholinergic drugs, immediate use of 0.6-1.2 mg atropine sulfate IV for adults, 0.01 mg/kg in infants, children <12 yrs.

NURSING IMPLICATIONS

BASELINE ASSESSMENT:

Have tissues readily available at pt's bedside. Assess vital signs before giving medication.

INTERVENTION/EVALUATION:

Assess vital signs q1-2h after oral dose, q15-30min following SubQ administration. Monitor B/P diligently. Assess for cholinergic reaction: GI discomfort/cramping, feeling of facial warmth, excessive salivation and sweating, lacrimation, pallor, urinary urgency, blurred vision. Assess eyes for pupillary contraction. Question for complaints of difficulty chewing, swallowing, progressive muscle weakness (See Adverse Reactions/Toxic Effects).

PATIENT/FAMILY TEACHING:

Report nausea, vomiting, diarrhea, sweating, increased salivary secretions, irregular heartbeat, muscle weakness, severe abdominal pain, or difficulty in breathing.

bisacodyl

bise-ah-code´ahl

(Dacody, Dulcolax)

CANADIAN AVAILABILITY:

Bisacolax, Dulcolax, Laxit

CLASSIFICATION

Laxative: Stimulant

PHARMACOKINETICS

	ONSET	PEAK	DURATION
PO	6-12 hrs	—	—
Rectal	15-60 min	—	—

Minimal absorption following oral, rectal administration. Absorbed drug excreted in urine; remainder eliminated in feces.

ACTION

Increases peristalsis by direct effect on colonic smooth musculature (stimulates intramural nerve plexi). Promotes fluid and ion accumulation in colon to increase laxative effect.

USES

Facilitates defecation in those w/ diminished colonic motor response; for evacuation of colon for rectal, bowel examination, elective colon surgery.

PO/RECTAL ADMINISTRATION

PO:

1. Give on empty stomach (faster action).
2. Offer 6-8 glasses of water/day (aids stool softening).
3. Administer tablets whole; do not chew or crush.
4. Avoid giving within 1 hr of antacids, milk, other oral medication.

RECTAL:

1. If suppository is too soft, chill for 30 min in refrigerator or run cold water over foil wrapper.
2. Moisten suppository w/cold water before inserting well up into rectum.

INDICATIONS/DOSAGE/ROUTES

Laxative:
PO: Adults: 10-15 mg as needed. **Children >6 yrs:** 5-10 mg (0.3 mg/kg) at bedtime or after breakfast.
RECTAL: Adults, children >2 yrs: 10 mg to induce bowel movement. **Children <2 yrs:** 5 mg.

Usual elderly dosage:
PO: Elderly: Initially, 5 mg/day.
RECTAL: Elderly: 5-10 mg/day.

PRECAUTIONS

CONTRAINDICATIONS: Abdominal pain, nausea, vomiting, appendicitis, intestinal obstruction. **CAUTIONS:** None significant. **PREGNANCY/LACTATION:** Unknown if drug crosses placenta or is distributed in breast milk. **Pregnancy Category C.**

INTERACTIONS

DRUG INTERACTIONS: Antacids, cimetidine, ranitidine, famotidine; milk may cause rapid dissolution of bisacodyl (produces abdominal cramping, vomiting). May decrease transit time of concurrently administered oral medication, decreasing absorption. **ALTERED LAB VALUES:** None significant.

SIDE EFFECTS

FREQUENT: Some degree of abdominal discomfort, nausea, mild cramps, griping, faintness. **OCCASIONAL:** Rectal administration may produce burning of rectal mucosa, mild proctitis.

ADVERSE REACTIONS/TOXIC EFFECTS

Long-term use may result in laxative dependence, chronic constipation, loss of normal bowel function. Chronic use or overdosage may result in electrolyte disturbances (hypokalemia, hypocalcemia, metabolic acidosis, or alkalosis), persistent diarrhea, malabsorption, weight loss. Electrolyte disturbance may produce vomiting, muscle weakness.

NURSING IMPLICATIONS

INTERVENTION/EVALUATION:

Encourage adequate fluid intake. Assess bowel sounds for peristalsis. Monitor daily bowel activity and stool consistency (watery, loose, soft, semi-solid, solid) and record time of evacuation. Assess for abdominal disturbances. Monitor serum electrolytes in those exposed to prolonged, frequent, or excessive use of medication.

PATIENT/FAMILY TEACHING:

Cola, unsalted crackers, dry toast may relieve nausea. Institute measures to promote defecation: increase fluid intake, exercise, high-fiber diet. Do not take antacids, milk, or other medication within 1 hr of taking medication (decreased effectiveness).

bismuth subsalicylate

bis'muth sub-sull-ih'sah-late

(Pepto-Bismol)

CANADIAN AVAILABILITY: Bismuth Liquid

CLASSIFICATION

Antidiarrheal, antinauseant

PHARMACOKINETICS

Hydrolyzed in stomach; nondissociated bismuth subsalicylate reacts to form insoluble bismuth salt; salicylate component rapidly, extensively absorbed from small intestine; bismuth poorly absorbed. Protein binding: high. Salicylate primarily excreted in urine; bismuth eliminated in feces.

ACTION

Absorbs fluid and electrolytes across intestinal wall; inhibits synthesis of prostaglandin responsible for intestinal inflammation and hypermotility. Binds toxins produced by *Escherichia coli.*

USES

Control of diarrhea, indigestion, nausea; relieves gas pain/abdominal cramps. *Helicobacter pylori*–associated duodenal ulcer, gastritis.

PO ADMINISTRATION

1. Shake suspension before administering.
2. Tablets may be chewed or dissolved in mouth.

INDICATIONS/DOSAGE/ROUTES

Diarrhea, gastric distress:

PO: Adults, elderly: 2 tablets (30 ml) q0.5-1h up to 8 doses/24 hrs. **Children 9-12 yrs:** 1 tablet or 15 ml q0.5-1h up to 8 doses/24 hrs. **Children 6-9 yrs:** 2/3 tablet or 10 ml q0.5-1h up to 8 doses/24 hrs. **Children 3-6 yrs:** 1/3 tablet or 5 ml q0.5-1h up to 8 doses/24 hrs.

H. pylori*–associated duodenal ulcer, gastritis:*

PO: Adults, elderly: 525 mg 3 times/day 1 hr before meals (w/ 500 mg amoxicillin and 500 mg metronidazole 3 times/day after meals) for 7-14 days.

PRECAUTIONS

CONTRAINDICATIONS: Bleeding ulcers, hemorrhagic states, gout, hemophilia, renal function impairment. **CAUTIONS:** Elderly, diabetic pts. **PREGNANCY/LAC-**

TATION: Readily crosses placenta. May increase risk of birth defects. Chronic, high-dose therapy during late pregnancy increases risk of long labor, complicated delivery, maternal or fetal hemorrhage. Excreted in breast milk. **Pregnancy Category C** (**Pregnancy Category D** during third trimester).

INTERACTIONS

DRUG INTERACTIONS: Anticoagulants, heparin, thrombolytics may increase risk of bleeding. Large dose may increase oral hypoglycemic, insulin effects. Other salicylates may increase toxicity. May decrease absorption of tetracyclines. **ALTERED LAB VALUES:** May alter SGPT (ALT), SGOT (AST), alkaline phosphatase, uric acid. May decrease potassium. May prolong prothrombin time.

SIDE EFFECTS

None significant.

ADVERSE REACTIONS/TOXIC EFFECTS

Debilitated pts and infants may develop impaction.

NURSING IMPLICATIONS

INTERVENTION/EVALUATION:

Encourage adequate fluid intake. Assess bowel sounds for peristaltic activity. Monitor stool frequency and consistency (watery, loose, soft, semi-solid, solid).

PATIENT/FAMILY TEACHING:

Stool may appear grey/black. If high fever accompanies diarrhea or if diarrhea continues longer than 2 days, contact physician. Dry crackers, cola may help relieve nausea. Chew tablets thoroughly before swallowing.

bisoprolol fumarate

bye-sew'prow-lol
(Zebeta)

FIXED-COMBINATION(S):
W/hydrochlorothiazide, a diuretic (Ziac)

CLASSIFICATION

Beta-adrenergic blocker

PHARMACOKINETICS

Well absorbed from GI tract. Protein binding: 30%. Metabolized in liver. Primarily excreted in urine. Half-life: 9-12 hrs (increased in decreased renal function).

ACTION

Selectively blocks $beta_1$-receptors, slowing sinus heart rate, decreasing cardiac output, decreasing B/P (exact mechanism unknown but may block peripheral adrenergic receptors, decrease sympathetic outflow from CNS or decrease renin release from kidney). Large doses may block $beta_2$-adrenergic receptors, increasing airway resistance.

USES

Management of hypertension, alone or in combination w/diuretics, other medications.

PO ADMINISTRATION

1. May give w/o regard to food.
2. Scored tablet may be crushed.

INDICATIONS/DOSAGE/ROUTES

Hypertension:
PO: Adults, elderly: Initially, 2.5-5 mg/day as single dose either alone or in combination w/di-

uretic. May increase gradually up to 20 mg/day.

PO: Renal impairment (<40 ml/min), hepatic impairment (cirrhosis, hepatitis): Initially, 2.5 mg.

PRECAUTIONS

CONTRAINDICATIONS: Overt cardiac failure, cardiogenic shock, heart block greater than first degree. **CAUTIONS:** Impaired renal or hepatic function, peripheral vascular disease, hyperthyroidism, diabetes, inadequate cardiac function, bronchospastic disease. **PREGNANCY/LACTATION:** Readily crosses placenta; distributed in breast milk. Avoid use during first trimester. May produce bradycardia, apnea, hypoglycemia, hypothermia during delivery, small birth weight infants. **Pregnancy Category C.**

INTERACTIONS

DRUG INTERACTIONS: Diuretics, other hypotensives may increase hypotensive effect; sympathomimetics, xanthines may mutually inhibit effects; may mask symptoms of hypoglycemia, prolong hypoglycemic effect of insulin, oral hypoglycemics; NSAIDs may decrease antihypertensive effect; cimetidine may increase concentration. **ALTERED LAB VALUES:** May increase ANA titer, BUN, creatinine, potassium, uric acid, lipoproteins, triglycerides.

SIDE EFFECTS

FREQUENT: Dizziness, fatigue, insomnia, bizarre dreams, paresthesia, visual disturbances, anxiety, peripheral edema, dyspnea, weight gain. **OCCASIONAL:** Nausea, GI distress, palpitation, coldness of extremities, syncope, tachycardia, chest pain, muscle or joint pain. **RARE:** Lethargy, hallucinations, diarrhea, vomiting, wheezing, rash, pruritus, urinary frequency, impotence.

ADVERSE REACTIONS/TOXIC EFFECTS

Abrupt withdrawal (particularly in those w/coronary artery disease) may produce angina or precipitate MI. May precipitate thyroid crisis in those w/thyrotoxicosis.

NURSING IMPLICATIONS

BASELINE ASSESSMENT:

Assess baseline renal/liver function tests. Assess B/P, apical pulse immediately before drug is administered (if pulse is 60/min or below, or systolic B/P is below 90 mm Hg, withhold medications, contact physician).

INTERVENTION/EVALUATION:

Assess pulse for strength/weakness, irregular rate, bradycardia. Monitor EKG for cardiac changes. Assist w/ambulation if dizziness occurs. Assess for peripheral edema of hands, feet (usually, first area of lower extremity swelling is behind medial malleolus in ambulatory, sacral area in bedridden). Monitor stool frequency and consistency. Assess skin for development of rash. Monitor any unusual changes in pt.

PATIENT/FAMILY TEACHING:

Do not abruptly discontinue medication. Compliance w/therapy regimen is essential to control hypertension. If dizziness occurs, sit or lie down immediately. Avoid tasks that require alertness, motor skills until response to drug is established. Teach pts how to properly take pulse before each dose and to report excessively slow pulse rate (<60 beats/min), peripheral numbness, dizziness. Do not use nasal decongestants, over-the-counter cold preparations (stimulants) w/o physician approval. Restrict salt, alcohol intake.

bitolterol mesylate

by-toll´ter-all
(Tornalate)

CLASSIFICATION

Bronchodilator

PHARMACOKINETICS

	ONSET	PEAK	DURATION
Inhalation	3-4 min	0.5-2 hrs	5-8 hrs 2.5-5 hrs (corticosteroid-dependent)

Hydrolyzed in tissue/blood to active compound. Excreted in urine, eliminated in feces. Half-life: 3 hrs.

ACTION

Stimulates beta$_2$-adrenergic receptors in lungs relaxing bronchial smooth muscle (increases production of cAMP))

USES

Prophylaxis, symptomatic treatment of bronchial asthma, acute bronchitis, reversible obstructive airway disease.

1. Shake container well, exhale completely then holding mouthpiece 1-inch away from lips, inhale and hold breath as long as possible before exhaling.

2. Wait 1-10 min before inhaling second dose (allows for deeper bronchial penetration).

3. Rinse mouth w/water immediately after inhalation (prevents mouth/throat dryness).

INDICATIONS/DOSAGE/ROUTES

Symptomatic relief:
INHALATION: Adults, elderly, children >12 yrs: 2 inhalations, separated by 1-3 min interval. Third inhalation may be needed.

Prophylaxis:
INHALATION: Adults, elderly, children >12 yrs: 2 inhalations q8h. Do not exceed 3 inhalations q6h, or 2 inhalations q4h.

PRECAUTIONS

CONTRAINDICATIONS: History of hypersensitivity to sympathomimetics. **CAUTIONS:** Hypertension, cardiovascular disorders, hyperthyroidism, seizure disorders, diabetes mellitus. **PREGNANCY/LACTATION:** Unknown if drug crosses placenta or is distributed in breast milk. May inhibit uterine contractility. **Pregnancy Category C.**

INTERACTIONS

DRUG INTERACTIONS: May decrease effects of beta-blockers. May increase risk of arrhythmias w/digoxin. **ALTERED LAB VALUES:** May decrease potassium.

SIDE EFFECTS

FREQUENT: Tremors, nervousness. **OCCASIONAL:** Throat irritation, coughing, headache, dizziness, lightheadedness, nausea, and palpitations. **RARE:** Chest discomfort, insomnia, tachycardia.

ADVERSE REACTIONS/TOXIC EFFECTS

Although tolerance to the bronchodilating effect has not been observed, prolonged or too-frequent use may lead to tolerance. Severe paradoxical bronchoconstriction may occur w/excessive use.

NURSING IMPLICATIONS

Baseline Assessment:

Offer emotional support (high incidence of anxiety due to difficulty in breathing and sympathomimetic response to drug).

Intervention/Evaluation:

Monitor rate, depth, rhythm, type of respiration; quality and rate of pulse. Assess lung sounds for wheezing. Monitor arterial blood gases. Observe lips, fingernails for blue or dusky color in light-skinned patients; gray in dark-skinned patients. Observe for clavicular retractions, hand tremor. Evaluate for clinical improvement (quieter, slower respirations, relaxed facial expression, cessation of clavicular retractions).

Patient/Family Teaching:

Increase fluid intake (decreases lung secretion viscosity). Instruct pt on proper administration technique. Do not exceed recommended dosage (excessive use may produce paradoxical bronchoconstriction, or a decreased bronchodilating effect). Rinsing mouth with water immediately after inhalation may prevent mouth/throat dryness. Avoid excessive use of caffeine derivatives (chocolate, coffee, tea, cola, cocoa). Do not take over-the-counter medications w/o consulting physician. Avoid smoking, smoke-filled environment. Notify physician of dizziness, palpitations/chest pain or lack of therapeutic response.

bleomycin sulfate

blee-oh-my´sin

(Blenoxane)

CANADIAN AVAILABILITY:

Blenoxane

CLASSIFICATION

Antineoplastic

PHARMACOKINETICS

Well absorbed after IM, SC administration; moderately absorbed following intrapleural or intraperitoneal administration. Protein binding <1%. Metabolized by enzyme degradation in tissues. Primarily excreted in urine. Half-life: 2 hrs (increased in decreased renal function).

ACTION

Exact mechanism unknown. May bind to DNA; decreases DNA, RNA, protein synthesis. Most effective in G_2 phase of cell division.

USES

Palliative treatment of lymphomas: Hodgkin's disease, reticulum cell sarcoma, lymphosarcoma. Squamous cell carcinomas: head and neck, including mouth, tongue, tonsil, nasopharynx, oropharynx, sinus, palate, lip, buccal mucosa, gingiva, epiglottis, larynx). Testicular carcinoma, choriocarcinoma. Treatment of malignant pleural effusions, prevention of recurrent pleural effusions.

STORAGE/HANDLING

NOTE: May be carcinogenic, mutagenic, or teratogenic. Handle w/extreme care during preparation/administration.

Refrigerate powder. After reconstitution with 5% dextrose or 0.9% NaCl injection, solution stable for 24 hours at room temperature.

SubQ/IM/IV ADMINISTRATION

SubQ/IM: Reconstitute 15 U vial w/1-5 ml sterile water for injection, 0.9% NaCl injection, 5% dextrose or bacteriostatic water for injection to provide concentration of 3-15 U/ml.

IV: Reconstitute 15 U vial w/at least 5 ml 0.9% NaCl injection, 5% dextrose and administer over at least 10 min.

INDICATIONS/DOSAGE/ROUTES

NOTE: Dosage individualized based on clinical response, tolerance to adverse effects. When used in combination therapy, consult specific protocols for optimum dosage, sequence of drug administration. Cumulative doses >400 U increase risk of pulmonary toxicity. Test doses of 2 units or less for first 2 doses recommended due to increased possibility of anaphylactoid reaction in lymphoma pts.

Squamous cell carcinoma, lymphosarcoma, reticulum cell sarcoma, testicular carcinoma, Hodgkin's disease:
SubQ/IM/IV: Adults, elderly: 0.25-0.50 U/kg (10-20 U/m^2) 1-2 times/wk.

Hodgkin's disease (maintenance dose after 50% response):
IM/IV: Adults, elderly: 1 U/day (or 5 U/wk).

PRECAUTIONS

CONTRAINDICATIONS: Previous allergic reaction. **EXTREME CAUTION:** Severe renal/pulmonary impairment. **PREGNANCY/LACTATION:** If possible, avoid use during pregnancy, especially first trimester. Breast feeding not recommended. **Pregnancy Category C.**

INTERACTIONS

DRUG INTERACTIONS: Other antineoplastics may increase toxicity. Cisplatin induced renal impairment may decrease clearance, increase toxicity. **ALTERED LAB VALUES:** None significant.

SIDE EFFECTS

FREQUENT: Anorexia, weight loss, erythematous skin swelling, urticaria, rash, striae (streaking), vesiculation (small blisters), hyperpigmentation (particularly at areas of pressure, skin folds, nail cuticles, IM injection sites, scars), mucosal lesions of lips, tongue. Usually evident 1-3 wks after initial therapy. May also be accompanied by decreased skin sensitivity followed by hypersensitivity of skin, nausea, vomiting, alopecia, fever/chills w/parenteral form (particularly noted few hours after large single dose, lasts 4-12 hrs). **OCCASIONAL:** Pain at tumor site, stomatitis, thrombophletibis w/IV administration.

ADVERSE REACTIONS/TOXIC EFFECTS

Interstitial pneumonitis occurs in 10% of pts, occasionally progressing to pulmonary fibrosis. Appears to be dose/age related (over 70 years, those receiving total dose more than 400 U). Severe bone marrow depression, renal, hepatic toxicity occur infrequently.

NURSING IMPLICATIONS

BASELINE ASSESSMENT:

Obtain chest x-rays q1-2wks.

INTERVENTION/EVALUATION:

Discontinue drug immediately if pulmonary toxicity (increased risk of toxicity if oxygen administered concurrently during therapy) occurs. Monitor lung sounds for pulmonary toxicity (dyspnea, fine lung rales). Monitor hematologic, pulmonary function studies, hepatic, renal function tests. Assess skin daily for cutaneous toxicity. Monitor for stomatitis (burning/erythema of oral mucosa at inner margin of lips), hematologic toxicity (fever, sore throat, signs of local infection, easy bruising, unusual bleeding), symptoms of anemia (excessive tiredness, weakness).

PATIENT/FAMILY TEACHING:

Fever/chills reaction occurs less frequently w/continued therapy. Improvement of Hodgkin's disease, testicular tumors noted within 2 wks, squamous cell carcinoma within 3 weeks. Do not have immunizations w/o doctor's approval (drug lowers body's resistance). Avoid contact w/those who have recently taken live virus vaccine. Contact physician if nausea/vomiting continues at home.

bretylium tosylate

bre-till'ee-um

(Bretylol)

CANADIAN AVAILABILITY:
Bretylate

CLASSIFICATION

Antiarrhythmic

PHARMACOKINETICS

	ONSET	PEAK	DURATION
IM	20 min-6 hrs	6-9 hrs	6-24 hrs
IV	20 min-6 hrs	6-9 hrs	6-24 hrs

Well absorbed after IM administration. Protein binding: 1-6%. Primarily excreted in urine. Removed by hemodialysis. Half-life: 4-17 hrs (increased in decreased renal function).

ACTION

Directly effects myocardial cell membrane. Initially, releases norepinephrine, then inhibits its release (contributes to suppression ventricular tachycardia).

USES

Prophylaxis and treatment of ventricular fibrillation in those w/life-threatening ventricular tachyarrhythmias who have not responded to conventional antiarrhythmic therapy.

STORAGE/HANDLING

Solution should appear clear after reconstitution. Discard if precipitate forms. Slight discoloration does not indicate loss of potency. Solution is stable for 48 hrs at room temperature, or 7 days if refrigerated.

IM/IV ADMINISTRATION

IM:

1. Do not dilute.
2. Do not give more than 5 ml into one site (over 3 ml may cause pain at injection site).
3. Rotate injection sites (same-site injection may cause muscular atrophy and necrosis).

IV:

1. For injection, give undiluted over 1 min.
2. For intermittent IV infusion (piggyback), dilute w/at least 50 ml 5% dextrose or 0.9% NaCl to provide concentration of 10 mg/ml.
3. Infuse over at least 8 min (too rapid IV produces nausea, vomiting).

INDICATIONS/DOSAGE/ROUTES

Ventricular arrhythmias, immediate, life-threatening:
IV: Adults, elderly: 5 mg/kg undiluted by rapid IV injection. May increase to 10 mg/kg, repeat as needed. **Maintenance:** 5-10 mg/kg diluted over >8 min, q6h or IV infusion at 1-2 mg/min. **Children:** 5 mg/kg, then 10 mg/kg at 15-30 min interval. **Maximum:** 30 mg/kg total dose. **Maintenance:** 5-10 mg/kg q6h.

Ventricular arrhythmias, other:
IM: Adults, elderly: 5-10 mg/kg undiluted, may repeat at 1-2 hr intervals. **Maintenance:** 5-10 mg/kg q6-8h.
IV: Adults, elderly: 5-10 mg/kg diluted over >8 min, may repeat at 1-2 hr intervals. **Maintenance:** 5-10 mg/kg q6h or IV infusion at 1-2 mg/min. **Children:** 5-10 mg/kg/dose diluted q6h.

PRECAUTIONS

CONTRAINDICATIONS: None significant. **EXTREME CAUTION:** Digitalis-induced arrhythmias, fixed cardiac output (severe pulmonary hypertension, aortic stenosis). **CAUTIONS:** Impaired renal function, sinus bradycardia. **PREGNANCY/LACTATION:** Unknown if drug crosses placenta. May decrease uterine blood flow, produce bradycardia in fetus. **Pregnancy Category C.**

INTERACTIONS

DRUG INTERACTIONS: May increase digoxin toxicity (due to initial norepinephrine release). Procainamide, quinidine may decrease inotropic effect, increase hypotension. **ALTERED LAB VALUES:** None significant.

SIDE EFFECTS

FREQUENT: Transitory hypertension followed by postural and supine hypotension in 50% of pts observed as dizziness, lightheadedness, faintness, syncope. **OCCASIONAL:** Diarrhea, loose stools, nasal stuffiness.

ADVERSE REACTIONS/TOXIC EFFECTS

Respiratory depression from possible neuromuscular blockade.

NURSING IMPLICATIONS

Baseline Assessment:

Have pt in area w/equipment and personnel for constant cardiac and B/P monitoring.

Intervention/Evaluation:

Assess for conversion of ventricular arrhythmias and absence of new arrhythmias. Constantly monitor B/P, pulse. Notify physician of systolic B/P <75 mm Hg (dopamine or norepinephrine may be needed, or blood, plasma or volume correction). Keep pt supine (risk of hypotension) during life-threatening therapy and during infusion until tolerance develops. When permitted, assist w/slow position change and ambulation. Put infusions on continuous infusion pumps. Monitor I&O. Provide emotional support to pt and family.

Patient/Family Teaching:

Tolerance to hypotensive effect usually occurs within several days after initial therapy. One hr after dose administration, may rise slowly from lying to sitting position and permit legs to dangle from bed for at least 5 min before standing.

bromocriptine

brom-oh-crip´teen
(Parlodel)

CANADIAN AVAILABILITY: Parlodel

CLASSIFICATION

Antiparkinson, prolactin inhibitor

PHARMACOKINETICS

	ONSET	PEAK	DURATION
PO	1-2 hrs	—	4-5 hrs
(growth hormone decrease)			
PO	2 hrs	8 hrs	24 hrs
(prolactin decrease)			

Minimal absorption from GI tract. Protein binding: 90-95%. Metabolized in liver. Excreted in feces via biliary secretion. Half-life: 15 hrs.

ACTION

Directly inhibits prolactin release from anterior pituitary. Stimulates presynaptic and postsynaptic dopamine receptors. Suppresses secretion, reduction of elevated growth hormone concentration.

USES

Treatment of hyperprolactinemia conditions (amenorrhea w/or w/o galactorrhea, prolactin secreting adenomas, infertility). Formerly used for prevention of lactation or when mother elects not to breast-feed; recommendation for this use was voluntarily withdrawn by manufacturer, August 1994. Treatment of Parkinson's disease, acromegaly.

PO ADMINISTRATION

1. Pt should be lying down before administering first dose.
2. Give after food intake (decreases incidence of nausea).

INDICATIONS/DOSAGE/ROUTES

Hyperprolactinemia:
PO: Adults, elderly: Initially, 1.25-2.5 mg/day. May increase by 2.5 mg/day at 3-7 day intervals. **Range:** 2.5-15 mg/day.

Parkinson's disease:
PO: Adults, elderly: Initially, 1.25 mg 2 times/day. Increase by 2.5 mg/day every 14-28 days. **Range:** 10-40 mg/day.

Acromegaly:
PO: Adults, elderly: Initially, 1.25-2.5 mg/day at bedtime for 3 days. May increase by 1.25-2.5 mg/day every 3-7 days. **Range:** 20-30 mg/day. **Max:** 100 mg/day.

PRECAUTIONS

CONTRAINDICATIONS: Pregnancy, peripheral vascular disease, severe ischemic heart disease, uncontrolled hypertension, hypersensitivity to ergot alkaloids. **CAUTIONS:** Impaired hepatic/cardiac function.

INTERACTIONS

DRUG INTERACTIONS: Disulfiram reaction may occur w/alcohol. Estrogens, progestins may decrease effects. Phenothiazines, haloperidol, MAO inhibitors may decrease prolactin effect. Hypotensive agents may increase hypotension. Levodopa may increase effects. **ALTERED LAB VALUES:** May elevate BUN, SGOT (AST), SGPT (ALT), CPK, alkaline phosphatase, uric acid.

SIDE EFFECTS

NOTE: Incidence of side effects is high, especially at beginning of therapy or w/high dosage. **FREQUENT:** Nausea, constipation, hypotension noted by dizziness, lightheadedness, anorexia, headache, abdominal cramps, vomiting, nasal stuffiness, constipation or diarrhea, peripheral vasoconstriction (Raynaud's phenomenon). **RARE:** Confusion, muscle cramping, visual hallucinations.

ADVERSE REACTIONS/TOXIC EFFECTS

Visual or auditory hallucinations noted in parkinsonism syndrome. Long-term, high-dose therapy may produce reversible pulmonary infiltrates, pleural effusion, thickening of pleura.

NURSING IMPLICATIONS

BASELINE ASSESSMENT:

Determine baseline, stability of vital signs. Evaluation of pituitary (R/O tumor) should be done prior to treatment for hyperprolactinemia w/amenorrhea/galactorrhea and infertility. Pregnancy test.

NTERVENTION/EVALUATION:

Assist w/ambulation if dizziness is noted after administration. Monitor B/P for evidence of hypotension, particularly during early therapy. Assess for therapeutic response (decrease in engorgement, decreases in parkinsonism symptoms). Monitor for constipation.

PATIENT/FAMILY TEACHING:

Take w/food. To reduce lightheadedness, rise slowly from lying to sitting position and permit legs to dangle momentarily before standing. Avoid sudden posture changes. Avoid tasks that require alertness, motor skills until response to drug is established. Must use contraceptive measures (other than oral) during treatment. Report any watery nasal discharge to physician. Do not suddenly discontinue the drug. Avoid alcohol.

brompheniramine maleate

brom-phen-err'ah-meen
(Bromphen, Dimetane)

FIXED COMBINATION(S): W/phenylpropanolamine, a nasal decongestant (Dimetapp); w/ phenylephrine, a nasal vasoconstrictor (Dimetane Decongestant). Dexbrompheniramine maleate is fixed-combination w/acetaminophen, pseudoephedrine (Drixoral Plus), w/pseudoephedrine (Drixoral).

CANADIAN AVAILABILITY: Dimetane

CLASSIFICATION

Antihistamine

PHARMACOKINETICS

	ONSET	PEAK	DURATION
PO	15-60 min	2-5 hrs	4-6 hrs
Ext-release	15-60 min	2-5 hrs	8-12 hrs
IM/IV	>15 min	2-5 hrs	4-6 hrs

Well absorbed from GI tract. Metabolized in liver. Primarily excreted in urine. Half-life: 25 hrs.

ACTION

Prevents, antagonizes most histamine effects (e.g., urticaria, pruritus). Anticholinergic effects cause drying of nasal mucosa.

USES

Symptomatic relief of allergic

conditions, allergic reaction to blood, plasma. Fixed-combination w/nasal decongestant used for relief of upper respiratory symptoms (nasal/sinus congestion, common cold).

STORAGE/HANDLING

Store tablets, elixir, parenteral form at room temperature. Parenteral form may produce crystals at temperatures colder than 32° F. (warm to 86° F to redissolve crystals).

PO/IM/IV ADMINISTRATION

PO:

1. Give w/o regard to meals. Scored tablets may be crushed. Do not crush or break extended-release capsules.

IM:

1. Give deep IM into large muscle mass.

IV:

1. Place pt in recumbent position.
2. Give undiluted but may be diluted with 5% dextrose, 0.9% NaCl injection (decreases incidence of side effects).
3. Administer IV injection at rate of 1 ml/min.

INDICATIONS/DOSAGE/ROUTES

Allergic condition:
PO: Adults, children >12 yrs: 4-8 mg 3-4 times/day. **Children 6-11 yrs:** 2-4 mg 3-4 times/day. **Children 2-5 yrs:** 1 mg q4-6h.
SubQ/IM/IV: Adults: 10 mg q6-12h. **Avg. dose:** 5-20 mg. **Maximum daily dose:** 40 mg. **Children <12 yrs:** 0.5 mg/kg or 15 mg/m^2 daily in 3-4 divided doses.

Usual elderly dosage:
PO: Elderly: Initially, 4 mg 1-2 times/day.

Extended-release:
PO: Adults, children >12 yrs: 8-12 mg q8-12h. **Children 6-11 yrs:** 8-12 mg q12h.

PRECAUTIONS

CONTRAINDICATIONS: Acute asthmatic attack, those receiving MAO inhibitors. **CAUTIONS:** Narrow-angle glaucoma, peptic ulcer, prostatic hypertrophy, pyloroduodenal or bladder neck obstruction, asthma, COPD, increased intraocular pressure, cardiovascular disease, hyperthyroidism, hypertension, seizure disorders. **PREGNANCY/LACTATION:** Crosses placenta; detected in breast milk (may produce irritability in nursing infants). Increased risk of seizures in neonates, premature infants if used during third trimester of pregnancy. May prohibit lactation. **Pregnancy Category B.**

INTERACTIONS

DRUG INTERACTIONS: Alcohol, CNS depressants may increase CNS depressant effects. MAO inhibitors may increase anticholinergic, CNS depressant effects. **ALTERED LAB VALUES:** May suppress wheal, flare reactions to antigen skin testing, unless antihistamines discontinued 4 days prior to testing.

SIDE EFFECTS

FREQUENT: Drowsiness, dizziness, muscular weakness, dry mouth/nose/throat/lips, urinary retention, thickening of bronchial secretions. Sedation, dizziness, hypotension more likely to be seen in elderly. **OCCASIONAL:** Epigastric distress, flushing, visual disturbances, hearing disturbances, paresthesia, sweating, chills. Fixed-combination form with pseudoephedrine may produce mild CNS stimulation.

ADVERSE REACTIONS/TOXIC EFFECTS

Children may experience dominant paradoxical reaction (restlessness, insomnia, euphoria, nervousness, tremors). Overdosage in children may result in hallucinations, convulsions, death. Hypersensitivity reaction (eczema, pruritus, rash, cardiac disturbances, photosensitivity) may occur. Overdosage may vary from CNS depression (sedation, apnea, cardiovascular collapse, death) to severe paradoxical reaction (hallucinations, tremor, seizures).

NURSING IMPLICATIONS

BASELINE ASSESSMENT:

If pt is undergoing allergic reaction, obtain history of recently ingested foods, drugs, environmental exposure, recent emotional stress. Monitor rate, depth, rhythm, type of respiration; quality and rate of pulse. Assess lung sounds for rhonchi, wheezing, rales.

INTERVENTION/EVALUATION:

Monitor B/P, especially in elderly (increased risk of hypotension). Monitor children closely for paradoxical reaction.

PATIENT/FAMILY TEACHING:

Tolerance to antihistaminic effect generally does not occur; tolerance to sedative effect may occur. Avoid tasks that require alertness, motor skills until response to drug is established. Dry mouth, drowsiness, dizziness may be an expected response of drug. Avoid alcoholic beverages during antihistamine therapy. Sugarless gum, sips of tepid water may relieve dry mouth. Coffee or tea may help reduce drowsiness.

---

budesonide (Rhinocort)
See supplement

---

bumetanide

byew-met´ah-nide
(Bumex)

CLASSIFICATION

Diuretic: Loop

PHARMACOKINETICS

	ONSET	PEAK	DURATION
PO	30-60 min	60-120 min	4-6 hrs
IM	40 min	60-120 min	4-6 hrs
IV	Rapid	15-30 min	2-3 hrs

Completely absorbed from GI tract (decreased in CHF, nephrotic syndrome). Protein binding: 94-96%. Partially metabolized in liver. Primarily excreted in urine. Half-life: 1-1.5 hrs.

ACTION

Enhances excretion of sodium, chloride, and to lesser degree, potassium, by direct action at ascending limb of loop of Henle.

USES

Treatment of edema associated w/CHF, chronic renal failure including nephrotic syndrome, hepatic cirrhosis w/ascites; treatment of acute pulmonary edema.

STORAGE/HANDLING

Store oral, parenteral form at room temperature.

PO/IM/IV ADMINISTRATION

PO:

1. Give w/food to avoid GI upset, preferably w/breakfast (may prevent nocturia).

IV:

1. May give undiluted but is compatible w/5% dextrose in water, 0.9% sodium chloride or lactated Ringer's.
2. Administer direct IV >1-2 min.
3. May give through Y tube or 3-way stopcock.

INDICATIONS/DOSAGE/ROUTES

Edema:
PO: Adults >18 yrs: 0.5-2 mg given as single dose in AM. May repeat at 4-5 hr intervals. May give in divided dose. **Maximum daily dose:** 10 mg. May use alternate day dosing or 3-4 day dosing w/1-2 day hiatus.

Usual elderly dosage:
PO: Elderly: 0.5 mg/day, increase as needed.

Acute pulmonary edema:
IM or IV: Adults, elderly: 0.5-1 mg given as single dose. May be repeated at 2-3 hr intervals. Do not exceed 10 mg daily.

PRECAUTIONS

CONTRAINDICATIONS: Anuria, hepatic coma, severe electrolyte depletion. **EXTREME CAUTION:** Hypersensitivity to sulfonamides. **CAUTIONS:** Impaired renal or hepatic function, diabetes mellitus, elderly/debilitated. **PREGNANCY/LACTATION:** Unknown if drug is distributed in breast milk. **Pregnancy Category C.**

INTERACTIONS

DRUG INTERACTIONS: Amphotericin, ototoxic, nephrotoxic agents may increase toxicity. May decrease effect of anticoagulants, heparin. Hypokalemia causing agents may increase risk hypokalemia. May increase risk of lithium toxicity. **ALTERED LAB VALUES:** May increase glucose, BUN, uric acid, urinary phosphate. May decrease calcium, chloride, magnesium, potassium, sodium.

SIDE EFFECTS

EXPECTED: Increase in urine frequency/volume. **OCCASIONAL:** Dizziness, hypotension. **RARE:** Nausea, headache, lightheadedness, vertigo, muscle cramps; rash, urticaria, pruritus, vomiting, diarrhea, impaired hearing, weakness, general body discomfort, breast tenderness, premature ejaculation, loss of erection.

ADVERSE REACTIONS/TOXIC EFFECTS

Vigorous diuresis may lead to profound water/electrolyte depletion, resulting in hypokalemia, hyponatremia, dehydration, coma, circulatory collapse. Acute hypotensive episodes may occur. Ototoxicity manifested as deafness, vertigo, tinnitus (ringing/roaring in ears) may occur, especially in those w/severe renal impairment or who are on other ototoxic drugs. Encephalopathy may occur in preexisting liver disease. Blood dyscrasias have been reported.

NURSING IMPLICATIONS

BASELINE ASSESSMENT:

Check vital signs, especially B/P for hypotension prior to administration. Assess baseline electrolytes, particularly check for low potassium. Assess edema, skin turgor, mucous membranes for hydration status. Assess muscle strength, mental status. Note skin temperature, moisture. Obtain baseline weight. Initiate I&O.

INTERVENTION/EVALUATION:

Continue to monitor B/P, vital signs, electrolytes, I&O, weight. Note extent of diuresis. Watch for changes from initial assessment (hypokalemia may result in muscle strength changes, tremor, muscle cramps, change in mental status, cardiac arrhythmias; hyponatremia may result in confusion, thirst, cold/clammy skin).

PATIENT/FAMILY TEACHING:

Expect increased frequency and volume of urination. Report irregular heartbeat, signs of electrolyte imbalances (see Adverse Reactions/Toxic Effects), hearing abnormalities (such as sense of fullness in ears, ringing/roaring in ears). Eat foods high in potassium such as whole grains (cereals), legumes, meat, bananas, apricots, orange juice, potatoes (white, sweet), raisins. Avoid sun/sunlamps.

bupivacaine

(Maraine, Sensorcaine)

(See Classifications section under Anesthetics: local)

buprenorphine hydrochloride

byew-pren-or′phen

(Buprenex)

CLASSIFICATION

Opioid analgesic **(Schedule V)**

PHARMACOKINETICS

	ONSET	PEAK	DURATION
IM	15 min	1 hr	<6 hrs
IV	Rapid	Rapid	<6 hrs

Rapidly absorbed from IM injection. Protein binding: high. Metabolized in liver, undergoes extensive first-pass metabolism. Primarily eliminated in feces via bile. Half-life: 2-3 hrs.

ACTION

Binds w/opioid receptors within CNS, altering processes affecting pain perception, emotional response to pain. May displace opioid agonists and competitively inhibit their action (may precipitate withdrawal symptoms).

USES

Relief of moderate to severe pain.

INDICATIONS/DOSAGE/ROUTES

NOTE: May be given IM or slow IV injection. Do not mix w/diazepam or lorazepam in same syringe.

Analgesia:
IM/IV: Adults, children >13 yrs: 0.3 mg q6h as needed; may repeat 30-60 min after initial dose. May increase to 0.6 mg and/or reduce dosing interval to q4h if necessary. **Children 2-12 yrs:** 2-6 mcg/kg q4-6h.

Usual elderly dosage:
IM/IV: Elderly: 0.15 mg q6h prn.

CONTRAINDICATIONS: None significant. **CAUTIONS:** Impaired hepatic/renal function, elderly, debilitated, head injury, respiratory disease, hypertension, hypothyroidism, Addison's disease, acute alcoholism, urethral stricture. **PREGNANCY/LACTATION:** Crosses placenta; unknown if distributed in breast milk (breast feeding not recommended). Prolonged use during pregnancy may produce withdrawal symptoms (irritability, excessive crying, tremors, hyperactive reflexes, fever, vomiting, diarrhea, yawning, sneezing, seizures) in neonate. **Pregnancy Category C.**

INTERACTIONS

DRUG INTERACTIONS: CNS depressants, MAO inhibitors may increase CNS, respiratory depression, hypotension. May decrease effects of other opioid analgesics. **ALTERED LAB VALUES:** May increase amylase, lipase.

SIDE EFFECTS

FREQUENT: Sedation, decreased respirations. **OCCASIONAL:** Sweaty palms, clammy skin, nausea, dizziness, dry mouth, headache. **RARE:** Restlessness, crying, euphoria, vomiting, bitter taste, urinary urgency, skin burning/itching, blurred vision.

ADVERSE REACTIONS/TOXIC EFFECTS

Overdosage results in severe respiratory depression, skeletal muscle flaccidity, cyanosis, extreme somnolence progressing to convulsions, stupor, coma.

NURSING IMPLICATIONS

BASELINE ASSESSMENT:

Obtain vital signs before giving medication. If respirations are 12/min or lower (20/min or lower in children), withhold medication, contact physician. Assess onset, type, location, duration of pain. Effect of medication is reduced if full pain recurs before next dose.

INTERVENTION/EVALUATION:

Monitor for change in respirations, B/P, change in rate/quality of pulse. Monitor stool frequency, consistency. Initiate deep breathing, coughing exercises, particularly in those w/impaired pulmonary function. Change pt's position q2-4h. Assess for clinical improvement and record onset of relief of pain.

PATIENT/FAMILY TEACHING:

Change positions slowly to avoid dizziness. Avoid tasks that require alertness, motor skills until response to drug is established. Avoid alcohol and benzodiazapines. Do not exceed prescribed dosage.

bupropion

byew-pro´peon

(Wellbutrin)

CLASSIFICATION

Antidepressant

PHARMACOKINETICS

Rapidly absorbed from GI tract. Crosses blood-brain barrier. Protein binding: 85%. Extensive first-pass metabolism in liver to active metabolite. Primarily excreted in urine. Half-life: 14 hrs.

ACTION

Weakly blocks neuronal re-uptake of serotonin, norepinephrine.

USES

Treatment of depression, particularly endogenous depression, exhibited as persistent and prominent dysphoria (occurring nearly every day for at least 2 wks) manifested by 4 of 8 symptoms: change in appetite, change in sleep pattern, increased fatigue, impaired concentration, feelings of guilt/worthlessness, loss of interest in usual activities, psychomotor agitation/retardation, or suicidal tendencies.

PO ADMINISTRATION

Avoid bedtime dosage (decreases risk of insomnia).

INDICATIONS/DOSAGE/ROUTES

NOTE: Reduce dosage in renal/hepatic impairment, elderly.

PO: Adults: Initially, 75 mg 3 times/day or 100 mg 2 times/day. May increase to 100 mg 3 times/day no sooner than 3 days after initial dosage. Do not exceed dose increase of 100 mg/day in 3-day period. **Maximum daily dose:** 150 mg 3 times/day. Do not exceed any single dose of 150 mg.

Usual elderly dosage:

PO: Elderly: Initially, 50-100 mg/day. May increase by 50-100 mg/day every 3-4 days.

PRECAUTIONS

CONTRAINDICATIONS: Those w/seizure disorder, current or prior diagnosis of bulimia or anorexia nervosa, concurrent use of MAO inhibitor. **EXTREME CAUTION:** History of seizure, cranial trauma; those currently taking antipsychotics, antidepressants. **CAUTIONS:** Impaired renal, hepatic function. **PREGNANCY/LACTATION:** Unknown if drug crosses placenta or is distributed in breast milk. **Pregnancy Category B.**

INTERACTIONS

DRUG INTERACTIONS: Alcohol, tricyclic antidepressants, lithium, trazodone may increase risk of seizures. May increase risk of acute toxicity w/MAO inhibitors. **ALTERED LAB VALUES:** May decrease WBCs.

SIDE EFFECTS

FREQUENT: Agitation, dry mouth, constipation, headache/migraine, weight loss/anorexia, excessive sweating, dizziness, tremor, sedation, insomnia, nausea. **OCCASIONAL:** Blurred vision, weight gain, tachycardia, confusion. **RARE:** Rash, diarrhea, cardiac disturbances (hyper/hypotension, palpitations), fatigue.

ADVERSE REACTIONS/TOXIC EFFECTS

Increased risk of seizures w/increase in dosage greater than 150 mg/dose, in those w/history of bulimia or seizure disorders, of discontinuing agents that may lower seizure threshold.

NURSING IMPLICATIONS

BASELINE ASSESSMENT:

For those on long-term therapy, liver/renal function tests should be performed periodically.

INTERVENTION/EVALUATION:

Supervise suicidal-risk patient closely during early therapy (as depression lessens, energy level improves, increasing suicide potential). Assess appearance, behavior, speech pattern, level of interest, mood. Monitor pattern of daily bowel activity, stool consistency. Monitor B/P, pulse for hypotension, arrhythmias.

PATIENT/FAMILY TEACHING:

Full therapeutic effect may be noted in 4 wks. Avoid alcohol (increases risk of seizure). Avoid tasks that require alertness, motor skills until response to drug is established. Dry mouth may be relieved by sugarless gum/sips of tepid water.

buspirone hydrochloride

byew´spear-own
(BuSpar)

CANADIAN AVAILABILITY:
Buspar

CLASSIFICATION

Antianxiety

PHARMACOKINETICS

Rapidly completely absorbed from GI tract. Undergoes extensive first-pass metabolism. Protein binding: 95%. Metabolized in liver to active metabolite. Primarily excreted in urine. Half-life: 2-3 hrs.

ACTION

Unknown. Binds to serotonin, dopamine receptors.

USES

Short-term relief (up to 4 wks); management of anxiety disorders.

PO ADMINISTRATION

1. Give w/o regard to meals.
2. Tablets may be crushed.

INDICATIONS/DOSAGE/ROUTES

PO: Adults: 5 mg 2-3 times daily. May increase in 5 mg increments/day at intervals of 2-4 days. **Maintenance:** 15-30 mg/day in 2-3 divided doses. Do not exceed 60 mg/day.

Usual elderly dosage:
PO: Elderly: Initially, 5 mg 2 times/day. May increase by 5 mg every 2-3 days. **Maximum:** 60 mg/day.

PRECAUTIONS

CONTRAINDICATIONS: Severe renal/hepatic impairment, MAO inhibitor therapy. **CAUTIONS:** Renal/hepatic impairment. **PREGNANCY/LACTATION:** Unknown if drug crosses placenta or is distributed in breast milk. **Pregnancy Category B.**

INTERACTIONS

DRUG INTERACTIONS: Alcohol, CNS depressants may increase sedation. MAO inhibitors may increase B/P. **ALTERED LAB VALUES:** May increase SGOT (AST), SGPT (ALT).

SIDE EFFECTS

FREQUENT: Dizziness, drowsiness, headache, nausea, lightheadedness, fatigue (particularly at dosage higher than 20 mg/day), insomnia and/or nervousness (particularly at very high dosage). **OCCASIONAL:** Paresthesia, excitement, tremors, dry mouth, tinnitus, nasal congestion, sore throat, redness/itching of eyes, abdominal distress, diarrhea/constipation, musculoskeletal aches/pains. **RARE:** Nightmares, blurred vision, tachycardia, palpitations.

ADVERSE REACTIONS/TOXIC EFFECTS

No evidence of tolerance or psychologic and/or physical dependence, no withdrawal syndrome. Overdosage may produce severe nausea, vomiting, dizziness, drowsiness, abdominal distention, excessive pupil contraction.

NURSING IMPLICATIONS

BASELINE ASSESSMENT:

Offer emotional support to anxious pt. Assess motor responses (agitation, trembling, tension) and autonomic responses (cold, clammy hands, sweating).

INTERVENTION/EVALUATION:

For those on long-term therapy, liver/renal function tests, blood counts should be performed periodically. Assist w/ambulation if drowsiness, lightheadedness occur. Evaluate for therapeutic response: calm, facial expression, decreased restlessness and/or insomnia.

PATIENT/FAMILY TEACHING:

Improvement may be noted in 7-10 days, but optimum therapeutic effect generally takes 3-4 wks. Drowsiness usually disappears during continued therapy. If dizziness occurs, change positions slowly from recumbent to sitting position before standing. Avoid tasks that require alertness, motor skills until response to drug is established. Avoid alcohol and other CNS depressants (unless ordered by physician). Do not discontinue drug abruptly.

busulfan

bew-sull'fan

(Myleran)

CANADIAN AVAILABILITY:
Myleran

CLASSIFICATION

Antineoplastic

PHARMACOKINETICS

Completely absorbed from GI tract. Metabolized in liver. Primarily excreted in urine. Half-life: 2.5 hrs.

ACTION

Cell cycle-phase nonspecific. Alkylates, cross-links DNA strands. Myelosuppressant.

USES

Palliative treatment of chronic myelogenous leukemia.

PO ADMINISTRATION

NOTE: May be carcinogenic, mutagenic, or teratogenic. Handle w/ extreme care during administration.

1. Give at same time each day.
2. Give on empty stomach if nausea/vomiting occur.

INDICATIONS/DOSAGE/ROUTES

NOTE: Dosage individualized based on clinical response, tolerance to adverse effects. When used in combination therapy, consult specific protocols for optimum dosage, sequence of drug administration.

Remission induction:
PO: Adults: 4-8 mg/day, withdraw drug when WBC falls below 15,000/mm^3.

Maintenance therapy:
PO: Adults: Induction dose (4-8 mg/day) when total leukocyte count reaches 50,000/mm^3. If remission <3 mos, 1-3 mg/day may produce satisfactory response.

Usual elderly dosage:
PO: Elderly: Initially, lowest dose for adults.

PRECAUTIONS

CONTRAINDICATIONS: Disease resistance to previous therapy w/drug. **EXTREME CAUTION:** Compromised bone marrow reserve. **PREGNANCY/LACTATION:** If possible, avoid use during pregnancy, esp. first trimester. May cause fetal harm. Unknown if distributed in breast milk. Breast feeding not recommended. **Pregnancy Category D.**

INTERACTIONS

DRUG INTERACTIONS: May decrease effect of antigout medications. Bone marrow depressant may increase risk of bone marrow depression. Live virus vaccines may potentiate virus replication, increase vaccine side effects, decrease antibody response to vaccine. **ALTERED LAB VALUES:** May increase blood/urine uric acid.

SIDE EFFECTS

FREQUENT: Hyperpigmentation of skin. **OCCASIONAL:** Nausea, vomiting, diarrhea, anorexia, weight loss.

ADVERSE REACTIONS/TOXIC EFFECTS

Major toxic effect is bone marrow depression resulting in hematologic toxicity (severe leukopenia, anemia, severe thrombocytopenia). Agranulocytosis occurs generally w/overdosage, may progress to pancytopenia. Very high doses may produce dizziness, blurred vision, muscle twitching, tonic-clonic seizures. Long-term therapy (>4 yrs) may produce pulmonary syndrome ("busulfan lung") characterized by persistent cough, congestion, rales, dyspnea. Hyperuricemia may produce uric acid nephropathy, renal stones, acute renal failure.

NURSING IMPLICATIONS

BASELINE ASSESSMENT:

Hgb, Hct, WBC, differential, platelet count, hepatic and renal functions studies should be performed weekly (dosage based on hematologic values).

INTERVENTION/EVALUATION:

Monitor WBC, differential, platelet count for evidence of bone marrow depression. Monitor for hematologic toxicity (fever, sore throat, easy bruising or unusual bleeding from any site), symptoms of anemia (excessive tiredness, weakness). Monitor lung sounds for pulmonary toxicity (dyspnea, fine lung rales).

PATIENT/FAMILY TEACHING:

Maintain adequate daily fluid intake (may protect against renal impairment). Report consistent cough, congestion, difficulty breathing. Promptly report fever, sore throat, signs of local infection, easy bruising or unusual bleeding from any site. Do not have immunizations w/o physician's approval (drug lowers body's resistance). Avoid contact w/those who have recently taken live virus vaccine. Contact physician if nausea/vomiting continues at home. Take on empty stomach if nausea and vomiting occurs. Take at same time each day. Contraception is recommended during therapy. Medication may cause darkening of skin.

butorphanol tartrate

byew-tore´phen-awl
(Stadol, Stadol NS)

CANADIAN AVAILABILITY:
Stadol

CLASSIFICATION

Opioid analgesic

PHARMACOKINETICS

	ONSET	PEAK	DURATION
IM	10-30 min	30-60 min	3-4 hrs
IV	<1 min	4-5 min	2-4 hrs
Nasal	15 min	1-2 hr	4-5 hrs

Rapidly absorbed from IM injection. Protein binding: 80%. Metabolized in liver, intestinal mucosa. Primarily excreted in urine. Half-life: 2.5-4 hrs.

ACTION

Binds w/opioid receptors within CNS, altering processes affecting pain perception, emotional response to pain. May displace opioid agonists and competitively inhibit their action (may precipitate withdrawal symptoms).

USES

Management of pain (including postop pain). *Nasal only:* Migraine headache pain. *Parenteral only:* Preop, preanesthetic medication, supplement balanced anesthesia, relief of pain during labor.

INDICATIONS/DOSAGE/ROUTES

NOTE: May be given by IM or IV injection.

Analgesia:
IM: Adults: 1-4 mg q3-4h as needed.
IV: Adults: 0.5-2 mg q3-4h as needed.
NASAL: Adults: 1 mg (1 spray in one nostril). May repeat in 60-90 min. May repeat 2 dose sequence q3-4h as needed. Alternatively, 2 mg (1 spray each nostril if pt remains recumbent), may repeat in 3-4h.

Usual elderly dosage:
IM/IV: Elderly: 1 mg q4-6h prn.

PRECAUTIONS

CONTRAINDICATIONS: None significant. **CAUTIONS:** Impaired hepatic/renal function, elderly, debilitated, head injury, respiratory disease, hypertension, prior to biliary tract surgery (produces spasm of sphincter of Oddi), MI w/nausea, vomiting. Not recommended for children <18 yrs. **PREGNANCY/LACTATION:** Readily crosses placenta; distributed in breast milk (breast feeding not recommended). **Pregnancy Category C.**

INTERACTIONS

DRUG INTERACTIONS: Alcohol, CNS depressants may increase CNS, respiratory depression, hypotension. MAO inhibitors may produce severe, fatal reaction (reduce dose to 1/4 usual dose). Effects may be decreased w/buprenorphine. **ALTERED LAB VALUES:** None significant.

SIDE EFFECTS

FREQUENT: Sedation, decreased respiration. *Nasal:* Vasodilation, constipation, insomnia, nasal congestion, unpleasant taste, dyspnea, epistaxis, nasal irritation, upper respiratory infection. **OCCASIONAL:** Sweaty palms, clammy skin, nausea, dizziness, dry mouth, headache. **RARE:** Restlessness, crying, euphoria, vomiting, bitter taste, urinary urgency, skin burning/itching, blurred vision.

ADVERSE REACTIONS/TOXIC EFFECTS

Abrupt withdrawal after prolonged use may produce symptoms of narcotic withdrawal (abdominal cramping, rhinorrhea, lacrimation, anxiety, increased temperature, piloerection [goosebumps]). Overdosage results in severe respiratory depression, skeletal muscle flaccidity, cyanosis, extreme somnolence progressing to convulsions, stupor, coma. Tolerance to analgesic effect, physical dependence may occur w/chronic use.

NURSING IMPLICATIONS

BASELINE ASSESSMENT:

Obtain vital signs before giving medication. If respirations are 12/min or lower (20/min or lower in children), withhold medication, contact physician. Assess onset, type, location, duration of pain. Effect of medication is reduced if full pain recurs before next dose. Protect from falls. During labor, assess fetal heart tones, uterine contractions.

INTERVENTION/EVALUATION:

Increase fluid intake and environmental humidity to improve viscosity of lung secretions. Monitor for change in respirations, B/P, change in rate/quality of pulse. Monitor pattern of daily bowel activity, stool consistency. Initiate deep breathing and coughing exercises, particularly in those w/impaired pulmonary function. Change pt's position q2-4h. Assess for clinical improvement and record onset of relief of pain.

PATIENT/FAMILY TEACHING:

Change positions slowly to avoid dizziness. Avoid tasks that require alertness, motor skills until response to drug is established. Instruct pt on proper use of nasal spray. Avoid use of alcohol or CNS depressants.

calcipotriene (Dovonex)
See supplement

calcitonin-salmon

kal-sih-toe´nin
(Calcimar, Miacalcin)

CANADIAN AVAILABILITY:
Calcimar

CLASSIFICATION

Calcium regulator

PHARMACOKINETICS

Rapidly metabolized (primarily in kidney). Primarily excreted in urine. Half-life: 70-90 minutes.

ACTION

Regulates serum calcium concentration. Decreases rate of bone turnover (initially blocks bone resorption). Decreases the number and function of osteoclasts.

USES

Management of moderate to severe Paget's disease of bone, early treatment of hypercalcemic emergencies. Management of postmenopausal osteoporosis to prevent progressive loss of bone mass (w/calcium, vitamin D).

STORAGE/HANDLING

Calcitonin-salmon: refrigerate; calcitonin-human: after reconstitution, use within 6 hrs.

SubQ/IM ADMINISTRATION

1. May be administered SubQ or IM. No more than 2 ml dose should be given IM.
2. Skin test should be performed before therapy.
3. Bedtime administration may reduce nausea, flushing.

INDICATIONS/DOSAGE/ROUTES

Skin testing: Prepare a 10 U/ml dilution; withdraw 0.05 ml from 200 IU/ml vial (0.1 ml from 100 IU/ml vial) solution in tuberculin syringe; fill up to 1 ml w/0.9% NaCl. Take 0.1 ml and inject intracutaneously on inner aspect of forearm. Observe after 15 min (positive response: appearance of more than mild erythema or wheal).

Paget's disease:
IM/SubQ: Adults, elderly: Initially, 100 IU/day (improvement in biochemical abnormalities, bone pain seen in first few months; in neurologic lesion, often longer than 1 yr). **Maintenance:** 50 IU/day or every other day.

Postmenopausal osteoporosis:
IM/SubQ: Adults, elderly: 100 IU/day (w/adequate calcium and vitamin D intake).

Hypercalcemia:
IM/SubQ: Adults, elderly: Initially, 4 IU/kg q12h; may increase to 8 IU/kg q12h if no response in 2 days; may further increase to 8 IU/kg q6h if no response in 2 days.

PRECAUTIONS

CONTRAINDICATIONS: Hypersensitivity to fish, calcitonin. Data does not support use in children. **CAUTIONS:** History of allergy, renal dysfunction. **PREGNANCY/LACTATION:** Drug does not cross placenta; unknown if distributed in breast milk. Safe usage during lactation not established (inhibits lactation in animals). **Pregnancy Category C.**

INTERACTIONS

DRUG INTERACTIONS: None significant. **ALTERED LAB VALUES:** None significant.

SIDE EFFECTS

FREQUENT: Nausea may occur in 30 min after injection, usually diminishes w/length of therapy. Anorexia, vomiting, diarrhea, flushing of face, ears, hands, and feet. **OCCASIONAL:** Tenderness/tingling of palms and soles, local inflammation at injection site, initial diuresis, unusual taste. **RARE:** Headache, chest pressure, nasal congestion, hypersensitivity (including rash, urticaria).

ADVERSE REACTIONS/TOXIC EFFECTS

Potential for hypocalcemic tetany or anaphylaxis w/protein allergy.

NURSING IMPLICATIONS

BASELINE ASSESSMENT:

Question for allergies, hypersensitivity to fish, calcitonin. Establish baseline electrolytes.

INTERVENTION/EVALUATION:

Assess for allergic response: rash, urticaria, swelling, shortness of breath, tachycardia, hypotension. Assure rotation of injection sites; check for inflammation. Monitor electrolytes.

PATIENT/FAMILY TEACHING:

Instruct pt/family on aseptic technique, proper injection of medication, including rotation of sites. Do not take any other medications w/o consulting physician. Nausea and flushing are transient; nausea and diuresis usually decrease w/continued therapy. Notify physician immediately if rash, urticaria, shortness of breath occur. Follow-up lab tests, office visits are necessary.

calcium acetate
(Phos-Ex, PhosLo)

calcium carbonate
(Dicarbasil, OsCal, Titralac, Tums)

calcium chloride

calcium citrate
(Citracal)

calcium glubionate
(NeoCalglucon)

calcium gluconate

CANADIAN AVAILABILITY: Apo-Cal, Calciject, Calsan, Caltrate, Calcium-Sandoz

CLASSIFICATION

Antacid, antihypocalcemic, nutritional supplement

PHARMACOKINETICS

Moderately absorbed from small intestine (dependent on presence of vitamin D metabolites, pH). Protein binding: 45%. Primarily eliminated in feces.

ACTION

Neutralizes or reduces gastric acid (increase pH). Essential for function, integrity of nervous, muscular, skeletal systems. Important role in normal cardiac, renal function, respiration, blood coagulation, and cell membrane and capillary permeability. Assists in regulating release/storage of neurotransmitter/hormones. *Calcium acetate:* Combines w/dietary phosphate forming insoluble calcium phosphate.

USES

Parenteral: Acute hypocalcemia (e.g., neonatal hypocalcemic tetany, alkalosis), electrolyte depletion, cardiac arrest (strengthens myocardial contractions), hyperkalemia (reverses EKG, cardiac depression), hypermagnesemia (aids in reversing CNS depression). *Oral:* Chronic hypocalcemia, calcium deficiency, antacid. *Calcium acetate:* Controls hyperphosphatemia in end stage renal disease.

PO/IV ADMINISTRATION

PO:

1. Take tablets w/full glass of water 0.5-1 hr after meals. Give syrup before meals (increases absorption), diluted in juice or water.
2. Chew chewable tablets well before swallowing.

IV:

1. Give by slow IV injection (0.5-1 ml/min for calcium chloride; 1.5-3 ml/min for calcium gluconate).
2. Maximum rate for intermittent infusion is 200 mg/min of calcium

gluconate (e.g., 10 ml/min when 1 Gm diluted w/50 ml diluent).

INDICATIONS/DOSAGE/ROUTES

CALCIUM ACETATE

Hypophosphatemia:
PO: Adults, elderly: 2 tablets 3 times/day w/meals.

CALCIUM CARBONATE

Antihypocalcemic, nutritional supplement:
PO: Adults, elderly: 1.25 Gm (500 mg calcium) 1-3 times/day.

Antacid:
PO: Adults, elderly: 0.5-1.25 Gm as needed.

CALCIUM CITRATE

Antihypocalcemic:
PO: Adults, elderly: 1-2 tablets 2-4 times/day.

Nutritional supplement:
PO: Adults, elderly: 4-8 tablets/day in 3-4 divided doses.

CALCIUM GLUBIONATE

Antihypocalcemic:
PO: Adults, elderly: 15 ml 3-4 times/day. **Children 1-4 yrs:** 10 ml 3 times/day. **Children <1 yr:** 5 ml 5 times/day.

CALCIUM CHLORIDE, CALCIUM GLUCONATE

Emergency increase of calcium:
IV: Adults, elderly: 7-14 mEq. **Children:** 1-7 mEq. **Infants:** <1 mEq. May repeat dose q1-3 days.

Hypocalcemic tetany:
IV: Adults, elderly: 4.5-16 mEq. May repeat until therapeutic response. **Children:** 0.5-0.7 mEq/kg 3-4 times/day. **Neonates:** 2.4 mEq/kg/day in divided doses.

Cardiopulmonary resuscitation:
IV: Adults, elderly: *Calcium gluconate:* 2.3-3.7 mEq. May repeat as needed. *Calcium chloride:* 2.7 mEq. May repeat as needed. **Children:** *Calcium chloride:* 0.27 mEq/kg. May repeat in 10 min if needed.

Hyperkalemia:
IV: Adults, elderly: 2.25-14 mEq. Monitor ECG. May repeat after 1-2 min if needed.

Magnesium intoxication:
IV: Adults, elderly: 7 mEq. May repeat based on pt response.

PRECAUTIONS

CONTRAINDICATIONS: Ventricular fibrillation, hypercalcemia, hypercalciuria, calcium renal calculi, sarcoidosis, digoxin toxicity. *Calcium acetate:* Hypoparathyroidism, decreased renal function. **CAUTIONS:** Dehydration, history of renal calculi, chronic renal impairment, decreased cardiac function, ventricular fibrillation during cardiac resuscitation. **PREGNANCY/LACTATION:** Distributed in breast milk. Unknown whether calcium chloride or gluconate is distributed in breast milk. **Pregnancy Category C.**

INTERACTIONS

DRUG INTERACTIONS: May antagonize etidronate effects. May decrease absorption of ketoconazole, phenytoin, tetracyclines. May decrease effects of methenamine, parenteral magnesium. May increase risk of arrhythmias w/digoxin. **ALTERED LAB VALUES:** May increase calcium gastrin, pH. May decrease phosphate, potassium.

SIDE EFFECTS

FREQUENT: *Parenteral:* Hypotension, flushing, feeling of warmth, nausea, vomiting; pain, rash, redness, burning at injection site; sweating, decreased B/P. **RARE:** Hypercalcemia: drowsiness, weakness, nausea, vomiting. *Oral:* Difficult or painful urination.

ADVERSE REACTIONS/TOXIC EFFECTS

Hypercalcemia: Early signs: Constipation, headache, dry mouth, increased thirst, irritability, decreased appetite, metallic taste, fatigue, weakness, depression. Later signs: Confusion, drowsiness, increased B/P, increased light sensitivity, irregular heartbeat, nausea, vomiting, increased urination.

NURSING IMPLICATIONS

BASELINE ASSESSMENT:

Assess B/P, EKG readings, renal function, magnesium, phosphate, potassium concentrations.

INTERVENTION/EVALUATION:

Monitor B/P, EKG, renal function, magnesium, phosphate, potassium, serum and urine calcium concentrations. Monitor for signs of hypercalcemia.

PATIENT/FAMILY TEACHING:

Stress importance of diet. Take tablets w/full glass of water, 1/2-1 hr after meals. Give liquid before meals. Do not take within 1-2 hrs of other oral medications, fiber-containing foods. Avoid excessive alcohol, tobacco, caffeine.

calcium carbonate

(Dicarbosil, Titralac, Tums)

FIXED-COMBINATION(S): W/aluminum and magnesium hydroxide, antacids (Camalox).

CANADIAN AVAILABILITY: Apo-Cal, Calcite 500, Calsan, Caltrate, Os-Cal

CLASSIFICATION

CLINICAL: Antacid, antihypocalcemic

PHARMACOKINETICS

Partially absorbed from intestine (determined by parathyroid hormone, vitamin D). Onset of action based on ability to solubilize in stomach and react w/hydrochloric acid. Duration of action based primarily on gastric emptying time (20 min when given before meals, up to 3 hrs given after meals).

ACTION

Neutralizes or reduces gastric acid by increasing gastric pH, inhibiting pepsin activity.

USES

Symptomatic relief of upset stomach associated w/hyperacidity (heartburn, acid indigestion, sour stomach). Hyperacidity associated w/gastric/duodenal ulcers. Symptomatic treatment of gastroesophageal reflux disease. Prophylactic treatment of GI bleeding secondary to gastritis and stress ulceration. Treatment of calcium depletion occurring in chronic hypoparathyroidism, osteomalacia, secondary to administration of anticonvulsant medication, vitamin D deficiency.

INDICATIONS/DOSAGE/ROUTES

Antacid:
PO: Adults: 0.5-1.5 Gm, as needed.

PRECAUTIONS

CONTRAINDICATIONS: Ventricular fibrillation, hypercalcemia, hypercalciuria, calcium renal calculi, sarcoidosis, digoxin toxicity. *Calcium acetate:* Hypoparathyroidism, decreased renal function. **CAUTIONS:** Dehydration, history of renal calculi, chronic renal impairment, decreased cardiac function, ventricular fibrillation during cardiac resuscitation. **PREGNANCY/LACTATION:** Distributed in breast milk. Unknown whether calcium chloride or gluconate is distributed in breast milk. **Pregnancy Category C.**

INTERACTIONS

DRUG INTERACTIONS: May antagonize etidronate effects. May decrease absorption of ketoconazole, phenytoin, tetracyclines. May decrease effects of methenamine, parenteral magnesium. May increase risk of arrhythmias w/digoxin. **ALTERED LAB VALUES:** May increase calcium gastrin, pH. May decrease phosphate, potassium.

SIDE EFFECTS

FREQUENT: *Parenteral:* Hypotension, flushing, feeling of warmth, nausea, vomiting; pain, rash, redness, burning at injection site; sweating, decreased B/P. **RARE:** Hypercalcemia: drowsiness, weakness, nausea, vomiting. *Oral:* Difficult or painful urination.

ADVERSE REACTIONS/TOXIC EFFECTS

Hypercalcemia: Early signs: Constipation, headache, dry mouth, increased thirst, irritability, decreased appetite, metallic taste, fatigue, weakness, depression. Later signs: Confusion, drowsiness, increased B/P, increased light sensitivity, irregular heartbeat, nausea, vomiting, increased urination.

NURSING IMPLICATIONS

BASELINE ASSESSMENT:

Assess B/P, EKG readings, renal function, magnesium, phosphate, potassium concentrations.

INTERVENTION/EVALUATION:

Assess for relief of gastric distress. Monitor B/P, EKG, renal function, magnesium, phosphate, potassium, serum and urine calcium concentrations. Monitor for signs of hypercalcemia.

PATIENT/FAMILY TEACHING:

Stress importance of diet. Take tablets w/full glass of water, 1/2-1 hr after meals. Give liquid before meals. Do not take within 1-2 hrs of other oral medications, fiber-containing foods. Avoid excessive alcohol, tobacco, caffeine.

capsaicin

cap-say´sin
(Axsain, Zostrix)

CANADIAN AVAILABILITY:
Zostrix

CLASSIFICATION

Topical analgesic

ACTION

Depletes and prevents reaccumulation of substance P in peripheral sensory neurons. (Substance P bnis believed to be the principal chemomediator of pain impulses from the periphery to the CNS). Substance P is also released into joint tissues and activates inflammatory mediators.

USES

Axsain: Temporary relief of neuralgia such as diabetic neuropathy and after trauma/surgery. *Zostrix:* Temporary relief of neuralgia following episodes of herpes zoster infections.

INDICATIONS/DOSAGE/ROUTES

Usual topical dosage:
TOPICAL: Adults, elderly, children >2 yrs: Apply directly to affected area 3-4 times/day. Continue for 14 to 28 days for optimal clinical response.

PRECAUTIONS

CONTRAINDICATIONS: Hypersensitivity to any component of the preparation. **CAUTIONS:** For external use only. **PREGNANCY/LACTATION: Pregnancy Category C.**

INTERACTIONS

DRUG INTERACTIONS: None significant. **ALTERED LAB VALUES:** None significant.

SIDE EFFECTS

OCCASIONAL: Burning, stinging, erythema at site of application.

NURSING IMPLICATIONS

PATIENT/FAMILY TEACHING:

For external use only. Avoid contact w/eyes, broken/irritated skin. Transient burning may occur on application, usually disappears after 72 hrs. Wash hands immediately after application. If there is no improvement or condition deteriorates after 28 days, discontinue use and consult physician.

captopril

cap toe-prill
(Capoten)

FIXED-COMBINATION(S): W/hydrochlorothiazide, a diuretic (Capozide)

CANADIAN AVAILABILITY: Capoten

CLASSIFICATION

Angiotensin converting enzyme (ACE) inhibitor

PHARMACOKINETICS

	ONSET	PEAK	DURATION
PO	0.25 hrs	0.5-1.5 hrs	Dose related

Rapid, well absorbed from GI tract (decreased in presence of food). Protein binding: 25-30%. Metabolized in liver. Primarily excreted in urine. Removed by hemodialysis. Half-life: <3 hrs (increased in decreased renal function).

ACTION

Suppresses renin-angiotensin-aldosterone system (prevents conversion of angiotensin I to angiotensin II, a potent vasoconstrictor; may inhibit angiotensin II at local vascular, renal sites). Decreases plasma angiotensin II; increases plasma renin activity; decreases aldosterone secretion. In hypertension, reduces peripheral arterial resistance. In CHF, increases cardiac output, decreases peripheral vascular resistance, B/P, pulmonary capillary wedge pressure, pulmonary vascular resistance.

USES

Treatment of hypertension alone

or in combination w/other antihypertensives. Adjunctive therapy for CHF (in combination w/cardiac glycosides, diuretics). Reduces development of severe heart failure following MI in pts w/impaired left ventricular (LV) function. Treat nephropathy/prevent kidney failure in Type I diabetes.

PO ADMINISTRATION

1. Best taken 1 hr before meals for maximum absorption (food significantly decreases drug absorption).
2. Tablets may be crushed.

INDICATIONS/DOSAGE/ROUTES

Hypertension:
PO: Adults, elderly: Initially, 12.5-25 mg 2-3 times/day. After 1-2 weeks, may increase to 50 mg 2-3 times/day. Diuretic may be added if no response in additional 1-2 wks. If taken in combination w/diuretic, may increase to 100-150 mg, 2-3 times/day after 1-2 wks. **Maintenance:** 25-150 mg 2-3 times/day. **Maximum:** 450 mg/day.

CHF:
PO: Adults, elderly: Initially, 6.25-25 mg 3 times/day. Increase to 50 mg 3 times/day. After at least 2 wks, may increase to 50-100 mg 3 times/day. **Maximum:** 450 mg/day.

Post MI, impaired LV function:
PO: Adults, elderly: 6.25 mg once, then 12.5 mg 3 times/day. Increase to 25 mg 3 times/day over several days up to 50 mg 3 times/day over several weeks.

Nephropathy/prevention of kidney failure:
PO: Adults, elderly: 25 mg 3 times/day.

PRECAUTIONS

CONTRAINDICATIONS: History of angioedema w/previous treatment w/ACE inhibitors. **CAUTIONS:** Renal impairment, those w/sodium depletion or on diuretic therapy, dialysis, hypovolemia, coronary/cerebrovascular insufficiency. **PREGNANCY/LACTATION:** Crosses placenta; distributed in breast milk. May cause fetal/neonatal mortality/morbidity. **Pregnancy Category C.**

INTERACTIONS

DRUG INTERACTIONS: Alcohol, diuretics, hypotensive agents may increase effect. NSAIDs may decrease effect. Potassium-sparing diuretics, potassium supplements may cause hyperkalemia. May increase lithium concentration, toxicity. **ALTERED LAB VALUES:** May increase potassium, SGOT (AST), SGPT (ALT), alkaline phosphatase, bilirubin, BUN, creatinine. May decrease sodium. May cause positive ANA titer.

SIDE EFFECTS

FREQUENT: Rash and/or urticaria, change/decrease in sense of taste, orthostatic hypotension during initial therapy. **OCCASIONAL:** Urinary frequency. **RARE:** Cough, proteinuria (mostly occurs in those w/history of renal disease), dry mouth, GI distress, headache, dizziness.

ADVERSE REACTIONS/TOXIC EFFECTS

Excessive hypotension ("first-dose syncope") may occur in those w/CHF, severely salt/volume depleted. Angioedema (swelling of face/lips), hyperkalemia occur rarely. Agranulocytosis, neutropenia may be noted in those w/impaired renal function or collagen vascular disease (systemic lupus erythematosus, scleroderma).

Nephrotic syndrome may be noted in those w/history of renal disease.

NURSING IMPLICATIONS

BASELINE ASSESSMENT:

Obtain B/P immediately before each dose, in addition to regular monitoring (be alert to fluctuations). If excessive reduction in B/P occurs, place pt in supine position w/legs elevated. Renal function tests should be performed before therapy begins. In those w/prior renal disease or receiving dosages higher than 150 mg/day, urine test for protein by dipstick method should be made w/first urine of day before therapy begins and periodically thereafter. In those w/renal impairment, autoimmune disease, or taking drugs that affect leukocytes or immune response, CBC and differential count should be performed before therapy begins and q2wks for 3 mos, then periodically thereafter.

INTERVENTION/EVALUATION:

Assess skin for rash, hives. Assess for peripheral edema of hands, feet (usually, first area of lower extremity swelling is behind medial malleolus in ambulatory, sacral area in bedridden). Assist w/ambulation if dizziness occurs. Check for urinary frequency. Assess lung sounds for rales, wheezing in those w/CHF. Monitor urinalysis for proteinuria. Assess for anorexia secondary to decreased taste perception. Monitor serum potassium levels in those on concurrent diuretic therapy.

PATIENT/FAMILY TEACHING:

To reduce hypotensive effect, rise slowly from lying to sitting position and permit legs to dangle from bed momentarily before standing. Report peripheral edema or any sign of infection (sore throat, fever). Several wks may be needed for full therapeutic effect of B/P reduction. Skipping doses or voluntarily discontinuing drug may produce severe, rebound hypertension. Avoid alcohol.

carbachol, intraocular

kar´bah-kole

(Miostat Intraocular)

carbachol, topical

(Isopto Carbachol)

CANADIAN AVAILABILITY:

Isopto-Carbachol, Miostat

CLASSIFICATION

Antiglaucoma

PHARMACOKINETICS

	ONSET	PEAK	DURATION
ORTHOP (IOP)	10-20 min	4 hrs	8 hrs

Miosis maximal in 2-5 min; persists for 24 hrs.

ACTION

Directly stimulates cholinergic receptors. Contracts iris sphincter muscle (miosis), ciliary muscle (increased accommodation), and decreases intraocular pressure (decrease resistance to aqueous humor outflow).

USES

To decrease elevated intraocular pressure in glaucoma (generally in pts who develop allergies or tolerance to pilocarpine); to counter the effects of cycloplegics and mydriatics after surgery or ophthalmoscopic examination.

OPHTHALMIC ADMINISTRATION

TOPICAL:

1. Instruct pt to lie down or tilt head backward and look up.
2. Gently pull lower lid down to form pouch and instill medication.
3. Do not touch tip of applicator to any surface.
4. When lower lid is released, have pt keep eye open w/o blinking for at least 30 sec.
5. Apply gentle finger pressure to lacrimal sac (bridge of the nose, inside corner of the eye) for 1-2 min.
6. Remove excess solution around eye w/tissue. Wash hands immediately to remove medication on hands.
7. Tell pt not to close eyes tightly or blink more often than necessary.
8. Never rinse dropper.
9. Do not use solution if discolored.

INTRAOCULAR:

1. Appropriate dose is drawn into dry, sterile syringe; needle is replaced w/suitable atraumatic cannula for intraocular irrigation.
2. Physician instills into anterior chamber of the eye during surgery.
3. Unused portions are discarded.

INDICATIONS/DOSAGE/ROUTES

Miosis in surgery:
OPHTHALMIC: Adults, elderly: Instill up to 0.5 ml into anterior chamber before or after securing sutures.

Glaucoma:
OPHTHALMIC: Adults, elderly: 1-2 drops up to 4 times/day.

PRECAUTIONS

CONTRAINDICATIONS: Hypersensitivity to any components; any condition where miosis is undesirable (e.g., acute iritis, some forms of secondary glaucoma, acute inflammatory disease of the anterior chamber). Safety in children not established. **CAUTIONS:** Corneal abrasions, bronchial asthma, spastic GI conditions, urinary tract obstruction, peptic ulcer, severe bradycardia, hypotension, epilepsy, hyperthyroidism, recent myocardial infarction. **PREGNANCY/LACTATION:** Safety during lactation not known. **Pregnancy Category C.**

INTERACTIONS

DRUG INTERACTIONS: May be ineffective following flurbiprofen. **ALTERED LAB VALUES:** None significant.

SIDE EFFECTS

FREQUENT: Difficulty in dark adaptation. **OCCASIONAL:** Headache, postop iritis following cataract extraction (w/intraocular use), ciliary spasm causing temporary decreased visual acuity. **RARE:** Bullous keratopathy. Systemic: excessive salivation, sweating, flushing, epigastric distress, vomiting, diarrhea, asthma, syncope, cardiac arrhythmias, urinary bladder contractions.

ADVERSE REACTIONS/TOXIC EFFECTS

Retinal detachment has occurred in susceptible individuals, those w/preexisting retinal disease or those predisposed to retinal tears.

NURSING IMPLICATIONS

BASELINE ASSESSMENT:

Question for hypersensitivity to components. Obtain baseline pulse, B/P. Assess physical appearance of eye and pt's perception of vision.

INTERVENTION/EVALUATION:

Evaluate therapeutic response. Assess for systemic reaction, esp. sweating, flushing, increased salivation. Check B/P, pulse, respiration.

PATIENT/FAMILY TEACHING:

Do not drive for several hours after administration. Avoid night driving or performing hazardous tasks in poor light. Blurred vision usually decreases w/prolonged use. W/glaucoma, probably will need medication for remainder of life. Important to remain under physician's care. Teach proper administration (see Ophthalmic Administration). Notify physician of difficulty breathing, change in vision, sweating, flushing.

carbamazepine

car-bah-maz´eh-peen

(Epitol, Tegretol)

CANADIAN AVAILABILITY:
Apo-Carbamazepine, Mazepine, Tegretol

CLASSIFICATION

Anticonvulsant

PHARMACOKINETICS

Slowly, completely absorbed from GI tract. Protein binding: 75-90%. Metabolized in liver to active metabolite. Primarily excreted in urine. Half-life: 25-65 hrs (decreased w/chronic use).

ACTION

Decreases synaptic transmission by blocking or inhibiting sodium channels.

USES

Management of generalized tonic-clonic seizures (grand mal), complex partial seizures (temporal lobe, psychomotor), mixed seizures; treatment of trigeminal neuralgia (tic douloureux).

STORAGE/HANDLING

Store oral suspension, tablets at room temperature.

PO ADMINISTRATION

1. Give w/meals to reduce risk of GI distress.
2. Shake oral suspension well.

INDICATIONS/DOSAGE/ROUTES

NOTE: When replacement by another anticonvulsant is necessary, decrease carbamazepine gradually as therapy begins w/low replacement dose. When transferring from tablets to suspension, divide total tablet daily dose into smaller, more frequent doses of suspension.

Seizure control:

PO: Adults, elderly, children >12 yrs: Initially, 200 mg 2 times/day. Increase dosage up to 200 mg/day at weekly intervals until response is attained. **Maintenance:** 800-1200 mg/day. Do not exceed 1,000 mg/day in children 12-15 yrs, 1,200 mg/day in pts >15 yrs. **Children 6-12 yrs:** Initially, 100 mg 2 times/day. Increase by 100 mg/day until response is attained. **Maintenance:** 400-800 mg/day. Give dosage 200 mg or greater/day in 3-4 equally divided doses. **Syrup: Children 6-12 yrs:** Initially, 50 mg

4 times/day. Increase dosage slowly (reduces sedation risk).

Trigeminal neuralgia:
PO: Adults, elderly: 100 mg 2 times/day on day 1. Increase by 100 mg q12h until pain is relieved. **Maintenance:** 200-1200 mg/day. Do not exceed 1200 mg/day.

PRECAUTIONS

CONTRAINDICATIONS: History of bone marrow depression, history of hypersensitivity to tricyclic antidepressants. **CAUTIONS:** Impaired cardiac, hepatic, renal function. **PREGNANCY/LACTATION:** Crosses placenta; distributed in breast milk. Accumulates in fetal tissue. **Pregnancy Category C.**

INTERACTIONS

DRUG INTERACTIONS: May decrease effect of steroids, anticoagulants. May increase metabolism of anticonvulsants, barbiturates, benzodiazepines, valproic acid. Tricyclic antidepressants, haloperidol, antipsychotics may increase CNS depressant effects. Cimetidine may increase concentration, toxicity. May decrease effects of estrogens, quinidine. Diltiazem, erythromycin, propoxyphene, verapamil may increase toxicity. May increase metabolism of isoniazid (hepatotoxicity). Isoniazid may increase concentration, toxicity. MAO inhibitors may cause hypertensive crises, convulsions. **ALTERED LAB VALUES:** May increase BUN, glucose, protein, SGOT (AST), SGPT (ALT), alkaline phosphatase, bilirubin, cholesterol, HDL, triglycerides. May decrease calcium, T_3, T_4, T_4 index.

SIDE EFFECTS

OCCASIONAL: Drowsiness, dizziness, nausea, vomiting, visual abnormalities (spots before eyes, difficulty focusing, blurred vision), dry mouth/pharynx, tongue irritation, headache, water retention, increased sweating, constipation/diarrhea.

ADVERSE REACTIONS/TOXIC EFFECTS

Toxic reactions appear as blood dyscrasias (aplastic anemia, agranulocytosis, thrombocytopenia, leukopenia, leukocytosis, eosinophilia), cardiovascular disturbances (CHF, hypo/hypertension, thrombophlebitis, arrhythmias), dermatologic effects (rash, urticaria, pruritus, photosensitivity). Abrupt withdrawal may precipitate status epilepticus.

NURSING IMPLICATIONS

Baseline Assessment:

Seizures: Review history of seizure disorder (intensity, frequency, duration, LOC). Provide safety precautions; quiet, dark environment. CBC, platelet count, serum iron determinations, urinalysis, BUN should be performed before therapy begins and periodically during therapy.

Intervention/Evaluation:

Seizures: Observe frequently for recurrence of seizure activity. Assess for clinical improvement (decrease in intensity/frequency of seizures). Monitor for therapeutic serum level (3-14 mcg/ml). Assess for clinical evidence of early toxic signs (fever, sore throat, mouth ulcerations, easy bruising, unusual bleeding, joint pain). *Neuralgia:* Avoid triggering tic douloureux (draft, talking, washing face, jarring bed, hot/warm/cold food or liquids).

PATIENT/FAMILY TEACHING:

Do not abruptly withdraw medication following long-term use (may precipitate seizures). Strict maintenance of drug therapy is essential for seizure control. Drowsiness usually disappears during continued therapy. Avoid tasks that require alertness, motor skills until response to drug is established. Report visual abnormalities. Blood tests should be repeated frequently during first 3 mos of therapy and at monthly intervals thereafter for 2-3 yrs.

carbamide peroxide

car′bah-mide
(Cankaid, Gly-Oxide Liquid, Orajel Brace-aid Rinse, Proxigel)

FIXED-COMBINATION(S):
W/glycerin (Murine Ear Drops, Murine Ear Wax Removal System, Auro Ear Drops, Debrox Drops, E. R. O. Ear Drops, Carbamide Peroxide Otic Drops)

CANADIAN AVAILABILITY:
Calmurid, Dermaflex, Onyvul, Uremol, Urisec.

CLASSIFICATION

Topical

ACTION

Releases oxygen with foaming action that provides cleansing effects, weak antibacterial action; w/glycerin, cerumen (ear wax) is softened by glycerin and loosened by carbamide peroxide for removal.

USES

Topical oral: Treatment of aphthous ulcers (canker sores), gingivitis, periodontitis, stomatitis, Vincent's infection, inflammation (due to dentures, mouth appliances, dental procedures); adjunct to oral hygiene. *Otic:* Adjunct to the removal of hardened, excessive cerumen from the external ear; aid in prevention of ceruminosis.

TOPICAL/OTIC ADMINISTRATION

NOTE: Keep all preparations away from eyes.

TOPICAL (ORAL):

1. Apply undiluted to area of mouth. Gel should be massaged gently into area w/swab.
2. Pt should expectorate after 1-3 min.
3. No rinsing or drinking for at least 5 min after application.

OTIC:

1. Tilt head sideways.
2. Instill drops keeping applicator outside of the ear canal.
3. Let solution remain in ear for 15 min or longer (keep head sideways or place cotton pledget in ear).
4. Irrigate gently with warm water, using a soft rubber-bulb syringe to remove softened cerumen. Take care not to obstruct flow of water leaving ear canal w/tip of ear syringe.

INDICATIONS/DOSAGE/ROUTES

Usual topical dosage:
SOLUTION: Adults, elderly: Several drops 4 times/day undiluted after meals and at bedtime.
GEL: Adults, elderly: 4 times/day undiluted.

Usual otic dosage:
OTIC: Adults, elderly: 5-10 drops 2 times/day for up to 4 days.

PRECAUTIONS

CONTRAINDICATIONS: Known or suspected injury, otic surgery (unless directed by physician), perforation of eardrum. Self-medication should not be used for children younger than 3 yrs for oral, younger than 12 yrs for otic. **PREGNANCY/LACTATION: Pregnancy Category C.**

INTERACTIONS

DRUG INTERACTIONS: None significant. **ALTERED LAB VALUES:** None significant.

SIDE EFFECTS

RARE: Redness, itching, irritation.

NURSING IMPLICATIONS

BASELINE ASSESSMENT:

Assess baseline discomfort and extent of topical involvement.

INTERVENTION/EVALUATION:

Monitor for therapeutic response or worsening of symptoms.

PATIENT/FAMILY TEACHING:

Teach proper administration (see Topical [Oral]/Otic Administration). Do not use oral preparations longer than 7 days, otic preparations longer than 4 days unless directed by physician. Notify physician if symptoms worsen. *Otic:* Do not use if there is ear drainage/discharge, ear pain, rash, dizziness; consult physician. Foaming is to be expected. Never use toothpicks, cotton swabs, hairpins, or other such instruments to remove wax from ear canal.

carbenicillin indanyl sodium

car-ben-ih-sill′in
(Geocillin)

CANADIAN AVAILABILITY:
Geopen Oral

CLASSIFICATION

Antibiotic: Penicillin

PHARMACOKINETICS

Moderately absorbed from GI tract. Protein binding: 50-60%. Primarily excreted unchanged in urine. Removed by hemodialysis. Half-life: 1-1.5 hrs (increased in decreased renal function).

ACTION

Bactericidal. Binds to bacterial membranes. Inhibits cell wall synthesis.

USES

Treatment of prostatitis, urinary tract infections; preop prophylaxis in transurethral resection.

PO ADMINISTRATION

1. Give 1 hr before or 2 hrs after food.
2. Space doses evenly around the clock.

INDICATIONS/DOSAGE/ROUTES

Urinary tract infections (including chronic UTI), asymptomatic bacteruria:
PO: Adults, elderly: 382-764 mg 4 times/day.

Prostatitis:
PO: Adults, elderly: 764 mg 4 times/day for 2-4 wks.

PRECAUTIONS

CONTRAINDICATIONS: Hypersensitivity to any penicillin. **CAUTIONS:** History of allergies, esp. cephalosporins. **PREGNANCY/LACTATION:** Crosses placenta; appears in cord blood, amniotic fluid. Distributed in breast milk in low concentrations. May lead to allergic sensitization, diarrhea, candidiasis, skin rash in infant. **Pregnancy Category B.**

INTERACTIONS

DRUG INTERACTIONS: None significant. **ALTERED LAB VALUES:** None significant.

FREQUENT: Bitter aftertaste and smell. **OCCASIONAL:** Nausea, vomiting, diarrhea, flatulence (directly proportional to dosage). **RARE:** Dry mouth.

ADVERSE REACTIONS/TOXIC EFFECTS

Hypersensitivity reactions, including anaphylaxis. Superinfections, potentially fatal antibiotic-associated colitis may result from bacterial imbalance.

NURSING IMPLICATIONS

BASELINE ASSESSMENT:

Question for history of allergies, esp. penicillins, cephalosporins. Obtain specimen for culture, sensitivity before giving first dose (therapy may begin before results are known).

INTERVENTION/EVALUATION:

Hold medication and promptly report rash (hypersensitivity) or diarrhea (w/fever, abdominal pain, blood and mucus in stool may indicate antibiotic-associated colitis). Check food tolerance. Provide mouth care, sugar-free gum/hard candy to offset taste, smell effects. Monitor I&O, urinalysis, renal function tests. Assess for superinfection: increased fever, sore throat onset, diarrhea, vomiting, genital/anal pruritus, vaginitis, ulceration of oral mucosa.

PATIENT/FAMILY TEACHING:

Space doses evenly. Continue antibiotic for full length of treatment. Notify physician in event of rash, diarrhea, vomiting, other new symptom.

carbidopa/levodopa

car′bih-dope-ah/lev′oh-dope-ah
(Sinemet)

CANADIAN AVAILABILITY:
Sinemet

CLASSIFICATION

Antiparkinson

PHARMACOKINETICS

Carbidopa: Rapid, completely absorbed from GI tract. Widely distributed. Protein binding: 36%. Excreted primarily in urine. Half-life: 1-2 hrs. *Levodopa:* Converted to dopamine. Excreted primarily in urine. Half-life: 1-3 hrs.

ACTION

Carbidopa: Inhibits peripheral decarboxylation of levodopa. *Levodopa:* Stimulates dopaminergic receptors in basal ganglia improving balance of cholinergic/dopaminergic activity, improving modulation of voluntary nerve impulse transmission to motor cortex.

USES

Treatment of idiopathic Parkinson's disease (paralysis agitans), postencephalitic parkinsonism, symptomatic parkinsonism following injury to nervous system by carbon monoxide poisoning, manganese intoxication.

PO ADMINISTRATION

1. Scored tablets may be crushed.
2. May be given w/o regard to meals.
3. Do not crush sustained-release tablet; may cut in half.

INDICATIONS/DOSAGE/ROUTES

PARKINSONISM:

Not receiving levodopa:
PO: Adults: 25/100 mg tablet 3 times/day or 10/100 mg tablet 3-4 times/day. May increase by 1 tablet every 1-2 days up to 8 tablets/day.

Usual elderly dosage:
PO: Elderly: Initially, 25/100 2 times/day, gradually increased as necessary.
SUSTAINED RELEASE: Adults: 1 tablet 2 times/day no closer than 6 hrs between doses. **Range:** 2-8 tablets at 4-8 hr intervals. May increase dose at intervals not less than 3 days.

Receiving only levodopa:
NOTE: Discontinue levodopa at least 8 hrs prior to carbidopa/levodopa. Initiate w/dose providing at least 25% of previous levodopa dosage.
PO: Adults (<1500 mg levodopa/day): 1 tablet (25/100 mg) 3-4 times/day.
PO: Adults (>1500 mg levodopa/day): 1 tablet (25/250 mg) 3-4 times/day.
SUSTAINED RELEASE: Adults: 1 tablet 2 times/day.

Receiving carbidopa/levodopa:
SUSTAINED RELEASE: Adults: Provide about 10% more levodopa; may increase up to 30% more at 4-8 hr dosing intervals.

PRECAUTIONS

CONTRAINDICATIONS: Narrow-angle glaucoma, those on MAO inhibitor therapy. **CAUTIONS:** History of MI, bronchial asthma (tartrazine sensitivity), emphysema; severe cardiac, pulmonary, renal, hepatic, endocrine disease; active peptic ulcer, treated open-angle glaucoma. **PREGNANCY/LACTATION:** Unknown if drug crosses placenta or is distributed in breast milk. May inhibit lactation. Do not nurse. **Pregnancy Category C.**

INTERACTIONS

DRUG INTERACTIONS: Anticonvulsants, benzodiazepines, haloperidol, phenothiazines may decrease effect. MAO inhibitors may increase risk of hypertensive crises. Selegiline may increase dyskinesias, nausea, orthostatic hypotension, confusion, hallucinations. **ALTERED LAB VALUES:** May increase alkaline phosphatase, SGOT (AST), SGPT (ALT), LDH, bilirubin, BUN.

SIDE EFFECTS

FREQUENT: Nausea, anorexia, dizziness, orthostatic hypotension, bradycardia, akinesia (temporary muscular weakness; lasts 1 min to 1 hr; also known as "on-off" phenomenon). **OCCASIONAL:** Dry mouth, blurred vision, nervousness, constipation, decreased sweating, mydriasis (pupil dilation), loss of taste, urinary hesitancy and/or retention, headache, dizziness, drowsiness, confusion. **RARE:** Palpitations, tachycardia.

ADVERSE REACTIONS/TOXIC EFFECTS

High incidence of involuntary choreiform, dystonic, dyskinetic movements may be noted in pts on long-term therapy. Mental changes (paranoid ideation, psychotic episodes, depression) may be noted. Numerous mild to severe CNS, psychiatric disturbances may include reduced attention span, anxiety, nightmares, daytime somnolence, euphoria, fatigue, paranoia, hallucinations.

NURSING IMPLICATIONS

BASELINE ASSESSMENT:

Instruct pt to void before giving medication (reduces risk of urinary retention).

INTERVENTION/EVALUATION:

Be alert to neurologic effects: headache, lethargy, mental confusion, agitation. Monitor for evidence of dyskinesia (difficulty w/ movement). Assess for clinical reversal of symptoms (improvement of tremor of head/hands at rest, mask-like facial expression, shuffling gait, muscular rigidity).

PATIENT/FAMILY TEACHING:

Avoid tasks that require alertness, motor skills until response to drug is established. Dry mouth, drowsiness, dizziness may be an expected response of drug. Avoid alcoholic beverages during therapy. Sugarless gum, sips of tepid water may relieve dry mouth. Coffee/tea may help reduce drowsiness.

carboplatin

car-bow-play′tin
(Paraplatin)

CANADIAN AVAILABILITY:
Paraplatin

CLASSIFICATION

Antineoplastic

PHARMACOKINETICS

Hydrolyzed in solution to active form. Protein binding: low. Primarily excreted in urine. Half-life: 2.6-5.9 hrs.

ACTION

Unknown. May be associated w/ cross-linking, interfering w/DNA function. Cell cycle-phase nonspecific.

USES

Treatment of recurrent ovarian carcinoma in those previously treated w/chemotherapy, including cisplatin. Initial treatment of advanced ovarian carcinoma.

STORAGE/HANDLING

NOTE: May be carcinogenic, mutagenic, or teratogenic. Handle w/ extreme care during preparation/ administration.

Store vials at room temperature. Reconstitute immediately before use. After reconstitution, solution stable for 8 hrs. Discard unused portions after 8 hrs.

IV ADMINISTRATION

1. Do not use aluminum needles or administration sets that come in contact w/drug (may produce black precipitate, loss of potency).

2. Reconstitute each 50 mg w/5 ml sterile water for injection, 5%

dextrose, or 0.9% NaCl to provide concentration of 10 mg/ml.

3. May be further diluted w/5% dextrose or 0.9% NaCl to provide concentration as low as 0.5 mg/ml.

4. Infuse over 15-60 min.

5. Rarely, anaphylactic reaction occurs minutes after administration. Use of epinephrine, corticosteroids alleviates symptoms.

INDICATIONS/DOSAGE/ROUTES

NOTE: Dosage individualized based on clinical response, tolerance to adverse effects.

Ovarian carcinoma (single agent):

IV: Adults: 360-400 mg/m^2 on day 1; q4wks. Do not repeat dose until neutrophil, platelet counts are within acceptable levels. Adjust dose in those previously treated based on lowest posttreatment platelet or neutrophil value.

NOTE: Make only one escalation, not >125% of starting dose.

Ovarian carcinoma (combination therapy):

IV: Adults: 300 mg/m^2 (w/cyclophosphamide) on day 1, q4wks. Do not repeat dose until neutrophil, platelet counts are within acceptable levels.

Dosage in renal impairment:

Initial dose based on creatinine clearance; subsequent doses based on pt's tolerance, degree of myelosuppression.

CREATININE CLEARANCE	DOSAGE DAY 1
>60 ml/min	360 mg/m^2
41-59 ml/min	250 mg/m^2
16-40 ml/min	200 mg/m^2

PRECAUTIONS

CONTRAINDICATIONS: History of severe allergic reaction to cisplatin, platinum compounds, mannitol; severe myelosuppression, severe bleeding. **PREGNANCY/LACTATION:** If possible, avoid use during pregnancy, esp. first trimester. May cause fetal harm. Unknown if distributed in breast milk. Breast feeding not recommended. **Pregnancy Category D.**

INTERACTIONS

DRUG INTERACTIONS: Bone marrow depressants may increase bone marrow depression. Nephrotoxic, ototoxic producing agents may increase toxicity. Live virus vaccines may potentiate virus replication, increase vaccine side effects, decrease antibody response to vaccine. **ALTERED LAB VALUES:** May decrease electrolytes (sodium, magnesium, calcium, potassium). High doses (above 4 times recommended dose) may elevate alkaline phosphatase, SGOT (AST), total bilirubin, BUN, serum creatinine concentrations.

SIDE EFFECTS

FREQUENT: Vomiting (may be severe), loss of energy, strength. **OCCASIONAL:** Nausea, generalized pain, diarrhea/constipation, peripheral neuropathies. **RARE:** Ototoxicity, visual disturbances, alopecia, allergic reaction.

ADVERSE REACTIONS/TOXIC EFFECTS

Bone marrow suppression may be severe, resulting in anemia, infection, bleeding (GI bleeding, sepsis, pneumonia). Prolonged treatment may result in peripheral neurotoxicity.

NURSING IMPLICATIONS

BASELINE ASSESSMENT:

Offer emotional support. Treatment should not be repeated until WBC, neutrophil, platelet count recovers from previous therapy. Transfusions may be needed in those receiving prolonged therapy (myelosuppression increased in those w/previous therapy, impaired kidney function).

INTERVENTION/EVALUATION:

Monitor lung sounds for pulmonary toxicity (dyspnea, fine lung rales). Monitor hematologic status, pulmonary function studies, hepatic and renal function tests. Monitor for fever, sore throat, signs of local infection, easy bruising or unusual bleeding from any site, symptoms of anemia (excessive tiredness, weakness).

PATIENT/FAMILY TEACHING:

Nausea, vomiting generally abates <24 hrs. Contact physician if nausea/vomiting continues at home. Do not have immunizations w/o physician's approval (drug lowers body's resistance). Avoid contact w/those who have recently received live virus vaccine. Teach signs of peripheral neuropathy.

carboprost

kar'boe-prost
(Hemabate)

CANADIAN AVAILABILITY:
Prostin/15M

CLASSIFICATION

Prostaglandin

PHARMACOKINETICS

Metabolized in liver and by enzymes in maternal lung tissues. Mean abortion time: 16 hrs. Primarily excreted in urine.

ACTION

Direct action on myometrium. Stimulates contraction in gravid uterus, produces cervical dilatation and softening.

USES

To induce abortion between the thirteenth and twentieth wk of pregnancy (as calculated from the first day of the last menstrual period), to treat postpartum hemorrhage related to uterine atony not responsive to conventional therapy.

STORAGE/HANDLING

Refrigerate.

IM ADMINISTRATION

1. Administer only in hospital setting w/emergency equipment available.
2. Give deep IM and rotate sites if subsequent doses necessary.
3. Avoid skin contact w/carboprost; if spilled on skin, wash thoroughly w/soap and water.

INDICATIONS/DOSAGE/ROUTES

Abortion:
IM: Adults: Initially, 100-250 mcg, may repeat at 1.5-3.5 hr intervals. May increase up to 500 mcg if uterine contractility inadequate. **Maximum:** 12 mg total dose or continuous administration >2 days.

Postpartum hemorrhage:
IM: Adults: Initially, 250 mcg, may repeat at 15-90 min intervals. **Maximum:** 2 mg total dose.

CONTRAINDICATIONS: Hypersensitivity to carboprost or other prostaglandins; acute pelvic inflammatory disease; active cardiac, pulmonary, renal, or hepatic disease. **CAUTIONS:** History of asthma, hypo/hypertension, anemia, jaundice, diabetes, epilepsy, compromised (scarred) uterus, cardiovascular, adrenal, or hepatic disease. **PREGNANCY/LACTATION:** Teratogenic, therefore abortion must be complete.

INTERACTIONS

DRUG INTERACTIONS: Oxytocin, oxytocics may cause uterine hypertonus, leading to uterine rupture or cervical lacerations. **ALTERED LAB VALUES:** None significant.

SIDE EFFECTS

FREQUENT: Nausea, vomiting, diarrhea. **OCCASIONAL:** Fever, chills, flushing/redness of face, headache, hyper/hypotension. **RARE:** Wheezing, troubled breathing, tightness in chest (esp. asthmatic patients). Stomach cramps/pain, increased uterine bleeding, foul-smelling lochia may indicate postabortion complications.

ADVERSE REACTIONS/TOXIC EFFECTS

Excessive dosage may cause uterine hypertonicity w/spasm and tetanic contraction, leading to cervical laceration/perforation, uterine rupture/hemorrhage.

NURSING IMPLICATIONS

Baseline Assessment:

Question for hypersensitivity to carboprost or other prostaglandins. Establish baseline B/P, temperature, pulse, respiration. Obtain orders for antiemetics and antidiarrheals, meperidine or other pain medication for abdominal cramps. Assess any uterine activity/vaginal bleeding.

Intervention/Evaluation:

Check strength, duration, frequency of contractions and monitor vital signs every 15 min until stable, then hourly until abortion complete. Check resting uterine tone. Administer medications for relief of GI effects if indicated, abdominal cramps. Provide emotional support as necessary.

Patient/Family Teaching:

Report fever, chills, foul-smelling/increased vaginal discharge, uterine cramps/pain promptly.

carisoprodol

care-is-pro´dol

(Soma, Rela)

FIXED COMBINATION(S): W/aspirin, nonnarcotic analgesic (Soma Compound); w/aspirin and codeine, narcotic analgesic (Soma Compound w/Codeine)

CANADIAN AVAILABILITY: Soma

CLASSIFICATION

Skeletal muscle relaxant

PHARMACOKINETICS

	ONSET	PEAK	DURATION
PO	30 min	—	4-6 hrs

Well absorbed from GI tract. Metabolized in liver. Excreted in urine. Half-life: 8 hrs.

ACTION

Muscle relaxant related to CNS depressant effects (sedation).

Blocks interneuronal activity in descending reticular formation and spinal cord.

USES

Adjunct to rest, physical therapy, other measures for relief of discomfort due to acute, painful musculoskeletal conditions.

PO ADMINISTRATION

May give w/food/milk if GI disturbances occur.

INDICATIONS/DOSAGE/ROUTES

Acute, painful, musculoskeletal spasm:
PO: Adults, elderly: 350 mg 3-4 times/day, last dose at bedtime.

PRECAUTIONS

CONTRAINDICATIONS: Acute intermittent porphyria, suspected porphyria, allergic/idiosyncratic reactions to meprobamate. **CAUTIONS:** Impaired renal/hepatic function, those w/tartrazine sensitivity. **PREGNANCY/LACTATION:** Unknown if drug crosses placenta; distributed in breast milk. **Pregnancy Category C.**

INTERACTIONS

DRUG INTERACTIONS: Potentiated effects when used w/other CNS depressants (including alcohol). **ALTERED LAB VALUES:** None significant.

SIDE EFFECTS

FREQUENT: Transient drowsiness, dizziness (postural hypotension). **OCCASIONAL:** Nausea, confusion, headache, insomnia, constipation, urinary frequency. **RARE:** Hypersensitivity reaction (rash, bronchospasm, pruritus), depression.

ADVERSE REACTIONS/TOXIC EFFECTS

Overdosage results in muscular hypotonia, respiratory depression, stupor, coma. Severe allergic reaction noted by dizziness, weakness, angioneurotic edema, hypotension, smarting eyes, anaphylactoid shock.

NURSING IMPLICATIONS

BASELINE ASSESSMENT:

Record onset, type, location, duration of muscular spasm. Check for immobility, stiffness, swelling.

INTERVENTION/EVALUATION:

Assist w/ambulation at all times. For those on long-term therapy, liver/renal function tests, blood counts should be performed periodically. Evaluate for therapeutic response: decreased intensity of skeletal muscle pain.

PATIENT/FAMILY TEACHING:

Drowsiness usually diminishes w/continued therapy. Avoid tasks that require alertness, motor skills until response to drug is established. Avoid alcohol or other depressants while taking medication. Avoid sudden changes in posture.

carmustine

car-muss′teen
(BiCNU)

CANADIAN AVAILABILITY:
BiCNU

CLASSIFICATION

Antineoplastic

PHARMACOKINETICS

Widely distributed (crosses blood-brain barrier, readily penetrates CSF). Metabolized in liver to active metabolite. Primarily excreted in urine.

ACTION

Inhibits DNA, RNA synthesis by cross-linking w/DNA, RNA strands, interfering w/nucleic acid function. Cell cycle-phase nonspecific.

USES

Palliative treatment of primary and metastatic brain tumors, multiple myeloma, disseminated Hodgkin's disease, non-Hodgkin's lymphoma.

STORAGE/HANDLING

NOTE: May be carcinogenic, mutagenic, or teratogenic. Handle w/ extreme care during preparation, administration.

Refrigerate unopened vials of dry powder. Reconstituted vials are stable for 8 hrs at room temperature or 24 hrs if refrigerated. Solutions further diluted to 0.2 mg/ml w/5% dextrose or 0.9% NaCl are stable for 48 hrs if refrigerated or an additional 8 hrs at room temperature. Solutions are clear, colorless to yellow. Discard if precipitate forms, color change occurs, or oily film develops on bottom of vial.

IV ADMINISTRATION

NOTE: Wear protective gloves during preparation of drug; may cause transient burning, hyperpigmentation to skin.

1. Reconstitute 100 mg vial w/3 ml sterile dehydrated (absolute) alcohol, followed by 27 ml sterile water for injection to provide concentration of 3.3 mg/ml.
2. Further dilute w/50-250 ml 5% dextrose or 0.9% NaCl. Infuse over 1-2 hrs (shorter duration may produce intense pain, burning at injection site).
3. Flush IV line w/5-10 ml 0.9% NaCl injection or 5% dextrose before and after administration to prevent irritation at injection site.
4. Rapid IV may produce intense flushing of skin, conjunctiva.

INDICATIONS/DOSAGE/ROUTES

NOTE: Dosage individualized based on clinical response, tolerance to adverse effects. When used in combination therapy, consult specific protocols for optimum dosage, sequence of drug administration.

Single agent in previously untreated pt:

IV: Adults, elderly, children: 150-200 mg/m^2 as single dose or 75-100 mg/m^2 on 2 successive days. Alternatively, give 40 mg/m^2 daily on 5 successive days. Repeat doses q6-8wks. Reduce dose if given in combination w/myelosuppressive drugs or if pt has compromised bone marrow function. Repeat courses not given until circulating blood elements return to acceptable levels and adequate number of neutrophils present on peripheral blood smear. Adjust dose based upon hematologic response to previous doses.

PRECAUTIONS

CONTRAINDICATIONS: None significant. **CAUTIONS:** Pts w/decreased platelet, leukocyte, erythrocyte counts. **PREGNANCY/LACTATION:** If possible, avoid use during pregnancy, esp. first trimester. May cause fetal harm. Unknown if distributed in breast milk. Breast feeding not recommended. **Pregnancy Category D.**

INTERACTIONS

DRUG INTERACTIONS: Bone marrow depressants, cimetidine may enhance myelosuppressive effect. Hepatotoxic, nephrotoxic drugs may enhance respective toxicities. Live virus vaccines may potentiate virus replication, increase vaccine side effects, decrease antibody response to vaccine. **ALTERED LAB VALUES:** May increase BUN, SGOT (AST), SGPT (ALT), alkaline phosphatase, bilirubin.

SIDE EFFECTS

FREQUENT: Pain at IV injection site, along course of vein; nausea and vomiting within min to 2 hrs (may last up to 6 hrs after administration). **OCCASIONAL:** Diarrhea, esophagitis, anorexia, dysphagia. **RARE:** Thrombophlebitis.

ADVERSE REACTIONS/TOXIC EFFECTS

Hematologic toxicity, due to bone marrow depression, occurs frequently. Thrombocytopenia occurs at about 4 wks, lasts 1-2 wks; leukopenia evident at about 5-6 wks, lasts 1-2 wks. Anemia occurs less frequently, is less severe. Mild, reversible hepatotoxicity also occurs frequently. Prolonged therapy w/high dosage may produce impaired renal function, pulmonary toxicity (pulmonary infiltrate and/or fibrosis).

NURSING IMPLICATIONS

BASELINE ASSESSMENT:

Perform pulmonary function tests before therapy begins and periodically during therapy. Perform liver function studies periodically during therapy. Perform blood counts weekly during and for at least 6 wks after therapy ends.

INTERVENTION/EVALUATION:

Monitor WBC, platelet count, BUN, Hct, serum transaminase, alkaline phosphatase, bilirubin; pulmonary, liver, renal function tests. Monitor for hematologic toxicity (fever, sore throat, signs of local infection, easy bruising, unusual bleeding from any site) or symptoms of anemia (excessive tiredness, weakness). Monitor lung sounds for pulmonary toxicity (dyspnea, fine lung rales).

PATIENT/FAMILY TEACHING:

Pain may occur w/IV administration. Maintain adequate daily fluid intake (may protect against renal impairment). Do not have immunizations w/o doctor's approval (drug lowers body's resistance). Avoid contact w/those who have recently received live virus vaccine. Contact physician if nausea/vomiting continues at home.

carteolol hydrochloride

cart-hee´oh-lol

(Cartrol)

CLASSIFICATION

Beta-adrenergic blocker

PHARMACOKINETICS

Well absorbed from GI tract. Protein binding: 25-30%. Minimally metabolized in liver. Primarily excreted unchanged in urine. Half-life: 6 hrs (increased in decreased renal function).

ACTION

Selectively blocks $beta_1$-adrenergic receptors, slowing sinus heart rate, decreasing cardiac output, decreasing B/P (exact mechanism unknown but may block peripheral adrenergic receptors, decrease sympathetic outflow from CNS or decrease renin release from kidney). Blocks $beta_2$-adrenergic receptors, increasing airway resistance. Decreases intraocular pressure by reducing aqueous humor production.

USES

Oral: Management of hypertension. *Ophthalmic:* Used alone or in combination w/other intraocular pressure reducing drugs to treat chronic open-angle glaucoma or intraocular hypertension.

PO/OPHTHALMIC ADMINISTRATION

PO: May give w/o regard to food.

OPHTHALMIC:

1. Place finger on lower eyelid and pull out until pocket is formed between eye and lower lid. Hold dropper above pocket and place prescribed number of drops in pocket.
2. Close eye gently. Apply digital pressure to lacrimal sac for 1-2 min (minimized drainage into nose and throat, reducing risk of systemic effects).
3. Remove excess solution w/ tissue.

INDICATIONS/DOSAGE/ROUTES

Hypertension:
PO: Adults, elderly: Initially, 2.5 mg/day as single dose either alone or in combination w/diuretic. May increase gradually to 5-10 mg/day as single dose. **Maintenance:** 2.5-5 mg/day.

Dosage in renal impairment:

CREATININE CLEARANCE	DOSAGE INTERVAL
>60 ml/min	24 hrs
20-60 ml/min	48 hrs
<20 ml/min	72 hrs

Usual ophthalmic dosage:
OPHTHALMIC: Adults, elderly: 1 drop 2 times/day.

PRECAUTIONS

CONTRAINDICATIONS: Bronchial asthma, COPD, bronchospasm, overt cardiac failure, cardiogenic shock, heart block greater than first degree, persistently severe bradycardia. **CAUTIONS:** Impaired renal/hepatic function, peripheral vascular disease, hyperthyroidism, diabetes, inadequate cardiac function. **PREGNANCY/LACTATION:** Readily crosses placenta; distributed in breast milk. Avoid use during first trimester. May produce bradycardia, apnea, hypoglycemia, hypothermia during delivery, small birth weight infants. **Pregnancy Category C.**

INTERACTIONS

DRUG INTERACTIONS: Diuretics, other hypotensives may increase hypotensive effect; sympathomimetics, xanthines may mutually inhibit effects; may mask symptoms of hypoglycemia, prolong hypoglycemic effect of insulin, oral hypoglycemics; NSAIDs may decrease antihypertensive effect; cimetidine may increase concentration. **ALTERED LAB VALUES:** May increase ANA titer, SGOT (AST), SGPT (ALT), alkaline phosphatase, LDH, bilirubin, BUN, creatinine, potassium, uric acid, lipoproteins, triglycerides.

SIDE EFFECTS

FREQUENT: Dizziness, fatigue, insomnia, bizarre dreams, paresthesia, visual disturbances, anxiety, peripheral edema, dyspnea, weight gain. **OCCASIONAL:** Nausea, GI distress, palpitation, coldness of extremities, syncope, tachycardia, chest pain, muscle/joint pain. **RARE:** Lethargy, hallucinations, diarrhea, vomiting, wheezing, rash, pruritus, urinary frequency, impotence.

ADVERSE REACTIONS/TOXIC EFFECTS

Abrupt withdrawal (particularly in those w/coronary artery disease) may produce angina or precipitate MI. May precipitate thyroid crisis in those w/thyrotoxicosis.

NURSING IMPLICATIONS

BASELINE ASSESSMENT:

Assess baseline renal/liver function tests. Assess B/P, apical pulse immediately before drug is administered (if pulse is 60/min or below, or systolic B/P is below 90 mm Hg, withhold medication, contact physician).

INTERVENTION/EVALUATION:

Assess pulse for strength/weakness, irregular rate, bradycardia. Monitor EKG for cardiac changes. Assist w/ambulation if dizziness occurs. Assess for peripheral edema of hands, feet (usually, first area of low extremity swelling is behind medial malleolus in ambulatory, sacral area in bedridden). Monitor pattern of daily bowel activity and stool consistency. Assess skin for development of rash. Monitor any unusual changes in pt. *Ophthalmic:* Monitor for potential systemic reaction.

PATIENT/FAMILY TEACHING:

Do not abruptly discontinue medication (compliance w/therapy regimen is essential to control hypertension). If dizziness occurs, sit or lie down immediately. Full therapeutic response may not occur for up to 2 wks. Avoid tasks that require alertness, motor skills until response to drug is established. Report excessively slow pulse rate (<60 beats/min), peripheral numbness, dizziness. Do not use nasal decongestants, over-the-counter cold preparations (stimulants) w/o physician approval. Outpatients should monitor B/P, pulse before taking medication. Restrict salt, alcohol intake. *Ophthalmic:* Instruct pt on proper administration of drops. Do not use after expiration date. Transient stinging or discomfort is common; notify physician of severe or continued discomfort.

cascara sagrada

cass-care´ah sah-graud´ah

(Cascara Sagrada)

FIXED-COMINBATION(S):

W/milk of magnesia, a saline laxative (Same)

CANADIAN AVAILABILITY:

Cascara Sagrada

CLASSIFICATION

Laxative: Stimulant

PHARMACOKINETICS

	ONSET	PEAK	DURATION
PO	6-12 hrs	—	—

Minimal absorption after oral administration. Hydrolyzed by enzymes of colonic flora to active form. Absorbed drug metabolized in liver, eliminated in feces via biliary system.

ACTION

Increases peristalsis by direct effect on colonic smooth musculature (stimulates intramural nerve plexi). Promotes fluid and ion accumulation in colon to increase laxative effect.

USES

Facilitates defecation in those w/ diminished colonic motor response, for evacuation of colon for rectal, bowel examination, elective colon surgery.

PO ADMINISTRATION

1. Give on empty stomach (faster results).
2. Offer 6-8 glasses water/day (aids softening stools).
3. Avoid giving within 1 hr of other oral medication (decreases drug absorption).

INDICATIONS/DOSAGE/ROUTES

Laxative:
PO: Adults, elderly: 1 tablet (or 5 ml) at bedtime.

PRECAUTIONS

CONTRAINDICATIONS: Abdominal pain, nausea, vomiting, appendicitis, intestinal obstruction. **CAUTIONS:** None significant. **PREGNANCY/LACTATION:** Distributed in breast milk (may produce loose stools in infant). **Pregnancy Category C.**

INTERACTIONS

DRUG INTERACTIONS: May decrease transit time of concurrently administered oral medication, decreasing absorption. **ALTERED LAB VALUES:** May increase blood glucose. May decrease potassium, calcium.

SIDE EFFECTS

FREQUENT: Pink-red, red-violet, red-brown, or yellow-brown discoloration of urine. **OCCASIONAL:** Some degree of abdominal discomfort, nausea, mild cramps, griping; faintness.

ADVERSE REACTIONS/TOXIC EFFECTS

Long-term use may result in laxative dependence, chronic constipation, loss of normal bowel function. Chronic use or overdosage may result in electrolyte disturbances (hypokalemia, hypocalcemia, metabolic acidosis or alkalosis), persistent diarrhea, malabsorption, weight loss. Electrolyte disturbance may produce vomiting, muscle weakness.

NURSING IMPLICATIONS

INTERVENTION/EVALUATION:

Encourage adequate fluid intake. Assess bowel sounds for peristalsis. Monitor daily bowel activity and stool consistency (watery, loose, soft, semisolid, solid) and record time of evacuation. Assess for abdominal disturbances. Monitor serum electrolytes in those exposed to prolonged, frequent, or excessive use of medication.

PATIENT/FAMILY TEACHING:

Urine may turn pink-red, red-violet, red-brown or yellow-brown (is only temporary and is not harmful). Institute measures to promote defecation: increase fluid intake, exercise, high-fiber diet. Laxative effect generally occurs in 6-12 hrs, but may take 24 hrs. Do not take other oral medication within 1 hr of taking this medicine (decreased effectiveness due to increased peristalsis).

castor oil

(Neoloid)

CANADIAN AVAILABILITY: Castor Oil

CLASSIFICATION

Laxative: Stimulant

PHARMACOKINETICS

	ONSET	PEAK	DURATION
PO	2-3 hrs	—	—

Minimal absorption. Converted to ricinoleic acid (active component) in GI tract.

ACTION

Increases peristalsis by direct effect on small bowel musculature (stimulates intramural nerve plexi). Promotes fluid and ion accumulation in colon to increase laxative effect.

USES

Facilitates defecation in those w/ diminished colonic motor response, for evacuation of colon for rectal, bowel examination, elective colon surgery.

PO ADMINISTRATION

1. Do not give late in day (acts in 2-6 hrs).
2. Chill, mix w/juice (improves taste).
3. Give on empty stomach (faster action).
4. Offer 6-8 glasses of water/day (aids stool softening).
5. Avoid giving within 1 hr of other oral medication (decreases drug absorption).

INDICATIONS/DOSAGE/ROUTES

Laxative:

PO: Adults, elderly: (liquid): 15-60 ml; (emulsion): 30-60 ml. **Children 6-12 yrs:** (liquid): 5-15 ml; (emulsion): 7.5-30 ml. **Infants:** (emulsion): 2.5-5 ml.

PRECAUTIONS

CONTRAINDICATIONS: Menstruating/pregnant women, abdominal pain, nausea, vomiting, appendicitis, intestinal obstruction. **CAUTIONS:** None significant. **PREGNANCY/LACTATION:** Contraindicated in pregnancy (may cause pelvic area engorgement, may initiate reflex stimulation of gravid uterus, inducing premature labor). **Pregnancy Category X.**

INTERACTIONS

DRUG INTERACTIONS: May decrease transit time of concurrently administered oral medication, decreasing absorption. **ALTERED LAB VALUES:** May increase blood glucose. May decrease potassium, calcium.

SIDE EFFECTS

FREQUENT: Some degree of abdominal discomfort, nausea, mild cramps, griping, faintness. **OCCASIONAL:** Excessive colon irritation producing violent purgation. **RARE:** Pelvic congestion.

ADVERSE REACTIONS/TOXIC EFFECTS

Long-term use may result in laxative dependence, chronic constipation, loss of normal bowel function. Chronic use or overdosage may result in electrolyte disturbances (hypokalemia, hypocalcemia, metabolic acidosis or alkalosis), persistent diarrhea, malabsorption, weight loss. Electrolyte disturbance may produce vomiting, muscle weakness.

NURSING IMPLICATIONS

BASELINE ASSESSMENT:

Question for possibility of pregnancy before initiating therapy (Pregnancy Category X)

INTERVENTION/EVAUATION:

Encourage adequate fluid intake. Assess bowel sounds for peristalsis. Monitor daily bowel activity and stool consistency (watery, loose, soft, semisolid, solid) and record time of evacuation. Assess for abdominal disturbances. Monitor serum electrolytes in those exposed to prolonged, frequent, or excessive use of medication.

PATIENT/FAMILY TEACHING:

Cola, unsalted crackers, dry toast may relieve nausea. Institute measures to promote defecation: increase fluid intake, exercise, high-fiber diet. Do not take other oral medication within 1 hr of taking this medicine (decreased effectiveness due to increased peristalsis).

cefaclor

sef'ah-klor
(Ceclor)

CANADIAN AVAILABILITY:
Ceclor

CLASSIFICATION

Antibiotic: Second-generation cephalosporin

PHARMACOKINETICS

Well absorbed from GI tract. Widely distributed. Protein binding: 25%. Primarily excreted unchanged in urine. Moderately removed by hemodialysis. Half-life: 0.6-0.9 hrs (increased in decreased renal function).

ACTION

Bactericidal. Binds to bacterial membranes, inhibiting bacterial cell wall synthesis.

USES

Treatment of respiratory, GU tract, skin, bone infections; septicemia, otitis media.

STORAGE/HANDLING

Oral suspension, after reconstitution, stable for 14 days if refrigerated.

PO ADMINISTRATION

1. Shake oral suspension well before using.
2. Give w/o regard to meals; if GI upset occurs, give w/food or milk.

INDICATIONS/DOSAGE/ROUTES

NOTE: Space doses evenly around the clock.

Mild to moderate infections:
PO: Adults, elderly: 250 mg q8h. **Children >1 mo:** 20 mg/kg/day in divided doses q8h.

Severe infections:
PO: Adults, elderly: 500 mg q8h. **Maximum:** 4 Gm/day. **Children >1 mo:** 40 mg/kg/day in divided doses q8h. **Maximum:** 1 Gm/day.

Otitis media:
PO: Children >1 mo: 40 mg/kg/day in divided doses q8h. **Maximum:** 1 Gm/day.

Dosage in renal impairment:
Reduced dosage may be necessary in those w/creatinine clearance <40 ml/min.

PRECAUTIONS

CONTRAINDICATIONS: History of hypersensitivity to cephalosporins, anaphylactic reaction to penicillins. **CAUTIONS:** Renal impairment, history of allergies or GI disease, concurrent use of nephrotoxic medications. **PREGNANCY/LACTATION:** Readily crosses placenta. Distributed in breast milk. **Pregnancy Category B.**

INTERACTIONS

DRUG INTERACTIONS: Probenecid may increase serum concentrations of cefaclor. **ALTERED LAB VALUES:** Positive direct/indirect Coombs' test may occur (interferes w/hematologic tests, cross-matching procedures). May increase BUN, serum creatinine, SGPT (ALT), SGOT (AST), alkaline phosphatase concentrations.

SIDE EFFECTS

FREQUENT: Nausea, vomiting, diarrhea. **OCCASIONAL:** Malaise, dizziness, headache, dyspepsia, abdominal pain, sore mouth and tongue.

ADVERSE REACTIONS/TOXIC EFFECTS

Antibiotic-associated colitis, other superinfections may result from altered bacterial balance, Nephrotoxicity may occur, esp. w/preexisting renal disease. Hypersensitivity reactions (ranging from rash, urticaria, fever to anaphylaxis) occur in fewer than 5%, particularly those w/history of allergies, esp. penicillin.

NURSING IMPLICATIONS

BASELINE ASSESSMENT:

Question for history of allergies, particularly cephalosporins, penicillins. Obtain culture and sensitivity test before giving first dose (therapy may begin before results are known).

INTERVENTION/EVALUATION:

Monitor for nausea, vomiting. Determine pattern of bowel activity and stool consistency. Assess skin for rash. Monitor I&O, urinalysis, renal function reports for nephrotoxicity if renal function impaired. Be alert for superinfection: genital/anal pruritus, vaginal discharge, ulceration or changes in oral mucosa, abdominal pain, moderate to severe diarrhea.

PATIENT/FAMILY TEACHING:

Continue therapy for full length of treatment. Doses should be evenly spaced. Notify physician in event of diarrhea or other new symptom.

cefadroxil

sef-ah-drocks´ill
(Duricef, Ultracef)

CANADIAN AVAILABILITY:
Duricef

CLASSIFICATION

Antibiotic: First-generation cephalosporin

PHARMACOKINETICS

Well absorbed from GI tract.

Widely distributed. Protein binding: 15-20%. Primarily excreted unchanged in urine. Removed by hemodialysis. Half-life: 1.2-1.5 hrs (increased in decreased renal function).

ACTION

Bactericidal. Binds to bacterial membranes, inhibiting bacterial cell wall synthesis.

USES

Treatment of respiratory and GU tract, skin and soft tissue infections; follow-up to parenteral therapy.

STORAGE/HANDLING

Oral suspension, after reconstitution, stable for 14 days if refrigerated.

PO ADMINISTRATION

1. Shake oral suspension well before using.
2. Give w/o regard to meals; if GI upset occurs, give w/food or milk.

INDICATIONS/DOSAGE/ROUTES

NOTE: Space doses evenly around the clock.

Urinary tract infections:
PO: Adults, elderly: 1-2 Gm/day in 1-2 divided doses.

Skin/skin structure infections, group A beta-hemolytic streptococcal pharyngitis, tonsillitis:
PO: Adults, elderly: 500 mg - 1 Gm/day as single or 2 divided doses.

Usual dosage for children:
PO: Children: 30 mg/kg/day as single or 2 divided doses.

Dosage in renal impairment:
Dose and/or frequency is based on degree of renal impairment and/or severity of infection. After initial 1 Gm dose:

CREATININE CLEARANCE	DOSAGE INTERVAL
25-50 ml/min	500 mg q12h
10-25 ml/min	500 mg q24h
0-10 ml/min	500 mg q36h

PRECAUTIONS

CONTRAINDICATIONS: History of hypersensitivity to cephalosporins, anaphylactic reaction to penicillins. **CAUTIONS:** Renal impairment, history of allergies or GI disease, concurrent use of nephrotoxic medications. **PREGNANCY/LACTATION:** Readily crosses placenta. Distributed in breast milk. **Pregnancy Category B.**

INTERACTIONS

DRUG INTERACTIONS: Probenecid increases serum concentrations of cefadroxil. **ALTERED LAB VALUES:** Positive direct/indirect Coombs' test may occur (interferes w/hematologic tests, cross-matching procedures).

SIDE EFFECTS

FREQUENT: Anorexia, nausea, vomiting, diarrhea. **OCCASIONAL:** Dyspepsia, abdominal pain, genital/anal pruritus, moniliasis.

ADVERSE REACTIONS/TOXIC EFFECTS

Antibiotic-associated colitis, other superinfections may result from altered bacterial balance. Nephrotoxicity may occur, esp. w/ preexisting renal disease. Hypersensitivity reactions (ranging from rash, urticaria, fever to anaphylaxis) occur in fewer than 5%, generally those w/history of allergies, esp. penicillin.

NURSING IMPLICATIONS

BASELINE ASSESSMENT:

Question history of allergies, particularly cephalosporins, penicillins. Obtain culture and sensitivity test before giving first dose (therapy may begin before results are known).

INTERVENTION/EVALUATION:

Monitor for anorexia, nausea, vomiting. Determine pattern of bowel activity and stool consistency. Assess skin for rash. Monitor I&O, urinalysis, renal function reports for nephrotoxicity. Be alert for superinfection: genital/anal pruritus, moniliasis, abdominal pain, sore mouth or tongue, moderate to severe diarrhea.

PATIENT/FAMILY TEACHING:

Continue therapy for full length of treatment. Doses should be evenly spaced. Notify physician in event of diarrhea or other new symptom.

cefamandole nafate

sef-a-man´dole

(Mandol)

CANADIAN AVAILABILITY:
Mandol

CLASSIFICATION

Antibiotic: Second-generation cephalosporin

PHARMACOKINETICS

Widely distributed. Protein binding: 70-80%. Primarily excreted unchanged in urine. Moderately removed by hemodialysis. Half-life: 0.5-1.2 hrs (increased in decreased renal function).

ACTION

Bactericidal. Binds to bacterial membranes, inhibiting bacterial cell wall synthesis.

USES

Treatment of respiratory, GU tract, skin, bone infections; septicemia, perioperative prophylaxis.

STORAGE/HANDLING

Solutions appear light yellow to amber. IV infusion (piggyback) stable for 24 hrs at room temperature, 96 hrs if refrigerated. Discard if precipitate forms or color change occurs.

IM/IV ADMINISTRATION

NOTE: Give IM, direct IV injection, intermittent IV infusion (piggyback).

IM:

1. Dilute each 1 Gm w/3 ml of sterile water for injection or 0.9% NaCl injection to provide concentration of 285 mg/ml.
2. To minimize discomfort, inject deep IM slowly. Less painful if injected into gluteus maximus rather than lateral aspect of thigh.

IV:

1. For direct IV injection, dilute w/10 ml sterile water for injection or 0.9% NaCl injection. Administer over 3-5 min.
2. For intermittent IV infusion (piggyback), further dilute w/50-100 ml 5% dextrose, 0.9% NaCl, or other compatible IV fluid. Infuse over 20 to 40 min.
3. Alternating IV sites, use large veins to reduce risk of phlebitis.

INDICATIONS/DOSAGE/ROUTES

NOTE: Space doses evenly around the clock.

Mild to moderate infections:
IM/IV: Adults, elderly: 500 mg to 1 Gm q4-8h.

Severe infections:
IM/IV: Adults, elderly: 1 Gm q4-6h.

Life-threatening infections:
IM/IV: Adults, elderly: 2 Gm q4h.

Perioperative prophylaxis:
IM/IV: Adults, elderly: 1-2 Gm 30-60 min before surgery and q6h for up to 24 hrs postop. **Children >3 mo:** 12.5-25 mg/kg 30-60 min before surgery and q6h for up to 24 hrs postop.

Usual dosage for children:
IM/IV: Children >1 mo: 50-150 mg/kg/day in divided doses q4-8h. **Maximum:** 12 Gm/day.

Dosage in renal impairment:
After initial loading dose of 1-2 Gm, dose and/or frequency is based on creatinine clearance and/or severity of infection.

CREATININE CLEARANCE	DOSAGE
50-80 ml/min	750 mg-2 Gm q6h
25-50 ml/min	750 mg-2 Gm q8h
10-25 ml/min	500 mg-1 Gm q6-8h
2-10 ml/min	500 mg-1 Gm q12h
<2 ml/min	250-500 mg q8-12h

PRECAUTIONS

CONTRAINDICATIONS: History of hypersensitivity to cephalosporins, anaphylactic reaction to penicillins. **CAUTIONS:** Renal impairment, history of allergies or GI disease, concurrent use of nephrotoxic medications. **PREGNANCY/LACTATION:** Readily crosses placenta. Distributed in breast milk. **Pregnancy Category B.**

INTERACTIONS

DRUG INTERACTIONS: Disulfiram reaction (facial flushing, nausea, sweating, headache, tachycardia) occurs if alcohol is ingested within 48-72 hrs after dose. Probenecid increases serum concentrations of cefamandole. May increase bleeding risk w/anticoagulants, heparin, thrombolytics. **ALTERED LAB VALUES:** Positive direct/indirect Coombs' test may occur (interferes w/hematologic tests, cross-matching procedures). False-positive urinary proteins after large doses of cefamandole. May prolong prothrombin times.

SIDE EFFECTS

OCCASIONAL: Pain, induration at IM site; phlebitis, thrombophlebitis if given IV; bleeding, esp. in debilitated, elderly; diarrhea. **RARE:** Nausea, vomiting.

ADVERSE REACTIONS/TOXIC EFFECTS

Nephrotoxicity has occurred w/ high dosages or preexisting renal impairment. Antibiotic-associated colitis, other superinfections may result from altered bacterial balance. Hypersensitivity reactions (ranging from rash, urticaria, fever to anaphylaxis) occur in fewer than 5%, particularly those w/history of allergies, esp. penicillin.

NURSING IMPLICATIONS

BASELINE ASSESSMENT:

Question for history of allergies, particularly cephalosporins, penicillins. Obtain culture and sensitivity test before giving first dose (therapy may begin before results are known).

INTERVENTION/EVALUATION:

Assess IV site for phlebitis (heat, pain, red streaking over vein). Check IM injection sites for induration, tenderness. Determine pattern of bowel activity and stool consistency. Assess skin for rash. Monitor I&O, urinalysis, renal function reports for nephrotoxicity. Be alert for superinfection: nausea, moderate to severe diarrhea, ulceration of oral mucosa, vaginal discharge, genital/anal pruritus. Monitor PT levels and be alert for signs of bleeding: overt bleeding, bruising or swelling of tissue.

PATIENT/FAMILY TEACHING:

Discomfort may occur w/IM injection. Doses should be evenly spaced. Continue antibiotic therapy for full length of treatment. Avoid alcohol and alcohol-containing preparations (salad dressings, sauces, cough syrups—read all labels carefully) during and for 72 hrs after last dose of cefamandole. Notify physician in event of diarrhea, bleeding, bruising, or onset of other new symptom.

cefazolin sodium

cef-ah-zoe´lin

(Ancef, Kefzol, Zolicef)

CANADIAN AVAILABILITY:

Ancef, Kefzol

CLASSIFICATION

Antibiotic: First-generation cephalosporin

PHARMACOKINETICS

Widely distributed. Protein binding: 85%. Primarily excreted unchanged in urine. Moderately removed by hemodialysis. Half-life: 1.4-1.8 hrs (increased in decreased renal function).

ACTION

Bactericidal. Binds to bacterial membranes, inhibiting bacterial cell wall synthesis.

USES

Treatment of respiratory tract, skin, soft tissue, bone and joint, GU tract, serious intra-abdominal, biliary infections; septicemia. Preferred first-generation cephalosporin for perioperative prophylaxis.

STORAGE/HANDLING

Solutions appear light yellow to yellow. IV infusion (piggyback) stable for 24 hrs at room temperature, 96 hrs if refrigerated. Discard if precipitate forms.

IM/IV ADMINISTRATION

NOTE: Give by IM injection, direct IV injection, intermittent IV infusion (piggyback).

IM:

1. Reconstitute each 250 mg or 500 mg vial w/2 ml (2.5 ml for 1 Gm vial) of sterile water for injection, bacteriostatic water for injection, or 0.9% NaCl injection to provide concentration of 125, 225, or 330 mg/ml, respectively.

2. To minimize discomfort, inject deep IM slowly. Less painful if injected into gluteus maximus rather than lateral aspect of thigh.

IV:

1. For direct IV injection, after

reconstitution, further dilute w/5-10 ml sterile water for injection. Administer over 3-5 min.

2. For intermittent IV infusion (piggyback), further dilute w/50-100 ml 5% dextrose, 0.9% NaCl, or other compatible IV fluid. Infuse over 20-40 min.

3. Alternating IV sites, use large veins to reduce risk of phlebitis.

INDICATIONS/DOSAGE/ROUTES

NOTE: Space doses evenly around the clock.

Uncomplicated UTI:
IM/IV: Adults, elderly: 1 Gm q12h.

Mild to moderate infections:
IM/IV: Adults, elderly: 250-500 mg q8-12h.

Severe infections:
IM/IV: Adults, elderly: 0.5-1 Gm q6-8h.

Life-threatening infections:
IM/IV: Adults, elderly: 1-1.5 Gm q6h. **Maximum:** 12 Gm/day.

Perioperative prophylaxis:
IM/IV: Adults, elderly: 1 Gm 30-60 min before surgery, 0.5-1 Gm during surgery, and q6-8h for up to 24 hrs post-op.

Usual dosage for children:
IM/IV: Children >1 mo: 25-100 mg/kg/day in 3-4 divided doses.

Dosage in renal impairment:

After initial loading dose of 500 mg, dose and/or frequency modified on basis of creatinine clearance and/or severity of infection.

CREATININE CLEARANCE	CHILDREN'S DOSAGE
40-70 ml/min	60% normal dose q12h
20-40 ml/min	25% normal dose q12h
5-20 ml/min	10% normal dose q24h

	ADULT DOSAGE
55 ml/min	250-1000 mg q6-8h
35-54 ml/min	250-1000 mg q8h
11-34 ml/min	125-500 mg q12h
10 ml/min	125-500 mg q24h

PRECAUTIONS

CONTRAINDICATIONS: History of hypersensitivity to cephalosporins, anaphylactic reaction to penicillins. **CAUTIONS:** Renal impairment, history of allergies or GI disease, concurrent use of nephrotoxic medications. **PREGNANCY/LACTATION:** Readily crosses placenta; distributed in breast milk. **Pregnancy Category B.**

INTERACTIONS

DRUG INTERACTIONS: Probenecid increases serum concentrations of cefazolin. **ALTERED LAB VALUES:** Positive direct/indirect Coombs' test may occur (interferes w/hematologic tests, cross-matching procedures).

SIDE EFFECTS

OCCASIONAL: Phlebitis, thrombophlebitis when given IV, esp. w/higher dosage/prolonged therapy; anorexia, diarrhea, genital/anal pruritus, oral candidiasis (thrush). **INFREQUENT:** Nausea, vomiting; pain and tenderness at IM injection site.

ADVERSE REACTIONS/TOXIC EFFECTS

Nephrotoxicity has occurred w/high dosage or preexisting renal impairment. Antibiotic-associated colitis, other superinfections may result from altered bacterial balance. Overdosage may produce seizures. Hypersensitivity reactions (ranging from rash, urticaria, fever to anaphylaxis) occur in fewer than 5%, particularly those w/history of allergies, esp. penicillin.

NURSING IMPLICATIONS

BASELINE ASSESSMENT:

Question for history of allergies, particularly cephalosporins, penicillins. Obtain culture and sensitivity test before giving first dose (therapy may begin before results are known).

INTERVENTION/EVALUATION:

Monitor IV site for phlebitis (heat, pain, red streaking over vein). Check IM injection sites for induration, tenderness. Determine pattern of bowel activity and stool consistency. Assess skin for rash. Monitor I&O, urinalysis, renal function reports for nephrotoxicity. Be alert for superinfection: nausea, diarrhea, vaginal discharge, anal pruritus, ulceration or changes in oral mucosa.

PATIENT/FAMILY TEACHING:

Discomfort may occur w/IM injection. Doses should be evenly spaced. Continue antibiotic therapy for full length of treatment. Notify physician in event of diarrhea, bleeding, bruising, or onset of other new symptoms.

cefepime

sef-eh-peem'
(Maxipime)

CLASSIFICATION

Antibiotic: Third-generation cephalosporin

PHARMACOKINETICS

Well absorbed after IM administration. Widely distributed. Protein binding: 16-19%. Primarily excreted unchanged in urine. Removed by hemodialysis. Half-life: 2-2.3 hrs (increased in decreased renal function, elderly).

ACTION

Bactericidal. Binds to bacterial membrane, inhibiting bacterial cell wall synthesis.

USES

Treatment of pneumonia, bronchitis, urinary tract, skin and skin structure, intra-abdominal infections, bacteremia, septicemia, fever and neutropenia in cancer pts.

STORAGE/HANDLING

Solutions stable for 24 hrs at room temperature or 7 days refrigerated.

IM/IV ADMINISTRATION

NOTE: May give by IM injection, IV injection, intermittent IV infusion (piggyback).

1. For IM injection, inject into a large muscle mass (e.g., upper gluteus maximus).
2. For direct IV injection, administer over 3-5 minutes.
3. For intermittent IV infusion, further dilute w/50-100 ml 5% dextrose or 0.9% NaCl. Infuse over 15-30 minutes.
4. Alternate IV sites, use large veins to reduce risk of phlebitis.

INDICATIONS/DOSAGE/ROUTES

NOTE: Space doses evenly around the clock.

Complicated, uncomplicated UTI:
IM/IV: Adults, elderly: 0.5-1.0 Gm q12h.

Moderate-severe infections:
IM/IV: Adults, elderly: 1 Gm q12h.

Severe infections:
IV: Adults, elderly: 2 Gm q12h.

Life-threatening infections:
IV: Adults, elderly: 2 Gm q8h.

Dosage in renal impairment:
Dose and/or frequency is based on degree of renal impairment (creatinine clearance) and/or severity of infection.

	CREATININE CLEARANCE 11-30 ML/MIN	<10 ML/MIN
Moderately severe infection	0.5 Gm q24h	0.25 Gm q24h
Severe infection	1 Gm q24h	0.5 Gm q24h
Life-threatening infection	1 Gm q12h	1 Gm q24h

PRECAUTIONS

CONTRAINDICATIONS: History of hypersensitivity to cephalosporins, anaphylactic reaction to penicillins. **CAUTIONS:** Renal impairment, history of allergies. **PREGNANCY/LACTATION:** Unknown whether distributed in breast milk. **Pregnancy Category B.**

INTERACTIONS

DRUG INTERACTIONS: Probenecid may increase concentration. **ALTERED LAB VALUES:** Positive direct/indirect Coombs' test may occur. May increase SGOT (AST), SGPT (ALT), alkaline phosphatase, LDH, bilirubin.

SIDE EFFECTS

OCCASIONAL: Headache, nausea, rash, diarrhea. **RARE:** Lightheadedness, phlebitis, dizziness, fever, anxiety, vomiting, constipation.

ADVERSE REACTIONS/TOXIC EFFECTS

Antibiotic-associated colitis, other superinfections may result from altered bacterial balance. Nephrotoxicity may occur, especially w/preexisting renal disease. Hypersensitivity reactions (ranging from rash, urticaria, fever to anaphylaxis) occur in less than 5%, generally those w/history of allergies, esp. penicillin.

NURSING IMPLICATIONS

BASELINE ASSESSMENT:

Question history of allergies, particularly cephalosporins, penicillins. Obtain culture and sensitivity test before giving first dose (therapy may begin before results are known).

INTERVENTION/EVALUATION:

Monitor for nausea, vomiting. Check stools for frequency, consistency. Assess skin for rash. Monitor I&O, urinalysis, renal function reports for nephrotoxicity. Be alert for superinfection: Genital/anal pruritus, moniliasis, sore mouth or tongue, moderate to severe diarrhea.

PATIENT/FAMILY TEACHING:

Discomfort may occur w/IM injection. Continue therapy for full length of treatment. Doses should be evenly spaced. Notify physician in event of diarrhea or other new symptom.

cefixime

sef´ih-zeem
(Suprax)

CANADIAN AVAILABILITY

Suprax

CLASSIFICATION

Antibiotic: Third-generation cephalosporin

PHARMACOKINETICS

Moderately absorbed from GI tract. Widely distributed. Protein binding: 60-70%. Primarily excreted unchanged in urine. Minimally removed by hemodialysis. Half-life: 3-4 hrs (increased in decreased renal function).

ACTION

Bactericidal. Binds to bacterial membranes, inhibiting bacterial cell wall synthesis.

USES

Otitis media, acute bronchitis and acute exacerbations of chronic bronchitis, pharyngitis, tonsillitis, uncomplicated UTI, uncomplicated gonorrhea.

STORAGE/HANDLING

Oral suspension, after reconstitution, stable for 14 days at room temperature. Do not refrigerate.

PO ADMINISTRATION

1. Give w/o regard to meals.
2. Shake oral suspension well before administering.

INDICATIONS/DOSAGE/RESULTS

NOTE: Use oral suspension to treat otitis media (achieves higher peak blood level).

Usual oral dosage:

PO: Adults, elderly, children >50 kg: 400 mg/day as single or 2 divided doses. **Children <50 kg:** 8 mg/kg/day as single or 2 divided doses.

Uncomplicated gonorrhea:

PO: Adults: 400 mg as single dose.

Dosage in renal impairment:

Creatinine clearance 21-60 ml/min, pt on renal dialysis: 300 mg/day as single or 2 divided doses.

Creatinine clearance <20 ml/min, pt on continuous ambulatory peritoneal dialysis: 200 mg/day as single or 2 divided doses.

PRECAUTIONS

CONTRAINDICATIONS: Hypersensitivity to cephalosporins. **CAUTIONS:** Hypersensitivity to penicillins or other drugs; allergies; history of GI disease (e.g., colitis); renal impairment. **PREGNANCY/LACTATION:** Not recommended during labor and delivery. Excretion in breast milk not known. **Pregnancy Category B.**

INTERACTIONS

DRUG INTERACTIONS: None significant. **ALTERED LAB VALUES:** None significant.

SIDE EFFECTS

FREQUENT: Diarrhea, abdominal pain, nausea, dyspepsia, flatulence. **OCCASIONAL:** Hypersensitivity reaction: skin rash, pruritus, urticaria, drug fever; headache, dizziness; genital pruritus; vaginitis.

ADVERSE REACTIONS/TOXIC EFFECTS

Superinfections, esp. antibiotic-associated colitis, may result from altered bacterial balance. Blood dyscrasias (transient leukopenia, thrombocytopenia, eosinophilia) occur rarely.

NURSING IMPLICATIONS

BASELINE ASSESSMENT:

Question for hypersensitivity to cefixime or other cephalosporins, penicillins, other drugs. Obtain specimens for culture and sensitivity test (therapy may begin before results are known).

INTERVENTION/EVALUATION:

Monitor bowel activity and stool consistency carefully; mild GI effects may be tolerable, but increasing severity may indicate onset of antibiotic-associated colitis. Report hypersensitivity reaction: skin rash, urticaria, pruritus, fever promptly. Be alert for superinfection (e.g., genital-anal pruritus, ulceration or changes in oral mucosa, moderate to severe diarrhea, new or increased fever). Provide symptomatic relief for nausea, flatulence. Monitor hematology reports.

PATIENT/FAMILY TEACHING:

Continue medication for full length of treatment; do not skip doses. Doses should be evenly spaced. Take cefixime w/meals if GI upset occurs. Notify physician promptly of onset of diarrhea, rash, bleeding or bruising, or other symptom.

cefmetazole sodium

cef-met´ah-zole

(Zefazone)

CLASSIFICATION

Antibiotic: Second-generation cephalosporin

PHARMACOKINETICS

Widely distributed. Protein binding: 65-85%. Primarily excreted unchanged in urine. Moderately removed by hemodialysis. Half-life: 0.8-1.8 hrs (increased in decreased renal function).

ACTION

Bactericidal. Binds to bacterial membranes, inhibiting bacterial cell wall synthesis.

USES

Treatment of GU, lower respiratory tract, skin and skin structure and intra-abdominal infections. Preop prophylaxis for certain clean, contaminated, or potentially contaminated surgical procedures (cesarean section, abdominal or vaginal hysterectomy, high-risk cholecystectomy, colorectal surgery).

STORAGE/HANDLING

After reconstitution, IV solution stable for 24 hrs at room temperature or 7 days if refrigerated.

IV ADMINISTRATION

1. Reconstitute 1 or 2 Gm vial w/4-15 ml sterile water for injection, bacteriostatic water for injection, or 0.9% NaCl.
2. Shake to dissolve, let stand until clear.
3. Plastic containers of frozen reconstituted solutions must be thawed at room temperature, not by microwave or water immersion. Do not refreeze.
4. Do not use if solution cloudy or insoluble precipitate noted.
5. For IV injection, administer over 3-5 min.
6. For IV infusion, further dilute w/50-100 ml 5% dextrose or 0.9% NaCl and infuse over 10-60 min.
7. Because of potential for hypersensitivity/anaphylaxis, start initial dose at few drops per minute, increase slowly to ordered rate; stay w/pt first 10-15 min, then check every 10 min for 1st hr.

8. Alternate IV sites, use large veins to reduce risk of phlebitis.

INDICATIONS/DOSAGE/ROUTES

Urinary tract infections:
IV: Adults, elderly: 2 Gm q12h.

Mild-moderate infections:
IV: Adults, elderly: 2 Gm q8h.

Severe infections:
IV: Adults, elderly: 2 Gm q6h.

Surgical prophylaxis:
IV: Adults, elderly: 2 Gm as single dose 30-90 min before surgery or after cord is clamped, or 1-2 Gm 30-90 min before surgery or after cord is clamped, and repeat 8 and 16 hrs later.

Dosage in renal impairment:

After loading dose of 1-2 Gm, dosage and/or frequency is modified on basis of creatinine clearance and/or severity of infection.

CREATININE CLEARANCE	DOSAGE
50-90 ml/min	1-2 Gm q12h
30-49 ml/min	1-2 Gm q16h
10-29 ml/min	1-2 Gm q24h
<10 ml/min	1-2 Gm q48h

PRECAUTIONS

CONTRAINDICATIONS: History of hypersensitivity to cefmetazole or cephalosporins. **CAUTIONS:** If given to penicillin-sensitive pt, use extreme caution; cross-sensitivity among beta-lactam antibiotics occurs in up to 10% of pts w/history of penicillin allergy. Concurrent use of nephrotoxic medications, history of allergies or GI disease (esp. colitis), renal impairment. Safety and effectiveness in children not established. **PREGNANCY/LACTATION:** Small amounts excreted in breast milk. **Pregnancy Category B.**

INTERACTIONS

DRUG INTERACTIONS: Disulfiram reaction (facial flushing, nausea, sweating, headache, tachycardia) occurs if alcohol is ingested within 48-72 hrs after dose. Probenecid increases half-life, duration of action. May increase bleeding risk w/anticoagulants, heparin, thrombolytics. **ALTERED LAB VALUES:** Positive direct/indirect Coombs' test may occur (interferes w/hematologic tests, cross-matching procedures). May prolong prothrombin times. May increase SGOT (AST), SGPT (ALT), alkaline phosphatase, bilirubin, LDH, BUN, serum creatinine.

SIDE EFFECTS

OCCASIONAL: Diarrhea (3.6%). **RARE:** Nausea, hypotension, headache, alteration in color perception, joint pain and inflammation, lymphocytopenia, thrombocytopenia.

ADVERSE REACTIONS/TOXIC EFFECTS

Antibiotic-associated colitis, other superinfections may result from altered bacterial balance. Hypersensitivity reactions (ranging from rash, urticaria, fever to anaphylaxis) may occur, particularly in those w/history of allergies (esp. penicillin).

NURSING IMPLICATIONS

BASELINE ASSESSMENT:

Question for history of allergies, esp. cefmetazole, cephalosporins, penicillins. Obtain culture and sensitivity test before giving first dose (therapy may begin before results are known).

INTERVENTION/EVALUATION:

Evaluate IV site for phlebitis

(heat, pain, red streaking over vein). Determine pattern of bowel activity and stool consistency. Assess for nausea, vomiting. Check skin for rash. Monitor I&O, urinalysis, renal function reports, particularly when nephrotoxic medications are given concurrently. Be alert for superinfection: ulceration or changes in oral mucosa, genital/anal pruritus, vaginal discharge, moderate to severe diarrhea. Monitor PT levels and be alert for signs of bleeding: overt bleeding, bruising or swelling of soft tissue. Check temperature and B/P at least 2 times/day.

PATIENT/FAMILY TEACHING:

Doses should be evenly spaced. Continue antibiotic therapy for full length of treatment. Report diarrhea, bleeding, bruising, swelling of tissue, or onset of other new symptoms. Do not take other medications w/o consulting physician.

Avoid alcohol and alcohol-containing preparations (salad dressings, sauces, cough syrups—read all labels carefully) during and for 72 hrs after last dose of cefmetazole.

cefonicid sodium

ce-fon´oh-sid

(Monocid)

CANADIAN AVAILABILITY

Monocid

CLASSIFICATION

Antibiotic: Second-generation cephalosporin

PHARMACOKINETICS

Widely distributed. Protein binding: 70-80%. Primarily excreted unchanged in urine. Moderately removed by hemodialysis. Half-life: 4.5 hrs (increased in decreased renal function).

ACTION

Bactericidal. Binds to bacterial membranes, inhibiting bacterial cell wall synthesis.

USES

Treatment of respiratory, GU tract, skin and bone infections, septicemia, perioperative prophylaxis.

STORAGE/HANDLING

Solutions appear colorless to light amber. Solutions may darken (slight yellow color change does not indicate loss of potency). IV infusion (piggyback) stable for 24 hrs at room temperature, 72 hrs if refrigerated. Discard if precipitate forms.

IM/IV ADMINISTRATION

NOTE: Give IM, direct IV injection, intermittent IV infusion (piggyback).

IM:

1. Reconstitute each 500 mg vial w/2 ml sterile water for injection (2.5 ml for 1 Gm vial) to provide concentration of 220 mg or 325 mg/ml, respectively.
2. Inject deep IM into gluteus maximus or lateral aspect of thigh. For 2 Gm dose, use 2 separate injection sites.

IV:

1. For direct IV injection, reconstitute as above. Administer over 3-5 min.
2. For intermittent IV infusion (piggyback), further dilute w/50-100 ml 5% dextrose, 0.9% NaCl, or

other compatible IV fluid. Infuse over 20-30 min.

3. Alternating IV sites, use large veins to reduce risk of phlebitis.

INDICATIONS/DOSAGE/ROUTES

NOTE: Space doses evenly around the clock.

Uncomplicated UTI:
IM/IV: Adults, elderly: 500 mg q24h.

Mild to moderate infections:
IM/IV: Adults, elderly: 1 Gm q24h.

Severe or life-threatening infections:
IM/IV: Adults, elderly: 2 Gm q24h.

Perioperative prophylaxis:
IM/IV: Adults, elderly: 1 Gm before surgery (in pts undergoing cesarean section, only after umbilical cord is clamped) up to 1 Gm daily for 2 days postop.

Dosage in renal impairment:
After loading dose of 7.5 mg/kg, dose and/or frequency based on creatinine clearance and/or severity of infection.

CREATININE CLEARANCE	MILD TO MODERATE INFECTIONS	SEVERE INFECTIONS
60-79 ml/min	10 mg/kg q24h	25 mg/kg q24h
40-59 ml/min	8 mg/kg q24h	20 mg/kg q24h
20-39 ml/min	4 mg/kg q24h	15 mg/kg q24h
10-19 ml/min	4 mg/kg q48h	15 mg/kg q48h
5-9 ml/min	4 mg/kg q3-5days	15 mg/kg q3-5days
<5 ml/min	3 mg/kg q3-5days	4 mg/kg q3-5days

PRECAUTIONS

CONTRAINDICATIONS: History of hypersensitivity to cephalosporins, anaphylactic reaction to penicillins. **CAUTIONS:** Renal impairment, history of allergies or GI disease, concurrent use of nephrotoxic medications. **PREGNANCY/LACTATION:** Readily crosses placenta; distributed in breast milk. **Pregnancy Category B.**

INTERACTIONS

DRUG INTERACTIONS: Probenecid increases serum concentrations of cefonicid. **ALTERED LAB VALUES:** Positive direct/indirect Coombs' test may occur (interferes w/hematologic tests, cross-matching procedures). May increase SGOT (AST), SGPT (ALT), alkaline phosphatase, bilirubin, LDH, BUN, serum creatinine concentrations.

SIDE EFFECTS

OCCASIONAL: Pain, tenderness, induration at IM injection site; phlebitis, thrombophlebitis w/IV administration. **RARE:** Nausea, vomiting, diarrhea.

ADVERSE REACTIONS/TOXIC EFFECTS

Nephrotoxicity has occurred w/ high dosages or preexisting renal impairment. Antibiotic-associated colitis, other superinfections may result from altered bacterial balance. Hypersensitivity reactions (ranging from rash, urticaria, fever to anaphylaxis) occur in fewer than 5%, particularly those w/history of allergies, esp. penicillin.

NURSING IMPLICATIONS

BASELINE ASSESSMENT:

Question for history of allergies, particularly cephalosporins, penicillins. Obtain culture and sensitivity test before giving first dose

INTERVENTION/EVALUATION:

Evaluate IV site for phlebitis (heat, pain, red streaking over vein). Check IM injection sites for induration, tenderness. Determine pattern of bowel activity and stool consistency. Assess skin for rash, Monitor I&O, urinalysis, renal function reports for nephrotoxicity. Be alert for superinfection: nausea, diarrhea, vaginal discharge, genital/anal pruritus, ulceration or changes in oral mucosa.

PATIENT/FAMILY TEACHING:

Discomfort may occur w/IM injection. Doses should be evenly spaced. Continue antibiotic therapy for full length of treatment. Notify physician in event of diarrhea, bleeding, bruising, or onset of other new symptoms.

cefoperazone

sef-o-pear´a-zone
(Cefobid)

CANADIAN AVAILABILITY:
Cefobid

CLASSIFICATION

Antibiotic: Third-generation cephalosporin

PHARMACOKINETICS

Widely distributed. Achieves high biliary concentration. Protein binding: 82-93%. Primarily excreted unchanged in bile (excreted primarily in urine in pts w/ severe liver impairment). Minimally removed by hemodialysis. Half-life: 1.6-2.6 hrs (increased in decreased liver and/or biliary function).

ACTION

Bactericidal. Binds to bacterial membranes, inhibiting bacterial cell wall synthesis.

USES

Treatment of intra-abdominal, biliary, pelvic inflammatory infections; respiratory, GU tract, skin and bone infections; septicemia.

STORAGE/HANDLING

Solutions appear colorless to light yellow. IV infusion (piggyback) stable for 24 hrs at room temperature, 5 days if refrigerated. Discard if precipitate forms.

IM/IV ADMINISTRATION

NOTE: Give by IM injection or intermittent IV infusion (piggyback).

IM:

1. Reconstitute each 1 Gm vial w/3.8 ml sterile water for injection (7.2 ml for 2 Gm vial) to provide concentration of 250 mg/ml.
2. Shake well. Allow to stand (dissipates resulting foam). Examine for clarity.
3. To minimize discomfort, inject deep IM slowly. Less painful if injected into gluteus maximus rather than lateral aspect of thigh.

IV:

1. Reconstitute each 1 Gm vial w/5 ml sterile water for injection.
2. Further dilute w/50 to 100 ml 5% dextrose, 0.9% NaCl, or other compatible IV fluid. Infuse over 15-30 min.
3. Alternating IV sites, use large veins to reduce risk of phlebitis.

INDICATIONS/DOSAGE/ROUTES

NOTE: Space doses evenly around the clock.

Mild to moderate infections:
IM/IV: Adults, elderly: 2-4 Gm/day in divided doses q12h.

Severe or life-threatening infections:
IM/IV: Adults, elderly: Total daily dose and/or frequency may be increased to 6-12 Gm/day divided into 2, 3, or 4 equal doses of 1.5-4 Gm per dose.

Dosage in renal and/or hepatic impairment:
Do not exceed 4 Gm/day in those w/liver disease and/or biliary obstruction. Modification of dose usually not necessary in those w/renal impairment. Dose should not exceed 1-2 Gm/day in those w/both hepatic and substantial renal impairment.

PRECAUTIONS

CONTRAINDICATIONS: History of hypersensitivity to cephalosporins, anaphylactic reaction to penicillins. **CAUTIONS:** History of allergies, GI disease, hepatic or renal impairment. **PREGNANCY/LACTATION:** Readily crosses placenta. Distributed in breast milk. **Pregnancy Category B.**

INTERACTIONS

DRUG INTERACTIONS: Disulfiram reaction (facial flushing, nausea, sweating, headache, tachycardia) may occur when alcohol is ingested. May increase bleeding risk w/anticoagulants, heparin, thrombolytics. **ALTERED LAB VALUES:** Positive direct/indirect Coombs' test may occur (interferes w/hematologic tests, cross-matching procedures). May produce false-positive urine glucose determination w/Benedict's solution or Clinitest. Prothrombin times may be increased. May increase BUN, serum creatinine, SGOT (AST), SGPT (ALT), alkaline phosphatase concentrations.

SIDE EFFECTS

OCCASIONAL: Diarrhea, nausea, vomiting, discomfort at IM injection site, phlebitis/thrombophlebitis w/IV administration. **RARE:** Bleeding.

ADVERSE REACTIONS/TOXIC EFFECTS

Antibiotic-associated colitis, other superinfections may result from altered bacterial balance. Nephrotoxicity may occur when administered concurrently w/aminoglycosides. Hypersensitivity reactions (ranging from rash, urticaria, fever to anaphylaxis) occur in fewer than 5%, particularly those w/history of allergies, esp. penicillin.

NURSING IMPLICATIONS

BASELINE ASSESSMENT:

Question for history of allergies, particularly cephalosporins, penicillins. Obtain culture and sensitivity test before giving first dose (therapy may begin before results are known).

INTERVENTION/EVALUATION:

Evaluate IV site for phlebitis (heat, pain, red streaking over vein). Check IM injection sites for tenderness, induration. Determine pattern of bowel activity and stool consistency. Assess skin for rash. Monitor PT results and be alert for bleeding: overt bleeding, bruising or swelling of soft tissue. Monitor I&O, urinalysis, renal function reports for nephrotoxicity when administering aminoglycosides concurrently. Be alert for superinfection: ulceration or other change in oral mucosa, genital/anal pruritus, moderate to severe diarrhea.

PATIENT/FAMILY TEACHING:

Discomfort may occur w/IM injection. Doses should be evenly spaced. Continue antibiotic therapy for full length of treatment. Avoid alcohol and alcohol-containing preparations (salad dressings, sauces, cough syrups—read all labels carefully) during and for 72 hrs after last dose of cefoperazone. Notify physician at once in event of diarrhea, bleeding, bruising, swelling of tissue, rash, or onset of other new symptoms.

cefotaxime sodium

seh-fo´tax-eem

(Claforan)

CANADIAN AVAILABILITY:
Claforan

CLASSIFICATION

Antibiotic: Third-generation cephalosporin

PHARMACOKINETICS

Widely distributed (including CSF). Protein binding: 38%. Partially metabolized in liver to active metabolite. Primarily excreted in urine. Moderately removed by hemodialysis. Half-life: 1 hr (increased in decreased renal function).

ACTION

Bactericidal. Binds to bacterial membranes, inhibiting bacterial cell wall synthesis.

USES

Treatment of respiratory, GU tract, skin and bone infections; septicemia, gonorrhea; gynecologic, intra-abdominal, biliary infections; meningitis; perioperative prophylaxis.

STORAGE/HANDLING

Solutions appear light yellow to amber. IV infusion (piggyback) may darken in color (does not indicate loss of potency). IV infusion (piggyback) stable for 24 hrs at room temperature, 5 days if refrigerated. Discard if precipitate forms.

IM/IV ADMINISTRATION

NOTE: Give by IM injection, direct IV injection, intermittent IV infusion (piggyback).

IM:

1. Reconstitute 1 Gm vial w/3 ml (5 ml for 2 Gm vial) sterile water for injection or bacteriostatic water for injection to provide concentration of 300 or 330 mg/ml, respectively.
2. To minimize discomfort, inject deep IM slowly. Less painful if injected into gluteus maximus rather than lateral aspect of thigh. For 2 Gm IM dose, give at 2 separate sites.

IV:

1. For direct IV injection, reconstitute 1 or 2 Gm vial w/10 ml sterile water for injection. Administer over 3-5 min.
2. For intermittent IV infusion (piggyback), further dilute w/50-100 ml 5% dextrose, 0.9% NaCl, or other compatible IV fluid. Infuse over 20-30 min.
3. Alternating IV sites, use large veins to reduce risk of phlebitis.

INDICATIONS/DOSAGE/ROUTES

NOTE: Space doses evenly around the clock.

Uncomplicated infections:
IM/IV: Adults, elderly: 1 Gm q12h.

Mild to moderate infections:
IM/IV: Adults, elderly: 1-2 Gm q8h.

Severe infections:
IM/IV: Adults, elderly: 2 Gm q6-8h.

Life-threatening infections:
IM/IV: Adults, elderly: 2 Gm q4h.

Uncomplicated gonorrhea:
IM: Adults: 1 Gm one time.

Perioperative prophylaxis:
IM/IV: Adults, elderly: 1 Gm 30-90 min before surgery.

Cesarean section:
IV: Adults: 1 Gm as soon as umbilical cord is clamped, then 1 Gm 6 and 12 hrs after first dose.

Usual dosage for children:
IM/IV: Children >1 mo: 50-180 mg/kg/day in 4 to 6 divided doses. **Neonates 1-4 wk:** 25-50 mg/kg q8h. **Neonates 0-7 days:** 25-50 mg/kg q12h.

Dosage in renal impairment:
Creatinine clearance <20 ml/min: give ½ dose at usual dosage intervals.

PRECAUTIONS

CONTRAINDICATIONS: History of hypersensitivity to cephalosporins, anaphylactic reaction to penicillins. **CAUTIONS:** Concurrent use of nephrotoxic medications, history of allergies or GI disease, renal impairment w/creatinine clearance <20 ml/min. **PREGNANCY/LACTATION:** Readily crosses placenta; distributed in breast milk. **Pregnancy Category B.**

INTERACTIONS

DRUG INTERACTIONS: Probenecid increases serum concentration of cefotaxime. **ALTERED LAB VALUES:** Positive direct/indirect Coombs' test may occur (interferes w/hematologic tests, cross-matching procedures).

SIDE EFFECTS

FREQUENT: Generally well tolerated. Pain, tenderness at IM injection site; phlebitis, thrombophlebitis when given IV. **OCCASIONAL:** Nausea, vomiting, diarrhea, abdominal pain. **RARE:** Bleeding.

ADVERSE REACTIONS/TOXIC EFFECTS

Antibiotic-associated colitis, other superinfections may result from altered bacterial balance. Hypersensitivity reactions (ranging from rash, urticaria, fever to anaphylaxis) occur in fewer than 5%, particularly those w/history of allergies, esp. penicillin.

NURSING IMPLICATIONS

BASELINE ASSESSMENT:

Question for history of allergies, particularly cephalosporins, penicillins. Obtain culture and sensitivity test before giving first dose (therapy may begin before results are known).

INTERVENTION/EVALUATION:

Evaluate IV site for phlebitis (heat, pain, red streaking over vein). Check IM injection sites for tenderness, induration. Determine pattern of bowel activity and stool consistency. Assess for nausea, vomiting. Check skin for rash.

Monitor I&O, urinalysis, renal function reports, particularly when nephrotoxic medications are given concurrently. Be alert for superinfection: ulceration or changes of oral mucosa, genital/anal pruritus, vaginal discharge, moderate to severe diarrhea. Monitor PT levels and be alert for signs of bleeding: overt bleeding, bruising or swelling of soft tissue.

PATIENT/FAMILY TEACHING:

Discomfort may occur w/IM injection. Doses should be evenly spaced. Continue antibiotic therapy for full length of treatment. Notify physician in event of diarrhea, bleeding, bruising, swelling of tissue, or onset of other new symptoms.

cefotetan disodium

seh-fo-teh´tan
(Cefotan)

CANADIAN AVAILABILITY:
Cefotan

CLASSIFICATION

Antibiotic: Second-generation cephalosporin

PHARMACOKINETICS

Widely distributed. Protein binding: 88%. Primarily excreted unchanged in urine. Minimally removed by hemodialysis. Half-life: 3-4.6 hrs (increased in decreased renal function).

ACTION

Bactericidal. Binds to bacterial membranes, inhibiting bacterial cell wall synthesis.

USES

Treatment of respiratory, GU tract, skin, bone, gynecologic, intra-abdominal infections; perioperative prophylaxis.

STORAGE/HANDLING

Solutions appear colorless to light yellow. Color change to deep yellow does not indicate loss of potency. IV infusion (piggyback) stable for 24 hrs at room temperature, 96 hrs if refrigerated. Discard if precipitate forms.

IM/IV ADMINISTRATION

NOTE: Give by IM injection, direct IV injection, intermittent IV infusion (piggyback).

IM:

1. Reconstitute each 1 Gm w/2 ml (3 ml for 2 Gm vial) sterile water for injection or 0.9% NaCl injection to provide concentration of 375 or 470 mg/ml, respectively.
2. To minimize discomfort, inject deep IM slowly. Less painful if injected into gluteus maximus rather than lateral aspect of thigh.

IV:

1. For direct IV injection, reconstitute each 1 Gm w/at least 10 ml sterile water for injection. Administer over 3-5 min.
2. For intermittent IV infusion (piggyback), further dilute w/50-100 ml 5% dextrose, 0.9% NaCl, or other compatible IV fluid. Infuse over 20-30 min.
3. Alternating IV sites, use large veins to reduce risk of phlebitis.

INDICATIONS/DOSAGE/ROUTES

NOTE: Space doses evenly around the clock.

Urinary tract infections:
IM/IV: Adults, elderly: 500 mg q12h, or 1-2 Gm q12-24h.

Mild to moderate infections:
IM/IV: Adults, elderly: 1-2 Gm q12h.

Severe infections:
IM/IV: Adults, elderly: 2 Gm q12h.

Life-threatening infections:
IM/IV: Adults, elderly: 3 Gm q12h.

Perioperative prophylaxis:
IV: Adults, elderly: 1-2 Gm 30-60 min before surgery.

Cesarean section:
IV: Adults: 1-2 Gm as soon as umbilical cord is clamped.

Dosage in renal impairment:
Dose and/or frequency modified on basis of creatinine clearance and/or severity of infection.

CREATININE CLEARANCE	DOSAGE INTERVAL
10-30 ml/min	Usual dose q24h
<10 ml/min	Usual dose q48h

PRECAUTIONS

CONTRAINDICATIONS: History of hypersensitivity to cephalosporins, anaphylactic reaction to penicillins. **CAUTIONS:** Renal impairment, history of allergies or GI disease, concurrent use of nephrotoxic medications. **PREGNANCY/LACTATION:** Readily crosses placenta. Distributed in breast milk. **Pregnancy Category B.**

INTERACTIONS

DRUG INTERACTIONS: Disulfiram reaction (facial flushing, nausea, sweating, headache, tachycardia) occurs if alcohol is ingested within 48-72 hrs after drug administration. May increase bleeding risk w/anticoagulants, heparin, thrombolytics. **ALTERED LAB VALUES:** May prolong PT. Positive direct/indirect Coombs' test may occur (interferes w/hematologic tests, cross-matching procedures). May falsely elevate serum, urine creatinine concentrations.

SIDE EFFECTS

FREQUENT: Nausea, diarrhea. **OCCASIONAL:** Tenderness, induration at IM injection site; phlebitis, thrombophlebitis w/IV administration. **RARE:** Bleeding, esp. in elderly, debilitated.

ADVERSE REACTIONS/TOXIC EFFECTS

Antibiotic-associated colitis and other superinfections may result from altered bacterial balance. Hypersensitivity reactions (ranging from rash, urticaria, fever to anaphylaxis) occur in fewer than 5%, particularly those w/history of allergies, esp. penicillin.

NURSING IMPLICATIONS

BASELINE ASSESSMENT:

Question for history of allergies, particularly cephalosporins, penicillins. Obtain culture and sensitivity test before giving first dose (therapy may begin before results are known).

INTERVENTION/EVALUATION:

Monitor for nausea. Determine pattern of bowel activity and stool consistency. Check IM injection sites for tenderness and induration. Evaluate IV sites for phlebitis (heat, pain, red streaking over vein). Assess skin for rash. Monitor I&O, urinalysis, renal function reports w/preexisting renal impairment or concurrent therapy w/

nephrotoxic medications. Be alert for superinfection: moderate to severe diarrhea, genital/anal pruritus, ulceration or change in oral mucosa. Monitor PT results and be alert for bleeding: overt bleeding, bruising or swelling of tissue.

PATIENT/FAMILY TEACHING:

Discomfort may occur w/IM injection. Doses should be evenly spaced. Continue antibiotic therapy for full length of treatment. Avoid alcohol and alcohol-containing preparations (salad dressings, sauces, cough syrups—read all labels carefully) during and for 72 hrs after last dose of cefotetan. Notify physician at once in event of diarrhea, bleeding, bruising, swelling of tissue, rash, onset of new symptoms.

cefoxitin sodium

seh-fox' ih-tin
(Mefoxin)

CANADIAN AVAILABILITY:
Mefoxin

CLASSIFICATION

Antibiotic: Second-generation cephalosporin

PHARMACOKINETICS

Widely distributed. Protein binding: 70-80%. Primarily excreted unchanged in urine. Moderately removed by hemodialysis. Half-life: 0.7-1.1 hrs (increased in decreased renal function).

ACTION

Bactericidal. Binds to bacterial membranes, inhibiting bacterial cell wall synthesis.

USES

Treatment of respiratory, GU tract, skin, bone, intra-abdominal, gynecologic infections; gonorrhea, septicemia, perioperative prophylaxis.

STORAGE/HANDLING

Solutions appear colorless to light amber but may darken (does not indicate loss of potency). IV infusion (piggyback) stable for 24 hrs at room temperature, 48 hrs if refrigerated. Discard if precipitate forms.

IM/IV ADMINISTRATION

NOTE: Give IM, direct IV injection, or intermittent IV infusion (piggyback).

IM:

1. Reconstitute each 1 Gm vial w/2 ml sterile water for injection to provide concentration of 400 mg/ml.
2. To minimize discomfort, inject deep IM slowly. Less painful if injected into gluteus maximus rather than lateral aspect of thigh.

IV:

1. For direct IV injection, reconstitute each 1 Gm w/at least 10 ml sterile water for injection. Administer over 3-5 min.
2. For intermittent IV infusion (piggyback), further dilute w/50 or 100 ml 5% dextrose, 0.9% NaCl, or other compatible IV fluid. Infuse over 30 min.
3. Alternating IV sites, use large veins to reduce potential for phlebitis.

INDICATIONS/DOSAGE/ROUTES

NOTE: Space doses evenly around the clock.

Mild to moderate infections:
IM/IV: Adults, elderly: 1-2 Gm q6-8h.

Severe infections:
IM/IV: Adults, elderly: 1 Gm q4h or 2 Gm q6-8h up to 2 Gm q4h.

Uncomplicated gonorrhea:
IM: Adults: 2 Gm one time w/1 Gm probenecid.

Perioperative prophylaxis:
IM/IV: Adults, elderly: 2 Gm 30-60 min before surgery and q6h up to 24 hrs postop. **Children >3 mo:** 30-40 mg/kg 30-60 min before surgery and q6h postop for no more than 24 hrs.

Cesarean section:
IV: Adults: 2 Gm as soon as umbilical cord is clamped, then 2 Gm 4 and 8 hrs after first dose, then q6h for no more than 24 hrs.

Usual dosage for children:
IM/IV: Children >3 mo: 80-160 mg/kg/day in 4-6 divided doses. **Maximum:** 12 Gm/day.

Dosage in renal impairment:
After loading dose of 1-2 Gm, dosage and/or frequency is modified on basis of creatinine clearance and/or severity of infection.

CREATININE CLEARANCE	DOSAGE
30-50 ml/min	1-2 Gm q8-12h
10-29 ml/min	1-2 Gm q12-24h
5-9 ml/min	500 mg-1 Gm q12-24h
<5 ml/min	500 mg-1 Gm q24-48h

PRECAUTIONS

CONTRAINDICATIONS: History of hypersensitivity to cephalosporins, anaphylactic reaction to penicillins. **CAUTIONS:** Renal impairment, history of allergies or GI disease, concurrent use of nephrotoxic medications. **PREGNANCY/LACTATION:** Readily crosses placenta. Distributed in breast milk. **Pregnancy Category B.**

INTERACTIONS

DRUG INTERACTIONS: Probenecid increases serum concentrations of cefoxitin. **ALTERED LAB VALUES:** Positive direct/indirect Coombs' test may occur (interferes w/hematologic tests, cross-matching procedures). May falsely elevate serum, urine creatinine concentrations.

SIDE EFFECTS

OCCASIONAL: Pain, induration at IM injection sites; phlebitis, thrombophlebitis w/IV administration. **RARE:** Nausea. vomiting, diarrhea, bleeding.

ADVERSE REACTIONS/TOXIC EFFECTS

Antibiotic-associated colitis, other superinfections may result from altered bacterial balance. Nephrotoxicity may occur, esp. w/ preexisting renal disease. Hypersensitivity reactions (ranging from rash, urticaria, fever to anaphylaxis) occur in fewer than 5%, particularly those w/history of allergies, esp. penicillin.

NURSING IMPLICATIONS

BASELINE ASSESSMENT:

Question for history of allergies, particularly cephalosporins, penicillins. Obtain culture and sensitivity test before giving first dose (therapy may begin before results are known).

INTERVENTION/EVALUATION:

Evaluate IV site for phlebitis (heat, pain, red streaking over vein). Check IM injection sites for induration, tenderness. Determine pattern of bowel activity and stool consistency. Monitor for nausea, vomiting. Assess skin for rash. Monitor I&O, urinalysis, renal function reports for nephrotoxicity. Be alert for superinfection: moderate to severe diarrhea, ulceration or change of oral mucosa, vaginal discharge, genital/anal pruritus. Monitor PT results and be alert for bleeding: overt bleeding, bruising or swelling of soft tissue.

PATIENT/FAMILY TEACHING:

Discomfort may occur w/IM injection. Doses should be evenly spaced. Continue antibiotic therapy for full length of treatment. Notify physician at once in event of diarrhea, bleeding, bruising, swelling of tissue, onset of other new symptoms.

cefpodoxime proxetil

sef-poe-docks'em

(Vantin)

CLASSIFICATION

Antibiotic: Second-generation cephalosporin

PHARMACOKINETICS

Well absorbed from GI tract (food increases absorption). Widely distributed. Protein binding: 21-33%. A prodrug de-esterified by intestinal wall esterases to active form. Primarily excreted unchanged in urine. Partially removed by hemodialysis. Half-life: 2.3 hrs (increased in decreased renal function, elderly).

ACTION

Bactericidal. Binds to bacterial membrane, inhibiting bacterial cell wall synthesis.

USES

Treatment of lower respiratory tract infections (pneumonia, chronic bronchitis), upper respiratory tract (otitis media, pharyngitis/tonsillitis), sexually transmitted diseases (urethral and cervical gonorrhea, anorectal infection), skin and skin structure, urinary tract infections.

STORAGE/HANDLING

Oral suspension, after reconstitution, stable for 14 days if refrigerated.

PO ADMINISTRATION

Administer w/food to enhance absorption.

INDICATIONS/DOSAGE/ROUTES

NOTE: Space doses evenly around the clock.

Pneumonia, chronic bronchitis:
PO: Adults, elderly, children >13 yrs: 200 mg q12h for 10-14 days.

Gonorrhea, rectal gonococcal infection (women only):
PO: Adults, children >13 yrs: 200 mg as single dose.

Skin/skin structure infections:
PO: Adults, elderly, children >13 yrs: 400 mg q12h for 7-14 days.

Pharyngitis/tonsillitis
PO: Adults, elderly, children >13 yrs: 100 mg q12h for 10 days. **Children 6 mo-12 yrs:** 5 mg/kg q12h for 10 days. **Maximum:** 100 mg/dose.

Urinary tract infection:
PO: Adults, elderly, children >13 yrs: 100 mg q12h for 7 days.

Acute otitis media:

PO: Children 6 mo-12 yrs: 5 mg/kg q12h for 10 days. **Maximum:** 200 mg/dose.

Dosage in renal impairment:

Dose and/or frequency is based on degree of renal impairment (creatinine clearance).

PRECAUTIONS

CONTRAINDICATIONS: History of hypersensitivity to cephalosporins, anaphylactic reaction to penicillins. **CAUTIONS:** Renal impairment, history of allergies or GI disease, concurrent use of nephrotoxic medications. **PREGNANCY/LACTATION:** Readily crosses placenta. Distributed in breast milk. **Pregnancy Category B.**

INTERACTIONS

DRUG INTERACTIONS: Antacids, H_2 antagonists may decrease absorption. Probenecid may increase concentration. **ALTERED LAB VALUES:** Positive direct/indirect Coombs' test may occur. May increase SGOT (AST), SGPT (ALT), alkaline phosphatase, LDH, bilirubin, prothrombin time, partial thromboplastin time. May alter blood glucose concentrations.

SIDE EFFECTS

FREQUENT: Abdominal pain, nausea, vomiting, diarrhea. **OCCASIONAL:** Vaginal fungal infections, rash, headache.

ADVERSE REACTIONS/TOXIC EFFECTS

Antibiotic-associated colitis, other superinfections may result from altered bacterial balance. Nephrotoxicity may occur, esp. w/ preexisting renal disease. Hypersensitivity reactions (ranging from rash, urticaria, fever to anaphylaxis) occur in less than 5%, generally those w/history of allergies, especially penicillin.

NURSING IMPLICATIONS

BASELINE ASSESSMENT:

Shake oral suspension well before using. Question history of allergies, particularly cephalosporins, penicillins. Obtain culture and sensitivity test before giving first dose (therapy may begin before results are known).

INTERVENTION/EVALUATION:

Monitor for anorexia, nausea, vomiting. Check stools for frequency, consistency. Assess skin for rash. Monitor I&O, urinalysis, renal function reports for nephrotoxicity. Be alert for superinfection: genital/anal pruritus, moniliasis, sore mouth or tongue, moderate to severe diarrhea.

PATIENT/FAMILY TEACHING:

Continue therapy for full length of treatment. Doses should be evenly spaced. Notify physician in event of diarrhea or other new symptom.

cefprozil

sef-proz´ill

(Cefzil)

CLASSIFICATION

Antibiotic: Second-generation cephalosporin

PHARMACOKINETICS

Well absorbed from GI tract. Widely distributed. Protein binding: 36%. Primarily excreted unchanged in urine. Moderately removed by hemodialysis. Half-life:

1.3 hrs (increased in decreased renal function).

ACTION

Bactericidal. Binds to bacterial membranes, inhibiting bacterial cell wall synthesis.

USES

Treatment of pharyngitis/tonsillitis, otitis media, secondary bacterial infection of acute bronchitis and acute bacterial exacerbation of chronic bronchitis, uncomplicated skin/skin structure infections.

STORAGE/HANDLING

Oral suspension, after reconstitution, stable for 14 days if refrigerated.

PO ADMINISTRATION

1. Shake oral suspension well before using.
2. Give w/o regard to meals; if GI upset occurs, give w/food or milk.

INDICATIONS/DOSAGE/ROUTES

NOTE: Space doses evenly around the clock.

Pharyngitis, tonsillitis:
PO: Adults, elderly: 500 mg q24h for 10 days. **Children: (2-12 yrs):** 7.5 mg/kg q12h for 10 days.

Secondary bacterial infection of acute bronchitis; acute bacterial exacerbation of chronic bronchitis:
PO: Adults, elderly: 500 mg q12h for 10 days.

Skin/skin structure infections:
PO: Adults, elderly: 250-500 mg q12h for 10 days.

Otitis media:
PO: Children (6 mo - 12 yrs): 15 mg/kg q12h for 10 days.

Dosage in renal impairment:

Dose and/or frequency is based on degree of renal impairment (creatinine clearance). Creatine clearance <30 ml/min: 50% dosage at usual interval.

PRECAUTIONS

CONTRAINDICATIONS: History of hypersensitivity to cephalosporins, anaphylactic reaction to penicillins. **CAUTIONS:** Renal impairment, history of allergies or GI disease, concurrent use of nephrotoxic medications. **PREGNANCY/LACTATION:** Readily crosses placenta. Distributed in breast milk. **Pregnancy Category C.**

INTERACTIONS

DRUG INTERACTIONS: Probenecid increases serum concentrations of cefprozil. **ALTERED LAB VALUES:** Positive direct/indirect Coombs' test may occur (interferes w/hematologic tests, cross-matching procedures).

SIDE EFFECTS

FREQUENT: Anorexia, nausea, vomiting, diarrhea. **OCCASIONAL:** Dyspepsia, abdominal pain, genital/anal pruritus, moniliasis.

ADVERSE REACTIONS/TOXIC EFFECTS

Antibiotic-associated colitis, other superinfections may result from altered bacterial balance. Nephrotoxicity may occur, esp. w/preexisting renal disease. Hypersensitivity reactions (ranging from rash, urticaria, fever to anaphylaxis) occur in fewer than 5%, generally those w/history of allergies, esp. penicillin.

NURSING IMPLICATIONS

BASELINE ASSESSMENT:

Question history of allergies,

particularly cephalosporins, penicillins. Obtain culture and sensitivity test before giving first dose (therapy may begin before results are known).

INTERVENTION/EVALUATION:

Monitor for anorexia, nausea, vomiting. Determine pattern of bowel activity and stool consistency. Assess skin for rash. Monitor I&O, urinalysis, renal function reports for nephrotoxicity. Be alert for superinfection: genital/anal pruritus, moniliasis, abdominal pain, sore mouth or tongue, moderate to severe diarrhea.

PATIENT/FAMILY TEACHING:

Continue therapy for full length of treatment. Doses should be evenly spaced. Notify physician in event of diarrhea or other new symptom.

ceftazidime

sef-taz´ih-deem

(Ceptaz, Fortaz, Tazicef, Tazidime)

CANADIAN AVAILABILITY:
Fortaz, Ceptaz

CLASSIFICATION

Antibiotic: Third-generation cephalosporin

PHARMACOKINETICS

Widely distributed (including CSF). Protein binding: <10%. Primarily excreted unchanged in urine. Removed by hemodialysis. Half-life: 2 hrs (increased in decreased renal function).

ACTION

Bactericidal. Binds to bacterial membranes, inhibiting bacterial cell wall synthesis.

USES

Treatment of intra-abdominal, biliary tract infections, respiratory, GU tract, skin, bone infections; meningitis, septicemia.

STORAGE/HANDLING

Solutions appear light yellow to amber, tend to darken (color change does not indicate loss of potency). IV infusion (piggyback) stable for 18 hrs at room temperture, 7 days if refrigerated. Discard if precipitate forms.

IM/IV ADMINISTRATION

NOTE: Give by IM injection, direct IV injection, intermittent IV infusion (piggyback).

IM:

1. Reconstitute each 500 mg w/1.5 ml sterile water for injection or bacteriostatic water for injection to provide concentration of 280 mg/ml.
2. To minimize discomfort, inject deep IM slowly. Less painful if injected into gluteus maximus rather than lateral aspect of thigh.

IV:

1. For direct IV injection, reconstitute each 500 mg vial w/5-10 ml sterile water for injection (10 ml for 1 or 2 Gm vial). Administer over 3-5 min.
2. For intermittent IV infusion (piggyback), further dilute w/50-100 ml 5% dextrose, 0.9% NaCl, or other compatible IV fluid. Infuse over 15-30 min.
3. Alternating IV sites, use large veins to reduce risk of phlebitis.

INDICATIONS/DOSAGE/ROUTES

NOTE: Space doses evenly around the clock.

Urinary tract infections:
IM/IV: Adults: 250-500 mg q8-12h.

Mild to moderate infections:
IM/IV: Adults: 1 Gm q8-12h.

Uncomplicated pneumonia, skin or skin structure infection:
IM/IV: Adults: 0.5-1 Gm q8h.

Bone and joint infection:
IM/IV: Adults: 2 Gm q12h.

Meningitis, serious gynecologic, intra-abdominal infections:
IM/IV: Adults: 2 Gm q8h.

Pseudomonal pulmonary infections in pts w/cystic fibrosis:
IV: Adults: 30-50 mg/kg q8h. **Maximum:** 6 Gm/day.

Usual elderly dosage:
IM/IV: Elderly: Normal renal function q12h.

Usual dosage for children:
IV: Children >1 mo: 30-50 mg/kg q8h. **Children <1 mo:** 30 mg/kg q12h (increase to 50 mg/kg for meningitis).

Dosage in renal impairment:
After initial 1 Gm dose, dose and/or frequency is modified on basis of creatinine clearance and/or severity of infection.

CREATININE CLEARANCE	DOSAGE
31-50 ml/min	1 Gm q12h
16-30 ml/min	1 Gm q24h
6-15 ml/min	500 mg q24h
<5 ml/min	500 mg q48h

PRECAUTIONS

CONTRAINDICATIONS: History of hypersensitivity to cephalosporins, anaphylactic reactions to penicillins. **CAUTIONS:** Renal impairment, history of GI disease or allergies, concurrent use of nephrotoxic medications. **PREGNANCY/LACTATION:** Readily crosses placenta. Distributed in breast milk. **Pregnancy Category B.**

INTERACTIONS

DRUG INTERACTIONS: None significant. **ALTERED LAB VALUES:** Positive direct/indirect Coombs' test may occur (interferes w/hematologic tests, cross-matching procedures). May increase BUN, serum creatinine, SGOT (AST), SGPT (ALT), alkaline phosphatase, LDH concentrations.

SIDE EFFECTS

Generally well tolerated. **FREQUENT:** Pain, induration at IM injection sites, phlebitis, thrombophlebitis w/IV administration. **OCCASIONAL:** Nausea, vomiting, diarrhea, and abdominal pain. **RARE:** Headache, dizziness.

ADVERSE REACTIONS/TOXIC EFFECTS

Antibiotic-associated colitis, other superinfections may result from altered bacterial balance. Nephrotoxicity may occur, especially w/preexisting renal disease. Hypersensitivity reactions (ranging from rash, urticaria, fever to anaphylaxis) occur in fewer than 5%, particularly those w/history of allergies, especially penicillin.

NURSING IMPLICATIONS

BASELINE ASSESSMENT:

Question for history of allergies, particularly cephalosporins, penicillins. Obtain culture and sensitivity test before giving the first dose (therapy may begin before results are known).

INTERVENTION/EVALUATION:

Evaluate IV site for phlebitis (heat, pain, red streaking over vein). Check IM injection sites for induration, tenderness. Determine pattern of bowel activity and stool consistency. Monitor for nausea and vomiting. Assess skin for rash. Monitor I&O, urinalysis, renal function reports for nephrotoxicity. Be alert for superinfection: moderate to severe diarrhea, ulceration or change in oral mucosa, vaginal discharge, genital/anal pruritus.

PATIENT/FAMILY TEACHING:

Discomfort may occur w/IM injection. Doses should be evenly spaced. Continue antibiotic therapy for full length of treatment. Notify physician at once in event of diarrhea, rash, or onset of other new symptoms.

ceftizoxime sodium

cef-tih-zox´eem

(Cefizox)

CANADIAN AVAILABILITY:

Cefizox

CLASSIFICATION

Antibiotic: Third-generation cephalosporin

PHARMACOKINETICS

Widely distributed (including CSF). Protein binding: 30%. Primarily excreted unchanged in urine. Moderately removed by hemodialysis. Half-life: 1.7 hrs (increased in decreased renal function).

ACTION

Bactericidal. Binds to bacterial membranes, inhibiting bacterial cell wall synthesis.

USES

Treatment of intra-abdominal, biliary tract, respiratory, GU tract, skin, bone infections; gonorrhea, meningitis, septicemia, pelvic inflammatory disease (PID).

STORAGE/HANDLING

Solutions appear clear to pale yellow. Color change from yellow to amber does not indicate loss of potency. IV infusion (piggyback) stable for 24 hrs at room temperature, 96 hrs if refrigerated. Discard if precipitate forms.

IM/IV ADMINISTRATION

NOTE: Give by IM injection, direct IV injection, intermittent IV infusion (piggyback).

IM:

1. Reconstitute each 1 Gm vial w/3 ml sterile water for injection to provide concentration of 270 mg/ml.
2. Inject deep IM slowly to minimize discomfort.
3. When giving 2 Gm dose, divide dose, give in different large muscle masses.

IV:

1. For direct IV injection, reconstitute each 1 Gm vial w/10-20 ml sterile water for injection. Administer over 3-5 min.
2. For intermittent IV infusion (piggyback), further dilute w/50-100 ml 5% dextrose, 0.9% NaCl, or other compatible IV fluid. Infuse over 15-30 min.
3. Alternating IV sites, use large veins to reduce risk of phlebitis.

INDICATIONS/DOSAGE/ROUTES

Uncomplicated UTI:
IM/IV: Adults, elderly: 500 mg q12h.

Mild to moderate to severe infection:
IM/IV: Adults, elderly: 1-2 Gm q8-12h.

PID:
IV: Adults: 2 Gm q4-8h.

Life-threatening infections:
IV: Adults, elderly: 3-4 Gm q8h, up to 2 Gm q4h.

Uncomplicated gonorrhea:
IM: Adults: 1 Gm one time.

Usual dosage for children:
IM/IV: Children >6 mo: 50 mg/kg q6-8h.

Dosage in renal impairment:
After loading dose of 0.5-1 Gm, dose and/or frequency is modified on basis of creatinine clearance and/or severity of infection.

CREATININE CLEARANCE	DOSAGE
50-79 ml/min	500 mg-1.5 Gm q8h
5-49 ml/min	250 mg-1 Gm q12h
<5 ml/min	250-500 mg q24h

PRECAUTIONS

CONTRAINDICATIONS: History of hypersensitivity to cephalosporins, anaphylactic reaction to penicillins. **CAUTIONS:** History of allergies, GI disease, hepatic and renal impairment. **PREGNANCY/LACTATION:** Readily crosses placenta; distributed in breast milk. **Pregnancy Category B.**

INTERACTIONS

DRUG INTERACTIONS: Probenecid increases serum concentration of ceftizoxime. **ALTERED LAB VALUES:** May increase BUN, serum creatinine, SGOT (AST), SGPT (ALT), alkaline phosphatase concentrations.

SIDE EFFECTS

Generally well tolerated. **FREQUENT:** Pain, induration at IM sites, phlebitis, thrombophlebitis w/IV administration. **OCCASIONAL:** Nausea, vomiting, diarrhea. **RARE:** Bleeding.

ADVERSE REACTIONS/TOXIC EFFECTS

Antibiotic-associated colitis, other superinfections may result from altered bacterial balance. Nephrotoxicity may occur when administered concurrently w/aminoglycosides. Hypersensitivity reactions (ranging from rash, urticaria, fever to anaphylaxis) occur in fewer than 5%, particularly those w/history of allergies, esp. penicillin.

NURSING IMPLICATIONS

BASELINE ASSESSMENT:

Question for history of allergies, particularly cephalosporins, penicillins. Obtain culture and sensitivity test before giving first dose (therapy may begin before results are known).

INTERVENTION/EVALUATION:

Evaluate IV site for phlebitis (heat, pain, red streaking over vein). Check IM injection sites for tenderness, induration. Determine pattern of bowel activity and stool consistency. Assess skin for rash. Monitor for nausea, vomiting. Monitor I&O, urinalysis, renal function reports for nephrotoxicity when administering aminoglycosides concurrently. Be alert to signs of superinfection: ulceration or other change in oral mucosa, genital/anal pruritus, vaginal discharge, moderate to severe diarrhea. Monitor PT results and assess for bleeding: overt bleeding, bruising or swelling of soft tissue.

PATIENT/FAMILY TEACHING:

Discomfort may occur w/IM injection. Doses should be evenly spaced. Continue antibiotic therapy for full length of treatment. Notify physician at once in event of bleeding, bruising, swelling of tissue, diarrhea, rash, onset of other new symptoms.

ceftriaxone sodium

cef-try-ox´zone
(Rocephin)

CANADIAN AVAILABILITY:
Rocephin

CLASSIFICATION

Antibiotic: Third-generation cephalosporin

PHARMACOKINETICS

Widely distributed (including CSF). Protein binding: 85-95%. Primarily excreted unchanged in urine. Not removed by hemodialysis. Half-life: 4.3-4.6 hrs IV; 5.8-8.7 hrs IM (increased in decreased renal function).

ACTION

Bactericidal. Binds to bacterial membranes, inhibiting bacterial cell wall synthesis.

USES

Treatment of respiratory, GU tract, skin, bone, intra-abdominal, biliary tract infections; septicemia, meningitis, gonorrhea, Lyme disease.

STORAGE/HANDLING

Solutions appear light yellow to amber. IV infusion (piggyback) stable for 3 days at room temperature, 10 days if refrigerated. Discard if precipitate forms.

IM/IV ADMINISTRATION

NOTE: Give by IM injection, intermittent IV infusion (piggyback).

IM:

1. Reconstitute each 250 mg vial w/0.9 ml sterile water for injection or 0.9% NaCl injection to provide concentration of 250 mg/ml.
2. To minimize discomfort, inject deep IM slowly. Less painful if injected into gluteus maximus rather than lateral aspect of thigh.

IV:

1. Reconstitute each 250 mg w/2.4 ml sterile water for injection or 0.9% NaCl injection to provide concentration of 100 mg/ml. Administer over 2-4 min.
2. For intermittent IV infusion (piggyback), further dilute in 50-100 ml 5% dextrose, 0.9% NaCl, or other compatible IV fluid. Infuse over 15-30 min for adults, 10-30 min in children, neonates.
3. Alternating IV sites, use large veins to reduce potential for phlebitis.

INDICATIONS/DOSAGE/ROUTES

Mild to moderate infections:
IM/IV: Adults, elderly: 1-2 Gm given as single dose or 2 divided doses.

Serious infections:
IM/IV: Adults, elderly: Up to 4

Gm/day in 2 divided doses. **Children:** 50-75 mg/kg/day in divided doses q12h. **Maximum:** 2 Gm/day.

Skin/skin structure infections:
IM/IV: Children: 50-75 mg/kg/day as single or 2 divided doses. **Maximum:** 2 Gm/day.

Meningitis:
IV: Children: Initially, 75 mg/kg, then 100 mg/kg/day as single or in divided doses q12h. **Maximum:** 4 Gm/day.

Lyme's disease:
IV: Adults, elderly: 2-4 Gm daily for 10-14 days.

Perioperative prophylaxis:
IM/IV: Adults, elderly: 1 Gm 0.5-2 hrs before surgery.

Uncomplicated gonorrhea:
IM: Adults: 250 mg one time plus doxycycline.

Dosage in renal impairment:
Dosage modification usually unnecessary, but should be monitored in those w/both renal and hepatic impairment or severe renal impairment.

PRECAUTIONS

CONTRAINDICATIONS: History of hypersensitivity to cephalosporins, anaphylactic reactions to penicillins. **CAUTIONS:** Renal or hepatic impairment, history of GI disease, concurrent administration of nephrotoxic medications. **PREGNANCY/LACTATION:** Readily crosses placenta; distributed in breast milk. **Pregnancy Category B.**

INTERACTIONS

DRUG INTERACTIONS: None significant. **ALTERED LAB VALUES:** Positive direct/indirect Coombs' test may occur (interferes w/hematologic tests, cross-matching procedures). May increase BUN, serum creatinine, SGOT (AST), SGPT (ALT), alkaline phosphatase, bilirubin concentrations.

SIDE EFFECTS

FREQUENT: Phlebitis, thrombophlebitis w/IV administration; pain, induration at IM injection site, diarrhea. **OCCASIONAL:** Nausea, vomiting, headache, dizziness. **RARE:** Bleeding.

ADVERSE REACTIONS/TOXIC EFFECTS

Antibiotic-associated colitis, other superinfections may result from altered bacterial balance. Nephrotoxicity has occurred w/high dosages or preexisting renal disease. Hypersensitivity reactions (ranging from rash, urticaria, fever to anaphylaxis) occur in fewer than 5%, particularly those w/history of allergies, esp. penicillin.

NURSING IMPLICATIONS

BASELINE ASSESSMENT:

Question for history of allergies, particularly cephalosporins, penicillins. Obtain culture and sensitivity test before giving first dose (therapy may begin before results are known).

INTERVENTION/EVALUATION:

Evaluate IV site for phlebitis (heat, pain, red streaking over vein). Check IM injection sites for tenderness, induration. Determine pattern of bowel activity and stool consistency. Monitor for nausea and vomiting. Assess skin for rash. Monitor I&O, urinalysis, renal function tests for nephrotoxicity. Monitor PT results and be alert for signs of bleeding: overt bleeding, bruising, swelling of tissue. Be alert for superinfection: ulceration or change in oral mucosa, genital/anal pruritus, vaginal discharge, moderate to severe diarrhea.

PATIENT/FAMILY TEACHING:

Discomfort may occur w/IM injection. Doses should be evenly spaced. Continue antibiotic therapy for full length of treatment. Notify physician at once in event of diarrhea, bleeding, bruising, swelling of tissue, rash, onset of other new symptom.

cefuroxime axetil

sef-yur-ox′ime

(Ceftin)

cefuroxime sodium

(Kefurox, Zinacef)

CANADIAN AVAILABILITY:
Zinacef

CLASSIFICATION

Antibiotic: Second-generation cephalosporin

PHARMACOKINETICS

Rapidly absorbed from GI tract. Oral form rapidly hydrolyzed to cefuroxime. Widely distributed (including CSF). Protein binding: 50%. Primarily excreted unchanged in urine. Moderately removed by hemodialysis. Half-life: 1.3 hrs (increased in decreased renal function).

ACTION

Bactericidal. Binds to bacterial membranes, inhibiting bacterial cell wall synthesis.

USES

Treatment of otitis media, impetigo, respiratory, GU tract, gynecologic, skin, bone infections; septicemia, bacterial meningitis, gonorrhea and other gonococcal infections; ampicillin-resistant influenza, perioperative prophylaxis.

STORAGE/HANDLING

Solutions appear light yellow to amber, may darken, but color change does not indicate loss of potency. IV infusion (piggyback) stable for 24 hrs at room temperature, 7 days if refrigerated. Discard if precipitate forms.

PO/IM/IV ADMINISTRATION

NOTE: Give orally, IM, direct IV injection, intermittent IV infusion (piggyback).

PO:

1. Give w/o regard to meals. If GI upset occurs, give w/food or milk.
2. Tablets may be crushed, mixed w/food.

IM:

1. Reconstitute each 750 mg vial w/3.6 ml sterile water for injection to provide concentration of 200 mg/ml. Shake gently.
2. To minimize discomfort, inject deep IM slowly. Less painful if injected into gluteus maximus rather than lateral aspect of thigh.

IV:

1. For direct IV injection, dilute 750 mg in 8 ml (1.5 Gm in 14 ml) sterile water for injection to provide a concentration of 100 mg/ml. Administer over 3-5 min.
2. For intermittent IV infusion (piggyback), further dilute w/50-100 ml 5% dextrose, 0.9% NaCl, or

other compatible IV fluid. Infuse over 15-60 min.

3. Alternating IV sites, use large veins to reduce risk of phlebitis.

INDICATIONS/DOSAGE/ROUTES

Pharyngitis/tonsillitis:
PO: Adults, elderly: 250 mg 2 times/day. **Children:** 125 mg 2 times/day or 20 mg/kg/day in 2 divided doses.

Acute otitis media:
PO: Children: 250 mg 2 times/day or 30 mg/kg/day in 2 divided doses.

Acute/chronic bronchitis:
PO: Adults: 250-500 mg 2 times/day.

Impetigo:
PO: Children: 30 mg/kg/day in 2 divided doses.

Skin/skin structure infections:
PO: Adults: 250-500 mg 2 times/day.
IM/IV: Adults: 750 mg-1.5 Gm q8h.

Urinary tract infections:
PO: Adults: 125-250 mg 2 times/day.
IM/IV: Adults: 750 mg-1.5 Gm q8h.

Pneumonia:
IM/IV: Adults: 750 mg-1.5 Gm q8h.

Uncomplicated gonorrhea:
PO: Adults: 1 Gm as single dose.
IM: Adults: 1.5 Gm as single dose.

Disseminated gonococcal infection:
IM/IV: Adults: 750 mg to 1.5 Gm q8h.

Bone/joint infections:
IM/IV: Adults, elderly: 1.5 Gm q8h.

Life-threatening infections:
IV: Adults, elderly: 1.5 Gm q6h. **Children:** 150 mg/kg/day in 3 divided doses.

Bacterial meningitis:
IV: Adults: Up to 3 Gm q8h. **Children:** Initially, 200-240 mg/kg/day in 3-4 divided doses; then, 100 mg/kg/day w/clinical improvement.

Perioperative prophylaxis:
IV: Adults, elderly: 1.5 Gm 30-60 min before surgery and 750 mg q8h postop.

Dosage in renal impairment:
Adult dosage is modified on basis of creatinine clearance and/or severity of infection.

CREATININE CLEARANCE	DOSAGE
10-20 ml/min	750 mg q12h
<10 ml/min	750 mg q24h

PRECAUTIONS

CONTRAINDICATIONS: History of hypersensitivity to cephalosporins, anaphylactic reaction to penicillins. **CAUTIONS:** Renal impairment, history of allergies or GI disease, concurrent use of nephrotoxic medications. **PREGNANCY/LACTATION:** Readily crosses placenta. Distributed in breast milk. **Pregnancy Category B.**

INTERACTIONS

DRUG INTERACTIONS: Probenecid increases serum concentration of cefuroxime. **ALTERED LAB VALUES:** Positive direct/indirect Coombs' test may occur (interferes w/hematologic tests, cross-matching procedures). May increase SGOT (AST), SGPT (ALT), alkaline phosphatase, bilirubin, LDH concentrations. May decrease hematocrit or hemoglobin concentrations.

SIDE EFFECTS

COMMON: Pain, induration at IM injection sites; phlebitis, thrombophlebitis w/IV administration. **OCCASIONAL:** Nausea, diarrhea.

ADVERSE REACTIONS/TOXIC EFFECTS

Antibiotic-associated colitis, other superinfections may result from altered bacterial balance. Nephrotoxicity may occur, esp. w/preexisting renal disease, concurrent nephrotoxic medications. Hypersensitivity reactions (ranging from rash, urticaria, fever to anaphylaxis) occur in fewer than 5%, particularly those w/history of allergies, esp. penicillin.

NURSING IMPLICATIONS

BASELINE ASSESSMENT:

Question for history of allergies, particularly cephalosporins, penicillins. Obtain culture and sensitivity test before giving first dose (therapy may begin before results are known).

INTERVENTION/EVALUATION:

Evaluate IV site for phlebitis (heat, pain, red streaking over vein).Check IM injection sites for tenderness, induration. Determine pattern of bowel activity and stool consistency. Monitor for nausea. Assess skin for rash. Monitor I&O, urinalysis, renal function reports for nephrotoxicity. Be alert for superinfection: moderate to severe diarrhea, genital/anal pruritus, vaginal discharge, moniliasis, ulceration or other change in oral mucosa.

PATIENT/FAMILY TEACHING:

Discomfort may occur w/IM injection. Doses should be evenly spaced. Continue antibiotic therapy for full length of treatment. Notify physician at once in event of diarrhea, rash, onset of other new symptoms.

---

celiprolol (Selecor)
See supplement

---

cephalexin

cef-ah-lex′in
(Keflet, Keflex)

cephalexin hydrochloride

(Keftab)

CANADIAN AVAILABILITY:
Apo-Cephalex, Ceporex, Keflex, Novolexin

CLASSIFICATION

Antibiotic: First-generation cephalosporin

PHARMACOKINETICS

Rapidly absorbed from GI tract. Widely distributed. Protein binding: 10-15%. Primarily excreted unchanged in urine. Moderately removed by hemodialysis. Half-life: 0.9-1.2 hrs (increased in decreased renal function).

ACTION

Bactericidal. Binds to bacterial membranes, inhibiting bacterial cell wall synthesis.

USES

Treatment of respiratory tract, GU tract, skin, soft tissue, bone infections; otitis media, rheumatic fever prophylaxis; follow-up to parenteral therapy.

STORAGE/HANDLING

Oral suspensions, after reconstitution, stable for 14 days if refrigerated.

PO ADMINISTRATION

1. Shake oral suspension well before using.
2. Give w/o regard to meals. If GI upset occurs, give w/food or milk.

INDICATIONS/DOSAGE/ROUTES

NOTE: Space doses evenly around the clock.

Usual dosage for adults:
PO: Adults, elderly: 250-500 mg q6h up to 4 Gm/day.

Streptococcal pharyngitis, skin/skin structure infections, uncomplicated cystitis:
PO: Adults, elderly: 500 mg q12h.

Usual dosage for children:
PO: Children: 25-100 mg/kg/day in 2-4 divided doses.

Otitis media:
PO: Children: 75-100 mg/kg/day in 4 divided doses.

Dosage in renal impairment:
After usual initial dose, dose and/or frequency is modified on basis of creatinine clearance and/or severity of infection.

CREATININE CLEARANCE	DOSAGE
11-40 ml/min	500 mg q8-12h
5-10 ml/min	250 mg q12h
<5 ml/min	250 mg q12-24h

PRECAUTIONS

CONTRAINDICATIONS: History of hypersensitivity to cephalosporins, anaphylactic reaction to penicillins. **CAUTIONS:** Renal impairment, history of allergies or GI disease, concurrent use of nephrotoxic medications. **PREGNANCY/LACTATION:** Readily crosses placenta; distributed in breast milk. **Pregnancy Category B.**

INTERACTIONS

DRUG INTERACTIONS: Probenecid increases serum concentration of cephalexin. **ALTERED LAB VALUES:** Positive direct/indirect Coombs' test may occur (interferes w/hematologic test, cross-matching procedures). May increase SGOT (AST), SGPT (ALT), alkaline phosphatase concentrations.

SIDE EFFECTS

FREQUENT: Anorexia, nausea, vomiting, diarrhea. **OCCASIONAL:** Dyspepsia, abdominal pain, genital/anal pruritus, moniliasis.

ADVERSE REACTIONS/TOXIC EFFECTS

Antibiotic-associated colitis, other superinfections may result from altered bacterial balance. Nephrotoxicity may occur, esp. w/preexisting renal disease. Hypersensitivity reactions (ranging from rash, urticaria, fever to anaphylaxis) occur in fewer than 5%, particularly those w/history of allergies, esp. penicillin.

NURSING IMPLICATIONS

BASELINE ASSESSMENT:

Question for history of allergies, particularly cephalosporins, penicillins. Obtain culture and sensitivity test before giving first dose (therapy may begin before results are known).

INTERVENTION/EVALUATION:

Assess for anorexia, nausea, vomiting. Determine pattern of bowel activity and stool consistency. Assess skin for rash. Monitor

I&O, urinalysis, renal function reports for nephrotoxicity. Be alert for superinfection: genital/anal pruritus, moniliasis, abdominal pain, sore mouth or tongue, moderate to severe diarrhea.

PATIENT/FAMILY TEACHING:

Continue antibiotic therapy for full length of treatment. Doses should be evenly spaced. Notify physician at once in event of diarrhea, rash, onset of other new symptoms.

cephalothin sodium

cef-ah-low´thin
(Keflin)

CANADIAN AVAILABILITY:
Ceporacin, Keflin

CLASSIFICATION

Antibiotic: First-generation cephalosporin

PHARMACOKINETICS

Widely distributed. Protein binding: 70%. Metabolized in liver. Primarily excreted in urine. Moderately removed by hemodialysis. Half-life: 0.5-1 hr (increased in decreased renal function).

ACTION

Bactericidal. Binds to bacterial membranes, inhibiting bacterial cell wall synthesis.

USES

Treatment of respiratory tract, skin, soft tissue, bone, joint, GI/GU tract infections; endocarditis, septicemia, perioperative prophylaxis in obstetric, orthopedic, cardiovascular, biliary procedures.

STORAGE/HANDLING

IV infusion (piggyback) stable for 12 hrs at room temperature, 96 hrs if refrigerated. Solution may darken (does not indicate loss of potency). If precipitate forms, redissolve by warming to room temperature and shaking.

IM/IV ADMINISTRATION

NOTE: Give by IM injection, IV injection, or intermittent IV infusion (piggyback).

IM:

1. Reconstitute each 1 Gm w/4 ml sterile water for injection to provide concentration of 225 mg/ml.
2. To minimize discomfort, inject deep IM slowly. Less painful if injected into gluteus maximus rather than lateral aspect of thigh.

IV:

1. For IV administration, reconstitute each 1 Gm vial w/10 ml sterile water for injection. Administer over 3-5 min.
2. For intermittent IV infusion (piggyback), further dilute w/50-100 ml 5% dextrose, 0.9% NaCl, or other compatible IV fluid. Infuse over 20-30 min.
3. Alternating IV sites, use large veins to reduce risk of phlebitis.

INDICATIONS/DOSAGE/ROUTES

NOTE: Space doses evenly around the clock.

Uncomplicated pneumonia, furunculosis w/cellulitis, most UTIs:
IM/IV: Adults, elderly: 500 mg q6h.

Severe infections:
IM/IV: Adults, elderly: 1 Gm q6h or 500 mg q4h.

Life-threatening infections:
IM/IV: Adults, elderly: Up to 2 Gm q4h.

Perioperative prophylaxis:
IM/IV: Adults, elderly: 1-2 Gm 30-60 min before surgery, during surgery, and q6h postop for 24 hrs. **Children:** 20-30 mg/kg 30-60 min before surgery, during surgery, and q6h postop for 24 hrs.

Usual dosage for children:
IM/IV: Children: 80-160 mg/kg/day in divided doses q4-6h.

Dosage in renal impairment:
After 1-2 Gm loading dose, dose and/or frequency is modified on basis of creatinine clearance and/or severity of infection.

CREATININE CLEARANCE	DOSE
50-80 ml/min	2 Gm q6h
25-50 ml/min	1.5 Gm q6h
10-25 ml/min	1 Gm q6h
2-10 ml/min	500 mg q6h
<2 ml/min	500 mg q8h

PRECAUTIONS

CONTRAINDICATIONS: History of hypersensitivity to cephalosporins, anaphylactic reaction to penicillins. **CAUTIONS:** Renal impairment, history of allergies or GI disease, concurrent use of nephrotoxic medications. **PREGNANCY/LACTATION:** Readily crosses placenta. Distributed in breast milk. **Pregnancy Category B.**

INTERACTIONS

DRUG INTERACTIONS: Probenecid increases serum concentration of cephalothin. Aminoglycosides, furosemide may increase risk of nephrotoxicity, in those w/preexisting renal disease. **ALTERED LAB VALUES:** May falsely elevate serum, urine creatinine concentrations. Positive direct/indirect Coombs' test may occur (interferes w/hematologic tests, cross-matching procedures). May increase BUN, SGOT (AST), SGPT (ALT), alkaline phosphatase concentrations.

SIDE EFFECTS

FREQUENT: Phlebitis, thrombophletbitis if given IV, esp. severe w/higher dosage/prolonged therapy. Pain, induration, tenderness w/IM injection. **OCCASIONAL:** GI upset, malaise, headache, dizziness.

ADVERSE REACTONS/TOXIC EFFECTS

Nephrotoxicity has occurred w/high dosage or preexisting renal impairment. Antibiotic-associated colitis, other superinfections may result from altered bacterial balance. Hypersensitivity reactions (ranging from rash, urticaria, fever to anaphylaxis) occur in fewer than 5%, particularly those w/history of allergies, esp. penicillin.

NURSING IMPLICATIONS

BASELINE ASSESSMENT:

Question for history of allergies, particularly cephalosporins, penicillins. Obtain culture and sensitivity test before giving first dose (therapy may begin before results are known).

INTERVENTION/EVALUATION:

Assess IV site for phlebitis (heat, pain, red streaking over vein). Check IM injection sites for induration, tenderness. Determine pattern of bowel activity and stool consistency. Assess skin for rash. Monitor I&O, urinalysis, renal function reports for nephrotoxicity. Be alert for superinfection: nausea, diarrhea, vaginal discharge, anal pruritus, ulceration or changes in oral mucosa. Monitor PT levels and be alert for signs of bleeding: overt bleeding, bruising or swelling of tissues.

PATIENT/FAMILY TEACHING:

Discomfort may occur w/IM injection. Doses should be evenly spaced. Continue antibiotic therapy for full length of treatment. Notify physician at once in event of diarrhea, bleeding, bruising, or onset of other new symptoms.

cetirizine (Reactine)
See supplement

charcoal, activated

(Actidose, Charcocaps)

CANADIAN AVAILABILITY:
Aqueous Charcodote

CLASSIFICATION

Antidote

PHARMACOKINETICS

Not absorbed or metabolized. Eliminated via intestinal tract.

ACTION

Adsorbs toxic substances, irritants, intestinal gas.

USES

Emergency antidote in treatment of poisoning. Reduces volume of intestinal gas, diarrhea.

PO ADMINISTRATION

1. Give 2 hrs before or 1 hr after other oral medication.
2. Shake suspension well before using.

INDICATIONS/DOSAGE/ROUTES

Antidote:
PO: Adults, elderly: Can give 30-100 Gm as slurry (30 Gm in at least 8 oz H_2O) or 12.5-50 Gm in aqueous or sorbital suspension. Usually given as single dose.

Antidiarrheal:
PO: Adults, elderly: 520 mg, repeat q½-1h up to 4.16 Gm/day.

Antiflatulent:
PO: Adults, elderly: 1.04-3.9 Gm 3 times/day after meals.

PRECAUTIONS

CONTRAINDICATIONS: None significant. **CAUTIONS:** None significant. **PREGNANCY/LACTATION:** Unknown whether drug crosses placenta or is distributed in breast milk. **Pregnancy Category C.**

INTERACTIONS

DRUG INTERACTIONS: May decrease absorption, effects of orally administered medications. **ALTERED LAB VALUES:** None significant.

SIDE EFFECTS

OCCASIONAL: Diarrhea, GI discomfort, intestinal gas.

ADVERSE REACTIONS/TOXIC EFFECTS

None significant.

NURSING IMPLICATIONS

INTERVENTION/EVALUATION:

Monitor bowel pattern, stool consistency. Assess bowel sounds for peristalsis. When using activated charcoal as an antidote, monitor vital signs, level of consciousness, and other clinical signs related to specific drug ingested.

chloral hydrate

klor´al-high´drate
(Noctec, Aquachloral Supprettes)

CANADIAN AVAILABILITY:
Noctec, Novochlorhydrate

CLASSIFICATION

Sedative, hypnotic

PHARMACOKINETICS

	ONSET	PEAK	DURATION
PO	30-60 min	—	4-8 hrs
Rectal	30-60 min	—	4-8 hrs

Readily absorbed from GI tract. Protein binding: 35-41%. Metabolized in liver, erythrocytes to active metabolite. Excreted in urine. Half-life: 7-10 hrs.

ACTION

Unknown. CNS depressant by action of active metabolite.

USES

Short-term treatment of insomnia (up to 2 wk). Also used for routine sedation, preop sedation, EEG testing, prevention/suppression of alcohol-withdrawal symptoms.

PO/RECTAL ADMINISTRATION

PO:

1. May be given w/o regard to meals.
2. Capsules may be emptied and mixed w/food.
3. Mix syrup form with 1/2 glass (4 oz) water, fruit juice, ginger ale.

RECTAL:

1. If suppository is too soft, chill for 30 min in refrigerator or run cold water over foil wrapper.
2. Moisten suppository w/cold water before inserting well up into rectum.

INDICATIONS/DOSAGE/ROUTES

Hypnotic:
PO/RECTAL: Adults: 500 mg-1 Gm 15-30 min before bedtime, or 30 min before surgery. **Elderly:** 250 mg at bedtime. **Children:** 50 mg/kg to maximum 1 Gm per single dose.

Sedative:
PO/RECTAL: Adults: 250 mg 3 times/day after meals. **Children:** 8.3 mg/kg 3 times/day.

Alcohol withdrawal:
PO/RECTAL: Adults: 500 mg-1 Gm q6h. Do not exceed 2 Gm daily.

EEG evaluation:
PO/RECTAL: Children: 20-25 mg/kg.

PRECAUTIONS

CONTRAINDICATIONS: Marked hepatic, renal impairment, severe cardiac disease, presence of gastritis. *Oral form:* Esophagitis, gastritis, gastric/duodenal ulcer. **CAUTIONS:** History of drug abuse, mental depression. **PREGNANCY/LACTATION:** Crosses placenta; small amount distributed in breast milk. Withdrawal symptoms may occur in neonates born to women who receive chloral hydrate during pregnancy. May produce sedation in nursing infants. **Pregnancy Category C.**

INTERACTIONS

DRUG INTERACTIONS: Alcohol, CNS depressants may increase effects. May increase effect of warfarin. IV furosemide given within 24 hrs following chloral hydrate may alter B/P, cause diaphoresis. **ALTERED LAB VALUES:** None significant.

SIDE EFFECTS

Generally well tolerated w/only mild and transient effects. **OCCASIONAL:** Gastric irritation (nausea, vomiting, flatulence, diarrhea), allergic skin rash, sleepwalking, disorientation, paranoid behavior. **RARE:** Residual hangover, headache, paradoxical CNS hyperactivity/nervousness in children, excitement/restlessness in elderly (particularly noted when given in presence of pain).

ADVERSE REACTIONS/TOXIC EFFECTS

Overdosage may produce somnolence, confusion, slurred speech, severe incoordination, respiratory depression, coma. Tolerance and psychological dependence may occur by second wk of therapy. Abrupt withdrawal of drug after long-term use may produce weakness, facial flushing, sweating, vomiting, tremor.

NURSING IMPLICATIONS

Baseline Assessment:

Assess B/P, pulse, respirations immediately before administration. Raise bedrails. Provide environment conducive to sleep (backrub, quiet environment, low lighting).

Intervention/Evaluation:

Assess sleep pattern of pt. Assess elderly/children for paradoxical reaction. Evaluate for therapeutic response to insomnia: a decrease in number of nocturnal awakenings, increase in length of sleep.

Patient/Family Teaching:

Do not abruptly withdraw medication after long-term use. Avoid tasks that require alertness, motor skills until response to drug is established. Tolerance/dependence may occur w/prolonged use of high doses.

chlorambucil

klor-am´bew-sill
(Leukeran)

CANADIAN AVAILABILITY:
Leukeran

CLASSIFICATION

Antineoplastic

PHARMACOKINETICS

Rapid, completely absorbed from GI tract. Protein binding: 99%. Rapidly metabolized in liver to active metabolite. Half-life: 1.5 hrs; metabolite: 2.5 hrs.

ACTION

Inhibits DNA, RNA synthesis by cross-linking w/DNA and RNA strands, interfering w/nucleic acid function. Cell cycle phase nonspecific. Has immunosuppressive activity.

USES

Palliative treatment of chronic lymphocytic leukemia, advanced malignant (non-Hodgkin's) lymphomas, lymphosarcoma, giant follicular lymphomas, advanced Hodgkin's disease.

INDICATIONS/DOSAGE/ROUTES

NOTE: May be carcinogenic, mutagenic, or teratogenic. Handle w/ extreme care during administration. Dosage individualized on basis of clinical response, tolerance to adverse effects. When used in combination therapy, consult specific protocols for optimum dosage, sequence of drug administration.

Usual dosage (initial or short-course therapy):
PO: Adults, elderly, children: 0.1-0.2 mg/kg/day as single or divided dose for 3-6 wk. **Avg. dose:** 4-10 mg/day. **Single daily dose q2wk:** 0.4 mg/kg initially. Increase by 0.1 mg/kg q2wk until response and/or myelosuppression.

Usual dosage (maintenance):
PO: Adults, elderly, children: 0.03-0.1 mg/kg/day. **Avg. dose:** 2-4 mg/day.

PRECAUTIONS:

CONTRAINDICATIONS: Previous allergic reaction, disease resistance to previous therapy w/ drug. **EXTREME CAUTION:** Within 4 weeks after full-course radiation therapy or myelosuppressive drug regimen. **PREGNANCY/LACTATION:** If possible, avoid use during pregnancy, especially first trimester. Breast feeding not recommended. **Pregnancy Category D.**

INTERACTIONS

DRUG INTERACTIONS: May decrease effect of antigout medications. Bone marrow depressants may increase bone marrow depression. Other immunosuppressants (e.g., steroids) may increase risk of infection or development of neoplasms. Live virus vaccines may potentiate virus replication, increase vaccine side effects, decrease antibody response to vaccine. **ALTERED LAB VALUES:** May increase SGOT (AST) alkaline phosphatase, uric acid.

SIDE EFFECTS

GI effects (nausea, vomiting, anorexia, diarrhea, abdominal distress) are generally mild, last less than 24 hrs, and occur only if single dose exceeds 20 mg. **OCCASIONAL:** Rash or dermatitis, itching, cold sores. **RARE:** Alopecia, hives, erythema, hyperuricemia.

ADVERSE REACTIONS/TOXIC EFFECTS

Bone marrow depression manifested as hematologic toxicity (neutropenia, leukopenia, progressive lymphopenia, anemia, thrombocytopenia). After discontinuation of therapy, thrombocytopenia, leukopenia usually occur at 1-3 wk and lasts 1-4 wk. Neutrophil count decreases up to 10 days after last dose. Toxicity appears to be less severe w/intermittent rather than continuous drug administration. Overdosage may produce seizures in children. Excessive uric acid level, hepatotoxicity occurs rarely.

NURSING IMPLICATIONS

BASELINE ASSESSMENT:

CBC should be performed each wk during therapy, WBC count performed 3-4 days after each weekly CBC during first 3-6 wk of therapy (4-6 wk if pt on intermittent dosing schedule).

INTERVENTION/EVALUATION:

Monitor serum uric acid concentration. Monitor for hematologic toxicity (fever, sore throat, signs of local infection, easy bruising, or unusual bleeding from any site), symptoms of anemia (excessive tiredness, weakness). Assess skin for rash, pruritus, urticaria. If there is abrupt fall in WBC count, or if WBC, platelet count are less than normal value, consult physician (dosage may be reduced). Dosage should be temporarily discontinued if further bone marrow depression occurs.

PATIENT/FAMILY TEACHING:

Increase fluid intake (may protect against hyperuricemia). Do not have immunizations w/o doctor's approval (drug lowers body's resistance). Avoid contact w/those who have recently received live virus vaccine. Promptly report fever, sore throat, signs of local infection, easy bruising, or unusual bleeding from any site. Contact physician if nausea/vomiting continues at home.

chloramphenicol

klor-am-fen´ih-call

(Chloromycetin, Chloroptic, Ophthoclor)

chloramphenicol palmitate

(Chloromycetin oral suspension)

chloramphenicol sodium succinate

(Chloromycetin, Mychel-S)

FIXED-COMBINATION(S):
W/polymyxin B, an antibiotic, and hydrocortisone, acetate (Ophthocort)

CANADIAN AVAILABILITY:
Ak-Chlor, Chloromycetin, Chloroptic, Sopamycetin

CLASSIFICATION

Antibiotic

PHARMACOKINETICS

Rapid, completely absorbed after oral, IM administration. Widely distributed (including CSF). Protein binding: 50-60%. Metabolized in liver. Primarily excreted in urine. Minimally removed by hemodialysis. Half-life: 1.5-3.5 hrs (increased in decreased renal, liver function, children, neonates).

ACTION

Bacteriostatic (may be bactericidal in high concentrations). Irreversibly binds to 50S subunit of bacterial ribosomes, inhibits protein synthesis.

USES

Intra-abdominal, soft tissue, or orofacial infections, typhoid fever, osteomyelitis, septic arthritis, cellulitis, septicemia, meningitis; adjunctive therapy for cerebral abscesses or other CNS infections, rickettsial infections when tetracyclines are contraindicated. Treatment of superficial ocular infections, superficial infections of external auditory canal, minor skin abrasions.

STORAGE/HANDLING

Store capsules, oral suspension at room temperature. Solution for injection is stable for 30 days at room temperature. Discard if cloudy or precipitate forms.

PO/IV/OPHTHALMIC ADMINISTRATION

PO:

1. Change therapy from IV to oral as soon as possible.
2. Administer oral doses on empty stomach 1 hr before or 2 hrs after meals (may give w/food if GI upset occurs).

IV:

NOTE: Give by IV injection or intermittent IV infusion (piggyback).

1. For IV injection, reconstitute each 1 Gm vial w/10 ml sterile water for injection to provide concentration of 100 mg/ml.

2. Administer dose over at least 1 min.

3. Dosage adjusted to maintain plasma concentration at 5-20 mcg/ml.

4. For intermittent IV infusion (piggyback), further dilute w/50-100 ml 5% dextrose, 0.9% NaCl, or other compatible IV fluid. Infuse >30 min.

5. Pts should be hospitalized during chloramphenicol therapy for close observation, adequate blood studies.

OPHTHALMIC:

1. Place finger on lower eyelid and pull out until a pocket is formed between eye and lower lid.

2. Hold dropper above pocket and place correct number of drops (¼-½ inch ointment) into pocket. Close eye gently.

3. *Solution:* Apply digital pressure to lacrimal sac for 1-2 min (minimizes drainage into nose and throat, reducing risk of systemic effects).

4. *Ointment:* Close eye for 1-2 min, rolling eyeball (increases contact area of drug to eye). Remove excess solution or ointment around eye w/tissue.

INDICATIONS/DOSAGE/ROUTES

NOTE: Space doses evenly around the clock.

Mild to moderate infections:
PO/IV: Adults, elderly, children: 50 mg/kg/day in divided doses q6h.

Severe infections, infections due to moderately resistant organisms:
PO/IV: Adults, elderly, children: 50-100 mg/kg/day in divided doses q6h.

Dosage in renal or hepatic impairment:

Dosage is reduced on basis of degree of renal impairment, plasma concentration of drug. Initially, 1 Gm, then 500 mg q6h.

Usual dosage for neonates:
IV/PO: Newborn infants: 25 mg/kg/day in 4 doses q6h. **Infants >2 wk:** 50 mg/kg/day in 4 doses q6h. **Neonates <2 kg:** 25 mg/kg once daily. **Neonates <7 days, >2 kg:** 25 mg/kg once daily. **Neonates >7 days, >2 kg:** 50 mg/kg/day in divided doses q12h.

Usual ophthalmic dosage:
OINTMENT: Adults, elderly, children: Apply thin strip to conjunctiva q3-4h.
DROPS: Adults, elderly, children: 1-2 drops 4-6 times/day.

Usual otic dosage:
OTIC: Adults, elderly, children: 2-3 drops into ear 3 times/day.

Usual topical dosage:
TOPICAL: Adults, elderly, children: Apply to affected area 3-4 times/day.

PRECAUTIONS

CONTRAINDICATIONS: Hypersensitivity to chloramphenicol or other components in fixed combination. Not for use in infections when less toxic drugs can be used. Prolonged treatment or frequent application should be avoided w/topical application. **CAUTIONS:** Hepatic or renal impairment, infants/children <2 yr. **PREGNANCY/LACTATION:** Crosses placenta; distributed in breast milk. Not recommended at term or during labor (potential "gray syndrome," bone marrow depression). **Pregnancy Category C.**

INTERACTIONS

DRUG INTERACTIONS: Anticonvulsants, bone marrow depressants may increase bone marrow depression. May increase effect of oral hypoglycemics. May antagonize effects of clindamycin, erythromycin. May increase concentration of phenobarbital, phenytoin, warfarin. **ALTERED LAB VALUES:** None significant.

SIDE EFFECTS

NOTE: Important to know side effects of components when chloramphenicol is used in fixed combination.
OCCASIONAL: Headache, depression, confusion. *Long-term therapy:* Optic and peripheral neuritis. Hypersensitivity reactions: fever, rash, urticaria. **RARE:** Nausea, vomiting, diarrhea, anaphylaxis; "gray syndrome" (toxic reaction in neonates to children 2 yr, evidenced by abdominal distention, pallid cyanosis, vasomotor collapse. Frequently reversible if treatment terminated at early symptoms). *Topical:* Hypersensitivity reaction (inflammation, itching, burning).

ADVERSE REACTIONS/TOXIC EFFECTS

Superinfection due to bacterial or fungal overgrowth. Narrow margin between effective therapy and toxic levels producing blood dyscrasias: Bone marrow depression w/resulting aplastic anemia, hypoplastic anemia, pancytopenia (may occur up to weeks or months later).

NURSING IMPLICATIONS

BASELINE ASSESSMENT:

Question pt for history of allergies, particularly to chloramphenicol. Avoid, if possible, other drugs that cause bone marrow depression. Obtain specimens for culture and sensitivity test before giving first dose (therapy may begin before results are known). Establish baseline blood studies before therapy.

INTERVENTION/EVALUATION:

Monitor hematology reports carefully. Coordinate w/lab for drawing of chloramphenicol plasma levels. Assess for appetite, vomiting. Evaluate mental status. Check for visual disturbances. Assess skin for rash. Determine pattern of bowel activity and stool consistency. Monitor I&O, renal function tests if indicated. Watch for superinfection: diarrhea, anal/genital pruritus, change in oral mucosa, increased fever. Be alert to signs of sensitivity w/topical use: burning, itching, inflammation. W/topical preparations containing corticosteroids, consider masking effect on clinical signs.

PATIENT/FAMILY TEACHING:

Continue therapy for full length of treatment; ophthalmic treatment should continue at least 48 hrs after eye returns to normal appearance. Doses should be evenly spaced. Take oral doses on empty stomach, 1 hr before or 2 hrs after meals (may take w/food if GI upset occurs, but not w/iron or vitamins). Notify physician in event of unusual bleeding or bruising, blurred vision, tired/weak feeling, or other new symptom; w/topical or ophthalmic use report any increased irritation, burning, itching.

chlordiazepoxide

klor-dye-az-eh-pox′eyd
(Libritabs)

chlordiazepoxide hydrochloride

(Librium, Lipoxide)

FIXED-COMBINATION(S):
W/clidinium bromide, an anticholinergic (Librax); w/estrogen (Menrium); w/amitriptyline hydrochloride, an antidepressant (Limbitrol)

CANADIAN AVAILABILITY:
Apo-Chlordiazepoxide, Librium, Medilium, Novopoxide

CLASSIFICATION

Antianxiety: Benzodiazepine

PHARMACOKINETICS

	ONSET	PEAK	DURATION
IV	1-5 min	—	15 min-1 hr

Well absorbed from GI tract; slow, erratic after IM administration. Protein binding: 96%. Metabolized in liver to active metabolite. Excreted in urine. Half-life: 5-30 hrs.

ACTION

Enhances action of inhibitory neurotransmitter gamma-aminobutyric acid (GABA). Depressant effects occur at all levels of CNS.

USES

Management of anxiety disorders, acute alcohol-withdrawal symptoms; short-term relief of symptoms of anxiety, preop anxiety, tension.

STORAGE/HANDLING

Store unreconstituted parenteral form at room temperature. Refrigerate diluent; do not use if hazy or opalescent. Prepare immediately before administration; discard unused portions. Do not mix w/infusion fluids.

PO/IM/IV ADMINISTRATION

PO:

1. Give w/o regard to meals.
2. Tablets may be crushed (do not crush combination form).
3. Capsules may be emptied and mixed w/food.

Parental form: Do not exceed 300 mg over a 6-hr period or 300 mg/24 hrs.

IM:

1. Do not use IV preparation for IM injection (produces pain at injection site).
2. Add 2 ml of diluent provided to 100 mg ampoule to yield 50 mg/ml. Add diluent carefully to minimize air bubbles. Agitate gently to dissolve.
3. Inject deep IM slowly into upper outer quadrant of gluteus maximus.

IV:

1. Do not use IM diluent solution for IV injection (air bubbles form during reconstitution of diluent).
2. Dilute each 100 mg ampoule w/5 ml of 0.9% NaCl or sterile water for injection administration to yield 20 mg/ml. Agitate gently until dissolved.
3. Use Y tube or 3-way stopcock to control infusion rate.
4. Administer 100 mg or fraction thereof over at least 1 min.
5. A too-rapid IV may produce hypotension, respiratory depression.

INDICATIONS/DOSAGE/ROUTES

NOTE: Use smallest effective dose in elderly or debilitated, those w/ liver disease, low serum albumin.

Mild to moderate anxiety:
PO: Adults: 5-10 mg 3-4 times/ day. **Elderly/debilitated:** 5 mg 2-4 times/day. Do not exceed 10 mg/ day initially. **Children >6 yr:** 5 mg 2-4 times/day. Do not exceed 10 mg/day initially.

Severe anxiety:
PO: Adults: 20-25 mg 3-4 times/ day.
IM/IV: Adults: Initially, 50-100 mg, then 25-50 mg 3-4 times/day. **Elderly:** 25-50 mg 3-4 times/day.

Preoperative:
IM/IV: Adults: 50-100 mg 1 hr before surgery. **Elderly/debilitated, children 12-18 yr:** 25-50 mg 1 hr before surgery.

Alcohol withdrawal:
PO: Adults: 50-100 mg followed by repeated doses until agitation is controlled. Do not exceed 300 mg/ day.
IM/IV: Adults: Initially, 50-100 mg. May repeat in 2-4 hrs, if necessary.

PRECAUTIONS

CONTRAINDICATIONS: Acute narrow-angle glaucoma, acute alcohol intoxication. **CAUTIONS:** Impaired kidney/liver function. **PREGNANCY/LACTATION:** Crosses placenta; distributed in breast milk. May increase risk of fetal abnormalities if administered during first trimester of pregnancy. Chronic ingestion during pregnancy may produce withdrawal symptoms, CNS depression in neonates. **Pregnancy Category D.**

INTERACTIONS

DRUG INTERACTIONS: Alcohol, CNS depressants may increase CNS depressant effect. **ALTERED LAB VALUES:** None significant.

SIDE EFFECTS

FREQUENT: Pain w/IM injection; drowsiness, ataxia, dizziness, confusion noted w/oral dose, particularly in elderly, debilitated. **OCCASIONAL:** Skin rash, edema, GI disturbances. **RARE:** Paradoxical CNS hyperactivity/nervousness in children, excitement/restlessness in elderly (generally noted during first 2 wk of therapy, particularly noted in presence of uncontrolled pain).

ADVERSE REACTIONS/TOXIC EFFECTS

IV route may produce pain, swelling, thrombophlebitis, carpal tunnel syndrome. Abrupt or too-rapid withdrawal may result in pronounced restlessness, irritability, insomnia, hand tremors, abdominal/muscle cramps, sweating, vomiting, seizures. Overdosage results in somnolence, confusion, diminished reflexes, coma.

NURSING IMPLICATIONS

BASELINE ASSESSMENT:

Assess B/P, pulse, respirations immediately before administration. Pt must remain recumbent for up to 3 hrs (individualized) after parenteral administration to reduce hypotensive effect. Assess autonomic response (cold, clammy hands, sweating) and motor response (agitation, trembling, tension). Offer emotional support to anxious pt.

INTERVENTION/EVALUATION:

Assess motor responses (agitation, trembling, tension) and autonomic responses (cold, clammy hands, sweating). Assess children, elderly for paradoxical reaction, particularly during early therapy. Assist w/ambulation if drowsiness, ataxia occur. For those on long-term therapy, liver/renal function tests, blood counts should be performed periodically.

PATIENT/FAMILY TEACHING:

Discomfort may occur w/IM injection. Drowsiness usually disappears during continued therapy. If dizziness occurs, change positions slowly from recumbent to sitting before standing. Avoid tasks that require alertness, motor skills until response to drug is established. Smoking reduces drug effectiveness. Do not abruptly withdraw medication after long-term therapy.

chloroprocaine hydrochloride

Klor-row′prow-cane

(Nesacaine)

(See Classifications section under Anesthetics: local)

chloroquine hydrochloride

klor′-oh-kwin

(Aralen hydrochloride)

chloroquine phosphate

(Aralen phosphate)

FIXED-COMBINATION(S):
W/primaquine phosphate, an antimalarial (Aralen w/primaquine)

CANADIAN AVAILABILITY:
Aralen

CLASSIFICATION

Antimalarial, Amebecide

PHARMACOKINETICS

Readily absorbed from GI tract. Widely distributed. Protein binding: 50-65%. Partially metabolized in liver to active metabolite. Excreted slowly in urine. Removed by hemodialysis. Half-life: 1-2 months.

ACTION

Concentrates in parasite acid vesicles, increases pH (inhibits parasite growth). May interfere w/ parasite protein synthesis.

USES

Treatment of *Plasmodium falciparum* malaria (terminates acute attacks, cures nonresistant strains), suppression of acute attacks, prolongation of interval between treatment/relapse in *P. vivax, P. ovale, P. malariae* malaria. Adjunctive therapy for extraintestinal amebiasis (including liver abscess). In combination w/primaquine cure for *P. vivax* and *P. ovale* malaria.

PO ADMINISTRATION

1. Administer w/meals to reduce adverse GI effects.
2. Tablets have bitter taste; may be crushed and mixed w/food or encased in gelatin capsule.

INDICATIONS/DOSAGE/ROUTES

NOTE: Chloroquine PO_4 500 mg = 300 mg base; chloroquine HCl 50 mg = 40 mg base.

CHLOROQUINE PHOSPHATE:

Treatment of malaria (acute attack): **Dose (mg base)**

DOSE	TIME	ADULTS	CHILDREN
Initial	Day 1	600 mg	10 mg/kg
Second	6 hrs later	300 mg	5 mg/kg
Third	Day 2	300 mg	5 mg/kg
Fourth	Day 3	300 mg	5 mg/kg

Suppression of malaria:
PO: Adults: 300 mg (base)/wk on same day each wk beginning 2 wk before exposure; continue for 6-8 wk after leaving endemic area. **Children:** 5 mg base/kg/wk. If therapy is not begun prior to exposure, then: **PO: Adults:** 600 mg base initially given in 2 divided doses 6 hrs apart. **Children:** 10 mg base/kg.

Amebiasis:
PO: Adults: 1 Gm (600 mg base) daily for 2 days; then, 500 mg (300 mg base)/day for at least 2-3 wk.

CHLOROQUINE HCL:

Treatment of malaria:
IM: Adults: Initially, 160-200 mg base (4-5 ml), repeat in 6 hrs. **Maximum:** 800 mg base in first 24 hrs. Begin oral therapy as soon as possible and continue for 3 days until approximately 1.5 Gm base given. **Children:** Initially, 5 mg base/kg, repeat in 6 hrs. Do not exceed 10 mg base/kg/24 hrs.

Amebiasis:
IM: Adults: 160-200 mg base (4-5 ml) daily for 10-12 days. Change to oral therapy as soon as possible.

PRECAUTIONS

CONTRAINDICATIONS: Hypersensitivity to 4-aminoquinolones, retinal or visual field changes, psoriasis, porphyria. **CAUTIONS:** Alcoholism, hepatic disease, G-6-PD deficiency. Children are esp. susceptible to chloroquine fatalities. **PREGNANCY/LACTATION:** Unknown if drug crosses placenta; small amount excreted in breast milk. Vestibular apparatus teratogenicity may occur. **Pregnancy Category C.**

INTERACTIONS

DRUG INTERACTIONS: May increase concentration of penicillamine, increase risk hematologic/renal or severe skin reaction. **ALTERED LAB VALUES:** Acute decrease in Hct, Hgb, RBC count may occur.

SIDE EFFECTS

FREQUENT: Mild transient headache, anorexia, nausea, vomiting. **OCCASIONAL:** Visual disturbances (blurring, difficulty focusing); nervousness, fatigue, pruritus esp. of palms, soles, scalp; bleaching of hair, irritability, personality changes, diarrhea, skin eruptions. **RARE:** Stomatitis, exfoliative dermatitis.

ADVERSE REACTIONS/TOXIC EFFECTS

Ocular toxicity (tinnitus), ototoxicity (reduced hearing). Prolonged therapy: peripheral neuritis and neuromyopathy, hypotension, ECG changes, agranulocytosis, aplastic anemia, thrombocytopenia, convulsions, psychosis. Overdosage: headache, vomiting, visual disturbance, drowsiness, convulsions, hypokalemia followed by cardiovascular collapse, death.

NURSING IMPLICATIONS

BASELINE ASSESSMENT:

Question for hypersensitivity to chloroquine or hydroxychloroquine sulfate. Evaluate CBC, hepatic function results.

INTERVENTION/EVALUATION:

Check for and promptly report any visual disturbances. Evaluate for GI distress: give dose w/food, discuss w/physician dividing dose into separate days during week. Monitor hepatic function tests and check for fatigue, jaundice, or other signs of hepatic effects. Assess skin and buccal mucosa, inquire about pruritus. Check vital signs and be alert to signs/symptoms of overdosage (esp. w/parental administration, children). Monitor CBC results for adverse hematologic effects. Notify physician of tinnitus, reduced hearing. W/prolonged therapy, test for muscle weakness. Parenteral therapy should be converted to oral therapy as soon as possible.

PATIENT/FAMILY TEACHING:

IM administration may cause local pain. Continue drug for full length of treatment. Notify physician of *any* new symptom, visual difficulties or decreased hearing, tinnitus immediately. Do not take any other medication w/o consulting physician. Periodic lab and visual tests are important part of therapy. Keep out of reach of children (small amount can cause serious effects, death).

chlorothiazide

chlor-oh-thigh´ah-zide
(Diuril)

chlorothiazide sodium

(Diuril)

FIXED-COMBINATION(S):
W/reserpine, an antihypertensive (Diupres); w/methyldopa, an antihypertensive (Aldoclor)

CLASSIFICATION

Diuretic: Thiazide

PHARMACOKINETICS

	ONSET	PEAK	DURATION
PO (Diuretic)	1-2 hrs	4 hrs	6-12 hrs
IV (Diuretic)	<15 min	30 min	2 hrs

Poorly absorbed from GI tract. Protein binding: 20-80%. Excreted unchanged in urine. Half-life: 1-2 hrs. Onset antihypertensive effect: 3-4 days; optimal therapeutic effect: 3-4 wk.

ACTION

Diuretic: Blocks reabsorption of sodium, potassium, chloride at distal convoluted tubule, increasing renal excretion. *Antihypertensive:* Reduces plasma, extracellular fluid volume. Decreases peripheral vascular resistance by direct effect on blood vessels.

USES

Adjunctive therapy in edema associated w/CHF, hepatic cirrhosis, corticoid or estrogen therapy, renal impairment. In treatment of hypertension, may be used alone or w/other antihypertensive agents.

STORAGE/HANDLING

Reconstituted parenteral solution is stable for 24 hrs at room temperature.

PO/IV ADMINISTRATION

PO:

1. May give w/food if GI upset occurs, preferably w/breakfast (may prevent nocturia).

IV:

NOTE: Do *not* give by SubQ or IM route.

1. Dilute each 500 mg vial w/18 ml sterile water for injection for IV injection.
2. May be further diluted w/dextrose or sodium chloride solution for IV infusion. Infuse over 15-30 min.
3. Do not give simultaneously w/whole blood or its derivatives.

INDICATIONS/DOSAGE/ROUTES

NOTE: Fixed-combination medication should not be used for initial therapy but for maintenance therapy.

Edema:
PO/IV: Adults: Initially, 500 mg-2 Gm as single dose or in 2 divided doses daily. When dry weight is achieved (weight w/o excessive fluid), reduce dosage to lowest maintenance level.

Hypertension:
PO: Adults: Initially, 250-500 mg as single dose or in 2 divided doses daily. Maintenance dose determined by B/P response. **Elderly:** 500 mg/day or 1 Gm 3 times/wk.

Pediatric:
PO: 2-12 yr: 20-22 mg/kg/day in 2 divided doses. **<2 yr:** 33 mg/kg/day in 2 divided doses. **Total daily dose 2-12 yr:** 375 mg-1 Gm/day in 2 divided doses, **Total daily dose <2 yr:** 125-375 mg/day in 2 divided doses.

PRECAUTIONS

CONTRAINDICATIONS: History of hypersensitivity to sulfonamides or thiazide diuretics, renal decompensation, anuria. **CAUTIONS:** Severe renal disease, impaired hepatic function, diabetes mellitus, elderly/debilitated, thyroid disorders. **PREGNANCY/LACTATION:** Crosses placenta; small amount distributed in breast milk—nursing not advised. **Pregnancy Category C.**

INTERACTIONS

DRUG INTERACTIONS: Cholestyramine, colestipol may decrease absorption, effects. May increase digoxin toxicity (due to hypokalemia). May increase lithium toxicity. **ALTERED LAB VALUES:** May increase bilirubin, serum calcium, LDL, cholesterol, triglycerides, creatinine, glucose, uric acid. May decrease urinary calcium, magnesium, potassium, sodium.

SIDE EFFECTS

EXPECTED: Increase in urine frequency/volume. **FREQUENT:** Potassium depletion (rarely produces symptoms). **OCCASIONAL:** Postural hypotension, headache, GI disturbances.

ADVERSE REACTIONS/TOXIC EFFECTS

Vigorous diuresis may lead to profound water loss and electrolyte depletion, resulting in hypokalemia, hyponatremia, dehydration. Acute hypotensive episodes may occur. Hyperglycemia may be noted during prolonged therapy. GI upset, pancreatitis, dizziness, paresthesias, headache, blood dyscrasias, pulmonary edema, allergic pneumonitis, dermatologic reactions occur rarely. Overdosage can lead to lethargy, coma w/o changes in electrolytes or hydration.

NURSING IMPLICATIONS

BASELINE ASSESSMENT:

Check vital signs, especially B/P for hypotension prior to administration. Assess baseline electrolytes, particularly check for low potassium. Evaluate edema, skin turgor, mucous membranes for hydration status. Assess muscle strength, mental status. Note skin temperature, moisture. Obtain weight. Initiate I&O.

INTERVENTION/EVALUATION:

Continue to monitor B/P, vital signs, electrolytes, I&O, weight. Note extent of diuresis. Watch for electrolyte disturbances (hypokalemia may result in weakness, tremor, muscle cramps, nausea, vomiting, change in mental status, tachycardia; hyponatremia may result in confusion, thirst, cold/clammy skin).

PATIENT/FAMILY TEACHING:

Expect increased frequency and volume of urination. To reduce hypotensive effect, rise slowly from lying to sitting position and permit legs to dangle momentarily before standing. Eat foods high in potassium, such as whole grains (cereals), legumes, meat, bananas, apricots, orange juice, potatoes (white, sweet), raisins.

chlorotrianisene

klor-oh-trye-an´ih-seen

(TACE)

CANADIAN AVAILABILITY:

TACE

CLASSIFICATION

Antineoplastic, estrogen

PHARMACOKINETICS

Well absorbed from GI tract. Widely distributed. Protein binding: 50-80%. Metabolized in liver. Primarily excreted in urine.

ACTION

Increases synthesis of DNA, RNA, and various proteins in responsive tissues. Reduces release of gonadotropin-releasing hormone, reducing follicle stimulating hormone (FSH) and leuteinizing hormone (LH). Promotes normal growth, development of female sex organs, maintaining genitourinary function, vasomotor stability. Inhibits LH, decreases serum concentration of testosterone.

USES

Management of moderate to severe vasomotor symptoms associated w/menopause. Treatment of atrophic vaginitis, kraurosis vulvae, female hypogonadism, postpartum breast engorgement. Palliative therapy for inoperable cancer of the prostate.

PO ADMINISTRATION

Give at the same time each day.

INDICATIONS/DOSAGE/ROUTES

Moderate-severe vasomotor symptoms associated w/ menopause, atrophic vaginitis, kraurosis vulvae:

PO: Adults: 12-25 mg/day for 21 days; rest 7 days; repeat.

Postpartum breast engorgement:

PO: Adults: 12 mg 4 times/day for

7 days or 50 mg q6h for 6 doses or 72 mg 2 times/day for 2 days.

Female hypogonadism:
PO: Adults: 12-25 mg/day for 21 days (may follow immediately w/ 100 mg progesterone IM or oral progestin during last 5 days of therapy). Further therapy begun on fifth day of induced uterine bleeding.

Cancer of prostate:
PO: Adults, elderly: 12-25 mg/day.

PRECAUTIONS

CONTRAINDICATIONS: Known or suspected breast cancer, estrogen-dependent neoplasia; undiagnosed abnormal genital bleeding; active thrombophlebitis or thromboembolic disorders; history of thrombophlebitis, thrombosis, or thromboembolic disorders w/previous estrogen use, hypersensitivity to estrogen. **CAUTIONS:** Conditions that may be aggravated by fluid retention: cardiac, renal, or hepatic dysfunction, epilepsy, migraine. Metabolic bone disease w/ potential hypercalcemia, mental depression, history of jaundice during pregnancy or strong family history of breast cancer, fibrocystic disease, or breast nodules, young pts in whom bone growth is not complete. **PREGNANCY/LACTATION:** Distributed in breast milk. May be harmful to fetus. Not for use during lactation. **Pregnancy Category X.**

INTERACTIONS

DRUG INTERACTIONS: May interfere w/effects of bromocriptine. May increase concentration cyclosporine, increase hepatic, nephrotoxicity. Hepatotoxic medications may increase hepatotoxicity. **ALTERED LAB VALUES:** May affect metapyrone, thyroid function tests. May decrease cholesterol, LDH. May increase calcium, glucose, HDL, triglycerides.

SIDE EFFECTS

FREQUENT: Anorexia, nausea, swelling of breasts, edema. **OCCASIONAL:** Vomiting (esp. w/ high dosages), intolerance to contact lenses, headache or migraine, increased blood pressure, changes in vaginal bleeding (spotting, breakthrough or prolonged bleeding), glucose intolerance, brown spots on exposed skin, libido changes. **RARE:** Chorea, cholestatic jaundice, hirsutism, loss of scalp hair, depression.

ADVERSE REACTIONS/TOXIC EFFECTS

Prolonged administration increases risk of gallbladder, thromboembolic disease, and breast, cervical, vaginal, endometrial, and liver carcinoma.

NURSING IMPLICATIONS

BASELINE ASSESSMENT:

Question hypersensitivity to estrogen or tartrazine, previous jaundice or thromboembolic disorders associated w/pregnancy or estrogen therapy. Establish baseline B/P, blood glucose.

INTERVENTION/EVALUATION:

Assess blood pressure at least daily. Monitor blood glucose 4 times/day in diabetic pts. Check for edema, weigh daily. Promptly report signs and symptoms of thromboembolic or thrombotic disorders: sudden severe headache, shortness of breath, vision or speech disturbance, weakness or numbness of an extremity, loss of coordination, pain in chest, groin, or leg. Estrogen therapy should be noted on specimens.

PATIENT/FAMILY TEACHING:

Importance of medical supervision. Avoid smoking because of increased risk of heart attack or blood clots. Do not take other medications w/o physician approval. Teach how to perform Homan's test, signs and symptoms of blood clots (report these to physician immediately). Notify physician of vaginal discharge or bleeding. Teach female patients to perform self-breast exam. Avoid exposure to sun or ultraviolet light. Decreased libido, gynecomastia relieved when medication stopped. Check weight daily; report weekly gain of 5 lb or more. Inform physician at once if pregnancy is suspected. Give labeling from drug package.

chlorpheniramine maleate

klor-phen-air´ah-meen
(Teldrin, Chlor-Trimeton)

FIXED-COMBINATION(S):
W/pseudoephedrine, a nasal decongestant (Co-pyronil, Deconamine SR, Isoclor, Novafed A, Sudafed); w/phenylephrine, a nasal vasoconstrictor (Novahistine); w/phenylephrine, methaxopolimine, an anticholinergic (Dallergy, Histaspan-D); w/phenylpropanolamine, a nasal decongestant (Contac, Demazin, Ornade, Triaminic); w/phenylephrine, phenylpropanolamine (nasal decongestants) and phenyltoloxamine, an antihistamine (Naldecon); w/acetaminophen (Coricidin); w/acetaminophen and pseudoephedrine (Sinutab); w/phenylpropanolamine, a nasal decongestant and phenindamine, an antihistamine (nolamine).

dexchlorpheniramine maleate

(Polaramine, Dexchlor, Polargen)

FIXED-COMBINATION(S):
W/guaifenesin, an expectorant, and pseudoephedrine, a nasal decongestant (Polaramine expectorant)

CANADIAN AVAILABILITY:
Polaramine

CLASSIFICATION

Antihistamine

PHARMACOKINETICS

	ONSET	PEAK	DURATION
PO	30-60 min	2-6 hrs	4-6 hrs
IM/IV	>15 min	—	4-6 hrs

Well absorbed from GI tract. Protein binding: 72%. Metabolized in liver. Primarily excreted in urine. Half-life: 14-25 hrs.

ACTION

Prevents, antagonizes most histamine effects (e.g., urticaria, pruritus). Anticholinergic effects cause drying of nasal mucosa.

USES

Symptomatic relief of allergic conditions, allergic reaction to blood, plasma. Fixed combination w/nasal decongestant used for relief of upper respiratory symptoms (nasal/sinus congestion, common cold).

PO/IM/IV ADMINISTRATION

PO:

1. May be given without regard to meals. Scored tablets may be crushed. Do not crush or chew extended-release or enteric-coated forms.

IM:

1. Give deep IM into large muscle mass.

IV:

1. May be given undiluted.
2. Administer at 10 mg/min rate of infusion.

INDICATIONS/DOSAGE/ROUTES

Allergic condition:
PO: Adults, children >12 yr: 4 mg q6h. Do not exceed 24 mg/24 hrs. **Children 6-11 yr:** 2 mg q4-6h. Do not exceed 12 mg/24 hrs. **Children 2-5 yr:** 1 mg q4-6h.
SubQ/IM: Adults, children >12 yr: 5-20 mg given as single dose. **Maximum daily dose:** 40 mg.

Extended-release:
PO: Adults, children >12 yr: 8-12 mg 2 times/day (morning, evening). Do not exceed 24 mg/day. **Children 6-11 yr:** 8 mg 1 time/day (bedtime or daytime).

Usual elderly dosage:
PO: Elderly: Initially, 4 mg 2 times/day or 8 mg (sustained release) at bedtime.

Allergic reaction to blood, plasma:
SubQ/IM/IV: Adults, children >12 yr: 10-20 mg.

Anaphylaxis:
IV: Adults, children >12 yr: 10-20 mg.

PRECAUTIONS

CONTRAINDICATIONS: Acute asthmatic attack, those receiving MAO inhibitors. **CAUTIONS:** Narrow-angle glaucoma, peptic ulcer, prostatic hypertrophy, pyloroduodenal or bladder neck obstruction, asthma, COPD, increased intraocular pressure, cardiovascular disease, hyperthyroidism, hypertension, seizure disorders. **PREGNANCY/LACTATION:** Crosses placenta; unknown if excreted in breast milk. Increased risk of seizures in neonates, premature infants if used during third trimester of pregnancy. May prohibit lactation. **Pregnancy Category B.**

INTERACTIONS

DRUG INTERACTIONS: Alcohol, CNS depressants may increase CNS depressant effects. MAO inhibitors may increase anticholinergic, CNS depressant effects. **ALTERED LAB VALUES:** May suppress wheal and flare reactions to antigen skin testing, unless antihistamines are discontinued 4 days before testing.

SIDE EFFECTS

FREQUENT: Drowsiness, dizziness, muscular weakness, dry mouth/nose/throat/lips, urinary retention, thickening of bronchial secretions. Sedation, dizziness, hypotension more likely to be seen in elderly. **OCCASIONAL:** Epigastric distress, flushing, visual disturbances, hearing disturbances, paresthesia, sweating, chills. Fixed-combination form with pseudoephedrine may produce mild CNS stimulation.

ADVERSE REACTIONS/TOXIC EFFECTS

Children may experience dominant paradoxical reaction (restlessness, insomnia, euphoria, nervousness, tremors). Overdosage in children may result in hallucinations, convulsions, death. Hypersensitivity reaction (eczema, pruritus, rash, cardiac disturbances, angioedema, photosensitivity) may occur. Overdosage may vary from CNS depression (sedation, apnea, cardiovascular collapse, death) to severe paradoxical reaction (hallucinations, tremor, seizures).

NURSING IMPLICATIONS

BASELINE ASSESSMENT:

If pt is undergoing allergic reaction, obtain history of recently ingested foods, drugs, environmental exposure, recent emotional stress. Monitor rate, depth, rhythm, type of respiration; quality and rate of pulse. Assess lung sounds for rhonchi, wheezing, rales.

INTERVENTION/EVALUATION:

Monitor B/P, especially in elderly (increased risk of hypotension). Monitor children closely for paradoxical reaction.

PATIENT/FAMILY TEACHING:

Tolerance to antihistaminic effect generally does not occur; tolerance to sedative effect may occur. Avoid tasks that require alertness, motor skills until response to drug is established. Dry mouth, drowsiness, dizziness may be an expected response of drug. Avoid alcoholic beverages during antihistamine therapy. Sugarless gum, sips of tepid water may relieve dry mouth. Coffee or tea may help reduce drowsiness.

chlorpromazine

klor-pro´mah-zeen
(Thorazine)

chlorpromazine hydrochloride

(Thorazine)

CANADIAN AVAILABILITY:
Chlorpromanyl, Largactil, Novo-Chlorpromazine

CLASSIFICATION

Antipsychotic

PHARMACOKINETICS

	ONSET	PEAK	DURATION
PO	30-60 min	—	4-6 hrs
Ext.-release	30-60 min	—	10-12 hrs
IM	Rapid	—	—
IV	Rapid	—	—
Rectal	>60 min	—	3-4 hrs

Variably absorbed after oral administration; well absorbed after IM administration. Protein binding: >90%. Metabolized in liver to some active metabolites. Excreted in urine, eliminated in feces. Half-life: 30 hrs.

ACTION

Blocks postsynaptic dopaminergic receptors in brain. Possesses strong alpha-adrenergic blocking, anticholinergic effects.

USES

Management of psychotic disorders, manic phase of manic-depressive illness, severe nausea or vomiting, preop sedation, severe behavioral disturbances in children. Relief of intractable hiccups, acute intermittent porphyria.

STORAGE/HANDLING

Store at room temperature (including suppositories), protect from light (darkens on exposure). Yellow discoloration of solution does not affect potency, but discard if markedly discolored or if precipitate forms.

PO/IM/IV/RECTAL ADMINISTRATION

PO:

1. Dilute oral concentrate solution w/tomato, fruit juice, milk, orange syrup, carbonated beverages, coffee, tea, water. May also mix w/semisolid food.

IM:

NOTE: After parenteral administration, pt must remain recumbent for 30-60 min in head-low position w/legs raised to minimize hypotensive effect.

1. Inject slow, deep IM. If irritation occurs, further injections may be diluted w/0.9% NaCl or 2% procaine hydrochloride.
2. Massage IM injection site to reduce discomfort.

IV:

NOTE: Give by direct IV injection or IV infusion.

1. Direct IV used only during surgery to control nausea and vomiting.
2. For direct IV, dilute w/0.9% NaCl to concentration not exceeding 1 mg/ml.
3. Administer direct IV at rate not exceeding 1 mg/min for adults and 0.5 mg/min for children.
4. IV infusion used only for intractable hiccups.
5. For IV infusion, add chlorpromazine hydrochloride to 500-1000 ml of 0.9% NaCl.

RECTAL:

1. If suppository is too soft, chill for 30 min in refrigerator or run cold water over foil wrapper.
2. Moisten suppository w/cold water before inserting well up into rectum.

INDICATIONS/DOSAGE/ROUTES

NOTE: Replace parenteral w/oral as soon as possible.

Outpatient: mild psychotic disorders, acute anxiety:
PO: Adults: 30-75 mg/day in 2-4 divided doses.
IM: Adults: 25 mg initially. May repeat in 1 hr.

Outpatient: moderate to severe psychotic disorders:
PO: Adults: 25 mg 3 times/day. Increase twice weekly by 20-25 mg until therapeutic response is achieved. Maintain dosage for 2 wk, then gradually reduce to maintenance level.

Hospitalized: acute psychotic disorders:
PO: Children: 0.55 mg/kg q4-6h.
IM: Adults: 25 mg. May give an additional 25-50 mg in 1 hr if needed. Gradually increase over several days to maximum 400 mg q4-6h.
RECTAL: Adults: 50-100 mg 3-4 times/day. **Children:** 1.1 mg/kg q6-8h (severe cases).

Nausea, vomiting:
PO: Adults: 10-25 mg q4-6h.
RECTAL: Adults: 50-100 mg q6-8h. **Children:** 1.1 mg/kg q6-8h.
IM: Adults: 25 mg. Give additional 25-50 mg q3-4h if hypotension does not occur. **Children:** 0.55 mg/kg q6-8h.

Porphyria:
PO: Adults: 25-50 mg 3-4 times/day.
IM: Adults: 25 mg 3-4 times/day.

Intractable hiccups:
PO: Adults: 25-50 mg 3 times/day. If symptoms continue, administer by IM or slow IV infusion.

Preop:
PO: Adults: 25-50 mg 2-3 hrs before surgery. **Children:** 0.55 mg/kg.
IM: Adults: 12.5-25 mg 1-2 hrs before surgery. **Children:** 0.55 mg/kg.

Usual elderly dosage (nonpsychotic):
PO: Elderly: Initially, 10-25 mg 1-2 times/day. May increase by 10-25 mg/day every 4-7 days. **Maximum:** 800 mg/day.

PRECAUTIONS

CONTRAINDICATIONS: Severe CNS depression, comatose states, severe cardiovascular disease, bone marrow depression, subcortical brain damage. **CAUTIONS:** Impaired respiratory/hepatic/renal/cardiac function, alcohol withdrawal, history of seizures, urinary retention, glaucoma, prostatic hypertrophy, hypocalcemia (increases susceptibility to dystonias). **PREGNANCY/LACTATION:** Crosses placenta; distributed in breast milk. **Pregnancy Category C.**

INTERACTIONS

DRUG INTERACTIONS: Alcohol, CNS depressants may increase CNS, respiratory depression, hypotensive effects. Tricyclic antidepressants, MAO inhibitors may increase sedative, anticholinergic effects. Antithyroid agents may increase risk of agranulocytosis. Increased risk of extrapyramidal symptoms (EPS) w/EPS-producing medications. Hypotensives may increase hypotension. May decrease levodopa effects. Lithium may decrease absorption, produce adverse neurologic effects. **ALTERED LAB VALUES:** May produce false-positive pregnancy test, phenylketonuria (PKU). EKG changes may occur, including Q and T wave disturbances.

SIDE EFFECTS

FREQUENT: Hypotension, dizziness, and fainting occur frequently after parenteral form is given, occasionally thereafter, and rarely w/oral dosage. **OCCASIONAL:** Drowsiness during early therapy, dry mouth, blurred vision, lethargy, constipation or diarrhea, nasal congestion, peripheral edema, urinary retention. **RARE:** Ocular changes, skin pigmentation (those on high doses for prolonged periods).

ADVERSE REACTIONS/TOXIC EFFECTS

Extrapyramidal symptoms appear dose related (particularly high dosage), and divided into 3 categories: akathisia (inability to sit still, tapping of feet, urge to move around), parkinsonian symptoms (mask-like face, tremors, shuffling gait, hypersalivation), and acute dystonias: torticollis (neck muscle spasm), opisthotonos (ridigity of back muscles), and oculogyric crisis (rolling back of eyes). Dystonic reaction may also produce profuse sweating, pallor. Tardive dyskinesia (protrusion of tongue, puffing of cheeks, chewing/puckering of the mouth) occurs rarely (may be irreversible). Abrupt withdrawal after long-term therapy may precipitate nausea, vomiting, gastritis, dizziness, tremors. Blood dyscrasias, particularly agranulocytosis, mild leukopenia may occur. May lower seizure threshold.

NURSING IMPLICATIONS

BASELINE ASSESSMENT:

Avoid skin contact w/solution

(contact dermatitis). *Antiemetic:* Assess for dehydration (poor skin turgor, dry mucous membranes, longitudinal furrows in tongue). *Antipsychotic:* Assess behavior, appearance, emotional status, response to environment, speech pattern, thought content.

INTERVENTION/EVALUATION:

Monitor B/P for hypotension. Assess for extrapyramidal symptoms. Monitor WBC, differential count for blood dyscrasias. Monitor for fine tongue movement (may be early sign of tardive dyskinesia). Supervise suicidal-risk pt closely during early therapy (as depression lessens, energy level improves, increasing suicide potential). Assess for therapeutic response (interest in surroundings, improvement in self-care, increased ability to concentrate, relaxed facial expression).

PATIENT/FAMILY TEACHING:

Full therapeutic response may take up to 6 wk. Urine may darken. Do not abruptly withdraw from long-term drug therapy. Report visual disturbances. Sugarless gum or sips of tepid water may relieve dry mouth. Drowsiness generally subsides during continued therapy. Avoid tasks that require alertness, motor skills until response to drug is established. Avoid alcohol.

chlorpropamide

klor-proe´pah-mide
(Diabinese, Glucamide)

CANADIAN AVAILABILITY:
Apo-Chlorpropamide, Diabinese, Novopropamide

CLASSIFICATION

Hypoglycemic: Oral

PHARMACOKINETICS

	ONSET	PEAK	DURATION
PO	1 hr	3-6 hrs	24 hrs

Well absorbed from GI tract. Protein binding: 90%. Metabolized in liver. Excreted in urine. Half-life: 36 hrs.

ACTION

Promotes release of insulin from beta cells of pancreas, decreases hepatic glycogenolysis and gluconeogenesis, increases insulin sensitivity at peripheral sites.

USES

As adjunct to diet/exercise in management of stable, mild to moderately severe non-insulin-dependent diabetes mellitus (type II, NIDDM). May be used to supplement insulin in pts w/type 1 diabetes mellitus.

PO ADMINISTRATION

May take w/food. Responses better if taken 15-30 min before meals.

INDICATIONS/DOSAGE/ROUTES

Diabetes mellitus:
PO: Adults: Initially, 100 mg/day up to 500 mg/day as single dose. **Maintenance:** 250 mg/day.

Usual elderly dosage:
PO: Elderly: Initially, 100 mg/day; gradually increased to optimal control of diabetes.

PRECAUTIONS

CONTRAINDICATIONS: Sole therapy for: type 1 diabetes mellitus, diabetic complications (ketosis, acidosis, diabetic coma), stress situations (severe infection, trauma, surgery); hypersensitivity to drug, severe renal, hepatic, or thyroid impairment. **CAUTIONS:** Elderly, malnourished or debilitated, those w/renal or hepatic dysfunction, cardiac disease, adrenal or pituitary insufficiency, history of hepatic porphyria. Cardiovascular risks may be increased. **PREGNANCY/LACTATION:** Insulin is drug of choice during pregnancy; chlorpropamide given within 1 month of delivery may cause neonatal hypoglycemia. Drug crosses placenta. Excreted in breast milk. **Pregnancy Category C.**

INTERACTIONS

DRUG INTERACTIONS: May have disulfiram reaction w/alcohol; may increase effect of oral anticoagulants; chloramphenicol, MAO inhibitors, salicylates, sulfonamides may increase effect; beta-blockers may impair hyperglycemic response; may increase effects of insulin, mask signs of hypoglycemia. **ALTERED LAB VALUES:** May increase alkaline phosphatase, SGOT (AST), LDH, creatinine, BUN.

SIDE EFFECTS

FREQUENT: Nausea, heartburn, epigastric fullness. **OCCASIONAL:** Anorexia, vomiting, diarrhea, pruritus. **INFREQUENT:** Skin reactions, headache, photosensitivity.

ADVERSE REACTIONS/TOXIC EFFECTS

Hypoglycemia may occur due to overdosage, insufficient food intake esp. w/increased glucose demands. Hepatic porphyria, cholestatic or mixed hepatic jaundice, leukopenia, thrombocytopenia, pancytopenia, agranulocytosis, aplastic or hemolytic anemia occur rarely.

NURSING IMPLICATIONS

BASELINE ASSESSMENT:

Question for hypersensitivity to chlorpropamide. Check blood glucose level. Discuss life-style to determine extent of learning, emotional needs.

INTERVENTION/EVALUATION:

Monitor blood glucose and food intake. Assess for hypoglycemia (cool wet skin, tremors, dizziness, anxiety, headache, tachycardia, numbness in mouth, hunger, diplopia) or hyperglycemia (polyuria, polyphagia, polydipsia, nausea and vomiting, dim vision, fatigue, deep rapid breathing). Measure I&O, assess for fluid retention. Monitor for diarrhea, bloody stools. Be alert to conditions altering glucose requirements: fever, increased activity or stress, surgical procedure. Check for adverse skin reactions, jaundice. Monitor hematology reports. Assess for bleeding or bruising.

PATIENT/FAMILY TEACHING:

Prescribed diet is principal part of treatment; do not skip or delay meals. Diabetes mellitus requires lifelong control. Check blood glucose/urine as ordered. Signs and symptoms, treatment of hypo/hyperglycemia. Carry candy, sugar packets, or other sugar supplements for immediate response to hypoglycemia. Wear, carry medical alert identification. Check w/physician when medication demands are altered (e.g., fever, infection, trauma, stress, heavy physical activity). Avoid alcoholic beverages. Do not take other medication w/o consulting physician. Weight control, exercise, hygiene (including foot care), and nonsmoking are essential part of therapy. Protect skin, limit sun exposure. Avoid exposure to infections. Select clothing, positions that do not restrict blood flow. Notify physician promptly of diarrhea, bleeding, shortness of breath, swelling, rash, yellow skin, dark urine. Inform dentist, physician, or surgeon of this medication before any treatment. (Assure follow-up instruction if patient/family does not thoroughly understand diabetes management or glucose testing techniques.)

chlorthalidone

klor-thal'ih-doan
(Hygroton)

FIXED-COMBINATION(S):
W/clonidine, an antihypertensive (Combipres); w/atenolol, an antihypertensive (Tenoretic); w/reserpine, an antihypertensive (Demi-Regroton, Regroton)

CANADIAN AVAILABILITY:
Apo-Chlorthalidone, Hygroton, Novo-Thalidone

CLASSIFICATION

Diuretic: Thiazide

PHARMACOKINETICS

	ONSET	PEAK	DURATION
PO (Diuretic)	2 hrs	2-6 hrs	Up to 36 hrs

Rapidly absorbed from GI tract. Protein binding: 75% (increased affinity to carbonic anhydrase in RBC). Excreted unchanged in urine. Half-life: 35-50 hrs. Onset antihypertensive effect: 3-4 days; optimal therapeutic effect: 3-4 wk.

ACTION

Diuretic: Blocks reabsorption of sodium, potassium, chloride at distal convoluted tubule, promoting renal excretion. *Antihypertensive:* Reduces plasma, extracellular fluid volume. Decreases PVR by direct effect on blood vessels.

USES

Adjunctive therapy in edema associated w/CHF, hepatic cirrhosis, corticoid or estrogen therapy, renal impairment. In treatment of hypertension, may be used alone or w/other antihypertensive agents.

PO ADMINISTRATION

1. Give w/food or milk if GI upset occurs, preferably w/breakfast (may prevent nocturia).
2. Scored tablets may be crushed.

INDICATIONS/DOSAGE/ROUTES

NOTE: Fixed-combination medication should not be used for initial therapy but for maintenance therapy.

Edema:
PO: Adults: 50-100 mg 1 time/day in morning or 100 mg every other day. May require 150-200 mg every day or every other day. Reduce dose to lowest maintenance level when dry weight is achieved (nonedematous state).

Hypertension:
PO: Adults: Initially, 25 mg/day. May increase to 50 mg/day. **Maintenance:** 25-50 mg/day.

Usual elderly dosage:
PO: Elderly: Initially, 12.5-25 mg/day or every other day.

PRECAUTIONS

CONTRAINDICATIONS: History of hypersensitivity to sulfonamides or thiazide diuretics, renal decompensation, anuria. **CAUTIONS:** Severe renal disease, impaired hepatic function, diabetes mellitus, elderly/debilitated, thyroid disorders. **PREGNANCY/LACTATION:** Crosses placenta; small amount distributed in breast milk—nursing not advised. **Pregnancy Category C.**

INTERACTIONS

DRUG INTERACTIONS: Cholestyramine, colestipol may decrease absorption, effects. May increase digoxin toxicity (due to hypokalemia). May increase lithium toxicity. **ALTERED LAB VALUES:** May increase bilirubin, serum calcium, LDL, cholesterol, triglycerides, creatinine, glucose, uric acid. May decrease urinary calcium, magnesium, potassium, sodium.

SIDE EFFECTS

EXPECTED: Increase in urine frequency/volume. **FREQUENT:** Potassium depletion (rarely produces symptoms). **OCCASIONAL:** Postural hypotension, headache, GI disturbances.

ADVERSE REACTIONS/TOXIC EFFECTS

Vigorous diuresis may lead to profound water loss and electrolyte depletion, resulting in hypokalemia, hyponatremia, dehydration. Acute hypotensive episodes may occur. Hyperglycemia may be noted during prolonged therapy. GI upset, pancreatitis, dizziness, paresthesias, headache, blood dyscrasias, pulmonary edema, allergic pneumonitis, dermatologic reactions occur rarely. Overdosage can lead to lethargy, coma w/o changes in electrolytes or hydration.

NURSING IMPLICATIONS

BASELINE ASSESSMENT:

Check vital signs, especially B/P for hypotension before administration. Assess baseline electrolytes, particularly check for low potassium. Assess edema, skin turgor, mucous membranes for hydration status. Evaluate muscle strength, mental status. Note skin temperature, moisture. Obtain baseline weight. Initiate I&O

INTERVENTION/EVALUATION:

Continue to monitor B/P, vital signs, electrolytes, I&O, weight. Note extent of diuresis. Watch for electrolyte disturbances (hypokalemia may result in weakness, tremor, muscle cramps, nausea, vomiting, change in mental status, tachycardia; hyponatremia may result in confusion, thirst, cold/clammy skin). Periodically check blood sugar for hyperglycemia in prolonged therapy.

PATIENT/FAMILY TEACHING:

Expect increased frequency and volume of urination. To reduce hypotensive effect, rise slowly from lying to sitting position and permit legs to dangle momentarily before standing. Eat foods high in potassium such as whole grains (cereals), legumes, meat, bananas, apricots, orange juice, potatoes (white, sweet), raisins.

chlorzoxazone

klor-zox′ah-sewn
(Paraflex, Parafon Forte DSC)

CLASSIFICATION

Skeletal muscle relaxant

PHARMACOKINETICS

	ONSET	PEAK	DURATION
PO	1 hr	—	3-4 hrs

Rapidly, completely absorbed from GI tract. Metabolized in liver. Excreted in urine. Half-life: 1-2 hrs.

ACTION

Muscle relaxant related to CNS depressant effects (sedation). Blocks interneuronal activity in descending reticular formation and spinal cord.

USES

Adjunct to rest, physical therapy, other measures for relief of discomfort due to acute, painful musculoskeletal conditions.

PO ADMINISTRATION

1. May give w/food or milk if GI disturbances occur.
2. Scored tablets may be crushed, mixed w/milk or fruit juice.

INDICATIONS/DOSAGE/ROUTES

Acute, painful musculoskeletal condition:
PO: Adults: 250-500 mg 3-4 times/day. May increase up to 750 mg 3-4 times/day. **Children:** 125-500 mg 3-4 times/day.

Usual elderly dosage:
PO: Elderly: Initially, 250 mg 2-4 times/day. May increase up to 750 mg 3-4 times/day.

PRECAUTIONS

CONTRAINDICATIONS: None significant. **CAUTIONS:** Impaired renal or hepatic function. **PREGNANCY/LACTATION:** Unknown whether drug crosses placenta or is distributed in breast milk. **Pregnancy Category C.**

INTERACTIONS

DRUG INTERACTIONS: Potentiated effects when used w/other CNS depressants (including alcohol). **ALTERED LAB VALUES:** May increase SGOT (AST), SGPT (ALT), alkaline phosphatase, bilirubin.

SIDE EFFECTS

FREQUENT: Urine discoloration (orange or purple-red), transient drowsiness, dizziness (postural hypotension). **OCCASIONAL:** Nausea, confusion, headache, insomnia, constipation, urinary frequency. **RARE:** Hypersensitivity reaction (rash, bronchospasm, pruritus), depression.

ADVERSE REACTIONS/TOXIC EFFECTS

Overdosage results in muscular hypotonia, respiratory depression, stupor, coma. Severe allergic reaction noted by dizziness, weakness, angioneurotic edema, hypotension, smarting eyes, anaphylactoid shock.

NURSING IMPLICATIONS

BASELINE ASSESSMENT:

Record onset, type, location, and duration of muscular spasm. Check for immobility, stiffness, swelling.

INTERVENTION/EVALUATION:

Assist w/ambulation at all times. For those on long-term therapy, liver/renal function tests, blood counts should be performed periodically. Evaluate for therapeutic response: decreased intensity of skeletal muscle pain.

PATIENT/FAMILY TEACHING:

Drowsiness usually diminishes w/continued therapy. Avoid tasks that require alertness, motor skills until response to drug is established. Avoid alcohol or other depressants while taking medication. Avoid sudden changes in posture. Urine may turn orange or purple-red.

cholestyramine resin

coal-es-tie´rah-mean
(Questran)

CANADIAN AVAILABILITY:
Questran

CLASSIFICATION

Antihyperlipoproteinemic

PHARMACOKINETICS

Not absorbed from GI tract. Decreases in LDL apparent in 5-7 days, serum cholesterol in 1 mo. Serum cholesterol returns to baseline levels about 1 mo after discontinuing drug.

ACTION

Binds w/bile acids in intestine forming insoluble complex. Binding increases bile acid synthesis from cholesterol, increases hepatic LDL receptor activity, increases LDL, cholesterol removal from plasma.

USES

Adjunct to dietary therapy to decrease elevated serum cholesterol levels in those w/primary hypercholesterolemia. Relief of pruritis associated w/partial biliary obstruction.

PO ADMINISTRATION

1. Give other drugs at least 1 hr before or 4-6 hrs after cholestyramine (capable of binding drugs in GI tract).
2. Do not give powder in dry form (highly irritating). Mix w/3-6 oz water, milk, fruit juice, soup. Place powder on surface for 1-2 min (prevents lumping), then mix thoroughly. Excessive foaming w/carbonated beverages; use extra large glass and stir slowly.
3. Administer before meals.

INDICATIONS/DOSAGE/ROUTES

Primary hypercholesterolemia:
PO: Adults, elderly: Initially: 4 Gm 3 times/day before meals. **Maintenance:** 4 Gm 1-6 times/day before meals and at bedtime.

PRECAUTIONS

CONTRAINDICATIONS: Hypersensitivity to cholestyramine or tartrazine (frequently seen in aspirin hypersensitivity), complete biliary obstruction. **CAUTIONS:** GI dysfunction (especially constipation), hemorrhoids, bleeding disorders, osteoporosis. **PREGNANCY/LACTATION:** Not systemically absorbed. May interfere w/maternal absorption of fat-soluble vitamins. **Pregnancy Category C.**

INTERACTIONS

DRUG INTERACTIONS: May increase effects of anticoagulants by decreasing vitamin K. May decrease warfarin absorption. May bind, decrease absorption of digoxin, thiazides, penicillins, propranolol, tetracyclines, folic acid, thyroid hormones, other medications. Binds, decreases effect of oral vancomycin. **ALTERED LAB VALUES:** May increase SGOT (AST), SGPT (ALT), alkaline phosphatase. May decrease calcium, potassium, sodium. May prolong prothrombin time.

SIDE EFFECTS

FREQUENT: Constipation. **OCCASIONAL:** Flatulence, anorexia, nausea, vomiting, diarrhea, abdominal pain/distention, rash, irritation of tongue/perianal area. **RARE:** Fecal impaction, hemorrhoids, bleeding tendency (vitamin K deficiency w/prolonged use), electrolyte imbalances: decreased calcium, increased magnesium, increased alkaline phosphatase.

ADVERSE REACTIONS/TOXIC EFFECT

GI tract obstruction, hyperchloremic acidosis, osteoporosis secondary to calcium excretion. High dosage may interfere w/fat absorption, resulting in steatorrhea.

NURSING IMPLICATIONS

BASELINE ASSESSMENT:

Question for history of hypersensitivity to cholestyramine, tartrazine, aspirin. Obtain specimens for baseline levels: serum cholesterol, serum triglyceride, electrolytes.

INTERVENTION/EVALUATION:

Determine pattern of bowel activity. Evaluate food tolerance, abdominal discomfort, and flatulence. Monitor lab results for electrolytes, serum cholesterol, and periodically serum triglyceride (may increase w/prolonged therapy). Assess skin and mucous membranes for rash/irritation. Encourage several glasses of water between meals.

PATIENT/FAMILY TEACHING:

Complete full course; do not omit or change doses. Take other drugs at least 1 hr before or 4 hrs after cholestyramine. Check w/physician before taking any other medication. Never take in dry form; mix w/3-6 oz water, milk, fruit juice, soup (place powder on surface for 1-2 min to prevent lumping, then mix well). Use extra large glass and stir slowly when mixing w/carbonated beverages due to foaming. Take before meals and drink several glasses of water between meals. Chew bars thoroughly. Reduce fats, sugars, and cholesterol per diet determined by physician. Eat high-fiber foods (whole grain cereals, fruits, vegetables) to reduce potential for constipation. Notify physician immediately of bleeding, constipation, or development of new symptom.

chorionic gonadotropin, HCG

kore-ee-on´ik
goe-nad´oh-troe-pin
(Pregnyl, APL, Profasai HP)

CANADIAN AVAILABILITY:
APL, Profasi HP

CLASSIFICATION

Gonadotropin

ACTION

Stimulates production of gonadal steroid hormones by stimulating interstitial cells (Leydig cells) of the testes to produce androgen, and the corpus luteum of the ovary to produce progesterone. Androgen stimulation in the male causes production of secondary sex characteristics and may stimulate descent of testes when no anatomic impediment exists. In women of child-bearing age w/normally functioning ovaries, causes maturation of corpus luteum and triggers ovulation.

USES

Treatment of prepubertal cryptorchidism w/o obstruction, selected cases of hypogonadotropic hypogonadism. To induce ovulation and pregnancy in women w/ secondary anovulation (after pretreatment w/menotropin).

IM ADMINISTRATION

1. For IM use only.
2. Follow manufacturer's directions for reconstitution.
3. Use completely or refrigerate after reconstitution.

INDICATIONS/DOSAGE/ROUTES

Prepubertal cryptorchidism, hypogonadotropic hypogonadism:
IM: Adults: Dosage is individualized based on indication, age and weight of pt, and physician preference.

Use w/menotropins:
IM: Adults: 5,000 IU 3 times/wk for 4-6 mos. After initiation of menotropin therapy, continue w/2,000 IU 2 times/wk.

Induction of ovulation and pregnancy:
IM: Adults: (After pretreatment w/menotropins), 5,000-10,000 IU 1 day after last dose of menotropins.

PRECAUTIONS

CONTRAINDICATIONS: Prior allergic reaction to chorionic gonadotropin, precocious puberty, carcinoma of the prostate or other androgen-dependent neoplasia. Not for adjunctive therapy in obesity. **CAUTIONS:** Prepubertal males, conditions aggravated by fluid retention (cardiac or renal disease, epilepsy, migraine, asthma). **PREGNANCY/LACTATION:** Caution: excretion in breast milk unknown. **Pregnancy Category C.**

INTERACTIONS

DRUG INTERACTIONS: None significant. **ALTERED LAB VALUES:** None significant.

SIDE EFFECTS

FREQUENT: Pain at injection site. **OCCASIONAL:** Edema, headache, irritability, depression, fatigue, gynecomastia. **RARE:** Precocious puberty (acne, deepening of voice, penile growth, pubic and axillary hair).

ADVERSE REACTIONS/TOXIC EFFECTS

When used w/menotropins: increased risk of arterial thromboembolism, ovarian hyperstimulation w/high incidence (20%) of multiple births (premature deliveries and neonatal prematurity), ruptured ovarian cysts.

NURSING IMPLICATIONS

BASELINE ASSESSMENT:

Question for prior allergic reaction to drug. Obtain baseline weight, B/P.

INTERVENTION/EVALUATION:

Assess for edema: weigh every 2-3 days, report >5 lb gain/wk;

monitor B/P periodically during treatment; check for decreased urinary output, swelling of ankles, fingers.

PATIENT/FAMILY TEACHING:

Report promptly abdominal pain, vaginal bleeding, signs of precocious puberty in males (deepening of voice; axillary, facial, and pubic hair; acne, penile growth) or signs of edema. In anovulation treatment, proper method of taking/recording daily basal temperature; advise intercourse daily beginning the day preceding HCG treatment. Possibility of multiple births.

ciclopirox olamine

sye-kloe-peer´ox
(Loprox)

CANADIAN AVAILABILITY:
Loprox

CLASSIFICATION

Antifungal

PHARMACOKINETICS

Absorbed portion rapidly absorbed. Protein binding: 94-97%. Metabolized in liver. Excreted in urine. Half-life: 1.7 hrs.

ACTION

Depletes essential intracellular components by inhibiting transport of potassium, other ions into cells; interferes w/synthesis of proteins, RNA, DNA. At high concentrations, alters cell membrane permeability causing leakage of cellular components.

USES

Treatment of tinea pedis, tinea cruris, tinea corporis, tinea versicolor (pityriasis), cutaneous candidiasis (moniliasis) caused by *Candida albicans.*

INDICATIONS/DOSAGE/ROUTES

Usual dosage:
TOPICAL: Adults, elderly: 2 times/day morning and evening. May take up to 4 wks for clinical improvement.

PRECAUTIONS

CONTRAINDICATIONS: Hypersensitivity to ciclopirox or components of preparation. **CAUTIONS:** Safety in children <10 yrs not established. **PREGNANCY/LACTATION:** Caution in lactation, unknown if distributed in milk. **Pregnancy Category B.**

INTERACTIONS

DRUG INTERACTIONS: None significant. **ALTERED LAB VALUES:** None significant.

SIDE EFFECTS

RARE: Increased irritation: burning, itching, swelling, oozing.

ADVERSE REACTIONS/TOXIC EFFECTS

None significant.

NURSING IMPLICATIONS

BASELINE ASSESSMENT:

Question for history of hypersensitivity to ciclopirox or components of preparation.

INTERVENTION/EVALUATION:

Assess improvement or increased irritation: burning, itching, swelling, oozing, redness of affected areas.

PATIENT/FAMILY TEACHING:

Rub well into affected, surrounding areas. Do not use occlusive covering or other preparations w/o consulting physician. Continue for full length of therapy; if no improvement after 4 wks see physician. Keep areas clean, dry; wear light clothing to promote ventilation. Keep personal items, linens separate. Avoid contact w/eyes. Inform physician of increased irritation.

cilazapril (Inhibace)
See supplement

cimetidine

sih-met´ih-deen
(Tagamet)

CANADIAN AVAILABILITY:

Apo-Cimetidine, Novocimetine, Peptol, Tagamet

CLASSIFICATION

H_2-receptor antagonist

PHARMACOKINETICS

Well absorbed from GI tract. Widely distributed. Protein binding: 15-20%. Metabolized in liver. Primarily excreted in urine. Half-life: 2 hrs (increased in decreased renal function).

ACTION

Inhibits histamine action at H_2 receptors of parietal cells, inhibiting basal and nocturnal gastric acid secretion.

USES

Short-term treatment of active duodenal ulcer. Prevention of duodenal ulcer recurrence, upper GI bleeding in critically ill pts. Treatment of active benign gastric ulcer, pathologic GI hypersecretory conditions, gastroesophageal reflux disease (GERD).

STORAGE/HANDLING

Store tablets, liquid, parenteral form at room temperature. Reconstituted IV is stable for 48 hrs at room temperature.

PO/IM/IV ADMINISTRATION

PO:

1. Give w/o regard to meals. Best given after meals and at bedtime.
2. Do not administer within 1 hr of antacids.

IM:

1. Administer undiluted.
2. Inject deep into large muscle mass.

IV:

1. For direct IV injection, dilute w/20 ml 0.9% NaCl or 5% dextrose. Administer over not less than 2 min (prevents arrhythmias, hypotension).
2. For intermittent IV (piggyback) administration, dilute w/50 ml 0.9% NaCl, 5% dextrose, or other compatible IV fluid. Infuse over 15-20 min.
3. For IV infusion, dilute w/100-1,000 ml 0.9% NaCl or 5% dextrose. Infuse over 24 hrs.

INDICATIONS/DOSAGE/ROUTES

Active duodenal ulcer:
PO: Adults, elderly: 300 mg 4 times/day, or 400 mg 2 times/day (morning and at bedtime), or 800 mg at bedtime.

Prophylaxis of recurrent duodenal ulcer:
PO: Adults, elderly: 400 mg at bedtime.

Benign active gastric ulcer:
PO: Adults, elderly: 300 mg 4 times/day or 800 mg at bedtime.

Pathologic gastric hypersecretory conditions:
PO: Adults, elderly: 300 mg 4 times/day up to 2,400 mg/day.

Gastroesophageal reflux disease:
PO: Adults, elderly: 1,600 mg/day in divided (800 mg 2 times/day or 400 mg 4 times/day) for 12 wks.

Usual parenteral dosage:
IM/IV: Adults, elderly: 300 mg q6-8h. **Maximum:** 2,400 mg/day.
IV INFUSION: Adults, elderly: 900 mg/day.

Prevent upper GI bleeding:
IV INFUSION: Adults, elderly: 1,200 mg/day (50 mg/hr).

Dosage in renal impairment:
PO/IM/IV: Adults, elderly: 300 mg q8-12h.

PRECAUTIONS

CONTRAINDICATIONS: None significant. **CAUTIONS:** Impaired renal/hepatic function, elderly. **PREGNANCY/LACTATION:** Crosses placenta; distributed in breast milk. In infants, may suppress gastric acidity, inhibit drug metabolism, produce CNS stimulation. **Pregnancy Category B.**

INTERACTIONS

DRUG INTERACTIONS: Antacids may decrease absorption (do not give within 1/2-1 hr). May decrease absorption of ketoconazole (give at least 2 hrs after). May decrease metabolism, increase concentration of oral anticoagulants, tricyclic antidepressants, oral hypoglycemics, metoprolol, metronidazole, phenytoin, propranolol, theophylline, calcium channel blockers, cyclosporine, lidocaine. **ALTERED LAB VALUES:** Interferes w/skin tests using allergen extracts. May increase creatinine, prolactin, transaminase. May decrease parathyroid hormone concentration.

SIDE EFFECTS

OCCASIONAL: Mental confusion, agitation, psychosis, depression, anxiety, disorientation, hallucinations, particularly in elderly, severely ill, those w/impaired renal, hepatic function (CNS effects reverse within 3-4 days after discontinuance of drug). **RARE:** Diarrhea, headache, gynecomastia, arthralgia, myalgia, jaundice, alopecia, rash, reversible impotence in those w/Zollinger-Ellison syndrome (particularly w/high dosage).

ADVERSE REACTIONS/TOXIC EFFECTS

Rapid IV may produce cardiac arrhythmias, hypotension.

NURSING IMPLICATIONS

BASELINE ASSESSMENT:

Do not administer antacids concurrently (separate by 1 hr).

INTERVENTION/EVALUATION:

Monitor B/P for hypotension during IV infusion. Assess for GI bleeding: Hematemesis, blood in stool. Check mental status in elderly, severely ill, those w/impaired renal function.

PATIENT/FAMILY TEACHING:

IM may produce transient discomfort at injection site. Do not take antacids within 1 hr of cimetidine administration. Avoid tasks that require alertness, motor skills until drug response is established.

Avoid smoking. Report any blood in vomitus or stool, or dark, tarry stool.

ciprofloxacin hydrochloride

sip-row-flocks´ah-sin
(Ciloxan, Cipro)

CANADIAN AVAILABILITY:
Cipro

CLASSIFICATION

Anti-infective: Quinolone

PHARMACOKINETICS

Well absorbed from GI tract (delayed by food). Widely distributed (including CSF). Protein binding: 20-40%. Metabolized in liver to active metabolite. Primarily excreted in urine. Minimal removal by hemodialysis. Half-life: 4-6 hrs (increased in decreased renal function, elderly).

ACTION

Inhibits DNA gyrase in susceptible microorganisms, interfering w/bacterial DNA replication and repair. Bactericidal.

USES

Treatment of infections of urinary tract, skin/skin structure, GI tract, bone/joint, lower respiratory tract, infectious diarrhea, uncomplicated gonorrhea. *Ophthalmic:* Conjunctival keratitis, keratoconjunctivitis, corneal ulcers, blepharitis, dacryocystitis, blepharoconjunctivitis, acute meibomianitis.

PO/IV/OPHTHALMIC ADMINISTRATION

PO:

1. May be given w/o regard to meals (preferred dosing time: 2 hrs after meals).
2. Do not administer antacids (aluminum, magnesium) within 2 hrs of ciprofloxacin.
3. Encourage cranberry juice, citrus fruits (to acidify urine).

IV:

1. Dilute preparation w/either 0.9% NaCl or 5% dextrose in water to final concentration of 1-2 mg/ml.
2. Discontinue any other solutions during infusion of ciprofloxacin.
3. Use large vein to reduce venous irritation.
4. Infuse over 60 min.

OPHTHALMIC:

1. Tilt pts head back; place solution in conjunctival sac.
2. Have pt close eyes; press gently on lacrimal sac for 1 min.
3. Do not use ophthalmic solutions for injection.
4. Unless infection very superficial, systemic administration generally accompanies ophthalmic.

INDICATIONS/DOSAGE/ROUTES

Mild to moderate urinary tract infections:
PO: Adults, elderly: 250 mg q12h.
IV: Adults, elderly: 200 mg q12h.

Complicated urinary tract/respiratory tract infections, skin/skin structure, bones and joint, infectious diarrhea:
PO: Adults, elderly: 500 mg q12h.
IV: Adults, elderly: 400 mg q12h.

Severe, complicated infections:
PO: Adults, elderly: 750 mg q12h.
IV: Adults, elderly: 400 mg q12h.

Uncomplicated gonorrhea:
PO: Adults: 250 mg as single dose.

Dosage in renal impairment:

The dose and/or frequency is modified in pts based on severity of infection and degree of renal impairment.

CREATININE CLEARANCE	DOSAGE
>50 ml/min (po); >30 ml/min (IV)	No change
30-50 ml/min	250-500 mg q12h
5-29 ml/min	250-500 mg po q18h; 200-400 mg IV q18-24h
Hemodialysis, peritoneal dialysis	250-500 mg q24h (after dialysis)

Usual ophthalmic dosage:
OPHTHALMIC: Adults, elderly: 1-2 drops 4-6 times/day.

PRECAUTIONS

CONTRAINDICATIONS: Hypersensitivity to ciprofloxacin, quinolones, any component of the preparation. Do not use in children <18 yrs of age. Ophthalmic: Vaccinia, varicella, epithelial herpes simplex, keratitis, mycobacterial infection, fungal disease of ocular structure. Not for use after uncomplicated removal of foreign body. **CAUTIONS:** Renal impairment, CNS disorders, seizures, those taking theophylline or caffeine. **PREGNANCY/LACTATION:** Unknown if distributed in breast milk. If possible, do not use during pregnancy/lactation (risk of arthropathy to fetus/infant). **Pregnancy Category C.**

INTERACTIONS

DRUG INTERACTIONS: Antacids, iron preparations, sucralfate may decrease absorption. Decreases clearance, may increase concentration, toxicity of theophylline. May increase effects of oral anticoagulants. **ALTERED LAB VALUES:** May increase SGOT (AST), SGPT (ALT), alkaline phosphatase, LDH, bilirubin, BUN, creatinine.

SIDE EFFECTS

FREQUENT: Nausea, vomiting, diarrhea, abdominal discomfort occur most often w/high dosage or in elderly; headache, restlessness, rash, bad taste (also w/ophthalmic). **OCCASIONAL:** Ophthalmic: After 1-7 days, may develop white crystalline precipitate on superficial portion of corneal defect (resolved in most pts in 2 wks). Transient irritation burning, stinging, itching, foreign body sensation. **RARE:** Dizziness, tremor, lethargy, seizures, dysphagia, GI bleeding, crystalluria, pruritus, photosensitivity, blurred vision, joint pain, chest pain, palpitations, hypertension. Ophthalmic: Lid edema, photophobia, tearing, allergic reactions.

ADVERSE REACTIONS/TOXIC EFFECTS

Superinfection (esp. enterococcal, fungal), nephropathy, cardiopulmonary arrest, cerebral thrombosis may occur. Arthropathy may occur if given to children <18 yrs. Ophthalmic: Sensitization may contraindicate later systemic use of ciprofloxacin.

NURSING IMPLICATIONS

BASELINE ASSESSMENT:

Question for history of hypersensitivity to ciprofloxacin, quinolones, any component of preparation. Obtain specimen for diagnostic tests before giving first dose (therapy may begin before results are known).

INTERVENTION/EVALUATION:

Evaluate food tolerance. Determine pattern of bowel activity; be alert to blood in feces. Check for dizziness, headache, visual difficulties, tremors. Monitor B/P at least twice daily. Assess for chest, joint pain. Ophthalmic: Check for therapeutic response, side effects (see Adverse Reactions/Toxic Effects).

PATIENT/FAMILY TEACHING:

Do not skip dose; take full course of therapy. Take w/8 oz water; drink several glasses of water between meals. Eat/drink high sources of ascorbic acid to prevent crystalluria (cranberry juice, citrus fruits). Do not take antacids (reduces/destroys effectiveness). Avoid tasks that require alertness, motor skills until response to drug is established. Avoid sunlight/ultraviolet exposure; wear sunscreen, protective clothing if photosensitivity develops. Sugarless gum or hard candy may relieve bad taste. Notify nurse/physician if new symptoms occur. Ophthalmic: Explain possibility of crystal precipitate forming, and usual resolution. Report any increased burning, itching, or other discomfort promptly.

cisapride

sis'ah-pride
(Propulsid)

CANADIAN AVAILABILITY:
Propulsid

CLASSIFICATION

GI stimulant

PHARMACOKINETICS

	ONSET	PEAK	DURATION
PO	30-60 min	—	—

Rapid, completely absorbed from GI tract. Widely distributed. Protein binding: 98%. Metabolized in liver. Excreted in urine, eliminated in feces. Half-life: 6-12 hrs.

ACTION

Enhances release of acetylcholine at myenteric plexus. Serotonin-4 receptor agonist (increase GI motility, cardiac rate, increases lower esophageal sphincter pressure, peristalsis). Accelerates gastric emptying.

USES

Treatment of nocturnal heartburn due to gastroesophageal reflux disease (GERD).

PO ADMINISTRATION

Tablets may be crushed.

INDICATIONS/DOSAGE/ROUTES

Symptomatic gastroesophageal reflux:
PO: Adults, elderly: 10 mg 4 times/day 15 min before meals and at bedtime. May increase up to 20 mg 4 times/day.

PRECAUTIONS

CONTRAINDICATIONS: GI hemorrhage, mechanical obstruction, perforation. **CAUTIONS:** None significant. **PREGNANCY/LACTATION:** May be embryotoxic, fetotoxic. Distributed in breast milk. **Pregnancy Category C.**

INTERACTIONS

DRUG INTERACTIONS: Anticholinergics may decrease effects.

ALTERED LAB VALUES: None significant.

SIDE EFFECTS

FREQUENT: Diarrhea, abdominal discomfort, headache. **OCCASIONAL:** Nausea, constipation, drowsiness. **RARE:** Rhinitis, flatulence, sinusitis.

ADVERSE REACTIONS/TOXIC EFFECTS

Acute overdosage results in tremors, convulsions, dyspnea, catatonia, hypotonia.

NURSING IMPLICATIONS

Baseline Assessment:

Consider effect of accelerated gastric emptying on rate of absorption of other drugs being administered.

Intervention/Evaluation:

Monitor stool frequency and consistency. Assess for periorbital edema.

Patient/Family Teaching:

Elevate head of bed to reduce potential for aspiration w/nocturnal gastroesophageal reflux. Sedative effects of alcohol may be accelerated.

cisplatin

sis-plah´tin
(Platinol, Platinol-AQ)

CANADIAN AVAILABILITY:
Abiplatin, Platinol

CLASSIFICATION

Antineoplastic

PHARMACOKINETICS

Widely distributed. Protein binding: >90%. Undergoes rapid nonenzymatic conversion to inactive metabolite. Excreted in urine. Half-life: 58-73 hrs (increase in decreased renal function).

ACTION

Inhibits DNA, and to lesser extent, RNA, protein synthesis by cross-linking w/DNA strands, preventing cellular division. Cell cycle phase nonspecific.

USES

Palliative treatment of metastatic testicular tumors, metastatic ovarian tumors, advanced bladder carcinoma.

STORAGE/HANDLING

NOTE: May be carcinogenic, mutagenic, or teratogenic. Handle w/ extreme care during preparation/ administration.

Following reconstitution, solutions should be clear and colorless. Protect from direct bright sunlight; do not refrigerate (may precipitate). Discard if precipitate forms. Stable for 20 hrs at room temperature.

IV ADMINISTRATION

NOTE: Wear protective gloves during handling of cisplatin. Do not use aluminum needles or administration sets that may come in contact w/drug; may cause formation of black precipitate, loss of potency.

1. Reconstitute 10 mg vial w/10 ml sterile water for injection (50 ml for 50 mg vial) to provide concentration of 1 mg/ml.
2. For IV infusion, dilute desired dose in up to 1,000 ml 5% dextrose, 0.33 or 0.45% NaCl containing 18.75

Gm mannitol/L. Infuse over 2-24 hrs.

3. Avoid rapid IV injection over 1-5 min (increases risk of nephrotoxicity, ototoxicity).

4. Monitor for anaphylactic reaction during first few min of IV infusion.

INDICATIONS/DOSAGE/ROUTES

NOTE: Dosage individualized based on clinical response, tolerance to adverse effects. When used in combination therapy, consult specific protocols for optimum dosage, sequence of drug administration. Repeat courses should not be given more frequently than q 3-4 wks. Do not repeat unless auditory acuity within normal limits, serum creatinine below 1.5 mg/dl, BUN below 25 mg/dl, circulating blood elements (platelets, WBC) are within acceptable levels.

Metastatic testicular tumors:
IV: Adults: (Combined w/bleomycin, vinblastine): 20 mg/m^2/day for 5 days q 3 wks for 3-4 courses of therapy.

Metastatic ovarian tumors:
IV: Adults: (Combined w/doxorubicin): 50 mg/m^2 once q 3-4 wks. *Single:* 100 mg/m^2 once q 4 wks.

Advanced bladder cancer:
IV: Adults: Single: 50-70 mg/m^2 q 3-4 wks.

PRECAUTIONS

CONTRAINDICATIONS: Myelosuppression, hearing impairment. **CAUTIONS:** Previous therapy w/other antineoplastic agents, radiation. **PREGNANCY/LACTATION:** If possible, avoid use during pregnancy, especially first trimester. Breast feeding not recommended. **Pregnancy Category D.**

INTERACTIONS

DRUG INTERACTIONS: May decrease effect of antigout medications. Bone marrow depressants may increase bone marrow depression. Nephrotoxic, ototoxic agents may increase toxicity. Live virus vaccines may potentiate virus replication, increase vaccine side effects, decrease patients antibody response to vaccine. **ALTERED LAB VALUES:** May cause positive Coombs test. May increase BUN, creatinine, uric acid, SGOT (AST). May decrease creatinine clearance, calcium, magnesium, phosphate, potassium, sodium.

SIDE EFFECTS

FREQUENT: Nausea, vomiting (begins 1-4 hrs after administration, generally last up to 24 hrs). Myelosuppression occurs in 25-30% of pts. Recovery can generally be expected in 18-23 days. Peripheral neuropathy (numbness, tingling of fingers, toes, face) may occur w/prolonged therapy (4-7 mo), but rarely noted at beginning of therapy. Loss of taste may occur.

ADVERSE REACTIONS/TOXIC EFFECTS

Anaphylactic reaction (facial edema, wheezing, tachycardia, hypotension) may occur in first few minutes of IV administration in those previously exposed to cisplatin. Nephrotoxicity in 28-36% of pts treated w/single dose of cisplatin, usually during second week of therapy. Ototoxicity (tinnitus, hearing loss) in 31% of pts treated w/single dose of cisplatin (more severe in children). May become more frequent, severe with repeated doses.

C

NURSING IMPLICATIONS

Baseline Assessment:

Pts should be well hydrated prior to and 24 hrs after medication to ensure good urinary output, decrease risk of nephrotoxicity. Give emotional support to pt and family.

Intervention/Evaluation:

Measure all vomitus (general guideline requiring immediate notification of physician: 750 ml/8 hrs, urinary output less than 100 ml/hr). Monitor I&O q1-2h beginning w/ pretreatment hydration, continue for 48 hrs after cisplatin therapy. Assess vital signs q1-2h during infusion. Monitor urinalysis, renal function reports for nephrotoxicity.

Patient/Family Teaching:

Report signs of ototoxicity (ringing/roaring in ears, hearing loss). Do not have immunizations w/o physician's approval (drug lowers body's resistance). Avoid contact w/those who have recently taken oral polio vaccine. Contact physician if nausea/vomiting continues at home. Teach signs of peripheral neuropathy.

citrates

potassium citrate

(Urocit K)

potassium citrate and citric acid

(Polycitra K)

sodium citrate and citric acid

(Bicitra)

tricitrates

(Polycitra syrup)

CANADIAN AVAILABILITY:
Oracit

CLASSIFICATION

Antiurolithic, alkalizer

PHARMACOKINETICS

Oxidized to form potassium or sodium bicarbonate. Primarily excreted in urine.

ACTION

Increases urinary pH, increasing solubility of cystine in urine and ionization of uric acid to urate ion. Increasing urinary pH and urinary citrate decreases calcium ion activity and decreases saturation of calcium oxalate. Increases plasma bicarbonate, buffers excess hydrogen ion concentration increasing blood pH and reversing acidosis.

USES

Treats/prevents uric acid/cystine lithiasis, prevents urate crystallization (increased urinary pH). Treats/prevents calcium phosphate, calcium oxalate or uric acid kidney stones (increase urinary citrate). Treats chronic metabolic acidosis. Neutralizes/buffers excess quantities gastric hydrochloric acid.

PO ADMINISTRATION

1. Take after meals.
2. *Tablets:* Swallow whole, do not crush, chew, take w/full glass of water or juice.
3. *Liquid:* Dilute w/6 ounces water or juice; chilling may increase palatability.

INDICATIONS/DOSAGE/ROUTES

POTASSIUM CITRATE

Antiurolithic, urinary alkalizer:
PO: Adults, elderly: 10 mEq 3 times/day up to 15 mEq 4 times/day or 20 mEq 3 times/day.

POTASSIUM CITRATE AND CITRIC ACID

Antiurolithic, urinary/systemic alkalizer:
PO: Adults, elderly: 20-30 mEq 4 times/day. **Children:** 10-30 mEq 4 times/day.

SODIUM CITRATE AND CITRIC ACID

Antiurolithic, urinary/systemic alkalizer:
PO: Adults, elderly: 10-30 mEq 4 times/day. **Maximum:** 150 mEq/day. **Children:** 5-15 mEq 4 times/day.

TRICITRATES

Antiurolithic, urinary alkalizer:
PO: Adults, elderly: 15-30 mEq 4 times/day. **Children:** 5-10 mEq 4 times/day.

PRECAUTIONS

CONTRAINDICATIONS: Aluminum toxicity, severe myocardial damage, heart failure, severe renal impairment, active urinary tract infection, hyperkalemia, peptic ulcer. **CAUTIONS:** Severe renal tubular acidosis. **PREGNANCY/LACTATION:** Unknown whether distributed in breast milk. **Pregnancy Category C.**

INTERACTIONS

DRUG INTERACTIONS: May increase quinidine excretion. Antacids may increase risk of systemic alkalosis. NSAIDs, angiotensin converting enzyme inhibitors, potassium-sparing diuretics, potassium-containing medication may increase risk of hyperkalemia. May decrease effect of methenamine. **ALTERED LAB VALUES:** None significant.

SIDE EFFECTS

OCCASIONAL: Diarrhea, loose bowel movements, mild abdominal pain, nausea, vomiting. **RARE:** Metabolic alkalosis, bowel obstruction/perforation, hyperkalemia, hypernatremia.

ADVERSE REACTIONS/TOXIC EFFECTS

None significant.

NURSING IMPLICATIONS

BASELINE ASSESSMENT:

Assess urinary pH determination, EKG in pts w/cardiac disease, serum acid-base balance, CBC, hemoglobin, hematocrit, serum creatinine.

INTERVENTION/EVALUATION:

Monitor urinary pH, EKG in pts w/cardiac disease, serum acid-base balance, CBC, hemoglobin, hematocrit, serum creatinine.

PATIENT/FAMILY TEACHING:

Take after meals. Mix in water or juice and follow w/additional liquid if desired. Notify physician if diarrhea, nausea/vomiting, abdominal pain, or seizures occur. Check w/physician if black, tarry stools or other signs of GI bleeding are observed.

cladribine

clad-rih-bean
(Leustatin)

CLASSIFICATION

Antineoplastic

PHARMACOKINETICS

Protein binding: 20%. Primarily excreted in urine. Half-life: 5.4 hrs.

ACTION

Disrupts cellular metabolism by incorporating into DNA of dividing cells. Cytotoxic to both actively dividing and quiescent lymphocytes and monocytes, preventing DNA synthesis and repair.

USES

Treatment for active hairy cell leukemia defined by clinically significant anemia, neutropenia, thrombocytopenia. Chronic multiple sclerosis.

STORAGE/HANDLING

Refrigerate unopened vials. Use diluted solutions immediately or refrigerate for no more than 8 hrs before administration. Solutions stable for at least 24 hrs at room temperature. Wear gloves and protective clothing during handling; if contact w/skin, rinse with copious amounts of water. Discard unused portion.

IV ADMINISTRATION

NOTE: Must dilute before administration. Do not mix w/other IV drugs, additives or infuse concurrently via a common IV line.

1. Add calculated dose (0.09 mg/kg) to 500 ml 0.9% NaCl. Avoid 5% dextrose (increases degradation of medication).
2. Monitor vital signs during infusion, especially during first hour. Observe for hypotension or bradycardia (usually both do not occur during same course).
3. Immediately discontinue administration if severe hypersensitivity reaction occurs.

INDICATIONS/DOSAGE/ROUTES

Hairy cell leukemia:
IV INFUSION: Adults: 0.09 mg/kg/day as continuous infusion for 7 days.

PRECAUTIONS

CONTRAINDICATIONS: None significant. **CAUTIONS:** Renal/hepatic impairment, bone marrow suppression. **PREGNANCY/LACTATION:** May produce fetal harm; may be embryotoxic and fetotoxic; potential for serious reactions in nursing infants. **Pregnancy Category D.**

INTERACTIONS

DRUG INTERACTIONS: Bone marrow depressants may increase bone marrow depression. High doses w/cyclophosphamide and total body irradiation may cause severe, irreversible neurologic toxicity, acute renal dysfunction. Nephrotoxic, neurotoxic medications may increase toxicity. Live virus vaccines may potentiate virus replication, increase vaccine side effects, decrease patients antibody response to vaccine. **ALTERED LAB VALUES:** None significant.

SIDE EFFECTS

FREQUENT: Fever (69% of pts), fatigue, mild nausea, headache, anorexia, rash, injection site reactions (redness, swelling, pain), mild to moderate infection. **OCCASIONAL:** Chills, diaphoresis, asthenia, vomiting, diarrhea/constipation, purpura, insomnia, edema, cough. **RARE:** Dizziness, tachycardia, shortness of breath, myalgia, arthralgia.

ADVERSE REACTIONS/TOXIC EFFECTS

Myelosuppression characterized as severe neutropenia (<500 cells/mm^3), severe anemia (hemoglobin <8.5 g/dl) and thrombocytopenia occur commonly. High dose treatment may produce acute nephrotoxicity and/or neurotoxicity manifested as irreversible motor weakness of upper or lower extremities.

NURSING IMPLICATIONS

BASELINE ASSESSMENT:

Give emotional support to pt and family. Perform neurologic function tests before chemotherapy. Obtain baseline temperature. Use strict asepsis and protect pt from infection. Check blood counts, particularly neutrophil, platelet count before each course of therapy and as clinically indicated.

INTERVENTION/EVALUATION:

Monitor temperature and report fever promptly. Assess for signs of infection or anemia (excessive tiredness, weakness). Avoid unnecessary trauma (rectal temperature, IM injections) when platelet counts decreased. Pt may require transfusions of RBCs or platelets.

PATIENT/FAMILY TEACHING:

Narrow margin between therapeutic and toxic response. Avoid crowds, persons w/known infections; report signs of infection at once (fever, flu-like symptoms). Do not have immunizations w/o physician's approval (drug lowers body's resistance). Avoid contact w/those who have recently received live virus vaccine. Women of childbearing potential should not become pregnant during treatment.

clarithromycin

clair-rith´row-my-sin
(Biaxin)

CLASSIFICATION

Antibiotic: Macrolide

PHARMACOKINETICS

Well absorbed from GI tract. Widely distributed. Protein binding: 65-75%. Metabolized in liver to active metabolite. Primarily excreted in urine. Half-life: 3-7 hrs, metabolite: 5-7 hrs (increased in decreased renal function).

ACTION

Binds to 50S ribosomal subunit of 70S ribosome. Inhibits bacterial RNA-dependent protein synthesis. Bacteriostatic.

USES

Treatment of mild to moderate infections of upper respiratory tract (pharyngitis, tonsillitis, sinusitis), lower respiratory tract (acute exacerbation chronic bronchitis, pneumonia), and uncomplicated skin/skin structure infections, disseminated mycobacterium complex in AIDS.

PO ADMINISTRATION

1. May give w/o regard to food.
2. Do not crush/break tablets.

INDICATIONS/DOSAGE/ROUTES

NOTE: Space doses evenly around the clock.

Lower respiratory tract infections:
PO: Adults, elderly: 250-500 mg q12h for 7-14 days.

Upper respiratory tract infections:
PO: Adults, elderly: 250-500 mg q12h for 10-14 days.

Uncomplicated skin/skin structure infections:
PO: Adults, elderly: 250 mg q12h for 7-14 days.

Usual pediatric dosage:
PO: Children (6 mo-12 yrs): 7.5 mg/kg q12h.

Disseminated mycobacterium complex:
PO: Adults: 500 mg q12h.

PRECAUTIONS

CONTRAINDICATIONS: Hypersensitivity to clarithromycin, erythromycins, any macrolide antibiotic. **CAUTIONS:** Hepatic and renal dysfunction. Elderly w/severe renal impairment. **PREGNANCY/LACTATION:** Unknown if distributed in breast milk. **Pregnancy Category C.**

INTERACTIONS

DRUG INTERACTIONS: May increase concentration, toxicity of theophylline. May decrease concentration of zidovudine. **ALTERED LAB VALUES:** May rarely increase SGOT (AST), SGPT (ALT), BUN.

SIDE EFFECTS

Mild transient effects. **FREQUENT:** Diarrhea, nausea, abnormal taste. **OCCASIONAL:** Headache, abdominal discomfort.

ADVERSE REACTIONS/TOXIC EFFECTS

Superinfections, esp. antibiotic-associated colitis may occur.

NURSING IMPLICATIONS

BASELINE ASSESSMENT:

Question pt for history of hepatitis or allergies to clarithromycin, erythromycins, hepatitis. Obtain specimens for culture and sensitivity before giving first dose (therapy may begin before results are known).

INTERVENTION/EVALUATION:

Check for GI discomfort, nausea. Determine pattern of bowel activity and stool consistency. Monitor hepatic function tests, assess for hepatotoxicity: malaise, fever, abdominal pain, GI disturbances. Evaluate for superinfection: genital/anal pruritus, sore mouth or tongue, moderate to severe diarrhea.

PATIENT/FAMILY TEACHING:

Continue therapy for full length of treatment. Doses should be evenly spaced. Take medication w/8 oz water w/o regard to food. Notify physician in event of GI upset, rash, diarrhea, or other new symptom.

clemastine fumarate

klem-ass´teen
(Tavist, Tavist-1)

FIXED-COMBINATION(S): W/phenylpropanolamine, a nasal decongestant (Tavist-D)

CANADIAN AVAILABILITY: Tavist

CLASSIFICATION

Antihistamine

PHARMACOKINETICS

	ONSET	PEAK	DURATION
PO	15-60 min	5-7 hrs	10-12 hrs

Well absorbed from GI tract. Metabolized in liver. Excreted primarily in urine.

ACTION

Prevents, antagonizes most histamine effects (e.g., urticaria, pruritus). Anticholinergic effects cause drying of nasal mucosa.

USES

Relief of allergic conditions (nasal allergies, allergic dermatitis), hypersensitivity reaction.

PO ADMINISTRATION

Give w/o regard to meals. Scored tablets may be crushed. Do not crush extended-release or film-coated forms.

INDICATIONS/DOSAGE/ROUTES

Allergic rhinitis:
PO: Adults, children >12 yrs: 1.34 mg 2 times/day. May increase dose to maximum 8.04 mg/day, if needed. **Children 6-11 yrs:** 0.67 mg 2 times/day. May increase dose to maximum 4.02 mg/day, if needed.

Allergic urticaria, angioedema:
PO: Adults, children >12 yrs: 2.68 1-3 times/day. Do not exceed 8.04 mg/day. **Children 6-11 yrs:** 1.34 mg 2 times/day. Do not exceed 4.02 mg/day.

Usual elderly dosage:
PO: Elderly: 1.34 mg 1-2 times/day.

PRECAUTIONS

CONTRAINDICATIONS: Acute asthmatic attack, those receiving MAO inhibitors. **CAUTIONS:** Narrow-angle glaucoma, peptic ulcer, prostatic hypertrophy, pyloroduodenal or bladder neck obstruction, asthma, COPD, increased intraocular pressure, cardiovascular disease, hyperthyroidism, hypertension, seizure disorders. **PREGNANCY/LACTATION:** Crosses placenta; detected in breast milk (may produce irritability in nursing infants). Increased risk of seizures in neonates, premature infants if used during third trimester of pregnancy. May prohibit lactation. **Pregnancy Category B.**

INTERACTIONS

DRUG INTERACTIONS: Alcohol, CNS depressants may increase CNS depressant effects. MAO inhibitors may increase anticholinergic, CNS depressant effects. **ALTERED LAB VALUES:** May suppress wheal, flare reactions to antigen skin testing, unless antihistamines discontinued 4 days prior to testing.

SIDE EFFECTS

FREQUENT: Drowsiness, dizziness, muscular weakness, dry mouth/nose/throat/lips, urinary retention, thickening of bronchial secretions. Sedation, dizziness, hypotension more likely noted in elderly. **OCCASIONAL:** Epigastric distress, flushing, visual disturbances, hearing disturbances, paresthesia, sweating, chills. Fixed-combination form with pseudoephedrine may produce mild CNS stimulation.

ADVERSE REACTIONS/TOXIC EFFECTS

Children may experience dominant paradoxical reaction (restlessness, insomnia, euphoria, nervousness, tremors). Overdosage in children may result in hallucinations, convulsions, death. Hypersensitivity reaction (eczema, pruritus, rash, cardiac disturbances, angioedema, photosensitivity) may occur. Overdosage may vary from CNS depression (sedation, apnea, cardiovascular collapse, death) to severe paradoxical reaction (hallucinations, tremor, seizures).

NURSING IMPLICATIONS

BASELINE ASSESSMENT:

If pt is undergoing allergic reaction, obtain history of recently ingested foods, drugs, environmental exposure, recent emotional stress. Monitor rate, depth, rhythm, type of respiration; quality and rate of pulse. Assess lung sounds for rhonchi, wheezing, rales.

INTERVENTION/EVALUATION:

Monitor B/P, especially in elderly (increased risk of hypotension). Monitor children closely for paradoxical reaction.

PATIENT/FAMILY TEACHING:

Tolerance to antihistaminic effect generally does not occur; tolerance to sedative effect may occur. Avoid tasks that require alertness, motor skills until response to drug is established. Dry mouth, drowsiness, dizziness may be an expected response of drug. Avoid alcoholic beverages during antihistamine therapy. Sugarless gum, sips of tepid water may relieve dry mouth. Coffee or tea may help reduce drowsiness.

clindamycin hydrochloride

klin-da-my′sin
(Cleocin HCL)

clindamycin palmitate hydrochloride

(Cleocin Pediatric)

clindamycin phosphate

(Cleocin phosphate, Cleocin T)

CANADIAN AVAILABILITY:
Dalacin

CLASSIFICATION

Antibiotic

PHARMACOKINETICS

Rapidly absorbed from GI tract. Widely distributed. Protein binding: 92-94%. Metabolized in liver to some active metabolites. Primarily excreted in urine. Not removed by hemodialysis. Half-life: 2.4-3 hrs (increased in decreased renal function, premature infants).

ACTION

Bacteriostatic. Binds to 50S subunits of bacterial ribosomes inhibiting protein synthesis. Topically, decreases fatty acid concentration on skin.

USES

Treatment of respiratory tract, skin/soft tissue, chronic bone/joint infections, septicemia, intra-abdominal, female genitourinary infections, bacterial vaginosis, endocarditis. *Topical:* Acne vulgaris.

STORAGE/HANDLING

Store capsules at room temperature. After reconstitution, oral solution is stable for 2 wks at room temperature. Do not refrigerate oral solution (avoids thickening). IV infusion (piggyback) stable for 16 days at room temperature, 32 days if refrigerated.

PO/IM/IV ADMINISTRATION

NOTE: Space doses evenly around the clock. May be given by IM injection, intermittent IV infusion (piggyback).

PO:

1. Give w/8 oz water.

IM:

1. Do not exceed 600 mg/dose.
2. Administer deep IM.

IV:

1. Dilute 300-600 mg w/50 ml 5% dextrose, 0.9% NaCl, or other compatible IV fluid (900-1,200 mg w/100 ml).
2. 50 ml piggyback is infused >10-20 min; 100 ml piggyback is infused >30-40 min.
3. No more than 1.2 Gm should be given in 1 infusion.
4. Do not administer IV push.
5. Alternating IV sites, use large veins to reduce risk of phlebitis.
6. Avoid prolonged use of indwelling IV catheters.

INDICATIONS/DOSAGE/ROUTES

Mild to moderate infections:
PO: Adults, elderly: 150-300 mg q6h. **Children:** 8-16 mg/kg/day in 3-4 divided doses.
IM/IV: Adults, elderly: 600-1,200 mg/day in 2-4 divided doses. **Children >1 mo:** 15-25 mg/kg/day in 3-4 divided doses. **Children <1 mo:** 15-20 mg/kg/day in 3-4 divided doses.

Serious infections:
PO: Adults, elderly: 300-450 mg q6h. **Children:** 13-25 mg/kg/day in 3-4 divided doses. **Children <10 kg:** Minimum: 37.5 mg 3 times/day.
IM/IV: Adults, elderly: 1.2-2.7 Gm/day in 2-4 divided doses. **Children:** 25-40 mg/kg/day in 3-4 divided doses.

Life-threatening infections:
IV: Adults, elderly: Up to 4.8 Gm/day in divided doses.

Bacterial vaginosis:
INTRAVAGINAL: Adults: One applicatorful at bedtime for 7 days.

Acne vulgaris:
TOPICAL: Adults: Apply thin film 2 times/day to affected area.

PRECAUTIONS

CONTRAINDICATIONS: Hypersensitivity to clindamycin or lincomycin, known allergy to tartrazine dye, history of ulcerative colitis, regional enteritis, or antibiotic-associated colitis. **CAUTIONS:** Allergies, particularly aspirin, severe renal or hepatic dysfunction, concomitant use of neuromuscular blocking agents, neonates. Initiate antifungal treatment for preexisting candidal, other fungal infections. Topical preparations should not be applied to abraded areas or near eyes. **PREGNANCY/LACTATION:** Readily crosses placenta; distributed in breast milk. **Pregnancy Category C.** *Topical/vaginal:* Unknown if distributed in breast milk. **Pregnancy Category B.**

INTERACTIONS

DRUG INTERACTIONS: Adsorbent antidiarrheals may delay absorption. Chloramphenicol, erythromycin may antagonize effects. May increase effect of neuromuscular blockers. **ALTERED LAB VALUES:** May increase SGOT (AST), SGPT (ALT), alkaline phosphatase.

SIDE EFFECTS

FREQUENT: Nausea, vomiting, diarrhea, abdominal pain. *Topical:* Rash, dry skin, contact dermatitis, irritation. **OCCASIONAL:** Phlebitis, thrombophlebitis w/IV administration; pain, induration at IM injection site; urticaria, pruritus, bloating, flatulence, esophagitis, metallic taste. *Topical:* Diarrhea, abdominal pain, GI disturbance.

ADVERSE REACTIONS/TOXIC EFFECTS

Antibiotic-associated colitis during and several weeks after therapy (including topical), superinfection (esp. fungal), due to bacterial imbalance may occur. Blood dyscrasias (leukopenia, thrombocytopenia), nephrotoxicity (proteinuria, azotemia, oliguria) occur rarely.

NURSING IMPLICATIONS

BASELINE ASSESSMENT:

Question pt for history of allergies, particularly to clindamycin, lincomycin, aspirin. Avoid, if possible, concurrent use of neuromuscular blocking agents. Obtain specimens for culture and sensitivity, Gram's stain for vaginitis, before giving first dose (therapy may begin before results are known).

INTERVENTION/EVALUATION:

Monitor bowel activity, stool consistency; report diarrhea promptly due to potential for serious colitis (even w/topical or vaginal). Monitor periodic renal, hepatic, blood cell reports. Assess for ability to swallow, vomiting. Check I&O. Assess skin for rash (dryness, irritation w/topical application). Observe for phlebitis: pain, heat, red streaking over vein. Check for pain, induration at IM sites. W/all routes of administration, assess for superinfection: severe diarrhea, anal/genital pruritus, increased fever, change of oral mucosa.

PATIENT/FAMILY TEACHING:

Continue therapy for full length of treatment. Doses should be evenly spaced. Take oral doses w/ 8 oz water. Caution should be used when applying topical clindamycin concurrently w/peeling, abrasive acne agents, soaps, or alcohol-containing cosmetics to avoid cumulative effect. Do not apply topical preparations near eyes or abraded areas. Notify physician immediately in event of diarrhea; report onset of new symptoms. *Vaginal:* Avoid contact w/eyes. In event of accidental contact w/ eyes, rinse w/copious amounts of cool tap water. Do not engage in sexual intercourse during treatment. Instruct pt on correct application (manufacturer's insert).

clobetasol propionate

cloe-bet´a-soh

(Temovate)

(See Classifications section under Corticosteroids, Topical)

clofibrate

clow-fih´brate

(Atromid-S)

CANADIAN AVAILABILITY: Atromid-S, Claripex, Novofibrate

CLASSIFICATION

Antihyperlipoproteinemic

PHARMACOKINETICS

Slow, completely absorbed from intestine. Protein binding: 96%. De-esterified in liver/GI tract to active form. Primarily excreted in urine. Half-life: 6-25 hrs (increased in decreased renal function).

ACTION

Lowers serum cholesterol and triglycerides (decreases VLDL, LDL; increases HDL). May accelerate catabolism of VLDL to LDL; decrease hepatic synthesis of VLDL; inhibit cholesterol formation; increase excretion of neutral sterols.

USES

Adjunct to diet therapy to decrease elevated serum triglyceride concentration (types IV and V hyperlipidemia) in selected pts who are at risk of developing abdominal pain or pancreatitis; primary dysbetalipoproteinemia (type III hyperlipidemia) not responding to diet.

PO ADMINISTRATION

Give w/o regard to meals. If GI upset occurs, take w/food.

INDICATIONS/DOSAGE/ROUTES

Hypertriglyceridemia:
PO: Adults, elderly: 2 Gm/day in divided doses.

PRECAUTIONS

CONTRAINDICATIONS: Hypersensitivity to clofibrate, clinically significant hepatic/renal dysfunction, biliary cirrhosis. **CAUTIONS:** Hypothyroidism, diabetes mellitus, peptic ulcer, anticoagulant therapy, history of jaundice or hepatic disease. **PREGNANCY/LACTATION:** Contraindicated in pregnancy/lactation. Discontinue several months before planned pregnancy; strict birth control indicated in women of childbearing potential. **Pregnancy Category C.**

INTERACTIONS

DRUG INTERACTIONS: May increase effects of oral anticoagulants, hypoglycemics. **ALTERED LAB VALUES:** May increase SGOT (AST), SGPT (ALT), amylase, creatine kinase. LDL, cholesterol may increase due to decreased VLDL. May decrease fibrinogen concentration.

SIDE EFFECTS

FREQUENT: Nausea (generally decreases as therapy continues). **OCCASIONAL:** Vomiting, diarrhea, flatulence, dyspepsia, abdominal distress. **RARE:** Headache, dizziness, rash, pruritus, dry skin/hair, alopecia, myalgia (aching, cramping, weak muscles), anemia, leukopenia, impotence, decreased libido.

ADVERSE REACTIONS/TOXIC EFFECTS

Cholelithiasis, cholecystitis, malignancy. Cardiac arrhythmias, intermittent claudication, angina, noncardiovascular deaths reported.

NURSING IMPLICATIONS

BASELINE ASSESSMENT:

Question for history of hypersensitivity to clofibrate, possibility of pregnancy. Assess baseline lab results: serum triglyceride, cholesterol, VLDL, LDL, CBC, and liver function tests.

INTERVENTION/EVALUATION:

Evaluate food tolerance. Determine pattern of bowel activity. Monitor LDL, VLDL, triglyceride, and cholesterol lab results for therapeutic response. Assess for rash, pruritus. Check for headache and dizziness. Monitor liver function and hematology tests. Assess for pain, especially right upper quadrant/epigastric pain suggestive of adverse gall bladder effects. Be alert to cramping, aching, weakness of muscles.

PATIENT/FAMILY TEACHING:

Follow special diet carefully (important part of treatment). Do not stop taking clofibrate w/o checking w/physician. Periodic lab tests are essential part of therapy. Take w/food if GI upset occurs. Do not take any other medication w/o physician's knowledge. Pregnancy must be avoided for several months after medication is discontinued. Impotence, decreased libido may occur during therapy w/ medication. Do not drive or perform other activities that require alert response if dizziness occurs. Notify physician promptly in event of any new symptom, particularly abdominal/epigastric pain, irregular heartbeat, chest pain, or shortness of breath.

clomipramine hydrochloride

klow-mih´prah-meen
(Anafranil)

CANADIAN AVAILABILITY:
Anafranil

CLASSIFICATION

Antidepressant: Tricyclic

PHARMACOKINETICS

Well absorbed from GI tract. Protein binding: 96-97%. Metabolized in liver, undergoes first-pass metabolism. Primarily excreted in urine. Minimal removal by hemodialysis. Half-life: 21-31 hrs.

ACTION

Increases synaptic concentration of norepinephrine and/or serotonin (inhibits re-uptake by presynaptic membrane).

USES

Treatment of obsessive-compulsive disorder manifested as repetitive tasks producing marked distress, time-consuming, or significantly interfering w/social or occupational behavior.

PO ADMINISTRATION

Give w/food or milk if GI distress occurs.

INDICATIONS/DOSAGE/ROUTES

Obsessive compulsive disorder:
PO: Adults: Initially, 25 mg/day. Gradually increase over 2 wks to 100 mg/day in divided doses. May further increase over several weeks to 250 mg/day in divided doses. After titration, may give as single bedtime dose (reduces daytime sedation). **Children >10 yrs:** Initially, 25 mg/day. Gradually increase over 2 wks to 3 mg/kg or 100 mg/day in divided doses (whichever is less). May then increase over several weeks up to 3 mg/kg or 200 mg (whichever is less). **Maintenance:** Lowest effective dose.

PRECAUTIONS

CONTRAINDICATIONS: Acute recovery period following MI, within 14 days of MAO inhibitor ingestion. **CAUTIONS:** Prostatic hypertrophy, history of urinary retention or obstruction, glaucoma, diabetes mellitus, history of seizures, hyperthyroidism, cardiac/hepatic/renal disease, schizophrenia, increased intraocular pressure, hiatal hernia. **PREGNANCY/LACTATION:** Crosses placenta; minimally distributed in breast milk. May produce neonatal withdrawal. **Pregnancy Category C.**

INTERACTIONS

DRUG INTERACTIONS: Alcohol, CNS depressants may increase CNS, respiratory depression, hypotensive effects. Antithyroid agents may increase risk of agranulocytosis. Phenothiazines may increase sedative, anticholinergic effects. Cimetidine may increase concentration, toxicity. May decrease effects of clonidine, guanadrel. May increase cardiac effects w/sympathomimetics. May increase risk of hypertensive crisis, hyperpyretic, convulsions w/ MAO inhibitors **ALTERED LAB VALUES:** May alter EKG readings, glucose.

SIDE EFFECTS

FREQUENT: Drowsiness, fatigue, dry mouth, blurred vision, constipation, sexual dysfunction (42%: ejaculatory failure, 20%: impotence), weight gain (18%), delayed micturition, postural hypotension, excessive sweating, disturbed concentration, increased appetite, urinary retention. **OCCASIONAL:** GI disturbances (nausea, GI distress, metallic taste sensation), asthenia, aggressiveness, muscle weakness. **RARE:** Paradoxical reaction (agitation, restlessness, nightmares, insomnia), extrapyramidal symptoms (particularly fine hand tremor), laryngitis, seizures.

ADVERSE REACTIONS/TOXIC EFFECTS

High dosage may produce cardiovascular effects (severe postural hypotension, dizziness, tachycardia, palpitations, arrhythmias) and seizures. May also result in altered temperature regulation (hyperpyrexia or hypothermia). Abrupt withdrawal from prolonged therapy may produce headache, malaise, nausea, vomiting, vivid dreams. Anemia has been noted.

NURSING IMPLICATIONS

BASELINE ASSESSMENT:

For those on long-term therapy, liver/renal function tests, blood counts should be performed periodically.

INTERVENTION/EVALUATION:

Supervise suicidal-risk pt closely during early therapy (as depression lessens, energy level improves, increasing suicide potential). Assess appearance, behavior, speech pattern, level of interest, mood. Monitor pattern of daily bowel activity and stool consistency. Monitor B/P, pulse for hypotension, arrhythmias. Assess for urinary retention by bladder palpation.

PATIENT/FAMILY TEACHING:

Change positions slowly to avoid hypotensive effect. Tolerance to postural hypotension, sedative, and anticholinergic effects usually develops during early therapy. Maximum therapeutic effect may be noted in 2-4 wks. Photosensitivity to sun may occur. Dry mouth may be relieved by sugarless gum, sips of tepid water. Report visual disturbances. Do not abruptly discontinue medication. Avoid tasks that require alertness, motor skills until response to drug is established. Avoid alcohol.

clonazepam

klon-nah'zih-pam
(Klonopin)

CANADIAN AVAILABILITY: Rivotril

CLASSIFICATION

Anticonvulsant

PHARMACOKINETICS

Well absorbed from GI tract. Protein binding: 85%. Metabolized in liver. Excreted in urine. Half-life: 18-50 hrs.

ACTION

Enhances presynaptic inhibition, suppresses spread of seizure activity.

USES

Adjunct in treatment of Lennox-Gastaut syndrome (petit mal variant epilepsy), akinetic, and myoclonic seizures, absence seizures (petit mal).

PO ADMINISTRATION

1. Give w/o regard to meals.
2. Tablets may be crushed.

INDICATIONS/DOSAGE/ROUTES

Anticonvulsant:
NOTE: When replacement by another anticonvulsant is necessary, decrease clonazepam gradually as therapy begins w/low-replacement dose.
PO: Adults, elderly: 1.5 mg daily. Dosage may be increased in 0.5-1 mg increments at 3-day intervals until seizures are controlled. Do not exceed maintenance dose of 20 mg daily. **Infants, children <10 yrs, or <66 lbs:** 0.01-0.03 mg/kg daily in 2-3 divided doses. Dosage may be increased in up to 0.5 mg increments at 3-day intervals until seizures are controlled. Do not exceed maintenance dose of 0.2 mg/kg daily.

PRECAUTIONS

CONTRAINDICATIONS: Significant liver disease, narrow-angle glaucoma. **CAUTIONS:** Impaired kidney/liver function, chronic respiratory disease. **PREGNANCY/LACTATION:** Crosses placenta, may be distributed in breast milk. Chronic ingestion during pregnancy may produce withdrawal symptoms, CNS depression in neonates. **Pregnancy Category C.**

INTERACTIONS

DRUG INTERACTIONS: Alcohol, CNS depressants may increase CNS depressant effect. **ALTERED LAB VALUES:** None significant.

SIDE EFFECTS

FREQUENT: Drowsiness, ataxia, behavioral disturbances (especially in children) manifested as aggressiveness, irritability, agitation. **OCCASIONAL:** Skin rash, ankle/facial edema, nocturia, dysuria, change in appetite/weight, dry mouth, sore gums, nausea, blurred vision, dry mouth. **RARE:** Paradoxical CNS hyperactivity/nervousness in children, excitement/restlessness in elderly (particularly noted in presence of uncontrolled pain).

ADVERSE REACTIONS/TOXIC EFFECTS

Abrupt withdrawal may result in pronounced restlessness, irritability, insomnia, hand tremors, abdominal/muscle cramps, sweating, vomiting, status epilepticus. Overdosage results in somnolence, confusion, diminished reflexes, coma.

NURSING IMPLICATIONS

BASELINE ASSESSMENT:

Review history of seizure disorder (frequency, duration, intensity, level of consciousness). Implement safety measures and observe frequently for recurrence of seizure activity.

INTERVENTION/EVALUATION:

Assess children, elderly for paradoxical reaction, particularly during early therapy. Assist w/ambulation if drowsiness, ataxia occur. For those on long-term therapy, liver/renal function tests, blood counts should be performed periodically. Evaluate for therapeutic response: a decrease in intensity/frequency of seizures.

PATIENT/FAMILY TEACHING:

Drowsiness usually diminishes w/continued therapy. Avoid tasks that require alertness, motor skills until response to drug is established. Smoking reduces drug effectiveness. Do not abruptly withdraw medication after long-term therapy. Strict maintenance of drug therapy is essential for seizure control. Avoid alcohol.

clonidine

klon´ih-deen

(Catapres TTS)

clonidine hydrochloride

(Catapres)

FIXED-COMBINATION(S):
W/chlorthalidone, a diuretic (Combipres)

CANADIAN AVAILABILITY:
Catapres, Dixarit

CLASSIFICATION

Antihypertensive

PHARMACOKINETICS

	ONSET	PEAK	DURATION
PO	0.5-1 hr	2-4 hrs	up to 8 hrs
Transdermal	—	—	—

Well absorbed from GI tract. Transdermal best absorbed from chest, upper arm, least absorbed from thigh. Protein binding: 20-40%. Metabolized in liver. Primarily excreted in urine. Minimal removal by hemodialysis. Half-life: 12-16 hrs (increased in decreased renal function).

ACTION

Stimulates alpha$_2$-adrenergic receptors in CNS (inhibits sympathetic cardioaccelerator and vasoconstrictor center). Decreases sympathetic outflow from CNS.

USES

Treatment of hypertension alone or in combination w/other antihypertensive agents.

PO/TRANSDERMAL ADMINISTRATION

PO:

1. May give w/o regard to food.
2. Tablets may be crushed.
3. Give last oral dose just before retiring.

TRANSDERMAL:

1. Apply transdermal system to dry, hairless area of intact skin on upper arm or chest.

2. Rotate sites (prevents skin irritation).

3. Do not trim patch to adjust dose.

INDICATIONS/DOSAGE/ROUTES

Hypertension:

PO: Adults: Initially, 0.1 mg 2 times/day. Increase by 0.1-0.2 mg q 2-4 days. **Maintenance:** 0.2-1.2 mg/day in 2-4 divided doses up to maximum of 2.4 mg/day. **Children:** 5-25 mcg/kg/day in divided doses q6h; increase at 5-7 day intervals. **TRANSDERMAL: Adults, elderly:** System delivering 0.1 mg/24 hrs up to 0.6 mg/24 hrs every 7 days.

Usual elderly dosage:

PO: Elderly: Initially, 0.1 mg at bedtime. May increase gradually.

PRECAUTIONS

CONTRAINDICATIONS: None significant. **CAUTIONS:** Severe coronary insufficiency, recent MI, cerebrovascular disease, chronic renal failure, Raynaud's disease, thromboangitis obliterans. **PREGNANCY/LACTATION:** Crosses placenta; distributed in breast milk. **Pregnancy Category C.**

INTERACTIONS

DRUG INTERACTIONS: Tricyclic antidepressants may decrease effect. Discontinuing concurrent beta-blockers may increase risk of clonidine-withdrawal hypertensive crisis. **ALTERED LAB VALUES:** None significant.

SIDE EFFECTS

FREQUENT: Drowsiness, dry mouth. **OCCASIONAL:** Constipation, dizziness, postural hypotension, transient weight gain, nausea, vivid dreams/nightmares, change in taste perception. **RARE:** Rash, parotid pain, palpitations, nocturia.

ADVERSE REACTIONS/TOXIC EFFECTS

Overdosage produces profound hypotension, irritability, bradycardia, respiratory depression, hypothermia, miosis (pupillary constriction), arrhythmias, apnea. Abrupt withdrawal may result in rebound hypertension associated w/nervousness, agitation, anxiety, insomnia, hand tingling, tremor, flushing, sweating.

NURSING IMPLICATIONS

BASELINE ASSESSMENT:

Obtain B/P immediately before each dose is administered, in addition to regular monitoring (be alert to B/P fluctuations).

INTERVENTION/EVALUATION:

Assist w/ambulation if dizziness occurs. Monitor pattern of daily bowel activity and stool consistency. If clonidine is to be withdrawn, discontinue concurrent beta-blocker therapy several days before discontinuing clonidine (prevents clonidine withdrawal hypertensive crisis). Slowly reduce clonidine dose over 2-4 days.

PATIENT/FAMILY TEACHING:

Sugarless gum, sips of tepid water may relieve dry mouth. If nausea occurs, unsalted crackers, noncola beverages, or dry toast may relieve effect. To reduce hypotensive effect, rise slowly from lying to sitting position and permit legs to dangle momentarily before standing. Skipping doses or voluntarily discontinuing drug may produce severe, rebound hypertension. Side effects tend to diminish during therapy.

clorazepate dipotassium

klor-az′eh-payt
(Traxene)

CANADIAN AVAILABILITY:
Novoclopate, Tranxene

CLASSIFICATION

Antianxiety, anticonvulsant

PHARMACOKINETICS

Rapidly, well absorbed from GI tract. Widely distributed. Protein binding: 97%. Metabolized in stomach and liver (first-pass metabolism) to active metabolites. Excreted in urine. Half-life: metabolite: 48-96 hrs.

ACTION

Enhances action of inhibitory neurotransmitter gamma-aminobutyric acid (GABA). Depressant effects occur at all levels of CNS. Suppresses spread of seizure activity.

USES

Management of anxiety disorders, short-term relief of anxiety symptoms, partial seizures, acute alcohol withdrawal symptoms.

PO ADMINISTRATION

1. Give w/o regard to meals.
2. Tablets may be crushed.
3. Capsules may be emptied and mixed w/food.

INDICATIONS/DOSAGE/ROUTES

NOTE: When replacement by another anticonvulsant is necessary, decrease clorazepate gradually as therapy begins w/low-replacement dose.

Anxiety:
PO: Adults: 30 mg daily in divided doses. **Elderly, debilitated:** 7.5-15 mg in divided doses or single bedtime dose. **Daily dose range:** 15-60 mg.

Partial seizures:
PO: Adults, children >12 yrs: Initially, up to 7.5 mg 3 times daily. Do not increase dosage more than 7.5 mg/wk or exceed 90 mg/day.

Alcohol withdrawal:
PO: Adults: Day 1: 30 mg followed by 30-60 mg in divided doses. **Day 2:** 45-90 mg in divided doses. **Day 3:** 22.5-45 mg in divided doses. **Day 4:** 15-30 mg in divided doses, then gradually reduce to 7.5-15 mg daily.

PRECAUTIONS

CONTRAINDICATIONS: Acute narrow-angle glaucoma, acute alcohol intoxication. **CAUTIONS:** Impaired renal/hepatic function. **PREGNANCY/LACTATION:** May cross placenta; distributed in breast milk. Chronic ingestion during pregnancy may produce withdrawal symptoms, CNS depression in neonates. **Pregnancy Category C.**

INTERACTIONS

DRUG INTERACTIONS: Alcohol, CNS depressants may increase CNS depressant effect. **ALTERED LAB VALUES:** None significant.

SIDE EFFECTS

FREQUENT: Drowsiness. **OCCASIONAL:** Dizziness, GI disturbances, nervousness, blurred vision, dry mouth, headache, confusion, ataxia, skin rash, irritability, slurred speech. **RARE:** Paradoxical CNS hyperactivity/nervousness in children, excitement/restlessness in elderly/debilitated (generally noted during first 2 wks of therapy, particularly noted in presence of uncontrolled pain).

ADVERSE REACTIONS/TOXIC EFFECTS

Abrupt or too-rapid withdrawal may result in pronounced restlessness, irritability, insomnia, hand tremors, abdominal/muscle cramps, sweating, vomiting, seizures. Overdosage results in somnolence, confusion, diminished reflexes, coma.

NURSING IMPLICATIONS

BASELINE ASSESSMENT:

Anxiety: Assess autonomic response (cold, clammy hands, sweating), and motor response (agitation, trembling, tension). Offer emotional support to anxious pt. *Seizures:* Review history of seizure disorder (intensity, frequency, duration, LOC). Observe frequently for recurrence of seizure activity. Initiate seizure precautions.

INTERVENTION/EVALUATION:

For those on long-term therapy, liver/renal function tests, blood counts should be performed periodically. Assess for paradoxical reaction, particularly during early therapy. Assist w/ambulation if drowsiness, dizziness occur. Evaluate for therapeutic response: *Anxiety:* A calm facial expression; decreased restlessness. *Seizures:* A decrease in intensity or frequency of seizures.

PATIENT/FAMILY TEACHING:

Do not abruptly withdraw medication following long-term use (may precipitate seizures). Strict maintenance of drug therapy is essential for seizure control. Drowsiness usually disappears during continued therapy. If dizziness occurs, change positions slowly from recumbent to sitting position before standing. Avoid tasks that require alertness, motor skills until response to drug is established. Smoking reduces drug effectiveness. Avoid alcohol.

clotrimazole

kloe-trim´a-zole

(Mycelex, Mycelex-G, Lotrimin, Gyne-Lotrimin)

FIXED-COMBINATION(S):

W/betamethasone dipropionate, a corticosteroid (Lotrisone)

CANADIAN AVAILABILITY:

Canesten, Clotrimaderm, Myclo

CLASSIFICATION

Antifungal

PHARMACOKINETICS

Poorly, erratically absorbed from GI tract. Bound to oral mucosa. Absorbed portion metabolized in liver. Eliminated in feces. *Topical:* Minimal systemic absorption (highest concentration in stratum corneum). *Intravaginal:* Small amount systemically absorbed.

ACTION

Binds w/phospholipids in fungal cell membrane to alter membrane permeability resulting in loss of potassium, other cellular components.

USES

Oral lozenges: Treatment/prophylaxis oropharyngeal candidiasis due to *Candida* sp. *Topical:* Treatment of tinea pedis, tinea cruris, tinea corporis, tinea versicolor, cutaneous candidiasis (moniliasis) due to *Candida albicans. In-*

travaginally: Treatment of vulvovaginal candidiasis (moniliasis) due to *Candida* sp.

Prophylaxis vs oropharyngeal candidiasis:
PO: Adults, elderly: 10 mg 3 times/day.

PO ADMINISTRATION

1. Lozenges must be dissolved in mouth >15-30 min for oropharyngeal therapy.
2. Swallow saliva.

INDICATIONS/DOSAGE/ROUTES

Oral-local/oropharyngeal:
PO: Adults, elderly: 10 mg 5 times/day for 14 days.

Topical:
TOPICAL: Adults, elderly: 2 times/day. Therapeutic effect may take up to 8 wks.

Vulvovaginal candidiasis:
VAGINAL: (Tablets) Adults, elderly: 1 tablet (100 mg) at bedtime for 7 days; 2 tablets (200 mg) at bedtime for 3 days; or 500 mg tablet one time.
VAGINAL: (Cream) Adults, elderly: 1 applicatorful at bedtime for 7-14 days.

PRECAUTIONS

CONTRAINDICATIONS: Hypersensitivity to clotrimazole or any ingredient in preparation, children <3 yrs. **CAUTIONS:** Hepatic disorder w/oral therapy. **PREGNANCY/LACTATION:** Cutaneous, vaginal: **Pregnancy Category B.** Oropharyngeal: **Pregnancy Category C.** Distribution in milk unknown.

INTERACTIONS

DRUG INTERACTIONS: None significant. **ALTERED LAB VALUES:** May increase SGOT (AST).

SIDE EFFECTS

OCCASIONAL: *Oral:* Nausea, vomiting. *Topical:* Itching, burning, stinging, erythema, urticaria *Vaginal:* Mild burning (tablets/cream); irritation, cystitis (cream). **RARE:** *Vaginal tablets:* Itching, rash, lower abdominal cramping.

ADVERSE REACTIONS/TOXIC EFFECTS

None significant.

NURSING IMPLICATIONS

BASELINE ASSESSMENT:

Question for history of hypersensitivity to clotrimazole. Assess pt's ability to understand and follow directions regarding use of oral lozenges.

INTERVENTION/EVALUATION:

W/oral therapy, assess for nausea, vomiting; monitor hepatic function tests esp. w/preexisting hepatic disorder. Check skin for erythema, urticaria, blistering; inquire about itching, burning, stinging. W/vaginal therapy, evaluate for vulvovaginal irritation, abdominal cramping, urinary frequency, discomfort.

PATIENT/FAMILY TEACHING:

Continue for full length of therapy. Inform physician of increased irritation. Avoid contact w/eyes. *Topical:* Rub well into affected, surrounding areas. Do not apply occlusive covering or other preparations w/o consulting physician. Keep areas clean, dry; wear light clothing to promote ventilation. Separate personal items, linens. *Vaginal:* Use vaginal applicator, insert high in vagina. Continue use during menses. Refrain from sexual intercourse or advise partner to use condom during therapy.

Oropharyngeal: Dissolve lozenges in mouth for 15-30 min.

cloxacillin sodium

clocks´ah-sill-in
(Cloxapen, Tegopen)

CANADIAN AVAILABILITY: ApoCloxi, Novocloxin, Orbenin, Tegopen

CLASSIFICATION

Antibiotic: Penicillin

PHARMACOKINETICS

Moderately absorbed from GI tract. Protein binding: 95-97%. Partially metabolized in liver. Primarily excreted in urine. Not removed by hemodialysis. Half-life: 0.5-1.1 hrs (increase in decreased renal function).

ACTION

Bactericidal. Binds to bacterial membranes. Inhibits cell wall synthesis.

USES

Treatment of mild to moderate infections of respiratory tract and skin/skin structure, chronic osteomyelitis, urinary tract infections; follow-up to parenteral therapy for acute, severe infections. Predominantly treatment of infections caused by penicillinase-producing staphylococci.

STORAGE/HANDLING

Store capsules at room temperature; oral solution, after reconstitution, is stable for 3 days at room temperature, 14 days if refrigerated.

PO ADMINISTRATION

1. Space doses evenly around clock.
2. Give 1 hr before or 2 hrs after meals.

INDICATIONS/DOSAGE/ROUTES

Mild to moderate upper respiratory, localized skin/skin structure infections:
PO: Adults, elderly, children >20 kg: 250 mg q6h. **Children <20 kg:** 50 mg/kg/day in divided doses q6h.

Severe infections, lower respiratory tract, disseminated infections:
PO: Adults, elderly, children >20 kg: 500 mg q6h. **Children <20 kg:** 100 mg/kg/day in divided doses q6h.

PRECAUTIONS

CONTRAINDICATIONS: Hypersensitivity to any penicillin. **CAUTIONS:** History of allergies, particularly cephalosporins. **PREGNANCY/LACTATION:** Readily crosses placenta, appears in cord blood and amniotic fluid; distributed in breast milk in low concentrations. May lead to allergic sensitization, diarrhea, candidiasis, skin rash in infant. **Pregnancy Category B.**

INTERACTIONS

DRUG INTERACTIONS: Probenecid may increase concentration, toxicity risk. **ALTERED LAB VALUES:** May increase SGOT (AST). May cause positive Coombs test.

SIDE EFFECTS

FREQUENT: Mild hypersensitivity reaction (fever, rash, pruritus), nausea, vomiting, diarrhea, flatulence.

ADVERSE REACTIONS/TOXIC EFFECTS

Superinfections, potentially fatal antibiotic-associated colitis may result from altered bacterial balance. Hematologic effects, severe hypersensitivity reactions, anaphylaxis occur rarely.

NURSING IMPLICATIONS

BASELINE ASSESSMENT:

Question for history of allergies, especially penicillins, cephalosporins. Obtain specimen for culture and sensitivity before giving first dose (therapy may begin before results are known).

INTERVENTION/EVALUATION:

Hold medication and promptly report rash (hypersensitivity) or diarrhea (w/fever, abdominal pain, mucous or blood in stool may indicate antibiotic-associated colitis). Assess food tolerance. Check hematology reports (esp. WBCs), periodic renal or hepatic reports in prolonged therapy. Be alert for superinfection: increased fever, onset sore throat, diarrhea, ulceration or changes of oral mucosa, vaginal discharge, anal/genital pruritus.

PATIENT/FAMILY TEACHING:

Space doses evenly. Continue antibiotic for full length of treatment. Notify physician in event of diarrhea, rash, other new symptom.

clozapine

klow'zah-peen
(Clozaril)

CANADIAN AVAILABILITY:
Clozaril

CLASSIFICATION

Antipsychotic

PHARMACOKINETICS

Rapid, almost completely absorbed from GI tract. Widely distributed. Protein binding: 95%. Extensively metabolized by first-pass liver metabolism. Primarily excreted in urine. Half-life: 8-12 hrs.

ACTION

Interferes w/binding of dopamine at dopaminergic receptors. Binds primarily to nondopaminergic sites (e.g., alpha-adrenergic, serotonergic, cholinergic).

USES

Management of severely ill schizophrenic pts who fail to respond to other antipsychotic therapy.

PO ADMINISTRATION

May give w/o regard to meals.

INDICATIONS/DOSAGE/ROUTES

Schizophrenic disorders:
PO: Adults: Initially, 25 mg 1-2 times/day. May increase by 25-50 mg/day over 2 wks until dose of 300-450 mg/day achieved. May further increase dose by 50-100 mg/day no more frequently than 1-2 times/wk. **Range:** 200-600 mg/day. **Maximum:** 900 mg/day.

Usual elderly dosage:
PO: Elderly: Initially, 25 mg/day. May increase by 25 mg/day. **Maximum:** 450 mg/day.

PRECAUTIONS

CONTRAINDICATIONS: Myeloproliferative disorders, history of clozapine-induced agranulocytosis or severe granulocytopenia, concurrent administration w/other drugs having potential to suppress bone marrow function, severe CNS depression, comatose state. **CAUTIONS:** History of seizures, cardiovascular disease, impaired respiratory, hepatic, renal function, alcohol withdrawal, urinary retention, glaucoma, prostatic hypertrophy. **PREGNANCY/LACTATION:** Crosses placenta; distributed in breast milk. **Pregnancy Category C.**

INTERACTIONS

DRUG INTERACTIONS: Alcohol, CNS depressants may increase CNS depressant effects. Bone marrow depressants may increase myelosuppression. Lithium may increase risk of seizures, confusion, dyskinesias. **ALTERED LAB VALUES:** None significant.

SIDE EFFECTS

FREQUENT: Drowsiness, salivation, constipation, dizziness, tachycardia. **OCCASIONAL:** Nausea, sweating, dry mouth, headache, hypotension, GI upset, weight gain. **RARE:** Visual disturbances, diarrhea, rash, urinary abnormalities.

ADVERSE REACTIONS/TOXIC EFFECTS

Most common symptoms include altered state of consciousness, CNS depression (drowsiness, coma, delirium), cardiac arrhythmias, hypotension, respiratory depression, increased salivation, seizures. Blood dyscrasias, particularly agranulocytosis, mild leukopenia may occur.

NURSING IMPLICATIONS

BASELINE ASSESSMENT:

Obtain baseline WBC and differential count before initiating treatment and WBC count every week during treatment and every week for 4 wks after treatment is discontinued. Assess behavior, appearance, emotional status, response to environment, speech pattern, thought content.

INTERVENTION/EVALUATION:

Monitor B/P for hypotension. Assess for extrapyramidal symptoms. Monitor WBC, differential count for blood dyscrasias. Monitor for fine tongue movement (may be early sign of tardive dyskinesia). Supervise suicidal-risk pt closely during early therapy (as depression lessens, energy level improves, increasing suicide potential). Assess for therapeutic response (interest in surroundings, improvement in self-care, increased ability to concentrate, relaxed facial expression).

PATIENT/FAMILY TEACHING:

Do not abruptly withdraw from long-term drug therapy. Report visual disturbances. Sugarless gum or sips of tepid water may relieve dry mouth. Drowsiness generally subsides during continued therapy. Avoid tasks that require alertness, motor skills until response to drug is established. Avoid alcohol.

cocaine

koe-kane´
(Cocaine HCl, Cocaine HCl Solvets)

CLASSIFICATION

Topical anesthetic

PHARMACOKINETICS

	ONSET	PEAK	DURATION
Topical	1 min	2-5 min	0.5-2 hrs

Readily absorbed from all mucous membranes. Hydrolyzed by plasma and liver cholinesterases to active metabolite. Primarily excreted in urine. Half-life: 1-1.5 hrs.

ACTION

Blocks initiation, conduction of nerve impulses by decreasing membrane permeability to sodium. Increases norepinephrine at postsynaptic receptor sites producing vasoconstriction.

USES

Topical anesthesia for mucous membranes of oral laryngeal, nasal areas.

TOPICAL ADMINISTRATION

1. Avoid inhalation of any sprays. Do not puncture spray container or use near open flame.
2. Do not get preparations near eyes.
3. When used for anesthesia of throat, NPO until sensation returns (failure to protect from aspiration, difficulty w/swallowing).

INDICATIONS/DOSAGE/ROUTES

Usual topical dosage:
TOPICAL: Adults, elderly: 1-10% solution. Maximum single dose: 1 mg/kg.

PRECAUTIONS

CONTRAINDICATIONS: Hypersensitivity to cocaine or local anesthetics. Systemic or ophthalmic use. **CAUTIONS:** History of drug sensitivities or drug abuse (can cause strong psychologic dependence and some tolerance); has been abused for cortical stimulant effect. Severe trauma or sepsis in area to be anesthetized. Limit to office and surgical procedures; prolonged use can cause ischemic damage to nasal mucosa. Safety in children not established. **PREGNANCY/LACTATION:** Safety during lactation not established. **Pregnancy Category C.**

INTERACTIONS

DRUG INTERACTIONS: Tricyclic antidepressants, digoxin, methyldopa may increase arrhythmias. May decrease effects of beta-blockers. Cholinesterase inhibitors may increase effects, risk of toxicity. CNS stimulation-producing agents may increase effects. Sympathomimetics increase CNS stimulation, risk of cardiovascular effects. **ALTERED LAB VALUES:** None significant.

SIDE EFFECTS

OCCASIONAL: W/systemic reaction to local application, effects are dose dependent. Small doses of cocaine may cause bradycardia. W/moderate doses: euphoria, reduced fatigue, sexual stimulation, increased mental acuity, increased sociality, hypertension, tachycardia, tachypnea. **RARE:** Hypersensitivity. Continued CNS stimulation may progress to tonic-clonic convulsions, vomiting and proceed to CNS depression.

ADVERSE REACTIONS/TOXIC EFFECTS

W/CNS depression, respiratory failure and death may occur.

NURSING IMPLICATIONS

BASELINE ASSESSMENT:

Question for hypersensitivity to cocaine. Obtain baseline vital signs.

INTERVENTION/EVALUATION:

Monitor for anesthetic response. Be alert to CNS stimulation: assess for euphoria, restlessness, increased B/P, pulse, respirations. Be prepared to provide ventilatory support and emergency medications in event of progression of CNS response—death from overdose will occur within minutes, up to 3 hours after initial reaction.

PATIENT/FAMILY TEACHING:

NPO until sensation returns when used for throat anesthesia. Onetime or infrequent use for procedures will not cause dependence. Report feelings of euphoria, restlessness, or rapid heartbeat if these develop during procedure.

codeine phosphate

koe´deen

codeine sulfate

FIXED-COMBINATION(S): W/aspirin, butalbital, a barbiturate, and caffeine (Fiorinal); w/acetaminophen (Phenaphen, Tylenol w/codeine); w/aspirin (Empirin w/codeine)

CANADIAN AVAILABILITY: Paveral, Penntuss

CLASSIFICATION

Opioid analgesic: **Schedule II;** fixed-combination form: **Schedule III**

PHARMACOKINETICS

	ONSET	PEAK	DURATION
PO	15-30 min	1-1.5 hrs	4-6 hrs
IM	15-30 min	30-60 min	4-6 hrs
SubQ	15-30 min	—	4-6 hrs

Moderately absorbed from GI tract; completely after IM administration. Widely distributed. Protein binding: low. Metabolized in liver. Excreted in urine. Half-life: 2.5-4 hrs.

ACTION

Binds at opiate receptor sites in CNS, reducing intensity of pain stimuli incoming from sensory nerve endings. Suppresses cough reflex by direct CNS action. Decreases intestinal motility.

USES

Relief of mild to moderate pain and/or nonproductive cough.

STORAGE/HANDLING

Store oral, parenteral form at room temperature.

PO/SubQ/IM ADMINISTRATTION

PO:

1. Give w/o regard to meals.
2. Shake oral suspension well.

SubQ/IM:

1. Parenteral form incompatible w/aminophylline, ammonium chloride, amobarbital, chlorothiazide, heparin, methicillin, nitrofurantoin, pentobarbital, phenobarbital, sodium bicarbonate, sodium iodide, thiopental.
2. Pt should be recumbent before drug is administered.
3. Assess for wheals at injection site (sign of local tissue irritation, induration).
4. Those w/circulatory impairment may experience overdosage due to delayed absorption of repeated administration.

INDICATIONS/DOSAGE/ROUTES

NOTE: Reduce initial dosage in those w/hypothyroidism, concurrent CNS depressants, Addison's disease, renal insufficiency, elderly/debilitated.

Analgesia:
PO/SubQ/IM: Adults, elderly: 30 mg q4-6h. **Range:** 15-60 mg daily. **Children:** 0.5 mg/kg q4-6h.

Antitussive:
PO: Adults, elderly, children >12 yrs: 10-20 mg q4-6h. **Children 6-11 yrs:** 5-10 mg q4-6h. **Children 2-5 yrs:** 2.5-5 mg q4-6h.

PRECAUTIONS

CONTRAINDICATIONS: None significant. **EXTREME CAUTION:** CNS depression, anoxia, hypercapnia, respiratory depression, seizures, acute alcoholism, shock, untreated myxedema, respiratory dysfunction. **CAUTIONS:** Increased intracranial pressure, impaired hepatic function, acute abdominal conditions, hypothyroidism, prostatic hypertrophy, Addison's disease, urethral stricture, COPD. **PREGNANCY/LACTATION:** Readily crosses placenta; distributed in breast milk. May prolong labor if administered in latent phase of first stage of labor, or before cervical dilation of 4-5 cm has occurred. Respiratory depression may occur in neonate if mother received opiates during labor. Regular use of opiates during pregnancy may produce withdrawal symptoms in the neonate (irritability, excessive crying, tremors, hyperactive reflexes, fever, vomiting, diarrhea, yawning, sneezing, seizures). **Pregnancy Category C.**

INTERACTIONS

DRUG INTERACTIONS: Alcohol, CNS depressants may increase CNS, respiratory depression, hypotension. MAO inhibitors may produce severe, fatal reaction (reduce dose to 1/4 usual dose). **ALTERED LAB VALUES:** None significant.

SIDE EFFECTS

NOTE: Effects dependent on dose amount, route of administration but occur infrequently w/oral antitussives. Ambulatory pts, those not in severe pain may experience dizziness, nausea, vomiting, hypotension more frequently than those in supine position or with severe pain. **FREQUENT:** Suppressed breathing depth. **OCCASIONAL:** Lightheadedness, mental clouding, dizziness, sedation, hypotension, nausea, vomiting, euphoria/dysphoria, constipation (drug delays digestion), sweating, flushing, feeling of facial and neck warmth, urinary retention.

ADVERSE REACTIONS/TOXIC EFFECTS

Too-frequent use may result in ileus. Overdosage results in respiratory depression, skeletal muscle flaccidity, cold, clammy skin, cyanosis, extreme somnolence progressing to convulsions, stupor, coma. Tolerance to analgesic effect, physical dependence may occur w/repeated use.

NURSING IMPLICATIONS

BASELINE ASSESSMENT:

Obtain vital signs before giving medication. If respirations are 12/min or lower (20/min or lower in children), withhold medication, contact physician. *Analgesic:* Assess onset, type, location, and duration of pain. Effect of medication is reduced if full pain recurs before next dose. *Antitussive:* Assess type, severity, frequency of cough, and production. Increase fluid intake and environmental humidity to lower viscosity of lung secretions.

INTERVENTION/EVALUATION:

Monitor vital signs q15-30min after parenteral administration (monitor for decreased B/P, change in rate or quality of pulse). Increase fluid intake and environmental humidity to improve viscosity of lung secretions. Palpate bladder for urinary retention. Monitor pattern of daily bowel activity and stool consistency. Initiate deep breathing and coughing exercises, particularly in those w/impaired pulmonary function. Assess for clinical improvement; record onset of relief of pain or cough.

PATIENT/FAMILY TEACHING:

Discomfort may occur w/injection. Change positions slowly to avoid orthostatic hypotension. Avoid tasks that require alertness, motor skills until response to drug is established. Tolerance/dependence may occur w/prolonged use of high doses. Avoid alcohol.

colchicine

coal´cheh-seen

(Colchicine)

CANADIAN AVAILABILITY:
Colchicine

CLASSIFICATION

Antigout

PHARMACOKINETICS

Rapidly absorbed from GI tract. Highest concentration in liver, spleen, kidney. Reenters intestinal tract (biliary secretion), reabsorbed from intestines. Partially metabolized in liver. Eliminated primarily in feces.

ACTION

Decreases urate crystal deposits, inflammatory process by decreasing leukocyte motility, phagocytosis, lactic acid production.

USES

Treatment of attacks of acute gouty arthritis, prophylaxis of recurrent gouty arthritis.

PO/IV ADMINISTRATION

PO:

1. May give w/o regard to meals.

IV:

NOTE: SubQ or IM administration produces severe local reaction. Use via IV route only.

1. Administer over 2-5 min.
2. May dilute w/0.9% NaCl or sterile water for injection.
3. Do not dilute w/5% dextrose.

INDICATIONS/DOSAGE/ROUTES

Acute gouty arthritis:
PO: Adults, elderly: 0.5-1.2 mg, then 0.5-0.6 mg q1-2h or 1-1.2 mg q2h until pain relieved or nausea, vomiting, or diarrhea occur. Total dose: 4-8 mg.
IV: Adults, elderly: Initially, 2 mg, then 0.5 mg q6h until satisfactory response. **Maximum:** 4 mg/24 hrs or 4 mg/one course of treatment.
Note: If pain recurs, may give 1-2 mg/day for several days but no sooner than 7 days after a full course of IV therapy (4 mg).

Chronic gouty arthritis:
PO: Adults, elderly: 0.5-0.6 mg once weekly up to once daily (de-

pendent on number of attacks per year).

PRECAUTIONS

CONTRAINDICATIONS: Severe gastrointestinal, renal, hepatic, or cardiac disorders; blood dyscrasias. **CAUTIONS:** Impaired hepatic function, elderly, debilitated. **PREGNANCY/LACTATION:** Unknown if drug crosses placenta or is distributed in breast milk. *Oral route:* **Pregnancy Category C.** *IV route:* **Pregnancy Category D.**

INTERACTIONS

DRUG INTERACTIONS: NSAIDs may increase risk of neutropenia, thrombocytopenia, bone marrow depression. Bone marrow depressants may increase risk of blood dyscrasias. **ALTERED LAB VALUES:** May decrease platelet count. May increase SGOT (AST), alkaline phosphatase.

SIDE EFFECTS

NOTE: Those w/impaired renal function may exhibit myopathy and neuropathy manifested as generalized weakness. **OCCASIONAL:** *Maximum dosage: or IV therapy:* Nausea, vomiting, diarrhea, abdominal pain. **RARE:** Thrombophlebitis at IV injection site.

ADVERSE REACTIONS/TOXIC EFFECTS

Toxic dosage produces severe diarrhea, generalized vascular damage, renal damage w/hematuria and oliguria. Bone marrow depression (aplastic anemia, agranulocytosis, thrombocytopenia) may occur w/long-term therapy.

NURSING IMPLICATIONS

BASELINE ASSESSMENT:

Instruct patient to drink 8-10 glasses (8 oz) of fluid daily while on medication. Medication should be discontinued if any GI symptoms occur. Periodic CBC should be performed routinely in those receiving long-term therapy.

INTERVENTION/EVALUATION:

Discontinue medication immediately if GI symptoms occur. Encourage high fluid intake (3,000 ml/day). Monitor I&O (output should be at least 2,000 ml/day). Assess CBC, serum uric acid levels. Assess for therapeutic response (reduced joint tenderness, swelling, redness, limitation of motion).

PATIENT/FAMILY TEACHING:

Encourage low-purine food intake, to drink 8-10 glasses (8 oz) of fluid daily while on medication. Contact physician, nurse if gastrointestinal disturbances, generalized weakness, or unusual bruising occurs.

colestipol hydrochloride

ko-less′tih-pole

(Cholestid)

CANADIAN AVAILABILITY: Cholestid

CLASSIFICATION

Antihyperlipoproteinemic

PHARMACOKINETICS

Not absorbed from GI tract. Decreases in LDL apparent in 5-7 days, serum cholesterol in 1 mo. Serum cholesterol returns to baseline levels about 1 mo after discontinuing drug.

ACTION

Binds w/bile acids in intestine forming insoluble complex. Binding increases bile acid synthesis from cholesterol, increases hepatic LDL receptor activity, increases LDL, cholesterol removal from plasma.

USES

Adjunct to dietary therapy to decrease elevated serum cholesterol in those w/primary hypercholesterolemia.

PO ADMINISTRATION

1. Give other drugs at least 1 hr before or 4 hrs after colestipol (capable of binding drugs in GI tract).
2. Do not give in dry form (highly irritating). Mix w/3-6 oz water, milk, fruit juice, soup. Place powder on surface for 1-2 min (prevents lumping), then mix thoroughly. W/carbonated beverages, there is excessive foaming; use extra large glass and stir slowly.
3. Administer before meals.
4. Swallow tablets whole; do not cut, chew, crush. Give w/water.

INDICATIONS/DOSAGE/ROUTE

Primary hypercholesterolemia:
PO: Adults, elderly: *(Granules):* 5-30 Gm/day; *(Tablets):* 2-16 Gm/day. Give as single or divided doses.

PRECAUTIONS

CONTRAINDICATIONS: Hypersensitivity to colestipol or any of its components, complete biliary obstruction. **CAUTIONS:** GI dysfunction (especially constipation), hemorrhoids, bleeding disorders. **PREGNANCY/LACTATION:** Not systemically absorbed, but may interfere w/maternal absorption of fat-soluble vitamins. **Pregnancy Category C.**

INTERACTIONS

DRUG INTERACTIONS: May increase effects of anticoagulants by decreasing vitamin K. May decrease warfarin absorption. May bind, decrease absorption of digoxin, thiazides, penicillins, propranolol, tetracyclines, thyroid hormones, other medications. Binds, decreases effect of oral vancomycin. **ALTERED LAB VALUES:** May increase SGOT (AST), SGPT (ALT), alkaline phosphatase. May decrease calcium, potassium, sodium. May prolong prothrombin time.

SIDE EFFECTS

FREQUENT: Constipation, nausea, vomiting, abdominal discomfort, flatulence, diarrhea. **OCCASIONAL:** Urticaria, dermatitis, fatigue, shortness of breath, muscle and joint pain. **RARE:** Headache, dizziness, anxiety, drowsiness.

ADVERSE REACTIONS/TOXIC EFFECTS

GI tract obstruction.

NURSING IMPLICATIONS

BASELINE ASSESSMENT:

Question for history of hypersensitivity to colestipol or components. Obtain specimens for serum cholesterol and triglyceride baselines.

INTERVENTION/EVALUATION:

Determine pattern of bowel activity. Evaluate food tolerance, abdominal discomfort, and flatulence. Monitor lab results for serum cholesterol and periodically for serum triglyceride. Assess skin and mucous membranes for rash/irritation. Check for headache and dizziness, muscle/joint pain. Encourage several glasses of water between meals.

PATIENT/FAMILY TEACHING:

Complete full course; do not omit or change doses. Take other drugs at least 1 hr before or 4 hrs after colestipol. Check w/physician before taking any other medication. Never take in dry form; mix w/3-6 oz water, milk, fruit juice, soup (place powder on surface for 1-2 min to prevent lumping, then mix well). Use extra large glass and stir slowly when mixing w/carbonated beverages due to foaming. Take before meals and drink several glasses of water between meals. Reduce fats, sugars, and cholesterol per diet determined by physician. Eat high-fiber foods (whole grain cereals, fruits, vegetables) to reduce potential for constipation. Notify physician immediately of bleeding, constipation, or development of new symptom.

colfosceril palmitate

kol-foss´er-ill

(Exosurf)

CLASSIFICATION

Lung surfactant

ACTION

Lowers surface tension on alveolar surfaces during respiration, stabilizes alveoli vs. collapse that may occur at resting transpulmonary pressures. Replenishes surfactant, restores surface activity to lungs.

USES

Prophylactic use in infants <1,350 Gm at risk of developing RDS, infants >1,350 Gm w/evidence of pulmonary immaturity; treatment in infants w/RDS.

STORAGE/HANDLING

Store vials at room temperature. After reconstitution, stable for 12 hrs.

INTRATRACHEAL ADMINISTRATION

1. Reconstitute immediately prior to use w/8 ml preservative-free sterile water for injection. Refer to manufacturer's instructions.
2. Do not use if vacuum in vial not present.
3. Instill through catheter inserted into infant's endotracheal tube. Do not instill into main stem bronchus.
4. Stop administration if reflux into endotracheal tube occurs. If needed, increase peak inspiratory pressure on ventilator by 4-5 cm H_2O until tube clears.
5. Stop administration if transcutaneous oxygen saturation decreases. If needed, increase peak inspiratory pressure on ventilator by 4-5 cm H_2O for 1-2 min. May also need to increase FiO_2 for 1-2 min.

INDICATIONS/DOSAGE/ROUTES

Prophylaxis for RDS:
INTRATRACHEAL: Neonates: 5 ml/kg given as two 2.5 ml/kg ½ doses as soon as possible after birth. May repeat at 12 and 24 hrs later in infants remaining on mechanical ventilator.

RDS rescue:
INTRATRACHEAL: Neonates: 5 ml/kg given as two 2.5 ml/kg ½ doses. Repeat in 12 hrs in all infants remaining on ventilator.

PRECAUTIONS

CONTRAINDICATIONS: None significant. **CAUTIONS:** Those at risk for circulatory overload.

INTERACTIONS

DRUG INTERACTIONS: None significant. **ALTERED LAB VALUES:** None significant.

SIDE EFFECTS

None significant.

ADVERSE REACTIONS/TOXIC EFFECTS

Failure to reduce peak ventilator inspiratory pressures after chest expansion after dosing may result in lung overdistention and fatal pulmonary air leak. Failure to reduce transcutaneous oxygen saturation if in excess of 95% by decreasing FiO_2 in small but repeated steps until saturation is 90% to 95% may result in hyperoxia. Failure to reduce ventilator if arterial or transcutaneous CO_2 measurements are <30, may result in hypocarbia, reducing brain blood flow.

NURSING IMPLICATIONS

BASELINE ASSESSMENT:

Drug must be administered in highly supervised setting. Clinicians in care of neonate must be experienced w/intubation, ventilator management. Give emotional support to parents. Suctioning infant before dosing may decrease chance of mucous plugs obstructing endotracheal tube.

INTERVENTION/EVALUATION:

Monitor infant w/arterial or transcutaneous measurement of systemic O_2 and CO_2. Maintain vigilant clinical attention to neonate prior to, during, and after drug administration. Assess lung sounds for rales and moist breath sounds. If chest expansion improves dramatically after dosing, reduce peak ventilator inspiratory pressures immediately (failure to do so may result in lung overdistention and fatal pulmonary air leak). If transcutaneous oxygen saturation >95% and neonate appears pink, reduce FiO_2 in small but repeated steps until saturation is 90% to 95% (failure to do so may result in hyperoxia). If arterial or transcutaneous CO_2 measurements are <30, reduce ventilator immediately (failure to do so may result in hypocarbia, reducing brain blood flow).

colistin sulfate

koh-listin

(Coly Mycin-S)

colistimethate sodium

(Coly Mycin-M)

CANADIAN AVAILABILITY: Coly-Mycin

CLASSIFICATION

Antibiotic

PHARMACOKINETICS

Poor absorption when given orally. After parenteral injection, widely distributed in tissue. Excreted in urine. Serum concentration increased, half-life prolonged in those w/renal impairment. Minimally removed by hemodialysis.

ACTION

Bactericidal in susceptible microorganisms due to alteration of cell membrane permeability w/ loss of essential elements.

USES

Colistimethate sodium (parenteral): Serious, acute, chronic infections due to susceptible gram-negative bacilli, especially *Pseudomonas aeruginosa.* **Colistin sulfate (oral):** Diarrhea in infants, children due to enteropathogenic *Escherichia coli, Shigella* gastroenteritis; superficial bacterial infections of external auditory canal, infections of mastoidectomy and fenestration cavities.

STORAGE/HANDLING

Oral suspension stable for 2 wks if refrigerated. Parenteral solution, once reconstituted, is stable for 24 hrs.

IM/IV ADMINISTRATION

NOTE: Give by IM injection, IV injection, intermittent IV infusion (piggyback).

IM:

1. Reconstitute each 150 mg vial w/2 ml sterile water for injection to provide concentration of 75 mg/ml.
2. Swirl vial gently to avoid frothing.

IV:

1. For IV injection, administer over 3-5 min (give q12h).
2. For intermittent IV infusion (piggyback), give one half of dose by IV injection, then further dilute second half of dose w/5% dextrose, or 0.9% NaCl (volume of diluent is dependent on patient requirements). Infuse at rate of 5-6 mg/hr. Give infusion 1-2 hrs after IV injection.

INDICATIONS/DOSAGE/ROUTES

NOTE: Space doses evenly around the clock.

Mild to severe infections:
IM/IV: Adults, children: 2.5-5 mg/kg/day in 2-4 divided doses.

Diarrhea, gastroenteritis:
PO: Adults, children: 5-15 mg/kg/day in 3 divided doses.

Dosage in renal impairment:
Dose and/or frequency may be modified based on serum creatinine and/or severity of infection.

SERUM CREATININE	DOSAGE
1.3-1.5 mg/dl	75-115 mg/day in two divided doses
1.6-2.5 mg/dl	66-150 mg/day in one or two divided doses
2.6-4 mg/dl	100-150 mg q36h

Usual otic dosage:
TOPICAL: Adults: 4 drops 3-4 times/day.

PRECAUTIONS

CONTRAINDICATIONS: Hypersensitivity to colistin, colistimethate, or polymyxin B. **CAUTIONS:** Renal impairment, concurrent use of anesthetics, or drugs w/neuromuscular blocking action. **PREGNANCY/LACTATION:** Crosses placenta; distributed in breast milk. **Pregnancy Category C.**

INTERACTIONS

DRUG INTERACTIONS: None significant. **ALTERED LAB VALUES:** May increase BUN, serum creatinine concentrations.

SIDE EFFECTS

No side effects reported w/oral administration. *Parenteral:* **OC-**

CASIONAL: Dizziness, blurred vision, slurred speech, tingling of extremities, circumoral numbness, paresthesia, muscular weakness, urticaria, decreased urine output, increased BUN, serum creatinine concentrations.

ADVERSE REACTIONS/TOXIC EFFECTS

Nephrotoxicity (usually reversible w/discontinuance of colistimethate) and neurotoxicity may occur especially w/high dosage and/or renal impairment. Prolonged therapy may result in superinfection. Apnea, anaphylaxis occur rarely.

NURSING IMPLICATIONS

BASELINE ASSESSMENT:

Question pt for history of allergies, especially to colistin, colistimethate, polymyxin B. Avoid, if possible, concurrent use of other medications that are neurotoxic or nephrotoxic. Obtain culture and sensitivity tests before giving first dose (therapy may begin before results are known).

INTERVENTION/EVALUATION:

Be alert to inability of infants, children to describe subjective symptoms. Monitor I&O, renal function tests for nephrotoxicity. Assess mental status. Take vital signs; assess for respiratory depression, vision, speech, steadiness with ambulation.

PATIENT/FAMILY TEACHING:

Continue therapy for full length of treatment. Do not drive or work w/hazardous machinery. Space doses evenly. Notify physician in event of dizziness, respiratory difficulty, decreased urine output, or other new symptom.

conjugated estrogens

ess´troe-jenz
(Premarin)

FIXED-COMBINATION(S):
W/meprobamate, a tranquilizer (Milprem), Premarin w/Methyltestosterone, an androgen, w/medroxyprogesterone, a progestin (Premphase, Prempro)

CANADIAN AVAILABILITY:
C.E.S., Congest, Premarin

CLASSIFICATION

Estrogen

PHARMACOKINETICS

Well absorbed from GI tract. Widely distributed. Protein binding: 50-80%. Metabolized in liver. Primarily excreted in urine.

ACTION

Increases synthesis of DNA, RNA, and various proteins in responsive tissues. Reduces release of gonadotropin-releasing hormone reducing follicle stimulating hormone (FSH) and leuteinizing hormone (LH). Promotes normal growth, development of female sex organs, maintaining genitourinary function, vasomotor stability. Prevents accelerated bone loss by inhibiting bone resorption, restoring balance of bone resorption and formation. Inhibits LH, decreases serum concentration of testosterone.

USES

Management of moderate to severe vasomotor symptoms associated w/menopause. Treatment of atrophic vaginitis, kraurosis vulvae, female hypogonadism and castration, primary ovarian failure.

Prevention of postpartum breast engorgement. Retardation of osteoporosis in postmenopausal women. Palliative treatment of inoperable, progressive cancer of the prostate in men and of the breast in postmenopausal women.

STORAGE/HANDLING

Keep tablets at room temperature. Refrigerate vials for IV use. Reconstituted solution stable for 60 days refrigerated. Do not use if solution darkens or precipitate forms.

PO/IV ADMINISTRATION

PO:

1. Administer at the same time each day.
2. Give w/milk or food if nausea occurs.

IV:

1. Reconstitute w/5 ml sterile water for injection containing benzyl alcohol (diluent provided).
2. Slowly add diluent, shaking gently. Avoid vigorous shaking.
3. Give slowly to prevent flushing reaction.

INDICATIONS/DOSAGE/ROUTES

Vasomotor symptoms associated w/menopause, atrophic vaginitis, kraurosis vulvae:
PO: Adults, elderly: 0.3-1.25 mg/day cyclically (21 days on; 7 days off). If pt is menstruating, begin on fifth day of cycle; if pt not menstruating within previous 2 mo, start arbitrarily.
INTRAVAGINALLY: Adults, elderly: 2-4 Gm/day cyclically.

Female hypogonadism:
PO: Adults: 2.5-7.5 mg/day in divided doses for 20 days; rest 10 days. If bleeding occurs prior to 10th drug-free day, a 20-day estrogen-progestin regimen given for 20 days w/progestin given during last 5 days of estrogen therapy. If menstruation begins prior to completing the estrogen-progestin regimen, discontinue therapy, reinstitute on 5th day of menstruation.

Female castration, primary ovarian failure:
PO: Adults: Initially, 1.25 mg/day cyclically.

Osteoporosis:
PO: Adults, elderly: 0.625 mg/day, cyclically.

Postpartum breast engorgement:
PO: Adults: 3.75 mg q4h × 5 doses (or 1.25 mg q4h × 5 days).

Breast cancer:
PO: Adults, elderly: 10 mg 3 times/day for at least 3 mo.

Prostate cancer:
PO: Adults, elderly: 1.25-2.5 mg 3 times/day.

Abnormal uterine bleeding:
IM/IV: Adults: 25 mg, may repeat once in 6-12 hrs.

PRECAUTIONS

CONTRAINDICATIONS: Known or suspected breast cancer (except select pts w/metastasis), estrogen-dependent neoplasia; undiagnosed abnormal genital bleeding; active thrombophlebitis or thromboembolic disorders; history of thrombophlebitis, thrombosis, or thromboembolic disorders w/previous estrogen use, hypersensitivity to estrogen. **CAUTIONS:** Conditions that may be aggravated by fluid retention: cardiac, renal or hepatic dysfunction, epilepsy, migraine, mental depression, metabolic bone disease w/potential hypercalcemia, history of jaundice during pregnancy, strong family history of breast cancer, fibrocystic disease or breast nodules, children in whom bone growth is not complete. **PREGNANCY/LACTATION:** Distributed in breast milk. May be harmful to fetus. Not for use during lactation. **Pregnancy Category X.**

INTERACTIONS

DRUG INTERACTIONS: May interfere w/effects of bromocriptine. May increase concentration of cyclosporine, increase hepatic, nephrotoxicity. Hepatotoxic medications may increase hepatotoxicity. **ALTERED LAB VALUES:** May affect metapyrone, thyroid function tests. May decrease cholesterol, LDH. May increase calcium, glucose, HDL, triglycerides.

SIDE EFFECTS

FREQUENT: Change in vaginal bleeding (spotting, breakthrough, heavy or prolonged bleeding). **OCCASIONAL:** Headache, increased B/P. *High dose therapy:* Anorexia, nausea. **RARE:** Chorea, cholestatic jaundice, hirsutism, loss of scalp hair, depression.

ADVERSE REACTIONS/TOXIC EFFECTS

Prolonged administration may increase risk of gall bladder, thromboembolic disease, and breast, cervical, vaginal, endometrial, and liver carcinoma.

NURSING IMPLICATIONS

BASELINE ASSESSMENT:

Question hypersensitivity to estrogen, previous jaundice, or thromboembolic disorders associated w/pregnancy or estrogen therapy. Establish baseline B/P, blood glucose.

INTERVENTION/EVALUATION:

Assess blood pressure periodically. Check for swelling, weigh daily. Monitor blood glucose q.i.d. for pts w/diabetes. Promptly report signs and symptoms of thromboembolic or thrombotic disorders: sudden severe headache, shortness of breath, vision or speech disturbance, weakness or numbness of an extremity, loss of coordination, pain in chest, groin, or leg. Note estrogen therapy on specimens.

PATIENT/FAMILY TEACHING:

Need for medical supervision. Avoid smoking due to increased risk of heart attack or blood clots. Explain importance of diet and exercise when taken to retard osteoporosis. Do not take other medications w/o physician approval. Teach how to perform Homan's test, signs and symptoms of blood clots (report these to physician immediately). Also notify physician of abnormal vaginal bleeding, depression, other symptoms. Teach female pts to perform self-breast exam. Avoid exposure to sun or ultraviolet light. Check weight daily; report weekly gain of ≥5 lbs. Stop taking medication and contact physician if suspect pregnancy. Give labeling from drug package.

corticotropin injection

kore-tih-koe-troe´pin

(ACTH, Acthar)

corticotropin repository

(Cortigel, Cortrophin-Gel, Acthar Gel)

corticotropin zinc hydroxide

(Cortrophin Zinc)

CANADIAN AVAILABILITY:
Acthar

CLASSIFICATION

Adrenocorticotropic hormone

PHARMACOKINETICS

Rapid absorption from IM/SubQ sites (respiratory forms have delayed absorption). Widely distributed.

ACTION

Increases endogenous corticoid synthesis. Stimulates initial reaction in synthesis of adrenal steroids from cholesterol. Other effects due to generated endogenous corticosteroids.

USES

Diagnostic testing of adrenocortical function. Limited therapeutic value in conditions responsive to corticosteroid therapy. May be used in hypercalcemia of cancer, acute exacerbations of multiple sclerosis, nonsuppurative thyroiditis.

STORAGE/HANDLING

Refrigerate repository dosage forms. After reconstitution, corticotropin injection is stable for 24 hrs if refrigerated.

IM/IV/SubQ ADMINISTRATION

Assess for hypersensitivity reaction during first 15 minutes of IV administration or immediately following IM or SubQ injection.

IM/SubQ:

1. Do *not* give corticotropin zinc hydroxide SubQ or IV; give deep IM in gluteal muscle.
2. Repository corticotropin may be given SubQ or IM for prolonged effects.
3. Reconstitute in 0.9% sodium chloride solution or sterile water for injection to produce final volume of 1-2 ml.

IV:

1. Give IV only for diagnostic use or in adults w/idiopathic thrombocytopenic purpura.
2. For IV infusion, further dilute in 0.9% sodium chloride, 5% dextrose, or 5% dextrose in 0.9% sodium chloride solutions.

INDICATIONS/DOSAGE/ROUTES

NOTE: May give IM, SubQ. IV only for corticotropin injection; IM only for corticotropin zinc hydroxide.

Diagnostic testing:
IV: Adults: 10-25 U in 500 ml D_5W infused over 8 hrs.
IM/SubQ: Adults: 20 U 4 times/day.

Acute exacerbation of multiple sclerosis:
IM: Adults: 80-120 U/day for 2-3 wks.

Infantile spasms:
IM: Infants: 20-40 U/day or 80 U every other day for 3 mo (or 1 mo after cessation of seizures).

Usual repository injection dosage:
IM/SubQ: Adults: 40-80 U q24-72h.

PRECAUTIONS

CONTRAINDICATIONS: Hypersensitivity to any corticosteroid or porcine proteins, systemic fungal infection, peptic ulcers (except life-threatening situations), scleroderma, primary adrenocortical insufficiency. Avoid live virus vaccine; long-term therapy in children. **CAUTIONS:** Thromboembolic disorders, history of tuberculosis (may reactivate disease), hypothyroidism, cirrhosis, nonspecific ulcerative colitis, CHF, hypertension, psychosis, renal insufficiency, seizures. Prolonged therapy should be discontinued slowly. **PREGNANCY/LACTATION:** Unknown if distributed in breast milk. May have embryocidal effects. Nursing contraindicated. **Pregnancy Category C.**

INTERACTIONS

DRUG INTERACTIONS: Aspirin may increase ulcerogenic effect. May decrease effect of insulin/oral hypoglycemics. May increase effect of diuretics (electrolyte loss). **ALTERED LAB VALUES:** None significant.

SIDE EFFECTS

FREQUENT: Increased appetite, exaggerated sense of well-being, abdominal distension, weight gain, insomnia, mood swings. *High dose, prolonged therapy:* **FREQUENT:** Increased susceptibility to infection (signs/symptoms masked); delayed wound healing; hypokalemia; hypocalcemia; GI distress, diarrhea or constipation; hypertension. **OCCASIONAL:** Headache, vertigo. **RARE:** Increased blood coagulability, tachycardia, frequency or urgency of urination, psychosis.

ADVERSE REACTIONS/TOXIC EFFECTS

Long-term therapy: Muscle wasting (esp. arms, legs), osteoporosis, spontaneous fractures, amenorrhea, cataracts, glaucoma, peptic ulcer, CHF. *Abrupt withdrawal following long-term therapy:* Anorexia, nausea, fever, headache, joint pain, rebound inflammation, fatigue, weakness, lethargy, dizziness, orthostatic hypotension.

NURSING IMPLICATIONS

BASELINE ASSESSMENT:

Question for hypersensitivity to any of the corticosteroids, porcine proteins. Obtain baselines for: height, weight, B/P, glucose, cholesterol, electrolytes. Check results of initial tests, e.g., TB skin test, X-rays, EKG.

INTERVENTION/EVALUATION:

Monitor I&O, daily weight; assess for edema. Check lab results for blood coagulability and clinical evidence of thromboembolism, thrombophlebitis. Evaluate food tolerance and bowel activity; report hyperacidity promptly. Check B/P, temperature, respirations, pulse at least b.i.d. Be alert to infection: sore throat, fever, or vague symptoms. Monitor electrolytes. Watch for hypocalcemia (muscle twitching, cramps, positive Trousseau's or Chvostek's signs) or hypokalemia (weakness and muscle cramps, numbness/tingling esp. lower extremities, nausea and vomiting, irritability, EKG changes). Assess emotional status, ability to sleep. Provide assistance w/ambulation.

PATIENT/FAMILY TEACHING:

Carry identification of drug and dose, physician's name and phone number. Do not change dose/schedule or stop taking drug; must taper off gradually under medical supervision. Notify physician of fever, sore throat, muscle weakness, sudden weight gain/swelling. W/dietician give instructions for prescribed diet (usually sodium restricted w/high vitamin D, protein, and potassium). Maintain careful personal hygiene, avoid exposure to disease or trauma. Severe stress (serious infection, surgery, or trauma) may require increased dosage. Do not take aspirin or any other medication w/o consulting physician. Follow-up visits, lab tests are necessary; children must be assessed for growth retardation. Inform dentist or other physicians of hydrocortisone therapy now or within past 12 months.

cortisone acetate

kore´tih-zone
(Cortone Acetate)

CANADIAN AVAILABILITY: Cortone

CLASSIFICATION

Corticosteroid

PHARMACOKINETICS

Rapid, complete absorption from GI tract, slow but complete absorption after IM administration. Widely distributed. Primarily metabolized in liver to hydrocortisone. Primarily excreted in urine. Half-life: 30 min.

ACTION

Decreases/prevents tissue response to inflammatory process. Inhibits accumulation of inflammatory cells at inflammation sites, phagocytosis, lysosomal enzyme release and synthesis and/or release of mediators of inflammation. Prevents/suppresses cell-mediated immune reactions.

USES

Substitution therapy in deficiency states: acute/chronic adrenal insufficiency, congenital adrenal hyperplasia, adrenal insufficiency secondary to pituitary insufficiency.

Nonendocrine disorders: arthritis, rheumatic carditis, allergic, collagen, intestinal tract, liver, ocular, renal, and skin diseases, bronchial asthma, cerebral edema, malignancies.

PO/IM ADMINISTRATION

PO:

1. Give w/milk or food (decreases GI upset).
2. Single doses given prior to 9 AM; multiple doses at evenly spaced intervals.

IM:

1. Inject deep IM; avoid deltoid.
2. Prevent accidental SubQ injection.

INDICATIONS/DOSAGE/ROUTES

NOTE: Individualize dose based on disease, pt, and response.

Usual oral dosage:
PO: Adults: Initially 25-300 mg/day. **Maintenance:** Lowest dosage that maintains adequate clinical response.

Usual elderly dosage:
PO: Elderly: Use lowest effective dosage.

Usual parenteral dosage:
IM: Adults: Initially, 20-300 mg/day.

PRECAUTIONS

CONTRAINDICATIONS: Hypersensitivity to any corticosteroid, systemic fungal infection, peptic ulcers (except life-threatening situations). Avoid live virus vaccine. **CAUTIONS:** Thromboembolic disorders, history of tuberculosis (may reactivate disease), hypothyroidism, cirrhosis, nonspecific ulcerative colitis, CHF, hypertension, psychosis, renal insufficiency, seizure disorders. Prolonged therapy should be discontinued slowly. **PREGNANCY/LACTATION:** Drug crosses placenta, distributed in breast milk. May cause cleft palate (chronic use first trimester). Nursing contraindicated. **Pregnancy Category C.**

INTERACTIONS

DRUG INTERACTIONS: Amphotericin may increase hypokalemia. May decrease effect of oral hypoglycemics, insulin, diuretics, potassium supplements. May increase digoxin toxicity (due to hypokalemia). Hepatic enzyme inducers may decrease effect. Live virus vaccines may potentiate virus replication, increase vaccine side effects, decrease pt's antibody response to vaccine. **ALTERED LAB VALUES:** May decrease calcium, potassium, thyroxine. May increase cholesterol, lipids, glucose, sodium, amylase.

SIDE EFFECTS

FREQUENT: Increased appetite, exaggerated sense of well-being, abdominal distension, weight gain, insomnia, mood swings. *High dose, prolonged therapy:* **FREQUENT:** Increased susceptibility to infection (signs/symptoms masked); delayed wound healing; hypokalemia; hypocalcemia; GI distress; diarrhea or constipation; hypertension. **OCCASIONAL:** Headache, vertigo. **RARE:** Increased blood coagulability, tachycardia, frequency or urgency of urination, psychosis.

ADVERSE REACTIONS/TOXIC EFFECTS

Long-term therapy: Muscle wasting (esp. arms, legs), osteoporosis, spontaneous fractures, amenorrhea, cataracts, glaucoma, peptic ulcer, CHF. *Abrupt withdrawal following long-term therapy:* Anorexia, nausea, fever, headache, joint pain, rebound inflammation, fatigue, weakness, lethargy, dizziness, orthostatic hypertension.

NURSING IMPLICATIONS

BASELINE ASSESSMENT:

Question for hypersensitivity to any of the corticosteroids. Obtain baseline values for: height, weight, B/P, glucose, cholesterol, electrolytes. Check results of initial tests, e.g., TB skin test, X-rays, EKG.

INTERVENTION/EVALUATION:

Monitor I&O, daily weight; assess for edema. Check lab results for blood coagulability and clinical evidence of thromboembolism, thrombophlebitis. Evaluate food tolerance and bowel activity; report hyperacidity promptly. Check B/P, temperature, respirations, pulse at least b.i.d. Be alert to infection: sore throat, fever, or vague symptoms. Monitor electrolytes. Watch for hypocalcemia (muscle twitching, cramps, positive Trousseau's or Chvostek's signs) or hypokalemia (weakness and muscle cramps, numbness/tingling esp. lower extremities, nausea and vomiting, irritability, EKG changes.) Assess emotional status, ability to sleep. Provide assistance w/ambulation.

PATIENT/FAMILY TEACHING:

Take w/food or milk. Carry identification of drug and dose,

physician's name and phone number. Do not change dose/schedule or stop taking drug, must taper off under medical supervision. Notify physician of fever, sore throat, muscle aches, sudden weight gain/swelling. W/dietician give instructions for prescribed diet (usually sodium restricted w/high vitamin D, protein, and potassium). Maintain careful personal hygiene, avoid exposure to disease or trauma. Severe stress (serious infection, surgery, or trauma) may require increased dosage. Do not take aspirin or any other medication w/o consulting physician. Follow-up visits, lab tests are necessary; children must be assessed for growth retardation. Inform dentist or other physicians of cortisone therapy now or within past 12 months.

cosyntropin

koe-syn-troe´pin
(Cortrosyn)

CANADIAN AVAILABILITY:
Cortrosyn, Synacthen Depot

CLASSIFICATION

Adrenocorticotropic hormone

PHARMACOKINETICS

Rapid absorption from IM/SubQ sites (respiratory forms have delayed absorption). Widely distributed.

ACTION

Increases endogenous corticoid synthesis. Stimulates initial reaction in synthesis of adrenal steroids from cholesterol. Other effects due to generated endogenous corticosteroids.

USES

Diagnostic testing of adrenocortical function.

IM/IV ADMINISTRATION

1. Reconstitute by adding 1 ml of 0.9% NaCl injection to a 0.25 mg vial of cosyntropin to produce solution of 0.25 mg/ml.
2. For IV infusion, dilute w/5% dextrose or 0.9% NaCl and infuse at rate of 0.04 mg/hr over 6 hrs.

INDICATIONS/DOSAGE/ROUTES

Screening test for adrenal function:
IM: Adults: 0.25-0.75 mg one time. **Children (<2 yrs):** 0.125 mg one time.
IV INFUSION: Adults: 0.25 mg in 5% dextrose or 0.9% NaCl, infuse at rate of 0.04 mg/hr.

PRECAUTIONS

CONTRAINDICATIONS: Hypersensitivity to cosyntropin or corticotropin. **CAUTIONS:** (Short duration for diagnostic use does not produce effects of long-term corticotropin therapy). **PREGNANCY/LACTATION:** Nursing not recommended. **Pregnancy Category C.**

INTERACTIONS

DRUG INTERACTIONS: None significant. **ALTERED LAB VALUES:** None significant.

SIDE EFFECTS

OCCASIONAL: Pruritus. **RARE:** Hypersensitivity reactions.

ADVERSE REACTIONS/TOXIC EFFECTS

None significant.

NURSING IMPLICATIONS

BASELINE ASSESSMENT:

Question for hypersensitivity to cosyntropin or corticotropin. Hold cortisone, hydrocortisone, or spironolactone on the test day. Assure that baseline plasma cortisol concentration has been drawn prior to start of test, or 24-hour urine for 17-KS or 17-OHCS is initiated.

INTERVENTION/EVALUATION:

Assess for pruritus, rash, or other sign of hypersensitivity reaction. Adhere to time frame for blood draws, monitor collection of urine if indicated.

PATIENT/FAMILY TEACHING:

Explain the procedure and purpose of the test.

co-trimoxazole (sulfamethoxazole-trimethoprim)

koe-try-mox´oh-zole

(Bactrim, Cotrim, Septra, Sulfamethoprim)

FIXED-COMBINATION(S):
W/sulfamethoxazole, a sulfonamide and trimethoprim, a folate antagonist

CANADIAN AVAILABILITY:
Apo-Sulfatrim, Bactrim, Novotrimel, Protrin, Septra

CLASSIFICATION

Anti-infective

PHARMACOKINETICS

Rapid, well absorbed from GI tract. Widely distributed. Protein binding: 60-70% (trimethoprim 40-70%). Metabolized in liver. Excreted in urine. Half-life: 6-12 hrs (trimethoprim 8-10 hrs). Half-life increased in decreased renal function.

ACTION

Usually bactericidal in susceptible microorganisms, blocking two steps in synthesis of essential nucleic acids: Sulfamethoxazole competes w/*p*-aminobenzoic acid to inhibit formation of dihydrofolic acid (bacteriostatic). Trimethoprim interferes w/production of tetrahydrofolic acid by inhibiting dihydrofolate reductase (usually bactericidal).

USES

Acute/complicated and recurrent/chronic urinary tract infection, *Pneumocystis carinii* pneumonia, shigellosis, enteritis, otitis media, chronic bronchitis, traveler's diarrhea. Prophylaxis of *Pneumocystis carinii* pneumonia.

STORAGE/HANDLING

Store tablets, suspension at room temperature. IV infusion (piggyback) stable for 2-6 hrs (use immediately); discard if cloudy or precipitate forms.

PO/IV ADMINISTRATION

NOTE: Space doses evenly around the clock.

PO:

1. Administer on empty stomach w/8 oz water.
2. Give several extra glasses of water/day.

IV:

1. For IV infusion (piggyback), each 5 ml of concentrate solution is diluted w/75-125 mg 5% dextrose.

2. Do not mix w/other drugs or solutions.

3. Infuse over 60-90 min. Must avoid bolus or rapid infusion.

4. Do not give IM.

5. Assure adequate hydration.

INDICATIONS/DOSAGE/ROUTES

NOTE: Potency expressed in terms of trimethoprim content.

UTI, enteritis, acute otitis media:
PO: Adults, elderly: 160 mg q12h for 7-14 days. **Children >2 mo:** 7.5-8 mg/kg/day q12h for 5-10 days.

Severe UTI, enteritis:
IV: Adults, elderly, children >2 mo: 8-10 mg/kg/day in 2-4 equally divided doses q6-12h for 5-14 days. **Maximum:** 960 mg/day.

Pneumocystis carinii pneumonia:
PO: Adults, elderly, children >2 mo: 20 mg/kg/day in 4 divided doses q6h.
IV: Adults, elderly, children >2 mo: 15-20 mg/kg/day in 3-4 divided doses q6-8h.

Prevention of Pneumocystis carinii pneumonia:
PO: Adults: 160 mg/day. **Children:** 150 mg/m^2/day on 3 consecutive days/wk.

Traveler's diarrhea:
PO: Adults, elderly: 160 mg q12h × 5 days.

Acute exacerbation of chronic bronchitis:
PO: Adults, elderly: 160 mg q12h for 14 days.

Dosage in renal impairment:
The dose and/or frequency is modified based on severity of infection, degree of renal impairment, and serum concentration of drug. For those w/creatinine clearance of 15-30 ml/min, a reduction in dose of 50% is recommended.

PRECAUTIONS

CONTRAINDICATIONS: Hypersensitivity to trimethoprim or any sulfonamides, megaloblastic anemia due to folate deficiency, infants <2 mo. Not for treatment of streptococcal pharyngitis. **CAUTIONS:** Elderly, impaired renal or hepatic function, history of severe allergy or bronchial asthma (allergic reaction to metabisulfite in injection more likely), AIDS (higher incidence of adverse reactions). **PREGNANCY/LACTATION:** Contraindicated during pregnancy at term and lactation. Readily crosses placenta; distributed in breast milk. May produce kernicterus in newborns. **Pregnancy Category C.**

INTERACTIONS

DRUG INTERACTIONS: May increase, prolong effects, increase toxicity w/warfarin, hydantoin anticonvulsants, oral hypoglycemics. May increase risk of toxicity w/other hemolytics. Hepatotoxic medications may increase risk of hepatotoxicity. Methenamine may form precipitate. May increase effect of methotrexate. **ALTERED LAB VALUES:** May increase SGOT (AST), SGPT (ALT), alkaline phosphatase, BUN, creatinine.

SIDE EFFECTS

FREQUENT: Anorexia, nausea, vomiting, rash (generally 7-14 days after therapy begins), urticaria. **OCCASIONAL:** Diarrhea, abdominal pain, pancreatitis, local pain/irritation at IV site. **RARE:** Headache, vertigo, insomnia, septic meningitis, convulsions, hallucinations, depression, thrombophlebitis, hypersensitivity, and hematologic reactions.

ADVERSE REACTIONS/TOXIC EFFECTS

Rash, fever, sore throat, pallor, purpura, cough, shortness of breath may be early signs of serious adverse reactions. Fatalities are rare but have occurred in sulfonamide therapy following Stevens-Johnson syndrome, toxic epidermal necrolysis, fulminant hepatic necrosis, agranulocytosis, aplastic anemia, other blood dyscrasias. Elderly are at increased risk of adverse reactions: bone marrow suppression, decreased platelets, severe dermatologic reactions.

NURSING IMPLICATIONS

BASELINE ASSESSMENT:

Check history for hypersensitivity to trimethoprim or any sulfonamide, sulfite sensitivity, severe allergy or bronchial asthma. Obtain specimens for diagnostic tests before giving first dose (therapy may begin before results are known). Determine renal, hepatic, hematologic baselines.

INTERVENTION/EVALUATION:

Evaluate food tolerance. Determine pattern of bowel activity. Assess skin for rash, pallor, purpura. Check IV site, flow rate. Monitor renal, hepatic, hematology reports. Assess I&O. Check for CNS symptoms: headache, vertigo, insomnia, hallucinations. Monitor vital signs at least twice a day. Watch for cough or shortness of breath. Assess for overt bleeding, bruising, or swelling.

PATIENT/FAMILY TEACHING:

Continue medication for full length of therapy. Space doses evenly around the clock. Take oral doses w/8 oz water and drink several extra glasses of water daily. Notify physician of new symptoms immediately, especially rash or other skin changes, bleeding or bruising, fever, sore throat.

C

cromolyn sodium

krom-awl´in

(Gastrocom, Intal, Nasalcrom, Opticrom)

CANADIAN AVAILABILITY:
Intal, Nalcrom, Opticrom, Rynacrom, Vistacrom

CLASSIFICATION

Antiasthmatic, antiallergic, mast cell stabilizer

PHARMACOKINETICS

Minimal absorption following oral, inhalation, or nasal administration. Absorbed portion excreted in urine or via biliary elimination.

ACTION

Exerts local effect on lung and nasal mucosa. Inhibits mast cell release after exposure to antigens, causing hypersensitivity reactions (e.g., histamine, SRS-A [a substance of anaphylaxsis]).

USES

Prophylactic management of severe bronchial asthma, exercise-induced bronchospasm, perennial or seasonal allergic rhinitis, symptomatic treatment of systemic mastocytosis.

INHALATION/NASAL ADMINISTRATION

INHALATION:

1. Shake container well, exhale

completely, then holding mouthpiece 1 inch away from lips; inhale and hold breath as long as possible before exhaling.

2. Wait 1-10 min before inhaling 2nd dose (allows for deeper bronchial penetration).

3. Rinse mouth w/water immediately after inhalation (prevents mouth/throat dryness).

NEBULIZATION, INHALATION CAPSULES:

1. Inhalation capsules are not to be swallowed; instruct patient on use of Spinhaler.

ORAL CAPSULES:

1. Give at least 30 min before meals.

2. Pour contents of capsule in hot water stirring until completely dissolved; add equal amount cold water while stirring.

3. Do not mix w/fruit juice, milk, or food.

NASAL:

1. Nasal passages should be clear (may require nasal decongestant).

2. Inhale through nose.

INDICATIONS/DOSAGE/ROUTES

Asthma:
ORAL INHALATION: Adults, elderly, children >2 yrs (oral solution), children >5 yrs (oral powder): 20 mg 4 times/day.

Prevention of bronchospasm:
ORAL INHALATION: Adults, elderly, children >2 yrs (oral solution), children >5 yrs (oral powder): 20 mg not longer than 1 hr before exercise or exposure to precipitating factor.

Allergic rhinitis:
INTRANASAL: Adults, elderly, children >6 yrs: 1 spray each nostril 3-4 times/day. May increase up to 6 times/day.

Systemic mastocytosis:
PO: Adults, elderly, children >12 yrs: 200 mg 4 times/day. **Children 2-12 yrs:** 100 mg 4 times/day. **Children <2 yrs:** 20 mg/kg/day in 4 divided doses.

PRECAUTIONS

CONTRAINDICATIONS: None significant. **CAUTIONS:** Impaired renal or hepatic function. **PREGNANCY/LACTATION:** Unknown if drug crosses placenta or is distributed in breast milk. **Pregnancy Category B.**

INTERACTIONS

DRUG INTERACTIONS: None significant. **ALTERED LAB VALUES:** None significant.

SIDE EFFECTS

OCCASIONALLY: Transient cough or bronchospasm following inhalation administration, nasal sting or sneezing following instillation of nasal solution. **RARE:** Headache, urinary frequency, rash, nausea, lacrimation, unusual taste sensation.

ADVERSE REACTIONS/TOXIC EFFECTS

None significant.

NURSING IMPLICATIONS

BASELINE ASSESSMENT:

Offer emotional support (high incidence of anxiety due to difficulty in breathing and sympathomimetic response to drug).

INTERVENTION/EVALUATION:

Monitor rate, depth, rhythm, type of respiration; quality and rate of pulse. Assess lung sounds for rhonchi, wheezing, rales. Monitor arterial blood gases. Observe lips, fingernails for blue or dusky color in light-skinned patients; gray in dark-skinned patients. Observe for clavicular retractions, hand tremor. Evaluate for clinical improvement (quieter, slower respirations, relaxed facial expression, cessation of clavicular retractions).

PATIENT/FAMILY TEACHING:

Increase fluid intake (decreases lung secretion viscosity). Do not take more than 2 inhalations at any one time (excessive use may produce paradoxical bronchoconstriction, or a decreased bronchodilating effect). Rinsing mouth with water immediately after inhalation may prevent mouth/throat dryness. Effect of therapy dependent on administration at regular intervals.

cyanocobalamin (vitamin B_{12})

sye-ah-no-koe-bal′a-min
(Rubramin PC, Crysti-12, Cyanoject, Cyomin)

hydroxocobalamin (vitamin $B_{12}a$)

(Hydrobexan, Hydro-Cobex)

FIXED-COMBINATION(S):
W/liver extract, 10 mcg/ml (liver injection); w/liver excrete crude, 2 mcg/ml; vitamin B_{12} w/intrinsic factor (Ciopar Forte)

CANADIAN AVAILABILITY:
Anacobin, Rubion, Rubramin

CLASSIFICATION

Vitamin, Antianemic

PHARMACOKINETICS

Absorbed in lower half of ileum in presence of calcium. Initially bound to intrinsic factor; this complex passes down intestine binding to receptor sites on ileal mucosa. In presence of calcium absorbed systemically. Protein binding: high. Metabolized in liver. Eliminated via biliary excretion. Half-life: 6 days.

ACTION

Coenzyme for metabolic functions (fat, carbohydrate metabolism, protein synthesis). Necessary for growth, cell replication, hematopoiesis, and myelin synthesis.

USES

Prophylaxis, treatment of pernicious anemia, vitamin B_{12} deficiency due to inadequate diet or intestinal malabsorption, hemolytic anemia, hyperthyroidism, malignancy of pancreas, bowel, gastrectomy, GI lesions, neurologic damage, malabsorption syndrome, vegetarians, breastfed infants, metabolic disorders, prolonged stress, chronic fever, renal disease. Deficiency generally occurs concurrently w/other B-vitamin deficiencies.

PO ADMINISTRATION

Give w/meals (increases absorption).

INDICATIONS/DOSAGE/ROUTES

Deficiency:
SubQ/IM: Adults, elderly: Initially, 100 mcg/day for 6-7 days, then every other day for 7 doses, then every 3-4 days for 2-3 wks. **Maintenance:** 100-200 mcg every month. **Children:** Initially, 30-50 mcg/day for at least 2 wks. **Maintenance:** 100 mcg every month.

Supplement:
PO: Adults, elderly: 1-25 mcg/day. **Children >1 yr:** 1 mcg/day. **Children <1 yr:** 0.3 mcg/day.

PRECAUTIONS

CONTRAINDICATIONS: History of allergy to cobalamin, folate deficient anemia, heredity optic nerve atrophy. **CAUTIONS:** Heart disease, history of gout, pulmonary disease, undiagnosed anemia, concurrent use of cardiac glycosides. **PREGNANCY/LACTATION:** Crosses placenta; excreted in breast milk. **Pregnancy Category C.**

INTERACTIONS

DRUG INTERACTIONS: Alcohol, colchicine may decrease absorption. Ascorbic acid may destroy vitamin B_{12}. Folic acid (large doses) may decrease concentration. **ALTERED LAB VALUES:** None significant.

SIDE EFFECTS

FREQUENT: Mild transient diarrhea, itching, skin eruptions, fever, urticaria, sensation of body swelling.

ADVERSE REACTIONS/TOXIC EFFECTS

Rare allergic reaction generally due to impurities in preparation. May produce peripheral vascular thrombosis, pulmonary edema, hypokalemia, CHF.

NURSING IMPLICATIONS

INTERVENTION/EVALUATION:

Assess for CHF, pulmonary edema, hypokalemia in cardiac pts receiving SubQ/IM therapy. Monitor potassium levels (3.5-5 mEq/L), serum B_{12} (200-800 pg/ml) rise in reticulocyte count (peaks in 5-8 days). Assess for reversal of deficiency symptoms: hyporeflexia, loss of positional sense, ataxia, fatigue, irritability, insomnia, anorexia, pallor, palpitation on exertion. Therapeutic response to treatment usually dramatic within 48 hrs.

PATIENT/FAMILY TEACHING:

Lifetime treatment may be necessary w/pernicious anemia. Report symptoms of infection. Foods rich in vitamin B_{12} include organ meats, clams, osyters, herring, red snapper, muscle meats, fermented cheese, dairy products, egg yolks.

cyclobenzaprine hydrochloride

cy-klow-benz´ah-preen
(Flexeril)

CANADIAN AVAILABILITY:
Flexeril

CLASSIFICATION

Skeletal muscle relaxant

PHARMACOKINETICS

	ONSET	PEAK	DURATION
PO	1 hr	3-4 hrs	12-24 hrs

Well (slow) absorbed from GI tract. Protein binding: 93% Metabolized in GI tract, liver. Primarily excreted in urine. Half-life: 1-3 days.

ACTION

Acts on brain stem reducing tonic somatic motor activity.

USES

For short-term (2-3 wks) use as

adjunct to rest, physical therapy, other measures for relief of discomfort due to acute, painful musculoskeletal conditions.

INDICATIONS/DOSAGE/ROUTES

NOTE: Do not use longer than 2-3 wks.

Acute, painful musculoskeletal conditions:

PO: Adults, elderly: 10 mg 3 times/day. **Range:** 20-40 mg/day in 2-4 divided doses. **Maximum:** 60 mg/day.

PRECAUTIONS

CONTRAINDICATIONS: Concurrent use of MAO inhibitors or within 14 days after their discontinuation, acute recovery phase of MI, those w/arrhythmias, heart blocks or conduction disturbances, CHF, hyperthyroidism. **CAUTIONS:** Impaired renal or hepatic function, history of urinary retention, angle-closure glaucoma, increased intraocular pressure. **PREGNANCY/LACTATION:** Unknown if drug crosses placenta or is distributed in breast milk. **Pregnancy Category B.**

INTERACTIONS

DRUG INTERACTIONS: Tricyclic antidepressants, CNS depression-producing medications may increase CNS depression. MAO inhibitors may increase risk of hypertensive crisis, severe seizures. **ALTERED LAB VALUES:** None significant.

SIDE EFFECTS

FREQUENT: Drowsiness, dry mouth, dizziness (postural hypotension). **OCCASIONAL:** Nausea, constipation, unpleasant taste sensation, blurred vision, headache, nervousness, confusion. **RARE:** Insomnia, anxiety, agitation, disorientation, urinary frequency or retention.

ADVERSE REACTIONS/TOXIC EFFECTS

Overdosage may result in visual hallucinations, hyperactive reflexes, muscle rigidity, vomiting, hyperpyrexia.

NURSING IMPLICATIONS

BASELINE ASSESSMENT:

Record onset, type, location, and duration of muscular spasm. Check for immobility, stiffness, swelling.

INTERVENTION/EVALUATION:

Assist w/ambulation at all times. Evaluate for therapeutic response: decreased intensity of skeletal muscle pain/tenderness, improved mobility, decrease in stiffness.

PATIENT/FAMILY TEACHING:

Drowsiness usually diminishes w/continued therapy. Avoid tasks that require alertness, motor skills until response to drug is established. Avoid alochol or other depressants while taking medication. Avoid sudden changes in posture.

cyclopentolate

sye-kloe-pen´toe-late

(Cyclogyl, Pentolair)

FIXED-COMBINATION(S): W/phenylephrine hydrochloride, a mydriatic (Cyclomydril); w/scopolamine hydrobromide, a mydriatic and cycloplegic, and phenylephrine, a mydriatic (Murocoll-2)

CANADIAN AVAILABILITY:
AK-Pentolate, Cyclogyl, Cyclopentolate Minims

CLASSIFICATION

Mydriatic, cycloplegic

PHARMACOKINETICS

	PEAK	RECOVERY
MYDRIASIS	30-60 min	1 day
CYCLOPLEGIA	25-75 min	0.25-1 day

ACTION

Blocks acetylcholine causing relaxation of the sphincter muscle of the iris; blocks cholinergic stimulation of the accommodative ciliary muscle of the lens. Dilation of the pupil and paralysis of accommodation are produced.

USES

To produce mydriasis and cycloplegic refraction during diagnostic procedures; the combination w/phenylephrine causes maximal mydriasis esp. useful in examination for retinal detachment.

OPHTHALMIC ADMINISTRATION

1. Instruct pt to lie down or tilt head backward and look up.
2. Gently pull lower lid down to form pouch and instill medication.
3. Do not touch tip of applicator to any surface.
4. When lower lid is released, have pt keep eye open w/o blinking for at least 30 sec.
5. Apply gentle finger pressure to lacrimal sac (bridge of the nose, inside corner of the eye) for 1-2 min.
6. Remove excess solution around eye w/tissue. Wash hands immediately to remove medication on hands.
7. Tell pt to shut eyes tightly/not blink more often than necessary.
8. Never rinse dropper.
9. Do not use solution if discolored.

INDICATIONS/DOSAGE/ROUTES

Mydriatic/cycloplegic diagnostic procedure:

OPHTHALMIC: Adults, elderly: 1 drop, repeat in 5-10 min. **Children:** 1 drop (0.5, 1, or 2%) repeat in 5-10 min (0.5 or 1%). **Note:** Pts w/heavily pigmented irides may require larger doses.

PRECAUTIONS

CONTRAINDICATIONS: Angle-closure glaucoma. Combination solutions should not be used in infants <1 yr of age. **CAUTIONS:** Extreme caution w/children due to potential psychotic reactions; w/phenylephrine risk of severe hypertension in children. Geriatric pts, those who may be predisposed to increased intraocular pressure. **PREGNANCY/LACTATION:** Caution during pregnancy or lactation: systemic absorption may occur. **Pregnancy Category C.**

INTERACTIONS

DRUG INTERACTIONS: None significant. **ALTERED LAB VALUES:** None significant.

SIDE EFFECTS

NOTE: When using combination solutions, consider effects of other medication in preparation.
FREQUENT: Transient, considerable burning w/1% or 2% solutions.
OCCASIONAL: W/repeated use, allergic reaction within minutes of instillation: irritation, diffuse redness, blurred vision.

ADVERSE REACTIONS/TOXIC EFFECTS

Psychotic reactions and behavioral disturbances (ataxia, incoherent speech, irrelevant talking, hallucinations, disorientation, failure to recognize people, tachycardia, amnesia) are rare in adults, but are more common in children, esp. w/2% solutions.

NURSING IMPLICATIONS

BASELINE ASSESSMENT:

Ask about hypersensitivity to cyclopentolate or components. Assess physical appearance of eye.

INTERVENTION/EVALUATION:

Check for allergic response: redness, irritation, blurred vision. In the event of psychotic reaction, provide protection to patient until physostigmine can be administered to counteract medication.

PATIENT/FAMILY TEACHING:

Burning sensation upon instillation is to be expected. Do not drive or operate machinery for 24 hrs unless otherwise directed by physician (administration of pilocarpine may reduce recovery time to 3-6 hrs). Wearing sunglasses until medication wears off may relieve photophobia. If sensitivity to light or other effects continue longer than 36 hrs, or blurred or diminished vision occurs, inform physician.

cyclophosphamide

sigh-klo-phos′fah-mide

(Cytoxan, Neosar)

CANADIAN AVAILABILITY:
Cytoxan, Procytox

CLASSIFICATION

Antineoplastic

PHARMACOKINETICS

Well absorbed from GI tract. Crosses blood-brain barrier. Protein binding: low. Metabolized in liver to active metabolites. Primarily excreted in urine. Half-life: 3-12 hrs.

ACTION

Cross-links strands of DNA, RNA. Inhibits protein synthesis. Potent immunosuppressant.

USES

Treatment of Hodgkin's disease, non-Hodgkin's lymphomas, multiple myeloma, leukemia (acute lymphoblastic, acute myelogenous, acute monocytic, chronic granulocytic, chronic lymphocytic), mycosis fungoides, disseminated neuroblastoma, adenocarcinoma of ovary, retinoblastoma, carcinoma of breast. Biopsy-proven "minimal change" nephrotic syndrome in children.

STORAGE/HANDLING

NOTE: May be carcinogenic, mutagenic, or teratogenic. Handle w/ extreme care during preparation/ administration.

Solutions prepared w/bacteriostatic water for injection for IV use are stable for 24 hrs at room temperature, 6 days if refrigerated.

PO/IV ADMINISTRATION

PO:

1. Give on an empty stomach. If GI upset occurs, give w/food.

IV:

1. For IV injection, reconstitute each 100 mg w/5 ml sterile water for injection or bacteriosatic water

for injection to provide concentration of 20 mg/ml.

2. Shake to dissolve. Allow to stand until clear.

3. May give by IV injection or further dilute w/5% dextrose, 0.9% NaCl, or other compatible fluid for IV infusion.

4. IV may produce faintness, facial flushing, diaphoresis, oropharyngeal sensation.

INDICATIONS/DOSAGE/ROUTES

NOTE: Dosage individualized based on clinical response, tolerance to adverse effects. When used in combination therapy, consult specific protocols for optimum dosage, sequence of drug administration.

Malignant diseases:
PO: Adults, children: 1-5 mg/kg/day.
IV: Adults, children: 40-50 mg/kg in divided doses over 2-5 days; or 10-15 mg/kg q7-10days or 3-5 mg/kg 2 times/wk.

Biopsy-proven "minimal change" nephrotic syndrome:
PO: Children: 2.5-3 mg/kg/day for 60-90 days.

PRECAUTIONS

CONTRAINDICATIONS: None significant. **CAUTIONS:** Severe leukopenia, thrombocytopenia, tumor infiltration of bone marrow, previous therapy w/other antineoplastic agents, radiation. **PREGNANCY/LACTATION:** If possible, avoid use during pregnancy. May cause malformations (limb abnormalities, cardiac anomalies, hernias). Distributed in breast milk. Breast feeding not recommended. **Pregnancy Category D.**

INTERACTIONS

DRUG INTERACTIONS: May decrease effect of antigout medications. Allopurinol, bone marrow depressants may increase bone marrow depression. Cytarabine may increase cardiomyopathy. Immunosuppressants may increase risk infection, develop neoplasms. Live virus vaccines may potentiate virus replication, increase vaccine side effects, decrease pt's antibody response to vaccine. **ALTERED LAB VALUES:** May increase uric acid.

SIDE EFFECTS

EXPECTED: Marked leukopenia 8-15 days after initial therapy. **FREQUENT:** Nausea, vomiting begins about 6 hrs after administration and lasts about 4 hrs. Alopecia occurs in 33% of pts. **OCCASIONAL:** Nonhemorrhagic colitis, diarrhea, darkening of skin and nails, mucosal irritation, oral ulceration.

ADVERSE REACTIONS/TOXIC EFFECTS

Major toxic effect is bone marrow depression resulting in hematologic toxicity (leukopenia, anemia, thrombocytopenia, hypoprothrombinemia). Thrombocytopenia may occur 10-15 days after drug initiation. Anemia generally occurs after large doses or prolonged therapy. Hemorrhagic cystitis occurs commonly in long-term therapy (esp. in children). Pulmonary fibrosis, cardiotoxicity noted w/high doses. Amenorrhea, azospermia, hyperkalemia may also occur.

NURSING IMPLICATIONS

BASELINE ASSESSMENT:

Obtain WBC count weekly during therapy or until maintenance dose is established, then at intervals of 2-3 wks.

INTERVENTION/EVALUATION:

Monitor serum uric acid concentration, hematologic status. Monitor WBC closely during initial therapy (at least 3,000-4,000 cells/mm^3 should be maintained). Assess urine output for hematuria (hemorrhagic cystitis). Assess pattern of daily bowel activity and stool consistency. Monitor for hematologic toxicity (fever, sore throat, signs of local infection, easy bruising or unusual bleeding from any site), symptoms of anemia (excessive tiredness, weakness). Recovery from marked leukopenia due to bone marrow depression can be expected in 17-28 days.

PATIENT/FAMILY TEACHING:

Encourage copious fluid intake and frequent voiding (assists in preventing cystitis) at least 24 hrs before, during, after therapy. Do not have immunizations w/o physician's approval (drug lowers body's resistance). Avoid contact w/those who have recently received live virus vaccine. Promptly report fever, sore throat, signs of local infection, easy bruising or unusual bleeding from any site. Alopecia is reversible, but new hair growth may have different color or texture. Contact physician if nausea/vomiting continue at home.

cyclosporine

sigh-klow-spore´in

(Sandimmune)

CANADIAN AVAILABILITY:

Sandimmune

CLASSIFICATION

Immunosuppressant

PHARMACOKINETICS

Variably absorbed from GI tract. Widely distributed. Protein binding: 90%. Metabolized in liver. Eliminated primarily by biliary/fecal excretion. Half-life: adults 10-27 hrs, children 7-19 hrs.

ACTION

Inhibits interleukin-2, a proliferative factor needed for T cell activity. Inhibits both cellular and humoral immune responses.

USES

Prevents rejection of kidney, liver, heart allografts in combination w/steroid therapy. Treat chronic allograft rejection in pts previously treated w/other immunosuppressives.

STORAGE/HANDLING

Store capsules, oral solution, parenteral form at room temperature. Protect IV solution from light. After diluted, stable for 24 hrs. Avoid refrigeration of oral solution (separation of solution may occur). Discard oral solution after 2 mo once bottle is opened.

PO/IV ADMINISTRATION

NOTE: Oral solution available in bottle form w/pipette. Oral form should replace IV administration as soon as possible.

PO:

1. Oral solution may be mixed in glass container w/milk, chocolate milk, or orange juice (preferably at room temperature). Stir well. Drink immediately.
2. Add more diluent to glass container and mix w/remaining

solution to ensure total amount is given.

3. Dry outside of pipette before replacing in cover. Do not rinse w/ water.

IV:

1. Dilute each ml concentrate w/20-100 ml 0.9% NaCl or 5% dextrose.
2. Infuse over 2-6 hrs.
3. Monitor patient continuously for first 30 min after instituting infusion and frequently thereafter for hypersensitivity reaction (see Side Effects).

INDICATIONS/DOSAGE/ROUTES

NOTE: May be given w/adrenal corticosteroids, but not w/other immunosuppressive agents (increases susceptibility to infection, development of lymphoma).

Prevention of allograft rejection:
PO: Adults, elderly, children: Initially, 15 mg/kg as single dose 4-12 hrs prior to transplantation, continue for 1-2 wks. Taper dose by 5%/wk over 6-8 wks. **Maintenance:** 5-10 mg/kg/day.
IV: Adults, elderly, children: Give about one-third of oral dose: 5-6 mg/kg as single dose 4-12 hrs prior to transplantation, continue until pt able to take oral medication.

PRECAUTIONS

CONTRAINDICATIONS: History of hypersensitivity to cyclosporine or polyoxyethylated castor oil. **CAUTIONS:** Impaired hepatic, renal, cardiac function, malabsorption syndrome. **PREGNANCY/LACTATION:** Readily crosses placenta, distributed in breast milk. Avoid nursing. **Pregnancy Category C.**

INTERACTIONS

DRUG INTERACTIONS: Cimetidine, danazol, diltiazem, erythromycin, ketoconazole may increase concentration, risk of hepatotoxicity, nephrotoxicity. ACE inhibitors, potassium-sparing diuretics, potassium supplements may cause hyperkalemia. Immunosuppressants may increase risk of infection, lymphoproliferative disorders. Lovastatin may increase risk rhabdomyolysis, acute renal failure. Live virus vaccines may potentiate virus replication, increase vaccine side effects, decrease pt's antibody response to vaccine. **ALTERED LAB VALUES:** May increase BUN, creatinine, SGOT (AST), SGPT (ALT), alkaline phosphatase, amylase, bilirubin, uric acid, potassium. May decrease magnesium.

SIDE EFFECTS

FREQUENT: Hypertension (most severe in children), hirsutism (abnormal hairiness especially in women), tremor, acne, gum hyperplasia. **OCCASIONAL:** Headache, blurred vision, diarrhea, nausea, paresthesia. **RARE:** Seizures, hypersensitivity reaction (flushing of face and thorax, wheezing, B/P changes), diabetes mellitus in renal transplantation.

ADVERSE REACTIONS/TOXIC EFFECTS

Mild nephrotoxicity occurs in 25% of renal transplants after transplantation, 38% in cardiac transplants, and 37% of liver transplants, respectively. Hepatotoxicity occurs in 4% of renal, 7% of cardiac, and 4% of liver transplants, respectively. Both toxicities usually responsive to dosage reduction. Severe hyperkalemia, hyperuricemia occur occasionally.

NURSING IMPLICATIONS

BASELINE ASSESSMENT:

Note that if nephrotoxicity occurs, mild toxicity is generally noted 2-3 mo after transplantation; more severe toxicity noted early after transplantation; hepatotoxicity may be noted during first month after transplantation.

INTERVENTION/EVALUATION:

Diligently monitor BUN, creatinine, bilirubin, SGOT (AST), SGPT (ALT), LDH blood serum levels for evidence of hepatotoxicity or nephrotoxicity (mild toxicity noted by slow rise in serum levels; more overt toxicity noted by rapid rise in levels. Hematuria also noted). Assess potassium level for evidence of hyperkalemia. Encourage diligent oral hygiene (gum hyperplasia). Monitor B/P for evidence of hypertension.

PATIENT/FAMILY TEACHING:

Essential to repeat blood testing on a routine basis while receiving medication. Headache, tremor may occur as a response to medication.

cyproheptadine hydrochloride

sigh-pro-hep′tah-deen
(Periactin)

CANADIAN AVAILABILITY:
Periactin

CLASSIFICATION

Antihistamine

PHARMACOKINETICS

Well absorbed from GI tract. Metabolized in liver. Primarily eliminated in feces.

ACTION

Prevents, antagonizes most histamine effects (e.g., urticaria, pruritus). Anticholinergic effects cause drying of nasal mucosa.

USES

Relief of nasal allergies, allergic dermatitis, cold urticaria, hypersensitivity reactions.

PO ADMINISTRATION

1. Give w/o regard to meals.
2. Scored tablets may be crushed.

INDICATIONS/DOSAGE/ROUTES

Allergic condition:
PO: Adults, children >15 yrs: 4 mg 3 times/day. May increase dose but do not exceed 0.5 mg/kg/day. **Children 7-14 yrs:** 4 mg 2-3 times/day, or 0.25 mg/kg daily in divided doses. **Children 2-6 yrs:** 2 mg 2-3 times/day, or 0.25 mg/kg daily in divided doses.

Usual elderly dosage:
PO: Elderly: Initially, 4 mg 2 times/day.

PRECAUTIONS

CONTRAINDICATIONS: Acute asthmatic attack, pts receiving MAO inhibitors. **CAUTIONS:** Narrow-angle glaucoma, peptic ulcer, prostatic hypertrophy, pyloroduodenal or bladder neck obstruction, asthma, COPD, increased intraocular pressure, cardiovascular disease, hyperthyroidism, hypertension, seizure disorders. **PREGNANCY/LACTATION:** Unknown if drug crosses placenta or is excreted in breast milk. Increased risk of seizures in neonates, premature infants if used during third trimester of pregnancy. May prohibit lactation. **Pregnancy Category B.**

INTERACTIONS

DRUG INTERACTIONS: Alcohol, CNS depressants may increase CNS depressant effects. MAO inhibitors may increase anticholinergic, CNS depressant effects. **ALTERED LAB VALUES:** May suppress wheal, flare reactions to antigen skin testing, unless antihistamines discontinued 4 days prior to testing.

SIDE EFFECTS

FREQUENT: Drowsiness, dizziness, muscular weakness, dry mouth/nose/throat/lips, urinary retention, thickening of bronchial secretions. Sedation, dizziness, hypotension more likely noted in elderly. **OCCASIONAL:** Epigastric distress, flushing, visual disturbances, hearing disturbances, paresthesia, sweating, chills.

ADVERSE REACTIONS/TOXIC EFFECTS

Children may experience dominant paradoxical reaction (restlessness, insomnia, euphoria, nervousness, tremors). Overdosage in children may result in hallucinations, convulsions, death. Hypersensitivity reaction (eczema, pruritus, rash, cardiac abnormalities, photosensitivity) may occur. Overdosage may vary from CNS depression (sedation, apnea, cardiovascular collapse, death) to severe paradoxical reaction (hallucinations, tremor, seizures).

NURSING IMPLICATIONS

BASELINE ASSESSMENT:

If pt is undergoing allergic reaction, obtain history of recently ingested foods, drugs, environmental exposure, recent emotional stress. Monitor rate, depth, rhythm, type of respiration; quality and rate of pulse. Assess lung sounds for rhonchi, wheezing, rales.

INTERVENTION/EVALUATION:

Monitor B/P, especially in elderly (increased risk of hypotension). Monitor children closely for paradoxical reaction.

PATIENT/FAMILY TEACHING:

Tolerance to antihistaminic effect generally does not occur; tolerance to sedative effect may occur. Avoid tasks that require alertness, motor skills until response to drug is established. Dry mouth, drowsiness, dizziness may be an expected response of drug. Avoid alcoholic beverages during antihistamine therapy. Sugarless gum, sips of tepid water may relieve dry mouth. Coffee or tea may help reduce drowsiness.

---

cysteamine (Cystagon)
See supplement

---

cytarabine

sigh-tar´ah-bean
(Cytosar-U)

CANADIAN AVAILABILITY:
Cytosar

CLASSIFICATION

Antineoplastic

PHARMACOKINETICS

Widely distributed, moderate amounts cross blood-brain barrier. Protein binding: 15%. Rapidly deaminated in blood, tissues. Primarily excreted in urine. Half-life: 1-3 hrs.

ACTION

Converted intracellularly to nucleotide, appears to inhibit DNA synthesis. Cell cycle specific for S phase of cell division. Potent immunosuppressive activity.

USES

Treatment of acute and chronic myelocytic leukemia, acute lymphocytic leukemia, meningeal leukemia, non-Hodgkin's lymphoma in children.

STORAGE/HANDLING

NOTE: May be carcinogenic, mutagenic, or teratogenic. Handle w/ extreme care during preparation/administration.

Reconstituted solution stable for 48 hrs at room temperature. IV infusion solutions at concentration up to 0.5 mg/ml stable for 7 days at room temperature. Discard if slight haze develops.

SubQ/IV/INTRATHECAL ADMINISTRATION

NOTE: May give SubQ, IV injection, IV infusion, or intrathecally.

1. Reconstitute 100 mg vial w/5 ml bacteriostatic water for injection w/benzyl alcohol (10 ml for 500 mg vial) to provide concentration of 20 mg/ml and 50 mg/ml, respectively.
2. Dose may be further diluted w/up to 1,000 ml 5% dextrose or 0.9% NaCl for IV infusion.
3. For intrathecal use, reconstitute vial w/preservative-free 0.9% NaCl or pts spinal fluid. Dose usually administered in 5-15 ml of solution, after equivalent volume of CSF removed.

INDICATIONS/DOSAGE/ROUTES

NOTE: Dosage individualized based on clinical response, tolerance to adverse effects. When used in combination therapy, consult specific protocols for optimum dosage, sequence of drug administration. Modify dose when serious hematologic depression occurs.

Acute nonlymphocytic leukemia:
IV INFUSION: Adults, children: (Combination): 100 mg/m^2/day, days 1 to 7.
IV: Adults: 100 mg/m^2 q12h, days 1-7.

Acute lymphocytic leukemia:
Refer to specific protocol.

Refractory acute leukemia:
IV: Adults: 3 Gm/m^2 q12h for 4-12 doses; repeat at 2-3 wk intervals.
INTRATHECAL: Adults: 5-75 mg/m^2/day for 4 days or once q 4 days, or 30 mg/m^2 once q 4 days until CSF findings normal, followed by one additional dose.

PRECAUTIONS

CONTRAINDICATIONS: None significant. **CAUTIONS:** Impaired hepatic function. **PREGNANCY/LACTATION:** If possible, avoid use during pregnancy, especially first trimester. May cause fetal harm. Unknown if distributed in breast milk. Breast feeding not recommended. **Pregnancy Category D.**

INTERACTIONS

DRUG INTERACTIONS: May decrease effect of antigout medications. Bone marrow depressants may increase bone marrow depression. Cyclophosphamide may increase cardiomyopathy. Live virus vaccines may potentiate virus replication, increase vaccine side effects, decrease patients antibody response to vaccine. **ALTERED LAB VALUES:** May increase SGOT (AST), bilirubin, alkaline phosphatase, uric acid.

SIDE EFFECTS

FREQUENT: Nausea and vomiting, particularly after IV injection rather than continuous IV infusion. **OCCASIONAL:** Diarrhea, anorexia, oral/anal inflammation, peripheral motor and sensory neuropathies w/high-dose therapy, abdominal pain, esophagitis, nausea, vomiting, fever, transient headache w/intrathecal administration.

ADVERSE REACTIONS/TOXIC EFFECTS

Major toxic effect is hematologic toxicity (leukopenia, anemia, thrombocytopenia, megaloblastosis, reticulocytopenia), occurring minimally after single IV dose, but leukopenia, anemia, thrombocytopenia should be expected w/daily or continuous IV. Cytarabine syndrome (fever, myalgia, rash conjunctivitis, malaise, chest pain), hyperuricemia may be noted. High-dose therapy may produce severe CNS, GI, pulmonary toxicity.

NURSING IMPLICATIONS

BASELINE ASSESSMENT:

Obtain WBC, platelet count before and periodically during therapy. Leukocyte count decreases within 24 hrs after initial dose, continues to decrease for 7-9 days followed by brief rise at 12 days, then decreases again at 15-24 days, then rises rapidly for next 10 days. Platelet count decreases 5 days after drug initiation to low count at 12-15 days, then rises rapidly for next 10 days.

INTERVENTION/EVALUATION:

Monitor WBC, differential, platelet count for evidence of bone marrow depression. Monitor for hematologic toxicity (fever, sore throat, signs of local infection, easy bruising, or unusual bleeding from any site), symptoms of anemia (excessive tiredness, weakness). Monitor for signs of neuropathy (gait disturbances, handwriting difficulties, numbness).

PATIENT/FAMILY TEACHING:

Increase fluid intake (may protect against hyperuricemia). Do not have immunizations w/o physician's approval (drug lowers body's resistance). Avoid contact w/those who have recently received live virus vaccine. Promptly report fever, sore throat, signs of local infection, easy bruising, or unusual bleeding from any site. Contact physician if nausea/vomiting continues at home.

dacarbazine

day-car´bah-zeen
(DTIC-Dome)

CANADIAN AVAILABILITY:
DTIC

CLASSIFICATION

Antineoplastic

PHARMACOKINETICS

Minimally crosses blood-brain barrier. Protein binding: low. Metabolized in liver. Excreted in urine. Half-life: 5 hrs (increased in decreased renal function).

ACTION

Cell-cycle phase nonspecific. May inhibit DNA, RNA synthesis.

USES

Treatment of metastatic malignant melanoma, refractory Hodgkin's disease.

STORAGE/HANDLING

NOTE: May be carcinogenic, mutagenic, or teratogenic. Handle w/ extreme care during preparation/ administration.

Protect from light; refrigerate vials. Color change from ivory to pink indicates decomposition; discard. Solutions containing 10 mg/ ml stable for 8 hrs at room temperature or 72 hrs if refrigerated. Solutions diluted w/up to 500 ml 5% dextrose or 0.9% NaCl stable for at least 8 hrs at room temperature or 24 hrs if refrigerated.

IV ADMINISTRATION

NOTE: May give by IV injection or IV infusion.

1. Reconstitute 100 mg vial w/ 9.9 ml sterile water for injection (19.7 ml for 200 mg vial) to provide concentration of 10 mg/ml.
2. Give IV injection over 1-2 min.
3. For IV infusion, further dilute w/up to 250 ml 5% dextrose or 0.9% NaCl. Infuse over 15-30 min.
4. Apply hot packs to relieve local pain, burning sensation, irritation at injection site.
5. Avoid extravasation (stinging, swelling, coolness, slight or no blood return at injection site).

INDICATIONS/DOSAGE/ROUTES

NOTE: Dosage individualized based on clinical response, tolerance to adverse effects. When used in combination therapy, consult specific protocols for optimum dosage, sequence of drug administration.

Malignant melanoma:

IV: Adults, elderly: 2-4.5 mg/kg/ day for 10 days, repeated at 4 wk intervals, or 250 mg/m^2 daily for 5 days, repeated q 3 wks.

Hodgkin's disease:

IV: Adults, elderly: Combination therapy: 150 mg/m^2 daily for 5 days, repeated q 4 wks, or 375 mg/ m^2 once, repeated q 15 days.

PRECAUTIONS

CONTRAINDICATIONS: Demonstrated hypersensitivity to drug. **CAUTIONS:** Impaired hepatic function. **PREGNANCY/LACTATION:** If possible, avoid use during pregnancy, especially first trimester. Breast feeding not recommended. **Pregnancy Category C.**

INTERACTIONS

DRUG INTERACTIONS: Bone marrow depressants may enhance myelosuppresion. Live virus vaccines may potentiate virus replication, increase vaccine side effects, decrease pt's antibody response to vaccine. **ALTERED LAB VALUES:** May increase SGOT (AST), SGPT (ALT), alkaline phosphatase, BUN.

SIDE EFFECTS

HIGH INCIDENCE: Nausea, vomiting, anorexia (occurs within 1 hr of initial dose, may last up to 12 hrs). **OCCASIONAL:** Facial flushing, paresthesia, alopecia, flulike syndrome (fever, myalgia, malaise), dermatologic reactions, CNS symptoms (confusion, blurred vision, headache, lethargy). **RARE:** Diarrhea, stomatitis, intractable nausea and vomiting, photosensitivity reaction.

ADVERSE REACTIONS/TOXIC EFFECTS

Bone marrow depression resulting in hematologic toxicity (leukopenia, thrombocytopenia) generally appears 2-4 wks after last drug dose. Hepatotoxicity occurs rarely.

NURSING IMPLICATIONS

BASELINE ASSESSMENT:

Some clinicians recommend food/fluids be restricted 4-6 hrs before treatment; other clinicians believe good hydration to within 1 hr of treatment will avoid dehydration due to vomiting. Conflicting reports of effectiveness of administering antiemetics for nausea, vomiting.

INTERVENTION/EVALUATION:

Monitor leukocyte, erythrocyte, platelet counts for evidence of bone marrow depression. Monitor for hematologic toxicity (fever, sore throat, signs of local infection, easy bruising, unusual bleeding from any site).

PATIENT/FAMILY TEACHING:

Tolerance to GI effects occurs rapidly (generally after 1-2 days treatment). Do not have immunizations w/o physician's approval (drug lowers body's resistance). Avoid contact w/those who have recently received live virus vaccine. Promptly report fever, sore throat, signs of local infection, easy bruising, unusual bleeding from any site. Contact physician if nausea/vomiting continues at home.

dactinomycin

dak-tin-oh-my'sin

(Cosmegen)

CANADIAN AVAILABILITY:
Cosmegen

CLASSIFICATION

Antineoplastic

PHARMACOKINETICS

Widely distributed. Does not cross blood-brain barrier. Extensive tissue binding. Primarily eliminated via biliary/fecal route. Half-life: 36 hrs.

ACTION

Inhibits DNA-dependent RNA synthesis by forming DNA-complex. Actively growing cells are most sensitive to drug's action. Cell cycle phase nonspecific.

USES

Treatment of Wilms' tumor, rhabdomyosarcoma, Ewing's sarcoma, advanced nonseminomatous testicular carcinoma, sarcoma botryoides, metastatic, and nonmetastatic choriocarcinoma.

STORAGE/HANDLING

NOTE: May be carcinogenic, mutagenic, or teratogenic. Handle w/ extreme care during preparation/administration.

Prepare solution immediately before use. Discard unused portion. Solution should be clear, gold color.

IV ADMINISTRATION

NOTE: Give by IV injection or IV infusion. Wear protective gloves when handling drug.

1. Reconstitute 500 mcg vial w/ 1.1 ml sterile water for injection w/o preservative (avoids precipitate) to provide concentration of 500 mcg/ml.
2. For IV injection, administer over 1-3 min into tubing of running IV. Withdraw dose from vial w/one

needle, use 2nd needle for injection.

3. For IV infusion, add up to 50 ml 5% dextrose or 0.9% NaCl and infuse over 20-30 min.

4. Extravasation usually produces immediate pain, severe local tissue damage. Aspirate as much infiltrated drug as possible, then infiltrate area w/hydrocortisone, sodium succinate injection (50-100 mg hydrocortisone) and/or isotonic sodium thiosulfate injection or ascorbic acid injection (1 ml of 5% injection). Apply cold compresses.

INDICATIONS/DOSAGE/ROUTES

NOTE: Dosage is individualized based on clinical response and tolerance to adverse effects. When used in combination therapy, consult specific protocols for optimum dosage and sequence of drug administration. Do not exceed 15 mcg/kg or 400-600 mcg/m^2/day. Dosage for obese or edematous pts based on surface area. Repeat dosage at least at 3 wk intervals, provided all signs of toxicity have disappeared.

Usual dosage:
IV: Adults, elderly: 500 mcg/day for maximum of 5 days. **Children:** 15 mcg/kg/day (up to maximum of 500 mcg/day) for 5 days, or total dosage of 2.5 mg/m^2 in divided doses over 1 wk.
ISOLATION PERFUSION:
Adults, elderly: 50 mcg/kg for lower extremity or pelvis; 35 mcg/kg for upper extremity.

PRECAUTIONS

CONTRAINDICATIONS: Those w/chickenpox or herpes zoster. **CAUTIONS:** Within first 2 mo of radiation therapy. **PREGNANCY/LACTATION:** If possible, avoid use during pregnancy, especially first trimester. Breast feeding not recommended. **Pregnancy Category C.**

D

INTERACTIONS

DRUG INTERACTIONS: May decrease effect of antigout medications. Bone marrow depressants may enhance myelosuppression. Live virus vaccines may potentiate virus replication, increase vaccine side effects, decrease pt's antibody response to vaccine. **ALTERED LAB VALUES:** May increase uric acid.

SIDE EFFECTS

FREQUENT: Nausea, vomiting, buccal/pharangeal/skin erythema, rash (particularly when combined with radiation). **OCCASIONAL:** Anorexia, alopecia, abdominal distress.

ADVERSE REACTIONS/TOXIC EFFECTS

Bone marrow depression resulting in hematologic toxicity (leukopenia, thrombocytopenia, and to lesser extent, anemia, pancytopenia, reticulopenia, agranulocytosis, aplastic anemia). GI and oral mucosal toxicity may result in diarrhea, oral/GI ulceration, stomatitis, glossitis, esophagitis, pharyngitis.

NURSING IMPLICATIONS

BASELINE ASSESSMENT:

Obtain baseline hematologic results. Nausea/vomiting occurs a few hours after dosing, can last up to 24 hrs. Decrease in platelet count generally appears 1-7 days after last drug dose, reaches lowest count at 14-21 days, returns to normal within 21-25 days.

INTERVENTION/EVALUATION:

Monitor hematologic status, renal/hepatic function studies, serum uric acid level. Assess pattern of daily bowel activity and stool consistency. Monitor for hematologic toxicity (fever, sore throat, signs of local infection, easy bruising, or unusual bleeding from any site), symptoms of anemia (excessive tiredness, weakness). Assess skin for dermatologic effects.

PATIENT/FAMILY TEACHING:

Alopecia is reversible, but new hair growth may have different color or texture. Pain, redness may occur at injection site. Do not have immunizations w/o physician's approval (drug lowers body's resistance). Avoid contact w/those who have recently received live virus vaccine. Promptly report fever, sore throat, signs of local infection, easy bruising, unusual bleeding from any site. Increase fluid intake. Contact physician if nausea/vomiting continues at home.

dalteparin (Fragmin)
See supplement

danazol

da´nah-zole
(Danocrine)

CANADIAN AVAILABILITY:
Cyclomen

CLASSIFICATION

Gonadotropin inhibitor

PHARMACOKINETICS

Metabolized in liver. Excreted in urine. Half-life: 4.5 hrs.

ACTION

Gonadotropin inhibitor that suppresses the pituitary-ovarian axis by inhibiting the output of pituitary gonadotropins. Follicle-stimulating hormone (FSH) and luteinizing hormone (LH) are depressed, reducing the ovarian production of estrogen. Causes atrophy of both normal and ectopic endometrial tissue, anovulation, and amenorrhea. Inhibits sex steroid synthesis and binding of steroids to their receptors in target tissues. Increases serum levels of C1 esterase inhibitor, causing increased serum levels of the C4 component of the complement system.

USES

Palliative treatment of endometriosis, fibrocystic breast disease; prophylactic treatment of hereditary angioedema.

INDICATIONS/DOSAGE/ROUTES

NOTE: Initiate therapy during menstruation or when pt not pregnant.

Endometriosis:
PO: Adults: 200-800 mg/day in 2 divided doses for 3-9 mo.

Fibrocystic breast disease:
PO: Adults: 100-400 mg/day in 2 divided doses.

Hereditary angioedema:
PO: Adults: Initially, 200 mg 2-3 times/day. Decrease dose by 50% or less at 1-3 mo intervals. If attack occurs, increase dose by up to 200 mg/day.

PRECAUTIONS

CONTRAINDICATIONS: Hypersensitivity to danazol or ingredients. Undiagnosed abnormal genital bleeding; severe hepatic, renal, or cardiac impairment. **CAUTIONS:** Conditions aggravated by fluid retention (cardiac or renal disease, epilepsy, migraine, asthma). Possibility of carcinoma of the breast should be excluded prior to therapy. **PREGNANCY/LACTATION:** Contraindicated during pregnancy, breast feeding. **Pregnancy Category X.**

INTERACTIONS

DRUG INTERACTIONS: May increase effect of oral anticoagulants. May decrease effect of insulin, oral hypoglycemics. May increase concentration, toxicity of cyclosporine. **ALTERED LAB VALUES:** May increase SGOT (AST), SGPT (ALT), glucose, LDL. May decrease HDL. May alter thyroid function tests.

SIDE EFFECTS

FREQUENT: Edema, acne, oily skin and hair, flushing, sweating, nervousness, emotional lability, fatigue. **OCCASIONAL:** Vaginitis (itching, dryness, burning, vaginal bleeding), hirsutism, deepening of the voice, decreased breast size, decreased testicular size, muscle cramps or spasms, sleep disorders, appetite changes. **RARE:** Enlarged clitoris, testicular atrophy, hepatic dysfunction.

ADVERSE REACTIONS/TOXIC EFFECTS

Jaundice may occur in those receiving 400 mg/day or more.

NURSING IMPLICATIONS

BASELINE ASSESSMENT:

Inquire about menstrual cycle; therapy should begin during menstruation. Establish baseline weight, B/P.

INTERVENTION/EVALUATION:

Weigh 2-3 times/week; report >5 lb/wk gain or swelling of fingers or feet. Monitor B/P periodically. Check for jaundice (yellow eyes or skin, dark urine, clay-colored stools).

PATIENT/FAMILY TEACHING:

Patient should use nonhormonal contraceptive during therapy. Do not take drug, check w/physician if suspect pregnancy (risk to fetus). Importance of full length of therapy, regular visits to physician office (hepatic function tests, etc.). Notify physician promptly of masculinizing effects (may not be reversible), weight gain, muscle cramps, or fatigue. Spotting or bleeding may occur in first months of therapy for endometriosis (does not mean lack of efficacy). In fibrocystic breast disease, irregular menstrual periods and amenorrhea may occur w/or w/o ovulation.

dantrolene sodium

dan´trow-lean

(Dantrium)

CANADIAN AVAILABILITY:
Dantrium

CLASSIFICATION

Skeletal muscle relaxant

PHARMACOKINETICS

Poorly absorbed from GI tract. Metabolized in liver. Primarily excreted in urine. Half-life: IV 4-8 hrs; oral 8.7 hrs.

ACTION

Reduces muscle contraction by direct action, dissociating excitation-contraction coupling. Interferes w/release of calcium, prevents increase in myoplasmic calcium which activates catabolic process associated w/malignant hyperthermic crisis.

USES

Oral: Relief of signs and symptoms of spasticity due to spinal cord injuries, stroke, cerebral palsy, multiple sclerosis, especially flexor spasms, concomitant pain, clonus, and muscular rigidity. *Parenteral:* Management of fulminant hypermetabolism of skeletal muscle due to malignant hyperthermia crisis.

STORAGE/HANDLING

Store oral, parenteral form at room temperature. Use within 6 hrs after reconstitution. Solution is clear, colorless. Discard if cloudy, precipitate formed.

PO/IV ADMINISTRATION

PO:

Give w/o regard to meals.

IV:

1. Diligently monitor for extravasation (high pH of IV preparation). May produce severe complications.
2. Reconstitute 20 mg vial w/60 ml sterile water for injection to provide concentration of 0.33 mg/ml.
3. For IV infusion, administer over 1 hr.

INDICATIONS/DOSAGE/ROUTES

Spasticity:
NOTE: Best to begin w/low-dose therapy, then increase gradually at 4-7 day intervals (reduces incidence of side effects).
PO: Adults, elderly: Initially, 25 mg/day. Increase to 25 mg 2-4 times/day, then by 25 mg increments up to 100 mg 2-4 times/day. **Children >5 yrs:** Initially, 0.5 mg/kg 2 times/day. Increase to 0.5 mg/kg 3-4 times/day, then increase by 0.5 mg/kg/day up to 3 mg/kg 2-4 times/day.

Prevention of malignant hyperthermia crisis:
PO: Adults, elderly, children: 4-8 mg/kg/day in 3-4 divided doses 1-2 days prior to surgery (last dose 3-4 hrs prior to surgery).
IV INFUSION: Adults, elderly, children: 2.5 mg/kg about 1.25 hrs prior to surgery.

Management of hyperthermia crisis:
IV: Adults, elderly, children: Initially (minimum) 1 mg/kg rapid IV; may repeat up to total maximum dose of 10 mg/kg. May follow w/ 4-8 mg/kg/day orally in 4 divided doses up to 3 days after crisis.

PRECAUTIONS

CONTRAINDICATIONS: *Oral:* Active liver disease (i.e., hepatitis, cirrhosis), when spasticity is needed to maintain upright posture and balance when walking or to achieve or support increased function, severely impaired cardiac function, previous liver disease/dysfunction. **CAUTIONS:** Females, those >35 years of age, impaired liver, or pulmonary function. **PREGNANCY/LACTATION:** Readily crossed placenta; do not use in breast-feeding mothers. **Pregnancy Category C.**

INTERACTIONS

DRUG INTERACTIONS: CNS depressants may increase CNS depression (short-term use). Hepatotoxic medications may increase risk of hepatotoxicity (chronic use). **ALTERED LAB VALUES:** May alter liver function tests.

SIDE EFFECTS

NOTE: Effects are generally transient and appears during early treatment.
FREQUENT: Drowsiness, dizzi-

ness, weakness, general malaise, diarrhea. **OCCASIONAL:** Fatigue, confusion, headache, insomnia, constipation, urinary frequency. **RARE:** Paradoxical CNS excitement/restlessness, paresthesia, tinnitus, slurred speech, tremor, blurred vision, dry mouth, diarrhea, nocturia, impotence.

ADVERSE REACTIONS/TOXIC EFFECTS

Risk of hepatotoxicity, most notably in females, those >35 years of age, those taking other medications concurrently. Overt hepatitis noted most frequently between 3rd and 12th mo of therapy. Overdosage results in vomiting, muscular hypotonia, muscle twitching, respiratory depression, seizures.

NURSING IMPLICATIONS

Baseline Assessment:

Obtain baseline liver function tests (SGOT [AST], SGPT [ALT], alkaline phosphatase, total bilirubin). Record onset, type, location, and duration of muscular spasm. Check for immobility, stiffness, swelling.

Intervention/Evaluation:

Assist w/ambulation at all times. For those on long-term therapy, liver/renal function tests, blood counts should be performed periodically. Evaluate for therapeutic response: decreased intensity of skeletal muscle pain.

Patient/Family Teaching:

Drowsiness usually diminishes w/continued therapy. Avoid tasks that require alertness, motor skills until response to drug is established. Avoid alcohol or other depressants while taking medication. Avoid sudden changes in posture.

dapiprazole hydrochloride

day-pip′rah-zoll
(Rev-Eyes)

CLASSIFICATION

Miotic

ACTION

Blocks the alpha-adrenergic receptors in smooth muscle; effect on dilator muscle of the iris produces miosis.

USES

Treatment of iatrogenically induced mydriasis produced by adrenergic (phenylephrine) or parasympatholytic (tropicamide) agents.

STORAGE/HANDLING

After reconstitution, stable at room temperature for 21 days. Discard any solution not clear and colorless.

OPHTHALMIC ADMINISTRATION

1. For topical ophthalmic use only.
2. Tear off aluminum seals, remove and discard rubber plugs from both drug and diluent vials. Pour diluent into drug vial. Remove dropper assembly from its wrapping without touching any surface and attach to drug vial. Shake container for 2-3 min until solution clear.
3. Do not use unless solution is clear and colorless.

4. Instruct pt to tilt head backward and look up.

5. Gently pull lower lid down to form pouch and instill medication.

6. Do not touch tip of applicator to lids or any surface.

7. When release lower lid, have pt keep eye open w/o blinking for at least 30 sec.

8. Apply gentle finger pressure to lacrimal sac (bridge of the nose, inside corner of the eye) for 1-2 min.

9. Remove excess solution around eye w/tissue. Wash hands immediately to remove medication on hands.

10. Administer additional drops 5 min later.

11. Do not use in same pt more often than once a week.

INDICATIONS/DOSAGE/ROUTES

Usual ophthalmic dosage:
OPHTHALMIC: Adults: 2 drops followed in 5 min w/additional 2 drops topically to conjunctiva of each eye after ophthalmic exam.

PRECAUTIONS

CONTRAINDICATIONS: When constriction undesirable, e.g., acute iritis; hypersensitivity to any component of preparation. Safety and efficacy in children not established. **PREGNANCY/LACTATION:** Use in pregnancy only if clearly needed. Excretion in breast milk unknown. **Pregnancy Category B.**

INTERACTIONS

DRUG INTERACTIONS: None significant. **ALTERED LAB VALUES:** None significant.

SIDE EFFECTS

FREQUENT: 80% or more of pts experience conjunctival irritation lasting 20 min; 50% have burning on instillation. From 10-40% of pts have ptosis, lid erythema, lid edema, chemosis, itching, photophobia, corneal edema, headache/browache, punctate keratitis. **OCCASIONAL:** Dryness of eyes, tearing, blurred vision.

ADVERSE REACTIONS/TOXIC EFFECTS

None significant.

NURSING IMPLICATIONS

INTERVENTION/EVALUATION:

Assess for side effects (see Effects).

PATIENT/FAMILY TEACHING:

Do not drive or engage in activity requiring visual acuity until adequate vision has been regained.

daunorubicin hydrochloride

dawn-oh-rue´bih-sin
(Cerubidine)

CANADIAN AVAILABILITY:
Cerubidine

CLASSIFICATION

Antineoplastic

PHARMACOKINETICS

Widely distributed. Does not cross blood-brain barrier. Metabolized in liver to active metabolite. Excreted in urine, eliminated by biliary excretion. Half-life: 18.5 hrs; metabolite: 55 hrs.

ACTION

Cell cycle-phase nonspecific. Most active in S phase of cell division. May bind to DNA, inhibit DNA, RNA synthesis.

USES

Remission induction in acute nonlymphocytic leukemia (myelogenous, monocytic, erythroid) of adults; acute lymphocytic leukemia of both children and adults.

STORAGE/HANDLING

NOTE: May be carcinogenic, mutagenic, or teratogenic. Handle w/ extreme care during preparation/ administration.

Reconstituted solution stable for 24 hrs at room temperature or 48 hrs if refrigerated. Color change from red to blue-purple indicates decomposition; discard.

IV ADMINISTRATION

NOTE: Give by IV injection, or IV infusion. IV infusion not recommended due to vein irritation, risk of thrombophlebitis. Avoid small veins, swollen or edematous extremities, areas overlying joints and tendons.

1. Reconstitute each 20 mg vial w/4 ml sterile water for injection to provide concentration of 5 mg/ ml.
2. Gently agitate vial until completely dissolved.
3. For IV injection, withdraw desired dose into syringe containing 10-15 ml 0.9% NaCl. Inject over 2-3 min into tubing of running IV solution of 5% dextrose or 0.9% NaCl.
4. For IV infusion, further dilute w/100 ml 5% dextrose or 0.9% NaCl. Infuse over 30-45 min.
5. Extravasation produces immediate pain, severe local tissue damage. Aspirate as much infiltrated drug as possible, then infiltrate area w/hydrocortisone sodium succinate injection (50-100 mg hydrocortisone) and/or isotonic sodium thiosulfate injection or ascorbic acid injection (1 ml of 5% injection). Apply cold compresses.

D

INDICATIONS/DOSAGE/ROUTES

NOTE: Dosage individualized based on clinical response, tolerance to adverse effects. When used in combination therapy, consult specific protocols for optimum dosage, sequence of drug administration. Do not exceed total dosage of 500-600 mg/m^2 in adults, 400-450 mg/m^2 in those who received irradiation of cardiac region, 300 mg/m^2 in children >2 yrs, 10 mg/kg in children <2 yrs (increases risk of cardiotoxicity). Reduce dosage in those w/liver and/ or renal impairment. Use body weight to calculate dose in children <2 yrs or surface area <0.5 m^2.

Acute nonlymphocytic leukemia (induction remission):
IV: Adults <60 yrs: Combined w/ cytosine: 45 mg/m^2/day for 3 successive days for first course of induction therapy. Give 45 mg/m^2/ day for 2 successive days on subsequent courses. **Adults >60 yrs:** 30 mg/m^2/day following same dosage regimen as above.

Acute lymphocytic leukemia (induction remission):
IV: Adults, elderly: Combination therapy: 45 mg/m^2/day first 3 days of induction therapy. **Children:** 25 mg/m^2 on day 1 q wk.

PRECAUTIONS

CONTRAINDICATIONS: None significant. **EXTREME CAUTION:** Preexisting bone marrow depression. **PREGNANCY/LACTATION:** If possible, avoid use during pregnancy, especially first trimester. May cause fetal harm. Breast feeding not recommended. **Pregnancy Category D.**

INTERACTIONS

DRUG INTERACTIONS: May decrease effect of antigout medications. Bone marrow depressants may enhance myelosuppression. Live virus vaccines may potentiate virus replication, increase vaccine side effects, decrease pt's antibody response to vaccine. **ALTERED LAB VALUES:** May increase serum bilirubin, SGOT (AST) and alkaline phosphatase levels. May raise blood uric acid level.

SIDE EFFECTS

FREQUENT: Complete alopecia (scalp, axillary, pubic hair), nausea, vomiting begins a few hours after administration, lasts 24-48 hrs. **OCCASIONAL:** Diarrhea, abdominal pain, esophagitis, stomatitis, transverse pigmentation of fingernails/toenails. **RARE:** Transient fever, chills.

ADVERSE REACTIONS/TOXIC EFFECTS

Bone marrow depression manifested as hematologic toxicity (generally severe leukopenia, anemia, thrombocytopenia). Decrease in platelet count, WBC occurs in 10-14 days, returns to normal level by third week.

Cardiotoxicity noted as either acute, transient, abnormal EKG findings and/or cardiomyopathy manifested as CHF (risk increases when cumulative dose exceeds 550 mg/m^2 in adults and 300 mg/m^2 in children >2 yrs, or total dosage more than 10 mg/kg in children <2 yrs).

NURSING IMPLICATIONS

BASELINE ASSESSMENT:

Obtain WBC, platelet, erythrocyte counts prior to and at frequent intervals during therapy. EKG should be obtained prior to therapy. Antiemetics may be effective in preventing, treating nausea.

INTERVENTION/EVALUATION:

Monitor for stomatitis (burning, erythema of oral mucosa). May lead to ulceration within 2-3 days. Assess skin, nailbeds for hyperpigmentation. Monitor hematologic status, renal/hepatic function studies, serum uric acid level. Assess pattern of daily bowel activity and stool consistency. Monitor for hematologic toxicity (fever, sore throat, signs of local infection, easy bruising, or unusual bleeding from any site), symptoms of anemia (excessive tiredness, weakness).

PATIENT/FAMILY TEACHING:

Urine may turn reddish color for 1-2 days after beginning therapy. Alopecia is reversible, but new hair growth may have different color or texture. New hair growth resumes about 5 wks after last therapy dose. Maintain fastidious oral hygiene. Do not have immunizations w/o physician's approval (drug lowers body's resistance). Avoid contact w/those who have recently received live virus vaccine. Promptly report fever, sore throat, signs of local infection, easy bruising, or unusual bleeding from any site. Increase fluid intake (may protect against hyperuricemia). Contact physician if nausea/vomiting continues at home.

deferoxamine mesylate

deaf-er-ox′ah-meen
(Desferal Mesylate)

CANADIAN AVAILABILITY:
Desferal

CLASSIFICATION

Antidote

PHARMACOKINETICS

Well absorbed after IM, SubQ administration. Widely distributed. Rapidly metabolized in tissues, plasma. Excreted in urine, eliminated in feces via biliary excretion. Removed by hemodialysis. Half-life: 6 hrs.

ACTION

Promotes excretion of acute iron poisoning by binding w/iron to form complex excreted in urine.

USES

Treatment of acute iron poisoning, chronic iron overload due to multiple transfusions.

STORAGE/HANDLING

Store parenteral powder at room temperature.

IM/SubQ/IV ADMINISTRATION

NOTE: Reconstitute each 500 mg vial w/2 ml sterile water to provide a concentration of 250 mg/ml.

SubQ:

1. Administer SubQ very slowly, may give undiluted.

IM:

1. Inject deeply into upper outer quadrant of buttock.
2. May give undiluted.

IV:

1. For IV infusion, further dilute w/0.9% NaCl, 5% dextrose, and administer at maximum rate of 15 mg/kg/hr.
2. A too-rapid IV administration may produce skin flushing, urticaria, hypotension, shock.

INDICATIONS/DOSAGE/ROUTES

NOTE: IM administration is preferred route; use except in cases of shock. Use IV administration only for those in cardiovascular collapse.

Acute iron intoxication:
IM/IV: Adults: Children: Initially, 1 Gm, then 500 mg q4h for 2 doses. May give subsequent doses of 500 mg q4-12h. **Maximum:** 6 Gm/day.

Chronic iron overload:
SubQ: Adults: Children: 1-2 Gm/day (20-40 mg/kg) over 8-24 hrs.
IM: Adults: Children: 0.5-1 Gm/day. Give 2 Gm w/but separate from, each unit of blood.

PRECAUTIONS

CONTRAINDICATIONS: Severe renal disease, anuria, primary hemochromatosis. **CAUTIONS:** None significant. **PREGNANCY/LACTATION:** Unknown if drug crosses placenta or is distributed in breast milk. Use only when absolutely necessary. Skeletal anomalies may present in neonate. **Pregnancy Category C.**

INTERACTIONS

DRUG INTERACTIONS: Vitamin C may increase effect. **ALTERED LAB VALUES:** None significant.

SIDE EFFECTS

OCCASIONAL: *IM, SubQ:* Pain, induration at injection site. **RARE:** *Long-term therapy:* Cataracts, impaired peripheral, color, and night vision; generalized itching, rash, blurred vision, abdominal discomfort, diarrhea, leg cramps. *SubQ therapy:* Pruritus, erythema, skin irritation, and swelling.

ADVERSE REACTIONS/TOXIC EFFECTS

Neurotoxicity, including high-frequency hearing loss, has been noted.

NURSING IMPLICATIONS

BASELINE ASSESSMENT:

Inform pt injection may produce discomfort at IM or SubQ injection site. Assess serum iron levels, iron binding capacity before and during therapy.

INTERVENTION/EVALUATION:

Question pt for evidence of hearing loss (neurotoxicity). Periodic slit-lamp ophthalmic exams should be obtained in those treated for chronic iron overload. If using SubQ technique, monitor for pruritus, erythema, skin irritation, and swelling.

PATIENT/FAMILY TEACHING:

Urine will appear reddish. Discomfort may occur at site of injection.

demecarium bromide

dem-eh-kare´ee-um

(Humorsol)

CLASSIFICATION

Miotic

PHARMACOKINETICS

	ONSET	PEAK	DURATION
OPHTH (Miosis)	15-60 min	2-4 hrs	3-10 days

Maximum reduction in IOP occurs within 24 hrs, and reduced IOP persists for at least 9 days.

ACTION

Prolongs effect of acetylcholine by inactivating cholinesterase causing constriction of iris sphincter muscle (miosis) and ciliary muscle. Improved aqueous humor outflow produces decreased IOP.

USES

Treatment of open-angle glaucoma and conditions obstructing aqueous outflow (e.g., synechial formation) that are responsive to miotic therapy; following iridectomy; in accommodative esotropia (convergent strabismus).

OPHTHALMIC ADMINISTRATION

1. For topical ophthalmic use only.
2. Administer at bedtime to reduce side effects.
3. Instruct pt to tilt head backward and look up.
4. Gently pull lower lid down to form pouch and instill medication.
5. Do not touch tip of applicator to lids or any surface.
6. When release lower lid, have pt keep eye open w/o blinking for at least 30 sec.
7. Apply gentle finger pressure to lacrimal sac (bridge of the nose, inside corner of the eye) for 1-2 min.
8. Remove excess solution around eye w/tissue. Wash hands immediately to remove medication on hands.

INDICATIONS/DOSAGE/ROUTES

Glaucoma:
OPHTHALMIC: Adults, elderly: Initially, 1-2 drops. **Children:** Initially, 1 drop. **Range:** 1-2 drops 2 times/wk, up to 1-2 drops 2 times/day.

Accommodative esotropia:
NOTE: Equal visual acuity of both eyes necessary for successful treatment.
OPHTHALMIC: Adults, children: (Diagnosis): 1 drop daily for 2 wks; then 1 drop q2days for 2-3 wks.
OPHTHALMIC: Adults: (Treatment): 1 drop both eyes daily for 2-3 wks; then 1 drop every other day for 3-4 wks. Reevaluate pt. Continue w/1 drop q2days or 2 times/wk. Evaluate q4-12wks. If improvement continues, 1 drop/wk; then no medication. If after 4 months, still giving 1 drop q2days, discontinue therapy.

PRECAUTIONS

CONTRAINDICATIONS: Hypersensitivity to cholinesterase inhibitors or any component of the preparation; active uveal inflammation; angle-closure (narrow-angle) glaucoma; glaucoma associated w/iridocyclitis. **CAUTIONS:** Bronchial asthma, gastrointestinal disturbances, peptic ulcer, bradycardia, hypotension, recent myocardial infarction, epilepsy, parkinsonism, and other disorders that may respond adversely to vagotonic effects. **PREGNANCY/LACTATION:** Contraindicated during pregnancy. Discontinue nursing during demecarium therapy. **Pregnancy Category X.**

INTERACTIONS

DRUG INTERACTIONS: Anticholinergics, antimyasthenics, cholinesterase inhibitors may increase toxicity. **ALTERED LAB VALUES:** None significant.

SIDE EFFECTS

FREQUENT: Stinging, burning, tearing, painful ciliary or accommodative spasm, blurred vision or myopia, poor vision in dim light. **OCCASIONAL:** Iris cysts (more frequent in children), increased visibility of floaters, headache, browache, photophobia, ocular pain, hypersensitivity reactions (including allergic conjunctivitis, dermatitis, or keratitis), potential hemorrhage during ocular surgery. **RARE:** Lens opacities, paradoxical increase in intraocular pressure, acute fibrinous iritis.

ADVERSE REACTIONS/TOXIC EFFECTS

Systemic toxicity, retinal detachment may occur.

NURSING IMPLICATIONS

INTERVENTION/EVALUATION:

Be alert for systemic toxicity: severe nausea, vomiting, diarrhea, frequent urination, excessive salivation, bradycardia (may trigger asthma attack in asthmatics). Assess vision acuity and provide assistance w/ambulation as needed.

PATIENT/FAMILY TEACHING:

Close observation is necessary for first 24 hrs. Teach proper administration. Do not use more often than directed due to risk of overdosage. Adverse effects often subside after the first few days of therapy. Avoid night driving, activities requiring visual acuity in dim light. Avoid insecticides, pesticides; inhalation or absorption through skin may add to systemic effects of demecarium. Report promptly any systemic effects (see Evaluation) or ocular problems. Inform dentist or physician of demecarium therapy.

demeclocycline hydrochloride

deh-meh-clo-sigh'clean
(Declomycin)

CANADIAN AVAILABILITY:
Declomycin

CLASSIFICATION

Antibiotic: Tetracycline

PHARMACOKINETICS

Readily absorbed from GI tract (food decreases absorption). Widely distributed. Protein binding: 91%. Primarily excreted unchanged in urine. Half-life: 10-17 hrs (increased in decreased renal function).

ACTION

Bacteriostatic due to binding to ribosomes, inhibiting protein synthesis. Inhibits ADH-induced water reabsorption (causes water diuresis).

USES

Treatment of respiratory and urinary tract infections, uncomplicated gonorrhea, brucellosis, rheumatic fever prophylaxis, trachoma, Rocky Mountain spotted fever, typhus, Q fever, rickettsialpox, psittacosis, ornithosis, granuloma inguinale, lymphogranuloma venereum. Treatment of syndrome of inappropriate ADH secretion (SIADH).

PO ADMINISTRATION

Give w/full glass of water 1 hr before or 2 hrs after meals/milk.

INDICATIONS/DOSAGE/ROUTES

NOTE: Space doses evenly around the clock.

Mild to moderate infections:
PO: Adults, elderly: 600 mg/day in 2-4 divided doses. **Children >8 yrs:** 6-12 mg/kg/day in 2-4 divided doses.

Uncomplicated gonorrhea:
PO: Adults: Initially, 600 mg, then 300 mg q12h for 4 days for total of 3 Gm.

Chronic form of SIADH:
PO: Adults, elderly: 600 mg-1.2 Gm/day in 3-4 divided doses, or 3.25-3.75 mg/kg q6h.

PRECAUTIONS

CONTRAINDICATIONS: Hypersensitivity to tetracyclines, last half of pregnancy, infants-8 yrs. **CAUTIONS:** Renal impairment, sun or ultraviolet exposure (severe photosensitivity reaction). **PREGNANCY/LACTATION:** Readily crosses placenta, distributed in breast milk. Avoid use during last half of pregnancy. May produce permanent teeth discoloration, enamel hypoplasia, inhibit fetal skeletal growth in children <8 yrs. **Pregnancy Category D.**

INTERACTIONS

DRUG INTERACTIONS: Antacids containing aluminum/calcium/magnesium, laxatives containing magnesium, oral iron preparations, dairy products impair absorption of tetracyclines (give 1-2 hrs before or after tetracyclines). Cholestyramine, colestipol may decrease absorption. May decrease effect of oral contraceptives. **AL-**

TERED LAB VALUES: May increase BUN, SGOT (AST), SGPT (ALT), aklaline phosphatase, amylase, bilirubin concentrations.

SIDE EFFECTS

FREQUENT: Anorexia, nausea, vomiting, diarrhea, dysphagia, exaggerated sunburn reaction w/ moderate to high dosage. **OCCASIONAL:** Urticaria, rash. Long-term therapy may result in diabetes insipidus syndrome: polydipsia, polyuria, weakness.

ADVERSE REACTIONS/TOXIC EFFECTS

Superinfection (especially fungal), anaphylaxis, increased intracranial pressure, bulging fontanelles occur rarely in infants.

NURSING IMPLICATIONS

BASELINE ASSESSMENT:

Question for history of allergies, especially to tetracyclines. Obtain culture, sensitivity test before giving first dose (therapy may begin before results are known).

INTERVENTION/EVALUATION:

Determine pattern of bowel activity and stool consistency. Check food intake, tolerance. Monitor I&O, renal function test results. Assess for rash. Be alert to superinfection: diarrhea, ulceration or changes of oral mucosa, tongue, anal/genital pruritus. Monitor B/P and LOC because of potential for increased intracranial pressure.

PATIENT/FAMILY TEACHING:

Continue antibiotic for full length of treatment. Space doses evenly. Take oral doses on empty stomach w/full glass of water. Avoid bedtime doses. Notify physician in event of diarrhea, rash, other new symptom. Avoid sun/ultraviolet light exposure. Consult physician before taking any other medication.

D

desipramine hydrochloride

deh-sip´rah-meen
(Norpramin, Pertofrane)

CANADIAN AVAILABILITY:
Norpramin, Pertofrane

CLASSIFICATION

Antidepressant: Tricyclic

PHARMACOKINETICS

Rapid, well absorbed from GI tract. Protein binding: 90-92%. Metabolized in liver. Primarily excreted in urine. Half-life: 12-27 hrs.

ACTION

Increases synaptic concentration of norepinephrine and/or serotonin (inhibits re-uptake by presynaptic membrane), producing antidepressant effect. Strong anticholinergic activity.

USES

Treatment of various forms of depression, often in conjunction w/ psychotherapy.

PO ADMINISTRATION

Give w/food or milk if GI distress occurs.

INDICATIONS/DOSAGE/ROUTES

Depression:
PO: Adults: Initially, 75-150 mg daily as single daily dose, or in divided doses. Gradually increase to lowest effective therapeutic level. Do not exceed 300 mg daily.

Usual elderly dosage:

PO: Elderly: Initially, 75 mg/day in divided doses. May gradually increase to 150-200 mg/day. **Maximum:** 300 mg/day.

PRECAUTIONS

CONTRAINDICATIONS: Acute recovery period following MI, within 14 days of MAO inhibitor ingestion. **CAUTIONS:** Prostatic hypertrophy, history of urinary retention or obstruction, glaucoma, diabetes mellitus, history of seizures, hyperthyroidism, cardiac/hepatic/renal disease, schizophrenia, increased intraocular pressure, hiatal hernia. **PREGNANCY/LACTATION:** Crosses placenta; minimally distributed in breast milk. **Pregnancy Category C.**

INTERACTIONS

DRUG INTERACTIONS: Alcohol, CNS depressants may increase CNS, respiratory depression, hypotensive effects. Antithyroid agents may increase risk of agranulocytosis. Phenothiazines may increase sedative, anticholinergic effects. Cimetidine may increase concentration, toxicity. May decrease effects of clonidine, guanadrel. May increase cardiac effects w/sympathomimetics. May increase risk of hypertensive crisis, hyperpyrexia, convulsions w/MAO inhibitors. Phenytoin may decrease concentrations. **ALTERED LAB VALUES:** May alter ECG readings, glucose.

SIDE EFFECTS

FREQUENT: Drowsiness, fatigue, dry mouth, blurred vision, constipation, delayed micturition, postural hypotension, excessive sweating, disturbed concentration, increased appetite, urinary retention. **OCCASIONAL:** GI disturbances (nausea, GI distress, metallic taste sensation). **RARE:** Paradoxical reaction (agitation, restlessness, nightmares, insomnia), extrapyramidal symptoms (particularly fine hand tremor).

ADVERSE REACTIONS/TOXIC EFFECTS

High dosage may produce cardiovascular effects (severe postural hypotension, dizziness, tachycardia, palpitations, arrhythmias) and seizures. May also result in altered temperature regulation (hyperpyrexia or hypothermia). Abrupt withdrawal from prolonged therapy may produce headache, malaise, nausea, vomiting, vivid dreams.

NURSING IMPLICATIONS

BASELINE ASSESSMENT:

For those on long-term therapy, liver/renal function tests, blood counts should be performed periodically.

INTERVENTION/EVALUATION:

Supervise suicidal-risk pt closely during early therapy (as depression lessens, energy level improves, increasing suicide potential). Assess appearance, behavior, speech pattern, level of interest, mood. Monitor pattern of daily bowel activity and stool consistency. Monitor B/P, pulse for hypotension, arrhythmias. Assess for urinary retention by monitoring I&O and by bladder palpation.

PATIENT/FAMILY TEACHING:

Change positions slowly to avoid hypotensive effect. Tolerance to postural hypotension, sedative, and anticholinergic effects usually develops during early therapy.

Maximum therapeutic effect may be noted in 2-4 wks. Photosensitivity to sun may occur. Dry mouth may be relieved by sugarless gum, or sips of tepid water. Do not abruptly discontinue medication. Report visual disturbances. Avoid tasks that require alertness, motor skills until response to drug is established. Avoid alcohol.

desmopressin

des-moe-press´-in

(DDAVP, Stimate)

CANADIAN AVAILABILITY:
DDAVP

CLASSIFICATION

Antidiuretic

PHARMACOKINETICS

	ONSET	PEAK	DURATION
INTRA-NASAL	0.25 -1 hr	1-5 hrs	5-21 hrs
IV	0.25-0.5 hr	1.5-3 hrs	—

Absorption 10-20% from nasal administration. Metabolized renally. Half-life: 75 minutes.

ACTION

Increases reabsorption of water by increasing permeability of collecting ducts of the kidneys; results in increased urine osmolality, decreased urinary output. Increases plasma factor VIII (antihemophilic factor), plasminogen activator.

USES

DDAVP *Intranasal:* Primary nocturnal enuresis, central cranial diabetes insipidus. *Parenteral:* Central cranial diabetes insipidus, hemophilia A, von Willebrand's disease (type I).

Stimate *Intranasal:* Hemophilia A, von Willebrand's disease (Type I).

STORAGE/HANDLING

Refrigerate nasal solution, injection. Nasal solution stable for up to 3 wks at room temperature.

SubQ/IV/INTRANASAL ADMINISTRATION

1. Evening dosage should consider satisfactory sleep response.
2. Morning and evening doses should be adjusted separately.

IV:

1. For preoperative use, administer 30 min before procedure.
2. Monitor B/P and pulse during IV infusion.
3. IV dose = 1/10 intranasal dose.
4. IV infusion: dilute in 10-50 ml 0.9% NaCl; infuse over 15-30 min.

INTRANASAL:

1. A calibrated catheter (rhinyle) is used to draw up a measured quantity of desmopressin; w/ one end inserted in the nose, the patient blows on the other end to deposit the solution deep in the nasal cavity.
2. For infants, young children, obtunded pts, an air-filled syringe may be attached to the catheter to deposit the solution.

INDICATIONS/DOSAGE/ROUTES

Primary nocturnal enuresis:
INTRANASAL: Adults, elderly: Initially, 20 mcg (0.2 ml) at bedtime (½ dose each nostril). Adjust up to 40 mcg.

Central cranial diabetes insipidus:
INTRANASAL: Adults, elderly:

0.1-0.4 ml/day as single or 2-3 divided doses. **Children (3 mos-12 yrs):** 0.05-0.3 ml/day as single or 2 divided doses.
SubQ/IV: Adults, elderly: 0.5-1 ml/day in 2 divided doses.

Hemophilia A, von Willebrand's disease (Type I):
IV INFUSION: Adults, elderly, children >10 kg: 0.3 mcg/kg diluted in 50 ml 0.9% NaCl. **Children <10 kg:** 0.3 mcg/kg diluted in 10 ml 0.9% NaCl.
INTRANASAL: Adults, elderly >50 kg: 300 mcg (1 spray each nostril). **Adults, elderly <50 kg:** 150 mcg as single spray.

PRECAUTIONS

CONTRAINDICATIONS: Hypersensitivity to desmopressin; type IIB or platelet-type von Willebrand's disease; nasal scarring, blockage, or other impairment w/intranasal administration. **CAUTIONS:** Coronary artery insufficiency, hypertensive cardiovascular disease, infants, and children. **PREGNANCY/LACTATION: Pregnancy Category B.**

INTERACTIONS

DRUG INTERACTIONS: Carbamazepine, chlorpropamide, clofibrate may increase effect. Demeclocycline, lithium, norepinephrine may decrease effect. **ALTERED LAB VALUES:** None significant.

SIDE EFFECTS

OCCASIONAL: Dose related w/ IV: transient headache; nausea; mild abdominal cramps; vulval pain; local erythema, swelling or burning pain at injection site; facial flushing; slight elevation of B/P. **RARE:** Dose related w/intranasal: transient headache, nausea, rhinitis, nasal congestion, flushing, slight elevation of B/P.

ADVERSE REACTIONS/TOXIC EFFECTS

Water intoxication may occur in overhydration; elderly, infants, and children are esp. at risk.

NURSING IMPLICATIONS

BASELINE ASSESSMENT:

Question for hypersensitivity to desmopressin. Establish baselines for B/P, pulse, weight, electrolytes, urine specific gravity. Check lab values for factor VIII coagulant concentration for hemophilia A and von Willebrand's disease; bleeding times, ristocetin cofactor, and Willebrand factor for von Willebrand's disease.

INTERVENTION/EVALUATION:

Monitor I&O closely, restrict intake as necessary to prevent water intoxication. Weigh daily if indicated. Check B/P and pulse q15min during IV administration, 2 times/day for other routes. Monitor electrolytes, urine specific gravity, and other lab results (see Assessment). Evaluate parenteral injection site for erythema, pain. Report side effects to physician for dose reduction. Assess bleeding as appropriate. Check for nasal mucosa changes w/intranasal route. Be alert for early signs of water intoxication: drowsiness, listlessness, headache.

PATIENT/FAMILY TEACHING:

Teach pt/family proper technique for intranasal administration. Report headache, nausea, shortness of breath, or other symptom promptly. Importance of I&O.

desonide

des´-oh´-nide
(Otic Tridesilon, Tridesilon)

CANADIAN AVAILABILITY:
Tridesilon

(See Classifications section under Corticosteroids: Topical)

desoximetasone

deh-sox´eh-meta-sewn
(Topicort)

CANADIAN AVAILABILITY:
Topicort

(See Classifications section under Corticosteroids: Topical)

dexamethasone

dex-a-meth´a-sone
(Decadron, Hexadrol)

dexamethasone acetate

(Dalalone L.A., Decadron L.A., Dexone L.A.)

dexamethasone sodium phosphate

(Decadron, Respihaler)

FIXED-COMBINATION(S):
Dexamethasone phosphate w/ neomycin sulfate, an anti-infective (Neodecadron); dexamethasone sodium phosphate w/lidocaine, a local anesthetic

CANADIAN AVAILABILITY:
Decadron, Dexasone, Hexadrol, Maxidex

CLASSIFICATION

Corticosteroid

PHARMACOKINETICS

Rapid, complete absorption from GI tract, after IM administration. Widely distributed. Protein binding: 69-90%. Metabolized in liver. Primarily excreted in urine. Half-life: 3-4.5 hrs.

ACTION

Decreases/prevents tissue response to inflammatory process. Inhibits accumulation of inflammatory cells at inflammation sites, phagocytosis, lysosomal enzyme release and synthesis and/or release of mediators of inflammation. Prevents/suppresses cell-mediated immune reactions.

USES

Substitution therapy in deficiency states: acute/chronic adrenal insufficiency, congenital adrenal hyperplasia, adrenal insufficiency secondary to pituitary insufficiency.

Nonendocrine disorders: arthritis, rheumatic carditis, allergic, collagen, intestinal tract, liver, ocular, renal, and skin diseases, bronchial asthma, cerebral edema, malignancies.

Ophthalmic: Treatment of responsive inflammatory conditions of palpebral, and bulbar conjunctiva, cornea, and anterior segment of globe. *Nasal:* Allergic/inflammatory nasal conditions and nasal polyps. *Topical:* Relief of inflammatory/pruritic conditions of steroid responsive dermatoses. *Respiratory:* Control bronchial asthma in patients requiring chronic steroid therapy.

PO/IM/IV/TOPICAL/ OPHTHALMIC ADMINISTRATION

PO:

1. Give w/milk or food.

IM:

1. Give deep IM, preferably in gluteus maximus.

IV: Dexamethasone sodium phosphate may be given by direct IV injection or IV infusion.

1. For IV infusion, mix w/0.9% NaCl or 5% dextrose.
2. For neonate, solution must be preservative free.
3. IV solution must be used within 24 hrs.

OPHTHALMIC:

1. Place finger on lower eyelid and pull out until a pocket is formed between eye and lower lid. Hold dropper above pocket and place correct number of drops (¼-½ inch ointment) into pocket. Close eye gently. *Solution:* Apply digital pressure to lacrimal sac for 1-2 min (minimizes drainage into nose and throat, reducing risk of systemic effects). *Ointment:* Close eye for 1-2 min, rolling eyeball (increases contact area of drug to eye). Remove excess solution or ointment around eye w/tissue.
2. Ointment may be used at night to reduce frequency of solution administration.
3. As w/other corticoids, taper dosage slowly when discontinuing.

TOPICAL:

1. Gently cleanse area prior to application.
2. Use occlusive dressings only as ordered.
3. Apply sparingly and rub into area thoroughly.

INDICATIONS/DOSAGE/ROUTES

Dexamethasone, oral:
PO: Adults, elderly: 0.75-9 mg/day.

Dexamethasone acetate:
IM: Adults, elderly: 8-16 mg, may repeat in 1-3 wks.
INTRALESIONAL: Adults, elderly: 0.8-1.6 mg.
INTRA-ARTICULAR AND SOFT TISSUES: Adults, elderly: 4-16 mg; may repeat q1-3wks.

Dexamethasone sodium phosphate:
IM/IV: Adults, elderly: Initially, 0.5-9 mg/day.
INTRA-ARTICULAR, INTRALESIONAL, OR SOFT TISSUE: 0.4-6 mg.

Usual topical dosage:
TOPICAL: Adults, elderly: 2-4 times/day.

Respiratory inhalant:
RESP. INH.: Adults, elderly: 3 inhalations 3-4 times/day; maximum: 12/day. **Children:** 2 inhalations 3-4 times/day; maximum: 8/day.

Usual intranasal dosage:
INTRANASAL: Adults, elderly: 2 sprays each nostril 2-3 times/day; maximum: 12/day. **Children:** 1-2 sprays 2 times/day; maximum 8/day.

PRECAUTIONS

CONTRAINDICATIONS: Hypersensitivity to any corticosteroid or components, systemic fungal infection, peptic ulcers (except life-threatening situations). Avoid live virus vaccine such as smallpox. *Topical:* Marked circulation impairment. Do not instill ocular solutions when topical corticosteroids are being used on eyelids or surrounding skin. **CAUTIONS:** Thromboembolic disorders, history of tuberculosis (may reactivate disease), hypothyroidism, cirrhosis, nonspecific ulcerative colitis, CHF, hypertension, psychosis, renal insufficiency, seizure disorders. Prolonged therapy should be discontinued slowly. *Topical:* Do not apply to extensive areas. **PREGNANCY/LACTATION:** Drug crosses placenta, distributed in breast milk. **Pregnancy Category C.**

INTERACTIONS

DRUG INTERACTIONS: Amphotericin may increase hypokalemia. May decrease effect of oral hypoglycemics, insulin, diuretics, potassium supplements. May increase digoxin toxicity (due to hypokalemia). Hepatic enzyme inducers may decrease effect. Live virus vaccines may potentiate virus replication, increase vaccine side effects, decrease pt's antibody response to vaccine. **ALTERED LAB VALUES:** May decrease calcium, potassium, thyroxine. May increase cholesterol, lipids, glucose, sodium, amylase.

SIDE EFFECTS

FREQUENT: Increased appetite, exaggerated sense of well-being, abdominal distension, weight gain, insomnia, mood swings. *High dose, prolonged therapy:* **FREQUENT:** Increased susceptibility to infection (signs/symptoms masked); delayed wound healing; hypokalemia; hypocalcemia; GI distress; diarrhea or constipation; hypertension. **OCCASIONAL:** Headache, vertigo. *Topical:* Itching, redness, irritation. **RARE:** Increased blood coagulability, tachycardia, frequency or urgency of urination, psychosis. *Topical:* Systemic absorption more likely w/occlusive dressings or extensive application, in young children.

ADVERSE REACTIONS/TOXIC EFFECTS

Long-term therapy: Muscle wasting (esp. arms, legs), osteoporosis, spontaneous fractures, amenorrhea, cataracts, glaucoma, peptic ulcer, CHF. *Abrupt withdrawal following long-term therapy:* Anorexia, nausea, fever, headache, joint pain, rebound inflammation, fatigue, weakness, lethargy, dizziness, orthostatic hypotension.

NURSING IMPLICATIONS

BASELINE ASSESSMENT:

Question for hypersensitivity to any of the corticosteroids, components. Obtain baselines for: height, weight, B/P, glucose, electrolytes. Check results of initial tests, e.g., TB skin test, X-rays, EKG.

INTERVENTION/EVALUATION:

Monitor I&O, daily weight; assess for edema. Check lab results for blood coagulability and clinical evidence of thromboembolism. Evaluate food tolerance and bowel activity; report hyperacidity promptly. Check B/P, temperature, respirations, pulse at least 2 times/day. Be alert to infection: sore throat, fever, or vague symptoms. Monitor electrolytes. Watch for hypercalcemia (muscle twitching, cramps, positive Trousseau's or Chvostek's signs) hypokalemia (weakness and muscle cramps, numbness/tingling esp. lower extremities, nausea and vomiting, irritability, EKG changes). Assess emotional status, ability to sleep. Provide assistance w/ambulation.

PATIENT/FAMILY TEACHING:

Take w/food or milk. Carry identification of drug and dose, physician's name and phone number. Do not change dose/schedule or stop taking drug, must taper off gradually under medical supervision. Notify physician of fever, sore throat, muscle aches, sudden weight gain/swelling. W/dietician give instructions for prescribed diet (usually sodium restricted w/ high vitamin D, protein, and potassium). Maintain careful personal hygiene, avoid exposure to disease or trauma. Severe stress (serious infection, surgery, or trauma) may require increased dosage. Do not take any other medication w/o consulting physician. Follow-up visits, lab tests are necessary; children must be assessed for growth retardation. Inform dentist or other physicians of dexamethasone therapy now or within past 12 mos. Caution against overuse of joints injected for symptomatic relief. *Topical:* Apply after shower or bath for best absorption. Do not cover unless physician orders; do not use tight diapers, plastic pants, or coverings. Avoid contact w/ eyes. Do not expose treated area to sunlight.

dexpanthenol

decks-pan´theh-nol
(Ilopan, Panthoderm)

FIXED-COMBINATION(S):

W/choline bitartrate, precusor to acetylcholine (Ilopan-choline)

CLASSIFICATION

GI stimulant, emollient

PHARMACOKINETICS

Readily absorbed. Converted to pantothenic acid. Widely distributed. Excreted in urine; eliminated in feces.

ACTION

IM: Stimulates formation of choline to acetylcholine (increases peristalsis). Important in metabolism of carbohydrates, proteins, lipids. *Topical:* Stimulates epithelialization and granulation. Essential for normal epithelial function.

USES

Stimulates intestinal peristalsis. Used prophylactically after abdominal surgery to relieve postoperative, postpartum flatus, paralytic ileus, postoperative delay in intestinal motility. *Topical:* Relieves itching, promotes healing of skin lesions or irritation.

INDICATIONS/DOSAGE/ROUTES

Prevention of postoperative adynamic ileus:
IM: Adults, elderly: 250-500 mg one time; may repeat in 2 hrs, then q6h until danger has passed.

Treatment of adynamic ileus:
IM: Adults, elderly: 500 mg one time; may repeat in 2 hrs, then q6h as needed.

Usual topical dosage:
TOPICAL: Adults, elderly: 1-2 times/day to affected area.

PRECAUTIONS

CONTRAINDICATIONS: Hemophilia, ileus due to mechanical obstruction. **CAUTIONS:** None significant. **PREGNANCY/LACTATION:** Unknown if drug crosses placenta or is distributed in breast milk. **Pregnancy Category C.**

INTERACTIONS

DRUG INTERACTIONS: Do not administer within 1 hr of succinylcholine (respiratory difficulty) or within 12 hrs of parasympathomimetic drugs (miotic effects). **ALTERED LAB VALUES:** May prolong bleeding time.

SIDE EFFECTS

None significant (nontoxic even in large doses). **RARE:** Itching, tingling, erythema, hypotension, agitation in elderly, temporary respiratory difficulty.

ADVERSE REACTIONS/TOXIC EFFECTS

None significant.

NURSING IMPLICATIONS

BASELINE ASSESSMENT:

Apply topically only to intact, dry skin.

INTERVENTION/EVALUATION:

Monitor bleeding time. When used as GI stimulant, monitor bowel sounds for return of peristalsis. Assess for soft abdomen. When administered topically, assess skin for rash, redness, itching.

PATIENT/FAMILY TEACHING:

Report any episodes of increased abdominal pain (ileus produces pain).

dextran, low molecular weight (dextran 40)

dex´tran

(Gentran, Rheomacrodex)

dextran, high molecular weight (dextran 75)

(Macrodex)

CANADIAN AVAILABILITY: Hyskon, Macrodex, Rheomacrodex

CLASSIFICATION

Plasma volume expander

PHARMACOKINETICS

Evenly distributed in vascular circulation. Enzymatically degraded to glucose. Excreted in urine, feces.

ACTION

Draws fluid from interstitial to intravascular space (colloidal osmotic effect) resulting in increased central venous pressure, cardiac output, stroke volume, B/P, urine output, capillary perfusion, pulse pressure, and decreased heart rate, peripheral resistance, blood viscosity, mean transit time. Reduces aggregation of erythrocytes. Enhances blood flow (corrects hypovolemia, improves microcirculation).

USES

Adjunctive treatment of shock or impending shock (due to burns, surgery, hemorrhage); primary fluid in pump oxygenation during extracorporeal circulation. Prophylaxis against deep vein thrombosis, pulmonary embolism in those having procedures associated w/high risk of thromboembolic complications.

STORAGE/HANDLING

Store at room temperature. Use only clear solutions. Discard partially used containers.

IV ADMINISTRATION

1. Give by IV infusion only.
2. Monitor patient closely during first minutes of infusion for anaphylactoid reaction. Monitor vital signs q5min.
3. Monitor urine flow rates during administration (if oliguria or anuria occurs, dextran 40 should be discontinued and osmotic diuretic given (minimizes vascular overloading).
4. Monitor central venous pressure (CVP) when given by rapid infusion. If there is a precipitous rise in CVP, immediately discontinue drug (overexpansion of blood volume).
5. Monitor B/P diligently during infusion; if marked hypotension occurs, stop infusion immediately (imminent anaphylactoid reaction).
6. If evidence of blood volume overexpansion occurs, discontinue IV until blood volume adjusts via urine output.

INDICATIONS/DOSAGE/ROUTES

Usual Low Molecular Weight Dextran Dosages:

Adjunct to shock therapy:
IV: Adults, elderly: Total dose for first 24 hrs not to exceed 20 ml/kg. Infuse first 10 ml/kg rapidly. Therapy beyond 24 hrs not to exceed 10 ml/kg/day or 5 days duration.

Hemodilution in extracorporeal solutions:
IV: Adults, elderly: 10-20 ml/kg added to perfusion circuit. Do not exceed 20 ml/kg.

Prophylactic use in deep vein thrombosis and pulmonary embolism:
IV: Adults, elderly: 500-1,000 ml (10 ml/kg) on day of surgery; continue 500 ml/day for 2-3 additional days. Thereafter, continue therapy at 500 ml q2-3days up to 2 wks (based on risk of complications).

Usual High Molecular Weight Dextran Dosages:

IV: Adults, elderly: 500-1,000 ml given up to 20-40 ml/min. Maximum dose 20 ml/kg in first 24 hrs, then 10 ml/kg/24 hrs thereafter. **Children:** 20 ml/kg in first 24 hrs, then 10 ml/kg/24 hrs.

PRECAUTIONS

CONTRAINDICATIONS: Marked hemostatic defects, including drug-induced, marked cardiac decompensation, renal disease with severe oliguria or anuria, hypervolemic conditions, severe bleeding disorders, when use of sodium or chloride could be detrimental. **CAUTIONS:** Those w/ thrombocytopenia, CHF, pulmonary edema, severe renal insufficiency, those on corticosteroids or corticotropin, presence of edema w/sodium retention, impaired renal clearance, chronic liver disease, pathologic abdominal conditions, those undergoing bowel surgery. **PREGNANCY/LACTATION:** Unknown if drug crosses placenta or is distributed in breast milk. **Pregnancy Category C.**

INTERACTIONS

DRUG INTERACTIONS: None

significant. **ALTERED LAB VALUES:** Prolongs bleeding time, increases bleeding tendency, depressed platelet count. Decreases factor VIII, factor V, factor IX.

SIDE EFFECTS

OCCASIONAL: Mild hypersensitivity reaction (urticaria, nasal congestion, wheezing).

ADVERSE REACTIONS/TOXIC EFFECTS

Severe or fatal anaphylaxis (marked hypotension, cardiac/respiratory arrest may occur, noted early during IV infusion, generally in those not previously exposed to IV dextran.

NURSING IMPLICATIONS

INTERVENTION/EVALUATION:

Monitor urine output closely (increase in output generally occurs in oliguric pts after dextran administration). If no increase is observed after 500 ml dextran is infused, discontinue drug until diuresis occurs. Monitor for fluid overload (peripheral and/or pulmonary edema, impending CHF symptoms). Assess lung sounds for rales. Monitor central venous pressure (detects overexpansion of blood volume). Observe closely for allergic reaction. Assess for bleeding esp. following surgery or in pts on anticoagulant therapy (overt bleeding esp. at surgical site and bruising, petechiae development).

dextroamphetamine sulfate

dex-tro-am-fet´ah-meen
(Dexedrine)

CANADIAN AVAILABILITY:
Dexedrine

CLASSIFICATION

CNS stimulant

PHARMACOKINETICS

	ONSET	PEAK	DURATION
PO	1-2 hrs	—	2-10 hrs

Well absorbed from GI tract. Widely distributed. Primarily excreted in urine. Half-life: 10-12 hrs (children 6-8 hrs).

ACTION

Enhances release, action of catecholamine (dopamine, norepinephrine) by blocking re-uptake, inhibiting MAO. Increases motor activity, mental alertness, decreases drowsiness, fatigue.

USES

Treatment of narcolepsy; treatment of attention deficit disorder in hyperactive children; short-term treatment to assist caloric restriction in exogenous obesity.

STORAGE/HANDLING

Store elixir form at room temperature.

PO ADMINISTRATION

1. Give single daily dose, initial daily dose upon awakening.
2. When given in 2-3 divided doses/day, give at 4-6 hr intervals.
3. Give last dose at least 6 hrs before retiring (prevents insomnia).
4. Give fixed-combination form (one capsule daily), 10-14 hrs before bedtime.
5. If used as anorexic, give dose 30-60 min before meals.
6. Do not break capsule or tablet form.

INDICATIONS/DOSAGE/ROUTES

Narcolepsy:

PO: Adults, children >12 yrs: Initially, 10 mg/day. Increase by 10 mg at weekly intervals until therapeutic response achieved. **Usual dose:** 5-60 mg/day. **Children 6-12 yrs:** Initially, 5 mg/day. Increase by 5 mg/day at weekly intervals until therapeutic response achieved.

Attention deficit disorder:

PO: Children >6 yrs: Initially, 5 mg 1-2 times/day. Increase by 5 mg/day at weekly intervals until therapeutic response achieved. Maximum daily dose: 40 mg. **Children 3-5 yrs:** Initially, 2.5 mg/day. Increase by 2.5 mg/day at weekly intervals until therapeutic response achieved.

Appetite suppressant:

PO: Adults: 5-30 mg daily in divided doses of 5-10 mg each dose, given 30-60 min before meals. **Extended-release:** 1 capsule in morning.

PRECAUTIONS

CONTRAINDICATIONS: Hyperthyroidism, advanced arteriosclerosis, agitated states, moderate to severe hypertension, symptomatic cardiovascular disease, history of drug abuse, glaucoma, history of hypersensitivity to sympathomimetic amines, within 14 days of MAO inhibitor ingestion. **CAUTIONS:** Elderly, debilitated, tartrazine-sensitive pts. **PREGNANCY/LACTATION:** Distributed in breast milk. Significant agitation in neonates of mothers dependent on amphetamines. **Pregnancy Category C.**

INTERACTIONS

DRUG INTERACTIONS: Tricyclic antidepressants may increase cardiovascular effects. Beta-blockers may increase risk of hypertension, bradycardia, heart block. CNS stimulants may increase effects. May increase risk of arrhythmias w/digoxin. Meperidine may increase risk of hypotension, respiratory depression, convulsions, vascular collapse. MAO inhibitors may prolong, intensify effects. May increase effects of thyroid hormone. Thyroid hormones may increase effects. **ALTERED LAB VALUES:** May increase plasma corticosteroid concentrations.

SIDE EFFECTS

FREQUENT: Increased motor activity, talkativeness, nervousness, mild euphoria, insomnia. **OCCASIONAL:** Headache, chilliness, dry mouth, GI distress, increased depression in depressed pts, tachycardia, palpitations, chest pain.

ADVERSE REACTIONS/TOXIC EFFECTS

Overdose may produce pallor or flushing, cardiac irregularities, psychotic syndrome. Abrupt withdrawal following prolonged administration of high dosage may produce psychosis, lethargy (may persist for weeks). Prolonged administration to children with attention-deficit disorder may produce a temporary suppression of weight and/or height patterns.

NURSING IMPLICATIONS

PATIENT/FAMILY TEACHING:

Normal dosage levels may produce tolerance to drug's anorexic, mood elevating effects within a few weeks. Avoid tasks that require alertness, motor skills until response to drug is established.

Dry mouth may be relieved by sugarless gum or sips of tepid water.

dextrothyroxine sodium

decks-trow-thigh-rocks´een
(Choloxin)

CANADIAN AVAILABILITY: Choloxin

CLASSIFICATION

Antihyperlipoproteinemic

PHARMACOKINETICS

Poorly absorbed from GI tract. Protein binding: high. Deiodinated in peripheral tissue. Excreted in urine, eliminated in feces. Half-life: 18 hrs.

ACTION

Stimulates liver to increase rate of cholesterol catabolism and excretion. Lowers serum cholesterol and low density lipoprotein (LDL).

USES

Adjunct to diet therapy to decrease elevated serum cholesterol (LDL) in euthroid pts w/no evidence of organic heart disease.

INDICATIONS/DOSAGE/ROUTES

Give as single daily dose. Increase dosage at no less than monthly intervals.

Hypercholesterolemia:
PO: Adults, elderly: Initially: 1-2 mg/day. Slowly increase dose (no more than 1-2 mg within 1 mo) to maximum of 4-8 mg/day. **Maintenance:** 4-8 mg/day. **Children:** Initially, 0.05 mg/kg/day. Slowly increase dose (no more than 0.05 mg/kg within 1 mo) to maximum of 0.4 mg/kg/day or 4 mg/day. **Maintenance:** 0.1 mg/kg/day.

PRECAUTIONS

CONTRAINDICATIONS: Hypersensitivity to dextrothyroxine or tartrazine (frequently seen in those hypersensitive to aspirin), organic heart disease (including angina pectoris), history of myocardial infarction, cardiac arrhythmias, CHF, rheumatic fever, hypertension, advanced hepatic or renal disease, iodism. **CAUTIONS:** Diabetes mellitus, impaired hepatic or renal function, concurrent sympathomimetic or anticoagulant therapy, those on dextrothyroxine therapy undergoing emergency surgery. Withdrawal of dextrothyroxine 2 wks prior to surgery is recommended (increased potential for cardiac arrhythmias). **PREGNANCY/LACTATION:** Contraindicated during pregnancy/lactation. Crosses placenta. May be distributed in breast milk. **Pregnancy Category C.**

INTERACTIONS

DRUG INTERACTIONS: May alter effects of oral anticoagulants. Cholestyramine, colestipol may decrease effects. **ALTERED LAB VALUES:** May increase SGOT (AST), alkaline phosphatase, bilirubin, glucose, T_4.

SIDE EFFECTS

Side effects generally due to increased metabolism, seen least in euthroid pts; minimized by maintaining dosage within recommended parameters. **FREQUENT:** Palpitation, sweating, tremors, flushing, insomnia, weight loss, hair loss, menstrual irregularities. **OCCASIONAL:** Nausea, vomiting, diarrhea, constipation, headache, dizziness, malaise, hoarseness, decreased libido, rash. **RARE:** Leukopenia, neutropenia, exophthalmos, retinopathy, angina pectoris, arrhythmias, decreased sensorium.

ADVERSE REACTIONS/TOXIC EFFECTS

Fatal and nonfatal myocardial infarctions have occurred.

NURSING IMPLICATIONS

Baseline Assessment:

Question for history of hypersensitivity to dextrothyroxine, tartrazine, or aspirin. Assess baseline ECG, cholesterol level, thyroxine, serum glucose (those w/diabetes mellitus), CBC.

Intervention/Evaluation:

Weigh daily. Monitor pulse at least twice/day. Assess for palpitations, chest pain, or shortness of breath. Check for headache, dizziness, level of mental acuity, visual disturbance. Evaluate food tolerance. Determine pattern of bowel activity. Assess for rash. Monitor cholesterol, thyroxine, blood cell counts, and ECG. Check sleep pattern.

Patient/Family Teaching:

Take as directed, do not stop taking dextrothyroxine. Consult physician before taking other medication. Do not drive or perform activities that require alert response if experience drowsiness, dizziness, nervousness. Notify physician immediately in event of chest pain, palpitations, or other new symptom. Follow special diet carefully (important part of treatment). Periodic tests are essential part of therapy. Menstrual irregularities, decreased libido may occur during dextrothyroxine therapy. Inform physician of any anticipated surgery, including dental surgery.

dezocine

dez´oh-seen
(Dalgan)

CLASSIFICATION

Opioid analgesic **(Schedule V)**

PHARMACOKINETICS

	ONSET	PEAK	DURATION
IM	<30 min	30-150 min	2-4 hrs
IV	<15 min	30 min	2-4 hrs

Rapid, complete absorption after IM administration. Metabolized in liver. Primarily excreted in urine. Half-life: IM 2.2 hrs; IV 2.4-2.6 hrs.

ACTION

Binds w/opiate receptors in CNS (probably in limbic system), producing impaired pain perception.

USES

Relief of moderate to severe pain.

STORAGE/HANDLING

Store parenteral form at room temperature. Discard if solution contains a precipitate.

INDICATIONS/DOSAGE/ROUTES

Analgesia:
IM: Adults, >18 yrs, elderly: 5-20 mg q3-6h as needed. **Maximum:** 120 mg/day.
IV: Adults, >18 yrs, elderly: 2.5-10 mg q2-4h as needed.

PRECAUTIONS

CONTRAINDICATIONS: None significant. **CAUTIONS:** Impaired hepatic/renal function, elderly, debilitated, head injury, respiratory disease, hypertension, hypothyroidism, acute alcoholism, urethral stricture. **PREGNANCY/LACTATION:** Unknown if drug crosses placenta or is distributed in breast milk (breast feeding not recommended). Prolonged use during pregnancy may produce withdrawal symptoms (irritability, excessive crying, tremors, hyperactive reflexes, fever, vomiting, diarrhea, yawning, sneezing, seizures) in neonate. **Pregnancy Category C.**

INTERACTIONS

DRUG INTERACTIONS: CNS depressants, MAO inhibitors may increase CNS, respiratory depression, hypotensive effects. May decrease effects of other opioid analgesics, may also precipitate withdrawal symptoms. **ALTERED LAB VALUES:** May increase SGOT (AST), alkaline phosphatase.

SIDE EFFECTS

FREQUENT: Sedation, reaction at injection site. **OCCASIONAL:** Nausea, vomiting, dizziness. **RARE:** Dry mouth, headache, hiccups, constipation or diarrhea, sweating, chills, flushing, hypotension, paradoxical reaction (anxiety, crying), blurred vision.

ADVERSE REACTIONS/TOXIC EFFECTS

Overdosage results in acute respiratory depression, skeletal muscle flaccidity, cyanosis, extreme somnolence progressing to convulsions, stupor, coma. Naloxone given as antidote.

NURSING IMPLICATIONS

BASELINE ASSESSMENT:

Raise bedrails. Obtain vital signs before giving medication. If respirations are 12/min or lower (20/min or lower in children), withhold medication, contact physician. Assess onset, type, location, and duration of pain. Effect of medication is reduced if full pain recurs before next dose.

INTERVENTION/EVALUATION:

Increase fluid intake and environmental humidity to improve viscosity of lung secretions. Monitor for change in respirations, B/P, change in rate or quality of pulse. Monitor daily bowel activity and prevent constipation. Initiate deep breathing and coughing exercises, particularly in those w/impaired pulmonary function. Change pts position q2-4h and ambulate w/assistance. Assess for clinical improvement and record onset of relief of pain.

PATIENT/FAMILY TEACHING:

Change positions slowly to avoid dizziness. Avoid tasks that require alertness, motor skills until response to drug is established.

diazepam

dye-az´eh-pam
(Valium, Valrelease)

CANADIAN AVAILABILITY:
Apo-Diazepam, Meval, Novodipam, Valium, Vivol

CLASSIFICATION

Antianxiety: Benzodiazepine **(Schedule IV)**

PHARMACOKINETICS

	ONSET	PEAK	DURATION
IV	1-5 min	—	15-60 min

Well absorbed from GI tract. Widely distributed. Protein binding: 98%. Metabolized in liver to active metabolite. Excreted in urine. Half-life: 20-70 hrs (increased in elderly, liver dysfunction).

ACTION

Enhances action of inhibitory neurotransmitter gamma-aminobutyric acid (GABA). Depressant effects occur at all levels of CNS. Enhances presynaptic inhibition, suppresses spread of seizure activity. Inhibits spinal polysynaptic pathways. Directly depresses motor nerve, muscle function.

USES

Short-term relief of anxiety symptoms, preanesthetic medication, relief of acute alcohol withdrawal. Adjunct for relief of acute musculoskeletal conditions, treatment of seizures (IV route used for termination of status epilepticus).

STORAGE/HANDLING

Store tablets, extended-release capsules, oral/parenteral solutions at room temperature.

PO/IM/IV ADMINISTRATION

PO:

1. Give w/o regard to meals.
2. Dilute oral concentrate w/ water, juice, carbonated beverages; may also be mixed in semisolid food (applesauce, pudding).
3. Tablets may be crushed.
4. Do not crush or break capsule.

Parenteral form: Do not mix w/ other injections (produces precipitate).

IM:

1. Injection may be painful. Inject deeply into deltoid muscle.

IV:

1. Give by direct IV injection.
2. Administer directly into a large vein (reduces risk of thrombosis/phlebitis). If not possible, administer into tubing of a flowing IV solution as close to the vein insertion point as possible. Do not use small veins (e.g., wrist/dorsum of hand).
3. Administer IV rate not exceeding 5 mg/min. For children, give over a 3-min period (a too-rapid IV may result in hypotension, respiratory depression).
4. Monitor respirations q5-15 min for 2h. May produce arrhythmias when used prior to cardioversion.

INDICATIONS/DOSAGE/ROUTES

NOTE: Use smallest effective dose in those w/liver disease, low serum albumin.

Anxiety:
PO/IM/IV: Adults: 2-10 mg 2-4 times/day. **Elderly/debilitated:** 2.5 mg 2 times/day. **Children >6 mo:** 1 to 2.5 mg 3-4 times/day.

Preanesthesia:
IV: Adults, elderly: 5-15 mg 5-10 min prior to procedure.

Alcohol withdrawal:
PO: Adults, elderly: 10 mg 3-4 times during first 24 hrs, then reduce to 5-10 mg 3-4 times/day as needed.

IM/IV: Adults, elderly: Initially, 10 mg, followed by 5-10 mg q3-4h.

Musculoskeletal spasm:
PO: Adults: 2-10 mg 2-4 times/day. **Elderly:** 2-5 mg 2-4 times/day.
IM/IV: Adults: 5-10 mg q3-4h.

Seizures:
PO: Adults: 2-10 mg 2-4 times/day. **Elderly, debilitated:** 2.5 mg 2 times/day.
IM/IV: Adults: 5-10 mg, repeated at 10-15 min intervals to total of 30 mg. **Elderly, debilitated:** 2-5 mg, increase gradually as needed.

PRECAUTIONS

CONTRAINDICATIONS: Acute narrow-angle glaucoma, acute alcohol intoxication. **CAUTIONS:** Impaired kidney/liver function. **PREGNANCY/LACTATION:** Crosses placenta; distributed in breast milk. May increase risk of fetal abnormalities if administered during first trimester of pregnancy. Chronic ingestion during pregnancy may produce withdrawal symptoms, CNS depression in neonates. **Pregnancy Category D.**

INTERACTIONS

DRUG INTERACTIONS: Alcohol, CNS depressants may increase CNS depressant effect. **ALTERED LAB VALUES:** None significant.

SIDE EFFECTS

FREQUENT: Pain w/IM injection, drowsiness, fatigue, ataxia (muscular incoordination). **OCCASIONAL:** Slurred speech, orthostatic hypotension, headache, hypoactivity, constipation, nausea, blurred vision. **RARE:** Paradoxical CNS hyperactivity/nervousness in children, excitement/restlessness in elderly/debilitated (generally noted during first 2 wks of therapy, particularly noted in presence of uncontrolled pain).

ADVERSE REACTIONS/TOXIC EFFECTS

IV route may produce pain, swelling, thrombophlebitis, carpal tunnel syndrome. Abrupt or too-rapid withdrawal may result in pronounced restlessness, irritability, insomnia, hand tremors, abdominal/muscle cramps, sweating, vomiting, seizures. Abrupt withdrawal in pts w/epilepsy may produce increase in frequency and/or severity of seizures. Overdosage results in somnolence, confusion, diminished reflexes, coma.

NURSING IMPLICATIONS

BASELINE ASSESSMENT:

Assess B/P, pulse, respirations immediately before administration. Pt must remain recumbent for up to 3 hrs (individualized) after parenteral administration to reduce hypotensive effect. *Anxiety:* Assess autonomic response (cold, clammy hands, sweating), and motor response (agitation, trembling, tension). Offer emotional support to anxious pt. *Musculoskeletal spasm:* Record onset, type, location, duration of pain. Check for immobility, stiffness, swelling. *Seizures:* Review history of seizure disorder (length, intensity, frequency, duration, LOC). Observe frequently for recurrence of seizure activity. Initiate seizure precautions.

INTERVENTION/EVALUATION:

Monitor IV site for swelling, phlebitis (heat, pain, red streaking of skin over vein, hardness to vein). Assess children, elderly for paradoxical reaction, particularly during early therapy. Assist w/ambulation if drowsiness, ataxia occur. For those on long-term therapy, liver/renal function tests, blood counts should be performed periodically. Evaluate for therapeutic response: a decrease in intensity/frequency of seizures; a calm, facial expression, decreased restlessness; decreased intensity of skeletal muscle pain.

PATIENT/FAMILY TEACHING:

Discomfort may occur w/IM injection. Drowsiness usually diminishes w/continued therapy. Avoid tasks that require alertness, motor skills until response to drug is established. Smoking reduces drug effectiveness. Do not abruptly withdraw medication after long-term therapy. Strict maintenance of drug therapy is essential for seizure control. Avoid alcohol.

diazoxide

dye-ah-zocks′eyd
(Hyperstat, Proglycem)

CANADIAN AVAILABILITY:
Hyperstat, Proglycem

CLASSIFICATION

Antihypertensive, Antihypoglycemic

PHARMACOKINETICS

	ONSET	PEAK	DURATION
PO: hypoglycemia	1 hr	—	Up to 8 hrs
IV: hypotensive	1 min	2-5 min	3-12 hrs

Readily absorbed from GI tract. Protein binding: >90%. Metabolized in liver. Excreted in urine. Removed by hemodialysis. Half-life: 21-36 hrs (increased in decreased renal function).

ACTION

Direct vasodilating effect on arterioles, decreasing peripheral resistance. Inhibits insulin release from pancreas.

USES

Emergency lowering of B/P in adults w/severe, nonmalignant and malignant hypertension; children w/acute severe hypertension. Management of hypoglycemia caused by hyperinsulinism associated w/islet cell adenoma, carcinoma, or extrapancreatic malignancy.

STORAGE/HANDLING

Store capsules, oral suspension at room temperature. Parenteral forms should appear clear, colorless. Discard darkened solution (may be subpotent), or if precipitate is present.

PO/IV ADMINISTRATION

PO:

1. Shake well before using oral suspension.
2. May give w/o regard to food.

IV:

NOTE: IV form frequently produces a feeling of warmth along injection vein. Extravasation produces severe burning, cellulitis, phlebitis.

1. Place pt in supine position during and for 1 hr after IV dosing, monitor B/P diligently, follow by standing B/P in ambulatory pts.
2. Administer only in peripheral vein.
3. Give over 30 sec or less.
4. Do not use longer than 10 days.

INDICATIONS/DOSAGE/ROUTES

Severe hypertension:

IV: Adults, elderly, children: 1-3 mg/kg (up to max of 150 mg). Repeat q5-15min until adequate decrease in B/P occurs. Thereafter, give at intervals of 4-24 hrs.

Hypoglycemia:

PO: Adults, elderly, children: Initially, 3 mg/kg/day in 3 divided doses q8h. **Maintenance:** 3-8 mg/kg/day in 2-3 divided doses at 12 or 8 hr intervals. **Maximum:** Up to 15 mg/kg/day. **Infants, neonates:** Initially, 10 mg/kg/day in 3 divided doses q8h. **Maintenance:** 8-15 mg/kg/day in 2-3 divided doses at 12 or 8 hr intervals.

PRECAUTIONS

CONTRAINDICATIONS: History of hypersensitivity to thiazide derivatives. *IV:* Hypertension associated w/aortic coarctation, arteriovenous shunt. *Oral:* management of functional hypoglycemia. **CAUTIONS:** Uremic pts (increases risk of excessive hypotension), impaired cardiac reserve, severely elevated B/P. **PREGNANCY/LACTATION:** Crosses placenta; unknown if distributed in breast milk. May produce fetal or neonatal hyperbilirubinemia, thrombocytopenia, altered carbohydrate metabolism, alopecia, hypertrichosis. May produce cessation of uterine contractions if given during labor via IV. **Pregnancy Category C.**

INTERACTIONS

DRUG INTERACTIONS: Beta-blockers, vasodilators, hypotension producing medications may increase hypotensive effect. **ALTERED LAB VALUES:** May increase SGOT (AST), alkaline phosphatase, free fatty acids, sodium, uric acid, glucose, BUN. May decrease hemoglobin, hematocrit, creatinine clearance.

SIDE EFFECTS

FREQUENT: *IV:* Hypotension, nausea, vomiting, dizziness, weakness, hyperglycemia. *IV; oral:* Edema, weight gain, diarrhea/constipation. *Oral:* Hirsutism (hair growth), particularly in women and children (regresses when drug is discontinued). **OCCASIONAL:** Orthostatic hypotension. **RARE:** Dry mouth, salivation, muscle cramps, chest discomfort, paresthesia, tinnitus, insomnia, dizziness, euphoria.

ADVERSE REACTIONS/TOXIC EFFECTS

Extrapyramidal symptoms (restlessness, rigidity, tremor) may occur. Symptoms disappear if dosage is reduced or drug is discontinued. IV form may produce seizures, paralysis, unconsciousness. Sensitivity reactions (rash, fever, leukopenia) noted w/IV or oral form.

NURSING IMPLICATIONS

BASELINE ASSESSMENT:

Establish baseline B/P, blood glucose. When adminstering IV, achieve desired B/P over as long a period of time as possible.

INTERVENTION/EVALUATION:

If excessive reduction in B/P occurs, place pt in supine position w/legs elevated. If parenteral form leaks in SubQ tissue, apply warm compresses to decrease pain sensation. Monitor for development of hyperglycemia, particularly in those w/renal disease, liver disease, diabetes mellitus, concurrent therapy that may increase blood glucose concentrations. Monitor blood glucose concentrations daily in those receiving IV therapy. Monitor serum uric acid in those w/history of gout, hyperuricemia.

PATIENT/FAMILY TEACHING:

Blood glucose or daily urine testing should be attained in those on chronic oral therapy.

dibucaine

dye´byoo-kane
(Nupercainal)

CANADIAN AVAILABILITY:
Nupercainal

CLASSIFICATION

Topical, Anesthetic

PHARMACOKINETICS

	ONSET	PEAK	DURATION
TOPICAL	—	<15 min	1-2 hrs

Readily absorbed through mucous membranes into systemic circulation. Metabolized in liver. Primarily excreted in urine.

ACTION

Inhibits conduction of nerve impulses from sensory nerves by altering cell membrane permeability to ions. Poorly absorbed through intact skin; readily absorbed from mucous membranes or when skin permeability has been increased by abrasions or ulcers.

USES

Skin application. For topical anesthesia: in pruritus and pain due to minor burns, fungus infections, chickenpox or other skin manifestations of systemic disease, abrasions, sunburn, insect bites, eczema, diaper rash, prickly heat, plant poisoning. *Mucous membranes.* Temporary relief of pain, itching, and burning due to hemorrhoids

TOPICAL ADMINSTRATION

NOTE: Do not get in or near eyes.

Skin:
1. Rub gently into affected areas only.
2. Cover w/light dressing for protection if necessary.
3. Cream is water soluble; reapply after swimming, bathing, sweating.

Mucous membranes:
OINTMENT:

1. Cleanse and dry area thoroughly before application.
2. Remove cap from tube; apply applicator to tube and squeeze tube until ointment begins to come through tip of applicator.
3. Use finger to lubricate the applicator w/ointment.
4. Insert entire applicator gently into rectum and squeeze enough ointment into rectum for comfort and lubrication.
5. Remove applicator from rectum and wipe clean.
6. Apply ointment to anal area.
7. After use, detach applicator, wash w/soap and water; recap tube.
8. Apply morning, evening, and after each bowel movement within dosage range.

INDICATIONS/DOSAGE/ROUTES

Usual topical dosage:
TOPICAL: Adults, elderly: Apply to area as needed (may apply to gauze/bandage prior to skin application).
MUCUS MEMBRANE: Adults, elderly: Dose varies based on area

to be anesthetized, vascularity, technique, pt tolerance.

PRECAUTIONS

CONTRAINDICATIONS: Hypersensitivity to dibucaine or amide-type local anesthetics, or any component of the preparation (sulfite sensitivity). **PREGNANCY/LACTATION:** Safety during pregnancy and lactation not established. **Pregnancy Category C.**

INTERACTIONS

DRUG INTERACTIONS: None significant. **ALTERED LAB VALUES:** None significant.

SIDE EFFECTS

OCCASIONAL: Redness, burning, stinging, tenderness, edema, urticaria, contact dermatitis.

ADVERSE REACTIONS/TOXIC EFFECTS

None significant.

NURSING IMPLICATIONS

BASELINE ASSESSMENT:

Question for hypersensitivity to dibucaine, amide-type anesthetics, components of preparation.

INTERVENTION/EVALUATION:

Discontinue if redness, rash, or irritation develop.

PATIENT/FAMILY TEACHING:

Do not apply to skin if blisters, ulcers, or abrasions present. Do not apply over large areas or use in large amounts. Not intended for prolonged use; consult physician for rash/irritation or if symptoms persist beyond 7 days. In event of rectal bleeding, do not apply ointment and notify physician. For treatment of hemorrhoids, maintain normal bowel function by proper diet, adequate fluid intake, and regular exercise. Adjunctive therapy w/stool softeners or bulk laxatives may be used (not excessive use) to avoid additional irritation to hemorrhoids.

D

diclofenac sodium

dye-klo´feh-nak

(Voltaren)

diclofenac potassium

(Cataflam)

CANADIAN AVAILABILITY: Voltaren

CLASSIFICATION

Nonsteroidal anti-inflammatory

PHARMACOKINETICS

	ONSET	PEAK	DURATION
PO	—	2-3 hrs	—

Completely absorbed from GI tract, penetrates cornea after ophthalmic administration (may be systemically absorbed). Widely distributed. Protein binding: 99%. Metabolized in liver. Primarily excreted in urine. Half-life: 1.2-2 hrs.

ACTION

Inhibits prostaglandin synthesis. Inhibits action of cyclooxygenase; decreases formation of prostaglandin, thromboxane precursors from arachidonic acid. Prevents, reduces miosis by relaxing iris sphincter.

USES

Symptomatic treatment of acute and/or chronic rheumatoid arthritis, osteoarthritis, ankylosing spondylitis; postoperative inflammation of cataract extraction; analgesic, primary dysmenorrhea.

PO/OPHTHALMIC ADMINISTRATION

PO:

1. Do not crush or break enteric-coated form.
2. May give w/food, milk, or antacids if GI distress occurs.

OPHTHALMIC:

1. Place finger on lower eyelid and pull out until pocket is formed between eye and lower lid. Hold dropper above pocket and place prescribed number of drops in pocket.
2. Close eye gently. Apply digital pressure to lacrimal sac for 1-2 min (minimized drainage into nose and throat, reducing risk of systemic effects).
3. Remove excess solution w/ tissue.

INDICATIONS/DOSAGE/ROUTES

Osteoarthritis:
PO: Adults, elderly: 100-150 mg/day in 2-3 divided doses.

Rheumatoid arthritis:
PO: Adults, elderly: 150-200 mg/day in 2-4 divided doses.

Ankylosing spondylitis:
PO: Adults, elderly: 100-125 mg/day in 4-5 divided doses.

Ophthalmic:
PO: Adults, elderly: Apply 1 drop to eye 4 times/day commencing 24 hrs after cataract surgery. Continue for 2 wks after surgery.

Analgesic, primary dysmenorrhea:
PO: Adults: 150 mg/day in 3 divided doses.

PRECAUTIONS

CONTRAINDICATIONS: Active peptic ulcer, GI ulceration, chronic inflammation of GI tract, GI bleeding disorders, history of hypersensitivity to aspirin or nonsteroidal anti-inflammatory agent. **CAUTIONS:** Impaired renal/hepatic function, history of GI tract disease, predisposition of fluid retention, those wearing soft-contact lenses, surgical pts w/bleeding tendencies. **PREGNANCY/LACTATION:** Crosses placenta; unknown if distributed in breast milk. Avoid use during last trimester (may adversely affect fetal cardiovascular system: premature closure of ductus arteriosus). **Pregnancy Category B.**

INTERACTIONS

DRUG INTERACTIONS: May increase effects of oral anticoagulants, heparin, thrombolytics. May decrease effect of antihypertensives, diuretics. Salicylates, aspirin may increase risk of GI side effects, bleeding. Bone marrow depressants may increase risk of hematologic reactions. May increase concentration, toxicity of lithium. May increase methotrexate toxicity. Probenecid may increase concentration. *Ophthalmic:* May decrease effect of acetylcholine, carbachol. May decrease antiglaucoma effect of epinephrine, other antiglaucoma medications. **ALTERED LAB VALUES:** May increase serum transaminase activity. May decrease uric acid.

SIDE EFFECTS

FREQUENT: *Ophthalmic:* Burning, stinging on instillation, keratitis, elevated intraocular pressure (IOP). **OCCASIONAL:** *Oral:* Dizziness, headache, dyspepsia (heartburn, indigestion, epigastric pain, diarrhea/constipation, cramping) occurs more frequently in elderly. **RARE:** *Oral:* Rash, peripheral edema/fluid retention, visual disturbances, vomiting, drowsiness.

ADVERSE REACTIONS/TOXIC EFFECTS

Overdosage may result in acute renal failure. In those treated chronically, peptic ulcer, GI bleeding, gastritis, severe hepatic reaction (jaundice), nephrotoxicity (hematuria, dysuria, proteinuria), severe hypersensitivity reaction (bronchospasm, angiofacial edema) occur rarely.

NURSING IMPLICATIONS

BASELINE ASSESSMENT:

Anti-inflammatory: Assess onset, type, location, and duration of pain or inflammation. Inspect appearance of affected joints for immobility, deformities, and skin condition.

INTERVENTION/EVALUATION:

Monitor for headache, dyspepsia. Monitor pattern of daily bowel activity and stool consistency. Evaluate for therapeutic response: relief of pain, stiffness, swelling, increase in joint mobility, reduced joint tenderness, improved grip strength.

PATIENT/FAMILY TEACHING:

Swallow tablet whole; do not crush or chew. Avoid aspirin, alcohol during therapy (increases risk of GI bleeding). If GI upset occurs, take w/food, milk. Report GI distress, visual disturbances, rash, edema, headache.

dicloxacillin sodium

dye´clocks-ah-sill-in

(Dynapen, Dycill, Pathocil)

CLASSIFICATION

Antibiotic: Penicillin

PHARMACOKINETICS

Moderately absorbed from GI tract (food decreases absorption). Protein binding: 95-97%. Metabolized in liver. Primarily excreted in urine. Not removed by hemodialysis. Half-life: 0.5-1.1 hrs (increase in decreased renal function).

ACTION

Bactericidal. Binds to bacterial membranes. Inhibits cell wall synthesis.

USES

Treatment of mild to moderate infections of respiratory tract and skin/skin structure, chronic osteomyelitis, urinary tract infection; follow-up to parenteral therapy for acute, severe infections. Predominantly treatment of infections caused by penicillinase-producing *Staphylococcus.*

STORAGE/HANDLING

Store capsules at room temperature. Oral solution, after reconstitution, is stable for 7 days at room temperature, 14 days if refrigerated.

PO ADMINISTRATION

1. Give 1 hr before or 2 hrs after meals.
2. Space doses evenly around the clock.

INDICATIONS/DOSAGE/ROUTES

Mild to moderate upper respiratory, localized skin/skin structure infections:
PO: Adults, elderly, children >40 kg: 125 mg q6h. **Children <40 kg:** 12.5 mg/kg/day in divided doses q6h.

Severe infections, lower respiratory tract, disseminated infections:
PO: Adults, elderly, children >40 kg: 250 mg q6h. **Maximum:** 4 Gm/day. **Children <40 kg:** 25 mg/kg/day in divided doses q6h.

PRECAUTIONS

CONTRAINDICATIONS: Hypersensitivity to any penicillin. **CAUTIONS:** History of allergies, particularly cephalosporins. **PREGNANCY/LACTATION:** Readily crosses placenta, appears in cord blood, amniotic fluid. Distributed in breast milk in low concentrations. May lead to allergic sensitization, diarrhea, candidiasis, skin rash in infant. **Pregnancy Category B.**

INTERACTIONS

DRUG INTERACTIONS: Probenecid may increase concentration, toxicity risk. **ALTERED LAB VALUES:** May increase SGOT (AST). May cause positive Coombs test.

SIDE EFFECTS

FREQUENT: Mild hypersensitivity reaction (fever, rash, pruritus), nausea, vomiting, diarrhea, flatulence.

ADVERSE REACTIONS/TOXIC EFFECTS

Superinfections, potentially fatal antibiotic-associated colitis may result from altered bacterial balance. Hematologic effects, severe hypersensitivity reactions, including anaphylaxis, occur rarely.

NURSING IMPLICATIONS

BASELINE ASSESSMENT:

Question for history of allergies, especially penicillins, cephalosporins. Obtain specimen for culture and sensitivity before giving first dose (therapy may begin before results are known).

INTERVENTION/EVALUATION:

Hold medication and promptly report rash (may indicate hypersensitivity) or diarrhea (w/fever, abdominal pain, mucous and blood in stool may indicate antibiotic-associated colitis). Assess food tolerance. Check hematology reports (esp. WBCs), periodic renal or hepatic reports in prolonged therapy. Be alert for superinfection: increased fever, onset sore throat, diarrhea, ulceration or changes of oral mucosa, vaginal discharge, anal/genital pruritus.

PATIENT/FAMILY TEACHING:

Continue antibiotic for full length of treatment. Space doses evenly. Notify physician in event of diarrhea, rash, other new symptom.

dicyclomine hydrochloride

dye-sigh´clo-meen
(Antispaz, Bentyl, Dibent, Di-Spaz, Neoquess, Or-Tyl, Spasmoject)

CANADIAN AVAILABILITY:
Bentylol, Formulex, Lomine

CLASSIFICATION

Antispasmodic

PHARMACOKINETICS

Readily absorbed from GI tract. Widely distributed. Metabolized in liver. Half-life: 9-10 hrs.

ACTION

Local, direct relaxant action on smooth muscle, reducing tone, motility of GI tract.

USES

Treatment of functional disturbances of GI motility (i.e., irritable bowel syndrome).

STORAGE/HANDLING

Store capsules, tablets, syrup, parenteral form at room temperature. Injection should appear colorless.

PO/IM ADMINSTRATION

PO:

1. Dilute oral solution w/equal volume of water just before administration.
2. May give w/o regard to meals (food may slightly decrease absorption).

IM:

1. Do not administer IV or SubQ.
2. Inject deep into large muscle mass.
3. Do not give longer than 2 days.

INDICATIONS/DOSAGE/ROUTES

Functional disturbances of GI motility:
PO: Adults: 10-20 mg 3-4 times/day up to 40 mg 4 times/day. **Children 6 mo-2 yrs:** 5-10 mg 3-4 times/day. **Children >2 yrs:** 10 mg 3-4 times/day.
IM: Adults: 20 mg q4-6h.

Usual elderly dosage:
PO: Elderly: 10-20 mg 4 times/day. May increase up to 160 mg/day.

PRECAUTIONS

CONTRAINDICATIONS: Narrow-angle glaucoma, severe ulcerative colitis, toxic megacolon, obstructive disease of GI tract, paralytic ileus, intestinal atony, bladder neck obstruction due to prostatic hypertrophy, myasthenia gravis in those not treated w/neostigmine, tachycardia secondary to cardiac insufficiency or thyrotoxicosis, cardiospasm, unstable cardiovascular status in acute hemorrhage. **EXTREME CAUTION:** Autonomic neuropathy, known or suspected GI infections, diarrhea, mild to moderate ulcerative colitis. **CAUTIONS:** Hyperthyroidism, hepatic or renal disease, hypertension, tachyarrhythmias, CHF, coronary artery disease, gastric ulcer, esophageal reflux or hiatal hernia associated w/reflux esophagitis, infants, elderly, those w/COPD. **PREGNANCY/LACTATION:** Unknown if drug crosses placenta or is distributed in breast milk. **Pregnancy Category C.**

INTERACTIONS

DRUG INTERACTIONS: Antacids, antidiarrheals may decrease absorption. Anticholinergics may increase effects. May decrease absorption of ketoconazole. May increase severity GI lesions with KCl (wax matrix). **ALTERED LAB VALUES:** None significant.

SIDE EFFECTS

FREQUENT: Dry mouth (sometimes severe), decreased sweating, constipation. **OCCASIONAL:** Blurred vision, bloated feeling, urinary hesitancy, drowsiness (w/high dosage), headache, intolerance to light, loss of taste, nervousness, flushing, insomnia, impotence, mental confusion/excitement (particularly in elderly, children). IM may produce temporary lightheadedness, local irritation. **RARE:** Dizziness, faintness.

ADVERSE REACTIONS/TOXIC EFFECTS

Overdosage may produce temporary paralysis of ciliary muscle, pupillary dilation, tachycardia, palpitation, hot/dry/flushed skin, absence of bowel sounds, hyperthermia, increased respiratory rate, EKG abnormalities, nausea, vomiting, rash over face/upper trunk, CNS stimulation, psychosis (agitation, restlessness, rambling speech, visual hallucination, paranoid behavior, delusions), followed by depression.

NURSING IMPLICATIONS

BASELINE ASSESSMENT:

Before giving medication, instruct pt to void (reduces risk of urinary retention).

INTERVENTION/EVALUATION:

Monitor daily bowel activity and stool consistency. Assess for urinary retention. Monitor changes in B/P, temperature. Assess skin turgor, mucous membranes to evaluate hydration status (encourage adequate fluid intake), bowel sounds for peristalsis. Be alert for fever (increased risk of hyperthermia).

PATIENT/FAMILY TEACHING:

Do not become overheated during exercise in hot weather (may result in heat stroke). Avoid hot baths, saunas. Avoid tasks that require alertness, motor skills until response to drug is established. Sugarless gum, sips of tepid water may relieve dry mouth. Do not take antacids or medicine for diarrhea within 1 hr of taking this medication (decreased effectiveness).

didanosine

dye-dan′oh-sin
(Videx)

CANADIAN AVAILABILITY:
Videx

CLASSIFICATION

Antiviral

PHARMACOKINETICS

Variably absorbed from GI tract. Rapidly metabolized intracellularly to active form. Primarily excreted in urine. Half-life: 1.5 hrs; metabolite: 8-24 hrs.

ACTION

Intracellularly converted into a triphosphate, interfering w/RNA-directed DNA polymerase (reverse transcriptase). Virustatic, inhibiting replication of retroviruses, including human immunodeficiency virus (HIV).

USES

Management (not cure) of advanced HIV disease in pts who cannot tolerate zidovudine or who have had clinically or immunologically significant deterioration during zidovudine therapy.

STORAGE/HANDLING

Store at room temperature. If tablets dispersed in water, stable for 1 hr at room temperature; after reconstitution of buffered powder, oral solution stable for 4 hrs at room temperature. Pediatric powder for oral solution after reconstitution as directed stable for 30 days refrigerated.

PO ADMINISTRATION

1. Give 1 hr before or 2 hrs after meals (food decreases rate and extent of absorption).
2. Chewable tablets: thoroughly crushed and dispersed in at least 30 ml water before swallowing. Mixture should be stirred well (2-3 min) and swallowed immediately.
3. Buffered powder for oral solution: reconstitute prior to administration by pouring contents of packet into about 4 oz water; stir until completely dissolved (up to 2-3 min). Do not mix w/fruit juice or other acidic liquid because didanosine is unstable at acidic pH.
4. Unbuffered pediatric powder: add 100-200 ml water to 2 or 4 Gm, respectively, to provide concentration of 20 mg/ml. Immediately mix w/equal amount of antacid to provide concentration of 10 mg/ml. Shake thoroughly prior to removing each dose.

INDICATIONS/DOSAGE/ROUTES

NOTE: Each dose consists of 2 tablets (prevents degradation of drug). Children <1 yr need only 1 tablet/dose.

HIV infections (adults):
PO (TABLETS): Adults ≥60 kg: 200 mg q12h. <**60 kg:** 125 mg q12h. **(BUFFERED ORAL SOLUTION): Adults ≥60 kg:** 250 mg q12h. <**60 kg:** 167 mg q12h.

HIV infections (children):
PO (TABLETS): Children BSA 1.1-1.4 m²: 100 mg q12h; **BSA 0.8-1.0 m²:** 75 mg q12h; **BSA 0.5-0.7 m²:** 50 mg q12h; **BSA <0.4 m²:** 25 mg q12h. **(PEDIATRIC ORAL SOLUTION): Children BSA 1.1-1.4 m²:** 125 mg q12h; **BSA 0.8-1.0 m²:** 94 mg q12h; **BSA 0.5-0.7 m²:** 62 mg q12h; **BSA <0.4 m²:** 31 mg q12h.

D

PRECAUTIONS

CONTRAINDICATIONS: Hypersensitivity to drug or any component of preparation; infants under 6 mo of age. **CAUTIONS:** Renal or hepatic dysfunction, alcoholism, elevated triglycerides, T cell counts less than 100 cells/mm³; extreme caution w/history of pancreatitis. Phenylketonuria and sodium-restricted diets due to phenylalanine and sodium content of preparations. **PREGNANCY/LACTATION:** Use during pregnancy only if clearly needed. Discontinue nursing during didanosine therapy. **Pregnancy Category B.**

INTERACTIONS

DRUG INTERACTIONS: May increase risk of pancreatitis, peripheral neuropathy w/medications producing pancreatitis, peripheral neuropathy respectively. May decrease concentration of quinolones (e.g., ciprofloxacin), tetracycline. **ALTERED LAB VALUES:** May increase alkaline phosphatase, SGOT (AST), SGPT (ALT), bilirubin, amylase, lipase, triglycerides, uric acid. May decrease potassium.

SIDE EFFECTS

Adults: **FREQUENT:** Diarrhea is the most common side effect. Headache, nausea, vomiting, abdominal pain, skin disorders. **OCCASIONAL:** Asthenia, insomnia, hypertension, dizziness, dry mouth, weight loss, confusion, seizures, myalgia. **RARE:** Less than 1% have taste loss, stomatitis, CNS depression, alopecia, facial edema, bronchitis, cerebrovascular disorders, herpes or acne, vision or hearing problems. *Children:* **FREQUENT:** Same as adults plus cough, dyspnea, stomatitis, asthenia, malaise, ecchymosis, liver abnormalities, ear pain, nervousness. **OCCASIONAL:** Weight loss, insomnia, dizziness, petechiae, hemorrhage, vision (including photophobia) or hearing problems, arrhythmias, dehydration, arthritis, myalgia. **RARE:** Diabetes mellitus or insipidus, seizures.

ADVERSE REACTIONS/TOXIC EFFECTS

Pneumonia, opportunistic infection occur occasionally. Peripheral neuropathy, potentially fatal pancreatitis are the major toxicities.

NURSING IMPLICATIONS

BASELINE ASSESSMENT:

Obtain baseline values for CBC, renal and hepatic function tests, vital signs, weight. Question for hypersensitivity to didanosine or components of preparation.

INTERVENTION/EVALUATION:

In event of abdominal pain and nausea, vomiting, or elevated serum amylase, triglycerides, contact physician before administering medication (potential pancreatitis). Be alert to burning feet, "restless leg syndrome" (unable to find comfortable position for legs and feet), lack of coordination and other signs of peripheral neuropathy. Check food intake and assure availability of desired foods. Monitor consistency and frequency of stools. Check skin for rash, eruptions. Assess temperature, respiration, pulse, B/P at least b.i.d. Assess for opportunistic infections: onset of fever, oral mucosa changes, cough, or other respiratory symptoms. Monitor lab values carefully. Assess children for epistaxis or other bleeding, petechiae. Evaluate for dehydration (esp. children): decreased skin turgor, dry skin and mucous membranes, decreased urinary output. Check weight at least twice a week. Assess for visual or hearing difficulty; provide protection from light if photophobia develops. Auscultate lungs and assess for difficult breathing. If dizziness occurs, provide assistance w/ambulation.

PATIENT/FAMILY TEACHING:

Explain correct administration of medication. Small, frequent meals of favorite foods to offset anorexia, vomiting. Accurate I&O record. Report development of fever or any new symptom promptly.

dienestrol

dye-en-ess´trole
(DV, Ortho Dienestrol, Estraguard)

CANADIAN AVAILABILITY:
Ortho Dienestrol

CLASSIFICATION

Estrogen

PHARMACOKINETICS

Extensively absorbed into systemic circulation. Widely distributed. Protein binding: 50-80%. Metabolized in liver. Primarily excreted in urine.

ACTION

Increases synthesis of DNA, RNA, and various proteins in responsive tissues, alleviating signs and symptoms of vulvovaginal epithelial atrophy (atrophic vaginitis), kraurosis vulvae associated w/ menopause.

USES

Treatment of atrophic vaginitis, kraurosis vulvae.

VAGINAL ADMINISTRATION

1. Apply at bedtime for best absorption.
2. Assemble and fill applicator per manufacturer's directions.
3. Insert end of applicator into vagina, direct slightly toward sacrum; push plunger down completely.
4. Avoid skin contact w/cream due to absorption.

INDICATIONS/DOSAGE/ROUTES

Atrophic vaginitis, kraurosis vulvae:
INTRAVAGINAL: Adults, elderly: Initially, 1-2 applicatorsful/day for 7-14 days. Reduce dose by ½ for additional 1-2 wks. **Maintenance:** 1 applicatorful 1-3 times/wk.

PRECAUTIONS

CONTRAINDICATIONS: Known or suspected breast cancer, estrogen-dependent neoplasia; undiagnosed abnormal genital bleeding; active thrombophlebitis or thromboembolic disorders; history of thrombophlebitis, thrombosis, or thromboembolic disorders w/previous estrogen use, hypersensitivity to estrogen or ingredients of cream. **CAUTIONS:** Conditions that may be aggravated by fluid retention: cardiac, renal or hepatic dysfunction, epilepsy, migraine. Mental depression, hypercalcemia, history of jaundice during pregnancy, or strong family history of breast cancer, fibrocystic disease or breast nodules. **PREGNANCY/LACTATION:** Possibly excreted in breast milk. May be harmful to fetus. **Pregnancy Category X.**

INTERACTIONS

DRUG INTERACTIONS: May interfere w/effects of bromocriptine. May increase concentration cyclosporine, increase hepatic, nephrotoxicity. Hepatotoxic medications may increase hepatotoxicity. **ALTERED LAB VALUES:** May affect metapyrone, thyroid function tests. May decrease cholesterol, LDH. May increase calcium, glucose, HDL, triglycerides.

SIDE EFFECTS

OCCASIONAL: Local irritation may occur w/initiation of vaginal therapy. Vaginal discharge, swelling of breasts. Systemic effects may include: **INFREQUENT:** Nausea, vomiting, headache, increased blood pressure, uterine bleeding, fluid retention, glucose intolerance, brown spots on exposed skin. **RARE:** Chorea, cholestatic jaundice, hirsutism, loss of scalp hair, depression.

ADVERSE REACTIONS/TOXIC EFFECTS

Prolonged administration increases risk of gall bladder, thromboembolic disease, and breast, cervical, vaginal, endometrial and liver carcinoma.

NURSING IMPLICATIONS

BASELINE ASSESSMENT:

Question hypersensitivity to estrogen or ingredients of cream, previous jaundice, or thromboembolic disorders associated w/ pregnancy or estrogen therapy.

Establish baseline B/P, blood glucose.

INTERVENTION/EVALUATION:

Initially assess B/P, weight daily. Monitor blood glucose 4 times/day for pts w/diabetes. Check for swelling. Assess for vaginal discharge, local irritation. Promptly report signs and symptoms of thromboembolic or thrombotic disorders: weakness, pain or numbness of an extremity, chest pain, shortness of breath. Note estrogen therapy on specimens.

PATIENT/FAMILY TEACHING:

Importance of medical supervision. W/systemic absorption, smoking may increase risk of heart attack or blood clots. Notify physician of abnormal vaginal bleeding, pain or numbness of an extremity, other symptoms. Teach self-breast exam. Use protection from sun or ultraviolet light. Check weight daily; report weekly gain of 5 lbs. or more. Remain recumbent at least 30 min after application and do not use tampons. Stop using dienestrol, contact physician at once if suspect pregnancy. Give labeling from drug package.

diethylstilbestrol

dye-eth-ill-still-bess′trole

(DES, Stilphostrol)

diethylstilbestrol diphosphate

(Stilphostrol)

CANADIAN AVAILABILITY:
Honvol

CLASSIFICATION

Antineoplastic, estrogen

PHARMACOKINETICS

Well absorbed from GI tract. Widely distributed. Protein binding: 50-80%. Metabolized in liver. Primarily excreted in urine.

ACTION

Increases synthesis of DNA, RNA, and various proteins in responsive tissues. Reduces release of gonadotropin-releasing hormone reducing follicle stimulating hormone (FSH) and leuteinizing hormone (LH), decreases serum concentration of testosterone.

USES

Treatment of atrophic vaginitis, kraurosis vulvae. Palliative therapy for inoperable cancer of the prostate and advanced metastatic cancer of the breast in men and postmenopausal women.

STORAGE/HANDLING

Injection is colorless to light-yellow solution. Discard if solution is cloudy or precipitate forms.

PO/IV ADMINISTRATION

PO:

1. Enteric tablets should not be crushed.
2. Give w/food to reduce nausea.

IV:

1. Dilute in 300 ml normal saline or 5% dextrose for injection.
2. Administer slowly (1-2 ml/min) the first 10-15 min, then increase rate to infuse over 1 hr.

INDICATIONS/DOSAGE/ROUTES

Breast carcinoma:
PO: Adults, elderly: 15 mg/day.

Prostatic carcinoma:
PO: Adults, elderly: Initially, 1-3 mg/day. **Maintenance:** 1 mg/day.

Usual dosage for diethylstilbestrol diphosphate:
PO: Adults, elderly: Initially, 50 mg 3 times/day; increase to 200 mg 3 times/day.
IV: Adults, elderly: Initially, 500 mg, then 1 Gm/day for 5 or more days. **Maintenance:** 250-500 mg 1-2 times/wk.

PRECAUTIONS

CONTRAINDICATIONS: Known or suspected breast cancer (except select cases), estrogen-dependent neoplasia; undiagnosed abnormal genital bleeding; active thrombophlebitis or thromboembolic disorders; history of thrombophlebitis, thrombosis, or thromboembolic disorders w/previous estrogen use, hypersensitivity to estrogen. Stilphostrol (diethylstilbestrol diphosphate) is not for use in women. **CAUTIONS:** Conditions that may be aggravated by fluid retention: cardiac, renal or hepatic dysfunction, epilepsy, migraine. Metabolic bone disease w/potential hypercalcemia, mental depression, history of jaundice during pregnancy, or strong family history of breast cancer, fibrocystic disease or breast nodules, young pts in whom bone growth is not complete. **PREGNANCY/LACTATION:** Not for use during lactation. May cause serious fetal toxicity (increased risk of congenital anomalies). **Pregnancy Category X.**

INTERACTIONS

DRUG INTERACTIONS: May interfere w/effects of bromocriptine. May increase concentration cyclosporine, increase hepatic, nephrotoxicity. Hepatotoxic medications may increase hepatotoxicity. **ALTERED LAB VALUES:** May affect metapyrone, thyroid function tests. May decrease cholesterol, LDH. May increase calcium, glucose, HDL, triglycerides.

SIDE EFFECTS

FREQUENT: Change in vaginal bleeding (spotting, breakthrough, heavy, or prolonged bleeding). **OCCASIONAL:** Headache, increased B/P. *High dose therapy:* Anorexia, nausea. **RARE:** Chorea, cholestatic jaundice, hirsutism, loss of scalp hair, depression.

ADVERSE REACTIONS/TOXIC EFFECTS

Prolonged administration may have possibility of increased risk of gall bladder, thromboembolic disease and cervical, vaginal, endometrial, and liver carcinoma.

NURSING IMPLICATIONS

Baseline Assessment:

Question for possibility of pregnancy before initiating therapy. Question hypersensitivity to estrogen, previous jaundice, or thromboembolic disorders associated w/pregnancy or estrogen therapy. Establish baseline B/P, blood glucose.

Intervention/Evaluation:

Assess B/P at least daily. Monitor blood glucose 4 times/day in diabetic pts. Check for swelling, weigh daily. Promptly report signs and symptoms of thromboembolic or thrombotic disorders: sudden severe headache, shortness of breath, vision or speech disturbance, weakness or numbness of an extremity, loss of coordination, pain in chest, groin or leg. Estrogen therapy should be noted on specimens.

PATIENT/FAMILY TEACHING:

Importance of medical supervision. Avoid smoking due to increased risk of heart attack or blood clots. Do not take other medications w/o physician approval. Teach how to perform Homan's test, signs and symptoms of blood clots (report these to physician immediately). Notify physician of vaginal discharge or bleeding, difficulty or discomfort w/urination, other symptoms. Teach female patients to perform self-breast exam. Cyclic treatment of atrophic vaginitis may take several years. Avoid exposure to sun or ultraviolet light. Check weight daily; report weekly gain of 5 lbs or more. Use nonhormonal contraceptive or inform physician if suspect pregnancy. Libido improves, gynecomastia is reduced when medication stopped.

diflunisal

dye-flew´neh-sol
(Dolobid)

CANADIAN AVAILABILITY:
Dolobid

CLASSIFICATION

Nonsteroidal anti-inflammatory

PHARMACOKINETICS

	ONSET	PEAK	DURATION
PO	1 hr	2-3 hrs	—

Completely absorbed from GI tract. Widely distributed. Protein binding: >99%. Metabolized in liver. Primarily excreted in urine. Half-life: 8-12 hrs.

ACTION

Peripherally acting agent that produces analgesic and anti-inflammatory effect by inhibiting prostaglandin synthesis.

USES

Treatment of acute or long-term mild to moderate pain associated w/acute and/or chronic rheumatoid arthritis, osteoarthritis.

PO ADMINISTRATION

1. May give w/water, milk, or meals.
2. Do not crush or break film-coated tablets.

INDICATIONS/DOSAGE/ROUTES

Mild to moderate pain:
PO: Adults, elderly: Initially, 0.5-1 Gm, then 250-500 mg q8-12h.

Rheumatoid arthritis, osteoarthritis:
PO: Adults, elderly: 0.5-1 Gm/day in 2 divided doses.

PRECAUTIONS

CONTRAINDICATIONS: Active peptic ulcer, GI ulceration, chronic inflammation of GI tract, GI bleeding disorders, history of hypersensitivity to aspirin or NSAIDs. **CAUTIONS:** Impaired renal/hepatic function, history of GI tract disease, hypertension or compromised cardiac function (those predisposed to fluid retention). **PREGNANCY/LACTATION:** Crosses placenta; distributed in breast milk. Avoid use during last trimester (may adversely affect fetal cardiovascular system: premature closure of ductus arteriosus). **Pregnancy Category C.**

INTERACTIONS

DRUG INTERACTIONS: May increase effects of oral anticoagulants, heparin, thrombolytics. May decrease effect of antihypertensives, diuretics. Salicylates, aspirin may increase risk of GI side effects, bleeding. Bone marrow depressants may increase risk of hematologic reactions. May increase concentration, toxicity of lithium. May increase methotrexate toxicity. Probenecid may increase concentration. **ALTERED LAB VALUES:** May increase serum transaminase activity. May decrease uric acid.

SIDE EFFECTS

Side effects appear less frequently w/short-term treatment. **OCCASIONAL:** Nausea, dyspepsia (heartburn, indigestion, epigastric pain), diarrhea, headache, rash. **RARE:** Vomiting, constipation, flatulence, dizziness, insomnia, fatigue, tinnitus.

ADVERSE REACTIONS/TOXIC EFFECTS

Overdosage may produce drowsiness, vomiting, nausea, diarrhea, hyperventilation, tachycardia, sweating, stupor, coma. Peptic ulcer, GI bleeding, gastritis, severe hepatic reaction (cholestasis, jaundice) occur rarely. Nephrotoxicity (dysuria, hematuria, proteinuria, nephrotic syndrome) and severe hypersensitivity reaction (bronchospasm, angiofacial edema) occur rarely.

NURSING IMPLICATIONS

BASELINE ASSESSMENT:

Assess onset, type, location, and duration of pain or inflammation. Inspect appearance of affected joints for immobility, deformities, and skin condition.

INTERVENTION/EVALUATION:

Monitor for nausea, dyspepsia. Assess skin for evidence of rash. Monitor pattern of daily bowel activity and stool consistency. Evaluate for therapeutic response: relief of pain, stiffness, swelling, increase in joint mobility, reduced joint tenderness, improved grip strength.

PATIENT/FAMILY TEACHING:

Swallow tablet whole; do not crush or chew. If GI upset occurs, take w/food, milk. Avoid aspirin, alcohol during therapy (increases risk of GI bleeding). Report GI distress, headache, rash.

digoxin

di-jox′in

(Lanoxin, Lanoxicaps)

CANADIAN AVAILABILITY:

Lanoxin, Novodigoxin

CLASSIFICATION

Antiarrhythmic, cardiotonic

PHARMACOKINETICS

Readily absorbed from GI tract. Widely distributed. Protein binding: 20-25%. Partially metabolized in liver. Primarily excreted in urine. Half-life: 36-48 hrs (increased in decreased renal function, elderly).

ACTION

Increases force, velocity of myocardial contraction. Decreases conduction rate through SA, AV node.

USES

Prophylactic management and treatment of CHF, control of ventricular rate in pts w/atrial fibrillation or flutter. Treatment and prevention of recurrent paroxysmal atrial tachycardia.

PO/IV ADMINISTRATION

NOTE: IM rarely used (produces severe local irritation, erratic absorption). If no other route possible, give deep into muscle followed by massage. Give no more than 2 ml at any one site.

PO:

1. May be given w/o regard to meals.
2. Tablets may be crushed.

IV:

1. May give undiluted or dilute w/at least a 4-fold volume of sterile water for injection, or 5% dextrose (less than this may cause a precipitate). Use immediately.
2. Give IV slowly over at least 5 min.

INDICATIONS/DOSAGE/ROUTES

NOTE: Adjust dose in elderly, patients w/renal dysfunction. Larger doses often required for adequate control of ventricular rate in patients w/atrial fibrillation or flutter. Administer loading dosage in several doses at 4-8 hr intervals.

USUAL DOSAGE FOR ADULTS:

Rapid loading dosage:
IV: Adults, elderly: 0.6-1 mg.
PO: Adults, elderly: 0.75-1.25 mg.

Maintenance dosage:
PO/IV: Adults, elderly: 0.125-0.375 mg/day.

USUAL DOSAGE FOR CHILDREN:

Rapid loading dosage:
IV: Children (>10 yrs): 8-12 mcg/kg; **(5-10 yrs):** 15-30 mcg/kg; **(2-5 yrs):** 25-35 mcg/kg; **(1-24 mo):** 30-50 mcg/kg; **(Full-term):** 20-30 mcg/kg; **(Premature):** 15-25 mcg/kg.
PO: Children (>10 yrs): 10-15 mcg/kg; **(5-10 yrs):** 20-35 mcg/kg; **(2-5 yrs):** 30-40 mcg/kg; **(1-24 mo):** 35-60 mcg/kg: **(Full-term):** 25-35 mcg/kg; **(Premature):** 20-30 mcg/kg.

Maintenance dosage:
PO/IV: Children: 25-35% loading dose (20-30% for premature).

PRECAUTIONS

CONTRAINDICATIONS: Ventricular fibrillation, ventricular tachycardia unrelated to CHF. **CAUTIONS:** Impaired renal function, impaired hepatic function, hypokalemia, advanced cardiac disease, acute myocardial infarction, incomplete AV block, cor pulmonale, hypothyroidism, pulmonary disease. **PREGNANCY/LACTATION:** Crosses placenta; distributed in breast milk. **Pregnancy Category C.**

INTERACTIONS

DRUG INTERACTIONS: Glucocorticoids, amphotericin, potassium depleting diuretics may increase toxicity (due to hypokalemia). Amiodarone may increase concentration, toxicity; additive effect on SA, AV nodes. Antiarrhythmics, parenteral calcium, sympathomimetics may increase risk of arrhythmias. Antidiarrheals, cholestyramine, colestipol may decrease absorption. Diltiazem, verapamil, quinidine may increase concentration. Parenteral magnesium may cause conduction changes, heart block. **ALTERED LAB VALUES:** None significant.

SIDE EFFECTS

None significant, however, there is a very narrow margin of safety between a therapeutic and toxic result.

ADVERSE REACTIONS/TOXIC EFFECTS

The most common early manifestations of toxicity are GI disturbances (anorexia, nausea, vomiting) and neurologic abnormalities (fatigue, headache, depression, weakness, drowsiness, confusion, nightmares). Facial pain, personality change, ocular disturbances (photophobia, light flashes, halos around bright objects, yellow or green color perception) may be noted.

NURSING IMPLICATIONS

BASELINE ASSESSMENT:

Assess apical-radial pulse for 60 sec (30 sec if on maintenance therapy). If pulse is 60/min or below (70/min or below for children), withhold drug and contact physician. Blood samples are best taken 6-8 hrs after dose or just prior to next dose.

INTERVENTION/EVALUATION:

Monitor pulse for bradycardia, EKG for arrhythmias for 1-2 hrs after administration (excessive slowing of pulse may be a first clinical sign of toxicity). Assess for GI disturbances, neurologic abnormalities (signs of toxicity) q2-4hrs during digitalization (daily during maintenance). Monitor serum potassium, magnesium levels. Monitor for therapeutic plasma level (0.5-2.0 ng/ml).

PATIENT/FAMILY TEACHING:

Importance of follow-up visits, tests. Teach pt to take pulse correctly and to report pulse below 60/min (or as indicated by physician). Assure pt understands signs of toxicity and need to notify physician if any occur. Wear/carry identification of digoxin therapy and inform dentist or other physician of taking digoxin. Take medication as directed; do not increase or skip doses. Do not take over-the-counter medications w/o consulting physician. Chronic therapy may produce mammary gland enlargement in women but is reversible when drug is withdrawn.

digoxin immune FAB

(Digibind)

CLASSIFICATION

Antidote

PHARMACOKINETICS

	ONSET	PEAK	DURATION
IV	30 min	—	3-4 days

Widely distributed into extracellular space. Excreted in urine. Half-life: 15-20 hrs.

ACTION

Binds molecules of digoxin, making digoxin unavailable for binding at its site of action on cells in the body. Acts in extracellular space.

USES

Treatment of potentially life-threatening digoxin intoxication.

STORAGE/HANDLING

Refrigerate vials. After reconstitution, stable for 4 hrs if refrigerated. Use immediately after reconstitution.

IV ADMINISTRATION

1. Reconstitute each 40 mg vial w/4 ml sterile water for injection to provide a concentration of 10 mg/ml.
2. Further dilute w/50 ml 0.9% NaCl and infuse over 30 min. (Recommended that solution be infused through a 0.22 μm filter).
3. If cardiac arrest imminent, may give IV push.

INDICATIONS/DOSAGE/ROUTES

NOTE: One 40 mg vial will bind approximate 0.6 mg digoxin or digitoxin, Dose (number of 40 mg vials) = (serum digoxin concentration) × (weight in kg) divided by 100.

PRECAUTIONS

CONTRAINDICATIONS: None significant. **CAUTIONS:** Impaired cardiac, renal function. **PREGNANCY/LACTATION:** Unknown if drug crosses placenta or is distributed in breast milk. **Pregnancy Category C.**

INTERACTIONS

DRUG INTERACTIONS: None significant. **ALTERED LAB VALUES:** May alter potassium concentration. Serum digoxin concentration may increase precipitously and persist for up to 1 wk (until FAB/digoxin complex is eliminated from body).

SIDE EFFECTS

None significant.

ADVERSE REACTIONS/TOXIC EFFECTS

As result digitalis intoxication, hyperkalemia may present (diarrhea, paresthesia of extremities, heaviness of legs, decreased B/P, cold skin, grayish pallor, hypotension, mental confusion, irritability, flaccid paralysis, tented T waves, widening QRS, ST depression). When effect of digitalis is reversed, hypokalemia may develop rapidly (muscle cramping, nausea, vomiting, hypoactive bowel sounds, abdominal distention, difficulty breathing, postural hypotension). Rarely, low cardiac output, CHF may occur.

NURSING IMPLICATIONS

BASELINE ASSESSMENT:

Obtain serum digoxin level before administering drug. If drawn <6 hrs before last digoxin dose, serum digoxin level may be unreliable. Those w/impaired renal function may require >1 wk before serum digoxin assay is reliable. Assess baseline electrolytes, particularly potassium levels. Assess muscle strength, mental status. Note skin temperature, moisture. Obtain baseline weight. Initiate I&O.

INTERVENTION/EVALUATION:

Closely monitor temperature, B/P, EKG, and potassium serum level during and after drug is administered. Watch for changes from initial assessment (hypokalemia may result in muscle strength changes, tremor, muscle cramps, change in mental status, cardiac arrhythmias; hyponatremia may result in confusion, thirst, cold/clammy skin).

diltiazem hydrochloride

dill-tea'ah-zem
(Cardizem, Dilacor XR)

CANADIAN AVAILABILITY:
Cardizem, Apo-Diltiazem

CLASSIFICATION

Calcium channel blocker

PHARMACOKINETICS

	ONSET	PEAK	DURATION
PO	30-60 min	—	—

Well absorbed from GI tract. Undergoes first-pass metabolism in liver. Protein binding: 70-80%. Metabolized in liver to active metabolite. Primarily excreted in urine. Not removed by hemodialysis. Half-life: 3-8 hrs.

ACTION

Inhibits calcium ion entry across cell membranes of cardiac and vascular smooth muscle (may dilate coronary arteries, peripheral arteries/arterioles); may decrease heart rate, myocardial contractility, slow SA and AV conduction. Decreases total peripheral vascular resistance by vasodilation.

USES

Oral: Treatment of angina due to coronary artery spasm (Prinzmetal's variant angina), chronic stable angina (effort-associated angina). *Extended release:* Treatment of essential hypertension, angina. *Parenteral:* Temporary control of rapid ventricular rate in atrial fibrillation/flutter. Rapid conversion of PSVT to normal sinus rhythm.

PO/IV ADMINISTRATION

PO:

1. Give before meals and bedtime.
2. Tablets may be crushed.
3. Do not crush sustained-release capsules.

IV:

1. Add 125 mg to 100 ml 5% dextrose, 0.9% NaCl, or 5% dextrose/0.45% NaCl to provide a concentration of 1 mg/ml. Add 250 mg to 250 or 500 ml diluent to provide a concentration of 0.83 mg/ml or 0.45 mg/ml, respectively.
2. After dilution, stable for 24 hrs.
3. Infuse per dilution/rate chart provided by manufacturer.
4. Do not mix directly w/furosemide.

INDICATIONS/DOSAGE/ROUTES

Angina:
PO: Adults, elderly: Initially, 30 mg 4 times/day. Increase up to 180-360 mg/day in 3-4 divided doses at 1-2 day intervals.
CD CAPSULE: Adults, elderly: Initially, 120-180 mg/day; titrate over 7-14 days. **Range:** up to 480 mg/day.

Essential hypertension:
EXTENDED RELEASE: Adults, elderly: Initially, 60-120 mg 2 times/day.
CD CAPSULES: Adults, elderly: Initially, 180-240 mg/day. **Range:** 240-360 mg in 2 divided doses.
DILACOR XR: Adults, elderly: Initially, 180-240 mg/day. **Range:** 180-480 mg/day.

Usual parenteral dosage:
IV PUSH: Adults, elderly: Initially, 0.25 mg/kg actual body weight

over 2 min. May repeat in 15 min at dose of 0.35 mg/kg actual body weight. Subsequent doses individualized.
IV INFUSION: Adults, elderly: After initial bolus injection, 5-10 mg/hr, may increase at 5 mg/hr up to 15 mg/hr. Maintain over 24 hrs. **Note:** Refer to manufacturer's information for dose concentration/infusion rates.

PRECAUTIONS

CONTRAINDICATIONS: Sick sinus syndrome/second- or third-degree AV block (except in presence of pacemaker), severe hypotension (<90 mm Hg, systolic), acute MI, pulmonary congestion. **CAUTIONS:** Impaired renal/hepatic function, CHF. **PREGNANCY/LACTATION:** Distributed in breast milk. **Pregnancy Category C.**

INTERACTIONS

DRUG INTERACTIONS: Beta-blockers may have additive effect. May increase digoxin concentration. Procainamide, quinidine may increase risk of QT interval prolongation. Carbamazepine, quinidine, theophylline may increase concentration, toxicity. **ALTERED LAB VALUES:** PR interval may be increased.

SIDE EFFECTS

Oral: **OCCASIONAL:** Peripheral edema, facial flushing, dizziness, headache, asthenia (loss of strength, weakness), bradycardia. **RARE:** Diarrhea/constipation, rash. *Parenteral:* **OCCASIONAL:** Hypotension, itching, burning at injection site, vasodilation, atrial flutter, bradycardia, CHF, pruritus, sweating, constipation, dizziness.

ADVERSE REACTIONS/TOXIC EFFECTS

Abrupt withdrawal may increase frequency/duration of angina. CHF, second- and third-degree AV block occur rarely. Overdosage produces nausea, drowsiness, confusion, slurred speech, profound bradycardia.

NURSING IMPLICATIONS

BASELINE ASSESSMENT:

Concurrent therapy of sublingual nitroglycerin may be used for relief of anginal pain. Record onset, type (sharp, dull, squeezing), radiation, location, intensity and duration of anginal pain, and precipitating factors (exertion, emotional stress). Assess baseline renal/liver function tests. Assess B/P, apical pulse immediately before drug is administered.

INTERVENTION/EVALUATION:

Assist w/ambulation if dizziness occurs. Assess for peripheral edema behind medial malleolus (sacral area in bedridden patients). Monitor pulse rate for bradycardia. Question for asthenia, headache.

PATIENT/FAMILY TEACHING:

Do not abruptly discontinue medication. Compliance w/therapy regimen is essential to control anginal pain. To avoid hypotensive effect, rise slowly from lying to sitting position, wait momentarily before standing. Avoid tasks that require alertness, motor skills until response to drug is established. Contact physician/nurse if irregular heart beat, shortness of breath, pronounced dizziness, nausea, or constipation occurs.

dinoprostone

dye-noe-prost´one
(Prostaglandin E_2, Prostin E_2)

CANADIAN AVAILABILITY:
Prepidil Gel, Prostin E_2

CLASSIFICATION

Prostaglandin

PHARMACOKINETICS

Undergoes rapid enzymatic deactivation primarily in maternal lungs. Primarily excreted in urine.

ACTION

Direct action on myometrium. Stimulates myometrial contractions in gravid uterus. Direct softening effect on cervix.

USES

To induce abortion from the 12th wk of pregnancy through the second trimester; to evacuate uterine contents in missed abortion or intrauterine fetal death up to 28 wks gestational age (as calculated from the first day of the last normal menstrual period), benign hydatidiform mole.

STORAGE/HANDLING

Keep frozen (<4°F); bring to room temperature just prior to use.

INTRAVAGINAL ADMINISTRATION

1. Administer only in hospital setting w/emergency equipment available.
2. Warm suppository to room temperature before removing foil wrapper.
3. Avoid skin contact because of risk of absorption.
4. Insert high in vagina.
5. Pt should remain supine for 10 min after administration.

INDICATIONS/DOSAGE/ROUTES

Abortifacient:
INTRAVAGINALLY: Adults: 20 mg (one suppository) high into vagina. May repeat at 3-5 hr intervals until abortion occurs. Do not administer >2 days.

PRECAUTIONS

CONTRAINDICATIONS: Hypersensitivity to dinoprostone or other prostaglandins; acute pelvic inflammatory disease; active cardiac, renal, hepatic, or pulmonary disease; fetal malpresentation or significant cephalopelvic disproportion. **CAUTIONS:** Cervicitis, infected endocervical lesions or acute vaginitis, history of asthma. hypo/hypertension, anemia, jaundice, diabetes, epilepsy, uterine fibroids, compromised (scarred) uterus, cardiovascular, renal, or hepatic disease. **PREGNANCY/LACTATION:** Teratogenic; therefore abortion must be complete.

INTERACTIONS

DRUG INTERACTIONS: Oxytocics may cause uterine hypertonus, possibly causing uterine rupture or cervical laceration. **ALTERED LAB VALUES:** None significant.

SIDE EFFECTS

FREQUENT: Nausea (25%), vomiting (50%), diarrhea (20%), fever, headache (10%), chills (10%), hypotension (10%). **OCCASIONAL:** Joint inflammation, flushing/redness of face. **RARE:** Wheezing, troubled breathing, tightness in chest (esp. asthmatic patients). Lower abdominal pain, increased uterine bleeding, foul smelling lochia may indicate postabortal complications.

ADVERSE REACTIONS/TOXIC EFFECTS

Excessive dosage may cause uterine hypertonicity w/spasm and tetanic contraction, leading to cervical laceration/perforation, uterine rupture or hemorrhage.

NURSING IMPLICATIONS

BASELINE ASSESSMENT:

Question for hypersensitivity to dinoprostone or other prostaglandins. Establish baseline B/P, temperature, respirations, pulse. Obtain orders for antiemetics and antidiarrheals, meperidine or other pain medication for abdominal cramps. Assess any uterine activity or vaginal bleeding.

INTERVENTION/EVALUATION:

Check strength, duration, and frequency of contractions and monitor vital signs q15min until stable, then hourly until abortion complete. Check resting uterine tone. Administer medications for relief of GI effects if indicated, abdominal cramps. Provide emotional support as necessary.

PATIENT/FAMILY TEACHING:

Report fever, chills, foul smelling/increased vaginal discharge, uterine cramps, or pain promptly.

dinoprostone gel (prostaglandin E_2 gel)

dye-noe-prost'one
(Prepidil Gel)

CLASSIFICATION

Prostaglandin

PHARMACOKINETICS

Rapidly absorbed after intracervical administration. Extensively metabolized in lung, liver, and kidney. Excreted in urine.

ACTION

Stimulates myometrium of gravid uterus to contract; stimulates smooth muscle of GI tract; local effect of cervical ripening (initiates softening, effacement, and dilation). Decreases duration of oxytocin administration (30-50% do not require oxytocin), induction to delivery interval, induction failure rate; increases Bishop score.

USES

Ripening unfavorable cervix in pregnant women at or near term w/medical or obstetrical need for labor induction.

STORAGE/HANDLING

Refrigerate.

INTRACERVICAL ADMINISTRATION

1. Use caution in handling, prevent skin contact. Wash hands thoroughly w/soap and water after administration.
2. Bring to room temperature just before use (avoid forcing the warming process).
3. Assemble dosing apparatus as described in manufacturer insert.
4. Have pt in dorsal position w/cervix visualized using a speculum.
5. Introduce gel into cervical canal just below level of internal os.
6. Have pt remain in supine po-

sition at least 15-30 min (minimizes leakage from cervical canal).

INDICATIONS/DOSAGE/ROUTES

Ripening unfavorable cervix:
INTRACERVICAL: Adults: Initially, 0.5 mg (2.5 ml); if no cervical/uterine response, may repeat 0.5 mg dose in 6 hrs. **Maximum:** 1.5 mg (7.5 ml) for a 24-hr period.

PRECAUTIONS

CONTRAINDICATIONS: Conditions where prolonged uterine contractions are inappropriate (e.g., history of cesarean section, major uterine surgery, history of difficult/traumatic labor). Ruptured membranes, hypersensitivity, placenta previa, unexplained vaginal bleeding during pregnancy. **CAUTIONS:** Asthma, glaucoma, increased intraocular pressures, renal/hepatic dysfunction. **PREGNANCY/LACTATION:** Sustained uterine hyperstimulation may affect fetus (e.g., abnormal heart rate). **Pregnancy Category C.**

INTERACTIONS

DRUG INTERACTIONS: May increase effect of other oxytocics (6-12 hr interval recommended when oxytocics follow prostaglandin E_2). **ALTERED LAB VALUES:** None significant.

SIDE EFFECTS

OCCASIONAL: Maternal: Nausea, vomiting, diarrhea, fever, pyrexia, warm feeling in vagina, back pain. **Fetus:** Heart rate abnormality (rare in absence of uterine hyperstimulation), bradycardia, deceleration.

ADVERSE REACTIONS/TOXIC EFFECTS

Overdosage produces uterine hypercontractility, uterine hypertonus, hyperstimulation. Treatment consists of nonspecific conservative management (e.g., maternal position change, administration of O_2 to mother). Beta adrenergics used to treat hyperstimulation.

NURSING IMPLICATIONS

BASELINE ASSESSMENT:

Question pt regarding conditions where prolonged uterine contractions are inappropriate. Assess Bishop score. Assess degree of effacement (determines size of shielded endocervical catheter).

INTERVENTION/EVALUATION:

Monitor uterine activity (onset of uterine contractions), fetal status (heart rate), character of cervix (dilation, effacement). Have pt remain recumbent 1-2 hrs after application w/continuous electronic monitoring of fetal heart rate and uterine activity. Record maternal vital signs at least hourly in presence of uterine activity. Reassess Bishop score.

diphenhydramine hydrochloride

dye-phen-high′dra-meen
(Benadryl, Benylin)

FIXED-COMBINATION(S):
W/calamine, an astringent, and camphor, a counter-irritant (Caladryl)

CANADIAN AVAILABILITY:
Allerdryl, Benadryl, Insomnal

CLASSIFICATION

Antihistamine

PHARMACOKINETICS

	ONSET	PEAK	DURATION
PO	15-30 min	1-4 hrs	4-6 hrs
IM/IV	<15 min	1-4 hrs	4-6 hrs

Well absorbed following oral, parenteral administration. Widely distributed. Protein binding: 98-99%. Metabolized in liver. Primarily excreted in urine. Half-life: 1-4 hrs.

ACTION

Prevents, antagonizes most histamine effects (e.g., urticaria, pruritus). Anticholinergic effects cause drying of nasal mucosa. Antidyskinetic effect related to central inhibition of acetylcholine, sedative effect. Antiemetic, antitussive through central effect.

USES

Treatment of allergic reactions, parkinsonism, prevention and treatment of nausea, vomiting, vertigo due to motion sickness; antitussive, short-term management of insomnia. Topical form used for relief of pruritus, insect bites, skin irritations.

STORAGE/HANDLING

Store oral, elixir, topical, parenteral form at room temperature. Powder slowly darkens on exposure to light (does not alter effectiveness).

PO/IM/IV ADMINISTRATION

PO:

1. Give w/o regard to meals. Scored tablets may be crushed. Do not crush capsules or film coated tablets.

IM:

1. Give deep IM into large muscle mass.

IV:

NOTE: Compatible w/most IV infusion solutions.

1. May be given undiluted.
2. Give IV injection over at least 1 min.

INDICATIONS/DOSAGE/ROUTES

Allergic reaction, parkinsonism, treatment of motion sickness:
PO: Adults: 25-50 mg 3-4 times/day q4-6h. **Elderly:** Initially, 25 mg 2-3 times/day. May increase as needed. **Children >20 lbs:** 5 mg/kg/24 hrs in divided doses 4 times/day.
IM/IV: Adults: 10-50 mg. **Maximum daily dose:** 400 mg. **Children >20 lbs:** 5 mg/kg/24 hrs 4 times/day.

Prevention of motion sickness:
PO: Adults: 25-50 mg 30 min before exposure to motion. Give subsequent doses q4-6h.

Nighttime sleep aid:
PO: Adults: 50 mg 20 min before bedtime.

Cough:
PO: Adults: 25 mg q4h.
SYRUP: Adults: 10-20 ml 3-4 times/day. **Children:** 5-10 ml 3-4 times/day.

Pruritus relief:
TOPICAL: Adults: Apply to affected area 3-4 times/day.

PRECAUTIONS

CONTRAINDICATIONS: Acute asthmatic attack, those receiving MAO inhibitors. **CAUTIONS:** Narrow-angle glaucoma, peptic ulcer, prostatic hypertrophy, pyloroduodenal or bladder neck obstruction, asthma, COPD, increased intraocular pressure, cardiovascular disease, hyperthyroidism, hypertension, seizure disorders. **PREG-**

NANCY/LACTATION: Crosses placenta; detected in breast milk (may produce irritability in nursing infants). Increased risk of seizures in neonates, premature infants if used during third trimester of pregnancy. May prohibit lactation. **Pregnancy Category B.**

INTERACTIONS

DRUG INTERACTIONS: Alcohol, CNS depressants may increase CNS depressant effects. MAO inhibitors may increase anticholinergic, CNS depressant effects. Anticholinergics may increase anticholinergic effects. **ALTERED LAB VALUES:** May suppress wheal and flare reactions to antigen skin testing unless antihistamines are discontinued 4 days prior to testing.

SIDE EFFECTS

FREQUENT: Drowsiness, dizziness, muscular weakness, dry mouth/nose/throat/lips, urinary retention, thickening of bronchial secretions. Sedation, dizziness, hypotension more likely noted in elderly. **OCCASIONAL:** Epigastric distress, flushing, visual disturbances, hearing disturbances, paresthesia, sweating, chills.

ADVERSE REACTIONS/TOXIC EFFECTS

Children may experience dominant paradoxical reactions (restlessness, insomnia, euphoria, nervousness, tremors). Overdosage in children may result in hallucinations, convulsions, death. Hypersensitivity reaction (eczema, pruritus, rash, cardiac disturbances, photosensitivity) may occur. Overdosage may vary from CNS depression (sedation, apnea, cardiovascular collapse, death) to severe paradoxical reaction (hallucinations, tremor, seizures).

NURSING IMPLICATIONS

BASELINE ASSESSMENT:

If pt is undergoing allergic reaction, obtain history of recently ingested foods, drugs, environmental exposure, recent emotional stress. Monitor rate, depth, rhythm, type of respiration and quality and rate of pulse. Assess lung sounds for rhonchi, wheezing, rales.

INTERVENTION/EVALUATION:

Monitor B/P, esp. in elderly (increased risk of hypotension). Monitor children closely for paradoxical reaction.

PATIENT/FAMILY TEACHING:

Tolerance to antihistaminic effect generally does not occur; tolerance to sedative effect may occur. Avoid tasks that require alertness, motor skills until response to drug is established. Dry mouth, drowsiness, dizziness may be an expected response of drug. Avoid alcoholic beverages during antihistamine therapy. Sugarless gum, sips of tepid water may relieve dry mouth. Coffee or tea may help reduce drowsiness.

diphenoxylate hydrochloride w/ atropine sulfate

dye-phen-ox′eh-late

(Lofene, Logen, Lomanate, Lomotil, Lonox)

CLASSIFICATION

Antidiarrheal

PHARMACOKINETICS

Well absorbed from GI tract. Metabolized in liver to active metabolite. Primarliy eliminated in feces.` Half-life: 2.5 hrs; metabolite: 12-24 hrs.

ACTION

Acts locally, centrally to reduce intestinal motility. Meperidine congener.

USES

Adjunctive treatment of acute, chronic diarrhea.

PO ADMINISTRATION

1. Give w/o regard to meals. If GI irritation occurs, give w/food or meals.
2. Use liquid for children under 12 yrs (use dropper for administration of liquids).

INDICATIONS/DOSAGE/ROUTES

Antidiarrheal:
PO: Adults, elderly: Initially, 2.5-5 mg 4 times/day. **Maintenance:** 2.5 mg 2-3 times/day. **Children:** Initially, 0.3-0.4 mg/kg/day in 4 divided doses. **Maintenance:** As low as ¼ initial dose (0.075-0.1 mg/kg/day in divided doses).

PRECAUTIONS

CONTRAINDICATIONS: Obstructive jaundice, diarrhea associated w/pseudomembranous enterocolitis due to broad-spectrum antibiotics or w/organisms that invade intestinal mucosa *(Escherichia* coli, *Shigella, Salmonella),* acute ulcerative colitis (may produce toxic megacolon). **CAUTIONS:** Advanced hepatorenal disease, abnormal liver function. **PREGNANCY/LACTATION:** Unknown if drug crosses placenta; distributed in breast milk. **Pregnancy Category C.**

INTERACTIONS

DRUG INTERACTIONS: Alcohol, CNS depressants may increase effect. Anticholinergics may increase effect of atropine. MAO inhibitors may precipitate hypertensive crisis. **ALTERED LAB VALUES:** May increase amylase.

SIDE EFFECTS

FREQUENT: Nausea, drowsiness, lightheadedness, dizziness, anorexia. **OCCASIONAL:** Headache, dry mouth. **RARE:** Flushing, tachycardia, urinary retention, constipation. Paradoxical reaction (restlessness, agitation), burning of eyes, blurred vision.

ADVERSE REACTIONS/TOXIC EFFECTS

Dehydration may predispose to toxicity. Delayed peristalsis may produce fluid retention, further aggravating dehydration, electrolyte imbalance. Addiction is possible w/high dosage (not w/recommended dosage). Symptoms of overdosage (dry skin/mucous membranes, hyperthermia, hypotonic reflexes) may not occur until 12-30 hrs after ingestion; may result in severe respiratory depression, coma, brain damage. Antidote: naloxone.

NURSING IMPLICATIONS

BASELINE ASSESSMENT:

Check baseline hydration status: skin turgor, mucous membranes for dryness, urinary status.

INTERVENTION/EVALUATION:

Encourage adequate fluid intake. Assess bowel sounds for peristalsis. Monitor daily bowel activity, stool consistency (watery, loose, soft, semisolid, solid) and record time of evacuation. Assess for abdominal disturbances. Discontinue medication if abdominal distention occurs. Check I&O. Monitor for paradoxical reaction.

PATIENT/FAMILY TEACHING:

Avoid tasks that require alertness, motor skills until response to drug is established. Do not ingest alcohol or barbiturates. Contact physician if fever, palpitations occur or diarrhea persists. Cola, unsalted crackers, dry toast may relieve nausea. Dry mouth may be relieved by sugarless gum, sips of tepid water.

dipivefrin

dye-pi-ver´inn

(Propine)

CANADIAN AVAILABILITY: Propine

CLASSIFICATION

Mydriatic

PHARMACOKINETICS

	ONSET	PEAK	DURATION
OPHTHALMIC	30 min	1 hr	12 hrs

Rapidly absorbed into aqueous humor, converted to epinephrine.

ACTION

Converted to epinephrine. Decreases aqueous production, enhances aqueous outflow.

USES

Initial or adjunctive therapy (w/ other antiglaucoma agents) for the control of intraocular pressure in chronic open-angle glaucoma.

STORAGE/HANDLING

Protect from light, discard if darkened or discolored.

OPHTHALMIC ADMINISTRATION

1. For topical ophthalmic use only.
2. Instruct pt to tilt head backward and look up.
3. Gently pull lower lid down to form pouch and instill medication.
4. Do not touch tip of applicator to lids or any surface.
5. When lower lid is released, have pt keep eye open w/o blinking for at least 30 sec.
6. Apply gentle finger pressure to lacrimal sac (bridge of the nose, inside corner of the eye) for 1-2 min.
7. Remove excess solution around eye w/a tissue. Wash hands immediately to remove medication on hands.

INDICATIONS/DOSAGE/ROUTES

Glaucoma:

OPHTHALMIC: Adults, elderly: 1 drop q12h.

NOTE: When replacing therapy w/dipivefrin, first day continue other medication, add dipivefrin; second day discontinue other medication.

PRECAUTIONS

CONTRAINDICATIONS: Hypersensitivity to any component; narrow-angle glaucoma. **CAUTIONS:** Sulfite sensitivity, aphakic pts (those w/o lens because of surgery, trauma, congenital defect), hypertension, cardiac disorders including dysrhythmias. **PREGNANCY/LACTATION:** Safety in pregnancy and lactation not established. **Pregnancy Category B.**

INTERACTIONS

DRUG INTERACTIONS: If significant systemic absorption occurs: tricyclic antidepressants may increase cardiovascular effects, digoxin may increase risk of arrhythmias, sympathomimetics may increase toxicity. Ophthalmic beta-blockers may increase effect. **ALTERED LAB VALUES:** None significant.

SIDE EFFECTS

OCCASIONAL: Conjunctival injection (6.5%), burning and stinging (6%). Blurred vision, ocular pain, headache. **INFREQUENT:** Follicular conjunctivitis and allergic reactions, photophobia.

ADVERSE REACTIONS/TOXIC EFFECTS

Unlike epinephrine, systemic effects (tachycardia, arrhythmias, hypertension) are rare w/dipivefrin.

NURSING IMPLICATIONS

BASELINE ASSESSMENT:

Question for hypersensitivity to dipivefrin or epinephrine (cross-sensitivity).

INTERVENTION/EVALUATION:

Assess for local or systemic reactions (see Adverse Reactions/Toxic Effects). Protect from light if photophobia occurs.

PATIENT/FAMILY TEACHING:

Teach proper administration. Slight burning, stinging may occur on initial instillation. Report any new symptoms (rapid pulse, shortness of breath, or dizziness immediately—may be systemic effects).

dipyridamole

die-pie-rid´ah-mole
(Persantine)

CANADIAN AVAILABILITY:
Apo-Dipyridamole, Novodipiradol, Persantine

CLASSIFICATION

Antiplatelet

PHARMACOKINETICS

Slow, variably absorbed from GI tract. Widely distributed. Protein binding: 91-99%. Metabolized in liver. Primarily eliminated via biliary excretion. Half-life: 10-15 hrs.

ACTION

Platelet adhesion inhibitor. May inhibit RBC uptake of adenosine, inhibit phosphodiesterase, or inhibit thromboxane A_2 formation.

USES

Adjunct to coumarin anticoagulant in prevention of postop thromboembolic complications of cardiac valve replacement. IV use: alternative to exercise in thallium myocardial perfusion imaging for evaluation of coronary artery disease.

PO/IV ADMINISTRATION

PO:

1. Best taken on empty stomach w/full glass of water.

IV:

1. Dilute to at least 1:2 ratio w/0.9% NaCl or 5% dextrose in water for total volume of 20-50 ml (undiluted may cause irritation).
2. Infuse over 4 min.

3. Inject thallium within 5 min after dipyridamole infusion.

INDICATIONS/DOSAGE/ROUTES

Prevention of thromboembolic disorders:
PO: Adults, elderly: 75-100 mg 4 times/day in combination w/other medications.

Diagnostic:
IV: Adults, elderly, (Based on weight): 0.142 mg/kg/min infused over 4 min; doses >60 mg not needed for any pt.

PRECAUTIONS

CONTRAINDICATIONS: None significant. **CAUTIONS:** Those w/hypotension. **PREGNANCY/LACTATION:** Excreted in breast milk. **Pregnancy Category B.**

INTERACTIONS

DRUG INTERACTIONS: May increase risk of bleeding w/anticoagulants, heparin, thrombolytics, aspirin, salicylates. **ALTERED LAB VALUES:** None significant.

SIDE EFFECTS

FREQUENT: Dizziness. **OCCASIONAL:** Headache, nausea, flushing, weakness/syncope, mild GI distress, rash.

ADVERSE REACTIONS/TOXIC EFFECTS

Overdosage produces peripheral vasodilation, resulting in hypotension.

NURSING IMPLICATIONS

BASELINE ASSESSMENT:

Assess chest pain, B/P, pulse. When used as antiplatelet, check hematologic levels.

INTERVENTION/EVALUATION:

Assist w/ambulation if dizziness occurs. Monitor heart sounds by auscultation. Assess B/P for hypotension. Assess skin for flushing, rash.

PATIENT/FAMILY TEACHING:

If nausea occurs, cola, unsalted crackers, or dry toast may relieve effect. Therapeutic response may not be achieved before 2-3 mos of continuous therapy.

disopyramide phosphate

dye-so-peer´ah-myd
(Norpace)

CANADIAN AVAILABILITY:
Norpace, Rythmodan

CLASSIFICATION

Antiarrhythmic

PHARMACOKINETICS

	ONSET	PEAK	DURATION
PO	0.5-3.5 hrs	—	1.5-8.5 hrs

Rapidly, completely absorbed from GI tract. Protein binding: 50%. Metabolized in liver. Primarily excreted in urine. Removed by hemodialysis. Half-life: 7 hrs (increased in decreased renal function).

ACTION

Prolongs refractory period by direct effect, decreasing myocardial excitability and conduction velocity. Depresses myocardial contractility. Has anticholinergic, negative inotropic effects.

USES

Suppression and prevention of unifocal/multifocal premature ventricular contractions (ectopic), paired ventricular contractions (couplets), episodes of ventricular tachycardia.

PO ADMINISTRATION

1. May be given w/o regard to meals but best absorbed 1 hr before or 2 hrs after meals.
2. Do not crush or break extended-release capsules.

INDICATIONS/DOSAGE/ROUTES

Usual dosage:
PO: Adults, elderly >50 kg: 150 mg q6h (300 mg q12h w/extended-release). **Adults, elderly <50 kg:** 100 mg q6h (200 mg q12h w/extended-release). **Children 12-18 yrs:** 6-15 mg/kg/day in divided doses q6h. **Children 4-12 yrs:** 10-15 mg/kg/day in divided doses q6h. **Children 1-4 yrs:** 10-20 mg/kg/day in divided doses q6h. **Children <1 yr:** 10-30 mg/kg/day in divided doses q6h.

Rapid control of arrhythmias:
NOTE: Do not use extended-release capsules.
PO: Adults, elderly >50 kg: Initially, 300 mg, then 150 mg q6h. **Adults, elderly <50 kg:** Initially, 200 mg, then 100 mg q6h.

Severe refractory arrhythmias:
PO: Adults, elderly: Up to 400 mg q6h.

Dosage in renal impairment:
W/or w/o loading dose of 150 mg:

CREATININE CLEARANCE	DOSAGE
>40 ml/min	100 mg q6h (extended-release 200 mg q12h)
30-40 ml/min	100 mg q8h
15-30 ml/min	100 mg q12h
<15 ml/min	100 mg q24h

Dosage in hepatic impairment:
100 mg q6h (200 mg q12h w/extended-release).

Dosage in cardiomyopathy, decompensated myocardium:
No loading dose, 100 mg q6-8h w/gradual dosage adjustments.

PRECAUTIONS

CONTRAINDICATIONS: Preexisting urinary retention, preexisting second- or third-degree AV block, cardiogenic shock, narrow-angle glaucoma, unless pt is undergoing cholinergic therapy. **CAUTIONS:** CHF, myasthenia gravis, narrow-angle glaucoma, prostatic hypertrophy, sick-sinus syndrome (bradycardia/tachycardia), Wolff-Parkinson-White syndrome, bundle-branch block, impaired renal/hepatic function. **PREGNANCY/LACTATION:** Crosses placenta; distributed in breast milk. May stimulate contractions of pregnant uterus. **Pregnancy Category C.**

INTERACTIONS

DRUG INTERACTIONS: Other antiarrhythmics (e.g., propranolol, diltiazem, verapamil) may prolong conduction, decrease cardiac output. Pimozide may increase cardiac arrhythmias. **ALTERED LAB**

VALUES: May decrease glucose. May cause ECG changes.

SIDE EFFECTS

FREQUENT: *Cholinergic effects:* Dry mouth, dry nose/eyes, urinary hesitancy, constipation, blurred vision, dizziness, fatigue, muscle weakness, headache, malaise. **OCCASIONAL:** Urinary retention, edema, weight gain. **RARE:** Nausea, vomiting, anorexia, diarrhea.

ADVERSE REACTIONS/TOXIC EFFECTS

May produce or aggravate CHF. May produce severe hypotension, compounded w/shortness of breath, chest pain, syncope (esp. in those w/primary cardiomyopathy or in inadequately compensated CHF). Hepatic toxicity occurs rarely.

NURSING IMPLICATIONS

BASELINE ASSESSMENT:

Assess baseline hepatic, renal function studies. Before giving medication, instruct pt to void (reduces risk of urinary retention).

INTERVENTION/EVALUATION:

Monitor EKG for cardiac changes, particularly widening of QRS complex, prolongation of PR and QT intervals. Notify physician of any significant interval changes. Assess pattern of daily bowel activity, stool consistency. Monitor I&O (be alert to urinary retention). Assess for evidence of CHF (cough, dyspnea [particularly on exertion], rales at base of lungs, fatigue). Assess for edema directly behind medial malleolus in ambulatory pts, sacral area in bedridden pts (usually first areas showing impending edema). Assist w/ambulation if dizziness occurs. Monitor for therapeutic serum level (2-8 mcg/ml).

PATIENT/FAMILY TEACHING:

Report shortness of breath, cough. Compliance w/therapy regimen is essential to control cardiac dysrhythmias. Do not use nasal decongestants, over-the-counter cold preparations (stimulants) w/o physician approval. Restrict salt, alcohol intake. Sugarless gum, sips of tepid water may relieve dry mouth. Report visual disturbances, headache, dizziness.

disulfiram

dye-sul´fi-ram
(Antabuse)

CANADIAN AVAILABILITY:
Antabuse

CLASSIFICATION

Alcohol deterrent

PHARMACOKINETICS

Slowly absorbed from GI tract. Metabolized in liver. Primarily excreted in urine. Up to 20% of dose remains in body for at least 1 week.

ACTION

Inhibits enzyme aldehyde dehydrogenase, responsible for breakdown of ethanol metabolite acetaldehyde. Increased acetaldehyde responsible for disulfiram reaction after alcohol ingestion.

USES

Adjunct in management of selected chronic alcoholic pts who want to remain in state of enforced sobriety.

PO ADMINISTRATION

1. Scored tablets may be crushed.
2. Give w/o regard to meals.

INDICATIONS/DOSAGE/ROUTES

NOTE: Pts must abstain from alcohol for at least 12 hrs before initial dose is administered.
PO: Adults, elderly: Initially, administer maximum of 500 mg daily given as a single dose for 1-2 wks. **Maintenance:** 250 mg daily (normal range: 125-500 mg). Do not exceed maximum daily dose of 500 mg.

PRECAUTIONS

CONTRAINDICATIONS: Severe heart disease, psychosis. **CAUTIONS:** Alcoholic disease.

INTERACTIONS

DRUG INTERACTIONS: Alcohol within 14 days results in disulfiram-alcohol reaction. Oral anticoagulant effect may increase. May increase concentration, toxicity of phenytoin. Isoniazid may increase CNS effects. Metronidazole may increase toxicity. **ALTERED LAB VALUES:** May increase cholesterol concentrations. May decrease VMA concentrations.

SIDE EFFECTS

Experienced during first 2 wks of therapy: mild drowsiness, fatigue, headache, metallic or garlic aftertaste, allergic dermatitis, acne eruptions. Symptoms disappear spontaneously w/continued therapy or w/reduced dosage.

ADVERSE REACTIONS/TOXIC EFFECTS

Disulfiram-alcohol reaction to ingestion of alcohol in any form: flushing/throbbing in head and neck, throbbing headache, nausea, copious vomiting, diaphoresis, dyspnea, hyperventilation, tachycardia, hypotension, marked uneasiness, vertigo, blurred vision, confusion. Can produce death.

NURSING IMPLICATIONS

INTERVENTION/EVALUATION:

Do not give w/o pt's knowledge. Fully inform pt of consequences of alcohol ingestion. Therapy cannot be started until a minimum of 12 hrs has elapsed since pt's last ingestion of alcohol.

PATIENT/FAMILY TEACHING:

Avoid cough syrups, vinegars, fluid extracts, elixirs because of their alcohol content. Even external application of liniments, shaving or body lotion may precipitate a crisis. Effects of medication may occur several days after discontinuance.

dobutamine hydrochloride

do-byew´ta-meen
(Dobutrex)

CANADIAN AVAILABILITY:
Dobutrex

CLASSIFICATION

Sympathomimetic

PHARMACOKINETICS

	ONSET	PEAK	DURATION
IV	1-2 min	10 min	length of infusion

Metabolized in liver. Primarily excreted in urine. Half-life: 2 minutes.

ACTION

Direct acting inotropic agent acting primarily on $beta_1$-adrenergic receptors (increases myocardial contractility, stroke volume, cardiac output). Decreases preload, afterload. Excessive doses increase heart rate. Improves renal blood flow, urine output.

USES

Short-term treatment of cardiac decompensation due to depressed myocardial contractility (due to organic heart disease, cardiac surgical procedures).

STORAGE/HANDLING

Store at room temperature. Freezing produces crystallization. Pink discoloration of solution (due to oxidation) does not indicate loss of potency if used within recommended time period. Reconstituted, concentrated solution maintains potency for 6 hrs at room temperature, 48 hrs if refrigerated. Further diluted solutions for infusion must be used within 24 hrs.

IV ADMINISTRATION

NOTE: Correct hypovolemia w/ volume expanders before dobutamine infusion. Those w/atrial fibrillation should be digitalized prior to infusion. Administer by IV infusion only.

IV:

1. Dilute 250 mg ampoule w/10 ml sterile water for injection or 5% dextrose for injection. Resulting solution: 25 mg/ml. Add additional 10 ml of diluent if not completely dissolved (resulting solution: 12.5 mg/ml).
2. Dilute further to at least 50 ml w/5% dextrose, 0.9% NaCl or sodium lactate injection before administration.
3. Use infusion pump to control flow rate.
4. Titrate dosage to individual response.

INDICATIONS/DOSAGE/ROUTES

NOTE: Dosage determined by pt response.

IV INFUSION: Adults, elderly: 2.5-10 mcg/kg/min. Rarely, infusion rate up to 40 mcg/kg/min may be required to increase cardiac output.

PRECAUTIONS

CONTRAINDICATIONS: Idiopathic hypertrophic subaortic stenosis, hypovolemic pts, sulfite sensitivity. **CAUTIONS:** Atrial fibrillation, hypertension. Safety in children not established. **PREGNANCY/LACTATION:** Unknown if drug crosses placenta or is distributed in breast milk. Has not been administered to pregnant women. **Pregnancy Category C.**

INTERACTIONS

DRUG INTERACTIONS: Beta blockers may antagonize effects. Nitroprusside may increase cardiac output, decrease pulmonary wedge pressure. **ALTERED LAB VALUES:** None significant.

SIDE EFFECTS

FREQUENT: Heart rate increase of 5-15 beats/min, and increase in systolic B/P of 10-20 mm Hg. **OCCASIONAL:** Chest pain, irregular heartbeat, shortness of breath, nausea, headache.

ADVERSE REACTIONS/TOXIC EFFECTS

Overdosage may produce marked increase in heart rate (30 beats/min or greater), marked increase in systolic B/P (50 mm Hg or greater), anginal pain, premature ventricular beats.

NURSING IMPLICATIONS

BASELINE ASSESSMENT:

Pt must be on continuous cardiac monitoring. Determine weight (for dosage calculation). Obtain initial B/P, heart rate, and respirations.

INTERVENTION/EVALUATION:

Continuously monitor for cardiac rate, arrhythmias. W/physician establish parameters for adjusting rate or stopping infusion. Maintain accurate I&O; measure urine output frequently. Assess potassium levels and dobutamine plasma level (therapeutic range = 40-190 ng/ml). Check cardiac output. Monitor B/P continuously (hypertension greater risk in pts w/ preexisting hypertension) and pulmonary wedge pressure or central venous pressure frequently. Immediately notify physician of decreased urine output, cardiac arrhythmias, significant increase in B/P or heart rate and, less commonly hypotension.

PATIENT/FAMILY TEACHING:

Explain rationale for therapy. Report chest pain, discomfort at IV site.

docusate calcium

dock´cue-sate

(Pro-Cal-Sof, Surfak)

docusate potassium

(Dialose, Diocto-K, Kasof)

docusate sodium

(Colace, Doxinate, Modane Soft)

FIXED-COMBINATION(S):
W/casanthranol, a stimulant laxative (Peri-colace); w/phenolphthalein, a laxative (Correctol, Doxidan)

CANADIAN AVAILABILITY:
Colace, Doxate-S

CLASSIFICATION

Laxative: Stool softener

PHARMACOKINETICS

Minimal absorption from GI tract. Acts in small/large intestine. Results occur 1-2 days after first dose (may take 3-5 days).

ACTION

Decreases surface film tension by interfacing liquid, contents of bowel, increases permeation of additional liquid to form a softer stool.

USES

Prophylaxis in those who should not strain during defecation.

PO ADMINISTRATION

Drink 6-8 glasses of water/day (aids stool softening). Give each dose w/glass of water or fruit juice.

INDICATIONS/DOSAGE/ROUTES

STOOL SOFTENER:

Calcium docusate:
PO: Adults, elderly: 240 mg/day until evacuation. **Children >6 yrs:** 50-150 mg/day.

Potassium docusate:
PO: Adults, elderly: 100-300 mg/day until evacuation. **Children >6 yrs:** 100 mg at bedtime.

Sodium docusate:
PO: Adults, elderly: 50-500 mg/day. **Children 6-12 yrs:** 40-120 mg/day. **Children 3-6 yrs:** 20-60

mg/day. **Children <3 yrs:** 10-40 mg/day.

PRECAUTIONS

CONTRAINDICATIONS: Abdominal pain, nausea, vomiting, appendicitis. **CAUTIONS:** None significant. **PREGNANCY/LACTATION:** Unknown if drug is distributed in breast milk. **Pregnancy Category C.**

INTERACTIONS

DRUG INTERACTIONS: May increase absorption of mineral oil, danthron, phenolphthalein. **ALTERED LAB VALUES:** None significant.

SIDE EFFECTS

RARE: Mild GI cramping, rash, throat irritation.

ADVERSE REACTIONS/TOXIC EFFECTS

None significant.

NURSING IMPLICATIONS

INTERVENTION/EVALUATION:

Encourage adequate fluid intake. Assess bowel sounds for peristalsis. Monitor daily bowel activity and stool consistency (watery, loose, soft, semisolid, solid) and record time of evacuation.

PATIENT/FAMILY TEACHING:

Institute measures to promote defecation: increase fluid intake, exercise, high-fiber diet.

dopamine hydrochloride

dope´a-meen

(Intropin, Dopastat)

CANADIAN AVAILABILITY: Intropin, Revimine

CLASSIFICATION

Sympathomimetic

PHARMACOKINETICS

	ONSET	PEAK	DURATION
IV	1-2 min	<5 min	<10 min

Widely distributed. Does not cross blood-brain barrier. Metabolized in liver, kidney, plasma by MAO, COMT. Primarily excreted in urine. Half-life: 2 minutes.

ACTION

Stimulates adrenergic receptors; effects are dose dependent. *Low doses:* Stimulates dopaminergic receptors causing renal vasodilation (increases renal blood flow, urine flow, sodium excretion). *Low-moderate doses:* Positive inotropic effect by direct action, release of norepinephrine (increases myocardial contractility, stroke volume, cardiac output). *High doses:* Stimulates alpha receptors (increased peripheral resistance, renal vasoconstriction, increases systolic and diastolic B/P).

USES

Treatment of shock due to myocardial infarction, trauma, open heart surgery, endotoxic septicemia, renal failure. Used in short-term treatment of severe CHF refractory to digitalis, diuretics.

STORAGE/HANDLING

Do not use solutions darker than slightly yellow or discolored to yellow, brown, or pink to purple (indicates decomposition of drug).

IV ADMINISTRATION

NOTE: Blood volume depletion must be corrected before administering dopamine (may be used concurrently with fluid replacement).

IV:

1. Dilute each 5 ml (200 mg) ampoule in 250-500 ml of compatible solution (concentration is dependent on dosage and fluid requirement of pt). 250 ml solution yields 800 mcg/ml; 500 ml solution yields 400 mcg/ml.
2. Administer into large vein (antecubital fossa) to prevent extravasation.
3. Use infusion pump to control rate of flow.
4. Titrate each pt to the desired hemodynamic or renal response.

INDICATIONS/DOSAGE/ROUTES

IV: Adults, elderly: Begin with rate of 1-5 mcg/kg/min in those likely to respond to minimal treatment. May be gradually increased in 1-4 mcg/kg/min increments at 10-30 min intervals until optimum response achieved. Most patients are maintained on dose of 20 mcq/kg/min or less.

Seriously ill:
IV: Adults, elderly: Begin with 5 mcg/kg/min rate; gradually increase in 5-10 mcg/kg/min increments up to rate of 20-50 mcg/kg/min. Those who do not respond may require further increments.

Pts with occlusive vascular disease:
IV: Adults, elderly: Begin with rate of 1 mcg/kg/min.

Pts on MAO inhibitors:
IV: Adults, elderly: Reduce dose to one-tenth the calculated amount.

PRECAUTIONS

CONTRAINDICATIONS: Pheochromocytoma, uncorrected tachyarrhythmias, ventricular fibrillation, sulfite sensitivity. **CAUTIONS:** Ischemic heart disease, occlusive vascular disease. Safety and efficacy for use in children has not been established. **PREGNANCY/LACTATION:** Unknown if drug crosses placenta or is distributed in breast milk. **Pregnancy Category C.**

INTERACTIONS

DRUG INTERACTIONS: Tricyclic antidepressants, may increase cardiovascular effects. Beta-blockers may decrease effects. May increase risk arrhythmias w/digoxin. Ergot alkaloids may increase vasoconstriction. MAO inhibitors may increase cardiac stimulation, vasopressor effects. **ALTERED LAB VALUES:** None significant.

SIDE EFFECTS

FREQUENT: Headache, ectopic beats, tachycardia, anginal pain, palpitations, vasoconstriction, hypotension, nausea, vomiting, dyspnea. **OCCASIONAL:** Piloerection (goosebumps), cardiac conduction abnormalities, bradycardia, widening of QRS complex, azotemia (urea nitrogen in blood).

ADVERSE REACTIONS/TOXIC EFFECTS

High doses may produce ventricular arrhythmias. Pts with occlusive vascular disease are high-risk candidates for further compromise of circulation to extremities, which may result in gangrene. Extravasation resulting in tissue necrosis with sloughing may occur w/IV administration.

NURSING IMPLICATIONS

BASELINE ASSESSMENT:

Check for MAO inhibitor therapy within last 2-3 wks (dosage reduction). Pt must be on continuous cardiac monitoring. Determine weight (for dosage calculation). Obtain initial B/P, heart rate, and respirations.

INTERVENTION/EVALUATION:

Continuously monitor for cardiac arrhythmias. W/physician, establish parameters for adjusting rate or stopping infusion. Maintain accurate I&O; measure urine output frequently. Assure proper placement of IV catheter; if extravasation occurs, immediately infiltrate the affected tissue w/10-15 ml 0.9% NaCl solution containing 5-10 mg phentolamine mesylate. Monitor B/P, heart rate, and respirations every 15 min during administration (or more often if indicated). Assess cardiac output, pulmonary wedge pressure or central venous pressure frequently. Assess peripheral circulation (palpate pulses, note color and temperature of extremities). Immediately notify physician of decreased urine output, cardiac arrhythmias, significant changes in B/P or heart rate (or failure to respond to increase/decrease in infusion rate), decreased peripheral circulation (cold, pale, or mottled extremities). Taper dosage before discontinuing because abrupt cessation of therapy may result in marked hypotension. Be alert to excessive vasoconstriction (as evidenced by decreased urine output, increased heart rate or arrhythmias and a disproportionate increase in diastolic blood pressure and decrease in pulse pressure); slow or temporarily stop the infusion and notify physician at once.

PATIENT/FAMILY TEACHING:

Explain rational for therapy. Report cold extremities, chest pain, difficulty breathing or discomfort at IV site.

D

dornase alfa

door'naze al'fah
(Pulmozyme)

CLASSIFICATION

Enzyme

PHARMACOKINETICS

	ONSET	PEAK	DURATION
Inhalant	15 min	3 days	—

Minimal systemic absorption after inhalation.

ACTION

Selectively cleaves DNA. Hydrolyzes DNA in sputum, reduces sputum visceoelasticity.

USES

Management (w/standard therapy) of cystic fibrosis pts to reduce frequency of respiratory infections, improve pulmonary function.

STORAGE/HANDLING

Refrigerate. Ampules are clear, colorless (discard if cloudy, discolored, or left at room temperature for a total time >24 hrs).

NEBULIZATION ADMINISTRATION

NOTE: Administer only w/compressed-air–driven nebulizers and compressors. Do not mix/dilute w/other drugs.

1. Wash hands thoroughly w/ soap and water before preparation.
2. Pour entire contents of one single-use ampule into nebulizer.
3. Hold tab at base of ampule

firmly, twist off top and squeeze contents into nebulizer cup (use full dose of drug).

4. Attach nebulizer cup, connect plastic T to nebulizer cup.

5. Connect open end to port of bottom of nebulizer cup.

6. Instruct pt to breathe normal by inhaling and exhaling through mouth only.

INDICATIONS/DOSAGE/ROUTES

Management of pulmonary function:

NEBULIZATION: Adults, children >5 yrs: 2.5 mg (1 ampule) once daily via recommended nebulizer. (Twice daily dosing may be beneficial for some pts.)

PRECAUTIONS

CONTRAINDICATIONS: None significant. **CAUTIONS:** None significant. **PREGNANCY/LACTATION:** Unknown whether drug crosses placenta or is distributed in breast milk. **Pregnancy Category B.**

INTERACTIONS

DRUG INTERACTIONS: None significant. **ALTERED LAB VALUES:** None significant.

SIDE EFFECTS

NOTE: Effects are generally mild and disappear within a few weeks after therapy begins.

OCCASIONAL: Voice alteration, pharyngitis, laryngitis, rash, conjunctivitis.

ADVERSE REACTIONS/TOXIC EFFECTS

None significant.

NURSING IMPLICATIONS

BASELINE ASSESSMENT:

Assess ABGs, lung sounds, dyspnea and fatigue, pulmonary secretions (amount, color, viscosity).

INTERVENTION/EVALUATION:

Provide emotional support to pt, family, parents. Encourage activity within limits of physical ability. Assess for relief of dyspnea, fatigue. Monitor ABGs, lung sounds, and observe for decreased viscosity of pulmonary secretions. Encourage fluid intake.

PATIENT/FAMILY TEACHING:

Refrigerate. Do not dilute/mix w/other medications. Treatment lasts 10-15 min. Inhale full-treatment dose. May have hoarseness or other upper airway irritation. Not a replacement for other components of therapy (e.g., antibiotics, bronchodilators, and daily physical exercise) or a cure.

dorzolamide (Trusopt)
See supplement

doxacurium chloride

doc´sah-cure-ee-um

(Nuromax)

(See Classifications section under Neuromuscular blockers)

doxapram hydrochloride

docks´ah-pram

(Dopram)

CANADIAN AVAILABILITY:
Dopram

CLASSIFICATION

Respiratory stimulant

PHARMACOKINETICS

	ONSET	PEAK	DURATION
PO	2 min	5 min	—

Widely distributed. Primarily eliminated in feces. Half-life: 3-4 hrs.

ACTION

Stimulates respirations by activity on peripheral carotid chemoreceptors. Higher doses stimulate central respiratory centers of medulla, increasing tidal volume.

USES

Treatment of respiratory depression associated w/CNS depressant drug overdosage, hypercapnia associated w/COPD; to reverse drug-induced postanesthesia respiratory depression.

STORAGE/HANDLING

Store parenteral form at room temperature.

IV ADMINISTRATION

NOTE: Give by IV injection or IV infusion.

1. For reconstitution for IV infusion, add 250 mg doxapram (12.5 ml) to 250 ml of 5 or 10% dextrose or 0.9% NaCl to provide solution containing 1 mg/ml.
2. Do not repeat use of any one IV injection site (reduces risk of irritation, thrombophlebitis).
3. Use IV infusion pump to prevent rapid IV infusion rate.
4. Maximum IV infusion length: 2 hrs.

INDICATIONS/DOSAGE/ROUTES

Drug-induced respiratory depression:

IV INJECTION: Adults, elderly: Initially, 2 doses at 5 min intervals of 1-2 mg/kg. If no response, repeat initial dose in 1-2 hrs until spontaneous breathing occurs, consciousness resumes, or maximum daily dose of 3 Gm is reached.

IV INFUSION: Adults, elderly: When spontaneous breathing occurs, may infuse at IV rate of 1-3 mg/min until pt awakens. **Max. IV infusion length:** 2 hrs. Resume IV infusion after rest period of 30 min-2 hrs. Do not exceed maximum daily dose.

Postanesthesia respiratory depression:

IV INJECTION: Adults, elderly: Initially, 0.5-1 mg/kg. Do not exceed single doses of 1.5 mg/kg. Repeat initial dose at 5 min intervals.

IV INFUSION: Adults, elderly: Give infusion containing 1 mg/ml IV infusion rate of 5 mg/min. When therapeutic response achieved, reduce rate to 1-3 mg/min. **Usual dose:** 0.5-4 mg/kg. **Max. total dose:** 3 Gm (4 mg/kg).

Hypercapnia due to COPD:

IV INFUSION: Adults: Infusion solution 2 mg/ml. Initially, administer 1-2 mg/min. If needed, increase rate of infusion to maximum of 3 mg/min.

PRECAUTIONS

CONTRAINDICATIONS: Epilepsy, history of head injury, coronary artery disease, frank uncompensated heart failure, severe hypertension, cerebrovascular accidents, respiratory insufficiency due to neuromuscular disorders, muscle paresis, flail chest, airway obstruction, suspected or confirmed pulmonary embolism, pneumothorax, pulmonary fibrosis, acute bronchial asthma, extreme dyspnea, hypoxia not associated with hypercapnia, in conjunction with mechanical ventilation. **CAUTIONS:** History of bronchial asthma, severe tachycardia, cardiac arrhythmias, cerebral edema, increased CSF pressure, hyperthyroidism, pheochromocytoma, profound metabolic disorders. **PREGNANCY/LACTATION:** Unknown if drug crosses placenta or is distributed in breast milk. **Pregnancy Category B.**

INTERACTIONS

DRUG INTERACTIONS: MAO inhibitors, vasopressors may increase effect. **ALTERED LAB VALUES:** None significant.

SIDE EFFECTS

OCCASIONAL: Disorientation, apprehension, pupillary dilation, flushing, sweating, pruritus, feeling of warmth in perineal or genital area, positive Babinski sign, nausea, vomiting, feeling of chest tightness or chest pain.

ADVERSE REACTIONS/TOXIC EFFECTS

Promptly discontinue drug if T waves are flattened or if sudden hypotension occurs. Early signs of overdosage are extreme B/P increase, cardiac arrhythmias, skeletal muscle hyperactivity with spasticity and involuntary movements, dyspnea. Excessive CNS stimulation may produce tonic-clonic seizures.

NURSING IMPLICATIONS

BASELINE ASSESSMENT:

Arterial blood gases should be obtained prior to and at 30 min intervals during IV administration.

INTERVENTION/EVALUATION:

Discontinue medication if arterial carbon dioxide tension increases, oxygen tension decreases, or mechanical ventilation is initiated. Monitor B/P, heart rate, deep tendon reflexes (increased activity reflects overdosage) diligently during therapy (dosage, rate of infusion based on these results). Assess pt closely for return of unconsciousness (narcosis) for at least 1 hr after pt is fully alert.

doxazosin mesylate

docks-ay´zoe-sin
(Cardura)

CANADIAN AVAILABILITY: Cardura

CLASSIFICATION

Antihypertensive

PHARMACOKINETICS

	ONSET	PEAK	DURATION
PO	—	2-6 hrs	—

Well absorbed from GI tract. Protein binding: 98-99%. Metabolized in liver. Primarily eliminated in feces. Half-life: 19-22 hrs.

ACTION

Selectively blocks alpha$_1$-adrenergic receptors, decreasing peripheral vascular resistance. Resulting peripheral vasodilation lowers B/P.

USES

Treatment of mild to moderate hypertension. Alone or in combination w/other antihypertensives. Treatment of benign prostatic hyperplasia.

PO ADMINISTRATION

May give w/o regard to food.

INDICATIONS/DOSAGE/ROUTES

Hypertension:
PO: Adults: Initially, 1 mg/day. May increase to 2, 4, 8, and 16 mg if necessary. **Elderly:** Initially, 0.5 mg/day.

NOTE: Doses >4 mg increase potential postural effects.

Benign prostatic hyperplasia: **PO: Adults, elderly:** 2-16 mg/day.

PRECAUTIONS

CONTRAINDICATIONS: None significant. **CAUTIONS:** Chronic renal failure, impaired hepatic function. **PREGNANCY/LACTATION:** Unknown if drug crosses placenta or is distributed in breast milk. **Pregnancy Category B.**

INTERACTIONS

DRUG INTERACTIONS: NSAIDs, estrogen may decrease effect. Hypotension-producing medications may increase effect. **ALTERED LAB VALUES:** None significant.

SIDE EFFECTS

FREQUENT: Dizziness, headache, peripheral edema. **OCCASIONAL:** Dry mouth, GI effects (diarrhea/constipation, abdominal discomfort), urinary urgency, nasal congestion, pharyngitis. **RARE:** Palpitations, abnormal vision, vertigo.

ADVERSE REACTIONS/TOXIC EFFECTS

First-dose syncope (hypotension w/sudden loss of consciousness) generally occurs 30-90 min after giving initial dose of 2 mg or greater, a too-rapid increase in dose, or addition of another hypotensive agent to therapy. May be preceded by tachycardia (120-160 beats/min).

NURSING IMPLICATIONS

BASELINE ASSESSMENT:

Give first dose at bedtime. If initial dose is given during daytime, pt must remain recumbent for 3-4 hrs. Assess B/P, pulse immediately before each dose, and q15-30min until stabilized (be alert to B/P fluctuations).

INTERVENTION/EVALUATION:

Monitor pulse diligently (first-dose syncope may be preceded by tachycardia). Monitor pattern of daily bowel activity and stool consistency. Assist w/ambulation if dizziness, lightheadedness occurs.

PATIENT/FAMILY TEACHING:

Dry mouth may be relieved by sugarless gum, sips of tepid water. Cola, unsalted crackers, dry toast may relieve nausea. Nasal congestion may occur. Full therapeutic effect may not occur for 3-4 wks.

doxepin hydrochloride

dox´eh-pin

(Adapin, Sinequan, Zonalon)

CANADIAN AVAILABILITY:
Sinequan, Triadapin

CLASSIFICATION

Antidepressant: Tricyclic

PHARMACOKINETICS

Rapid, well absorbed from GI tract. Protein binding: 80-85%. Metabolized in liver to active metabolite. Primarily excreted in urine. Half-life: 11-23 hrs.

ACTION

Increases synaptic concentration of norepinephrine and/or serotonin (inhibits re-uptake by presynaptic membrane). Has strong anticholinergic activity.

USES

Treatment of various forms of depression, often in conjunction w/

psychotherapy. Treatment of anxiety. *Topical:* Pruritus.

PO ADMINISTRATION

1. Give w/food or milk if GI distress occurs.
2. Dilute concentrate in 8-oz glass of water, milk, orange, grapefruit, tomato, prune, pineapple juice. Incompatible w/carbonated drinks.

INDICATIONS/DOSAGE/ROUTES

Mild to moderate depression/anxiety:
PO: Adults: 25 mg 3 times/day (75 mg/day). **Usual therapeutic range:** 75-150 mg/day. Alternately, 150 mg/day as single dose at bedtime.

Severe depression/anxiety:
PO: Adults: 50 mg 3 times/day. Gradually increase to 300 mg/day, if needed.

Emotional symptoms accompanying organic brain disease:
PO: Adults: 25-50 mg/day.

Usual elderly dosage:
PO: Elderly: Initially, 10-25 mg at bedtime. May increase by 10-25 mg/day every 3-7 days. **Maximum:** 75 mg/day.

Usual topical dosage:
TOPICAL: Adults, elderly: Apply thin film 4 times/day.

PRECAUTIONS

CONTRAINDICATIONS: Acute recovery period following MI, within 14 days of MAO inhibitor ingestion. **CAUTIONS:** Prostatic hypertrophy, history of urinary retention/obstruction, glaucoma, diabetes mellitus, history of seizures, hyperthyroidism, cardiac/hepatic/renal disease, schizophrenia, increased intraocular pressure, hiatal hernia. **PREGNANCY/LACTATION:** Crosses placenta; distributed in breast milk. **Pregnancy Category C.**

INTERACTIONS

DRUG INTERACTIONS: Alcohol, CNS depressants may increase CNS, respiratory depression, hypotensive effects. Antithyroid agents may increase risk of agranulocytosis. Phenothiazines may increase sedative, anticholinergic effects. Cimetidine may increase concentration, toxicity. May decrease effects of clonidine, guanadrel. May increase cardiac effects w/sympathomimetics. May increase risk of hypertensive crisis, hyperpyretic, convulsions w/MAO inhibitors. **ALTERED LAB VALUES:** May alter ECG readings, glucose.

SIDE EFFECTS

FREQUENT: Drowsiness, fatigue, dry mouth, blurred vision, constipation, delayed micturition, postural hypotension, excessive sweating, disturbed concentration, increased appetite, urinary retention. **OCCASIONAL:** GI disturbances (nausea, GI distress, metallic taste sensation). **RARE:** Paradoxical reaction (agitation, restlessness, nightmares, insomnia), extrapyramidal symptoms (particularly fine hand tremor).

ADVERSE REACTIONS/TOXIC EFFECTS

High dosage may produce cardiovascular effects (severe postural hypotension, dizziness, tachycardia, palpitations, arrhythmias) and seizures. May also result in altered temperature regulation (hyperpyrexia or hypothermia). Abrupt withdrawal from prolonged therapy may produce headache, malaise, nausea, vomiting, vivid dreams.

NURSING IMPLICATIONS

BASELINE ASSESSMENT:

For those on long-term therapy, liver/renal function tests, blood counts should be performed periodically.

INTERVENTION/EVALUATION:

Supervise suicidal-risk pt closely during early therapy (as depression lessens, energy level improves, increasing suicide potential). Assess appearance, behavior, speech pattern, level of interest, mood. Monitor pattern of daily bowel activity, stool consistency. Monitor B/P, pulse for hypotension, arrhythmias. Assess for urinary retention by bladder palpation. Avoid alcohol.

PATIENT/FAMILY TEACHING:

Change positions slowly to avoid hypotensive effect. Tolerance to postural hypotension, sedative and anticholinergic effects usually develops during early therapy. Therapeutic effect may be noted within 2-5 days, maximum effect within 2-3 wks. Photosensitivity to sun may occur. Dry mouth may be relieved by sugarless gum, sips of tepid water. Report visual disturbances. Do not abruptly discontinue medication. Avoid tasks that require alertness, motor skills until response to drug is established.

doxorubicin hydrochloride

dox-o-roo´bi-sin

(Adriamycin, Rubex)

CANADIAN AVAILABILITY:
Adriamycin

CLASSIFICATION

Antineoplastic

PHARMACOKINETICS

Widely distributed. Does not cross blood-brain barrier. Protein binding: high. Metabolized rapidly in liver to active metabolite. Primarily eliminated via biliary system. Half-life: 16 hrs; metabolite: 32 hrs.

ACTION

Cell cycle-specific for S phase of cell division. May bind DNA, inhibit DNA, RNA synthesis. Has immunosuppressant activity.

USES

Produces regression in breast, ovarian, thyroid, transitional cell bladder, bronchogenic, gastric carcinoma; soft-tissue and bone sarcomas, neuroblastoma, Wilms' tumor, lymphomas of Hodgkin's and non-Hodgkin's type, acute lymphoblastic and myeloblastic leukemia.

STORAGE/HANDLING

NOTE: May be carcinogenic, mutagenic, or teratogenic. Handle w/ extreme care during preparation/administration.

Reconstituted solution stable for 24 hrs at room temperature or 48 hrs if refrigerated. Protect from prolonged exposure to sunlight; discard unused solution.

IV ADMINISTRATION

NOTE: Give by IV injection. Wear gloves. If powder or solution comes in contact w/skin, wash thoroughly. Avoid small veins, swollen or edematous extremities, and areas overlying joints, tendons.

1. Reconstitute each 10 mg vial w/5 ml preservative-free 0.9% NaCl injection (10 ml for 20 mg; 25 ml for 50 mg) to provide concentration of 2 mg/ml.

2. Shake vial; allow contents to dissolve.

3. Withdraw appropriate volume of air from vial during reconstitution (avoids excessive pressure buildup).

4. For IV injection, administer into tubing of freely running IV infusion of 5% dextrose or 0.9% NaCl, preferably via butterfly needle, at rate no faster than 3-5 min (avoids local erythematous streaking along vein and facial flushing).

5. Extravasation produces immediate pain, severe local tissue damage. Terminate immediately; flood site w/normal saline.

INDICATIONS/DOSAGE/ROUTES

NOTE: Dosage individualized based on clinical response, tolerance to adverse effects. When used in combination therapy, consult specific protocols for optimum dosage, sequence of drug administration.

Usual dose:
IV: Adults: 60-75 mg/m^2 single dose every 21 days, 20 mg/m^2 once weekly, or 25-30 mg/m^2 daily on 2-3 successive days q4wks. Due to cardiotoxicity, do not exceed cumulative dose of 550 mg/m^2 (400-450 mg/m^2 for those whose previous therapy included related compounds or irradiation of cardiac region).

Dosage in hepatic impairment:

SERUM BILIRUBIN CONCENTRATION	DOSAGE
1.2-3 mg/dl	50% usual dose
>3 mg/dl	25% usual dose

PRECAUTIONS

CONTRAINDICATIONS: Preexisting myelosuppression, impaired cardiac function, previous treatment w/complete cumulative doses of doxorubicin and/or daunorubicin. **CAUTIONS:** Impaired hepatic, renal function. **PREGNANCY/LACTATION:** If possible, avoid use during pregnancy, esp. first trimester. Breast feeding not recommended. **Pregnancy Category C.**

INTERACTIONS

DRUG INTERACTIONS: May decrease effect of antigout medication. Bone marrow depressants may increase bone marrow depression. May increase cardiotoxicity w/daunorubicin. Live virus vaccines may potentiate virus replication, increase vaccine side effects, decrease pt's antibody response to vaccine. **ALTERED LAB VALUES:** May cause ECG changes. May increase uric acid.

SIDE EFFECTS

FREQUENT: Complete alopecia (scalp, axillary, pubic hair), nausea, vomiting, stomatitis, esophagitis (esp. if drug given daily on several successive days). **OCCASIONAL:** Anorexia, diarrhea, hyperpigmentation of nailbeds, phalangeal and dermal creases. **RARE:** Fever, chills, conjunctivitis, lacrimation.

ADVERSE REACTIONS/TOXIC EFFECTS

Bone marrow depression manifested as hematologic toxicity (principally leukopenia, and to lesser extent anemia, thrombocytopenia). Generally occurs within 10-15 days, returns to normal levels by third week. Cardiotoxicity noted as either acute, transient abnormal EKG findings and/or cardiomyopathy manifested as CHF.

NURSING IMPLICATIONS

BASELINE ASSESSMENT:

Obtain WBC, platelet, erythrocyte counts before and at frequent intervals during therapy. Obtain EKG prior to therapy, liver function studies prior to each dose. Antiemetics may be effective in preventing, treating nausea.

INTERVENTION/EVALUATION:

Monitor for stomatitis (burning/erythema of oral mucosa at inner margin of lips, sore throat, difficulty swallowing). May lead to ulceration within 2-3 days. Assess skin, nailbeds for hyperpigmentation. Monitor hematologic status, renal/hepatic function studies, serum uric acid levels. Assess pattern of daily bowel activity, stool consistency. Monitor for hematologic toxicity (fever, sore throat, signs of local infection, easy bruising, unusual bleeding from any site), symptoms of anemia (excessive tiredness, weakness).

PATIENT/FAMILY TEACHING:

Alopecia is reversible, but new hair growth may have different color or texture. New hair growth resumes 2-3 mos after last therapy dose. Maintain fastidious oral hygiene. Do not have immunizations w/o physician's approval (drug lowers body's resistance). Avoid contact w/those who have recently received live virus vaccine. Promptly report fever, sore throat, signs of local infection, easy bruising or unusual bleeding from any site. Contact physician if nausea/vomiting continues at home. Avoid alcohol.

doxycycline calcium

dock-see-sigh´clean

(Vibramycin Calcium syrup)

doxycycline hyclate, monohydrate

(Doryx, Vibra-Tabs, Vibramycin)

CANADIAN AVAILABILITY:

Apo-Doxy, Doxycin, Vibramycin, Vibra-Tabs

CLASSIFICATION

Antibiotic: Tetracycline

PHARMACOKINETICS

Well absorbed from GI tract (may give w/food). Widely distributed. Protein binding: 99%. Partially inactivated in intestine. Excreted in urine, eliminated in feces via biliary secretion. Not removed by hemodialysis. Half-life: 12-22 hrs.

ACTION

Bacteriostatic because of binding to ribosomes, inhibiting protein synthesis.

USES

Treatment of respiratory, skin/soft-tissue, urinary tract infections, syphilis, uncomplicated gonorrhea, pelvic inflammatory disease, rheumatic fever prophylaxis, brucellosis, trachoma, Rocky Mountain spotted fever, typhus, Q fever, rickettsialpox, psittacosis, ornithosis, granuloma inguinale, lymphogranuloma venereum, adjunctive treatment of intestinal amebiasis.

STORAGE/HANDLING

Store capsules, tablets at room temperature. Oral suspension stable for 2 wks at room temperature. After reconstitution, IV infusion (piggyback) is stable for 12 hrs at room temperature, 72 hrs if refrigerated. Protect from direct sunlight. Discard if precipitate forms.

PO/IV ADMINISTRATION

NOTE: Do not administer IM or SubQ. Space doses evenly around clock.

PO:

Give w/full glass of fluid.

IV:

NOTE: Give by intermittent IV infusion (piggyback).

1. Reconstitute each 100 mg vial w/10 ml sterile water for injection for concentration of 10 mg/ml.
2. Further dilute each 100 mg w/ at least 100 ml 5% dextrose, 0.9% NaCl or other compatible IV fluid. Infuse >1-4 hrs.

INDICATIONS/DOSAGE/ROUTES

Usual dosage:
PO: Adults, elderly: Initially, 200 mg (100 mg q12h), then 100 mg/day as single dose or in 2 divided doses (100 mg q12h in severe infections). **Children >8 yrs, >45 kg:** Initially, 4.4 mg/kg divided in 2 doses, then 2.2 mg/kg as single dose or in 2 divided doses (4.4 mg/kg in severe infections).
IV: Adults, elderly: Initially, 200 mg as 1-2 infusions; then 100-200 mg/day (200 mg as 1-2 infusions). **Children:** Initially, 4.4 mg/kg on first day as 1-2 infusions; then 2.2-4.4 mg/kg as 1-2 infusions.

Acute gonococcal infections:
PO: Adults: Initially, 200 mg, then 100 mg at bedtime on first day; then 100 mg 2 times/day for 3 days.

Syphilis:
PO/IV: Adults: 300 mg/day in divided doses for 10 days.

Traveler's diarrhea:
PO: Adults, elderly: 100 mg daily during a period of risk (up to 14 days) and for 2 days after returning home.

PRECAUTIONS

CONTRAINDICATIONS: Hypersensitivity to tetracyclines, sulfite, last half of pregnancy, children <8 yrs. **CAUTIONS:** Sun/ultraviolet light exposure (severe photosensitivity reaction). **PREGNANCY/LACTATION:** Readily crosses placenta; distributed in breast milk. Avoid use in women during last half of pregnancy. May produce permanent teeth discoloration, enamel hypoplasia, inhibit fetal skeletal growth in children <8 yrs. **Pregnancy Category D.**

INTERACTIONS

DRUG INTERACTIONS: Antacids containing aluminum/calcium/magnesium, laxatives containing magnesium, oral iron preparations impair absorption of tetracyclines (give 1-2 hrs before or after tetracyclines). Barbiturates, phenytoin, carbamazepine may decrease doxycycline concentrations. Cholestyramine, colestipol may decrease absorption. May decrease effect of oral contraceptives. Carbamazepine, phenytoin may decrease concentrations. **ALTERED LAB VALUES:** May increase SGOT (AST), SGPT (ALT), alkaline phosphatase, amylase, bilirubin concentrations.

SIDE EFFECTS

FREQUENT: Anorexia, nausea, vomiting, diarrhea, dysphagia. **OCCASIONAL:** Rash, urticaria, hemolytic anemia.

ADVERSE REACTIONS/TOXIC EFFECTS

Superinfection (esp. fungal), anaphylaxis, increased intracranial pressure, bulging fontanelles rare in infants.

NURSING IMPLICATIONS

BASELINE ASSESSMENT:

Question for history of allergies, esp. to tetracyclines, sulfite. Obtain culture and sensitivity test before giving first dose (therapy may begin before results are known).

INTERVENTION/EVALUATION:

Check IV site for phlebitis (heat, pain, red streaking over vein). Determine pattern of bowel activity, stool consistency. Monitor food intake, tolerance. Assess skin for rash. Monitor B/P and LOC because of potential for increased intracranial pressure. Be alert for superinfection: diarrhea, ulceration or changes of oral mucosa, anal/genital pruritus.

PATIENT/FAMILY TEACHING:

Continue antibiotic for full length of treatment. Space doses evenly. Drink full glass of water w/capsules/tablets. Notify physician in event of diarrhea, rash, or other new symptom. Protect skin from sun/ultraviolet light exposure. Consult physician before taking any other medication.

dronabinol

drow-nab´in-all)
(Marinol)

CLASSIFICATION

Antinausea, antiemetic

PHARMACOKINETICS

Poorly absorbed from GI tract. Metabolized in liver. Primarily eliminated via biliary excretion. Half-life: 15-18 hrs (metabolite).

ACTION

May inhibit vomiting control mechanisms in medulla oblongata.

USES

Prevention, treatment of nausea, vomiting due to cancer chemotherapy; appetite stimulant in AIDS pts.

INDICATIONS/DOSAGE/ROUTES

Nausea, vomiting:
PO: Adults: Initially, 5 mg/m^2, 1-3 hrs before chemotherapy, then q2-4h after chemotherapy for total of 4-6 doses/day. May increase by 2.5 mg/m^2 up to 15 mg/m^2/dose.

Appetite stimulant:
PO: Adults: Initially, 2.5 mg 2 times/day (before lunch, dinner). **Range:** 2.5-20 mg/day.

PRECAUTIONS

CONTRAINDICATIONS: Nausea, vomiting other than due to chemotherapy. **CAUTIONS:** Hypertension, heart disease; manic, depressive, or schizophrenic pts. Not recommended in children. **PREGNANCY/LACTATION:** Unknown if drug crosses placenta. Distributed in breast milk. **Pregnancy Category B.**

INTERACTIONS

DRUG INTERACTIONS: CNS depressants may enhance sedative effects. **ALTERED LAB VALUES:** None significant.

SIDE EFFECTS

FREQUENT: Mood changes, drowsiness, euphoria, dizziness, anxiety, impaired thinking, perception difficulty, incoordination, irritability, depression, fatigue, headache, memory lapse, dry mouth, tingling, visual distortions, disturbance of sleep for several wks after discontinuing medication. **OCCASIONAL:** Unsteadiness, paranoia. **RARE:** Confusion, tachycardia, postural hypotension.

ADVERSE REACTIONS/TOXIC EFFECTS

Overdosage may produce combination of CNS stimulation and depressant effects.

NURSING IMPLICATIONS

BASELINE ASSESSMENT:

Assess for dehydration if excessive vomiting occurs (poor skin turgor, dry mucous membranes, decreased urine output).

INTERVENTION/EVALUATION:

Provide emotional support. Supervise closely for serious mood and behavior responses. Do not continue drug after a psychotic episode until pt and situation have been fully evaluated.

PATIENT/FAMILY TEACHING:

Potentially abusable drug—take only as directed. Report visual disturbances. Dry mouth is expected response to medication. Relief from nausea/vomiting generally occurs within 15 min of drug administration. Avoid alcohol, barbiturates. Avoid tasks that require alertness, motor skills until response to drug is established. Remain under supervision of a responsible adult because mood alterations and adverse behavioral effects can occur. For appetite stimulation take before lunch and dinner.

droperidol

droe-pear′ih-dall

(Inapsine)

FIXED-COMBINATION(S): W/fentanyl, a narcotic (Innovar)

CANADIAN AVAILABILITY: Inapsine

CLASSIFICATION

Antiemetic

PHARMACOKINETICS

	ONSET	PEAK	DURATION
IM	3-10 min	30 min	2-4 hrs
IV	3-10 min	30 min	2-4 hrs

Well absorbed after IM administration. Crosses blood-brain barrier. Metabolized in liver. Primarily excreted in urine.

ACTION

Antagonizes dopamine neurotransmission at synapses by blocking postsynaptic dopamine receptor sites; partially blocks adrenergic receptor binding sites.

USES

Tranquilization, control of nausea, vomiting during surgical, diagnostic procedures. Used preoperatively w/opiate analgesics during general anesthesia as anxiolytic, to increase analgesic effect of opiate.

STORAGE/HANDLING

Store parenteral form at room temperature.

IM/IV ADMINISTRATION

PARENTERAL ADMINISTRATION: Pt must remain recumbent for 30-60 min in head-low position w/legs raised, to minimize hypotensive effect.

IM:

Inject slow, deep IM into upper outer quadrant of gluteus maximus.

IV:

Dose for high-risk pts should be added to 5% dextrose or lactated Ringer's injection, give by slow IV infusion.

INDICATIONS/DOSAGE/ROUTES

Preop:
IM/IV: Adults, elderly: 2.5-10 mg 30-60 min before induction of general anesthesia. **Children 2-12 yrs:** 0.088-0.165 mg/kg.

Adjunct for induction of general anesthesia:
IV: Adults, elderly: 0.22-0.275 mg/kg. **Children 2-12 yrs:** 0.088-0.165 mg/kg.

Adjunct for maintenance of general anesthesia:
IV: Adults, elderly: 1.25-2.5 mg.

Diagnostic procedures w/o general anesthesia:
IM: Adults, elderly: 2.5-10 mg 30-60 min before procedure. If needed, may give additional doses of 1.25-2.5 mg (usually by IV injection).

Adjunct to regional anesthesia:
IM/IV: Adults, elderly: 2.5-5 mg.

PRECAUTIONS

CONTRAINDICATIONS: Known intolerance to drug. **CAUTIONS:** Impaired hepatic/renal/cardiac function. **PREGNANCY/LACTATION:** Crosses placenta; unknown if drug is distributed in breast milk. **Pregnancy Category C.**

INTERACTIONS

DRUG INTERACTIONS: CNS depressants may increase CNS depressant effect. Hypotensives may increase hypotension. **ALTERED LAB VALUES:** None significant.

SIDE EFFECTS

FREQUENT: Mild to moderate hypotension. **OCCASIONAL:** Tachycardia, postop drowsiness, dizziness, chills, shivering. **RARE:** Postop nightmares, facial sweating, bronchospasm.

ADVERSE REACTIONS/TOXIC EFFECTS

Extrapyramidal symptoms may appear as akathisia (motor restlessness), and dystonias: torticollis (neck muscle spasm), opisthotonus (rigidity of back muscles), and oculogyric crisis (rolling back of eyes).

NURSING IMPLICATIONS

BASELINE ASSESSMENT:

Assess vital signs. Have pt void. Prepare for surgery. Raise side rails. Instruct to remain recumbent.

INTERVENTION/EVALUATION:

Monitor B/P and pulse diligently

for hypotensive reaction during and after procedure. Assess pulse for tachycardia. Monitor for extrapyramidal symptoms. Evaluate for therapeutic response from anxiety: a calm, facial expression, decreased restlessness.

echothiophate iodide

ek-oh-thye′-oh-fate
(Phospholine Iodide)

CANADIAN AVAILABILITY:
Phospholine Iodide

CLASSIFICATION

Miotic

PHARMACOKINETICS

	ONSET	PEAK	DURATION
OPHTHALMIC (Miosis)	2 min	1-2 hrs	12-48 hrs

Decrease in intraocular pressure seen in 4-8 hrs, peak in 24 hrs, persists for 1-4 wks.

ACTION

Prolongs effect of acetylcholine by inactivating cholinesterase causing constriction of iris sphincter muscle (miosis) and ciliary muscle. Lowers resistance to outflow of aqueous humor.

USES

Treatment of open-angle glaucoma and conditions obstructing aqueous outflow (e.g., synechial formation) that are responsive to miotic therapy; following iridectomy; in accommodative esotropia (convergent strabismus).

STORAGE/HANDLING

Protect from light. After reconsituation, solution stable for 6 mos refrigerated; 1 mo at room temperature.

OPHTHALMIC ADMINISTRATION

1. For topical ophthalmic use only.
2. Place pt in supine position, looking up.
3. Gently pull lower lid down to form pouch and instill medication.
4. Do not touch tip of applicator to lids or any surface.
5. When lower lid is released, have pt keep eye open w/o blinking for at least 30 sec.
6. Apply gentle finger pressure to lacrimal sac (bridge of the nose, inside corner of the eye) for 1-2 min.
7. Remove excess solution around eye w/tissue. Wash hands immediately to remove medication on hands.

INDICATIONS/DOSAGE/ROUTES

Glaucoma:
OPHTHALMIC: Adults, elderly: 2 doses/day; may administer once daily or every other day.

Accommodative esotropia (diagnosis):
OPHTHALMIC: Adults, elderly: 1 drop (0.125% solution) daily at bedtime for 2-3 wks.

Accommodative esotropia (treatment):
OPHTHALMIC: Adults, elderly: 1 drop (0.125% solution) every other day or 1 drop (0.06% solution) daily. **Maximum:** 1 drop (0.125% solution) daily.

PRECAUTIONS

CONTRAINDICATIONS: Hypersensitivity to cholinesterase inhibitors or any component of the preparation; active uveal inflammation; angle-closure (narrow-angle) glaucoma; glaucoma associated w/ iridocyclitis. **CAUTIONS:** Bronchial asthma, GI disturbances, peptic ulcer, bradycardia, hypotension, recent MI, epilepsy, parkinsonism, and other disorders that may respond adversely to vagotonic effects. **PREGNANCY/LACTATION:** Safety during pregnancy and nursing has not been established. **Pregnancy Category C.**

INTERACTIONS

DRUG INTERACTIONS: Anticholinergics, antimyasthenics, cholinesterase inhibitors may increase toxicity. Physostigmine given before echothiophate may decrease effect. **ALTERED LAB VALUES:** None significant.

SIDE EFFECTS

FREQUENT: Stinging, burning, tearing, painful ciliary or accommodative spasm, blurred vision or myopia, poor vision in dim light. **OCCASIONAL:** Iris cysts (more frequent in children), increased visibility of floaters, headache, browache, photophobia, ocular pain, hypersensitivity reactions (including allergic conjunctivitis, dermatitis, keratitis), potential hemorrhage during ocular surgery. **RARE:** Lens opacities, paradoxical increase in intraocular pressure, acute fibrinous iritis.

ADVERSE REACTIONS/TOXIC EFFECTS

Systemic toxicity, retinal detachment may occur.

NURSING IMPLICATIONS

INTERVENTION/EVALUATION:

Be alert for systemic toxicity: severe nausea, vomiting, diarrhea, frequent urination, excessive salivation, bradycardia (may trigger asthma attack in asthmatics). Assess vision acuity and provide assistance w/ambulation as needed.

PATIENT/FAMILY TEACHING:

Close observation is necessary for first 24 hrs. Teach proper administration. Do not use more often than directed because of risk of overdosage. Adverse effects often subside after the first few days of therapy. Avoid night driving, activities requiring visual acuity in dim light. Avoid insecticides, pesticides; inhalation or absorption through skin may add to systemic effects of echothiophate. Report promptly any systemic effects (see Evaluation) or ocular problems. Inform dentist or physician of echothiophate therapy.

edetate calcium disodium (calcium EDTA)

ed'eh-tate

(Calcium Disodium Versenate)

CLASSIFICATION

Antidote

PHARMACOKINETICS

	ONSET	PEAK	DURATION
IV	1 hr	24-48 hrs	—

Well absorbed after parenteral administration. Primarily distributed in extracellular fluid. Excreted unchanged in urine. Half-life: 20-90 minutes.

ACTION

Reduces blood concentration, depot stores of lead. Calcium is replaced by divalent, trivalent metals, esp. lead, forming stable complexes, allowing excretion in urine.

USES

Acute and chronic lead poisoning, lead encephalopathy.

STORAGE/HANDLING

Store parenteral form at room temperature.

IM/IV ADMINISTRATION

IM:

Add 1 ml 1% procaine to each ml calcium EDTA prior to administration.

IV:

1. Dilute each calcium EDTA ampoule (1 Gm) w/5% dextrose or 0.9% NaCl to provide a concentration of 2-4 mg/ml.
2. For intermittent IV administration, solution containing ½ daily dose infused over 1-2 hrs; second dose infused at least 6 hrs after first infusion.
3. For IV infusion, give over 12-24 hrs. **NOTE:** Interrupt infusion for 1 hr before blood lead concentration measured (avoids falsely elevated reading).

INDICATIONS/DOSAGE/ROUTES

NOTE: When administered IV, calcium EDTA may be given in 2 divided doses at 12 hr intervals or 12-24 hr infusions; when administered IM and used alone may be given in divided doses at 8-12 hr intervals; when given IM w/dimercaprol in divided doses, administer at 4 hr intervals.

Diagnosis of lead poisoning:
IM/IV INFUSION: Adults, elderly: 500 mg/m^2. **Maximum:** 1 Gm.
IV INFUSION: Children: 500 mg/m^2.
IM: Children: 500 mg/m^2 as single dose or 500 mg/m^2 each at 12 hr intervals.

Lead poisoning (w/o encephalopathy):
NOTE: Total dose dependent on severity of lead poisoning, pt response/tolerance to medication. Consult specific protocols.
IM/IV: Adults, elderly, children: 1-1.5 Gm/m^2 daily for 3-5 days. (If blood lead concentration >100 mcg/dl, calcium edetate usually given w/dimercaprol.) Allow at least 2-4 days up to 2-3 wks between courses of therapy. Adults should not be given more than 2 courses of therapy.

Lead poisoning (w/ encephalopathy):
IM: Adults, elderly, children: Initially, dimercaprol 4 mg/kg; then 4 hrs later and q4h for 5 days give dimercaprol 4 mg/kg and calcium EDTA 250 mg/m^2.

PRECAUTIONS

CONTRAINDICATIONS: Anuria. **CAUTIONS:** None significant. **PREGNANCY/LACTATION:** Unknown if drug crosses placenta or is distributed in breast milk. Do not use in pregnancy unless benefits outweigh potential risk to fetus. **Pregnancy Category C.**

INTERACTIONS

DRUG INTERACTIONS: May decrease effects of zinc. **ALTERED LAB VALUES:** None significant.

SIDE EFFECTS

None significant.

ADVERSE REACTIONS/TOXIC EFFECTS

Renal tubular necrosis.

NURSING IMPLICATIONS

BASELINE ASSESSMENT:

Assure urine flow before start of therapy. Determine serum and urine, lead levels, BUN. Assess family members for lead poisoning.

INTERVENTION/EVALUATION:

Monitor EKG during therapy. Assess vital signs, neurologic status. Maintain careful I&O. Avoid rapid IV infusion (may be lethal due to increased ICP). Periodically check serum and urine lead levels, BUN; obtain daily urinalysis. Stop drug immediately and notify physician of anuria or urinalysis report of increased proteinuria, increased erythrocytes, or presence of large renal epithelial cells.

PATIENT/FAMILY TEACHING:

Necessity of follow-up visits for tests and possible further therapy. Evaluation of home to prevent future poisoning.

enalapril maleate

en-awl'ah-prill

(Vasotec)

FIXED-COMBINATION(S):
W/hydrochlorothiazide, a diuretic (Vaseretic)

CANADIAN AVAILABILITY:
Vasotec

CLASSIFICATION

Angiotensin converting enzyme (ACE) inhibitor.

PHARMACOKINETICS

	ONSET	PEAK	DURATION
P.O.	1 hr	4-6 hrs	24 hrs
IV	15 min	1-4 hrs	6 hrs

Readily absorbed from GI tract (not affected by food). Protein binding: 50-60%. Converted to active metabolite enalaprit. Primarily excreted in urine. Removed by hemodialysis. Half-life: 11 hrs (increased in decreased renal function).

ACTION

Suppresses renin-angiotensin-aldosterone system (prevents conversion of angiotensin I to angiotensin II, a potent vasoconstrictor; may inhibit angiotensin II at local vascular, renal sites). Decreases plasma angiotensin II, increases plasma renin activity, decreases aldosterone secretion. In hypertension, reduces peripheral arterial resistance. In CHF, increases cardiac output, decreases peripheral vascular resistance, B/P, pulmonary capillary wedge pressure, heart size.

USES

Treatment of hypertension alone or in combination w/other antihypertensives. Adjunctive therapy for CHF (in combination w/cardiac glycosides, diuretics).

STORAGE/HANDLING

Store tablets, parenteral form at room temperature. For parenteral form, use only clear, colorless solution. Diluted IV solution is stable for 24 hrs at room temperature.

PO/IV ADMINISTRATION

PO:

1. May give w/o regard to food.
2. Tablets may be crushed.

IV:

1. For direct IV, give undiluted over 5 min.
2. May dilute w/5% dextrose or 0.9% NaCl. Infuse over 10-15 min.

INDICATIONS/DOSAGE/ROUTES

Hypertension (used alone):
PO: Adults, elderly: Initially, 5 mg/day. **Maintenance:** 10-40 mg/day as single or in 2 divided doses.
IV: Adults, elderly: 1.25 mg q6h.

Hypertension (w/diuretics):
NOTE: Discontinue diuretic 2-3 days before initiating enalapril therapy; if unable, initiate w/2.5 mg enalapril (0.625 mg IV).

Dose in renal impairment:
(Based on creatinine clearance).
PO: Adults, elderly: Initially, 2.5-5 mg/day titrate up to maximum of 40 mg/day.
IV: Adults, elderly (Ccr <30ml/min): Initially, 0.625 mg. May repeat in 1 hr if no response, then 1.25 mg q6h.

CHF
PO: Adults, elderly: Initially, 2.5-5 mg/day. **Maintenance:** 5-20 mg/day in 2 divided doses. **Maximum:** 40 mg/day in 2 divided doses.

Dosage in renal impairment, hyponatremia (Na <130, Creat >1.6):
Initially, 2.5 mg/day, increase to 2.5 mg 2 times/day, then 5 mg 2 times/day at 4-day intervals (minimum) up to 40 mg/day.

PRECAUTIONS

CONTRAINDICATIONS: History of angioedema w/previous treatment w/ACE inhibitors. **CAUTIONS:** Renal impairment, those w/sodium depletion or on diuretic therapy, dialysis, hypovolemia, coronary/cerebrovascular insufficiency. **PREGNANCY/LACTATION:** Crosses placenta; distributed in breast milk. May cause fetal/neonatal mortality/morbidity. **Pregnancy Category D.**

INTERACTIONS

DRUG INTERACTIONS: Alcohol, diuretics, hypotensive agents may increase effects. NSAIDs may decrease effect. Potassium sparing diuretics, potassium supplements may cause hyperkalemia. May increase lithium concentration, toxicity. **ALTERED LAB VALUES:** May increase potassium, SGOT (AST), SGPT (ALT), alkaline phosphatase, bilirubin, BUN, creatinine. May decrease sodium. May cause positive ANA titer.

SIDE EFFECTS

FREQUENT: Headache, dizziness, fatigue. **OCCASIONAL:** Rash, diarrhea, nausea, cough, loss of taste perception. **RARE:** Postural hypotension, insomnia, nervousness, paresthesia, nightmares, cold extremities, palpitations.

ADVERSE REACTIONS/TOXIC EFFECTS

Excessive hypotension ("first-dose syncope") may occur in those w/CHF, severely salt/volume depleted. Angioedema (swelling of face/lips), hyperkalemia occur rarely. Agranulocytosis, neutropenia may be noted in those w/impaired renal function or collagen vascular disease (systemic lupus erythematosus, scleroderma). Nephrotic syndrome may be noted in those w/history of renal disease.

NURSING IMPLICATIONS

BASELINE ASSESSMENT:

Obtain B/P immediately before each dose in addition to regular monitoring (be alert to fluctuations). Renal function tests should be performed before therapy begins. In those w/renal impairment, autoimmune disease, or taking drugs that affect leukocytes or immune response, CBC and differential count should be performed before therapy begins and q2wks for 3 mos, then periodically thereafter.

INTERVENTION/EVALUATION:

Assist w/ambulation if dizziness occurs. Assess skin for development of rash. Monitor serum potassium, BUN, serum creatinine levels. Monitor pattern of daily bowel activity, stool consistency. Assess for anorexia due to decreased taste sensation. If excessive reduction in B/P occurs, place pt in supine position w/legs elevated.

PATIENT/FAMILY TEACHING:

To reduce hypotensive effect, rise slowly from lying to sitting position and permit legs to dangle from bed momentarily before standing. If nausea occurs, noncaffeinated carbonated beverages, unsalted crackers, or dry toast may relieve effect. Report any sign of infection (sore throat, fever). Several wks may be needed for full therapeutic effect of B/P reduction. Skipping doses or voluntarily discontinuing drug may produce severe, rebound hypertension.

enoxacin

en-ox'ah-sin
(Penetrex)

E

CLASSIFICATION

Anti-infective: quinolone

PHARMACOKINETICS

Well absorbed from GI tract. Protein binding: 40%. Partially metabolized in liver. Primarily excreted in urine. Half-life: 3-6 hrs.

ACTION

Inhibits DNA-gyrase in susceptible microorganisms, interfering w/bacterial DNA replication and repair.

USES

Treatment of uncomplicated urethral or cervical gonorrhea, uncomplicated (cystitis) or complicated urinary tract infections.

PO ADMINISTRATION

Give 1 hr before or 2 hrs after meals.

INDICATIONS/DOSAGE/ROUTES

Uncomplicated (cystitis) urinary tract infection:
PO: Adults >18 yrs, elderly: 200 mg q12h for 7 days.

Complicated urinary tract infection:
PO: Adults >18 yrs, elderly: 400 mg q12h for 14 days.

Uncomplicated gonorrhea:
PO: Adults >18 hrs: 400 mg given as single dose.

Dosage in renal impairment:
The dose and/or frequency is modified based on degree of renal impairment.

CREATININE CLEARANCE	DOSAGE
<30 ml/min	Normal initial dose, then 1/2 regular dose q12h

PRECAUTIONS

CONTRAINDICATIONS: Do not use in children <18 years of age. **CAUTIONS:** Impaired renal function, any predisposition to seizures. **PREGNANCY/LACTATION:** May produce maternal toxicity (weight loss, venous irritation), fetal toxicity. Unknown whether distributed in breast milk. Should not be used in pregnant women. **Pregnancy Category C.**

INTERACTIONS

DRUG INTERACTIONS: Antacids, bismuth subsalicylate, sucralfate may decrease absorption (give at least 4 hrs before or 2 hrs after enoxacin). Decreases clearance, may increase concentration, toxicity of theophylline. May increase effects of oral anticoagulants. **ALTERED LAB VALUES:** May increase SGOT (AST), SGPT (ALT), alkaline phosphatase, bilirubin. May decrease hemoglobin, hematocrit. May alter potassium, platelets.

SIDE EFFECTS

OCCASIONAL: Nausea, vomiting, photosensitivity. **RARE:** Dizziness, abdominal discomfort, diarrhea.

ADVERSE REACTIONS/TOXIC EFFECTS

Superinfection (particularly enterococcal, fungal). Hypersensitivity reactions, serious and occasionally fatal, have occurred in pts receiving quinolone therapy. Arthropathy may occur if given to children <18 yrs.

NURSING IMPLICATIONS

BASELINE ASSESSMENT:

Question for history of hypersensitivity to fluoroquinolones, quinolone group of antibacterials (cinoxacin, nalidixic acid).

INTERVENTION/EVALUATION:

Monitor stool frequency and consistency. Be alert for superinfection, e.g., genital pruritus, vaginitis, fever, sores and discomfort in mouth.

PATIENT/FAMILY TEACHING:

Drink fluids liberally. Complete full course of therapy. Instruct pt regarding meals/medications (see PO Administration). Do not drive or perform activities requiring alertness or dexterity if dizziness occurs. Avoid sunlight/ultraviolet exposure, wear sun screen and protective clothing.

enoxaparin sodium

en-ox'ah-pear-in
(Lovenox)

CLASSIFICATION

Anticoagulant

PHARMACOKINETICS

	ONSET	PEAK	DURATION
SubQ	—	3-5 hr	12 hr

Well absorbed after SubQ administration. Eliminated primarily in urine. Half-life: 4.5 hrs.

ACTION

Antithrombin; in presence of low-molecular-weight heparin, produces anticogulation by inhibition of factor Xa. Enoxaparin causes less inactivation of thrombin, inhibition of platelets, and bleeding than standard heparin. Does not significantly influence bleeding time, prothrombin time (PT), activated partial thromboplastin time (APTT).

USES

Prevention of postoperative deep vein thrombosis (DVT) following hip replacement surgery.

STORAGE/HANDLING

Parenteral form appears clear and colorless to pale yellow. Store at room temperature.

SubQ ADMINISTRATION

NOTE: Do not mix w/other injections or infusions. Do *not* give IM.

SubQ:

1. After withdrawal of enoxaparin from vial, change needle before injection (prevents leakage along needle track).
2. Instruct pt to lie down before administering by deep SubQ injection.
3. Inject between left and right anterolateral and left and right posterolateral abdominal wall.
4. Introduce entire length of needle (½ inch) into skin fold held between thumb and forefinger, holding skin fold during injection.

INDICATIONS/DOSAGE/ROUTES

NOTE: Give initial dose as soon as possible after surgery but not more than 24 hrs after surgery.

Prevent deep vein thrombosis:
SubQ: Adults, elderly: 30 mg twice daily, generally for 7-10 days.

PRECAUTIONS

CONTRAINDICATIONS: Active major bleeding, concurrent heparin therapy, thrombocytopenia associated w/positive in vitro test for antiplatelet antibody, hypersensitivity to heparin or pork products. **CAUTIONS:** Conditions w/increased risk of hemorrhage, history of heparin-induced thrombocytopenia, impaired renal function, elderly, uncontrolled arterial hypertension, history of recent GI ulceration and hemorrhage. **PREGNANCY/LACTATION:** Use w/caution, particularly during last trimester, immediate postpartum period (increased risk of maternal hemorrhage). Unknown whether it is excreted in breast milk. **Pregnancy Category B.**

INTERACTIONS

DRUG INTERACTIONS: Anticoagulants, platelet inhibitors may increase bleeding (use w/care). **ALTERED LAB VALUES:** Reversible increases in SGOT (AST), SGPT (ALT), alkaline phosphatase, lactate dehydrogenase (LDH).

SIDE EFFECTS

OCCASIONAL: Mild, local skin irritation, pain, erythema at injection site. **RARE:** Hypersensitivity reaction (chills, fever, pruritus, urticaria, asthma, rhinitis, lacrimation, headache).

ADVERSE REACTIONS/TOXIC EFFECTS

Accidental overdosage may lead to bleeding complications ranging from local ecchymoses to major hemorrhage. **Antidote:** Dose of protamine sulfate (1% solution) should be equal to the dose of enoxaparin injected. One mg protamine sulfate neutralizes 1 mg enoxaparin. A second dose of 0.5 mg/mg protamine sulfate may be given if APTT tested 2-4 hrs after the first infusion remains prolonged.

NURSING IMPLICATIONS

BASELINE ASSESSMENT:

Assess complete blood count, including platelet count. Determine initial B/P.

INTERVENTION/EVALUATION:

Periodically monitor CBC, platelet count, stool for occult blood (no need for daily monitoring in pts w/ normal presurgical coagulation parameters). Assess for any sign of bleeding: bleeding at surgical site, hematuria, blood in stool, bleeding from gums, petechiae, bruising, bleeding from injection sites; monitor B/P for hypotension.

PATIENT/FAMILY TEACHING:

Usual length of therapy is 7-10 days. Report any sign of bleeding (as above). Do not take any over-the-counter medication (esp. aspirin) w/o consulting physician.

epinephrine

eh-pih-nef´rin

(Adrenalin, Sus-Phrine, Primatene, Bronkaid, AsthmaHaler, Bronitin, Medihaler-Epi, EpiPen)

CANADIAN AVAILABILITY:

Adrenalin, Bronkaid, Epi-Pen, Medihaler-Epi

CLASSIFICATION

Sympathomimetic

PHARMACOKINETICS

	ONSET	PEAK	DURATION
SubQ	5-10 min	20 min	1-4 hrs
IM	5-10 min	20 min	1-4 hrs
Inhalation	3-5 min	20 min	1-3 hrs
Ophthalmic	1 hr	4-8 hrs	12-24 hrs

Minimal absorption after inhalation, well absorbed after parenteral administration. Metabolized in liver, other tissues, sympathetic nerve endings. Excreted in urine. *Ophthalmic:* May have systemic absorption from drainage into nasal pharyngeal passages. Mydriasis occurs within several min, persists several hrs; vasoconstrtiction occurs within 5 min, last <1 hr.

ACTION

Stimulates alpha-adrenergic receptors (vasoconstriction, pressor effects), $beta_1$-adrenergic receptors (cardiac stimulation) and $beta_2$-adrenergic receptors (bronchial dilation, vasodilation) resulting in relaxation of smooth muscle of bronchial tree, peripheral vasculature. *Ophthalmic:* Increases outflow of aqueous humor from anterior eye chamber, dilates pupils (constricts conjuctival blood vessels).

USES

Treatment of acute bronchial asthma attacks, reversible bronchospasm in pts w/chronic bronchitis, emphysema, hypersensitivity reactions. Restores cardiac rhythm in cardiac arrest. *Ophthalmic:* Management of chronic open-angle glaucoma alone or in combination w/other agents.

STORAGE/HANDLING

Store parenteral forms at room temperature. Do not use if solution appears discolored or contains a precipitate.

INHALATION/OPHTHALMIC/SubQ/IV ADMINISTRATION

INHALATION:

1. Shake container well, exhale completely then holding mouthpiece 1 inch away from lips, inhale and hold breath as long as possible before exhaling.
2. Wait 1-10 min before inhaling second dose (allows for deeper bronchial penetration).
3. Rinse mouth w/water immediately after inhalation (prevents mouth/throat dryness).

OPHTHALMIC:

1. For topical ophthalmic use only.
2. Instruct pt to tilt head backward and look up.
3. Gently pull lower lid down to form pouch and instill medication.
4. Do not touch tip of applicator to lids or any surface.
5. When lower lid is released, have pt keep eye open w/o blinking for at least 30 sec.
6. Apply gentle finger pressure to lacrimal sac (bridge of the nose, inside corner of the eye) for 1-2 min.
7. Remove excess solution around eye w/a tissue. Wash hands immediately to remove medication on hands.

SubQ:

1. Shake ampoule thoroughly.
2. Use tuberculin syringe for SubQ into lateral deltoid region.
3. Massage injection site (minimizes vasoconstriction effect).

IV:

1. For injection, dilute each 1 mg of 1:1,000 solution w/10 ml normal saline to provide 1:10,000 solution.
2. For infusion, further dilute w/5% dextrose in water.

INDICATIONS/DOSAGE/ROUTES

Cardiac arrest:

IV: Adults, elderly: 0.1-1 mg (1-10 ml of 1:10,000 concentration). May repeat q5min (or may be followed by 0.3 mg SubQ or IV infusion initially at 1 mcg/min up to 4 mcg/min. **Children:** 0.01 mg/kg (0.1 ml/kg of 1:10,000 concentration). May repeat q5min (or may give IV infusion initially at 0.1 mcg/kg/min increased at 0.1 mcg/kg/min increments up to maximum of 1 mcg/kg/min. **Neonates:** 0.01-0.03 mg/kg (0.1-0.3 ml/kg of 1:10,000 concentration). May repeat q5min.

INTRACARDIAC: Adults, elderly: 0.1-1 mg (1-10 ml of 1:10,000 concentration). **Children:** 0.005-0.01 mg/kg (0.05-0.1 ml/kg of 1:10,000 concentration).

Severe anaphylaxis or asthma:

SubQ/IM: Adults, elderly: 0.1-0.5 mg (0.1-0.5 ml of 1:1,000 concentration). May repeat at 10-15 min intervals for anaphylaxis; 20 min-4 hrs for asthma.

SubQ: Children: 0.01 mg/kg (0.01 ml/kg of 1:1,000 concentration). **Maximum single dose:** 0.5 mg. May repeat at 20 min-4 hr intervals.

Asthma (prolonged effect):

SubQ: Adults, elderly: Initially, 0.5 mg (0.1 ml of 1:200 concentration). May repeat w/0.5-1.5 mg no sooner than 6 hrs from previous dose. **Children:** 0.02-0.025 mg/kg (0.004-0.005 ml/kg of 1:200 concentration). **Maximum single dose:** 0.75 mg. May repeat no sooner than 6 hrs from previous dose.

Severe anaphylactic shock:

IV: Adults, elderly: 0.1-0.25 mg

(1-2.5 ml of 1 : 10,000 concentration) over 5-10 min. May repeat q5-15min, or continuous IV infusion initially at 1 mcg/min up to 4 mcg/min. **Children:** 0.1 mg (10 ml of 1 : 100,000 concentration) over 5-10 min followed w/IV infusion of 0.1 mcg/kg/min up to 1.5 mcg/kg/min.

Usual inhalation dosage:
INHALATION: Adults, elderly, children >4 yrs: 1 inhalation, may repeat in at least 1 min; subsequent doses no sooner than 3 hrs.
NEBULIZER: Adults, elderly, children >4 yrs: 1-3 deep inhalations; subsequent doses no sooner than 3 hrs.

Glaucoma:
OPHTHALMIC: Adults, elderly: 1-2 drops 1-2 times/day.

PRECAUTIONS

CONTRAINDICATIONS: Hypertension, hyperthroidism, ischemic heart disease, cardiac arrhythmias, cerebrovascular insufficiency, narrow-angle glaucoma, shock. **CAUTIONS:** Elderly, diabetes mellitus, angina pectoris, tachycardia, MI, severe renal/hepatic impairment, psychoneurotic disorders, hypoxia. **PREGNANCY/LACTATION:** Crosses placenta; distributed in breast milk. **Pregnancy Category C.**

INTERACTIONS

DRUG INTERACTIONS: Tricyclic antidepressants may increase cardiovascular effects. May decrease effects of beta-blockers. Ergonovine, *methergine*, oxytocin may increase vasoconstriction. Digoxin, sympathomimetics may increase risk of arrhythmias. **ALTERED LAB VALUES:** May decrease serum potassium levels.

SIDE EFFECTS

FREQUENT: Restlessness, anxiety, tremor, headache, tachycardia w/palpitations; tissue blanching (due to vascular constriction) at injection site.

ADVERSE REACTIONS/TOXIC EFFECTS

Excessive doses may cause acute hypertension, arrhythmias. Prolonged or excessive use may result in metabolic acidosis (due to increased serum lactic acid concentrations). Observe for disorientation, weakness, hyperventilation, headache, nausea, vomiting, diarrhea.

NURSING IMPLICATIONS

BASELINE ASSESSMENT:

Offer emotional support (high incidence of anxiety due to difficulty in breathing and sympathomimetic response to drug).

INTERVENTION/EVALUATION:

Monitor B/P; rate, depth, rhythm, type of respiration; quality and rate of pulse. Assess lung sounds for rhonchi, wheezing, rales. Monitor arterial blood gases. Observe lips, fingernails for blue or dusky color in light-skinned patients; gray in dark-skinned patients. In cardiac arrest, monitor EKG, B/P, pulse. Evaluate for clinical improvement (quieter, slower respirations, relaxed facial expression, cessation of clavicular retractions).

PATIENT/FAMILY TEACHING:

Increase fluid intake (decreases lung secretion viscosity). Avoid excessive use of caffeine derivatives (chocolate, coffee, tea, cola, cocoa). *Ophthalmic:* Teach proper administration. Slight burning, stinging may occur on initial instillation. Report any new symptoms (rapid pulse, shortness of breath, or dizziness immediately—may be systemic effects).

epoetin alfa

eh-poy´tin

(Epogen, Procrit)

CANADIAN AVAILABILITY

Eprex

CLASSIFICATION

Erythropoietin

PHARMACOKINETICS

Well absorbed after SubQ administration. After administration, an increase in reticulocyte count seen within 10 days; increases in Hgb, Hct and RBC count within 2-6 wks. Half-life: 4-13 hrs.

ACTION

Induces erythropoiesis by stimulating division, differentiation of erythroid progenitor cells in bone marrow. Induces release of reticulocytes from marrow.

USES

Treatment of anemia associated w/chronic renal failure or related to zidovudine (AZT) therapy in HIV-infected pts or to chemotherapy in cancer pts.

STORAGE/HANDLING

Refrigerate; stable for up to 14 days at room temperature. Use 1 dose/vial; do not reenter vial. Discard unused portion.

INDICATIONS/DOSAGE/ROUTES

NOTE: May give IV or SubQ. *IV:* Hemodialysis (may give into venous line at end of procedure); *SubQ:* Peritoneal dialysis; *IV or SubQ:* nondialysis pt.

Chronic renal failure:
IV/SubQ: Adults, elderly: Initially 50-100 U/kg 3 times/wk. Target Hct range: 30-36%. Dosage adjustments not earlier than 1 mo intervals unless clinically indicated. *Decrease dose:* Hct increasing and approaching 36% (temporarily hold doses if Hct continues to rise, reinstate lower dose when Hct begins to decrease); Hct increases by >4 points in 2 wk period (monitor Hct 2 times/wk for 2-6 wks). *Increase dose:* Hct does not increase 5-6 points after 8 wks (w/iron stores adequate) and Hct below target range. **Maintenance:** *(Dialysis):* 75 U/kg 3 times/wk. **Range:** 12.5-525 U/kg. *(Nondialysis):* 75-150 U/kg/wk.

AZT-treated, HIV-infected patients:
NOTE: Pt receiving AZT w/serum erythropoietin levels >500 mU likely not to respond to therapy.
IV/SubQ: Adults: Initially, 100 U/kg 3 times/wk for 8 wks; may increase by 50-100 U/kg 3 times/wk. Evaluate response q4-8wks thereafter; adjust dose by 50-100 U/kg 3 times/wk. If doses >300 U/kg 3 times/wk are not eliciting response, unlikely pt will respond. **Maintenance:** Titrate to maintain desired Hct.

Chemotherapy patients:
SubQ: Adults, elderly: Initially, 150 units/kg 3 times/wk up to 300 U/kg 3 times/wk.

PRECAUTIONS

CONTRAINDICATIONS: Uncontrolled hypertension, history of sensitivity to mammalian cell–derived products or human albumin. **CAUTIONS:** Those w/known porphyria (impairment of erythrocyte formation in bone marrow or responsible for liver impairment). **PREGNANCY/LACTATION:** Unknown if drug crosses placenta or is distributed in breast milk. **Pregnancy Category C.**.

INTERACTIONS

DRUG INTERACTIONS: May need to increase heparin (increase in RBC volume may enhance blood clotting). **ALTERED LAB VALUES:** May decrease bleeding time, iron concentration, serum ferritin. May increase BUN, creatinine, phosphorus, potassium, sodium, uric acid.

SIDE EFFECTS

NOTE: Generally well tolerated. **FREQUENT:** Improved sense of well-being. **OCCASIONAL:** Hypertension, headache, arthralgia, tachycardia, nausea. **RARE:** Rash, urticaria (generally mild, transient), diarrhea, shortness of breath (SOB). *AZT-treated HIV-infected:* **FREQUENT:** Fever, headache, cough, rash, respiratory congestion, nausea, SOB, skin reaction at injection site.

ADVERSE REACTIONS/TOXIC EFFECTS

Hypertensive encephalopathy, thrombosis, cerebrovascular accident, MI, seizures have occurred rarely. Hyperkalemia occurs occasionally, usually in those who do not conform to medication compliance, dietary guidelines, frequency of dialysis.

NURSING IMPLICATIONS

BASELINE ASSESSMENT:

Assess B/P before drug initiation (80% of those w/CRF have history of hypertension). B/P often rises during early therapy in those w/history of hypertension. Consider that all pts will eventually need supplemental iron therapy. Assess serum iron (transferrin saturation: should be >20%) and serum ferritin (>100 ng/ml) prior to and during therapy. Establish baseline CBC, differential and platelet counts (esp. note hematocrit). Monitor B/P aggressively for increased B/P (25% of those on medication require antihypertension therapy, dietary restrictions).

INTERVENTION/EVALUATION:

Monitor Hct level diligently (if level increases >4 points in 2 wk period, dosage should be reduced); assess CBC, differential, platelet counts routinely. Monitor temperature, esp. in cancer pts on chemotherapy and zidovudine-treated HIV pts, and BUN, uric acid, creatinine, phosphorus, potassium, esp. in CRF patients. Evaluate food tolerance and stool frequency, consistency. Provide assistance for dizziness, fatigue, and safety for possible seizures.

PATIENT/FAMILY TEACHING:

Compliance w/dietary guidelines and frequency of dialysis is essential (improved sense of well-being may be misleading in CRF pts). Evidence of response to epoetin alfa may be seen in increased reticulocyte count within 10 days; however, Hct changes take 2-6 wks. Does not substitute for emergency transfusions. Avoid tasks that require alertness, motor skills until response to drug is established.

ergoloid mesylates

ur´go-loyd mess-ah´lates
(Gerimal, Hydergine)

CANADIAN AVAILABILITY: Hydergine

CLASSIFICATION

Psychotherapeutic

PHARMACOKINETICS

Rapid, incompletely absorbed from GI tract. Metabolized in liver. Eliminated primarily in feces. Half-life: 2-5 hrs.

ACTION

Central action decreases vascular tone, slows HR. Peripheral action blocks alpha adrenergic receptors. May improve O_2 uptake and improve cerebral metabolism.

USES

Treatment of age-related (those >60 yrs) mental capacity decline (cognitive and interpersonal skills, mood, self-care, apparent motivation).

PO ADMINISTRATION

1. Instruct pt to allow sublingual tablets to completely dissolve under tongue; do not crush or chew.
2. Do not break capsule or tablet form.

INDICATIONS/DOSAGE/ROUTES

Age-related decline in mental capacity:
PO: Adults, elderly: Initially, 1 mg 3 times/day. **Range:** 1.5-12 mg/day.

PRECAUTIONS

CONTRAINDICATIONS: Acute or chronic psychosis, regardless of etiology. **CAUTIONS:** None significant.

INTERACTIONS

DRUG INTERACTIONS: None significant. **ALTERED LAB VALUES:** None significant.

SIDE EFFECTS

OCCASIONAL: GI distress, transient nausea, sublingual irritation.

ADVERSE REACTIONS/TOXIC EFFECTS

None significant.

NURSING IMPLICATIONS

BASELINE ASSESSMENT:

Exclude possibility that pt's signs and symptoms arise from a possibly reversible and treatable condition secondary to systemic disease, neurological disease, or primary disturbance of mood before administering medication.

INTERVENTION/EVALUATION:

Periodically reassess benefit of current therapy.

PATIENT/FAMILY TEACHING:

Elimination of symptoms appears gradual; results may not be noted for 3-4 wks.

ergonovine maleate

er-goe-noe´veen
(Ergotrate)

E

CANADIAN AVAILABILITY:
Ergotrate

CLASSIFICATION

Uterine stimulant

PHARMACOKINETICS

	ONSET	PEAK	DURATION
PO	10 min	—	>3 hrs
IM	3-5 min	—	>3 hrs
IV	40 sec	—	>45 min

Rapidly absorbed after oral/IM administration. Distributed to plasma, extracellular fluid. Metabolized in liver. Excreted in urine.

ACTION

Directly stimulates uterine muscle (increases force, frequency of contractions). Induces cervical contractions. Stimulates alpha adrenergic, serotonin receptors producing arterial vasoconstriction. Causes vasospasm of coronary arteries.

USES

To prevent and treat postpartum, postabortal hemorrhage due to atony or involution. (Not for induction or augmentation of labor).

STORAGE/HANDLING

Refrigerate parenteral form; protect from light.

PO/IM/IV ADMINISTRATION

1. Initial dose may be given parenterally (IM preferred), followed by oral regimen.
2. IV use in life-threatening emergencies only; may dilute to volume of 5 ml w/0.9% NaCl injection; give over at least 1 min, carefully monitoring B/P.

INDICATIONS/DOSAGE/ROUTES

Oxytocic:
PO: Adults: 1-2 tabs q6-12h for 2-7 days.
IM/IV: Adults: Initially, 0.2 mg. May repeat no more often than q2-4h for no more than 5 doses total.

PRECAUTIONS

CONTRAINDICATIONS: Hypersensitivity to ergot, hypertension, pregnancy, toxemia, untreated hypocalcemia. **CAUTIONS:** Renal/hepatic impairment, coronary artery disease, occlusive peripheral vascular disease, sepsis. **PREGNANCY/LACTATION:** Contraindicated during pregnancy. Small amounts in breast milk.

INTERACTIONS

DRUG INTERACTIONS: Vasoconstrictors, vasopressors may increase effect. **ALTERED LAB VALUES:** May decrease prolactin concentration.

SIDE EFFECTS

OCCASIONAL: Nausea, vomiting, esp. w/IV administration. **RARE:** Dizziness, diaphoresis, tinnitus, foul taste, palpitations, temporary chest pain, headache, pruritus; pale/cold hands or feet; pain in arms, legs, lower back; weakness in legs.

ADVERSE REACTIONS/TOXIC EFFECTS

Severe hypertensive episodes may result in cerebrovascular accident, serious arrhythmias, seizures; hypertensive effects more frequent w/pt susceptibility, rapid IV administration, concurrent regional anesthesia or vasoconstrictors. Peripheral ischemia may lead to gangrene.

NURSING IMPLICATIONS

Baseline Assessment:

Question for hypersensitivity to any ergot derivatives. Determine calcium, B/P and pulse baselines. Assess bleeding prior to administration.

Intervention/Evaluation:

Monitor uterine contractions (frequency, strength, duration), bleeding, B/P, and pulse every 15 min until stable (about 1-2 hrs). Assess extremities for color, warmth, movement, pain. Report chest pain promptly. Provide support w/ambulation if dizziness occurs.

Patient/Family Teaching:

Avoid smoking because of added vasoconstriction. Report increased cramping, bleeding, or foul-smelling lochia. Pale, cold hands/feet should be reported because may mean decreased circulation.

ergotamine tartrate

er-go´tah-meen
(Ergostat Medihaler-Ergotamine)

FIXED-COMBINATION(S):
W/caffeine, a stimulant (Cafergot, Wigraine)

CANADIAN AVAILABILITY:
Ergomar, Gynergen

CLASSIFICATION

Antimigraine

PHARMACOKINETICS

Slow, incomplete absorption from GI tract, rapid, extensive absorption rectally. Protein binding: 93-98%. Undergoes extensive first-pass metabolism in liver. Metabolized to active metabolite. Eliminated in feces via biliary system. Half-life: 21 hrs.

ACTION

May have agonist/antagonist actions w/alpha adrenergic, serotonergic, dopaminergic receptors. Directly stimulates vascular smooth muscle constricting arteries and veins. May inhibit re-uptake of norepinephrine.

USES

Prevents or aborts vascular headaches (e.g., migraine, cluster headaches).

SUBLINGUAL/INHALATION ADMINISTRATION

SUBLINGUAL:

1. Place under tongue; do not swallow.

INHALATION:

1. Shake container well; exhale completely; then holding mouthpiece 1 inch away from lips, inhale and hold breath as long as possible before exhaling.
2. Wait at least 5 min before inhaling second dose, if needed.
3. Rinse mouth w/water immediately after inhalation (prevents mouth/throat dryness).

INDICATIONS/DOSAGE/ROUTES

NOTE: Initiate therapy as soon as possible after first signs of attack.

Vascular headaches:
SUBLINGUAL: Adults, elderly: Initially, 2 mg (1 tablet). May repeat at 30 min intervals. **Maximum:** 3 tablets/24 hrs or 5 tablets/wk.
AEROSOL: Adults, elderly: Initially, 1 inhalation. May repeat in 5

min. **Maximum:** 6 inhalations/24 hrs or 15 inhalations/wk.

PRECAUTIONS

CONTRAINDICATIONS: Hypersensitivity to ergot alkaloids, peripheral vascular disease (thromboangiitis obliterans, syphlitic arteritis, severe arteriosclerosis, thrombophlebitis, Raynaud's disease), impaired renal/hepatic function, severe pruritus, coronary artery disease, hypertension, sepsis, malnutrition. **CAUTIONS:** None significant. **PREGNANCY/LACTATION:** Contraindicated in pregnancy (produces uterine stimulant action, resulting in possible fetal death or retarded fetal growth); increases vasoconstriction of placental vascular bed. Drug distributed in breast milk. May produce diarrhea, vomiting in neonate. May prohibit lactation. **Pregnancy Category X.**

INTERACTIONS

DRUG INTERACTIONS: Beta blockers, erythromycin may increase risk vasospasm. May decrease effect of nitroglycerin. Ergot alkaloids, systemic vasoconstrictors may increase pressor effect. **ALTERED LAB VALUES:** None significant.

SIDE EFFECTS

None significant.

ADVERSE REACTIONS/TOXIC EFFECTS

Prolonged administration or excessive dosage may produce ergotamine poisoning: nausea, vomiting, weakness of legs, pain in limb muscles, numbness and tingling of fingers/toes, precordial pain, tachycardia or bradycardia, hyper/hypotension. Localized edema, itching due to vasoconstriction of peripheral arteries and arterioles. Feet, hands will become cold, pale, numb. Muscle pain occurs when walking and later, even at rest. Gangrene may occur. Occasionally confusion, depression, drowsiness, convulsions appear.

NURSING IMPLICATIONS

BASELINE ASSESSMENT:

Question pt regarding history of peripheral vascular disease, renal/hepatic impairment, or possibility of pregnancy. Contact physician w/findings before administering drug. Question pt regarding onset, location, and duration of migraine and possible precipitating symptoms.

INTERVENTION/EVALUATION:

Monitor closely for evidence of ergotamine overdosage as result of prolonged administration or excessive dosage (see Adverse Reactions/Toxic Effects). Notify physician of any signs and symptoms of ergotamine poisoning.

PATIENT/FAMILY TEACHING:

Initiate therapy at first sign of migraine attack. Report if there is need to progressively increase dose to relieve vascular headaches or if irregular heartbeat, nausea, vomiting, numbness/tingling of fingers/toes, or pain or weakness of extremities is noted. Discuss contraception w/physician; report suspected pregnancy immediately.

erythrityl tetranitrate

eh-rith´rih-till

(Cardilate)

CANADIAN AVAILABILITY:
Cardilate

CLASSIFICATION

Nitrate

PHARMACOKINETICS

	ONSET	PEAK	DURATION
PO	15-30 min	60 min	6 hrs
Sublingual/chew	5 min	15 min	3 hrs

Readily absorbed from GI tract. Undergoes extensive first-pass metabolism. Metabolized in liver, blood (enzymatic). Primarily excreted in urine.

ACTION

Decreases myocardial O_2 demand. Reduces left ventricular preload and afterload. Dilates coronary arteries, improves collateral blood flow to ischemic areas within myocardium.

USES

Prophylaxis, long-term treatment of angina.

PO/SUBLINGUAL ADMINISTRATION

PO:

1. May crush scored tablets.
2. Take on empty stomach.

SUBLINGUAL:

1. Dissolve under tongue; do not swallow.
2. Administer while seated.
3. Hold tablet in mouth for 1-2 min (absorption through buccal tissue).

INDICATIONS/DOSAGE/ROUTES

Prophylaxis, treatment of angina:
SUBLINGUAL: Adults, elderly: Initially, 5-10 mg prior to anticipated physical/emotional stress.
PO: Adults, elderly: 10 mg before meals, midmorning, and midafternoon. In pts w/nocturnal attacks, 10 mg at bedtime. **Maximum:** 100 mg/day.

PRECAUTIONS

CONTRAINDICATIONS: Hypersensitivity to nitrates, severe anemia, closed-angle glaucoma, postural hypotension, head trauma, increased intracranial pressure. **CAUTIONS:** Acute MI, hepatic/renal disease, glaucoma (contraindicated in closed-angle glaucoma), blood volume depletion from diuretic therapy, systolic B/P below 90 mm Hg. **PREGNANCY/LACTATION:** Unknown if drug crosses placenta or is distributed in breast milk. **Pregnancy Category C.**

INTERACTIONS

DRUG INTERACTIONS: Alcohol, antihypertensives, vasodilators may increase risk of orthostatic hypotension. **ALTERED LAB VALUES:** May increase urine catecholamines, urine VMA.

SIDE EFFECTS

FREQUENT: Headache (may be severe) occurs mostly in early therapy, diminishes rapidly in intensity, usually disappears during continued treatment; transient flushing of face and neck, dizziness (esp. if pt is standing immobile or is in a warm environment), weakness, postural hypotension. *Sublingual:* Burning, tingling sensation at oral point of dissolution. **OCCASIONAL:** GI upset.

ADVERSE REACTIONS/TOXIC EFFECTS

Drug should be discontinued if

blurred vision, dry mouth occur. Severe postural hypotension manifested by fainting, pulselessness, cold/clammy skin, profuse sweating. Tolerance may occur w/repeated, prolonged therapy (minor tolerance w/intermittent use of sublingual tablets). High dose tends to produce severe headache.

NURSING IMPLICATIONS

BASELINE ASSESSMENT:

Record onset, type (sharp, dull, squeezing), radiation, location, intensity, and duration of anginal pain and precipitating factors (exertion, emotional stress).

INTERVENTION/EVALUATION:

Assist w/ambulation if lightheadedness, dizziness occurs. Assess for facial/neck flushing. Monitor B/P for hypotension.

PATIENT/FAMILY TEACHING:

Rise slowly from lying to sitting position and dangle legs momentarily before standing. Take oral form on empty stomach (however, if headache occurs during management therapy, take medication w/meals). Dissolve sublingual tablet under tongue; do not swallow. Take at first sign of angina. If not relieved within 5 min, dissolve second tablet under tongue. Repeat if no relief in another 5 min. If pain continues, contact physician. Expel from mouth any remaining sublingual tablet after pain is completely relieved. Do not change from one brand of drug to another. Avoid alcohol (intensifies hypotensive effect). If alcohol is ingested soon after taking nitroglycerin, possible acute hypotensive episode (marked drop in B/P, vertigo, pallor) may occur.

erythromycin base

eh-rith-row-my´sin

(E-Mycin, Eryc, Ery-tab, PCE Dispertab, Ilotycin)

erythromycin estolate

(Ilosone)

erythromycin ethylsuccinate

(EES, Pediamycin, EryPed)

erythromycin lactobionate

(Erythrocin)

erythromycin stearate

(Erythrocin, Wyamycin)

erythromycin topical

(Akne-mycin, Eryderm, Erymax)

FIXED-COMBINATION(S):

Erythromycin ethylsuccinate combined w/sulfisoxazole, a sulfonamide (Pediazole)

CANADIAN AVAILABILITY:

E-mycin, Eryc, Erythromid, Novorythro, PCE, Ilotycin

CLASSIFICATION

Antibiotic: Macrolide

PHARMACOKINETICS

Variably absorbed from GI tract (affected by dosage form used). Widely distributed. Protein binding: 75-90%. Metabolized in liver. Primarily eliminated in feces via bile. Not removed by hemodialysis. Half-life: 1.4-2 hrs (increased in decreased renal function).

ACTION

Bacteriostatic. Penetrates bacterial cell membrane and reversibly binds to 50S subunit of bacterial ribosomes inhibiting protein synthesis.

USES

Respiratory infections, otitis media, pertussis, inflammatory acne vulgaris, diphtheria (adjunctive therapy), Legionnaires' disease, intestinal amebiasis, preop intestinal antisepsis. Prophylaxis for rheumatic fever, bacterial endocarditis, respiratory tract surgery/invasive procedures, gonococcal ophthalmia neonatorum; if penicillin, tetracycline is contraindicated: gonorrheal pelvic inflammatory disease, coexisting chlamydial infections, uncomplicated urogenital infections, Lyme disease (younger than 9 yrs).

STORAGE/HANDLING

Store capsules, tablets at room temperature. Oral suspension stable for 14 days at room temperature. Diluted IV solutions stable for 8 hrs at room temperature, 24 hrs if refrigerated. Discard if precipitate forms.

PO/IV/OPHTHALMIC ADMINISTRATION

PO:

1. Administer erythromycin base, stearate 1 hr before or 2 hrs after food. Erythromycin estolate, ethylsuccinate may be given w/o regard to meals, but optimal absorption occurs when given on empty stomach.
2. Give w/8 oz water.
3. If swallowing difficulties exist, sprinkle capsule contents on tsp applesauce, follow w/water.
4. Do not swallow chewable tablets whole.

IV:

1. Reconstitute each 500 mg vial w/10 ml sterile water for injection (20 ml for 1 Gm) to provide concentration of 50 mg/ml.
2. After mixing w/diluent, immediately shake vial to dissolve medication.
3. For intermittent IV infusion, further dilute w/100-250 ml 5% dextrose, 0.9% NaCl or other compatible IV fluid. Infuse over 20-60 min.
4. Alternating IV sites, use large veins to reduce risk of phlebitis.

OPHTHALMIC:

1. Place finger on lower eyelid and pull out until a pocket is formed between eye and lower lid. Place ¼-½ inch ointment into pocket.
2. Have pt close eye gently for 1-2 min, rolling eyeball (increases contact area of drug to eye).
3. Remove excess ointment around eye w/tissue.

INDICATIONS/DOSAGE/ROUTES

NOTE: Space doses evenly around the clock. 400 mg erythromycin ethylsuccinate = 250 mg erythromycin base, stearate, or estolate.

Usual parenteral dosage:
IV: Adults, elderly, children: 15-20 mg/kg/day in divided doses. **Maximum:** 4 Gm/day.

Usual oral dosage:
PO: Adults, elderly: 250 mg q6h; 500 mg q12h; or 333 mg q8h. Increase up to 4 Gm/day. **Children:** 30-50 mg/kg/day in divided doses up to 60-100 mg/kg/day for severe infections.

Preop intestinal antisepsis:
PO: Adults, elderly: Give 1 Gm at 1, 2, and 11 PM on day prior to surgery (w/neomycin).

Acne vulgaris:
TOPICAL: Adults: Apply to skin 2 times/day.

Gonococcal ophthalmia neonatorum:
OPHTHALMIC: Neonates: 0.5-2 cm no later than 1 hr after delivery.

PRECAUTIONS

CONTRAINDICATIONS: Hypersensitivity to erythromycins, preexisting liver disease, history of hepatitis due to erythromycins. Do not administer Pediazole to infants <2 mo. **CAUTIONS:** Hepatic dysfunction. If combination used (Pediazole), consider precautions of sulfonamides. **PREGNANCY/LACTATION:** Crosses placenta, distributed in breast milk. Erythromycin estolate may increase liver function test results in pregnant women. **Pregnancy Category B.**

INTERACTIONS

DRUG INTERACTIONS: May inhibit metabolism of carbamazepine. May decrease effects of chloramphenicol, clindamycin. May increase concentration, nephrotoxicity of cyclosporine. Hepatotoxic medications may increase hepatotoxicity. May increase risk of cardiotoxicity w/terfenadine. May increase risk of toxicity w/theophylline. May increase effect of warfarin. **ALTERED LAB VALUES:** May increase SGOT (AST), SGPT (ALT), alkaline, phosphatase, bilirubin.

SIDE EFFECTS

FREQUENT: Abdominal discomfort/cramping, phlebitis/thrombophlebitis w/IV administration. *Topical:* Dry skin (50%). **OCCASIONAL:** Nausea, vomiting, diarrhea, rash, urticaria. **RARE:** *Ophthalmic:* Sensitivity reaction w/increased irritation, burning, itching, inflammation. *Topical:* Urticaria.

ADVERSE REACTIONS/TOXIC EFFECTS

Superinfections, esp. antibiotic-associated colitis, reversible cholestatic hepatitis may occur. High dosage in renal impairment may lead to reversible hearing loss. Anaphylaxis occurs rarely.

NURSING IMPLICATIONS

BASELINE ASSESSMENT:

Question pt for history of allergies (particularly erythromycins), hepatitis. Obtain specimens for culture and sensitivity before giving first dose (therapy may begin before results are known.)

INTERVENTION/EVALUATION:

Check for GI discomfort, nausea, vomiting. Determine pattern of bowel activity, stool consistency. Assess skin for rash. Monitor hepatic function tests, assess for hepatotoxicity: malaise, fever, abdominal pain, GI disturbances. Evaluate for superinfection: genital/anal pruritus, sore mouth or tongue, moderate to severe diarrhea. Check for phlebitis (heat, pain, red streaking over vein).

PATIENT/FAMILY TEACHING:

Continue therapy for full length of treatment. Doses should be evenly spaced. Do NOT swallow chewable tablets whole. Take medication w/8 oz water 1 hr before or 2 hrs after food/beverage. Notify physician in event of GI upset, rash, diarrhea, or other new symptom. *Ophthalmic:* Report burning, itching, or inflammation; inquire about use of eye make-up. *Topical:* Report excessive dryness, itching, burning. Improvement of acne may not occur for 1-2 mos, maximum benefit may take 3 mos; therapy may last months or years. Use caution in use of other topical acne preparations containing peeling or abrasive agents, medicated or abrasive soaps, cosmetics containing alcohol (e.g. astringents, aftershave lotion).

esmolol hydrochloride

ez´moe-lol

(Brevibloc)

CLASSIFICATION

Beta$_1$-adrenergic blocker

PHARMACOKINETICS

Widely distributed. Protein binding: 55%. Rapidly hydrolyzed by esterases in RBCs. Primarily excreted in urine. Half-life: 9 minutes.

ACTION

Selectively blocks beta$_1$-adrenergic receptors, slowing sinus heart rate, decreasing cardiac output, decreasing B/P (exact mechanism unknown but may block peripheral adrenergic receptors, decrease sympathetic outflow from CNS or decrease renin release from kidney). Antiarrhythmic activity due to blocking stimulation of cardiac pacemaker potentials.

USES

Rapid, short-term control of ventricular rate in those w/supraventricular arrhythmias, sinus tachycardia.

STORAGE/HANDLING

Use only clear and colorless to light yellow solution. After dilution, solution is stable for 24 hrs. Discard solution if it is discolored or if precipitate forms.

IV ADMINISTRATION

NOTE: Give by IV infusion. Avoid butterfly needles, very small veins.

1. Must be diluted to concentration of 10 mg/ml or less (prevents vein irritation).
2. For IV infusion, remove 20 ml from 500 ml container of 5% dextrose, 0.9% NaCl, or other compatible IV fluid and dilute 5 GM vial esmolol hydrochloride w/remaining 480 ml to provide concentration of 10 mg/ml.
3. Administer by controlled infusion device set at rate judged by tolerance and response. Hypotension (systolic B/P below 90 mm Hg) is greatest during first 30 min of IV infusion.

INDICATIONS/DOSAGE/ROUTES

IV: Adults, elderly: Initially, loading dose of 500 mcg/kg/min for 1 min, followed by 50 mcg/kg/min for 4 min. If optimum response is not attained in 5 min, give second loading dose of 500 mcg/kg/min for 1 min, followed by infusion of 100 mcg/kg/min for 4 min. Additional loading doses can be given and infusion increased by 50 mcg/kg/min (up to 200 mcg/kg/min) for 4 min. Once desired response is attained, cease loading dose and increase infusion by no more than 25 mcg/kg/min. Interval between doses may be increased to 10 min. Infusion usually administered over 24-48 hrs in most pts.

PRECAUTIONS

CONTRAINDICATIONS: Overt cardiac failure, cardiogenic shock, heart block greater than first degree, sinus bradycardia. **CAUTIONS:** Impaired renal function, peripheral vascular disease, hyperthyroidism, diabetes, inadequate cardiac function, bronchospastic disease. **PREGNANCY/LACTATION:** Unknown if drug crosses placenta or is distributed in breast milk. **Pregnancy Category C.**

INTERACTIONS

DRUG INTERACTIONS: Sympathomimetics, xanthines may mutually inhibit effects. May mask symptoms of hypoglycemia, prolong hypoglycemic effect of insulin, oral hypoglycemics. MAO inhibitors may cause significant hypertension. **ALTERED LAB VALUES:** None significant.

SIDE EFFECTS

Generally well tolerated, w/ transient and mild side effects. **FREQUENT:** Hypotension (systolic B/P below 90 mm Hg) manifested as dizziness, nausea, diaphoresis, headache, cold extremities, fatigue. **OCCASIONAL:** Induration and inflammation at IV site, somnolence, confusion. **RARE:** Bradycardia, peripheral ischemia, bronchospasm.

ADVERSE REACTIONS/TOXIC EFFECTS

Excessive dosage may produce profound hypotension, bradycardia. May potentiate insulin-induced hypoglycemia in diabetic pts.

NURSING IMPLICATIONS

BASELINE ASSESSMENT:

Assess B/P, apical pulse immediately before drug is administered (if pulse is 60/min or below, or systolic B/P is below 90 mm Hg, withhold medication, contact physician).

INTERVENTION/EVALUATION:

Monitor B/P for hypotension, development of diaphoresis or dizziness (usually first sign of impending hypotension). Assess pulse for strength/weakness, irregular rate, bradycardia. Monitor EKG for cardiac changes, particularly shortening of QT interval, prolongation of PR interval. Assess extremities for coldness. Assist w/ambulation if dizziness occurs. Assess for nausea, diaphoresis, headache, fatigue.

estazolam

es-tah´zoe-lam
(ProSom)

CLASSIFICATION

Sedative-hypnotic

PHARMACOKINETICS

Well absorbed from GI tract. Crosses blood-brain barrier. Protein binding: 93%. Metabolized in liver. Primarily excreted in urine. Half-life: 10-24 hrs.

ACTION

Enhances action of inhibitory neurotransmitter gamma-aminobutyric acid (GABA). Depressant effects occur at all levels of CNS.

USES

Short-term treatment of insomnia (up to 6 wks). Reduces sleep-induction time, number of nocturnal awakenings; increases length of sleep.

PO ADMINISTRATION

1. Give w/o regard to meals.
2. Tablet may be crushed.

INDICATIONS/DOSAGE/ROUTES

NOTE: Use smallest effective dose in those w/liver disease, low serum albumin.

Insomnia:
PO: Adults >18 yrs: 1-2 mg at bedtime. **Elderly/debilitated:** 0.5-1 mg at bedtime.

PRECAUTIONS

CONTRAINDICATIONS: Acute narrow-angle glaucoma, acute alcohol intoxication. **CAUTIONS:** Impaired renal/hepatic function. **PREGNANCY/LACTATION:** Crosses placenta; may be distributed in breast milk. Chronic ingestion during pregnancy may produce withdrawal symptoms, CNS depression in neonates. **Pregnancy Category X.**

INTERACTIONS

DRUG INTERACTIONS: Alcohol, CNS depressants may increase CNS depressant effect. **ALTERED LAB VALUES:** None significant.

SIDE EFFECTS

FREQUENT: Drowsiness, sedation, rebound insomnia (may occur for 1-2 nights after drug is discontinued), dizziness, confusion, euphoria. **OCCASIONAL:** Weakness, anorexia, diarrhea. **RARE:** Paradoxical CNS excitement, restlessness (particularly noted in elderly/debilitated).

ADVERSE REACTIONS/TOXIC EFFECTS

Abrupt or too-rapid withdrawal may result in pronounced restlessness, irritability, insomnia, hand tremors, abdominal/muscle cramps, sweating, vomiting, seizures. Overdosage results in somnolence, confusion, diminished reflexes, coma.

NURSING IMPLICATIONS

BASELINE ASSESSMENT:

Assess B/P, pulse, respirations immediately before administration. Raise bedrails. Provide environment conductive to sleep (backrub, quiet environment, low lighting).

INTERVENTION/EVALUATION:

Assess sleep pattern of pt. Assess elderly/debilitated for paradoxical reaction, particularly during early therapy. Evaluate for therapeutic response: a decrease in number of nocturnal awakenings, increase in length of sleep.

PATIENT/FAMILY TEACHING:

Smoking reduces drug effectiveness. Do not abruptly withdraw medication following long-term use. Rebound insomnia may occur when drug is discontinued after short-term therapy. Do not use during pregnancy.

---

estradiol

ess-tra-dye´ole
(Estrace, Estraderm, Vivelle)

estradiol cypionate

(Depo-Estradiol, Depogen)

estradiol valerate

(Delestrogen, Dioval, Valergen-10)

ethinyl estradiol

(Estinyl)

FIXED-COMBINATION(S):
Estradiol cypionate w/testosterone cypionate, an androgen (Depo-Testadiol); estradiol valerate w/testosterone enanthate, an androgen (Deladumone, Estra-Testrin); ethinyl estradiol w/fluoxymesterone, an androgen (Halodrin).

CANADIAN AVAILABILITY:
Estrace, Estraderm, Delestrogen, Femogex

CLASSIFICATION

Antineoplastic, Estrogen

PHARMACOKINETICS

Well absorbed from GI tract. Widely distributed. Protein binding: 50-80%. Metabolized in liver. Primarily excreted in urine. Half-life: 50-60 minutes.

ACTION

Increases synthesis of DNA, RNA and various proteins in responsive tissues. Reduces release of gonadotropin-releasing hormone reducing follicle stimulating hormone (FSH) and leuteinizing hormone (LH). Promotes normal growth, development of female sex organs, maintaining GU function, vasomotor stability. Prevents accelerated bone loss by inhibiting bone resorption, restoring balance of bone resorption and formation. Inhibits LH, decreases serum concentration of testosterone.

USES

Management of moderate to severe vasomotor symptoms associated w/menopause, female hypogonadism. Palliative treatment of advanced, inoperable metastatic carcinoma of the breast in postmenopausal women (estradiol, ethinyl estradiol), prostate in men (estradiol, estradiol valerate, ethinyl estradiol). Prevention of postpartum breast engorgement (estradiol valerate). Treatment of atrophic vaginitis, kraurosis vulvae (estradiol, estradiol valerate). Treatment of postmenopausal osteoporosis (estradiol transdermal system). Prevention of osteoporosis.

PO/IM/VAGINAL/TRANSDERMAL ADMINISTRATION

PO:

1. Administer at the same time each day.
2. Give w/milk or food if nausea occurs.

TRANSDERMAL:

1. Remove old patch; select new site (buttocks an alternative application site).
2. Peel off protective strip to expose adhesive surface.
3. Apply immediately to clean, dry, intact skin on the trunk of the body (area w/as little hair as possible).
4. Press in place for at least 10 sec.
5. Do not apply to the breasts or waistline.

IM:

1. Rotate vial to disperse drug in solution.
2. Inject deep IM in gluteus maximus.

VAGINAL:

1. Apply at bedtime for best absorption.
2. Assemble and fill applicator per manufacturer's directions.

3. Insert end of applicator into vagina, directed slightly toward sacrum; push plunger down completely.

4. Avoid skin contact w/cream because of absorption.

INDICATIONS/DOSAGE/ROUTES

ESTRADIOL ORAL, INTRAVAGINAL, TRANSDERMAL

Vasomotor symptoms, atrophic vaginitis, kraurosis vulvae, female hypogonadism, castration, primary ovarian failure:
PO: Adults, elderly: Initially, 1-2 mg/day cyclically.
INTRAVAGINALLY: Adults, elderly: Initially, 2-4 Gm/day for 1-2 wks; reduce dose by ½ over 1-2 wks. **Maintenance:** 1 Gm 1-3 times/wk cyclically.
TOPICAL: Adults, elderly: Initially, 0.05 mg/24 hrs 2 times/wk cyclically; maintenance dose adjusted to pt's needs.

Breast cancer:
PO: Adults, elderly: 10 mg 3 times/day.

Prostate cancer:
PO: Adults, elderly: 1-2 mg 3 times/day.

Osteoporosis prevention:
PO: Adults, elderly: 0.5 mg/day (3 wks on, 1 wk off).

ESTRADIOL CYPIONATE

Vasomotor symptoms:
IM: Adults, elderly: 1-5 mg q3-4wks.

Female hypogonadism:
IM: Adults, elderly: 1.5-2 mg every month.

ESTRADIOL VALERATE

Vasomotor symptoms, atrophic vaginitis, kraurosis vulvae, female hypogonadism, castration, primary ovarian failure:
IM: Adults, elderly: 10-20 mg q4h.

Prevention of postpartum breast engorgement:
IM: Adults, elderly: 10-25 mg as single dose at end of first stage of labor.

Prostate cancer:
IM: Adults, elderly: 30 mg or more q1-2wks.

ETHINYL ESTRADIOL

Vasomotor symptoms:
PO: Adults, elderly: 0.02-0.15 mg/day cyclically.

Female hypogonadism:
PO: Adults, elderly: 0.05 mg 1-3 times/day during first 2 wks menstrual cycle.

Breast cancer:
PO: Adults, elderly: 1 mg 3 times/day.

Prostate cancer:
PO: Adults, elderly: 0.15-0.2 mg/day.

PRECAUTIONS

CONTRAINDICATIONS: Known or suspected breast cancer (except select pts w/metastasis), estrogen-dependent neoplasia; undiagnosed abnormal genital bleeding; active thrombophlebitis or thromboembolic disorders; history of thrombophlebitis, thrombosis or thromboembolic disorders w/previous estrogen use, hypersensitivity to estrogen. **CAUTIONS:** Conditions which may be aggravated by fluid retention: cardiac, renal/hepatic dysfunction, epilepsy, migraine. Mental depression, metabolic bone disease w/potential hypercalcemia, history of jaundice during pregnancy or strong family history of breast cancer, fibrocystic disease or breast nodules, children in whom bone growth is not complete. **PREGNANCY/LACTATION:** Distributed in breast milk. May be harmful to offspring. Not for use during lactation. **Pregnancy Category X.**

INTERACTIONS

DRUG INTERACTIONS: May interfere w/effects of bromocriptine. May increase concentration cyclosporine, increase hepatic, nephrotoxicity. Hepatotoxic medications may increase hepatotoxicity. **ALTERED LAB VALUES:** May affect metapyrone, thyroid function tests. May decrease cholesterol, LDH. May increase calcium, glucose, HDL, triglycerides.

SIDE EFFECTS

FREQUENT: Anorexia, nausea, swelling of breasts, peripheral edema evidenced by swollen ankles, feet. *Transdermal route:* Skin irritation, redness. **OCCASIONAL:** Vomiting (esp. w/high dosages), headache (may be severe), intolerance to contact lenses, increased B/P, glucose intolerance, brown spots on exposed skin. *Vaginal route:* Local irritation, vaginal discharge, changes in vaginal bleeding (spotting, breakthrough or prolonged bleeding). **RARE:** Chorea, cholestatic jaundice, hirsutism, loss of scalp hair, depression.

ADVERSE REACTIONS/TOXIC EFFECTS

Prolonged administration increases risk of gallbladder, thromboembolic disease and breast, cervical, vaginal, endometrial, and liver carcinoma.

NURSING IMPLICATIONS

BASELINE ASSESSMENT:

Question hypersensitivity to estrogen, previous jaundice or thromboembolic disorders associated w/pregnancy or estrogen therapy. Establish baseline B/P, blood glucose.

INTERVENTION/EVALUATION:

Assess B/P at least daily. Check for swelling, weigh daily. Monitor blood glucose 4 times/day for pts w/diabetes. Promptly report signs and symptoms of thromboembolic or thrombotic disorders: sudden severe headache, shortness of breath, vision or speech disturbance, weakness or numbness of an extremity, loss of coordination, pain in chest, groin, or leg. Assess skin for irritation due to transdermal application or brown blotches. Note estrogen therapy on specimens.

PATIENT/FAMILY TEACHING:

Importance of medical supervision. Avoid smoking due to increased risk of heart attack or blood clots. Do not take other medications w/o physician approval. Teach how to perform Homan's test, signs and symptoms of blood clots (report these to physician immediately). Notify physician of abnormal vaginal bleeding, depression, other symptoms. Teach female pts to perform self-breast exam. Avoid exposure to sun/ultraviolet light. Check weight daily; report weekly gain of 5 lbs or more. W/vaginal application:

remain recumbent at least 30 min after application and do not use tampons. Stop taking the medication and contact physician at once if pregnancy is suspected. Give labeling from drug package.

estramustine phosphate sodium

es-trah-mew´steen

(Emcyt)

CANADIAN AVAILABILITY: Emcyt

CLASSIFICATION

Antineoplastic

PHARMACOKINETICS

Well absorbed from GI tract. Highly localized in prostatic tissue. Rapidly dephosphorylated during absorption into peripheral circulation. Metabolized in liver. Primarily eliminated in feces via biliary system. Half-life: 20 hrs.

ACTION

Exact mechanism unknown. Combinations of estradiol and mechlorethamine, action may be due to direct effect of estrogen component or antimitotic activity. Reduces serum testosterone concentration.

USES

Treatment of metastatic or progressive carcinoma of prostate gland.

STORAGE/HANDLING

NOTE: May be carcinogenic, mutagenic, or teratogenic. Handle w/ extreme care during administration.

Refrigerate capsules (may remain at room temperature for 24-48 hrs w/o loss of potency).

PO ADMINISTRATION

Give w/water 1 hr before or 2 hrs after meals.

INDICATIONS/DOSAGE/ROUTES

Prostatic carcinoma:
PO: Adults, elderly: 10-16 mg/kg/day (140 mg for each 10 kg weight) in 3-4 doses/day.

PRECAUTIONS

CONTRAINDICATIONS: Hypersensitivity to estradiol or nitrogen mustard, active thrombophlebitis or thrombolic disorders unless tumor is cause for thrombolic disorders and benefits outweigh risk. **CAUTIONS:** History of thrombophlebitis, thrombosis, or thromboembolic disorders, cerebrovascular or coronary artery disease, impaired hepatic function, metabolic bone disease in those w/hypercalcemia or renal insufficiency. **PREGNANCY/LACTATION: Pregnancy Category C.**

INTERACTIONS

DRUG INTERACTIONS: Hepatotoxic drugs may increase risk of hepatotoxicity. **ALTERED LAB VALUES:** May increase SGOT (AST), LDH, bilirubin, cortisol, glucose, phospholipids, prolactin, prothrombin, sodium, triglycerides. May decrease antithrombin 3, folate, pregnanediol excretion, phosphate. May alter thyroid function tests.

SIDE EFFECTS

FREQUENT: Peripheral edema of lower extremities, breast tenderness or enlargement, diarrhea, flatulence, nausea. **OCCASIONAL:** Increase in B/P, thirst, dry skin, easy bruising, flushing, thinning hair, night sweats. **RARE:** Headache, rash, fatigue, insomnia, vomiting.

ADVERSE REACTIONS/TOXIC EFFECTS

May exacerbate CHF, pulmonary emboli, thrombophlebitis, cerebrovascular accident.

NURSING IMPLICATIONS

INTERVENTION/EVALUATION:

Monitor B/P periodically.

PATIENT/FAMILY TEACHING:

Do not take with milk, milk products or calcium-rich food, calcium-containing antacids. Use contraceptive measures during therapy. If headache (migraine or severe), vomiting, disturbed speech or vision, dizziness, numbness, shortness of breath, calf pain, heaviness in chest, unexplained cough occurs, contact physician. Do not have immunizations w/o physician's approval (drug lowers body's resistance). Avoid contact w/those who have recently received live virus vaccine. Contact physician if nausea/vomiting continues at home.

estropipate

ess-troe-pye´pate
(Ogen)

CANADIAN AVAILABILITY:
Ogen

CLASSIFICATION

Estrogen

PHARMACOKINETICS

Well absorbed from GI tract. Widely distributed. Protein binding: 50-80%. Metabolized in liver. Primarily excreted in urine.

ACTION

Increases synthesis of DNA, RNA, and various proteins in responsive tissues. Reduces release of gonadotropin-releasing hormone reducing follicle stimulating hormone (FSH) and leuteinizing hormone (LH). Promotes normal growth, development of female sex organs, maintaining GU function, vasomotor stability. Prevents accelerated bone loss by inhibiting bone resorption, restoring balance of bone resorption and formation.

USES

Management of moderate to severe vasomotor symptoms associated w/menopause. Treatment of atrophic vaginitis, kraurosis vulvae, female hypogonadism and castration, primary ovarian failure. Prevention of osteoporosis.

PO/VAGINAL ADMINISTRATION

PO:

Administer at the same time each day.

VAGINAL:

1. Apply at bedtime for best absorption.
2. Assemble and fill applicator per manufacturer's directions.
3. Insert end of applicator into vagina, directed slightly toward sacrum; push plunger down completely.
4. Avoid skin contact w/cream because of absorption.

INDICATIONS/DOSAGE/ROUTES

Vasomotor symptoms, atrophic vaginitis, kraurosis vulvae:
PO: Adults, elderly: 0.625-5 mg/day cyclically.

Atrophic vaginitis, kraurosis vulvae:
INTRAVAGINALLY: Adults, elderly: 2-4 Gm/day cyclically.

Female hypogonadism, castration, primary ovarian failure:
PO: Adults, elderly: 1.25-7.5 mg/day × 21 days; off 8-10 days. Repeat if bleeding does not occur by end of rest period.

Osteoporosis prevention:
PO: Adults, elderly: 0.625 mg/day (25 days of 31 day cycle/month).

PRECAUTIONS

CONTRAINDICATIONS: Known or suspected breast cancer, estrogen-dependent neoplasia; undiagnosed abnormal genital bleeding; active thrombophlebitis or thromboembolic disorders; history of thrombophlebitis, thrombosis, or thromboembolic disorders w/previous estrogen use, hypersensitivity to estrogen. **CAUTIONS:** Conditions that may be aggravated by fluid retention: cardiac, renal, or hepatic dysfunction, epilepsy, migraine. Mental depression, hypercalcemia, history of jaundice during pregnancy or strong family history of breast cancer, fibrocystic disease or breast nodules, children in whom bone growth is not complete. **PREGNANCY/LACTATION:** Distributed in breast milk. May be harmful to fetus. Not for use during lactation. **Pregnancy Category X.**

INTERACTIONS

DRUG INTERACTIONS: May interfere w/effects of bromocriptine. May increase concentration cyclosporine, increase hepatic/nephrotoxicity. Hepatotoxic medications may increase hepatotoxicity. **ALTERED LAB VALUES:** May affect metapyrone, thyroid function tests. May decrease cholesterol, LDH. May increase calcium, glucose, HDL, triglycerides.

SIDE EFFECTS

FREQUENT: Anorexia, nausea, swelling of breasts, peripheral edema evidenced by swollen ankles, feet. **OCCASIONAL:** Vomiting (esp. w/high dosages), headache (may be severe), intolerance to contact lenses, increased B/P, glucose intolerance, brown spots on exposed skin. *Vaginal route:* Local irritation, vaginal discharge, changes in vaginal bleeding (spotting, breakthrough, or prolonged bleeding). **RARE:** Chorea, cholestatic jaundice, hirsutism, loss of scalp hair, depression.

ADVERSE REACTIONS/TOXIC EFFECTS

Prolonged administration increases risk of gallbladder, thromboembolic disease and breast, cervical, vaginal, endometrial, and liver carcinoma.

NURSING IMPLICATIONS

BASELINE ASSESSMENT:

Question for hypersensitivity to estrogen, previous jaundice or thromboembolic disorders associated w/pregnancy or estrogen therapy. Establish baseline B/P, blood glucose.

INTERVENTION/EVALUATION:

Assess B/P at least daily. Check

for swelling, weigh daily. Check blood glucose 4 times/day for pts w/diabetes. Promptly report signs and symptoms of thromboembolic or thrombotic disorders: sudden severe headache, shortness of breath, vision or speech disturbance, weakness or numbness of an extremity, loss of coordination, pain in chest, groin, or leg. Note estrogen therapy on specimens.

PATIENT/FAMILY TEACHING:

Importance of medical supervision. Avoid smoking because of increased risk of heart attack or blood clots. Do not take other medications w/o physician approval. Teach how to perform Homan's test, signs and symptoms of blood clots (report these to physician immediately). Also notify physician of abnormal vaginal discharge or bleeding, depression. Teach self-breast exam. Avoid exposure to sun/ultraviolet light. Check weight daily; report weekly gain of 5 lbs or more. W/vaginal application: remain recumbent at least 30 min after application and do not use tampons. Stop taking estropipate and contact physician if pregnancy suspected. Give labeling from drug package.

ethacrynic acid

eth-ah-krin´ick
(Edecrin)

ethacrynate sodium

eth-ah-krin´ate
(Edecrin Sodium)

CANADIAN AVAILABILITY:
Edecrin

CLASSIFICATION

Diuretic: Loop

PHARMACOKINETICS

	ONSET	PEAK	DURATION
PO	<30 min	2 hrs	6-8 hrs
IV	<5 min	15-30 min	2 hrs

Rapidly absorbed from GI tract. Protein binding: high. Metabolized in liver to active metabolite. Primarily excreted in urine.

ACTION

Enhances excretion of sodium and chloride by inhibiting reabsorption at ascending limb of loop of Henle and potassium at distal renal tubule.

USES

Treatment of edema associated w/CHF, severe renal impairment, nephrotic syndrome, hepatic cirrhosis; short-term management of ascites, children w/congenital heart disease.

STORAGE/HANDLING

Store oral, parenteral form at room temperature. Discard if parenteral form appears hazy or opalescent. Discard unused reconstituted solution after 24 hrs.

PO/IV ADMINISTRATION

PO:

1. Give w/food to avoid GI upset, preferably w/breakfast (may prevent nocturia).

IV:

1. For direct IV, administer slowly over several min.
2. For IV infusion, reconstitute each 50 mg ethacrynate sodium w/ 50 ml 5% dextrose injection or sodium chloride injection.
3. Infuse slowly, over 20-30 min,

through tubing of running IV infusion.

INDICATIONS/DOSAGE/ROUTE

Edema:

PO: Adults: 50-100 mg daily. Dosage may be increased in 25-50 mg increments until therapeutic response is achieved. **Elderly:** Initially, 25-50 mg/day; increase as needed. **Children:** Initially, 25 mg. Dosage may be increased in increments of 25 mg until therapeutic response is achieved. Alternate-day scheduling may be used for maintenance therapy.

IV: Adults >18 yrs, elderly: 0.5-1.0 mg/kg or 50 mg for average-sized adult. Single IV dose should not exceed 100 mg.

PRECAUTIONS

CONTRAINDICATIONS: Anuria. **CAUTIONS:** Hepatic cirrhosis, ascites, history of gout, systemic lupus erythematosus, diabetes mellitus, elderly, debilitated. **PREGNANCY/LACTATION:** Unknown if drug crosses placenta or is distributed in breast milk. **Pregnancy Category B.**

INTERACTIONS

DRUG INTERACTIONS: Amphotericin, ototoxic and nephrotoxic agents may increase toxicity. May decrease effect of anticoagulants, heparin. Hypokalemia causing agents may increase risk hypokalemia. May increase risk lithium toxicity. **ALTERED LAB VALUES:** May increase glucose, BUN, uric acid, urinary phosphate. May decrease calcium, chloride, magnesium, potassium, sodium.

SIDE EFFECTS

EXPECTED: Increase in urine frequency/volume. **OCCASIONAL:** Nausea, gastric upset w/cramping, diarrhea, headache, fatigue, apprehension. **RARE:** Severe, watery diarrhea.

ADVERSE REACTIONS/TOXIC EFFECTS

Vigorous diuresis may lead to profound water loss and electrolyte depletion, resulting in hypokalemia, hyponatremia, dehydration, coma, circulatory collapse. Acute hypotensive episodes may also occur, sometimes several days after beginning of therapy. Ototoxicity manifested as deafness, vertigo, tinnitus (ringing/roaring in ears) may occur, especially in those w/severe renal impairment. Can exacerbate diabetes mellitus, systemic lupus erythematosus, gout, pancreatitis. Blood dyscrasias have been reported.

NURSING IMPLICATIONS

BASELINE ASSESSMENT:

Check vital signs, esp. B/P for hypotension prior to administration. Obtain baseline electrolytes, particularly check for low potassium. Check edema, skin turgor, mucous membranes for hydration status. Assess muscle strength, mental status. Note skin temperature, moisture. Obtain baseline weight. Initiate I&O.

INTERVENTION/EVALUATION:

Monitor B/P, vital signs, electrolytes, I&O, weight. Note extent of diuresis. Watch for changes from initial assessment (hypokalemia may result in muscle strength changes, tremor, muscle cramps, change in mental status, cardiac arrhythmias; hyponatremia may result in confusion, thirst, cold/clammy skin).

PATIENT/FAMILY TEACHING:

Expect increased frequency

E

and volume of urination. Report irregular heartbeat, signs of electrolyte imbalances (noted above), hearing abnormalities (such as sense of fullness in ears, ringing/roaring in ears). Eat foods high in potassium such as whole grains (cereals), legumes, meat, bananas, apricots, orange juice, potatoes (white, sweet), raisins. Avoid sun/sunlamps.

ethambutol

ee-tham´byoo-tole

(Myambutol)

CANADIAN AVAILABILITY: Etibi, Myambutol

CLASSIFICATION

Antitubercular

PHARMACOKINETICS

Rapidly, well absorbed from GI tract. Widely distributed. Protein binding: 20-30%. Metabolized in liver. Primarily excreted in urine. Removed by hemodialysis. Half-life: 3-4 hrs (increased in decreased renal function).

ACTION

Bacteriostatic. Interferes w/cell metabolism and multiplication by inhibiting one or more metabolites in susceptible bacteria. Active only during cell division.

USES

In conjunction w/at least one other antitubercular agent for initial treatment and retreatment of clinical tuberculosis.

PO ADMINISTRATION

1. Give w/food (decreases GI upset).
2. Give once q24h.

INDICATIONS/DOSAGE/ROUTES

Tuberculosis:

PO: Adults, elderly: Initially (no prior anti-TB medication): 15 mg/kg q24h. (Prior anti-TB medication): 25 mg/kg/day q24h for 60 days then decrease to 15 mg/kg/day.

NOTE: When used in combination therapy and given 2 times/wk, dose is 50 mg/kg. Decrease dose in those w/renal impairment.

PRECAUTIONS

CONTRAINDICATIONS: Hypersensitivity to ethambutol, optic neuritis. **CAUTIONS:** Renal dysfunction, gout, ocular defects: diabetic retinopathy, cataracts, recurrent ocular inflammatory conditions. Not recommended for children under 13 yrs of age. **PREGNANCY/LACTATION:** Crosses placenta; excreted in breast milk. **Pregnancy Category C.**

INTERACTIONS

DRUG INTERACTIONS: Neurotoxic medications may increase risk of neurotoxicity. **ALTERED LAB VALUES:** May increase uric acid.

SIDE EFFECTS

OCCASIONAL: Anorexia, nausea, vomiting, headache, dizziness, malaise, mental confusion, joint pain, dermatitis.

ADVERSE REACTIONS/TOXIC EFFECTS

Optic neuritis (occurs more often w/high dosage, long-term therapy), peripheral neuritis, thrombocytopenia, anaphylactoid reaction occur rarely.

NURSING IMPLICATIONS

BASELINE ASSESSMENT:

Question for hypersensitivity to ethambutol. Assure collection of specimens for culture, sensitivity. Evaluate initial CBC, renal and hepatic test results.

INTERVENTION/EVALUATION:

Assess for vision changes (altered color perception, decreased visual acuity may be first signs); discontinue drug and notify physician immediately. Give w/food if GI distress occurs. Monitor uric acid concentrations and assess for hot/painful/swollen joints, esp. big toe, ankle, or knee (gout). Check CBC, culture and sensitivity tests, renal and hepatic function results. Monitor I&O in event of renal dysfunction. Report numbness, tingling, burning of extremities (peripheral neuritis). Assess for dizziness and assure assistance w/ambulation. Check mental status. Evaluate skin for rash.

PATIENT/FAMILY TEACHING:

Do not skip doses; take for full length of therapy (may take months, years). Not affected by food. Office visits, vision and lab tests are essential part of treatment. Do not take *any* other medication w/o consulting physician. Notify physician *immediately* of *any* visual problem (visual effects generally reversible w/discontinuation of ethambutol, but in rare cases may take up to a yr to disappear or may be permanent); promptly report rash, swelling and pain of joints, numbness/tingling/burning of hands or feet. Do not drive or use machinery if visual problems or dizziness occur.

ethosuximide

eth-oh-sucks′ih-myd
(Zarontin)

CANADIAN AVAILABILITY:
Zarontin

CLASSIFICATION

Anticonvulsant

PHARMACOKINETICS

Rapid, completely absorbed from GI tract. Protein binding: low. Metabolized in liver. Primarily excreted in urine. Half-life: adults: 56-60 hrs; children: 30-36 hrs.

ACTION

Increases seizure threshold, reduces synaptic response in nerve transmission, suppressing paroxysmal spike, wave pattern noted w/absence (petit mal) seizures.

USES

Management of absence (petit mal) seizures, as adjunct w/phenytoin and phenobarbital, in treatment of mixed seizures (absence seizures w/tonic-clonic seizures).

STORAGE/HANDLING

Store capsules, syrup at room temperature.

PO ADMINISTRATION

Give w/o regard to meals.

INDICATIONS/DOSAGE/ROUTES

Seizures:
PO: Adults, children >6 yrs: Initially, 500 mg daily in divided doses. **Children 3-6 yrs:** 250 mg

daily given as single dose. **Maintenance:** Increase daily dose by 250 mg q4-7days until control is achieved. **Usual maintenance dose:** 20 mg/kg daily. Do not exceed 1.5 Gm daily, given in divided doses.

PRECAUTIONS

CONTRAINDICATIONS: Hypersensitivity to succinimides. **EXTREME CAUTION:** Hepatic/renal disease. **PREGNANCY/LACTATION:** Unknown if drug crosses placenta or is distributed in breast milk. **Pregnancy Category C.**

INTERACTIONS

DRUG INTERACTIONS: Alcohol, CNS depressants may increase CNS depression. Tricyclic antidepressants, antipsychotics may decrease seizure threshold effects, increase CNS depression. May decrease concentration of haloperidol (may change pattern/frequency of epileptiform seizures). **ALTERED LAB VALUES:** None significant.

SIDE EFFECTS

FREQUENT: GI disturbances (nausea, anorexia, vague gastric upset, cramps, weight loss, diarrhea, abdominal and epigastric distress). **OCCASIONAL:** Headache, hiccups, dizziness, drowsiness, irritability, tiredness.

ADVERSE REACTIONS/TOXIC EFFECTS

Psychiatric/psychologic disturbances (sleep disturbances, nightmares, aggressiveness, inability to concentrate) may be noted. Blood dyscrasias, systemic lupus erythematosus occur rarely. Abrupt withdrawal may precipitate status epilepticus. Skin eruptions appear as hypersensitivity reaction.

NURSING IMPLICATIONS

BASELINE ASSESSMENT:

Review history of seizure disorder (intensity, frequency, duration, LOC). Initiate seizure precautions. Liver function tests, CBC, platelet count should be performed before therapy begins and periodically during therapy.

INTERVENTION/EVALUATION:

Observe frequently for recurrence of seizure activity. Monitor for therapeutic serum level (40-100 mcg/ml). Assess for clinical improvement (decrease in intensity or frequency of seizures).

PATIENT/FAMILY TEACHING:

Do not abruptly withdraw medication following long-term use (may precipitate seizures). Strict maintenance of drug therapy is essential for seizure control. Drowsiness usually disappears during continued therapy. Avoid tasks that require alertness, motor skills until response to drug is established.

etidronate disodium

eh-tih-droe´nate

(Didronel)

CANADIAN AVAILABILITY:
Didronel

CLASSIFICATION

Calcium regulator

PHARMACOKINETICS

Minimally absorbed from GI tract (1-6%). Chemically adsorbed to bone in areas of elevated osteogenesis. Absorbed dose excreted in urine; unabsorbed dose eliminated in feces. Half-life: 5-7 hrs.

ACTION

Binds to calcium phosphate surface of calcium hydroxyapatite crystals retarding mineralization, growth of heterotropic ossification. May also retard bone resorption and accelerated rate of bone turnover in Paget's disease.

USES

Orally: treatment of symptomatic Paget's disease of the bone, prevention and treatment of heterotopic ossification following hip replacement or due to spinal injury. Parenteral (IV): treatment of hypercalcemia associated w/malignant neoplasms inadequately managed by dietary modification or oral hydration; treatment of hypercalcemia of malignancy persisting after adequate hydration has been restored.

STORAGE/HANDLING

Store tablets at room temperature. After dilution, IV stable for at least 48 hrs.

PO/IV ADMINISTRATION

PO:

1. Give on empty stomach, 2 hrs before meals.
2. Do not give within 2 hrs of vitamins w/mineral supplements, antacids, or medications high in calcium, magnesium, iron, or aluminum.

IV INFUSION:

1. Dilute in at least 250 ml 0.9% NaCl.
2. Infuse slowly, over a *minimum* of 2 hrs regardless of volume of solution.

INDICATIONS/DOSAGE/ROUTES

ORAL:

Paget's disease:
PO: Adults, elderly: Initially, 5-10 mg/kg/day not to exceed 6 mos or 11-20 mg/kg/day not to exceed 3 mos. Retreat only after drug-free period of at least 90 days.

Heterotopic ossification (due to spinal cord injury):
PO: Adults, elderly: 20 mg/kg/day for 2 wks; then 10 mg/kg/day for 10 wks.

Heterotopic ossification (complicating total hip replacement):
PO: Adults, elderly: 20 mg/kg/day for 1 mo preop; follow w/20 mg/kg/day for 3 mos postop.

PARENTERAL:

Usual parenteral dosage:
IV: Adults, elderly: 7.5 mg/kg/day × 3 days; retreatment no sooner than 7-day intervals between courses. Follow w/oral therapy on day after last infusion (20 mg/kg/day for 30 days; may extend up to 90 days).

PRECAUTIONS

CONTRAINDICATIONS: Children, severe renal function. **CAUTIONS:** Enterocolitis, renal impairment, pts unable to maintain adequate intake of vitamin D or calcium. **PREGNANCY/LACTATION:** Unknown if drug crosses placenta or is distributed in breast milk. **Pregnancy Category B** (oral). **Pregnancy Category C** (parenteral).

INTERACTIONS

DRUG INTERACTIONS: Antacids w/calcium, magnesium, aluminum, foods w/calcium, mineral supplements may decrease absorption.

ALTERED LAB VALUES: None significant.

SIDE EFFECTS

FREQUENT: Nausea, diarrhea increased, continuing or more frequent bone pain in those with Paget's disease. **OCCASIONAL:** Bone fractures (esp. femur). *Parenteral:* Metallic, altered, or loss of taste. **RARE:** Hypersensitivity reaction, (rash, pruritus, urticaria, angioedema).

ADVERSE REACTIONS/TOXIC EFFECTS

Nephrotoxicity (hematuria, dysuria, proteinuria) noted w/parenteral route.

NURSING IMPLICATIONS

BASELINE ASSESSMENT:

Obtain lab baselines, esp. electrolytes, renal function.

INTERVENTION/EVALUATION:

Assess food tolerance. Check for diarrhea. Monitor electrolytes. Check I&O, BUN, creatinine in pts w/impaired renal function. Evaluate pain in pts w/Paget's disease. Assess skin for eruptions.

PATIENT/FAMILY TEACHING:

May take up to 3 mos for therapeutic response; do not stop taking medication, discuss w/physician. Taste may be altered, usually disappears w/continuation of therapy. Assure milk, dairy products in diet for calcium, vitamin D. Do not take any other medications w/o physician approval. Take medication on empty stomach, 2 hrs from food, vitamins, antacids. Report nausea, diarrhea, rash, or other symptoms. Follow-up office visits are necessary even when therapy is discontinued.

etodolac

eh-toe´doe-lack

(Lodine)

CANADIAN AVAILABILITY: Lodine

CLASSIFICATION

Nonsteroidal anti-flammatory

PHARMACOKINETICS

	ONSET	PEAK	DURATION
PO (analgesic)	30 min	—	4-12 hrs

Completely absorbed from GI tract. Widely distributed. Protein binding: 99%. Metabolized in liver. Primarily excreted in urine. Half-life: 6-7 hrs.

ACTION

Inhibits prostaglandin synthesis. Inhibits action of cyclooxygenase, decreases formation of prostaglandin, thromboxane precursors from arachidonic acid.

USES

Acute and long-term treatment of osteoarthritis, management of pain.

PO ADMINISTRATION

1. Do not crush or break capsules.
2. May give w/food, milk, or antacids if GI distress occurs.

INDICATIONS/DOSAGE/ROUTES

NOTE: Reduce dosage in elderly; maximum dose for pts weighing <60 kg: 20 mg/kg.

Osteoarthritis:

PO: Adults, elderly: Initially, 800-1,200 mg/day in 2-4 divided doses. **Maintenance:** 600-1,200 mg/day.

Analgesia:
PO: Adults, elderly: 200-400 mg q6-8h as needed. **Maximum:** 1,200 mg/day.

PRECAUTIONS

CONTRAINDICATIONS: Active peptic ulcer, GI ulceration, chronic inflammation of GI tract, GI bleeding disorders, history of hypersensitivity to aspirin or nonsteroidal anti-inflammatory agent. **CAUTIONS:** Impaired renal/hepatic function, history of GI tract disease, predisposition to fluid retention. **PREGNANCY/LACTATION:** Unknown if drug crosses placenta or is distributed in breast milk. Avoid use during last trimester (may adversely affect fetal cardiovascular system: premature closure of ductus arteriosus). **Pregnancy Category C.**

INTERACTIONS

DRUG INTERACTIONS: May increase effects of oral anticoagulants, heparin, thrombolytics. May decrease effect of antihypertensives, diuretics. Salicylates, aspirin may increase risk of GI side effects, bleeding. Bone marrow depressants may increase risk of hematologic reactions. May increase concentration, toxicity of lithium. May increase methotrexate toxicity. Probenecid may increase concentration. **ALTERED LAB VALUES:** May increase bleeding time, creatinine, liver function tests. May decrease uric acid.

SIDE EFFECTS

OCCASIONAL: Dyspepsia (heartburn, indigestion, epigastric pain, diarrhea/constipation, cramping, flatulence), headache occurs more frequently in elderly. **RARE:** Rash, peripheral edema/fluid retention, visual disturbances, vomiting, drowsiness.

ADVERSE REACTIONS/TOXIC EFFECTS

Overdosage may result in acute renal failure. In those treated chronically, peptic ulcer, GI bleeding, gastritis, severe hepatic reaction (jaundice), nephrotoxicity (hematuria, dysuria, proteinuria), severe hypersensitivity reaction (bronchospasm, angiofacial edema) occur rarely.

NURSING IMPLICATIONS

BASELINE ASSESSMENT:

Assess onset, type, location, duration of pain or inflammation. Inspect appearance of affected joints for immobility, deformities, skin condition.

INTERVENTION/EVALUATION:

Monitor for headache, dyspepsia. Monitor pattern of daily bowel activity, stool consistency. Evaluate for therapeutic response: relief of pain, stiffness, swelling, increase in joint mobility, reduced joint tenderness, improved grip strength.

PATIENT/FAMILY TEACHING:

Swallow tablet whole; do not crush or chew. Avoid aspirin, alcohol during therapy (increases risk of GI bleeding). If GI upset occurs, take w/food, milk. Report GI distress, visual disturbances, rash, edema, headache.

etoposide, VP-16

eh-toe´poe-side

(VePesid)

CANADIAN AVAILABILITY:
VePesid

CLASSIFICATION

Antineoplastic

PHARMACOKINETICS

Variably absorbed from GI tract. Rapidly distributed. Low concentrations in CSF. Protein binding: 97%. Metabolized in liver. Primarily excreted in urine. Half-life: 3-12 hrs.

ACTION

Cell cycle-dependent and phase-specific w/maximum effect on S, G_2 phase of cell division. Inhibits DNA synthesis.

USES

Treatment of refractory testicular tumors, small cell lung carcinoma.

STORAGE/HANDLING

NOTE: May be carcinogenic, mutagenic, or teratogenic. Handle w/ extreme care during preparation/ administration.

Refrigerate gelatin capsules. Concentrate for injection is clear, yellow. Diluted solutions of 0.2-0.4 mg/ml stable for at least 48 hrs at room temperature. Discard if crystallization occurs.

IV ADMINISTRATION

NOTE: Administer by slow IV infusion. Wear gloves when preparing solution. If powder or solution come in contact w/skin, wash immediately and thoroughly w/soap, water.

1. Syringes w/Luer-Lock fittings should be used for handling concentrate (prevents displacement of needle from syringe).
2. Dilute concentrate (20 mg/ ml) w/50 ml 5% dextrose or 0.9% NaCl to provide concentration of 0.4 mg/ml (100 ml for concentration of 0.2 mg/ml). Avoid concentrations above 0.4 mg/ml (solutions may precipitate).
3. Infuse slowly, over 30-60 min (rapid IV may produce transient hypotension, local pain).
4. Monitor for anaphylactic reaction during infusion (chills, fever, dyspnea, sweating, lacrimation, sneezing, throat/back/chest pain).

INDICATIONS/DOSAGE/ROUTES

NOTE: Dosage individualized based on clinical response, tolerance to adverse effects. When used in combination therapy, consult specific protocols for optimum dosage, sequence of drug administration. Treatment repeated at 3-4 wk intervals.

Refractory testicular tumors:
IV: Adults: Combination therapy: 50-100 mg/m²/day on days 1 to 5 up to 100 mg/m²/day on days 1, 3, 5.

Small cell lung carcinoma:
PO: Adults: 2 times IV dose rounded to nearest 50 mg.
IV: Adults: Combination therapy: 35 mg/m² daily for 4 consecutive days up to 50 mg/m² daily for 5 consecutive days.

PRECAUTIONS

CONTRAINDICATIONS: None significant. **CAUTIONS:** Impaired hepatic function. **PREGNANCY/ LACTATION:** If possible, avoid use during pregnancy, esp. first trimester. May cause fetal harm. Breast feeding not recommended. **Pregnancy Category D.**

INTERACTIONS

DRUG INTERACTIONS: Bone marrow depressants may increase bone marrow depression. Live virus vaccines may potentiate virus replication, increase vaccine side effects, decrease patients antibody response to vaccine. **ALTERED LAB VALUES:** None significant.

SIDE EFFECTS

FREQUENT: Mild to moderate nausea and vomiting, anorexia, alopecia. **OCCASIONAL:** Diarrhea, somnolence, fatigue, peripheral neuropathy. **RARE:** Headache, vertigo, intermittent muscle cramps, rash, hyperpigmentation.

ADVERSE REACTIONS/TOXIC EFFECTS

Bone marrow depression manifested as hematologic toxicity (principally leukopenia, thrombocytopenia, anemia, and to lesser extent, pancytopenia). Leukopenia occurs within 7-14 days after drug administration, thrombocytopenia occurs within 9-16 days after administration. Bone marrow recovery occurs by day 20. Hepatotoxicity occurs occasionally.

NURSING IMPLICATIONS

BASELINE ASSESSMENT:

Obtain hematology tests prior to and at frequent intervals during therapy. Antiemetics readily control nausea, vomiting.

INTERVENTION/EVALUATION:

Monitor Hgb, Hct, WBC, differential, platelet count. Assess pattern of daily bowel activity and stool consistency. Monitor for hematological toxicity (fever, sore throat, signs of local infection, easy bruising, unusual bleeding from any site), symptoms of anemia (excessive tiredness, weakness). Assess for paresthesias (peripheral neuropathy).

PATIENT/FAMILY TEACHING:

Alopecia is reversible, but new hair growth may have different color or texture. Do not have immunizations w/o physician's approval (drug lowers body's resistance). Avoid contact w/those who have recently received live virus vaccine. Promptly report fever, sore throat, signs of local infection, easy bruising, or unusual bleeding from any site. Contact physician if nausea/vomiting continues at home. Teach signs of peripheral neuropathy.

factor IX complex (human)

(Konyne, Profilnine, Heat-treated Propex T)

CLASSIFICATION

Antihemophilic

ACTION

Increases blood levels of blood clotting factors II, VII, IX, and X. Raises plasma levels of factor IX, restores hemostasis in pts w/factor IX deficiency.

USES

NOTE: Only Propex T controls bleeding in pts w/factor VII deficiency. Treatment of bleeding caused by hemophilia B (deficiency of factor IX is demonstrated). Treatment of bleeding in pts w/hemophilia A who have factor VIII inhibitors. Reversal of anticoagulant effect of coumarin anticoagulants.

STORAGE/HANDLING

Store in refrigerator. Do not freeze. Reconstituted solutions stable for 12 hrs at room temperature. Begin administration within 3 hrs. Do not refrigerate reconstituted solutions.

IV ADMINISTRATION

1. Administer by slow IV injection or IV infusion.
2. Filter before administration.
3. Before reconstitution, warm diluent to room temperature.
4. Gently agitate vial until powder is completely dissolved (prevents removal of active components during administration through filter).
5. Infuse slowly, not to exceed 3 ml/min. A too-rapid IV rate may produce headache, flushing, change in B/P and pulse rate, tingling sensation. Discontinuing infusion will eliminate effects immediately. Resume IV at slower rate.
6. If evidence of disseminated intravascular coagulation (DIC) occurs (change in B/P and pulse rate, respiratory distress, chest pain, cough), stop infusion immediately.

INDICATIONS/DOSAGE/ROUTES

NOTE: Amount of factor IX required is individualized. Dosage depends on degree of deficiency, level of each factor desired, weight of pt, severity of bleeding. Give sufficient drug to achieve/maintain plasma level of at least 20% of normal until hemostasis achieved.

PRECAUTIONS

CONTRAINDICATIONS: All factor IX complex (human) except Propex T: Factor VII deficiencies. Liver impairment w/evidence of intravascular coagulation or fibrinolysis. **CAUTIONS:** Impaired hepatic function. **PREGNANCY/LACTATION:** Unknown if drug crosses placenta or is distributed in breast milk. **Pregnancy Category C.**

INTERACTIONS

DRUG INTERACTIONS: Aminocaproic acid may increase risk of thrombosis. **ALTERED LAB VALUES:** None significant.

SIDE EFFECTS

RARE: Mild hypersensitivity reaction (fever, chills, change in B/P and pulse rate, rash, tingling, urticaria [hives]).

ADVERSE REACTIONS/TOXIC EFFECTS

High risk of venous thrombosis during postop period. Acute hypersensitivity reaction, anaphylactoid reaction may occur. *Antidote:* Epinephrine 1 : 1,000. High dosage may produce DIC, MI, thrombosis, pulmonary embolism. There is a risk of transmitting viral hepatitis, other viral diseases.

NURSING IMPLICATIONS

BASELINE ASSESSMENT:

When monitoring B/P, avoid overinflation of cuff. Remove adhesive tape from any pressure dressing very carefully and slowly. Assess results of coagulation studies and extent of existing bleeding (overt bleeding, bruising, joint pain, and swelling).

INTERVENTION/EVALUATION:

Monitor vital signs, I&O. Assess for hypersensitivity reaction (slow infusion and notify physician). Monitor results of coagulation studies closely. Avoid IM or SubQ injections or rectal temperatures. After IV administration, apply direct pressure to venipuncture site for a full 5 min or longer to assure bleeding has stopped. Monitor IV site for oozing q5-15min for 1-2 hrs after administration. Report any evidence of hematuria or change in vital signs immediately. Assess for decrease in B/P, increase in pulse rate, complaint of abdominal/back pain, severe headache (may be evidence of hemorrhage). Question for increase in amount of discharge during menses. Assess peripheral pulses; skin for bruises, petechiae. Check for excessive bleeding from minor cuts, scratches. Assess gums for erythema, gingival bleeding. Evaluate for therapeutic relief of pain, reduction of swelling, and restricted joint movement.

PATIENT/FAMILY TEACHING:

Use electric razor, soft toothbrush to prevent bleeding. Report any sign of red/dark urine, black/red stool, coffee-ground vomitus, red-speckled mucus from cough. Do not use any over-the-counter medication w/o physician approval (may interfere w/platelet aggregation). Carry identification that indicates disease.

famciclovir (Famvir)
See supplement

famotidine

fah-mow´tih-deen
(Pepcid)

CANADIAN AVAILABILITY:
Pepcid

CLASSIFICATION

H_2 receptor antagonist

PHARMACOKINETICS

Rapid, incompletely absorbed from GI tract. Protein binding: 15-20%. Partially metabolized in liver. Primarily excreted in urine. Half-life: 2.5-3.5 hrs (increased in decreased renal function).

ACTION

Inhibits histamine action at H_2 receptors of parietal cells, inhibiting basal and nocturnal gastric acid secretion.

USES

Short-term treatment of active duodenal ulcer. Prevention of duodenal ulcer recurrence. Treatment of active benign gastric ulcer, pathologic GI hypersecretory conditions. Short-term treatment of gastroesophageal reflux disease including erosive esophagitis.

STORAGE/HANDLING

Store tablets, suspension at room temperature. After reconstitution, suspension is stable for 30 days at room temperature. Refrigerate unreconstituted vials. IV solution appears clear, colorless. After dilution, IV solution is stable for 48 hrs at room temperature.

PO/IV ADMINISTRATION

PO:

1. Give w/o regard to meals or antacids. Best given after meals or at bedtime.
2. Shake suspension well before use.

IV:

1. For direct IV injection, dilute 20 mg vial w/5-10 ml 0.9% NaCl or other compatible IV solution. Inject over not less than 2 min.
2. For intermittent IV infusion (piggyback), dilute w/100 ml 5% dextrose or other compatible IV fluid. Infuse over 15-30 min.

F

INDICATIONS/DOSAGE/ROUTES

Acute therapy—duodenal ulcer:
PO: Adults, elderly: 40 mg at bedtime or 20 mg q12h. **Maintenance:** 20 mg at bedtime.

Acute therapy—benign gastric ulcer:
PO: Adults, elderly: 40 mg at bedtime.

Gastroesophageal reflux disease:
PO: Adults, elderly: 20 mg 2 times/day up to 6 wks; 20-40 mg 2 times/day up to 12 wks in pts w/ esophagitis (including erosions, ulcerations).

Pathologic hypersecretory conditions:
PO: Adults, elderly: Initially, 20 mg q6h up to 160 mg q6h.

Usual parenteral dosage:
IV: Adults, elderly: 20 mg q12h.

Dosage in renal impairment:
Creatinine clearance equal or less than 10 ml/min: decrease dose to 20 mg at bedtime or increase dosage interval to 36-48 hrs.

PRECAUTIONS

CONTRAINDICATIONS: None significant. **CAUTIONS:** Impaired renal/hepatic function. **PREGNANCY/LACTATION:** Unknown if drug crosses placenta or is distributed in breast milk. **Pregnancy Category B.**

INTERACTIONS

DRUG INTERACTIONS: Antacids may decrease absorption (do not give within 1/2-1 hr). May decrease absorption of ketoconazole (give at least 2 hrs after). **ALTERED LAB VALUES:** Interferes w/skin tests using allergen extracts. May increase liver function tests.

SIDE EFFECTS

FREQUENT: Headache. **OCCASIONAL:** Dizziness, diarrhea/constipation.

ADVERSE REACTIONS/TOXIC EFFECTS

None significant.

NURSING IMPLICATIONS

INTERVENTION/EVALUATION:

Monitor daily bowel activity and stool consistency. Assess for abdominal pain, GI bleeding signs. Monitor for diarrhea/constipation.

PATIENT/FAMILY TEACHING:

IV may produce transient discomfort at injection site. May take w/o regard to meals or antacids. Report headache. Avoid tasks that require alertness, motor skills until drug response is established. Avoid smoking (decreases effectiveness). Do not use over-the-counter medications/alcohol w/o consulting physician.

felbamate

fell-bah'mate
(Felbatol)

CLASSIFICATION

Anticonvulsant

PHARMACOKINETICS

Well absorbed from GI tract. Binds to plasma proteins (22-25%). Excreted in urine. Food does not affect absorption. Half-life: 20-23 hrs.

ACTION

Exact mechanism unknown. May reduce seizure spread, may increase seizure threshold. Possesses weak inhibitory effects on

GABA-receptor and benzodiazepine receptor binding.

USES

Monotherapy and adjunctive therapy in treatment of partial and secondary generalized seizures in adults; adjunctive therapy in treatment of partial and generalized seizures associated w/Lennox-Gastaut syndrome in children.

PO ADMINISTRATION

1. Scored tablets may be crushed.
2. May give w/food to avoid or reduce GI upset.

INDICATIONS/DOSAGE/ROUTES

Monotherapy:
PO: Adults, elderly, children >14 yrs: Initially, 1,200 mg/day in divided doses 3-4 times daily. Increase dosage in 600 mg increments every 2 wks to 2,400 mg/day based on clinical response and thereafter to 3,600 mg/day if clinically indicated.

Conversion to monotherapy:
PO: Adults, elderly, children >14 yrs: 1,200 mg/day in divided doses 3-4 times daily and reduce concurrent antiepileptic drug (AED) by one third at initial felbamate therapy. At week 2, increase felbamate dosage to 2,400 mg/day while reducing AED up to an additional third of its original dosage. At week 3, increase felbamate dosage up to 3,600 mg/day and continue to reduce AED as clinically indicated.

Adjunctive therapy:
PO: Adults, elderly, children >14 yrs: Add 1,200 mg/day in divided doses 3-4 times daily while reducing present AEDs by 20%. Increase felbamate by 1,200 mg/day increments at weekly intervals to 3,600 mg/day.

Children w/Lennox-Gastaut syndrome (adjunctive therapy):
PO: Children 2-14 yrs: Add 15 mg/kg/day in divided doses 3-4 times daily while reducing present AED by 20%. Increase felbamate by 15 mg/kg/day increments at weekly intervals to 45 mg/kg/day.

PRECAUTIONS

CONTRAINDICATIONS: None significant. **CAUTIONS:** Previous hypersensitivity reaction to carbamates. **PREGNANCY/LACTATION:** Unknown whether drug crosses placenta; detected in breast milk. **Pregnancy Category C.**

INTERACTIONS

DRUG INTERACTIONS: May increase carbamazepine, phenytoin, valproate serum concentrations. Carbamazepine, phenytoin may increase clearance of felbamate. **ALTERED LAB VALUES:** None significant.

SIDE EFFECTS

Side effects appear mild and transient. **OCCASIONAL: (Monotherapy):** Anorexia, nausea, insomnia, headache. **(Adjunctive therapy):** Anorexia, nausea, insomnia, headache, dizziness, somnolence. **RARE:** Rash, photosensitivity.

ADVERSE REACTIONS/TOXIC EFFECTS

Abrupt withdrawal may precipitate seizure status. May cause aplastic anemia or acute liver failure.

NURSING IMPLICATIONS

BASELINE ASSESSMENT:

Review history of seizure disorder (intensity, frequency, duration, level of consciousness). Initiate safety measures. Unnecessary to routinely monitor clinical laboratory parameters (unprecedented safety profile).

INTERVENTION/EVALUATION:

Observe frequently for recurrence of seizure activity. Assess for clinical improvement (decrease in intensity/frequency of seizures).

PATIENT/FAMILY TEACHING:

Do not abruptly withdraw medication following long-term use (may precipitate seizures). Strict maintenance of drug therapy is essential for seizure control. Avoid tasks that require alertness, motor skills until response to drug is established. Avoid sunlight until sensitivity established. Carry ID card/bracelet indicating anticonvulsant therapy.

felodipine

fell-oh´dih-peen
(Plendil)

CANADIAN AVAILABILITY:
Plendil, Renedil

CLASSIFICATION

Calcium channel blocker

PHARMACOKINETICS

	ONSET	PEAK	DURATION
PO	2-5 hrs	—	—

Rapid, completely absorbed from GI tract. Undergoes first-pass metabolism in liver. Protein binding: 99%. Metabolized in liver. Primarily excreted in urine. Half-life: 11-16 hrs.

ACTION

Potent peripheral vasodilator; does not depress SA, AV nodes. Reflex increased heart rate masks negative inotropic effect.

USES

Management of hypertension. May be used alone or w/other antihypertensives.

PO ADMINISTRATION

1. May take w/o regard to food.
2. Do not crush or break tablets.

INDICATIONS/DOSAGE/ROUTES

Hypertension:
PO: Adults, elderly: Initially, 5 mg/day as single dose. Adjust dosage at no less than 2 wk intervals. **Maintenance:** 5-10 mg/day. **Maximum:** 20 mg/day.

PRECAUTIONS

CONTRAINDICATIONS: Sick sinus syndrome/second- or third-degree AV block (except in presence of pacemaker). ,**CAUTIONS:** Impaired renal/hepatic function, CHF. **PREGNANCY/LACTATION:** Unknown if drug crosses placenta or is distributed in breast milk. **Pregnancy Category C.**

INTERACTIONS

DRUG INTERACTIONS: Beta-blockers may have additive effect. May increase digoxin concentration. Procainamide, quinidine may increase risk of QT interval prolongation. Hypokalemia producing agents may increase risk of arrhythmias. **ALTERED LAB VALUES:** None significant.

SIDE EFFECTS

COMMON: Peripheral edema, headache. **FREQUENT:** Dizziness/lightheadedness (hypotensive effect), asthenia (loss of strength, weakness), facial flushing. **OCCASIONAL:** Dyspepsia, paresthesia, cough, respiratory infection.

RARE: Palpitations, nausea, diarrhea/constipation, muscle cramps.

ADVERSE REACTIONS/TOXIC EFFECTS

Overdosage produces nausea, drowsiness, confusion, slurred speech.

NURSING IMPLICATIONS

BASELINE ASSESSMENT:

Assess baseline renal/liver function tests. Assess B/P, apical pulse immediately before drug is administered (if pulse is 60/min or below, or systolic B/P is below 90 mm Hg, withhold medication, contact physician).

INTERVENTION/EVALUATION:

Assist w/ambulation if lightheadedness, dizziness occur. Assess for peripheral edema behind medial malleolus (sacral area in bedridden pts). Monitor pulse rate for bradycardia. Assess skin for flushing. Monitor liver enzyme tests. Question for headache, asthenia.

PATIENT/FAMILY TEACHING:

Do not abruptly discontinue medication. Compliance w/therapy regimen is essential to control hypertension. To avoid hypotensive effect, rise slowly from lying to sitting position, wait momentarily before standing. Avoid tasks that require alertness, motor skills until response to drug is established. Contact physician/nurse if irregular heart beat, shortness of breath, pronounced dizziness, or nausea occurs.

fenofibrate (Lipidil)
See supplement

fenoprofen calcium

fen-oh-pro′fen
(Nalfon)

CANADIAN AVAILABILITY:
Nalfon

CLASSIFICATION

Nonsteroidal anti-inflammatory

PHARMACOKINETICS

	ONSET	PEAK	DURATION
PO (anti-rheumatic)	2 days	—	2-3 wks

Rapidly absorbed from GI tract. Widely distributed. Protein binding: 99%. Metabolized in liver. Primarily excreted in urine. Half-life: 3 hrs.

ACTION

Inhibits prostaglandin synthesis. Inhibits action of cyclooxygenase, decreases formation of prostaglandin, thromboxane precursors from arachidonic acid. Prevents, reduces miosis by relaxing iris sphincter.

USES

Treatment of acute or long-term mild to moderate pain, symptomatic treatment of acute and/or chronic rheumatoid arthritis, osteoarthritis.

PO ADMINISTRATION

May give w/food, milk or antacids if GI distress occurs.

INDICATIONS/DOSAGE/ROUTES

NOTE: Do not exceed 3.2 Gm/day.

Mild to moderate pain:
PO: Adults, elderly: 200 mg q4-6h as needed.

Rheumatoid arthritis, osteoarthritis:
PO: Adults, elderly: 300-600 mg 3-4 times/day.

PRECAUTIONS

CONTRAINDICATIONS: Active peptic ulcer, GI ulceration, chronic inflammation of GI tract, GI bleeding disorders, history of hypersensitivity to aspirin/NSAIDs, history of significantly impaired renal function. **CAUTIONS:** Impaired renal/hepatic function, history of GI tract diseases, predisposition to fluid retention. **PREGNANCY/LACTATION:** Distributed in low concentration in breast milk. Avoid use during last trimester (may adversely affect fetal cardiovascular system: premature closure of ductus arteriosus). **Pregnancy Category C.**

INTERACTIONS

DRUG INTERACTIONS: May increase effects of oral anticoagulants, heparin, thrombolytics. May decrease effect of antihypertensives, diuretics. Salicylates, aspirin may increase risk of GI side effects, bleeding. Bone marrow depressants may increase risk of hematologic reactions. May increase concentration, toxicity of lithium. May increase methotrexate toxicity. Probenecid may increase concentrations. **ALTERED LAB VALUES:** May increase serum transaminases, LDH, alkaline phosphatase, BUN, creatinine, potassium, glucose, protein, bleeding time.

SIDE EFFECTS

FREQUENT: Headache, somnolence/drowsiness, dyspepsia (heartburn, indigestion, epigastric pain), nausea, vomiting, constipation. **OCCASIONAL:** Dizziness, pruritus, nervousness, asthenia (loss of strength), diarrhea, abdominal cramps, flatulence, tinnitus, blurred vision, peripheral edema/fluid retention.

ADVERSE REACTIONS/TOXIC EFFECTS

Overdosage may result in acute hypotension, tachycardia. Peptic ulcer, GI bleeding, nephrotoxicity (dysuria, cystitis, hematuria, proteinuria, nephrotic syndrome), gastritis, severe hepatic reaction (cholestasis, jaundice), severe hypersensitivity reaction (bronchospasm, angiofacial edema) occur rarely.

NURSING IMPLICATIONS

BASELINE ASSESSMENT:

Assess onset, type, location, duration of pain or inflammation. Inspect appearance of affected joints for immobility, deformities, skin condition.

INTERVENTION/EVALUATION:

Assist w/ambulation if somnolence/drowsiness/dizziness occurs. Monitor for evidence of dyspepsia. Monitor pattern of daily bowel activity, stool consistency. Check behind medial malleolus for fluid retention (usually first area noted). Evaluate for therapeutic response: relief of pain, stiffness, swelling, increase in joint mobility, reduced joint tenderness, improved grip strength.

PATIENT/FAMILY TEACHING:

Swallow capsule whole; do not crush or chew. Avoid tasks that require alertness, motor skills until response to drug is established. If GI upset occurs, take w/food, milk. Avoid aspirin, alcohol during therapy (increases risk of GI bleeding).

Report headache, GI distress, visual disturbances, edema.

fentanyl

fen´tah-nil
(Duragesic)

fentanyl citrate

(Fentanyl Oralet, Sublimaze)

FIXED-COMBINATION(S):
W/droperidol, an antianxiety, antiemetic (Innovar)

CANADIAN AVAILABILITY:
Sublimaze

CLASSIFICATION

Opioid: Analgesic **(Schedule II)**

PHARMACOKINETICS

	ONSET	PEAK	DURATION
IM	7-15 min	20-30 min	1-2 hrs
IV	1-2 min	3-5 min	0.5-1 hr

Well absorbed after topical, IM administration. Transmucosal absorbed through mucosal tissue of mouth, GI tract. Protein binding: 80-90%. Metabolized in liver. Primarily eliminated via biliary system. Half-life: 3.6 hrs (increased in elderly).

ACTION

Binds to specific receptors within CNS altering processes affecting pain perception, emotional response to pain. Altering neurotransmitters may contribute to action.

USES

Analgesic action for short-duration surgery, outpatient minor surgery, diagnostic procedures requiring pt to be awake or lightly anesthesized; during surgery, immediately after surgery to prevent/relieve tachypnea, postop delirium, adjunct to general/regional anesthesia. Transdermal for management of chronic pain. Transmucosal for anesthetic premedication.

F

STORAGE/HANDLING

Store parenteral form at room temperature.

IM/IV/TRANSDERMAL/ TRANSMUCOSAL ADMINISTRATION

IV/IM:

NOTE: Incompatible w/methohexital, pentobarbital, thiopental.

1. For initial anesthesia induction dosage, give small amount, give via tuberculin syringe.
2. Give by slow IV injection (over 1-2 min).
3. Too-rapid IV increases risk of severe adverse reactions (skeletal and thoracic muscle rigidity resulting in apnea, laryngospasm, bronchospasm, peripheral circulatory collapse, anaphylactoid effects, cardiac arrest).
4. Opiate antagonist (naloxone) should be readily available.

TRANSDERMAL:

1. Apply to nonhairy area of intact skin of upper torso.
2. Use flat, nonirritated site.
3. Firmly press evenly for 10-20 sec assuring adhesion is in full contact w/skin and edges are completely sealed.
4. Use only water to cleanse site prior to application (soaps, oils, etc., may irritate skin).
5. Rotate sites of application.
6. Used patches are carefully

folded so system adheres to itself; discard in toilet.

TRANSMUCOSAL:

1. Suck lozenge vigorously.

INDICATIONS/DOSAGE/ROUTES

NOTE: Reduce initial dose by 25-33% in those receiving CNS depressants. Reduce dose in elderly, debilitated. Obese (>20% ideal body weight): adjust dosage based on lean body weight.

PREOP:

IM: Adults, elderly: 50-100 mcg (0.05-0.1 mg) 30-60 min before surgery.

PRIMARY AGENT ANESTHESIA:

IV: Adults, elderly: 50-100 mcg/kg, administered w/oxygen and skeletal muscle relaxant. **Children 2-12 yrs:** 1.7-3.3 mcg/kg.

ADJUNCT TO LOCAL ANESTHESIA:

IM/IV: Adults, elderly: 50-100 mcg.

ADJUNCT TO GENERAL ANESTHESIA:

Total low dose:
IV: Adults, elderly: 2 mcg/kg one time.

Total moderate dose:
IV/IM: Adults, elderly: Initially, 2-20 mcg/kg IV, then 25-100 mcg IM/IV as necessary.

Total high dose:
IV: Adults, elderly: Initially, 20-50 mcg/kg. May give additional doses ranging from 25 mcg up to one-half initial dose.

POSTOP (RECOVERY ROOM):

IM: Adults, elderly: 50-100 mcg q1-2h, as needed.

USUAL TRANSDERMAL DOSAGE:

TRANSDERMAL: Adults, elderly: Individualized. Use lowest effective dose based on previous analgesics given, opioid tolerance, pt condition, medical status.

USUAL TRANSMUCOSAL DOSAGE:

TRANSMUCOSAL: Adults, children: 200-400 mcg.

PRECAUTIONS

CONTRAINDICATIONS: None significant. **EXTREME CAUTION:** Bradyarrhythmias, severe CNS depression, anoxia, hypercapnia, respiratory depression, seizures, acute alcoholism, shock, untreated myxedema, respiratory dysfunction. **CAUTIONS:** Increased intracranial pressure; impaired hepatic, renal function. **PREGNANCY/LACTATION:** Readily crosses placenta; unknown if distributed in breast milk. May prolong labor if administered in latent phase of first stage of labor, or before cervical dilation of 4-5 cm has occurred. Respiratory depression may occur in neonate if mother received opiates during labor. **Pregnancy Category C.**

INTERACTIONS

DRUG INTERACTIONS: Benzodiazepines, may increase risk of hypotension, respiratory depression. Buprenorphine may decrease effect. CNS depressants may increase CNS, respiratory depression, hypotension. **ALTERED LAB VALUES:** May increase amylase, lipase plasma concentrations.

SIDE EFFECTS

NOTE: Respiratory depressant effect lasts longer than analgesic effect. **FREQUENT:** Suppressed breathing depth, decreased B/P (particularly w/moderate to high dosage), sweating. *Transmucosal:*

Hypoventilation, nausea, vomiting, dizziness, pruritus. **OCCASIONAL:** Bradycardia, nausea, vomiting, constipation. **RARE:** Postop confusion, hives, pruritus, paradoxical reaction, blurred vision, chills, seizures.

ADVERSE REACTIONS/TOXIC EFFECTS

Overdosage or too-rapid IV results in severe respiratory depression, skeletal and thoracic muscle rigidity resulting in apnea, laryngospasm, bronchospasm, cold and clammy skin, cyanosis, coma. Tolerance to analgesic effect may occur w/repeated use.

NURSING IMPLICATIONS

BASELINE ASSESSMENT:

Resuscitative equipment and opiate antagonist (naloxone, 0.5 mcg/kg) must be available. Establish baseline B/P and respirations. Assess type, location, intensity, and duration of pain.

INTERVENTION/EVALUATION:

Monitor B/P and respirations closely. Assist w/ambulation. Encourage pt to turn, cough, and deep breathe q2h. Check for constipation; increase fluids, bulk, and exercise as appropriate. Assess for relief of pain.

PATIENT/FAMILY TEACHING:

Avoid alcohol; do not take other medications w/o consulting physician. Do not drive or perform other activities requiring alertness, coordination. Teach pt proper application of transdermal. Use as directed to avoid overdosage; potential for physical dependence w/prolonged use. After long-term use, must be discontinued slowly.

ferrous fumarate

fair´us fume´ah-rate

(Feostat)

ferrous gluconate

fair´us glue´kuh-nate

(Fergon, Ferralet, Simron)

ferrous sulfate

fair´us sul´fate

(Feosol, Slow-Fe)

FIXED-COMBINATION(S):
W/docusate sodium, a stool softener (Ferro-Sequels); w/aluminum and magnesium hydroxide, antacids (Fermalox)

CANADIAN AVAILABILITY:
Apo-Ferrous Gluconate, Apo-Ferrous Sulfate, Fertinic, Neo-Fer, Novoferrogluc, Palafer

CLASSIFICATION

Iron preparation

PHARMACOKINETICS

Absorption increased when iron stores depleted. Primarily absorbed in duodenum, proximal jejunum and stored in hepatocytes and reticuloendothelial system. Protein binding: 90%. No physiologic system of elimination (small amounts lost daily in shedding skin, hair, nails). Half-life: 6 hrs.

ACTION

Essential component in formation of hemoglobin, myoglobin, and enzymes necessary for effective erythropoiesis and for transport and utilization of oxygen.

USES

Prevention and treatment of iron deficiency anemia due to inadequate diet, malabsorption, pregnancy, and/or blood loss.

STORAGE/HANDLING

Store all forms (tablets, capsules, suspension, drops) at room temperature.

PO ADMINISTRATION

1. Ideally, give between meals w/water but may give w/meals if GI discomfort occurs.
2. Transient staining of mucous membranes and teeth will occur w/liquid iron preparation. Place liquid on back of tongue w/dropper or straw.
3. Avoid simultaneous administration of antacids or tetracycline.
4. Do not crush sustained-release preparations.

INDICATIONS/DOSAGE/ROUTES

NOTE: Dosage expressed in terms of elemental iron. Elemental iron content: ferrous fumarate: 33% (99 mg iron/300 mg tablet); ferrous gluconate: 11.6% (35 mg iron/300 mg tablet); ferrous sulfate: 20% (60 mg iron/300 mg tablet).

Deficiency:
PO: Adults, elderly: 2-3 mg/kg/day in 3 divided doses. **Children 2-12 yrs:** 3 mg/kg/day in 3-4 divided doses. **Children 6 mo - 2 yrs:** Up to 6 mg/kg/day in 3-4 divided doses. **Infants:** 10-25 mg/day in 3-4 divided doses.

PRECAUTIONS

CONTRAINDICATIONS: Hemochromatosis, hemosiderosis, hemolytic anemias, those w/peptic ulcer, regional enteritis, or ulcerative colitis. **CAUTIONS:** Those w/bronchial asthma, aspirin hypersensitivity. **PREGNANCY/LACTATION:** Crosses placenta; excreted in breast milk. **Pregnancy Category A.**

INTERACTIONS

DRUG INTERACTIONS: Antacids, calcium supplements, pancreatin, pancrelipase may decrease absorption. May decrease absorption of quinolones, etidronate, tetracyclines. **ALTERED LAB VALUES:** May increase bilirubin. May decrease calcium. May obscure occult blood in stools.

SIDE EFFECTS

OCCASIONAL: Mild, transient nausea. **RARE:** Heartburn, anorexia, constipation, or diarrhea.

ADVERSE REACTIONS/TOXIC EFFECTS

Large doses may aggravate existing GI tract disease (peptic ulcer, regional enteritis, ulcerative colitis). Severe iron poisoning occurs mostly in children and is manifested as vomiting, severe abdominal pain, diarrhea, dehydration, followed by hyperventilation, pallor or cyanosis, cardiovascular collapse.

NURSING IMPLICATIONS

BASELINE ASSESSMENT:

To prevent mucous membrane and teeth staining w/liquid preparation, use dropper or straw and allow solution to drop on back of tongue. Eggs, milk inhibit absorption. Obtain Hgb, Hct results.

INTERVENTION/EVALUATION:

Those w/normal iron balance should not take iron preparation routinely. Monitor daily pattern of bowel activity and stool consistency. Assess for clinical improvement and record relief of iron deficiency symptoms (fatigue, irritability, pallor, paresthesia of extremities, headache). Monitor Hgb, Hct results.

PATIENT/FAMILY TEACHING:

Expect stools to darken in color. Take on empty stomach. If GI discomfort occurs, take after meals or w/food. Do not take antacids (prevents absorption).

filgrastim

fill-grass´tim

(Neupogen)

CANADIAN AVAILABILITY:
Neupogen

CLASSIFICATION

Colony stimulating factor

PHARMACOKINETICS

Readily absorbed after SubQ administration. Half-life: 3.5 hrs.

ACTION

Regulates production of neutrophils within bone marrow. Primarily affects neutrophil progenitor proliferation, differentiation, and selected end-cell functional activation (e.g., increased phagocytic ability, antibody-dependent killing).

USES

Decrease infection incidence in pt w/nonmyeloid malignancies receiving myelosuppressive therapy associated w/severe neutropenia, fever. Reduce neutropenia duration (and sequelae) in pt w/nonmyeloid malignancies having myeloablative therapy followed by bone marrow transplant (BMT).

STORAGE/HANDLING

Refrigerate. Do not shake vial. Use 1 dose/vial, do not re-enter vial. Stable for up to 24 hrs at room temperature (provided vial contents are clear, contain no particulate matter).

INDICATIONS/DOSAGE/ROUTES

NOTE: Begin at least 24 hrs after last dose of chemotherapy, discontinue at least 24 hrs prior to next dose of chemotherapy.

Myelosuppressive:
SubQ/IV or SubQ INFUSION: Adults, elderly: Initially, 5 mcg/kg/day. May increase by 5 mcg/kg for each chemotherapy cycle based on duration/severity of absolute neutrophil count (ANC) nadir.
NOTE: Begin at least 24 hrs after last dose of chemotherapy and at least 24 hrs after bone marrow infusion.

BMT:
IV or SubQ INFUSION: Adults, elderly: 10 mcg/kg/day. Adjust dose daily during period of neutrophil recovery based on neutrophil response.

PRECAUTIONS

CONTRAINDICATIONS: Hypersensitivity to *Escherichia coli*-derived proteins, 24 hrs before or after cytotoxic chemotherapy, use w/other drugs that may result in lowered platelet count. **CAUTIONS:** Concurrent use w/myeloid properties. **PREGNANCY/LACTATION:** Unknown if drug crosses placenta or is distributed in breast milk. **Pregnancy Category C.**

INTERACTIONS

DRUG INTERACTIONS: None significant. **ALTERED LAB VALUES:** May increase alkaline phosphatase, LDH, uric acid, leukocyte (LAP) scores.

F

SIDE EFFECTS

FREQUENT: Bone pain, mild to severe (occurs more frequently in those receiving high dose via IV form, less frequently in low dose, SubQ form), nausea, vomiting, alopecia, diarrhea, fever, fatigue. **OCCASIONAL:** Anorexia, dyspnea, headache, cough, skin rash. **RARE:** Psoriasis, hematuria/proteinuria, osteoporosis.

ADVERSE REACTIONS/TOXIC EFFECTS

Chronic administration occasionally produces chronic neutropenia, splenomegaly. Thrombocytopenia, MI, arrhythmias occur rarely. Adult respiratory distress syndrome may occur in septic pts.

NURSING IMPLICATIONS

BASELINE ASSESSMENT:

A CBC, platelet count (differential) should be obtained before initiation of therapy and twice weekly thereafter.

INTERVENTION/EVALUATION:

In septic pts, be alert to adult respiratory distress syndrome. Closely monitor those w/preexisting cardiac conditions. Monitor B/P (transient decrease in B/P may occur).

finasteride

fin-ah'stir-eyd
(Proscar)

CLASSIFICATION

5-alpha reductase inhibitor

PHARMACOKINETICS

	ONSET	PEAK	DURATION
PO	24 hr	1-2 days	5-7 days

Rapidly absorbed from GI tract. Widely distributed. Protein binding: 90%. Metabolized in liver. Half-life: 6-8 hrs.

ACTION

Inhibits steroid 5-alpha reductase, an intracellular enzyme that converts testosterone into dihydrotestosterone (DHT) in the prostate gland, providing a reduction in serum DHT, regressing the enlarged prostate gland.

USES

Treatment of symptomatic benign prostatic hyperplasia (BPH). Most improvement noted in hesitancy, feeling of incomplete bladder emptying, interruption of urinary stream, difficulty initiating flow, dysuria, impaired size and force of urinary stream.

PO ADMINISTRATION

1. Do not break or crush film-coated tablets.
2. May take w/o regard to meals.

INDICATIONS/DOSAGE/ROUTES

Benign prostatic hypertrophy:
PO: Adults, elderly: 5 mg once daily (minimum 6 mo).

PRECAUTIONS

CONTRAINDICATIONS: Physical handling of tablet in those who may become, or are, pregnant, exposure to semen in those who may become pregnant. **CAUTIONS:** Liver function abnormalities. **PREGNANCY/LACTATION:** Physical handling of tablet in those who may become, or are, pregnant. Exposure to semen in those who may become pregnant may harm male fetus. **Pregnancy Category X.**

INTERACTIONS

DRUG INTERACTIONS: None significant. **ALTERED LAB VALUES:** Produces decrease in serum prostate-specific antigen (PSA) levels (even in presence of prostate cancer).

SIDE EFFECTS

OCCASIONAL: Impotence, decreased libido, decreased volume of ejaculate.

ADVERSE REACTIONS/TOXIC EFFECTS

None significant.

NURSING IMPLICATIONS

BASELINE ASSESSMENT:

Digital rectal exam, serum PSA determination should be performed in those w/BPH before initiating therapy and periodically thereafter.

INTERVENTION/EVALUATION:

Diligent monitoring of I&O, especially in those w/large residual urinary volume or severely diminished urinary flow for obstructive uropathy.

PATIENT/FAMILY TEACHING:

Pt should be aware of potential impotence, may not notice improved urinary flow even if prostate gland shrinks, need to take medication >6 mo, and it is not known if medication decreases need for surgery. Regular visits to physician and monitoring tests are necessary. Because of potential risk to male fetus, a woman who is or may become pregnant should not handle tablets or be exposed to pt semen. Volume of ejaculate may be decreased during treatment (decrease does not interfere w/sexual function).

F

flavoxate

flay-vocks'ate
(Urispas)

CANADIAN AVAILABILITY:
Urispas

CLASSIFICATION

Antispasmodic

PHARMACOKINETICS

Well absorbed from GI tract. Primarily excreted in urine.

ACTION

Direct antispasmodic effect on urinary tract smooth muscle.

USES

Symptomatic relief of dysuria, urgency, nocturia, frequency, incontinence associated w/cystitis, prostatitis, urethritis, urethrocystitis, or urethrotrigonitis.

PO ADMINISTRATION

1. Take on empty stomach. May take w/food (decreases GI irritation).

INDICATIONS/DOSAGE/ROUTES

Urinary antispasmodic:
PO: Adults, elderly, adolescent: 100-200 mg 3-4 times/day.

PRECAUTIONS

CONTRAINDICATIONS: GI tract obstructive disease, GI hemorrhage, paralytic ileus, obstructive uropathy. **CAUTIONS:** None significant. **PREGNANCY/LACTATION: Pregnancy Category B.**

INTERACTIONS

DRUG INTERACTIONS: None significant. **ALTERED LAB VALUES:** None significant.

SIDE EFFECTS

Generally well tolerated. Side effects usually mild and transient. **FREQUENT:** Drowsiness, dry mouth, throat. **OCCASIONAL:** Constipation, difficult urination, blurred vision, dizziness, headache, increased light sensitivity, nausea, vomiting, stomach pain. **RARE:** Confusion (primarily in elderly), hypersensitivity, increase intraocular pressure, leukopenia.

ADVERSE REACTIONS/TOXIC EFFECTS

Anticholinergic effect w/overdose (unsteadiness, severe dizziness, drowsiness, fever, flushed face, shortness of breath, nervousness, irritability).

NURSING IMPLICATIONS

BASELINE ASSESSMENT:

Assess dysuria, urgency, frequency, incontinence, or suprapubic pain.

INTERVENTION/EVALUATION:

Monitor for symptomatic relief. Observe elderly esp. for mental confusion.

PATIENT/FAMILY TEACHING:

Avoid driving or other tasks requiring alertness, coordination, or manual dexterity (blurred vision, drowsiness). Dry mouth may be relieved by sips of water, sugarless gum, or hard candy.

flecainide acetate

fleh′kun-eyed

(Tambocor)

CANADIAN AVAILABILITY:
Tambocor

CLASSIFICATION

Antiarrhythmic

PHARMACOKINETICS

Completely absorbed from GI tract. Widely distributed. Protein binding: 40%. Metabolized in liver. Primarily excreted in urine. Minimal removal by hemodialysis. Half-life: 12-27 hrs (increased in decreased renal, liver function, CHF).

ACTION

Slows atrial, AV, His-Purkinje, intraventricular conduction (decreases excitability, conduction velocity, automaticity). Greatest effect on His-Purkinje system.

USES

Prevention of documented life-threatening ventricular arrhythmias, paroxysmal supraventricular tachycardias (PSVT) without structural heart disease, and paroxysmal atrial fibrillation (PAF).

PO ADMINISTRATION

1. Scored tablets may be crushed.
2. Monitor EKG for cardiac changes, particularly, widening of QRS, prolongation of PR interval. Notify physician of any significant interval changes.

INDICATIONS/DOSAGE/ROUTES

Life-threatening ventricular arrhythmias, sustained ventricular tachycardia:
PO: Adults, elderly: Initially, 100

mg q12h, increased by 100 mg (50 mg 2 times/day) every 4 days until effective dose or maximum of 400 mg/day attained.

PSVT, PAF:

PO: Adults, elderly: Initially, 50 mg q12h, increased by 100 mg (50 mg 2 times/day) every 4 days until effective dose or maximum of 300 mg/day attained. **Dose in patients w/CHF or myocardial dysfunction:** Initially, 50-100 mg q12h. Increase by 50 mg 2 times/day every 4 days up to 200 mg q12h (400 mg/day). **Dose in those w/renal or hepatic impairment:** Initially, 100 mg q12h increased at intervals greater than 4 days. Creatinine clearance <35 ml/min/m^2 dose is reduced by 25-50%.

PRECAUTIONS

CONTRAINDICATIONS: Cardiogenic shock, preexisting second- or third-degree AV block, right bundle branch block (w/o presence of pacemaker). **CAUTIONS:** Impaired myocardial function, second- or third-degree AV block (w/pacemaker), CHF, sick sinus syndrome. **PREGNANCY/LACTATION:** Unknown if drug crosses placenta. May be distributed in breast milk. **Pregnancy Category C.**

INTERACTIONS

DRUG INTERACTIONS: Urinary acidifiers may increase excretion; urinary alkalizers may decrease excretion. Other antiarrhythmics may have additive effects. Beta-blockers may increase negative inotropic effects. May increase digoxin concentrations. **ALTERED LAB VALUES:** None significant.

SIDE EFFECTS

NOTE: Most effects appear mild, transient. **FREQUENT:** Dizziness, visual disturbances (blurred vision, spots before eyes), dyspnea, headache, nausea, fatigue, palpitations, tremor, constipation, edema, abdominal pain. **OCCASIONAL:** Eye pain, photophobia, dyspepsia, anorexia. **RARE:** Hypotension, bradycardia, urinary retention, hypersensitivity reaction (rash, pruritus).

ADVERSE REACTIONS/TOXIC EFFECTS

Has ability to worsen existing arrhythmias or produce new ones. May also produce or worsen CHF. Overdosage may increase QRS duration, QT interval and conduction disturbances, reduce myocardial contractility, conduction disturbances, hypotension.

NURSING IMPLICATIONS

INTERVENTION/EVALUATION:

Assess pulse for strength/weakness, irregular rate. Monitor EKG for cardiac changes, particularly, widening of QRS, prolongation of PR interval. Notify physician of any significant interval changes. Question for visual disturbances, headache, GI upset. Monitor fluid and electrolyte serum levels. Assess for evidence of CHF: dyspnea (particularly on exertion or lying down), night cough, peripheral edema, distended neck veins. Monitor I&O (increase in weight, decrease in urine output may indicate CHF). Assess hand movement for sign of tremor. Monitor for therapeutic serum level (0.2-1 mcg/ml).

PATIENT/FAMILY TEACHING:

Side effects generally disappear w/continued use or decreased dosage. Do not abruptly discontinue medication. Compliance w/ therapy regimen is essential to control arrhythmias. Do not use nasal decongestants, over-the-counter cold preparations (stimulants) w/o physician approval. Restrict salt, alcohol intake.

fleroxacin (Megalone)
See supplement

floxuridine

flocks-your′ih-deen
(FUDR)

CLASSIFICATION

Antineoplastic

PHARMACOKINETICS

Metabolized in liver, tissues to active metabolites. After continuous intra-arterial infusion primarily converted to FUDR-MP; converted to 5-fluorouracil after IV or intra-arterial injection. Partially crosses blood brain barrier. Active metabolites localized intracellularly. Excreted via lungs, urine.

ACTION

Cell cycle specific for S-phase cell division. Inhibits DNA, RNA synthesis by inhibiting action of thymidylate synthetase.

USES

Palliative management of GI adenocarcinoma metastatic to liver.

STORAGE/HANDLING

NOTE: May be carcinogenic, mutagenic, or teratogenic. Handle w/ extreme care during preparation/administration.

Reconstituted solutions stable for 2 wks, if refrigerated.

INTRA-ARTERIAL ADMINISTRATION

NOTE: Give by continuous intra-arterial infusion via catheter inserted into arterial blood supply of tumor.

1. Reconstitute each 500 mg vial w/5 ml sterile water for injection to provide concentration of 100 mg/ml.
2. Further dilute w/5% dextrose or 0.9% NaCl to volume appropriate for specific infusion apparatus used.

INDICATIONS/DOSAGE/ROUTES

NOTE: Dosage individualized based on clinical response, tolerance to adverse effects. When used in combination therapy, consult specific protocols for optimum dosage, sequence of drug administration.

INTRA-ARTERIAL INFUSION:
Adults: 0.1-0.6 mg/kg/day (0.4-0.6 mg/kg/day for hepatic artery infusion). Continue therapy until toxicity or as long as response continues.

PRECAUTIONS

CONTRAINDICATIONS: Poor nutritional state, depressed bone marrow function (WBC less than 5,000/mm^3 and/or platelet count less than 100,000/mm^3, serious infection. **EXTREME CAUTION:** Previous high-dose pelvic irradiation therapy or alkylating agents, impaired liver, kidney function. **PREGNANCY/LACTATION:** If possible, avoid use during pregnancy, especially first trimester. Breast feeding not recommended. **Pregnancy Category D.**

INTERACTIONS

DRUG INTERACTIONS: Bone marrow depressants may increase

bone marrow depression. Live virus vaccines may potentiate virus replication, increase vaccine side effects, decrease pt's antibody response to vaccine. **ALTERED LAB VALUES:** May increase SGOT (AST), SGPT (ALT), alkaline phosphatase, LDH, bilirubin. Interferes w/BSP, prothrombin, sedimentation rate assays.

SIDE EFFECTS

FREQUENT: Nausea, vomiting, diarrhea, leukopenia, anemia, localized erythema, anorexia, abdominal cramping, thrombocytopenia, alopecia, rash, pruritus. **OCCASIONAL:** Duodenal ulcer, gastritis, glossitis, pharyngitis, ataxia, blurred vision, vertigo, weakness, mental depression, lethargy.

ADVERSE REACTIONS/TOXIC EFFECTS

Toxicity manifested as stomatitis, enteritis. Hepatic arterial infusion associated w/sclerosis of bile ducts, cirrhosis of liver.

NURSING IMPLICATIONS

BASELINE ASSESSMENT:

Notify physician if WBC falls below 3500 mm^3 or rapidly decreases, platelet count falls below 100,000/mm^3, intractable vomiting, diarrhea, stomatitis, GI bleeding occurs (drug may need to be discontinued).

INTERVENTION/EVALUATION:

Monitor leukocyte, platelet counts diligently. Check for stomatitis (burning/erythema of oral mucosa at inner margin of lips, sore throat, difficulty swallowing). May lead to ulceration within 2-3 days. Avoid IM and SubQ injections or rectal temperatures; other trauma. Apply direct pressure to venipuncture sites for full 5 min. Assess intra-arterial site for signs of bleeding, infection, or catheter displacement. Monitor I&O, food tolerance, and stool frequency/consistency. Assess vital signs. Use infusion pump to overcome pressure and provide consistent rate of infusion.

PATIENT/FAMILY TEACHING:

Maintain fastidious but gentle oral hygiene. Do not have immunizations w/o physician's approval (drug lowers body's resistance). Avoid contact w/those who have recently received live virus vaccine. Promptly report fever, sore throat, signs of local infection, easy bruising, unusual bleeding from any site. Increase fluids. Do not take medications or alcohol w/o consulting physician. Contact physician if nausea/vomiting continue at home.

fluconazole

flu-con´ah-zole
(Diflucan)

CANADIAN AVAILABILITY:
Diflucan

CLASSIFICATION

Antifungal

PHARMACOKINETICS

Well absorbed from GI tract. Widely distributed (including CSF). Protein binding: 11%. Partially metabolized in liver. Primarily excreted unchanged in urine. Partially removed by hemodialysis. Half-life: 20-50 hrs (increased in decreased renal function).

ACTION

Fungistatic. Interferes w/cytochrome (necessary for ergosterol formation). Alters cell membrane function. Directly damages fungal membrane, triglycerides, phospholipids. Inhibits enzyme activity.

USES

Treatment of oropharyngeal and esophageal candidiasis, serious systemic candidal infections (e.g., urinary tract infections, peritonitis, pneumonia), *Cryptococcus neoformans* meningitis, vaginal candidiasis. Prevent candidiasis in bone marrow transplants.

STORAGE/HANDLING

Store at room temperature. Do not use parenteral form if solution is cloudy, precipitate forms, seal is not intact, or it is discolored.

PO/IV ADMINISTRATION

PO:

1. Give w/o regard to meals.
2. Not affected by gastric pH.
3. Oral and IV therapy equally effective; IV therapy for pt intolerant of the drug or unable to take orally.

IV:

1. Do not remove from outer wrap until ready to use.
2. Squeeze inner bag to check for minute leaks.
3. Discard if solution is cloudly or precipitate is noted.
4. Do not add supplementary medication.
5. Plastic containers are not to be used in series connections (could cause air embolism).
6. Maximum flow rate is 200 mg/hr.

INDICATIONS/DOSAGE/ROUTES

Oropharyngeal candidiasis:
PO/IV: Adults, elderly: Initially, 200 mg once, then 100 mg/day for at least 14 days.

Esophageal candidiasis:
PO/IV: Adults, elderly: 200 mg once, then 100 mg/day (up to 400 mg/day) for 21 days and at least 14 days following resolution of symptoms.

Candidiasis prevention:
PO: Adults: 400 mg/day.

Systemic candidiasis:
PO/IV: Adults, elderly: Initially, 400 mg once, then 200 mg/day (up to 400 mg/day) for at least 28 days and at least 14 days following resolution of symptoms.

Cryptococcal meningitis:
PO/IV: Adults, elderly: Initially, 400 mg once, then 200 mg/day (up to 400 mg/day). Continue for 10-12 wks after CSF becomes negative. (200 mg/day for suppression of relapse in pts w/AIDS.)

Dosage in renal impairment:
After loading dose of 400 mg, daily dose based on creatinine clearance:

CREATININE CLEARANCE	% OF RECOMMENDED DOSE
>50	100
21-50	50
11-20	25
Dialysis	Dose after dialysis

Vaginal candidiasis:
PO: *Adults, elderly:* 150 mg as a single dose.

PRECAUTIONS

CONTRAINDICATIONS: Hypersensitivity to fluconazole or any component of preparation. **CAUTIONS:** Hepatic impairment. Hypersensitivity to other triazoles (e.g., itraconazole, terconazole) or imidazoles (butoconazole, ketoconazole, etc.). Safety and efficacy in children under 13 years of age not established. **PREGNANCY/**

LACTATION: Unknown if excreted in breast milk. **Pregnancy Category C.**

INTERACTIONS

DRUG INTERACTIONS: May increase concentration, effects of oral hypoglycemics. High doses increase cyclosporine concentration. May decrease metabolism of phenytoin, warfarin. Rifampin may increase metabolism. **ALTERED LAB VALUES:** May increase SGOT (AST), SGPT (ALT), alkaline phosphatase, bilirubin.

SIDE EFFECTS

FREQUENT: Nausea, vomiting, abdominal pain, diarrhea, rash, pruritus. **OCCASIONAL:** Headache, dizziness. **RARE:** Somnolence, fever, fatigue, arthralgia/myalgia, psychiatric disturbances, seizures.

ADVERSE REACTIONS/TOXIC EFFECTS

Exfoliative skin disorders, serious hepatic effects, blood dyscrasias (eosinophilia, thrombocytopenia, anemia, leukopenia) have been reported rarely.

NURSING IMPLICATIONS

BASELINE ASSESSMENT:

Question for hypersensitivity to fluconazole or components of preparation. Confirm that a culture or histologic test was done for accurate diagnosis; therapy may begin before results are known. Establish baselines for CBC, potassium.

INTERVENTION/EVALUATION:

Monitor hepatic function tests; be alert for hepatotoxicity: dark urine, pale stools, anorexia/nausea/vomiting, yellow skin or sclera. Report rash, itching promptly. Check CBC and potassium lab results. Evaluate food tolerance. Monitor temperature at least daily. Determine pattern of bowel activity, stool consistency. Assess for dizziness and provide assistance as needed.

PATIENT/FAMILY TEACHING:

Do not drive car, machinery if dizziness, drowsiness occur. Notify physician of dark urine, pale stool, yellow skin/eyes or rash w/or w/o itching. Pts w/oropharyngeal infections should be taught good oral hygiene. Consult physician before taking any other medication.

fludarabine phosphate

flew-dare´ah-bean

(Fludara)

CLASSIFICATION

Antineoplastic

PHARMACOKINETICS

Rapidly dephosphorylated in serum, then phosphorylated intracellularly to active triphosphate. Primarily excreted in urine. Half-life: 10 hrs.

ACTION

Interferes w/DNA polymerase alpha, ribonucleotide reductase, and DNA primase, inhibiting DNA synthesis.

USES

Treatment of chronic lymphocytic leukemia in pt who has not responded to or has progressed w/another standard alkylating agent.

STORAGE/HANDLING

Store in refrigerator. Handle w/ extreme care during preparation and administration. If contact w/ skin or mucous membranes, wash thoroughly w/soap and water; rinse eyes profusely w/plain water. After reconstitution, use within 8 hrs; discard unused portion.

IV ADMINISTRATION

NOTE: Give by IV infusion. Do not add to other IV infusions. Avoid small veins, swollen or edematous extremities, areas overlying joints, tendons.

1. Reconstitute 50 mg vial w/2 ml sterile water for injection to provide a concentration of 25 mg/ml.
2. Further dilute w/100-125 ml 0.9% NaCl or 5% dextrose and infuse over 30 min.

INDICATIONS/DOSAGE/ROUTES

NOTE: Dosage is individualized on basis of clinical response and tolerance to adverse effects. When used in combination therapy, consult specific protocols for optimum dosage, sequence of drug administration. Dosage based on pt's actual weight. Use ideal body weight in obese or edematous pts.

Chronic lymphocytic leukemia:
IV: Adults: 25 mg/m^2 daily for 5 consecutive days. Continue up to 3 additional cycles. Begin each course of treatment every 28 days.

PRECAUTIONS

CONTRAINDICATIONS: None significant. **CAUTIONS:** Impaired renal function. **PREGNANCY/LACTATION:** If possible, avoid use during pregnancy, esp. first trimester. May cause fetal harm. Not known whether distributed in breast milk. Breast feeding not recommended. **Pregnancy Category D.**

INTERACTIONS

DRUG INTERACTIONS: May decrease effect of antigout medications. Bone marrow depressants may increase risk of bone marrow depression. Live virus vaccines may potentiate virus replication, increase vaccine side effects, decrease pt's antibody response to vaccine. **ALTERED LAB VALUES:** May increase uric acid, alkaline phosphatase, SGOT (AST).

SIDE EFFECTS

OCCASIONAL: Anorexia, nausea, diarrhea, peripheral edema, dry skin, rash, erythema, aches/pains, confusion, chilliness, fatigue, weakness, sinusitis. **RARE:** Paresthesia, headaches, hearing loss, visual disturbances, urinary difficulties, GI bleeding.

ADVERSE REACTIONS/TOXIC EFFECTS

Pneumonia occurs frequently. Severe bone marrow toxicity (anemia, thrombocytopenia, neutropenia) may occur, evidenced by fever, chills, infection, nausea, vomiting, fatigue, anorexia, weakness. High dosage may produce acute leukemia, blindness, coma.

NURSING IMPLICATIONS

BASELINE ASSESSMENT:

Drug should be discontinued if intractable vomiting, diarrhea, stomatitis, GI bleeding occurs.

INTERVENTION/EVALUATION:

Monitor CBC, platelet, differential count, serum creatinine routinely. Assess for weakness, agitation, confusion, visual disturbances, peripheral neuropathy.

Assess lung sounds for evidence of pneumonia. Monitor for dyspnea, cough, rapidly falling WBC and/or intractable diarrhea, GI bleeding (bright red or tarry stool). Avoid IM, SubQ injections; protect from trauma; do not take rectal temperatures. Apply direct pressure to IV sites for full 5 min. Assess oral mucosa for mucosal erythema, ulceration at inner margin of lips, sore throat, difficulty swallowing (stomatitis). Assess skin for rash. Monitor for and report diarrhea. Check food tolerance, provide antiemetics as needed. Be alert to possible tumor lysis syndrome (onset w/ flank pain and hematuria). This syndrome may include hypercalcemia, hyperphosphatemia, hyperuricemia and result in renal failure.

PATIENT/FAMILY TEACHING:

Avoid crowds and exposure to infection. Do not take alcohol or other medications w/o consulting physician. Maintain fastidious oral hygiene. Do not have immunizations w/o physician's approval (drug lowers body's resistance). Promptly report fever, sore throat, signs of local infection, easy bruising, unusual bleeding from any site. Contact physician if nausea/vomiting continues at home.

fludrocortisone

floo-droe-kore´tih-sone
(Florinef)

CANADIAN AVAILABILITY:
Florinef

CLASSIFICATION

Mineralocorticoid

PHARMACOKINETICS

Well absorbed from GI tract. Widely distributed. Protein binding: 42%. Metabolized in liver, kidney. Primarily excreted in urine. Half-life: 3.5 hrs.

ACTION

High mineralocorticoid, moderate glucocorticoid activity. Acts at distal tubules to increase potassium, hydrogen ion excretion, sodium reabsorption, and water retention.

USES

Partial replacement therapy for primary and secondary adrenocortical insufficiency in Addison's disease. Adjunctive treatment of salt-losing forms of congenital adrenogenital syndrome.

PO ADMINISTRATION

1. Give w/food or milk.
2. Administer w/glucocorticoid.

INDICATIONS/DOSAGE/ROUTES

Addison's disease:
PO: Adults, elderly: 0.05-0.1 mg/day. **Range:** 0.1 mg 3 times/wk-0.2 mg/day. Administration w/cortisone/hydrocortisone preferred.

Salt-losing adrenogenital syndrome:
PO: Adults, elderly: 0.1-0.2 mg/day.

PRECAUTIONS

CONTRAINDICATIONS: Hypersensitivity to fludrocortisone, any condition except those requiring high mineralocorticoid activity.

CAUTIONS: CHF, hypertension, renal insufficiency. Prolonged therapy should be discontinued slowly. **PREGNANCY/LACTATION:** Not known whether drug crosses placenta or is distributed in breast milk. **Pregnancy Category C.**

INTERACTIONS

DRUG INTERACTIONS: May increase digoxin toxicity (hypokalemia). Hepatic enzyme inducers (e.g., phenytoin) may increase metabolism. Hypokalemia causing medications may increase effect. Sodium containing medication may increase sodium, edema, B/P. **ALTERED LAB VALUES:** May increase sodium. May decrease potassium, hematocrit.

SIDE EFFECTS

FREQUENT: Increased appetite, exaggerated sense of well-being, abdominal distention, weight gain, insomnia, mood swings. *High dose, prolonged therapy, too rapid withdrawal:* Increased susceptibility to infection (signs/symptoms masked); delayed wound healing, hypokalemia, hypocalcemia, GI distress, diarrhea or constipation, hypertension. **OCCASIONAL:** Headache (frontal or occipital), dizziness, menstrual difficulty or amenorrhea, ulcer development. *Topical:* Itching, redness, irritation. **RARE:** Hypersensitivity reaction.

ADVERSE REACTIONS/TOXIC EFFECTS

Long-term therapy: muscle wasting (esp. arms, legs), osteoporosis, spontaneous fractures, amenorrhea, cataracts, glaucoma, peptic ulcer, CHF. Abrupt withdrawal following long-term therapy: anorexia, nausea, fever, headache, joint pain, rebound inflammation, fatigue, weakness, lethargy, dizziness, orthostatic hypotension.

NURSING IMPLICATIONS

BASELINE ASSESSMENT:

Question for hypersensitivity to any corticosteroids. Obtain baselines for weight, B/P, blood glucose, electrolytes, chest x-ray, EKG.

INTERVENTION/EVALUATION:

Monitor I&O, daily weight. Check B/P, pulse at least 2 times/day. Assess for signs of edema. Monitor blood glucose and electrolytes. Provide assistance w/ambulation, notify physician of dizziness. Be alert to signs/symptoms of hypokalemia (weakness and muscle cramps, numbness/tingling, esp. lower extremities, nausea and vomiting, irritability, EKG changes). Evaluate food tolerance and bowel activity; report hyperacidity promptly. Assess emotional status, ability to sleep. Assess for infection: fever, sore throat, vague symptoms.

PATIENT/FAMILY TEACHING:

Take w/food or milk. Usually given in conjunction w/glucocorticoids, electrolytes. Carry identification of drug and dose, physician name and phone number. Do not change dose/schedule or stop taking drug; must taper off gradually under medical supervision. Notify physician of fever, sore throat, muscle aches, sudden weight gain/swelling, continuing headaches. W/dietician give instructions for prescribed diet (usually high-potassium). Maintain careful personal hygiene, avoid exposure to disease or trauma. Severe stress (serious infection, surgery, or trauma) may require increased dosage. Do not take aspirin or any other medication w/o consulting physician. Follow-up visits, lab tests are necessary; children must be assessed for growth retardation. Inform dentist or other physicians of fludrocortisone therapy now or within past 12 mo.

flumazenil

flew-maz´ah-nil

(Romazicon)

CLASSIFICATION

Benzodiazepine receptor antagonist

PHARMACOKINETICS

	ONSET	PEAK	DURATION
IV	1-2 min	6-10 min	—

Duration, degree of benzodiazepine reversal related to dosage, plasma concentration. Metabolized by liver; excreted in urine.

ACTION

Antagonizes sedation, impairment of recall and psychomotor impairment due to benzodiazepine activity on CNS.

USES

Complete or partial reversal of sedative effects of benzodiazepines when general anesthesia has been induced and/or maintained w/benzodiazepines, when sedation has been produced w/benzodiazepines for diagnostic and therapeutic procedures, management of benzodiazepine overdosage.

STORAGE/HANDLING

Store parenteral form at room temperature. Discard after 24 hrs once medication is drawn into syringe, is mixed w/any solutions, or if particulate or discoloration is noted.

IV ADMINISTRATION

NOTE: Compatible w/5% dextrose in water, lactated Ringer's, 0.9% NaCl solutions.

1. Rinse spilled medication from skin w/cool water.
2. Administer through freely running IV infusion into large vein (local injection produces pain, inflammation at injection site).

INDICATIONS/DOSAGE/ROUTES

Reversal of conscious sedation, in general anesthesia:

IV: Adults, elderly: Initially, 0.2 mg (2 ml) over 15 sec; may repeat 0.2 mg dose in 45 sec; then at 60 sec intervals. **Maximum:** 1 mg (10 ml total dose).

NOTE: If resedation occurs, repeat dose at 20 min intervals. **Maximum:** 1 mg (given as 0.2 mg/min) at any one time, 3 mg in any 1 hr.

Benzodiazepine overdose:

IV: Adults, elderly: Initially, 0.2 mg (2 ml) over 30 sec; may repeat after 30 sec w/0.3 mg (3 ml) over 30 sec if desired level of consciousness not achieved. Further doses of 0.5 mg (5 ml) over 30 sec may be administered at 60 sec intervals. **Maximum:** 3 mg (30 ml) total dose.

NOTE: If resedation occurs, repeat dose at 20 min intervals. **Maximum:** 1 mg (given as 0.5 mg/min) at any one time, 3 mg in any 1 hr.

PRECAUTIONS

CONTRAINDICATIONS: History of hypersensitivity to benzodiazepines, in those who have been given a benzodiazepine for control of a potentially life-threatening condition (control of intracranial pressure, status epilepticus), those showing signs of serious cyclic antidepressant overdose manifested by motor abnormalities, dysrhythmias, anticholinergic signs, cardiovascular collapse. **CAUTIONS:** Head injury, impaired hepatic function, alcoholism, drug dependency. **PREGNANCY/LACTATION:** Not known whether drug crosses placenta or is distributed in breast milk. Not recommended during labor, delivery. **Pregnancy Category C.**

INTERACTIONS

DRUG INTERACTIONS: None significant. **ALTERED LAB VALUES:** None significant.

SIDE EFFECTS

FREQUENT: Dizziness, nausea, vomiting, headache, blurred vision, agitation (anxiety, nervousness, dry mouth, tremor, palpitations, insomnia, dyspnea, hyperventilation). **OCCASIONAL:** Flushing, increased sweating, hiccups, shivering.

ADVERSE REACTIONS/TOXIC EFFECTS

May produce onset of seizures (particularly those on long-term benzodiazepine use), overdosage, concurrent sedative-hypnotic drug withdrawal, recent therapy w/repeated doses of parenteral benzodiazepine, myoclonic jerking, concurrent cyclic antidepressant poisoning. May provoke panic attack in those w/history of panic disorder.

NURSING IMPLICATIONS

BASELINE ASSESSMENT:

Arterial blood gases should be obtained before and at 30 min intervals during IV administration. Prepare to intervene in reestablishing airway, assisting ventilation (drug may not fully reverse ventilatory insufficiency induced by benzodiazepines). Note that effects of flumazenil may wear off before effects of benzodiazepines.

INTERVENTION/EVALUATION:

Properly manage airway, assisted breathing, circulatory access and support, internal decontamination by lavage and charcoal, adequate clinical evaluation. Monitor for reversal of benzodiazepine effect. Assess for possible resedation, respiratory depression, hypoventilation. Assess closely for return of unconsciousness (narcosis) for at least 1 hr after pt is fully alert.

PATIENT/FAMILY TEACHING:

Avoid tasks that require alertness, motor skills, ingestion of alcohol, or taking nonprescription drugs until at least 18-24 hrs after discharge.

flunisolide

flew-nis′oh-lide
(AeroBid, Nasalide)

CANADIAN AVAILABILITY:
Bronalide aerosol, Rhinalar

CLASSIFICATION

Corticosteroid

PHARMACOKINETICS

Minimally absorbed from pulmonary, nasal, and GI tissue. Protein binding: 65-90%. Primarily metabolized in liver, lung. Primarily excreted in urine. Half-life: 1-1.5 hrs (nasal: 1-2 hrs).

ACTION

Decreases immediate and late phase allergic reactions. Reduces influx of inflammatory cells.

USES

Inhalation: Control of bronchial asthma in those requiring chronic steroid therapy. *Intranasal:* Relief of symptoms of seasonal/perennial rhinitis.

INHALATION/INTRANASAL ADMINISTRATION

INHALATION:

1. Shake container well; exhale completely; holding mouthpiece 1 inch away from lips, inhale and hold breath as long as possible before exhaling; then exhale slowly.
2. Wait 1 min between inhalations when multiple inhalations ordered (allows for deeper bronchial penetration).
3. Rinse mouth w/water immediately after inhalation (prevents mouth/throat dryness).

INTRANASAL:

1. Clear nasal passages before use (topical nasal decongestants may be needed 5-15 min before use).
2. Tilt head slightly forward.
3. Insert spray tip up in 1 nostril, pointing toward inflamed nasal turbinates, away from nasal septum.
4. Pump medication into 1 nostril while holding other nostril closed and concurrently inspire through nose.
5. Discard used nasal solution after 3 months.

INDICATIONS/DOSAGE/ROUTES

Usual inhalation dosage:
INHALATION: Adults, elderly: 2 inhalations 2 times/day, morning and evening. **Maximum:** 4 inhalations 2 times/day. **Children (6-15 yrs):** 2 inhalations 2 times/day.

Usual intranasal dosage:
NOTE: Improvement seen within few days; may take 3 wk. Do not continue beyond 3 wk if no significant improvement occurs.
INTRANASAL: Adults, elderly: Initially, 2 sprays each nostril 2 times/day, may increase to 2 sprays 3 times/day. **Maximum:** 8 sprays each nostril/day. **Children (6-14 yr):** Initially, 1 spray 3 times/day or 2 sprays 2 times/day. **Maximum:** 4 sprays each nostril/day. **Maintenance:** Smallest amount to control symptoms.

PRECAUTIONS

CONTRAINDICATIONS: Hypersensitivity to any corticosteroid or components, primary treatment of status asthmaticus, systemic fungal infections, persistently positive sputum cultures for *Candida albicans.* **CAUTIONS:** Adrenal insufficiency. **PREGNANCY/LACTATION:** Not known whether drug crosses placenta or is distributed in breast milk. **Pregnancy Category C.**

INTERACTIONS

DRUG INTERACTIONS: None significant. **ALTERED LAB VALUES:** None significant.

SIDE EFFECTS

OCCASIONAL: *Inhalation:* Throat irritation, hoarseness, dry mouth, coughing, temporary wheezing, localized fungal infection in mouth, pharynx, larynx (particularly if mouth is not rinsed w/water after each administration). *Intranasal:* Mild nasopharyngeal irritation; nasal irritation, burning, stinging, dryness, rebound congestion, bronchial asthma, rhinorrhea, loss of sense of taste.

ADVERSE REACTIONS/TOXIC EFFECTS

Acute hypersensitivity reaction (urticaria, angioedema, severe bronchospasm) occurs rarely. Transfer from systemic to local steroid therapy may unmask previously suppressed bronchial asthma condition.

NURSING IMPLICATIONS

BASELINE ASSESSMENT:

Question for hypersensitivity to any corticosteroids, components. Offer emotional support (high incidence of anxiety due to difficulty in breathing and sympathomimetic response to drug).

INTERVENTION/EVALUATION:

In those receiving bronchodilators by inhalation concomitantly w/steroid inhalation therapy, advise pts to use bronchodilator several min before corticosteroid aerosol (enhances penetration of steroid into bronchial tree). Monitor rate, depth, rhythm, type of respiration; quality and rate of pulse. Assess lung sounds for rhonchi, wheezing, rales. Monitor arterial blood gases. Observe lips, fingernails for blue or dusky color in light-skinned pts; gray in dark-skinned pts. Observe for clavicular retractions, hand tremor. Evaluate for clinical improvement (quieter, slower respirations, relaxed facial expression, cessation of clavicular retractions).

PATIENT/FAMILY TEACHING:

Do not change dose schedule or stop taking drug; must taper off gradually under medical supervision. Maintain careful mouth hygiene. Rinse mouth w/water immediately after inhalation (prevents mouth/throat dryness, fungal infection of mouth). Contact physician/nurse if sore throat/mouth occurs. Increase fluid intake (decreases lung secretion viscosity). Do not take more than 2 inhalations at any one time (excessive use may produce paradoxical bronchoconstriction or a decreased bronchodilating effect). Avoid excessive use of caffeine derivatives (chocolate, coffee, tea, cola).

fluocinolone acetonide

floo-oh-sin′oh-lone

(Flurosyn, Synalar, Synemol)

fluocinonide

floo-oh-sin′oh-nide

(Lidex, Vasoderm)

CANADIAN AVAILABILITY:
Dermalar, Fluoderm, Fluonide, Lidemol, Lidex, Lydern, Synalar

(See Classifications section under Corticosteroids: topical)

fluoride

flur′ide

(Fluoritab, Luride)

CANADIAN AVAILABILITY:
Fluor-A-Day, Fluotic

CLASSIFICATION

Dietary supplement

PHARMACOKINETICS

Rapid, completely absorbed from GI tract. Concentrated primarily in bone, developing teeth. Primarily excreted in urine.

ACTION

Incorporated into, stabilizes apatite crystal of bone, teeth. Promotes remineralization of decalcified enamel, may interfere w/ growth development, of dental plaque bacteria, increases resistance to development of caries.

USES

Dietary supplement for prevention of dental caries in children. Treatment of osteoporosis.

PO ADMINISTRATION

1. May take w/o regard to food.
2. May crush chewable tablets. Liquid: avoid glass (causes etching of glass), may mix w/cereal, juice, food.

INDICATIONS/DOSAGE/ROUTES

Dietary supplement:

WATER FLUORIDE	AGE	MG/DAY
$<$0.3 ppm	$<$2 yrs	0.25 mg/day
	2-3 yrs	0.5 mg/day
	3-13 yrs	1 mg/day
0.3-0.7 ppm	$<$2 yrs	None
	2-3 yrs	0.25 mg/day
	3-13 yrs	0.5 mg/day
$>$0.7 ppm	None	None

Osteoporosis:
PO: Adults, elderly: 50-75 mg/day in divided doses.

PRECAUTIONS

CONTRAINDICATIONS: Arthralgia, GI ulceration, severe renal insufficiency. **CAUTIONS:** None significant. **PREGNANCY/LACTATION:** Readily crosses placenta; minimal amount distributed in breast milk.

INTERACTIONS

DRUG INTERACTIONS: Aluminum hydroxide, calcium may decrease absorption. **ALTERED LAB VALUES:** May increase SGOT (AST), alkaline phosphatase.

SIDE EFFECTS

Generally well tolerated. Side effects usually mild and transient. **RARE:** Oral mucus membrane ulceration.

ADVERSE REACTIONS/TOXIC EFFECTS

Hypocalcemia, tetany, bone pain (esp. ankles, feet), electrolyte disturbances, arrhythmias, may cause cardiac failure, respiratory arrest. May cause skeletal fluorosis, osteomalacia, osteosclerosis.

NURSING IMPLICATIONS

PATIENT/FAMILY TEACHING:

Use only as directed and keep out of reach of children to avoid overdosage. Do not take w/milk or other dairy products (decreases absorption). Rinses and gels should be used at bedtime after brushing or flossing. Expectorate excess—do not swallow. Do not eat, drink, or rinse mouth after application.

fluorometholone

flure-oh-meth′oh-loan
(FML)

FIXED-COMBINATION(S): W/sulfacetamide sodium 10%, an anti-infective (FML-S Liquifilm)

CANADIAN AVAILABILITY: Flarex, FML

CLASSIFICATION

Corticosteroid, ophthalmic

PHARMACOKINETICS

After administration distributed to aqueous humor, cornea, iris, ciliary body, retina. Systemic absorption in children receiving high doses.

ACTION

Diffuses across cell membrane. Stimulates protein synthesis of enzymes responsible for anti-inflammatory effects. Provide local anti-inflammatory effect.

USES

Symptomatic relief of inflammatory conditions of the conjunctiva, cornea, lid, and anterior segment of the globe (e.g., allergic conjunctivitis, superficial punctate keratitis, herpes zoster keratitis, iritis, and cyclitis). Also used to help prevent fibrosis, scarring, and potential visual impairment due to chemical, radiation, or thermal burns or penetration of foreign bodies.

OPHTHALMIC ADMINISTRATION

1. For topical ophthalmic use only.
2. Position pt w/head tilted back, looking up.
3. Gently pull lower lid down to form pouch and instill drops (or apply thin strip of ointment).
4. Do not touch tip of applicator to lids or any surface.
5. When lower lid is released, have pt keep eye open w/o blinking for at least 30 sec for solution; for ointment, have pt close eye and roll eyeball around to distribute medication.
6. Apply gentle finger pressure to lacrimal sac (bridge of the nose, inside corner of eye) for 1-2 min after administration of solution.
7. Remove excess solution around eye w/tissue. Wash hands immediately to remove medication on hands.

INDICATIONS/DOSAGE/ROUTES

Usual ophthalmic dosage:
OPHTHALMIC: Adults, elderly: Instill 1-2 drops into conjunctival sac qh during day and q2h at night. First 24-48 hrs after favorable response, decrease to 1 drop q4h, then 1 drop 3-4 times/day.

PRECAUTIONS

CONTRAINDICATIONS: Hypersensitivity to any component of preparation, acute superficial herpes simplex keratitis, fungal diseases of ocular structure. In pts w/vaccinia, varicella, or most other viral diseases of the cornea and conjunctiva. **CAUTIONS:** Safety and efficacy in children <2 yrs of age not established. **PREGNANCY/LACTATION:** Safety during pregnancy, lactation not established. **Pregnancy Category C.**

INTERACTIONS

DRUG INTERACTIONS: None significant. **ALTERED LAB VALUES:** None significant.

SIDE EFFECTS

OCCASIONAL: Transient stinging, burning on instillation. Increased intraocular pressure, mydriasis, ptosis, infection. In high doses, may slow corneal healing.

RARE: Filtering blebs after cataract surgery; hypersensitivity.

ADVERSE REACTIONS/TOXIC EFFECTS

Systemic reactions occur rarely w/extensive use.

NURSING IMPLICATIONS

BASELINE ASSESSMENT:

Question for hypersensitivity to any components of preparation.

INTERVENTION/EVALUATION:

Assess for therapeutic response, superinfection, delayed healing, or irritation.

PATIENT/FAMILY TEACHING:

Explain possible burning or stinging on application. Visual acuity may be decreased after administration, esp. w/ointment; avoid driving or working with machinery. Do not discontinue use w/o consulting physician. Notify physician if no improvement in 7-8 days, if condition worsens, or if pain, itching, or swelling of eye occurs. Sensitivity to bright light may occur; wear sunglasses to minimize discomfort.

fluorouracil

phlur-oh-your´ah-sill
(Adrucil, Efudex, Fluoroplex)

CANADIAN AVAILABILITY:
Adrucil, Efudex

CLASSIFICATION

Antineoplastic

PHARMACOKINETICS

Crosses blood-brain barrier. Widely distributed. Rapidly metabolized in tissues to active metabolite which is localized intracellularly. Primarily excreted via lungs as carbon dioxide. Half-life: 20 hrs.

ACTION

Cell cycle specific for S phase of cell division. Inhibits DNA, RNA synthesis. *Topical:* Destroys rapidly proliferating cells.

USES

Parenteral: Treatment of carcinoma of colon, rectum, breast, stomach, pancreas. Used in combination w/levamisole after surgical resection in patients w/Duke's stage C colon cancer. *Topical:* Treatment of multiple actinic or solar keratoses, superficial basal cell carcinomas.

STORAGE/HANDLING

NOTE: May be carcinogenic, mutagenic, or teratogenic. Handle w/extreme care during preparation/administration.

Solution appears colorless to faint yellow. Slight discoloration does not adversely affect potency or safety. If precipitate forms, redissolve by heating, shaking vigorously, allow to cool to body temperature.

IV ADMINISTRATION

NOTE: Give by IV injection or IV infusion. Do not add to other IV infusions. Avoid small veins, swollen or edematous extremities, areas overlying joints, tendons.

1. IV injection does not need to be diluted or reconstituted.
2. Give IV injection slowly over 1-2 min.
3. Apply prolonged pressure to IV injection site if thrombocyto-

penia is demonstrated by platelet count.

4. For IV infusion, further dilute with 5% dextose or 0.9% NaCl and infuse over 30 min-24 hrs.

5. Extravasation produces immediate pain, severe local tissue damage. Notify physician and apply ice packs to area.

INDICATIONS/DOSAGE/ROUTES

NOTE: Dosage is individualized on basis of clinical response and tolerance to adverse effects. When used in combination therapy, consult specific protocols for optimum dosage, sequence of drug administration. Dosage based on pt's actual weight. Use ideal body weight in obese or edematous pts.

Initial course:
IV: Adults: 12 mg/kg daily for 4 consecutive days; if no toxicity, then 6 mg/kg on days 6, 8, 10, and 12. Do not exceed 800 mg/day. **Adults, poor risk:** 6 mg/kg daily for 3 consecutive days; if no toxicity, then 3 mg/kg on days 5, 7, and 9. Do not exceed 400 mg/day. Repeat at 30-day intervals after last dose of previous schedule.

Maintenance:
IV: Adults: 10-15 mg/kg 1 time/week not to exceed 1 Gm/week. Reduce dosage in poor-risk pts.

Usual topical dosage:
TOPICAL: Adults: Apply 2 times/day to cover lesions.

PRECAUTIONS

CONTRAINDICATIONS: Poor nutritional status, depressed bone marrow function, potentially serious infections, major surgery within previous month. **CAUTIONS:** History of high-dose pelvic irradiation, metastatic cell infiltration of bone marrow, impaired hepatic, renal function. **PREGNANCY/LACTATION:** If possible, avoid use during pregnancy, esp. first trimester. May cause fetal harm. Not known whether distributed in breast milk. Breast feeding not recommended. **Pregnancy Category D.**

INTERACTIONS

DRUG INTERACTIONS: Bone marrow depressant may increase risk of bone marrow depression. Live virus vaccines may potentiate virus replication, increase vaccine side effects, decrease pt's antibody response to vaccine. **ALTERED LAB VALUES:** May decrease albumin. May increase excretion of 5-HIAA in urine. *Topical:* May cause eosinophilia, leukocytosis, thrombocytopenia, toxic granulation.

SIDE EFFECTS

OCCASIONAL: Anorexia, diarrhea, minimal alopecia, fever, dry skin, fissuring, scaling, erythema. *Topical:* pain, pruritus, hyperpigmentation, irritation, inflammation, burning at application site. **RARE:** Nausea, vomiting, anemia, esophagitis, proctitis, GI ulcer, confusion, headache, lacrimation, visual disturbances, angina, allergic reactions.

ADVERSE REACTIONS/TOXIC EFFECTS

Earliest sign of toxicity (4-8 days after beginning of therapy) is stomatitis (dry mouth, burning sensation, mucosal erythema, ulceration at inner margin of lips). Most common dermatologic toxicity is pruritic rash (generally appears on extremities, less frequently on trunk). Leukopenia generally occurs within 9-14 days after drug administration (may occur as late as

25th day). Thrombocytopenia occasionally occurs within 7-17 days after administration. Hematologic toxicity may also manifest itself as pancytopenia, agranulocytosis.

NURSING IMPLICATIONS

BASELINE ASSESSMENT:

Monitor hematology tests results. Drug should be discontinued if intractable vomiting, diarrhea, stomatitis, GI bleeding occurs.

INTERVENTION/EVALUATION:

Monitor for rapidly falling WBC and/or intractable diarrhea, GI bleeding (bright red or tarry stool). Assess oral mucosa for mucosal erythema, ulceration of inner margin of lips, sore throat, difficulty swallowing (stomatitis). Assess skin for rash, check for diarrhea.

PATIENT/FAMILY TEACHING:

Transient alopecia may occur. Contraceptive measures should be used during therapy. Drink plenty of fluids. Maintain fastidious oral hygiene. Do not have immunizations w/o physician's approval (drug lowers body's resistance). Avoid contact w/those who have recently taken oral polio vaccine. Promptly report fever, sore throat, signs of local infection, easy bruising, unusual bleeding from any site. Contact physician if diarrhea, nausea/vomiting continue at home. Avoid ultraviolet rays w/topical or parenteral therapy. *Topical:* Apply only to affected area. Do not use occlusive coverings. Be careful near eyes, nose, and mouth. Wash hands thoroughly after application. Treated areas may be unsightly for several weeks after therapy.

fluoxetine hydrochloride

flew-ox´eh-teen

(Prozac)

F

CANADIAN AVAILABILITY:
Prozac

CLASSIFICATION

Antidepressant

PHARMACOKINETICS

Well absorbed from GI tract. Crosses blood-brain barrier. Protein binding: 94%. Metabolized in liver to active metabolite. Primarily excreted in urine. Half-life: 2-3 days; metabolite: 7-9 days.

ACTION

Selectively inhibits serotonin (5-HT) uptake in CNS enhancing serotonergic function.

USES

Outpatient treatment of major depression exhibited as persistent, prominent dysphoria (occurring nearly every day for at least 2 wk) manifested by 4 of 8 symptoms: change in appetite, change in sleep pattern, increased fatigue, impaired concentration, feelings of guilt or worthlessness, loss of interest in usual activities, psychomotor agitation or retardation, or suicidal tendencies. Treatment of obsessive-compulsive disorder (OCD).

PO ADMINISTRATION

Give w/food or milk if GI distress occurs.

INDICATIONS/DOSAGE/ROUTES

NOTE: Use lower or less frequent doses in those w/renal, hepatic impairment, elderly, those w/concurrent disease or on multiple medications.

Depression, OCD:
PO: Adults: Initially, 20 mg each morning. If therapeutic improvement does not occur after 2 wk, gradually increase dose to maximum 80 mg/day in 2 equally divided doses in morning, noon. **Elderly:** Initially, 10 mg/day. May increase by 10-20 mg q2wks. Avoid administration at night.

PRECAUTIONS

CONTRAINDICATIONS: Within 14 days of MAO inhibitor ingestion. **CAUTIONS:** Impaired renal or hepatic function. **PREGNANCY/LACTATION:** Not known whether drug crosses placenta or is distributed in breast milk. **Pregnancy Category B.**

INTERACTIONS

DRUG INTERACTIONS: Alcohol, CNS depressants antagonize CNS depressant effect. May displace highly protein-bound medications from protein binding sites (e.g., oral anticoagulants). MAO inhibitors may produce serotonin syndrome. May increase phenytoin concentration, toxicity. **ALTERED LAB VALUES:** None significant.

SIDE EFFECTS

FREQUENT: Headache, nervousness, insomnia, drowsiness, excessive sweating, anxiety, tremor, anorexia, nausea, diarrhea, dry mouth. **OCCASIONAL:** Dizziness, fatigue, constipation, rash, pruritus, vomiting, back pain, visual disturbances.

ADVERSE REACTIONS/TOXIC EFFECTS

Overdosage may produce seizures, nausea, vomiting, excessive agitation, restlessness.

NURSING IMPLICATIONS

BASELINE ASSESSMENT:

For those on long-term therapy, liver/renal function tests, blood counts should be performed periodically.

INTERVENTION/EVALUATION:

Supervise suicidal-risk pt closely during early therapy (as energy level improves, suicide potential increases). Assess appearance, behavior, speech pattern, level of interest, mood. Assist w/ambulation if dizziness occurs. Monitor stool frequency and consistency. Assess skin for appearance of rash.

PATIENT/FAMILY TEACHING:

Change positions slowly to avoid hypotensive effect. Maximum therapeutic response may require 4 or more wks of therapy. Photosensitivity to sun may occur. Dry mouth may be relieved by sugarless gum, or sips of tepid water. Report visual disturbances. Do not abruptly discontinue medication. Avoid tasks that require alertness, motor skills until response to drug is established. Avoid alcohol.

fluoxymesterone

floo-ox-ih-mes′teh-rone
(Android-F, Halotestin)

FIXED-COMBINATION(S):
W/ethinyl estradiol, an estrogen (Halodrin)

CANADIAN AVAILABILITY:
Halotestin

CLASSIFICATION

Androgen

PHARMACOKINETICS

Metabolized in liver. Primarily excreted in urine. Half-life: 9.2 hrs.

ACTION

Stimulates spermatogenesis, development of male secondary sex characteristics, sexual maturation at puberty. Stimulates production of RBCs.

USES

Treatment of delayed puberty; testicular failure due to cryptorchidism, bilateral orchism, orchitis, vanishing testis syndrome, or orchidectomy; hypogonadotropic hypogonadism due to pituitary/hypothalamic injury (tumors, trauma, or radiation), idiopathic gonadotropin or LHRH deficiency. Palliative therapy in women 1-5 years past menopause w/advancing, inoperable metastatic breast cancer or premenopausal women who have benefited from oophorectomy and have a hormone-responsive tumor. Prevention of postpartum breast pain and engorgement. In combination w/estrogens for management of moderate to severe vasomotor symptoms associated w/ menopause when estrogens alone are not effective.

PO ADMINISTRATION

Take w/food if GI upset occurs.

INDICATIONS/DOSAGE/ROUTES

Males (hypogonadism):
PO: Adults: 5-20 mg/day.

Males (delayed puberty):
PO: Adults: 2.5-20 mg/day for 4-6 months.

Females (inoperable breast cancer):
PO: Adults: 10-40 mg/day in divided doses for 1-3 months.

Females (prevent postpartum breast pain/engorgement):
PO: Adults: Initially, 2.5 mg shortly after delivery, then 5-10 mg/day in divided doses for 4-5 days.

PRECAUTIONS

CONTRAINDICATIONS: Hypersensitivity to drug or components of preparation, serious cardiac, renal, or hepatic dysfunction. Do not use for men w/carcinomas of the breast or prostate. **CAUTIONS:** Epilepsy, migraine, or other conditions aggravated by fluid retention; metastatic breast cancer or immobility increases risk of hypercalcemia. Extreme caution in children because of bone maturation effects. **PREGNANCY/LACTATION:** Contraindicated during lactation. **Pregnancy Category X.**

INTERACTIONS

DRUG INTERACTIONS: May increase effect of oral anticoagulants. Hepatotoxic medications may increase hepatotoxicity. **ALTERED LAB VALUES:** May increase alkaline phosphatase, SGOT (AST), bilirubin, calcium, potassium, sodium, Hgb, Hct, LDL. May decrease HDL.

SIDE EFFECTS

FREQUENT: Gynecomastia, acne, amenorrhea or other menstrual irregularities. Females: hirsutism, deepening of voice, clitoral enlargement (may not be reversible when drug is discontinued). **OCCASIONAL:** Edema, nausea, insomnia, oligospermia, priapism, male pattern of baldness, bladder irritability, hypercalcemia in immobilized pts or those w/breast cancer, hypercholesterolemia. **RARE:** Polycythemia w/high dosage, cholestatic jaundice, hypersensitivity, and anaphylactoid reactions.

ADVERSE REACTIONS/TOXIC EFFECTS

Peliosis hepatitis (liver, spleen replaced w/blood-filled cysts), hepatic neoplasms, and hepatocellular carcinoma have been associated w/prolonged high dosage.

NURSING IMPLICATIONS

BASELINE ASSESSMENT:

Question for hypersensitivity to drug or components (sensitivity to aspirin may indicate tartrazine sensitivity). Establish baseline weight, B/P, Hgb, Hct. Check liver function test results, electrolytes, and cholesterol if ordered. Wrist x-rays may be ordered to determine bone maturation in children.

INTERVENTION/EVALUATION:

Weigh daily and report weekly gain of more than 5 lb; evaluate for edema. Monitor I&O. Check B/P at least 2 times/day. Assess electrolytes, cholesterol, Hgb, Hct (periodically for high dosage), liver function test results. W/breast cancer or immobility, check for hypercalcemia (lethargy, muscle weakness, confusion, irritability). Assure adequate intake of protein, calories. Be alert to signs of virilization. Monitor sleep patterns. Assess for hepatitis: nausea, yellowing of eyes and skin, dark urine, light stools.

PATIENT/FAMILY TEACHING:

Regular visits to physician and monitoring tests are necessary. Do not take any other medications w/o consulting physician. Teach diet high in protein, calories. Food may be tolerated better in small, frequent feedings. Weigh daily, report weekly gain of 5 lb or more. Teach signs of jaundice; notify physician if these, nausea, vomiting, acne, ankle swelling occur. *Female:* Promptly report menstrual irregularities, hoarseness, deepening of voice. *Male:* Report frequent erections, difficulty urinating, gynecomastia.

fluphenazine decanoate

flew-phen´ah-zeen

(Prolixin)

fluphenazine enanthate

(Prolixin)

fluphenazine hydrochloride

(Prolixin, Permitil)

CANADIAN AVAILABILITY:

Apo-Fluphenazine, Modecate, Moditen, Permitil

CLASSIFICATION

Antipsychotic

PHARMACOKINETICS

Variably absorbed after oral administration; well absorbed after IM administration. Protein binding: >90%. Metabolized in liver to active metabolites. Primarily excreted in urine. Half-life: 33 hrs.

ACTION

Blocks postsynaptic dopaminergic receptors in brain. Produces weak anticholinergic, sedative, antiemetic effects, strong extrapyramidal activity.

USES

Management of psychotic disturbances (schizophrenia, delusions, hallucinations).

STORAGE/HANDLING

Store oral and parenteral form at room temperature. Yellow discoloration of solution does not affect potency, but discard if markedly discolored or if precipitate forms.

PO/IM ADMINISTRATION

PO:

1. Mix oral concentrate w/water, 7-Up, carbonated orange drink, milk, V-8, pineapple, apricot, prune, orange, tomato, grapefruit juice.
2. Do not mix oral concentrate w/caffeine (coffee, cola), tea, apple juice because of physical incompatibility.

IM:

NOTE: Pt must remain recumbent for 30-60 min in head-low position w/legs raised, to minimize hypotensive effect.

1. Use a dry 21-gauge needle, syringe for administering fluphenazine decanoate or enanthate (wet needle and syringe turn solution cloudy).
2. Inject slow, deep IM into upper outer quadrant of gluteus maximus. If irritation occurs, further injections may be diluted w/0.9% NaCl or 2% procaine hydrochloride.
3. Massage IM injection site to reduce discomfort.

INDICATIONS/DOSAGE/ROUTES

Psychotic disorders:
PO: Adults: Initially, 0.5-10 mg/day fluphenazine HCl in divided doses q6-8h. Increase gradually until therapeutic response is achieved (usually under 20 mg daily); decrease gradually to maintenance level (1-5 mg/day). **Elderly:** Initially, 1-2.5 mg/day.
IM: Adults: Initially, 1.25 mg, followed by 2.5-10 mg/day in divided doses q6-8h.

Chronic schizophrenic disorder:
IM: Adults: Initially, 12.5-25 mg of fluphenazine decanoate q1-6wk, or 25 mg fluphenazine enanthate q2wk.

Usual elderly dosage (nonpsychotic):
PO: Elderly: Initially, 1-2.5 mg/day. May increase by 1-2.5 mg/day q4-7 days. **Maximum:** 20 mg/day.

PRECAUTIONS

CONTRAINDICATIONS: Severe CNS depression, comatose states, severe cardiovascular disease, bone marrow depression, subcortical brain damage. **CAUTIONS:** Impaired respiratory/hepatic/renal/cardiac function, alcohol withdrawal, history of seizures, urinary retention, glaucoma, prostatic hypertrophy, hypocalcemia (increased susceptibility to dystonias). **PREGNANCY/LACTATION:** Crosses placenta; distributed in breast milk. **Pregnancy Category C.**

INTERACTIONS

DRUG INTERACTIONS: Alcohol, CNS depressants may increase CNS, respiratory depression, hypotensive effects. Tricyclic antidepressants, MAO inhibitors may increase sedative, anticholinergic effects. Antithyroid agents may increase risk of agranulocytosis. Extrapyramidal symptoms (EPS) may increase w/EPS-producing medications. Hypotensives may increase hypotension. May decrease levodopa effects. Lithium may decrease absorption, produce adverse neurologic effects. **ALTERED LAB VALUES:** May produce false-positive pregnancy test, PKU. EKG changes may occur, including Q and T wave disturbances.

SIDE EFFECTS

FREQUENT: Hypotension, dizziness, and fainting occur frequently after first injection, occasionally after subsequent injections, and rarely w/oral dosage. **OCCASIONAL:** Drowsiness during early therapy, dry mouth, blurred vision, lethargy, constipation or diarrhea, nasal congestion, peripheral edema, urinary retention. **RARE:** Ocular changes, skin pigmentation (those on high doses for prolonged periods).

ADVERSE REACTIONS/TOXIC EFFECTS

Extrapyramidal symptoms appear dose related (particularly high dosage); divided into 3 categories: akathisia (inability to sit still, tapping of feet, urge to move around); parkinsonian symptoms (mask-like face, tremors, shuffling gait, hypersalivation); and acute dystonias—torticollis (neck muscle spasm), opisthotonos (rigidity of back muscles), and oculogyric crisis (rolling back of eyes). Dystonic reaction may also produce profuse sweating, pallor. Tardive dyskinesia (protrusion of tongue, puffing of cheeks, chewing/puckering of the mouth) occurs rarely (may be irreversible). Abrupt withdrawal after long-term therapy may precipitate nausea, vomiting, gastritis, dizziness, tremors. Blood dyscrasias, particularly agranulocytosis, mild leukopenia (sore mouth/gums/throat) may occur. May lower seizure threshold.

NURSING IMPLICATIONS

BASELINE ASSESSMENT:

Avoid skin contact w/solution (contact dermatitis). Assess behavior, appearance, emotional status, response to environment, speech pattern, thought content.

INTERVENTION/EVALUATION:

Monitor B/P for hypotension. Assess for extrapyramidal symptoms. Monitor WBC, differential count for blood dyscrasias. Monitor for fine tongue movement (may be early sign of tardive dyskinesia). Supervise suicidal-risk pt closely during early therapy (as depression lessens, energy level improves, increasing suicide potential). Assess for therapeutic response (interest in surroundings, improvement in self-care, increased ability to concentrate, relaxed facial expression).

PATIENT/FAMILY TEACHING:

Full therapeutic effect may take up to 6 wk. Urine may darken. Do not abruptly withdraw from long-term drug therapy. Report visual disturbances. Sugarless gum or sips of tepid water may relieve dry mouth. Drowsiness generally subsides during continued therapy. Avoid tasks that require alertness, motor skills until response to drug is established. Avoid alcohol.

flurandrenolide

flure-an-dren´oh-lide
(Cordran)

FIXED-COMBINATION(S):
W/neomycin sulfate, an aminoglycoside (Cordran-N)

CANADIAN AVAILABILITY:
Drenison

(See Classifications section under Corticosteroids: topical)

flurazepam hydrochloride

flur-a´zah-pam
(Dalmane)

CANADIAN AVAILABILITY:
Apo-Flurazepam, Dalmane, Novoflupam

CLASSIFICATION

Sedative-hypnotics **(Schedule IV)**

PHARMACOKINETICS

	ONSET	PEAK	DURATION
PO	15-45 min	—	7-8 hrs

Well absorbed from GI tract. Crosses blood-brain barrier. Widely distributed. Protein binding: 97%. Metabolized in liver to active metabolite. Primarily excreted in urine. Half-life: 2.3 hrs; metabolite: 40-114 hrs.

ACTION

Enhances action of inhibitory neurotransmitter gamma-aminobutyric acid (GABA). Depressant effects occur at all levels of CNS.

USES

Short-term treatment of insomnia (up to 4 wk). Reduces sleep-induction time, number of nocturnal awakenings; increases length of sleep.

PO ADMINISTRATION

1. Give w/o regard to meals.
2. Capsules may be emptied and mixed w/food.

INDICATIONS/DOSAGE/ROUTES

PO: Adults: 15-30 mg at bedtime. **Elderly/debilitated/liver disease/low serum albumin:** 15 mg at bedtime.

PRECAUTIONS

CONTRAINDICATIONS: Acute narrow-angle glaucoma, acute alcohol intoxication. **CAUTIONS:** Impaired renal/hepatic function. **PREGNANCY/LACTATION:** Crosses placenta; may be distributed in breast milk. Chronic ingestion during pregnancy may produce withdrawal symptoms, CNS depression in neonates. **Pregnancy Category C.**

INTERACTIONS

DRUG INTERACTIONS: Alcohol, CNS depressants may increase CNS depressant effect. **ALTERED LAB VALUES:** None significant.

SIDE EFFECTS

FREQUENT: Drowsiness, dizziness, ataxia, sedation. Morning drowsiness may occur initially. **OCCASIONAL:** Dizziness, GI disturbances, nervousness, blurred vision, dry mouth, headache, confusion, skin rash, irritability, slurred speech. **RARE:** Paradoxical CNS excitement/restlessness (particularly noted in elderly/debilitated).

ADVERSE REACTIONS/TOXIC EFFECTS

Abrupt or too-rapid withdrawal may result in pronounced restlessness and irritability, insomnia, hand tremors, abdominal/muscle cramps, sweating, vomiting, seizures. Overdosage results in somnolence, confusion, diminished reflexes, coma.

NURSING IMPLICATIONS

BASELINE ASSESSMENT:

Assess B/P, pulse, respirations immediately before administration. Raise bed rails. Provide environment conducive to sleep (back rub, quiet environment, low lighting).

INTERVENTION/EVALUATION:

Assist w/ambulation. Assess for paradoxical reaction, particularly during early therapy. Evaluate for therapeutic response: a decrease in number of nocturnal awakenings, increase in length of sleep duration.

PATIENT/FAMILY TEACHING:

Smoking reduces drug effectiveness. Do not abruptly withdraw medication after long-term use. Avoid alcohol.

flurbiprofen

fleur'bih-pro-fen

(Ansaid)

flurbiprofen sodium

(Ocufen)

CANADIAN AVAILABILITY:
Ansaid, Froben, Ocufen

CLASSIFICATION

Nonsteroidal anti-inflammatory

PHARMACOKINETICS

Well absorbed from GI tract, penetrates cornea after ophthalmic administration (may be systemically absorbed). Widely distributed. Protein binding: 99%. Metabolized in liver. Primarily excreted in urine. Half-life: 3-4 hrs.

ACTION

Inhibits prostaglandin synthesis. Inhibits action of cyclooxygenase, decreases formation of prostaglandin, thromboxane precursors from arachidonic acid. Prevents, reduces miosis by relaxing iris sphincter.

USES

Symptomatic treatment of acute and/or chronic rheumatoid arthritis, osteoarthritis; inhibits intraoperative miosis.

PO/OPHTHALMIC ADMINISTRATION

PO:

1. Do not crush or break enteric-coated form.
2. May give w/food, milk, or antacids if GI distress occurs.

OPHTHALMIC:

1. Place finger on lower eyelid and pull out until pocket is formed between eye and lower lid. Hold dropper above pocket and place prescribed number of drops into pocket. Close eye gently. Apply digital pressure to lacrimal sac for 1-2 min (minimizes drainage into nose and throat, reducing risk of systemic effects). Remove excess solution w/tissue.

INDICATIONS/DOSAGE/ROUTES

Rhemuatoid arthritis, osteoarthritis:

PO: Adults, elderly: 200-300 mg/day in 2-4 divided doses. Do not give >100 mg/dose or 300 mg/day.

Ophthalmic:

PO: Adults, elderly: Apply 2 drops into conjunctival sac 3, 2, and 1 hr before surgery or 2 drops q4h while pt is awake day before surgery.

PRECAUTIONS

CONTRAINDICATIONS: Active peptic ulcer, GI ulceration, chronic inflammation of GI tract, GI bleeding disorders, history of hypersensitivity to aspirin or nonsteroidal anti-inflammatory agent. **CAUTIONS:** Impaired renal/hepatic function, history of GI tract disease, predisposition to fluid retention, those wearing soft-contact lenses, surgical pts w/bleeding tendencies. **PREGNANCY/LACTATION:** Crosses placenta; not known whether distributed in breast milk. Avoid use during last trimester (may adversely affect fetal cardiovascular system: premature closure of ductus arteriosus). **Pregnancy Category B.** *Ophthalmic:* **Pregnancy Category C.**

INTERACTIONS

DRUG INTERACTIONS: May increase effects of oral anticoagulants, heparin, thrombolytics. May decrease effect of antihypertensives, diuretics. Salicylates, aspirin may increase risk of GI side effects, bleeding. Bone marrow depressants may increase risk of hematologic reactions. May increase concentration, toxicity of lithium. May increase methotrexate toxicity. Probenecid may increase concentration. *Ophthalmic:* May decrease effect of acetylcholine, carbachol. May decrease antiglaucoma effect of epinephrine, other antiglaucoma medications. **ALTERED LAB VALUES:** May increase serum transaminases, alkaline phosphatase, LDH, bleeding time.

SIDE EFFECTS

FREQUENT: *Ophthalmic:* Burning, stinging on instillation, keratitis, elevated intraocular pressure. **OCCASIONAL:** *Oral:* Dizziness, headache, dyspepsia (heartburn, indigestion, epigastric pain, diarrhea/constipation, cramping) occurs more frequently in elderly. **RARE:** *Oral:* Rash, peripheral edema/fluid retention, visual disturbances, vomiting, drowsiness.

ADVERSE REACTIONS/TOXIC EFFECTS

Overdosage may result in acute renal failure. In those treated chronically, peptic ulcer, GI bleeding, gastritis, severe hepatic reaction (jaundice), nephrotoxicity (hematuria, dysuria, proteinuria), severe hypersensitivity reaction (bronchospasm, angiofacial edema) occur rarely.

NURSING IMPLICATIONS

BASELINE ASSESSMENT:

Anti-inflammatory: Assess onset, type, location, and duration of pain or inflammation. Inspect appearance of affected joints for immobility, deformities, and skin condition.

INTERVENTION/EVALUATION:

Monitor for headache, dyspepsia. Monitor pattern of daily bowel activity and stool consistency. Evaluate for therapeutic response:

relief of pain, stiffness, swelling, increase in joint mobility, reduced joint tenderness, improved grip strength.

PATIENT/FAMILY TEACHING:

Swallow tablet whole; do not crush or chew. Avoid aspirin, alcohol during therapy (increases risk of GI bleeding). If GI upset occurs, take w/food, milk. Report GI distress, visual disturbances, rash, edema, headache. *Ophthalmic:* Eye burning may occur w/instillation.

flutamide

flew´tah-myd
(Eulexin)

CANADIAN AVAILABILITY: Euflex

CLASSIFICATION

Antineoplastic

PHARMACOKINETICS

Completely absorbed from GI tract. Protein binding: 94-96%. Metabolized in liver to active metabolite. Primarily excreted in urine. Half-life: 6 hrs (increase in elderly).

ACTION

Inhibits androgen uptake and/or binding of androgen in tissues. Interferes w/testosterone at cellular level (complements leuprolide, suppressing testicular androgen production by inhibiting LH secretion).

USES

Treatment of metastatic prostatic carcinoma (in combination w/ LHRH agonistic analogues (i.e., leuprolide). Treatment w/both drugs must be started at same time.

INDICATONS/DOSAGE/ROUTES

Prostatic carcinoma:
PO: Adults, elderly: 250 mg q8h.

PRECAUTIONS

CONTRAINDICATIONS: None significant. **CAUTIONS:** None significant. **PREGNANCY/LACTATION:** May cause fetal harm. **Pregnancy Category D.**

INTERACTIONS

DRUG INTERACTIONS: None significant. **ALTERED LAB VALUES:** May increase estradiol, testosterone, SGOT (AST), SGPT (ALT), bilirubin, creatinine.

SIDE EFFECTS

FREQUENT: Hot flashes, loss of libido, impotence, diarrhea, nausea/vomiting, gynecomastia. **OCCASIONAL:** Rash, anorexia. **RARE:** Photosensitivity.

ADVERSE REACTIONS/TOXIC EFFECTS

Hepatitis, hypertension may be noted.

NURSING IMPLICATIONS

INTERVENTION/EVALUATION:

Monitor B/P periodically and hepatic function tests in long-term therapy. Check for diarrhea, nausea, and vomiting.

PATIENT/FAMILY TEACHING:

Do not stop taking medication (both drugs must be continued). Explain side effects and action on carcinoma. Contact physician if nausea/vomiting continues at home.

fluticasone

flu-tih-kay´sun

(Cutivate)

(See Classifications section under Corticosteroids: topical)

fluticasone (Flonase)

See supplement

fluvastatin

flu-vah-stah'tin

(Lescol)

CANADIAN AVAILABILITY: Lescol

CLASSIFICATION

Antihyperlipoproteinemic

PHARMACOKINETICS

Well absorbed from GI tract (unaffected by food). Does not cross blood-brain barrier. Protein binding: 98%. Primarily eliminated in feces.

ACTION

Inhibits HMG-CoA, preventing conversion of HMG-CoA to mevalonate (early step in cholesterol synthesis). Decreases LDL cholesterol, VLDL, plasma triglycerides. Increases HDL concentration slightly.

USES

Adjunct to diet therapy to decrease elevated total and LDL cholesterol concentrations in those w/primary hypercholesterolemia (types IIa and IIb) and in those w/ combined hypercholesterolemia, hypertriglyceridemia.

PO ADMINISTRATION

1. May take w/o regard to food.

INDICATIONS/DOSAGE/ROUTES

Hyperlipoproteinemia:

PO: Adults, elderly: Initially: 20 mg/day in the evening. May increase up to 40 mg/day. **Maintenance:** 20-40 mg/day in single or divided doses.

PRECAUTIONS

CONTRAINDICATIONS: Hypersensitivity to fluvastatin, active liver disease, unexplained increased serum transaminases. **CAUTIONS:** Anticoagulant therapy, history of liver disease, substantial alcohol consumption. Withholding/discontinuing fluvastatin may be necessary when pt at risk for renal failure (secondary to rhabdomyolysis); major surgery, severe acute infection, trauma, hypotension, severe metabolic, endocrine or electrolyte disorders, or uncontrolled seizures. **PREGNANCY/LACTATION:** Contraindicated in pregnancy (suppression of cholesterol biosynthesis may cause fetal toxicity) and lactation. Unknown whether drug is distributed in breast milk. **Pregnancy Category X.**

INTERACTIONS

DRUG INTERACTIONS: Increased risk of rhabdomyolysis, acute renal failure w/cyclosporine, erythromycin, gemfibrozil, niacin, other immunosuppressants. **ALTERED LAB VALUES:** May increase creatinine kinase (CK), serum transaminase concentrations.

SIDE EFFECTS

Generally well tolerated. Side effects usually mild and transient. **FREQUENT:** GI complaints (e.g., nausea, dyspepsia, diarrhea, constipation, flatulence, abdominal pain, heartburn), dizziness, skin rash. **OCCASIONAL:** Myalgia (fever, muscle aches, unusual tiredness, weakness), insomnia.

ADVERSE REACTIONS/TOXIC EFFECTS

Myositis, w/ or w/o increased CK, muscle weakness. May progress to frank rhabdomyolysis and renal impairment.

NURSING IMPLICATIONS

BASELINE ASSESSMENT:

Question for possibility of pregnancy before initiating therapy **(Pregnancy Category X).** Question history of hypersensitivity to fluvastatin. Assess baseline lab results: cholesterol, triglycerides, liver function tests.

INTERVENTION/EVALUATION:

Evaluate food tolerance. Determine pattern of bowel activity. Check for headache, dizziness, blurred vision. Assess for rash, pruritus. Monitor cholesterol and triglyceride lab results for therapeutic response. Be alert for malaise, muscle cramping or weakness. Monitor temperature at least twice a day.

PATIENT/FAMILY TEACHING:

Follow special diet (important part of treatment). Periodic lab tests are essential part of therapy. Do not take other medications w/o physician knowledge. Do not stop medication w/o consulting physician. Report promptly any muscle pain or weakness, esp. if accompanied by fever or malaise. Do not drive or perform activities that require alert response if dizziness occurs.

---

fluvoxamine (Luvox)
See supplement

---

folic acid (vitamin B_9)

foh´lick ah´sid
(Folvite)

sodium folate

(Folvite - parenteral)

CANADIAN AVAILABILITY:
Apo-Folic, Folvite

CLASSIFICATION

Coenzyme

PHARMACOKINETICS

Almost completely absorbed from GI tract (upper duodenum). Protein binding: extensive. Metabolized in liver, plasma to active form. Excreted in urine. Removed by hemodialysis.

ACTION

Stimulates production of red and white blood cells and platelets, essential for nucleoprotein synthesis, maintenance of normal erythropoiesis.

USES

Treatment of megaloblastic, macrocytic anemia associated w/ pregnancy, infancy, childhood, inadequate dietary intake.

PO/SubQ/IM/IV ADMINISTRATION

NOTE: Parenteral form used in acutely ill, parenteral or enteral alimentation, those unresponsive to oral route in GI malabsorption syndrome. Dosage >0.1 mg daily may conceal pernicious anemia.

INDICATIONS/DOSAGE/ROUTES

Deficiency:
PO/IM/IV: Adults, children: Up to 1 mg/day.

Supplement:
PO/IM/IV: Adults, elderly, children >4 yr: 0.4 mg/day. **Children <4 yr:** 0.3 mg/day. **Children <1 yr:** 0.1 mg/day. **Pregnancy:** 0.8 mg/day.

PRECAUTIONS

CONTRAINDICATIONS: Anemias (pernicious, aplastic, normocytic, refractory). **CAUTIONS:** None significant. **PREGNANCY/LACTATION:** Distributed in breast milk. **Pregnancy Category A.** If more than RDA: **Pregnancy Category C.**

INTERACTIONS

DRUG INTERACTIONS: May decrease effects of hydantoin anticonvulsants. Analgesics, anticonvulsants, carbamazepine, estrogens may increase folic acid requirements. Antacids, cholestyramine may decrease absorption. Methotrexate, triamterene, trimethoprim may antagonize effects. **ALTERED LAB VALUES:** May decrease vitamin B_{12} concentration.

SIDE EFFECTS

None significant.

ADVERSE REACTIONS/TOXIC EFFECTS

Allergic hypersensitivity occurs rarely w/parenteral form. Oral folic acid is nontoxic.

NURSING IMPLICATIONS

BASELINE ASSESSMENT:

Pernicious anemia should be ruled out by Schilling test and vitamin B_{12} blood level before therapy is initiated (may produce irreversible neurologic damage). Resistance to treatment may occur if decreased hematopoiesis, alcoholism, antimetabolic drugs or deficiency of vitamin B_6, B_{12}, C, or E is evident.

INTERVENTION/EVALUATION:

Assess for therapeutic improvement: improved sense of well-being, relief from iron-deficiency symptoms (fatigue, shortness of breath, sore tongue, headache, pallor).

PATIENT/FAMILY TEACHING:

Take only under medical supervision. Follow diet as ordered. Foods rich in folic acid including fruits, vegetables and organ meats. Report rash or hives promptly.

foscarnet sodium

fos-car´net
(Foscavir)

CLASSIFICATION

Antiviral

PHARMACOKINETICS

Sequestered into bone, cartilage. Protein binding: 14-17%. Primarily excreted unchanged in urine. Removed by hemodialysis. Half-life: 3.3-6.8 hrs (increased in decreased renal function).

ACTION

Inhibits replication of herpes virus. Provides selective inhibition at the pyrophosphate binding site on virus-specific DNA polymerases and reverse transcriptases.

USES

Treatment of CMV retinitis in pts w/AIDS.

STORAGE/HANDLING

Store parenteral vials at room temperature. After dilution, stable for 24 hrs at room temperature.

IV ADMINISTRATION

1. Do not give IV injection or rapid infusion (increases toxicity).
2. Administer only by IV infusion over a minimum of 1 hr (no more than 1 mg/kg/min).
3. To minimize toxicity and phlebitis, use central venous lines or veins w/adequate blood to permit rapid dilution and dissemination of foscarnet.
4. Use IV infusion pump to prevent accidental overdose.
5. The standard 24 mg/ml solution may be used w/o dilution when central venous catheter is used for infusion; 24 mg/ml solution *must* be diluted to 12 mg/ml when peripheral vein catheter is being used. Only 5% dextrose in water or normal saline solution for injection should be used for dilution.
6. Since dosage is calculated on body weight, unneeded quantity may be removed before start of infusion to avoid overdosage. Aseptic technique must be used and solution administered within 24 hrs of first entry into sealed bottle.
7. Do not use if solution is discolored or contains particulate material.

INDICATIONS/DOSAGE/ROUTES

NOTE: Individualized dosage based on renal function, pt, clinical response.

HIV retinitis:
IV: Adults: Initially, 60 mg/kg q8h for 2-3 wk. **Maintenance:** 90 mg/kg/day; may increase up to 120 mg/kg/day if retinitis progresses.

Dosage in renal impairment:
Dosage individualized according to pt's creatinine clearance. Refer to dosing guide provided by manufacturer.

PRECAUTIONS

CONTRAINDICATIONS: Hypersensitivity to foscarnet sodium. **CAUTIONS:** Neurologic or cardiac abnormalities, history of renal impairment, altered calcium or other electrolyte levels. **PREGNANCY/LACTATION:** Excreted in milk of lactating rats. **Pregnancy Category C.**

INTERACTIONS

DRUG INTERACTIONS: Nephrotoxic medications may increase risk of renal toxicity. Pentamidine (IV) may cause reversible hypocalcemia, hypomagnesemia, nephrotoxicity. Zidovudine may increase anemia. **ALTERED LAB VALUES:** May increase SGOT (AST), SGPT (ALT), alkaline phosphatase, bilirubin, creatinine. May decrease magnesium, potassium. May alter calcium, phosphate concentrations.

SIDE EFFECTS

FREQUENT: Fever (65%), nausea (47%), vomiting, diarrhea (30%), abnormal renal functioning, anemia (33%), bone marrow suppression, headache, seizures (10%), mineral and electrolyte imbalances. **OCCASIONAL:** Pain and inflammation at injection site, back and chest pain, hyper/hypotension, tachycardia, ulcerative stomatitis, rash or urticaria, taste perversions, insomnia, bronchospasm, pneumonia, urinary retention or polyuria. **RARE:** Ascites, hemoptysis, hypothermia, abnormal crying, earache, deafness, retinal detachment, photophobia, alopecia, abnormal gait, speech disorders, cholestatic hepatitis, cholecystitis.

ADVERSE REACTIONS/TOXIC EFFECTS

Renal impairment is a major toxicity that occurs to some extent in most pts. Seizures and mineral/electrolyte imbalances may be life-threatening.

NURSING IMPLICATIONS

BASELINE ASSESSMENT:

Question for hypersensitivity to foscarnet. Obtain baseline mineral and electrolyte levels, vital signs, CBC values, renal functioning.

INTERVENTION/EVALUATION:

Monitor electrolyte results closely; assess for signs of electrolyte imbalance, esp. hypocalcemia (perioral tingling, numbness/paresthesia of extremities) or hypokalemia (weakness, muscle cramps, numbness/tingling of extremities, irritability). Maintain accurate I&O, provide adequate hydration to assure diuresis before and during dosing, and monitor renal function tests to avoid or identify promptly renal impairment. Assess for tremors; provide safety measures for potential seizures. Evaluate vital signs at least 2 times/day. Provide small, attractive meals; avoid unattractive sights, smells, esp. at mealtimes, and administer ordered antiemetics to support nutrition. Monitor number, consistency of stools. Assess for bleeding, anemia, or developing superinfections.

PATIENT/FAMILY TEACHING:

Foscarnet is not a cure for CMV retinitis; regular ophthalmologic examinations are part of therapy. Dose modifications may be necessary, esp. w/regard to controlling side effects; close medical supervision is essential. Infusion rate must be controlled to prevent overdosage (no more than 1 mg/kg/min). Important to report perioral tingling, numbness in the extremities, or paresthesias during or after infusion (may indicate electrolyte abnormalities). Risk of renal impairment can be reduced by sufficient fluid intake to assure diuresis before and during dosing. Tremors should be reported promptly because of potential for seizures.

fosinopril

foh-sin´oh-prill

(Monopril)

CLASSIFICATION

Angiotensin-converting enzyme (ACE) inhibitor

PHARMACOKINETICS

	ONSET	PEAK	DURATION
PO	1 hr	2-6 hrs	24 hrs

Slowly absorbed from GI tract. Protein binding: 97-98%. Metabolized in liver, GI mucosa to active metabolite. Primarily excreted in urine. Minimal removal by hemodialysis. Half-life: 11.5 hrs.

ACTION

Suppresses renin-angiotensin-aldosterone system (prevents conversion of angiotensin I to angiotensin II, a potent vasoconstrictor; may also inhibit angiotensin II at local vascular and renal sites). Decreases plasma angiotensin II, increases plasma renin activity, decreases aldosterone secretion. Reduces peripheral arterial resistance.

USES

Treatment of hypertension. Used alone or in combination w/ other antihypertensives.

PO ADMINISTRATION

1. May give w/o regard to food.
2. Tablets may be crushed.

INDICATIONS/DOSAGE/ROUTES

Hypertension (used alone):
PO: Adults, elderly: Initially, 10 mg/day. **Maintenance:** 20-40 mg/day. **Maximum:** 80 mg/day.

Hypertension (w/diuretic):
NOTE: Discontinue diuretic 2-3 days before initiation of fosinopril therapy.
PO: Adults, elderly: Initially, 10 mg/day titrated to pt's needs.

PRECAUTIONS

CONTRAINDICATIONS: History of angioedema w/previous treatment w/ACE inhibitors. **CAUTIONS:** Renal impairment, those w/sodium depletion or on diuretic therapy, dialysis, hypovolemia, coronary or cerebrovascular insufficiency. **PREGNANCY/LACTATION:** Crosses placenta; distributed in breast milk. May cause fetal/neonatal mortality/morbidity. **Pregnancy Category D.**

INTERACTIONS

DRUG INTERACTIONS: Alcohol, diuretics, hypotensive agents may increase effects. NSAIDs may decrease effect. Potassium-sparing diuretics, potassium supplements may cause hyperkalemia. May increase lithium concentration, toxicity. **ALTERED LAB VALUES:** May increase potassium, SGOT (AST), SGPT (ALT), alkaline phosphatase, bilirubin, BUN, creatinine. May decrease sodium. May cause positive ANA titer.

SIDE EFFECTS

OCCASIONAL: Headache, cough. **RARE:** Orthostatic hypotension, dizziness, fatigue, diarrhea, GI distress.

ADVERSE REACTIONS/TOXIC EFFECTS

Excessive hypotension ("first-dose syncope") may occur in those w/CHF, severely salt/volume depleted. Angioedema (swelling of face/lips), hyperkalemia occur rarely. Agranulocytosis, neutropenia may be noted in those w/ impaired renal function or collagen vascular disease (systemic lupus erythematosus, scleroderma). Nephrotic syndrome may be noted in those w/history of renal disease.

NURSING IMPLICATIONS

BASELINE ASSESSMENT:

Obtain B/P immediately before each dose, in addition to regular monitoring (be alert to fluctuations). Renal function tests should be performed before therapy begins. In those w/renal impairment, autoimmune disease, or taking drugs that affect leukocytes or immune response, CBC and differential count should be performed before therapy begins and q2wk for 3 months, then periodically thereafter.

INTERVENTION/EVALUATION:

If excessive reduction in B/P occurs, place pt in supine position w/ legs elevated. Assist w/ambulation if dizziness occurs. Assess for urinary frequency. Auscultate lung sounds for rales, wheezing in those w/CHF. Monitor urinalysis for proteinuria. Monitor serum potassium levels in those on concurrent diuretic therapy. Monitor pattern of daily bowel activity and stool consistency.

PATIENT/FAMILY TEACHING:

Report any sign of infection (sore throat, fever). Several weeks may be needed for full therapeutic effect of B/P reduction. Skipping doses or voluntarily discontinuing drug may produce severe, rebound hypertension. To reduce hypotensive effect, rise slowly from lying to sitting position and permit legs to dangle from bed momentarily before standing.

furazolidone

fur-ah-zoe´lih-dun
(Furoxone)

CANADIAN AVAILABILITY:
Furoxone

CLASSIFICATION

Antibacterial, antiprotozoal

PHARMACOKINETICS

Poorly absorbed from GI tract. Distributed to tissues. Rapidly, extensively metabolized. Primarily excreted in urine.

ACTION

Interferes w/several bacterial enzyme systems inhibiting bacterial carbohydrate metabolism; MAO inhibitor. Bactericidal.

USES

Treatment of diarrhea/enteritis caused by susceptible bacteria or protozoa.

PO ADMINISTRATION

1. May give w/o regard to meals.
2. Scored tablets may be crushed.

INDICATIONS/DOSAGE/ROUTES

Diarrhea, enteritis:
PO: Adults, elderly: 100 mg 4 times/day. **Children >5 yr:** 25-50 mg 4 times/day. **Children 1-4 yr:** 17-25 mg 4 times/day. **Children 1-12 mo:** 8-17 mg 4 times/day. Do not exceed 8.8 mg/kg/day (increases possibility of nausea, vomiting).

PRECAUTIONS

CONTRAINDICATIONS: History of hypersensitivity to furazolidone. Do not administer to infants <1 mo of age (risk of hemolytic anemia). **CAUTIONS:** Those w/G-6-PD deficiency. **PREGNANCY/LACTATION:** Not known whether drug crosses placenta or is distributed in breast milk. **Pregnancy Category C.**

INTERACTIONS

DRUG INTERACTIONS: Alcohol may rarely cause disulfiram reaction. Tricyclic antidepressants, MAO inhibitors, sympathomimetics may increase B/P. **ALTERED LAB VALUES:** None significant.

SIDE EFFECTS

COMMON: Nausea, vomiting. **OCCASIONAL:** Diarrhea, abdominal pain, headache, malaise. **RARE:** Hypoglycemia, hypersensitivity reactions: hypotension, angioedema, urticaria, arthralgia, fever, rash.

ADVERSE REACTIONS/TOXIC EFFECTS

Erythema multiforme, hemolytic

anemia. Potential for hypertensive crisis w/high dosage or prolonged therapy.

NURSING IMPLICATIONS

BASELINE ASSESSMENT:

Question for history of hypersensitivity to furazolidone. Obtain specimens for diagnostic tests before giving first dose (therapy may begin before results are known).

INTERVENTION/EVALUATION:

Evaluate food tolerance. Determine pattern of bowel activity. Assess skin for rash, urticaria. Monitor hematology and blood glucose results. Check for signs of hypoglycemia: sweating, nervousness, tremor, light-headedness, palpitations.

PATIENT/FAMILY TEACHING:

Complete full course of therapy. Do not take any medications w/o checking w/physician. Avoid alcohol intake (e.g., alcoholic beverages, cough syrups, elixirs, tonics) during therapy and for at least 4 days after completion (read food labels). Avoid tyramine-containing foods/beverages (e.g., bananas, avocados, strong unpasteurized cheeses, yogurt, fermented products). Reduce caffeine intake: coffee, tea, colas, chocolate. In event of nausea, vomiting, diarrhea, rash headache, notify nurse/physician.

furosemide

feur-oh´sah-mide

(Lasix)

CANADIAN AVAILABILITY:

Apo-Furosemide, Lasix, Novosemide

CLASSIFICATION

Diuretic: Loop

PHARMACOKINETICS

	ONSET	PEAK	DURATION
PO	30-60 min	1-2 hrs	6-8 hrs
IM	—	30 min	—
IV	5 min	20-60 min	2 hrs

Well absorbed from GI tract. Protein binding: 91-97%. Partially metabolized in liver. Primarily excreted in urine (in severe renal impairment, nonrenal clearance increases). Half-life: 30-90 min (increased in decreased renal, liver function, neonates).

ACTION

Enhances excretion of sodium, chloride, potassium by direct action at ascending limb of loop of Henle.

USES

Treatment of edema associated w/CHF, chronic renal failure including nephrotic syndrome, hepatic cirrhosis, acute pulmonary edema. Treats hypertension, either alone or in combination w/ other antihypertensives.

STORAGE/HANDLING

Solution appears clear, colorless. Discard yellow injections or discolored tablet.

PO/IM/IV ADMINISTRATION

PO:

1. Give w/food to avoid GI upset, preferably w/breakfast (may prevent nocturia).

IM:

Temporary pain at injection site may be noted.

IV:

1. May give undiluted but is compatible w/5% dextrose in water, 0.9% NS or lactated Ringer's solutions.
2. Administer direct IV over 1-2 min, preferably through Y tube or 3-way stopcock.
3. Do not exceed administration rate of 4 mg/min in those w/renal impairment.

INDICATIONS/DOSAGE/ROUTE

Edema:
PO: Adults: 20-80 mg daily given as single dose in morning. May increase in 20-40 mg increments q6-8h. Give effective dose 1-2 times/day. **Maximum:** 600 mg.
IM/IV: Adults: 20-40 mg given as single injection. May increase in 20 mg increments no sooner than 2 hr after previous dose. May give effective dose 1-2 times/day.

Acute pulmonary edema:
IV: Adults: 40 mg slow IV, given over 1-2 min. If satisfactory response is not reached in 1 hr, may increase to 80 mg slow IV, given over 1-2 min.

Hypertension:
PO: Adults: Initially 40 mg 2 times/day based on pt response.

Usual elderly dosage:
IM/IV/PO: Elderly: Initially, 20 mg/day. May increase slowly to desired response.

Usual dosage for children:
PO: Children: 2 mg/kg given as single dose. May be increased in 1-2 mg/kg increments q6-8h. **Maximum:** 6 mg/kg/day.
IV/IM: Children: 1 mg/kg given as single dose. May increase by 1 mg/kg no sooner than 2 hrs after previous dose. **Maximum:** 6 mg/kg/day.

PRECAUTIONS

CONTRAINDICATIONS: Anuria, hepatic coma, severe electrolyte depletion. **CAUTIONS:** Acute MI, oliguria, hepatic cirrhosis, history of gout, diabetes, systemic lupus erythematosus, pancreatitis. **PREGNANCY/LACTATION:** Crosses placenta; distributed in breast milk. **Pregnancy Category C.**

INTERACTIONS

DRUG INTERACTIONS: Amphotericin, ototoxic, nephrotoxic agents may increase toxicity. May decrease effect of anticoagulants, heparin. Hypokalemia-causing agents may increase risk of hypokalemia. May increase risk of lithium toxicity. Probenecid may increase concentrations. **ALTERED LAB VALUES:** May increase glucose, BUN, uric acid. May decrease calcium, chloride, magnesium, potassium, sodium.

SIDE EFFECTS

EXPECTED: Increase in urinary frequency/volume. **FREQUENT:** Nausea, gastric upset w/cramping, diarrhea, or constipation, electrolyte disturbances. **OCCASIONAL:** Dizziness, light-headedness, headache, blurred vision, paresthesia, photosensitivity, rash, weakness, urinary frequency/bladder spasm, restlessness, diaphoresis. **RARE:** Flank pain, loin pain.

ADVERSE REACTIONS/TOXIC EFFECTS

Vigorous diuresis may lead to profound water loss and electrolyte depletion, resulting in hypokalemia, hyponatremia, dehydration. Sudden volume depletion may result in increased risk of thrombosis, circulatory collapse, sudden death. Acute hypotensive episodes may also occur, sometimes several days after beginning of therapy. Ototoxicity manifested as deafness, vertigo, tinnitus (ringing/roaring in ears) may occur, especially in those w/severe renal impairment. Can exacerbate diabetes mellitus, systemic lupus erythematosus, gout, pancreatitis. Blood dyscrasias have been reported.

NURSING IMPLICATIONS

BASELINE ASSESSMENT:

Check vital signs, especially B/P for hypotension before administration. Assess baseline electrolytes, particularly check for low potassium. Assess edema, skin turgor, mucous membranes for hydration status. Assess muscle strength, mental status. Note skin temperature, moisture. Obtain baseline weight. Initiate I&O monitoring.

INTERVENTION/EVALUATION:

Monitor B/P, vital signs, electrolytes, I&O, weight. Note extent of diuresis. Watch for changes from initial assessment (hypokalemia may result in changes in muscle strength, tremor, muscle cramps, change in mental status, cardiac arrhythmias). Hyponatremia may result in confusion, thirst, cold/clammy skin.

PATIENT/FAMILY TEACHING:

Expect increased frequency and volume of urination. Report irregular heartbeat, signs of electrolyte imbalances (noted above), hearing abnormalities (such as sense of fullness in ears, ringing/roaring in ears). Eat foods high in potassium such as whole grains (cereals), legumes, meat, bananas, apricots, orange juice, potatoes (white, sweet) raisins. Avoid sun/sunlamps.

gabapentin

gah-bah-pen'tin

(Neurontin)

CLASSIFICATION

Anticonvulsant

PHARMACOKINETICS

Well absorbed from GI tract (not affected by food). Widely distributed. Crosses blood-brain barrier. Protein binding: <3%. Primarily excreted unchanged in urine. Removed by hemodialysis. Half-life: 5-7 hrs (increased in decreased renal function, elderly).

ACTION

Exact mechanism unknown. May be due to increased GABA synthesis rate, increased GABA accumulation, or binding to as yet undefined receptor in brain tissue.

USES

Adjunctive therapy in treatment of partial seizures and partial seizures w/secondary generalization in adults.

PO ADMINISTRATION

1. May be given w/o regard to meals; may give w/food to avoid or reduce GI upset.
2. If treatment is discontinued or anticonvulsant therapy is added, do so gradually over at least 1

week (reduces risk of loss of seizure control).

INDICATIONS/DOSAGE/ROUTES

Seizure control:

NOTE: Maximum time between doses should not exceed 12 hrs.

PO: Adults, elderly: 900-1800 mg/day given in divided doses q8h. May titrate to effective dose rapidly: *Day 1:* 300 mg (give at bedtime). *Day 2:* 300 mg q12h. *Day 3:* 300 mg q8h.

Renal function impairment:

Based on creatinine clearance:

CREATININE CLEARANCE	DOSAGE
>60 ml/min	400 mg q8h
30-60 ml/min	300 mg q12h
15-30 ml/min	300 mg daily
<15 ml/min	300 mg every other day
Hemodialysis	200-300 mg after each 4 hr hemodialysis

PRECAUTIONS

CONTRAINDICATIONS: None significant. **CAUTIONS:** Renal impairment. Discontinue/add anticonvulsant therapy gradually (reduces loss of seizure control). Children <18 yrs of age. **PREGNANCY/LACTATION:** Unknown whether it is distributed in breast milk. **Pregnancy Category C.**

INTERACTIONS

DRUG INTERACTIONS: None significant. **ALTERED LAB VALUES:** May decrease WBCs.

SIDE EFFECTS

FREQUENT: Ataxia, dizziness, fatigue, nystagmus, somnolence. **OCCASIONAL:** Increased weight, dyspepsia, myalgia, tremor, nervousness, rhinitis, pharyngitis, blurred vision, nausea, vomiting.

ADVERSE REACTIONS/TOXIC EFFECTS

Abrupt withdrawal may increase seizure frequency. Overdosage may result in double vision, slurred speech, drowsiness, lethargy, diarrhea.

NURSING IMPLICATIONS

BASELINE ASSESSMENT:

Assess type, onset, duration, intensity, and frequency of seizures. Routine laboratory monitoring of blood serum levels unnecessary for safe use.

INTERVENTION/EVALUATION:

Provide safety measures as needed. Assess for seizure activity.

PATIENT/FAMILY TEACHING:

Take gabapentin only as prescribed; do not abruptly stop taking drug because seizure frequency may be increased. Do not drive, operate machinery, or perform activities requiring mental acuity due to potential dizziness, somnolence. Avoid alcohol. Carry identification card/bracelet to note anticonvulsant therapy.

gallium nitrate

gal'lee-um

(Ganite)

CLASSIFICATION

Antihypercalcemic

PHARMACOKINETICS

Primarily excreted in urine. Half-life: 24 hrs.

ACTION

Inhibits abnormal bone resorption, reduces flow of calcium from resorbing bone into blood (decreases total and ionized serum calcium).

USES

Treatment of hypercalcemia or malignancy that is inadequately managed by oral hydration alone. Use concomitantly w/saline (increases urine output) and diuretics (increases rate of calcium excretion).

STORAGE/HANDLING

Store undiluted vials at room temperature. After dilution, stable for 48 hrs at room temperature or up to 7 days refrigerated.

IV ADMINISTRATION

1. Must dilute daily dose in 1000 ml 0.9% NaCl or 5% dextrose.

INDICATIONS/DOSAGE/ROUTES

Hypercalcemia:
IV INFUSION: Adults, elderly: 100-200 mg/m^2/day over 24 hrs for 5 days. May repeat after waiting 3-4 wks.

PRECAUTIONS

CONTRAINDICATIONS: Decreases renal function when serum creatinine >2.5 mg/dl. **CAUTIONS:** Renal function when serum creatinine 2-2.5 mg/dl. **PREGNANCY/LACTATION:** Unknown whether excreted in breast milk. **Pregnancy Category C.**

INTERACTIONS

DRUG INTERACTIONS: Calcium-containing medications, products, vitamin D may decrease effect. Nephrotoxic medications may increase nephrotoxicity. **ALTERED LAB VALUES:** None significant.

SIDE EFFECTS

FREQUENT: Hypophosphatemia (e.g., bone pain, muscle weakness, anorexia), nephrotoxicity (blood in urine, nausea, vomiting), diarrhea, metallic taste. **OCCASIONAL:** Hypocalcemia (abnormal cramps, confusion, muscle spasms). **RARE:** Anemia.

ADVERSE REACTIONS/TOXIC EFFECTS

None significant.

NURSING IMPLICATIONS

BASELINE ASSESSMENT:

Assure no other nephrotoxic drugs are being given concurrently. Determine initial serum calcium and creatinine levels. Establish adequate hydration w/oral or IV fluids, preferably saline, to counteract dehydration (caused by hypercalcemia) and increase excretion of calcium. Assure satisfactory urine output (2L/day recommended) before starting gallium therapy.

INTERVENTION/EVALUATION:

Throughout therapy maintain adequate hydration w/o overhydrating pt w/compromised cardiovascular status. Monitor urinary output. Assess serum calcium, phosphorus, creatinine, and BUN frequently (therapy should be discontinued if serum creatinine level exceeds 2.5 mg/dl).

PATIENT/FAMILY TEACHING:

Explain rationale of therapy and importance of fluids, I&O.

ganciclovir sodium

gan-sye′klo-vir
(Cytovene)

CANADIAN AVAILABILITY:
Cytovene

CLASSIFICATION

Antiviral

PHARMACOKINETICS

Widely distributed. Protein binding: 1%. Undergoes minimal metabolism. Primarily excreted unchanged in urine. Removed by hemodialysis. Half-life: 2.5-3.6 hrs (increased in decreased renal function).

ACTION

Converted intracellularly, inhibits viral DNA synthesis by competition w/viral DNA polymerases and by direct incorporation into growing viral DNA chains. Congener of acyclovir.

USES

Treatment of cytomegalovirus (CMV) retinitis in immunocompromised pts (e.g., AIDS, bone marrow recipients); prevention of CMV in transplant pts.

STORAGE/HANDLING

Store vials at room temperature. Reconstituted solution in vial stable for 12 hrs at room temperature. Do not refrigerate. After dilution, refrigerate, use within 24 hrs. Discard if precipitate forms, discoloration occurs. Avoid exposure to skin, eyes, mucus membranes. Wear latex gloves.

IV ADMINISTRATION

IV:

1. Latex gloves and safety glasses should be used during preparation and handling of solution. Avoid inhalation. (If solution contacts skin, mucous membrane wash carefully w/soap and water; rinse eyes thoroughly w/plain water).
2. Reconstitute 500 mg vial w/10 ml sterile water for injection to provide a concentration of 50 mg/ml; do *not* use bacteriostatic water (contains parabens, which is incompatible w/ganciclovir).
3. Further dilute w/100 ml D5W, 0.9% NaCl, or other compatible fluid to provide a concentration of 5 mg/ml.
4. Administer only by IV infusion over 1 hr.
5. Do not give IV injection or rapid infusion (increases toxicity).
6. Do not give IM or subQ; protect from infiltration (high pH causes severe tissue irritation).
7. Use veins w/adequate blood to permit rapid dilution and dissemination of ganciclovir (minimize phlebitis); central venous catheters tunneled under subcutaneous tissue may reduce catheter-associated infection.

INDICATIONS/DOSAGE/ROUTES

NOTE: Do not give if neutrophil count <500 cells/mm^3 or platelets $<25{,}000$/mm^3.

CMV retinitis treatment:
IV: Adults: Initially, 5 mg/kg q12h for 14-21 days.

CMV disease prevention:
IV: Adults: Initially, 5 mg/kg q12h for 7-14 days.

Maintenance:
IV: Adults: 5 mg/kg/day for 7 days or 6 mg/kg 5 days.

Dosage in renal impairment:

CREATININE CLEARANCE	DOSAGE	DOSING INTERVAL
≥ 80 ml/min	5 mg/kg	12 hrs
50-79 ml/min	2.5 mg/kg	12 hrs
25-49 ml/min	2.5 mg/kg	24 hrs
<25 ml/min	1.25 mg/kg	24 hrs

PRECAUTIONS

CONTRAINDICATIONS: Hypersensitivity to ganciclovir or acyclovir. Not for use in immunocompetent persons or those w/congenital or neonatal CMV disease. **CAUTIONS:** Extreme caution in children because of long-term carcinogenicity, reproductive toxicity. Renal impairment, preexisting cytopenias or history of cytopenic reactions to other drugs, elderly (at greater risk of renal impairment). **PREGNANCY/LACTATION:** Effective contraception should be used during therapy; ganciclovir should not be used during pregnancy. Nursing should be discontinued. May be resumed no sooner than 72 hrs after the last dose of ganciclovir. **Pregnancy Category C.**

INTERACTIONS

DRUG INTERACTIONS: Bone marrow depressants may increase bone marrow depression. May increase risk of seizures w/imipenem-cilastatin. May increase hematologic toxicity w/zidovudine. **ALTERED LAB VALUES:** May increase SGOT (AST), SGPT (ALT), alkaline phosphatase, bilirubin.

SIDE EFFECTS

FREQUENT: Neutropenia (up to 50% of pts), thrombocytopenia (20% of pts), platelets reduced below 20,000/mm^3 (10% of pts). **OCCASIONAL:** Retinal detachment, nausea/vomiting, fever, rash, confusion, increased creatinine clearance. **RARE:** Headache, dizziness, thought disorders, behavioral changes, psychosis, coma, seizures, abnormal dreams, intention tremor, chills, malaise, cardiac arrhythmias, hyper/hypotension, pruritus, hematuria, diarrhea, paresthesia, ataxia, edema alopecia.

ADVERSE REACTIONS/TOXIC EFFECTS

Hematologic toxicity, GI hemorrhage occur rarely.

NURSING IMPLICATIONS

BASELINE ASSESSMENT:

Question for hypersensitivity to ganciclovir or acyclovir. Evaluate hematologic baseline. Obtain specimens for support of differential diagnosis (urine, feces, blood, throat) because usually retinal infection due to hematogenous dissemination.

INTERVENTION/EVALUATION:

Monitor I&O and assure adequate hydration (minimum 1500 ml/24 hrs). Check IV site, rate of infusion every 15 min during dosage administration. Diligently evaluate hematology reports for potentially life-threatening neutropenia, thrombocytopenia, decreased platelets (hold ganciclovir and notify physician immediately of neutrophil count less than 500/mm^3, platelet count less than 25,000/mm^3). Monitor B/P at least 2 times/day for hyper/hypotension. Check temperature at least 2 times/day for onset or increase in fever. Assess pt carefully for change (i.e., increased bleeding tendency, signs of infection). Question pt regarding vision, therapeutic improvement, or complications. Be alert for behavior changes, thought disorders, confusion, or other nervous system effects and report promptly. Assess for rash, pruritus.

PATIENT/FAMILY TEACHING:

Ganciclovir provides suppression, not cure of CMV retinitis. Frequent blood tests and eye exams are necessary during therapy because of toxic nature of drug. It is essential to report any new symptom promptly. May temporarily or permanently inhibit sperm production in men, suppress fertility in women. Barrier contraception should be used during and for 90 days after therapy because of mutagenic potential.

gemfibrozil

gem-fie´bro-zill

(Lopid)

CANADIAN AVAILABILITY:
Lopid

CLASSIFICATION

Antihyperlipoproteinemic

PHARMACOKINETICS

Well absorbed from GI tract. Metabolized in liver. Primarily excreted in urine. Half-life: 1.5 hrs.

ACTION

Lowers serum cholesterol and triglycerides (decreases VLDL, LDL, increases HDL). Inhibits lipolysis of fat in adipose tissue; decreases liver uptake of free fatty acids (reduces hepatic triglyceride production). Inhibits synthesis of VLDL carrier apolipoprotein B.

USES

Adjunct to diet therapy to decrease elevated serum triglyceride concentration in selected pts w/increased risk of pancreatitis or recurrent abdominal pain typical of pancreatitis.

PO ADMINISTRATION

Give 30 min before morning and evening meals.

INDICATIONS/DOSAGE/ROUTES

Hypertriglyceridemia:
PO: Adults, elderly: 900 mg to 1.5 Gm/day in 2 divided doses.

PRECAUTIONS

CONTRAINDICATIONS: Hypersensitivity to gemfibrozil, hepatic dysfunction (including primary biliary cirrhosis), severe renal dysfunction, preexisting gallbladder disease. **CAUTIONS:** Hypothyroidism, diabetes mellitus, estrogen or anticoagulant therapy. **PREGNANCY/LACTATION:** Not known whether drug crosses placenta or is distributed in breast milk. Decision to discontinue nursing or drug should be based on potential for serious adverse effects. **Pregnancy Category B.**

INTERACTIONS

DRUG INTERACTIONS: May increase effect of warfarin. May cause rhabdomyolysis, leading to acute renal failure w/lovastatin. **ALTERED LAB VALUES:** May increase SGOT (AST), SGPT (ALT), alkaline phosphatase, bilirubin, creatinine kinase, LDH. May decrease Hgb, Hct, potassium, leukocyte counts.

SIDE EFFECTS

FREQUENT: Abdominal/epigastric pain, diarrhea. **OCCASIONAL:** Nausea, vomiting, flatulence, headache, dizziness, blurred vision, rash, pruritus. **RARE:** Head, neck, or extremity pain, anemia, leukopenia, hyperglycemia (particularly in those receiving insulin or oral antihyperglycemics).

ADVERSE REACTIONS/TOXIC EFFECTS

Cholelithiasis, cholecystitis, acute appendicitis, pancreatitis, malignancy occur rarely.

NURSING IMPLICATIONS

BASELINE ASSESSMENT:

Question for history of hypersensitivity to gemfibrozil. Assess baseline lab results: serum glucose, triglyceride, cholesterol levels, liver function tests, CBC.

INTERVENTION/EVALUATION:

Evaluate food tolerance. Determine pattern of bowel activity. Monitor LDL, VLDL, serum triglyceride, and cholesterol lab results for therapeutic response. Assess for rash, pruritus. Check for headache and dizziness, blurred vision. Monitor liver function and hematology tests. Assess for pain, esp. right upper quadrant/epigastric pain suggestive of adverse gallbladder effects. Monitor serum glucose for those receiving insulin or oral antihyperglycemics.

PATIENT/FAMILY TEACHING:

Follow special diet (important part of treatment). Do not take other medication w/o checking w/ physician. Do not stop medication w/o physician's knowledge. Periodic lab tests are essential part of therapy. Notify physician in event of new symptoms, particularly abdominal/epigastric pain. Do not drive or perform other activities that require alert response if dizziness occurs.

gentamicin sulfate

jen-tah-my´sin

(Garamycin, Genoptic, Gentacidin, Jenamicin)

CANADIAN AVAILABILITY:

Alcomicin, Cidomycin, Garamycin, Gentrasul

CLASSIFICATION

Antibiotic: Aminoglycoside

PHARMACOKINETICS

Rapid, complete absorption after IM administration. Widely distributed (does not cross blood-brain barrier, low concentrations in CSF). Protein binding: 10%. Excreted unchanged in urine. Removed by hemodialysis. Half-life: 2-4 hrs (increased in decreased renal function, neonates; decreased in cystic fibrosis, burn or febrile pts).

ACTION

Bactericidal. Irreversibly binds to protein on 30S subunit of bacterial ribosome, interfering in protein synthesis of susceptible microorganisms.

USES

Parenteral: Treatment of skin/skin structure, bone, joint, respiratory tract, intra-abdominal, complicated urinary tract, and acute pelvic infections; postop, burns, septicemia, meningitis. *Ophthal-*

mic: Ointment/solution for superficial eye infections. *Topical:* Cream/ointment for superficial skin infections. Ophthalmic or topical applications may be combined w/systemic administration for serious, extensive infections.

STORAGE/HANDLING

Store vials, ophthalmic, topical preparations at room temperature. Solutions appear clear or slightly yellow. Intermittent IV infusion (piggyback) stable for 24 hrs at room temperature. Discard if precipitate forms. Use intrathecal forms immediately after preparation. Discard unused portion.

IM/IV/INTRATHECAL/ OPHTHALMIC ADMINISTRATION

NOTE: Coordinate peak and trough lab draws w/administration times.

IM:

1. To minimize discomfort, give deep IM slowly. Less painful if injected into gluteus maximus rather than lateral aspect of thigh.

IV:

1. Dilute w/50-200 ml 5% dextrose, 0.9% NaCl, or other compatible fluid. Amount of diluent for infants, children depends on individual needs.
2. Infuse over 30-60 min for adults, older children, and over 60-120 min for infants, young children.
3. Alternating IV sites, use large veins to reduce risk of phlebitis.

INTRATHECAL:

1. Use only 2 mg/ml intrathecal preparation w/o preservative.
2. Mix w/10% estimated CSF volume or sodium chloride.
3. Give over 3-5 min.

OPHTHALMIC:

1. Place finger on lower eyelid and pull out until a pocket is formed between eye and lower lid.
2. Hold dropper above pocket and place correct number of drops (¼-½ inch ointment) into pocket. Close eye gently.
3. *Solution:* Apply digital pressure to lacrimal sac for 1-2 min (minimizes drainage into nose and throat, reducing risk of systemic effects). *Ointment:* Close eye for 1-2 min, rolling eyeball (increases contact area of drug to eye).
4. Remove excess solution or ointment around eye w/tissue.

INDICATIONS/DOSAGE/ROUTES

NOTE: Space parenteral doses evenly around the clock. Dosage based on ideal body weight. Peak, trough level determined periodically to maintain desired serum concentrations (minimizes risk of toxicity). *Recommended peak level:* 4-10 mcg/ml; *trough level:* 1-2 mcg/ml.

Moderate to severe infections:
IM/IV Adults, elderly: 3 mg/kg/day in divided doses q8h. **Children:** 6-7.5 mg/kg/day in divided doses q8h. **Infants, neonates:** 7.5 mg/kg/day in divided doses q8h. **Premature or full-term neonates <7 days:** 5/mg/kg/day in divided doses q12h.

Life-threatening infections:
IM/IV: Adults, elderly: Up to 5 mg/kg/day in divided doses 3-4 times/day.
INTRATHECAL: Adults, elderly: 4-8 mg as single daily dose (w/IM/IV doses). **Children >3 mo:** 1-2 mg as single daily dose (w/IM/IV doses).

Dosage in renal impairment:
Dose and/or frequency is mod-

G

ified according to degree of renal impairment, serum concentration of drug. After loading dose of 1-2 mg/kg, maintenance dose/frequency based on serum creatinine or creatinine clearance.

Usual ophthalmic dosage:
OPHTHALMIC OINTMENT:
Adults, elderly: Thin strip to conjunctiva q6-12h.
OPHTHALMIC SOLUTION:
Adults, elderly: 1 drop q4-8h to conjunctiva.

Usual topical dosage:
TOPICAL: Adults, elderly: Apply 3-4 times/day.

PRECAUTIONS

CONTRAINDICATIONS: Hypersensitivity to gentamicin, other aminoglycosides (cross-sensitivity). Sulfite sensitivity may result in anaphylaxis, especially in asthmatics. **CAUTIONS:** Elderly, neonates because of renal insufficiency or immaturity; neuromuscular disorders (potential for respiratory depression), prior hearing loss, vertigo, renal impairment. Cumulative effects may occur w/concurrent systemic administration and topical application to large areas. **PREGNANCY/LACTATION:** Readily crosses placenta, not known whether distributed in breast milk. May produce fetal nephrotoxicity. **Pregnancy Category C.**

INTERACTIONS

DRUG INTERACTIONS: Other aminoglycosides, nephrotoxic, ototoxic producing medications may increase toxicity. May increase effects of neuromuscular blocking agents. **ALTERED LAB VALUES:** May increase BUN, SGPT (ALT), SGOT (AST), bilirubin, creatinine, LDH concentrations; may decrease serum calcium, magnesium, potassium, sodium concentrations.

SIDE EFFECTS

OCCASIONAL: Pain, induration at IM injection site; phlebitis, thrombophlebitis w/IV administration; hypersensitivity reactions: rash, fever, urticaria, pruritus. *Ophthalmic:* Burning, tearing, itching. **RARE:** Alopecia, hypertension, weakness. *Topical:* Redness, itching.

ADVERSE REACTIONS/TOXIC EFFECTS

Nephrotoxicity (evidenced by increased BUN and serum creatinine, decreased creatinine clearance) may be reversible if drug stopped at first sign of symptoms; irreversible otoxicity (tinnitus, dizziness, ringing/roaring in ears, reduced hearing) and neurotoxicity (headache, dizziness, lethargy, tremors, visual disturbances) occur occasionally. Risk is greater w/ higher dosages, prolonged therapy, or if solution is applied directly to mucosa. Superinfections, particularly w/fungi, may result from bacterial imbalance via any route of administration. Ophthalmic application may cause paresthesia of conjunctiva, mydriasis.

NURSING IMPLICATIONS

BASELINE ASSESSMENT:

Dehydration must be treated before parenteral therapy is begun. Establish baseline hearing acuity. Question for history of allergies, especially to aminoglycosides and sulfite (and parabens for topical/ophthalmic routes). Obtain specimens for culture, sensitivity before giving first dose (therapy may begin before results are known).

INTERVENTION/EVALUATION:

Monitor I&O (maintain hydration), urinalysis (casts, RBCs, WBCs, decrease in specific gravity). Monitor results of peak/trough blood tests. Be alert to ototoxic and neurotoxic symptoms (see Adverse Reactions/Toxic Effects). Check IM injection site for pain, induration. Evaluate IV site for phlebitis (heat, pain, red streaking over vein). Assess for rash (*ophthalmic*—assess for redness, burning, itching, tearing; *topical*—assess for redness, itching). Be alert for superinfection, particularly genital/anal pruritus, changes in oral mucosa, diarrhea. When treating those w/neuromuscular disorders, assess respiratory response carefully.

PATIENT/FAMILY TEACHING:

Continue antibiotic for full length of treatment. Space doses evenly. Discomfort may occur w/IM injection. Blurred vision or tearing may occur briefly after each ophthalmic dose. Notify physician in event of any hearing, visual, balance, urinary problems, even after therapy is completed. *Ophthalmic:* Contact physician if tearing, redness, or irritation continues. *Topical:* Cleanse area gently before applying; notify physician if redness, itching occurs. Do not take other medication w/o consulting physician. Lab tests are an essential part of therapy.

glipizide

glip ih-zide
(Glucotrol)

CLASSIFICATION

Hypoglycemic: Oral

PHARMACOKINETICS

	ONSET	PEAK	DURATION
PO	10-30 min	0.5-2 hrs	24 hrs

Well absorbed from GI tract. Protein binding: 98-99%. Metabolized in liver. Excreted in urine. Half-life: 2-4 hrs.

ACTION

Promotes release of insulin from beta cells of pancreas, decreases hepatic glycogenolysis and gluconeogenesis, increases insulin sensitivity at peripheral sites.

USES

Adjunct to diet/exercise in management of stable, mild to moderately severe non-insulin-dependent diabetes mellitus (type II, NIDDM). May be used to supplement insulin in those w/type I diabetes mellitus.

PO ADMINISTRATION

May take w/food (response better if taken 15-30 min before meals).

INDICATIONS/DOSAGE/ROUTES

Diabetes mellitus:
PO: Adults: Initially, 5 mg/day (2.5 mg in geriatric/those w/liver disease). Adjust dosage in 2.5-5 mg increments at intervals of several days. **Maximum single dose:** 15 mg. **Maximum dose/day:** 40 mg. **Maintenance:** 10 mg/day.

Usual elderly dosage:
PO: Elderly: Initially, 2.5-5 mg/day. May increase by 2.5-5 mg/day q1-2wks.

PRECAUTIONS

CONTRAINDICATIONS: Sole

therapy for type I diabetes mellitus, diabetic complications (ketosis, acidosis, diabetic coma), stress situations (severe infection, trauma, surgery), hypersensitivity to drug, severe renal or hepatic impairment. **CAUTIONS:** Elderly, malnourished, or debilitated, those w/renal or hepatic dysfunction, cardiac disease, adrenal or pituitary insufficiency, history of hepatic porphyria. **PREGNANCY/LACTATION:** Insulin is drug of choice during pregnancy; glipizide given within 1 mo of delivery may produce neonatal hypoglycemia. Drug crosses placenta; distributed in breast milk. **Pregnancy Category C.**

INTERACTIONS

DRUG INTERACTIONS: May increase effect of oral anticoagulants; chloramphenicol, MAO inhibitor, salicylates, sulfonamides may increase effect; beta-blockers may increase hypoglycemic effect; mask signs of hypoglycemia; may increase effects of insulin. **ALTERED LAB VALUES:** May increase alkaline phosphatase, SGOT (AST), LDH, creatinine, BUN.

SIDE EFFECTS

FREQUENT: Nausea, heartburn, stomach pain. **OCCASIONAL:** Anorexia, vomiting, diarrhea, constipation, pruritus. **INFREQUENT:** Skin reactions (may be transient), dizziness, drowsiness, headache. **RARE:** Proctocolitis.

ADVERSE REACTIONS/TOXIC EFFECTS

Hypoglycemia may occur because of overdosage, insufficient food intake esp. w/increased glucose demands, GI hemorrhage, cholestatic hepatic jaundice, leukopenia, thrombocytopenia, pancytopenia, agranulocytosis, aplastic or hemolytic anemia occur rarely.

NURSING IMPLICATIONS

BASELINE ASSESSMENT:

Question for hypersensitivity to glipizide. Check blood glucose level. Discuss life-style to determine extent of learning, emotional needs. Assure follow-up instruction if pt/family do not thoroughly understand diabetes management or glucose-testing technique.

INTERVENTION/EVALUATION:

Monitor blood glucose and food intake. Assess for hypoglycemia (cool wet skin, tremors, dizziness, anxiety, headache, tachycardia, numbness in mouth, hunger, diplopia) or hyperglycemia (polyuria, polyphagia, polydipsia, nausea, vomiting, dim vision, fatigue, deep rapid breathing). Check for adverse skin reactions, jaundice. Monitor hematology reports. Assess for bleeding or bruising. Be alert to conditions that alter glucose requirements: fever, increased activity or stress, surgical procedure.

PATIENT/FAMILY TEACHING:

Prescribed diet is principal part of treatment; do not skip or delay meals. Diabetes mellitus requires lifelong control. Check blood glucose/urine as ordered. Carry candy, sugar packets, or other sugar supplements for immediate response to hypoglycemia. Wear medical alert identification. Check w/physician when glucose demands are altered (e.g., fever, infection, trauma, stress, heavy physical activity). Avoid alcoholic beverages. Do not take other medication w/o consulting physician. Weight control, exercise, hygiene (including foot care) and nonsmoking are essential part of therapy. Protect skin, limit sun exposure. Avoid exposure to infections. Select clothing, positions that do not restrict blood flow. Notify physician promptly of skin eruptions, itching, bleeding, yellow skin, dark urine. Inform dentist, physician, or surgeon of this medication before any treatment.

glucagon hydrochloride

glōō´ka-gon

(Glucagon Emergency Kit)

CANADIAN AVAILABILITY:
Glucagon Emergency Kit

CLASSIFICATION

Antihypoglycemic

PHARMACOKINETICS

Well absorbed after IM, SubQ administration. Undergoes enzymatic proteolysis in liver/kidney. Half-life: 10 minutes. Peak hyperglycemia occurs within 30 min, lasting 1-2 hrs. Return to consciousness in 5-20 min.

ACTION

Promotes hepatic glycogenolysis, gluconeogenesis. Stimulates enzyme to increase production of c-AMP. This results in increased plasma glucose concentration, relaxant effect on smooth muscle and inotropic myocardial effect.

USES

Treatment of severe hypoglycemia in diabetic pts. Not for use in chronic hypoglycemia or hypoglycemia due to starvation, adrenal insufficiency since liver glycogen unavailable. Diagnostic aid in radiographic examination of GI tract.

STORAGE/HANDLING

Store vial at room temperature. After reconstitution, stable for 48 hrs if refrigerated. If reconstituted w/sterile water for injection, use immediately. Do not use glucagon solution unless clear.

SubQ/IM/IV ADMINISTRATION

NOTE: Place pt on side to avoid potential aspiration (glucagon, as well as hypoglycemia, may produce nausea and vomiting).

1. Reconstitute powder w/manufacturer's diluent when preparing 2 mg doses or less. For doses exceeding 2 mg, dilute w/sterile water for injection.
2. To provide 1 mg glucagon/ml, use 1 ml diluent. For 1 mg vial of glucagon, use 10 ml diluent for 10 mg vial.
3. Pt will usually awaken in 5-20 min. Although 1-2 additional doses may be administered, the concern for effects of continuing cerebral hypoglycemia requires consideration of parenteral glucose.
4. When pt awakens, give supplemental carbohydrate to restore liver glycogen and prevent secondary hypoglycemia. If pt fails to respond to glucagon, IV glucose is necessary.

INDICATIONS/DOSAGE/ROUTES

NOTE: Administer IV dextrose if pt fails to respond to glucagon.

Hypoglycemia:
SubQ/IM/IV: Adults, elderly: 0.5-1 mg (0.5-1 unit). May repeat 1-

G

2 additional doses if response is delayed.

Diagnostic aid:
IM: Adults, elderly: 1-2 mg (1-2 units).
IV: Adults, elderly: 0.25-2 mg (0.25-2 units).

PRECAUTIONS

CONTRAINDICATIONS: Pheochromocytoma, hypersensitivity to glucagon (protein). **CAUTIONS:** History of insulinoma or pheochromocytoma. **PREGNANCY/LACTATION:** Not known whether drug crosses placenta or is distributed in breast milk. **Pregnancy Category B.**

INTERACTIONS

DRUG INTERACTIONS: May increase anticoagulant effect. **ALTERED LAB VALUES:** May decrease potassium.

SIDE EFFECTS

OCCASIONAL: Nausea, vomiting. **RARE:** Allergic reaction (urticaria, respiratory distress, hypotension).

ADVERSE REACTIONS/TOXIC EFFECTS

None significant.

NURSING IMPLICATIONS

BASELINE ASSESSMENT:

Obtain immediate assessment, including history, clinical signs, and symptoms. If hypoglycemic coma is established, give glucagon promptly as described above.

INTERVENTION/EVALUATION:

Monitor response time carefully. Have IV dextrose readily available in event pt does not awaken within 5-20 min. Assess for possible allergic reaction (urticaria, respiratory difficulty, hypotension). When pt is conscious, give carbohydrate and review insulin/diet needs w/ physician.

PATIENT/FAMILY TEACHING:

Recognize significance of recognizing symptoms of hypoglycemia: pale, cool skin; anxiety, difficulty concentrating, headache, hunger, nausea, nervousness, shakiness, sweating, unusual tiredness, weakness, unconsciousness. Instruct pt, family, or friend to give sugar form first (orange juice, honey, hard candy, sugar cubes, or table sugar dissolved in water or juice) if symptoms of hypoglycemia develop, followed by cheese and crackers or half a sandwich or glass of milk. Inform physician of hypoglycemic episode and use of glucagon so that regimen can be regulated appropriately. Replace glucagon as soon as possible.

glyburide

glye´byoo-ride
(Diabeta, Micronase)

CANADIAN AVAILABILITY:
Diabeta, Euglucon

CLASSIFICATION

Hypoglycemic: Oral

PHARMACOKINETICS

	ONSET	PEAK	DURATION
PO	0.25-1 hr	1-2 hrs	24 hrs

Well absorbed from GI tract. Protein binding: 90%. Metabolized in liver to weakly active metabolite. Primarily excreted in urine. Half-life: 10 hrs.

ACTION

Promotes release of insulin from beta cells of pancreas; decreases hepatic glycogenolysis and gluconeogenesis; increases insulin sensitivity at peripheral sites.

USES

Adjunct to diet/exercise in management of stable, mild to moderately severe non-insulin-dependent diabetes mellitus (type II, NIDDM). May be used to supplement insulin in those w/type I diabetes mellitus.

PO ADMINISTRATION

May take w/food (response better if taken 15-30 min before meals).

INDICATIONS/DOSAGE/ROUTES

Diabetes mellitus:
PO: Adults: Initially, 2.5 mg up to 20 mg/day. **Range:** 1.25-20 mg/day as a single or in divided doses. **Maintenance:** 7.5 mg/day.

Usual elderly dosage:
PO: Elderly: Initially, 1.25-2.5 mg/day. May increase by 1.25-2.5 mg/day q1-3wks.

PRECAUTIONS

CONTRAINDICATIONS: Sole therapy for type I diabetes mellitus, diabetic complications (ketosis, acidosis, diabetic coma), stress situations (severe infection, trauma, surgery), hypersensitivity to drug, severe renal or hepatic impairment. **CAUTIONS:** Elderly, malnourished or debilitated, those w/renal or hepatic dysfunction, cardiac disease, severe endocrine disorders, adrenal or pituitary insufficiency, history of hepatic porphyria. **PREGNANCY/LACTATION:** Crosses placenta, distributed in breast milk. May produce neonatal hypoglycemia if given within 2 weeks of delivery. **Pregnancy Category B.**

INTERACTIONS

DRUG INTERACTIONS: May increase effect of oral anticoagulants; chloramphenicol, MAO inhibitors, salicylates, sulfonamides may increase effect; beta-blockers may increase hypoglycemic effect; mask signs of hypoglycemia; may increase effects of insulin. **ALTERED LAB VALUES:** May increase alkaline phosphatase, SGOT (AST), LDH, creatinine, BUN.

SIDE EFFECTS

FREQUENT: Nausea, heartburn, epigastric fullness, skin eruptions (may be transient), pruritus. **OCCASIONAL:** Photosensitivity, **RARE:** Disulfiram-like reaction.

ADVERSE REACTIONS/TOXIC EFFECTS

Overdosage, insufficient food intake may produce hypoglycemia, esp. w/increased glucose demands. Cholestatic jaundice, leukopenia, thrombocytopenia, pancytopenia, agranulocytosis, aplastic or hemolytic anemia occur rarely.

NURSING IMPLICATIONS

BASELINE ASSESSMENT:

Question for hypersensitivity to glyburide. Check blood glucose level. Discuss life-style to determine extent of learning, emotional needs. Assure follow-up instruction if pt/family does not thoroughly understand diabetes management or glucose-testing techniques.

INTERVENTION/EVALUATION:

Monitor blood glucose and food

intake. Assess for hypoglycemia (cool wet skin, tremors, dizziness, anxiety, headache, tachycardia, numbness in mouth, hunger, diplopia) or hyperglycemia (polyuria, polyphagia, polydipsia, nausea and vomiting, dim vision, fatigue, deep rapid breathing). Be alert to conditions altering glucose requirements: fever, increased activity or stress, surgical procedure. Check for adverse skin reactions, jaundice. Monitor hematology reports. Assess for bleeding or bruising.

PATIENT/FAMILY TEACHING:

Prescribed diet is principal part of treatment; do not skip or delay meals. Diabetes mellitus requires lifelong control. Check blood glucose/urine as ordered. Signs and symptoms, treatment of hypo/hyperglycemia. Carry candy, sugar packets, or other sugar supplements for immediate response to hypoglycemia, wear medical alert identification. Check w/physician when glucose demands change (e.g., fever, infection, trauma, stress, heavy physical activity). Avoid alcoholic beverages. Do not take other medication w/o consulting physician. Weight control, exercise, hygiene (including foot care) and nonsmoking are essential part of therapy. Protect skin, limit sun exposure. Avoid exposure to infections. Select clothing, positions that do not restrict blood flow. Notify physician promptly of skin eruptions, itching, bleeding, yellow skin, dark urine. Inform dentist, physician, or surgeon of this medication before any treatment.

glycopyrrolate

gly-ko-pie´roll-ate
(Robinul)

CANADIAN AVAILABILITY:
Robinul

CLASSIFICATION

Anticholinergic

PHARMACOKINETICS

Incompletely absorbed from GI tract. Well absorbed after IM administration. Metabolized in liver. Primarily excreted in urine. Half-life: 1.7 hrs.

ACTION

Inhibits action of acetylcholine on structures innervated by postganglionic sites: smooth, cardiac muscle, SA, AV nodes, exocrine glands. Larger doses may decrease motility, secretory activity of GI system, tone of ureter, urinary bladder.

USES

Treatment of peptic ulcer disease. Pre-op medication to reduce salivation and excessive secretions of respiratory tract; reduces gastric secretions, acidity. Prevents cholinergic effect during surgery (i.e., arrhythmias). Given concurrently w/anticholinesterase agents to block adverse muscarinic effects. Blocks vagal inhibitory reflexes during anesthesia induction and intubation. Used intraoperatively to counter vagal reflexes w/arrhythmias. Protects against peripheral muscarinic effects (bradycardia, secretions) of cholinergic agents.

PO/SubQ/IM/IV ADMINISTRATION

PO:

Administer before meals (food decreases absorption) and bedtime.

IM:

For preop, may be given in same syringe w/other compatible preop medication.

IV:

1. Give by direct IV injection.
2. May be given via tubing or running IV infusion of compatible solution.
3. When used concurrently w/ neostigmine or physostigmine, may be administered via same syringe.

INDICATIONS/DOSAGE/ROUTES

Peptic ulcer disease:
PO: Adults, elderly: Initially, 1 mg 3 times/day. **Maintenance:** 1 mg 2 times/day. **Maximum:** 8 mg/ day.
IM/IV: Adults, elderly: 0.1-0.2 mg q4h (3-4 times/day). **Maximum:** 4 doses/day.

Preop:
IM: Adults, elderly, children >2 yr: 0.004 mg/kg 30-60 min before anesthesia. **Children <2 yr:** Up to 0.004 mg/lb.

Intraoperative (prevent cholinergic effects):
IV: Adults, elderly, children: 0.1 mg (0.5 ml). May repeat at 2-3 min intervals.

Block effects of anticholinesterase agents:
IV: Adults, elderly: 0.2 mg for each 1 mg neostigmine or 5 mg pyridostigmine.

PRECAUTIONS

CONTRAINDICATIONS: Narrow-angle glaucoma, severe ulcerative colitis, toxic megacolon, obstructive disease of GI tract, paralytic ileus, intestinal atony, bladder neck obstruction due to prostatic hypertrophy, myasthenia gravis in those not treated w/neostigmine, tachycardia secondary to cardiac insufficiency or thyrotoxicosis, cardiospasm, unstable cardiovascular status in acute hemorrhage. **EXTREME CAUTION:** Autonomic neuropathy, known or suspected GI infections, diarrhea, mild to moderate ulcerative colitis. **CAUTIONS:** Hyperthyroidism, hepatic or renal disease, hypertension, tachyarrhythmias, CHF, coronary artery disease, gastric ulcer, esophageal reflux or hiatal hernia associated w/reflux esophagitis, infants, elderly, those w/COPD. **PREGNANCY/LACTATION:** Not known whether drug crosses placenta or is distributed in breast milk. **Pregnancy Category C.**

INTERACTIONS

DRUG INTERACTIONS: Antacids, antidiarrheals may decrease absorption. Anticholinergics may increase effects. May decrease absorption of ketoconazole. May increase severity GI lesions with potassium chloride (wax matrix). **ALTERED LAB VALUES:** May decrease uric acid.

SIDE EFFECTS

FREQUENT: Dry mouth (sometimes severe), decreased sweating, constipation. **OCCASIONAL:** Blurred vision, bloated feeling, urinary hesitancy, drowsiness (w/ high dosage), headache, intolerance to light, loss of taste, nervousness, flushing, insomnia, impotence, mental confusion/excitement (particularly in elderly, children). Parenteral form may produce temporary light-headedness, local irritation. **RARE:** Dizziness, faintness.

ADVERSE REACTIONS/TOXIC EFFECTS

Overdosage may produce temporary paralysis of ciliary muscle, pupillary dilation, tachycardia, palpitation, hot/dry/flushed skin, absence of bowel sounds, hyperthermia, increased respiratory rate, EKG abnormalities, nausea, vomiting, rash over face/upper trunk, CNS stimulation, psychosis (agitation, restlessness, rambling speech, visual hallucination, paranoid behavior, delusions), followed by depression.

NURSING IMPLICATIONS

BASELINE ASSESSMENT:

Before giving medication, instruct pt to void (reduces risk of urinary retention).

INTERVENTION/EVALUATION:

Monitor daily bowel activity and stool consistency. Palpate bladder for urinary retention. Monitor changes in B/P, temperature. Assess skin turgor, mucous membranes to evaluate hydration status (encourage adequate fluid intake), bowel sounds for peristalsis. Be alert for fever (increased risk of hyperthermia).

PATIENT/FAMILY TEACHING:

Take 30 min before meals (food decreases absorption of medication). Use care not to become overheated during exercise in hot weather (may result in heat stroke). Avoid hot baths, saunas. Avoid tasks that require alertness, motor skills until response to drug is established. Sugarless gum, sips of tepid water may relieve dry mouth. Do not take antacids or medicine for diarrhea within 1 hr of taking this medication (decreased effectiveness).

gold sodium thiomalate

gold sodium thigh-oh′mah-late
(Myochrysine)

CANADIAN AVAILABILITY:
Myochrysine

CLASSIFICATION

Antirheumatic, anti-inflammatory

PHARMACOKINETICS

Rapidly absorbed after IM administration. Widely distributed. Protein binding: 95-99%. Metabolic fate unknown. Primarily excreted in urine. Half-life: 3-27 days after single dose up to 168 days w/multiple doses.

ACTION

Exact mechanism unknown (may alter cellular mechanisms, enzyme systems, immune responses, collagen biosynthesis; may suppress phagocytic activity).

USES

Management of rheumatoid arthritis in those w/insufficient therapeutic response to nonsteroidal anti-inflammatory agents.

IM ADMINISTRATION

1. Give in upper outer quadrant of gluteus maximus.

2. Pt to be lying down when administered.

INDICATIONS/DOSAGE/ROUTES

Rheumatoid arthritis:
NOTE: Give as weekly injections. **IM: Adults, elderly:** Initially, 10 mg, then 25 mg for second dose. Follow w/25 mg/wk until improvement noted or total of 1 Gm administered. **Maintenance:** 25-50 mg q2wk for 2-20 wk; if stable, may increase to q3-4wk intervals. **Children:** Initially, 10 mg, then 1 mg/kg/wk. **Maximum single dose:** 50 mg.

PRECAUTIONS

CONTRAINDICATIONS: History of gold-induced pathoses (necrotizing enterocolitis, exfoliative dermatitis, pulmonary fibrosis, blood dyscrasias), hepatic dysfunction or history of hepatitis, uncontrolled diabetes or CHF, urticaria, eczema, colitis, hemorrhagic conditions, systemic lupus erythematosus, recent radiation therapy. **CAUTIONS:** Renal/hepatic disease, inflammatory bowel disease. **PREGNANCY/LACTATION:** Crosses placenta, distributed in breast milk. Use only when benefits outweigh hazard to fetus. **Pregnancy Category C.**

INTERACTIONS

DRUG INTERACTIONS: Bone marrow depressants, hepatotoxic, nephrotoxic medications may increase toxicity. Penicillamine may increase risk hematologic or renal adverse effects. **ALTERED LAB VALUES:** May decrease Hgb, Hct, platelets, WBCs. May alter liver function tests. May increase urine protein.

SIDE EFFECTS

FREQUENT: Diarrhea/loose stools, rash, pruritus, abdominal pain, nausea. **OCCASIONAL:** Vomiting, anorexia, flatulence, dyspepsia, conjunctivitis, photosensitivity. **RARE:** Constipation, urticaria, rash.

ADVERSE REACTIONS/TOXIC EFFECTS

Signs of gold toxicity: decreased hemoglobin, leukopenia (WBC below 4000 mm^3), reduced granulocyte counts (below 150,000/mm^3), proteinuria, hematuria, stomatitis, blood dyscrasias (anemia, leukopenia, thrombocytopenia, eosinophilia), glomerulonephritis, nephrotic syndrome, cholestatic jaundice.

NURSING IMPLICATIONS

BASELINE ASSESSMENT:

Rule out pregnancy before beginning treatment, CBC, urinalysis, platelet and differential, renal and liver function tests should be performed before therapy begins.

INTERVENTION/EVALUATION:

Monitor daily bowel activity and stool consistency. Assess urine tests for proteinuria or hematuria. Monitor WBC, hemoglobin, differential, platelet count, renal and hepatic function studies. Question for skin pruritus (may be first sign of impending rash). Assess skin daily for rash, purpura, or ecchymoses. Assess oral mucous membranes, borders of tongue, palate, pharynx for ulceration, complaint of metallic taste sensation (signs of stomatitis). Evaluate for therapeutic response: relief of pain, stiffness, swelling, increase in joint mobility, reduced joint tenderness, improved grip strength.

PATIENT/FAMILY TEACHING:

Therapeutic response may take

6 months or longer. Avoid exposure to sunlight (gray to blue pigment may appear). Contact physician/nurse if pruritus, rash, sore mouth, indigestion, or metallic taste occurs. Maintain diligent oral hygiene.

gonadorelin acetate

go-nad-oh-rell′in

(Lutrepulse)

gonadorelin hydrochloride

(Factrel)

CANADIAN AVAILABILITY:
Factrel

CLASSIFICATION

Gonadotropin-releasing hormone

PHARMACOKINETICS

Rapidly metabolized. Primarily excreted in urine. Half-life: 10-40 min.

ACTION

Stimulates synthesis, release of luteinizing hormone (LH), follicle stimulating hormone (FSH) from anterior pituitary. Stimulates release of gonadotropin-releasing hormone from hypothalamus.

USES

As a single dose, to evaluate the functional capacity and response of gonadotropes of anterior pituitary in suspected gonadotropic deficiency (does not differentiate between hypothalamus or pituitary disorders). Multiple injection testing is used to evaluate residual gonadotropic function of pituitary after removal of a pituitary tumor by surgery and/or irradiation. Induction of ovulation in women w/ primary hypothalamic amenorrhea.

STORAGE/HANDLING

Solution should appear clear, colorless, free of particulate matter. Do not use if discolored/precipitate formed. Discard unused portion.

SubQ/IV ADMINISTRATION

Gonadorelin Acetate:

1. Reconstitute vial w/8 ml diluent immediately before use. Inject diluent onto dry product cake.
2. Shake a few seconds.
3. Transfer solution to plastic reservoir.
4. Set Lutrepulse pump to deliver appropriate volume/pulse over 1 min q90min.
5. Solution will supply doses for approximately 7 days.

Gonadorelin Hydrochloride:

1. Reconstitute 100 mcg w/1.0 ml of sterile diluent supplied.
2. Reconstitute 500 mcg w/2.0 ml of sterile diluent supplied.
3. Prepare solution immediately before use.

INDICATIONS/DOSAGE/ROUTES

NOTE: Test should be conducted in the absence of other drugs that affect pituitary secretion of gonadotropins.

Gonadorelin Acetate:

Primary hypothalamic amenorrhea:

IV PUMP: Adults: 5 mcg q90min (range 1-20 mcg) treatment interval 21 days. Refer to manufacturer's manual for proper dilutions/settings on pump. Response usually occurs in 2-3 wk after initiation. Continue additional 2 wk after ovulation occurs (maintains corpus luteum).

GONADORELIN HYDROCHLORIDE:

Diagnostic agent:
IV/SubQ: Adults: 100 mcg. In females, perform test in early follicular phase of menstrual cycle.

PRECAUTIONS

CONTRAINDICATIONS: Hypersensitivity to gonadorelin, components. *Gonadorelin acetate:* Women w/any condition exacerbated by pregnancy, ovarian cysts, or causes of anovulation other than hypothalamic in origin. **CAUTIONS:** None significant. **PREGNANCY/LACTATION: Pregnancy Category B.**

INTERACTIONS

DRUG INTERACTIONS: None significant. **ALTERED LAB VALUES:** None significant.

SIDE EFFECTS

OCCASIONAL: *Gonadorelin acetate:* Multiple pregnancy, inflammation, infection, mild phlebitis, hematoma at catheter site. *Gonadorelin hydrochloride:* Swelling, pain, or itching at injection site w/ SubQ administration. Local or generalized skin rash w/chronic SubQ administration. **RARE:** *Gonadorelin acetate:* Ovarian hyperstimulation. *Gonadorelin hydrochloride:* Headache, nausea, light-headedness, abdominal discomfort, hypersensitivity reactions (bronchospasm, tachycardia, flushing, urticaria), induration at injection site.

ADVERSE REACTIONS/TOXIC EFFECTS

Anaphylactic reaction occurs rarely.

NURSING IMPLICATIONS

BASELINE ASSESSMENT:

Before test is started, assure that pt understands procedure. Question for hypersensitivity to gonadorelin or components. *Gonadorelin acetate:* Pt instructions included w/kit from manufacturer. *Gonadorelin hydrochloride:* Venous blood sample (for LH) to be drawn immediately before gonadorelin hydrochloride administration.

INTERVENTION/EVALUATION:

Gonadorelin acetate: W/baseline pelvic ultrasound, follow-up studies. *Gonadorelin hydrochloride:* At 7 and 14 days of therapy. Change cannula and IV site at 48 hr intervals. Assure protocol for test is maintained: usually venous blood samples (for LH) drawn after administration at intervals of 15, 30, 45, 60, and 120 min.

goserelin acetate

gos-er´ah-lin
(Zoladex)

CANADIAN AVAILABILITY:
Zoladex

CLASSIFICATION

Antineoplastic

PHARMACOKINETICS

Well absorbed (slower first 8 days after injection than remainder of 28 day cycle). Half-life: 4.2 hrs.

ACTION

Synthetic luteinizing hormone–releasing hormone analog. Stimulates release of luteinizing hormone (LH), follicle stimulating hormone (FSH) from anterior pituitary (increases testosterone concentrations). After initial increase, decreases release of LH, FSH, testosterone.

USES

Treatment of advanced carcinoma of prostate as alternative when orchiectomy or estrogen therapy is either not indicated or unacceptable to pt. Management of endometriosis. Treatment of advanced breast cancer in premenopausal and perimenopausal women.

STORAGE/HANDLING

Store at room temperature.

SubQ ADMINISTRATION

Administer into upper abdominal wall (local anesthesia acceptable).

INDICATIONS/DOSAGE/ROUTES

Prostatic carcinoma, endometriosis:
SubQ IMPLANT: Adults >18 yr, elderly: 3.6 mg q28d into upper abdominal wall.

PRECAUTIONS

CONTRAINDICATIONS: Pregnancy. **CAUTIONS:** None significant. **PREGNANCY/LACTATION:** Produces atrophic secondary sex organs, implantation loss; suppresses ovarian function, ovarian weight and size. Not known whether drug is distributed in breast milk. Do not use during pregnancy or in those who may become pregnant. **Pregnancy Category X.**

INTERACTIONS

DRUG INTERACTIONS: None significant. **ALTERED LAB VALUES:** May increase serum acid phosphatase, testosterone concentrations.

SIDE EFFECTS

FREQUENT: Hot flashes, sexual dysfunction, decreased erections, lower urinary tract symptoms, lethargy, pain, edema, upper respiratory infection, rash, sweating, anorexia, dizziness, insomnia, nausea. **OCCASIONAL:** Transient worsening of symptoms of prostatic cancer, particularly bone pain.

ADVERSE REACTIONS/TOXIC EFFECTS

Arrhythmias, CHF, hypertension occur rarely. Ureteral obstruction, spinal cord compression observed (immediate orchiectomy may be necessary).

NURSING IMPLICATIONS

INTERVENTION/EVALUATION:

Monitor pt closely for worsening signs and symptoms of prostatic cancer, especially during first month of therapy.

PATIENT/FAMILY TEACHING:

Use contraceptive measures during therapy. Do not have immunizations w/o doctor's approval (drug lowers body's resistance). Avoid contact w/those who have recently received live virus vaccine.

granisetron

gran-is'eh-tron
(Kytril)

CLASSIFICATION

Antiemetic

PHARMACOKINETICS

Rapid, widely distributed to tissues. Protein binding: 65%. Metabolized in liver to active metabolite.

Excreted in urine, eliminated in feces. Half-life: 10-12 hrs (increased in elderly).

ACTION

Selectively antagonizes serotonin at 5-HT_3 receptors on abdominal vagal afferent nerve and chemoreceptor trigger zone. Blocks serotonin stimulation and vomiting after emetogenic stimulus.

USES

Prevents nausea, vomiting associated w/emetogenic cancer therapy (includes high-dose cisplatin).

STORAGE/HANDLING

Clear, colorless solution. Store at room temperature. After dilution, stable for at least 24 hrs at room temperature. Inspect for particulates, discoloration.

IV ADMINISTRATION

1. Dilute calculated dose w/20-50 ml 0.9% NaCl or 5% dextrose. Do not mix w/other medications.
2. Infuse IV over 5 minutes.

INDICATIONS/DOSAGE/ROUTES

Antiemetic:
IV: Adults, elderly, children >2 yrs: 10 mcg/kg over 5 min beginning within 30 min before initiating chemotherapy. Give only on days that chemotherapy is administered.

PRECAUTIONS

CONTRAINDICATIONS: None significant. **CAUTIONS:** Safety in children <2 yrs of age not established. **PREGNANCY/LACTATION:** Unknown whether it is distributed in breast milk. **Pregnancy Category B.**

INTERACTIONS

DRUG INTERACTIONS: Hepatic enzyme inducers may decrease effect. **ALTERED LAB VALUES:** May increase SGOT (AST), SGPT (ALT).

SIDE EFFECTS

FREQUENT: Headache. **OCCASIONAL:** Constipation, somnolence, diarrhea, asthenia, taste disorders, fever.

ADVERSE REACTIONS/TOXIC EFFECTS

None significant.

NURSING IMPLICATIONS

BASELINE ASSESSMENT:

Assure granisetron is given within 30 min before start of chemotherapy.

INTERVENTION/EVALUATION:

Monitor for therapeutic effect. Assess for headache. Monitor frequency and consistency of stools.

PATIENT/FAMILY TEACHING:

Granisetron is effective shortly after administration; prevents nausea, vomiting. Explain that transitory taste disorder may occur.

griseofulvin

griz-ee-oh-full´vin
(Fulvicin, Grisactin, GrisPEG)

CANADIAN AVAILABILITY:
Fulvicin, Grisovin-FP

CLASSIFICATION

Antifungal

PHARMACOKINETICS

Microsize: Variably absorbed from GI tract. *Ultra microsize:*

Completely absorbed from GI tract. Primarily deposited in keratin layer of skin, hair, nails. Metabolized in liver. Primarily excreted in urine. Half-life: 24 hrs.

ACTION

Fungistatic. Inhibits fungal cell mitosis by disrupting mitotic spindle structure. Arrests metaphase of cell division.

USES

Treatment of tineas (ringworm): t. capitis, t. corporis, t. cruris, t. pedis, t. unguium.

PO ADMINISTRATION

1. Take w/or after meals (decreases GI irritation, increases absorption).
2. Shake suspension well before administration.
3. Distinguish carefully between microsize and ultramicrosize doses.

INDICATIONS/DOSAGE/ROUTES

NOTE: Give orally as a single dose or in 2-4 divided doses. Dosage is individualized.

Tinea corporis, tinea cruris, tinea capitis:
PO: Adults, elderly: Ultramicrosize: 330-375 mg/day. **Microsize:** 500 mg/day.

Tinea pedis, tinea unguium:
PO: Adults, elderly: Ultramicrosize: 660-750 mg/day. **Microsize:** 750 mg to 1 Gm/day. **Children >2yr: Ultramicrosize:** 7.3 mg/kg/day. **Microsize:** 10-11 mg/kg/day.

PRECAUTIONS

CONTRAINDICATIONS: Hypersensitivity to griseofulvin, porphyria, hepatocellular failure. **CAUTIONS:** Exposure to sun or ultraviolet light (photosensitivity), hypersensitivity to penicillins. **PREGNANCY/LACTATION:** Not known whether drug crosses placenta or is distributed in breast milk. **Pregnancy Category C.**

INTERACTIONS

DRUG INTERACTIONS: May decrease effects of warfarin, oral contraceptives. **ALTERED LAB VALUES:** None significant.

SIDE EFFECTS

OCCASIONAL: Hypersensitivity reaction (rash, pruritus, urticaria), headache, nausea, diarrhea, excessive thirst, flatulence, oral thrush, dizziness, insomnia. **RARE:** Paresthesia of hands/feet, proteinuria.

ADVERSE REACTIONS/TOXIC EFFECTS

Granulocytopenia should cause discontinuation of drug.

NURSING IMPLICATIONS

BASELINE ASSESSMENT:

Question for history of allergies, especially to griseofulvin, penicillins. Confirm that a culture/histologic test was done for accurate diagnosis.

INTERVENTION/EVALUATION:

Assess skin for rash and response to therapy. Evaluate food intake, tolerance. Determine pattern of bowel activity and stool consistency. Question presence of headache: onset, location, type of discomfort. Assess mental status for dizziness and provide ambulation assistance when necessary.

PATIENT/FAMILY TEACHING:

Prolonged therapy (weeks or months) is usually necessary. Do not miss a dose; continue therapy as long as ordered. Avoid alcohol (may produce tachycardia, flushing). Maintain good hygiene (prevents superinfection). Separate personal items in direct contact w/ affected areas. Do not apply other preparations or take other medications w/o consulting physician. Avoid exposure to sunlight. Keep areas dry; wear light clothing for ventilation. Take w/foods high in fat such as milk, ice cream (reduces GI upset and assists absorption).

guaifenesin (glyceryl guaiacolate)

guay-fen´ah-sin

(Glycotuss, Humibid, Robitussin)

FIXED-COMBINATION(S): W/phenylephrine and phenylpropanolamine, sympathomimetics (Entex)

CANADIAN AVAILABILITY: Balminil, Resyl, Robitussin

CLASSIFICATION

Expectorant

PHARMACOKINETICS

Well absorbed from GI tract. Metabolized in liver. Excreted in urine.

ACTION

Enhances fluid output of respiratory tract by decreasing adhesiveness and surface tension, promoting removal of viscous mucus.

USES

Symptomatic relief of cough in presence of mucus in respiratory tract. Not for use w/persistent cough due to smoking, asthma, emphysema or cough accompanied by excessive secretions.

STORAGE/HANDLING

Store syrup, liquid, capsules at room temperature.

PO ADMINISTRATION

1. Give w/o regard to meals.
2. Do not crush or break sustained-release capsule.

INDICATIONS/DOSAGE/ROUTES

Expectorant:

PO: Adults, elderly, children >12 yr: 200-400 mg q4h. **Maximum:** 2.4 Gm/day. **Children 6-12 yr:** 100-200 mg q4h. **Maximum:** 1.2 Gm/day. **Children 2-6 yr:** 50-100 mg q4h. **Maximum:** 600 mg/day.

PRECAUTIONS

CONTRAINDICATIONS: None significant. **CAUTIONS:** None significant. **PREGNANCY/LACTATION:** Not known whether drug crosses placenta or is distributed in breast milk. **Pregnancy Category C.**

INTERACTIONS

DRUG INTERACTIONS: None significant. **ALTERED LAB VALUES:** None significant.

SIDE EFFECTS

RARE: Dizziness, headache, rash.

ADVERSE REACTIONS/TOXIC EFFECTS

Excessive dosage may produce nausea, vomiting.

NURSING IMPLICATIONS

BASELINE ASSESSMENT:

Assess type, severity, frequency of cough and productions. Increase fluid intake and environmental humidity to lower viscosity of lung secretions.

INTERVENTION/EVALUATION:

Initiate deep breathing and coughing exercises, particularly in those w/impaired pulmonary function. Assess for clinical improvement and record onset of relief of cough.

PATIENT/FAMILY TEACHING:

Avoid tasks that require alertness, motor skills until response to drug is established.

guanabenz acetate

gwan´ah-benz

(Wytensin)

CLASSIFICATION

Antihypertensive

PHARMACOKINETICS

	ONSET	PEAK	DURATION
PO	1 hr	2-4 hrs	6-8 hrs

Well absorbed from GI tract. Widely distributed. Protein binding: 90%. Metabolized in liver. Primarily excreted in urine. Half-life: 7-10 hrs.

ACTION

Stimulates central alpha$_2$-adrenergic receptors. Decreases sympathetic outflow to heart, kidneys, peripheral vasculature. Decreases systolic, diastolic B/P. Chronic use decreases peripheral vascular resistance.

USES

Treatment of hypertension. Used alone or in combination w/thiazide-type diuretics.

PO ADMINISTRATION

1. May give w/food if GI distress occurs.
2. Tablets may be crushed.
3. Give last dose at bedtime (ensures control of B/P at night, minimizing daytime drowsiness).

INDICATIONS/DOSAGE/ROUTES

Hypertension:

PO: Adults: Initially, 4 mg 2 times/day. Increase by 4-8 mg at 1-2 wk intervals. **Elderly:** Initially, 4 mg/day. May increase q1-2wks. **Maintenance:** 8-16 mg/day. **Maximum:** 32 mg/day.

PRECAUTIONS

CONTRAINDICATIONS: None significant. **CAUTIONS:** Severe coronary insufficiency, recent MI, cerebrovascular disease, severe hepatic, renal failure. **PREGNANCY/LACTATION:** Not known whether drug crosses placenta or is distributed in breast milk. May cause fetal harm. **Pregnancy Category C.**

INTERACTIONS

DRUG INTERACTIONS: Beta-adrenergic blockers, hypotension producing medications may increase antihypertensive effect. **ALTERED LAB VALUES:** May decrease cholesterol, total triglyceride concentrations.

SIDE EFFECTS

FREQUENT: Extreme dry mouth, drowsiness, tiredness, dizziness, weakness, headache. **OCCASIONAL:** Edema, GI distress, diarrhea, blurred vision, rash, pruritus, muscle aches, urinary frequency, unusual taste sensation, irritability, insomnia, paresthesias, palpitations, bradycardia. **RARE:** Orthostatic hypotension, exacerbation of asthma.

ADVERSE REACTIONS/TOXIC EFFECTS

Abrupt withdrawal may result in rebound hypertension manifested as nervousness, agitation, anxiety, insomnia, hand tingling, tremor, flushing, sweating. Overdosage produces hypotension, somnolence, lethargy, irritability, bradycardia, miosis (pupillary constriction).

NURSING IMPLICATIONS

Baseline Assessment:

Obtain B/P immediately before each dose administration, in addition to regular monitoring (be alert to B/P fluctuations).

Intervention/Evaluation:

Sedative effect, drowsiness may require assistance w/ambulation, especially during early therapy. Assess for peripheral edema of hands, feet (usually, first area of low extremity swelling is behind medial malleolus). Assess skin for development of rash. If excessive reduction in B/P occurs, place pt in supine position w/legs elevated. Assess for anorexia secondary to decreased taste perception. Monitor pattern of daily bowel activity and stool consistency.

Patient/Family Teaching:

Side effects may occur during first 2 wk of therapy but generally diminish or disappear during continued therapy. Sugarless gum, sips of tepid water may relieve dry mouth. Skipping doses or voluntarily discontinuing drug may produce severe, rebound hypertension.

guanadrel sulfate

gwan´ah-drel

(Hylorel)

CLASSIFICATION

Antihypertensive

PHARMACOKINETICS

	ONSET	PEAK	DURATION
PO	2 hrs	4-6 hrs	—

Rapid, completely absorbed from GI tract. Widely distributed. Protein binding: 20%. Metabolized in liver. Primarily excreted in urine. Half-life: 10 hrs.

ACTION

Reduces B/P by depleting norepinephrine from adrenergic nerve endings. Prevents release of norepinephrine normally produced by nerve stimulation.

USES

Treatment of hypertension in those not controlled w/thiazide-type diuretic. Combine w/diuretic therapy for optimum control of B/P.

PO ADMINISTRATION

1. May give w/o regard to food.
2. Tablets may be crushed.

INDICATIONS/DOSAGE/ROUTES

Hypertension:

PO: Adults: Initially, 5 mg 2 times/day. Increase at 1-4 wk intervals by 10-40 mg/day. **Elderly:** Initially, 5 mg/day. May gradually increase at 1-4 wk intervals. **Maintenance:** 20-75 mg/day in 2 divided doses.

PRECAUTIONS

CONTRAINDICATIONS: Frank CHF, pheochromocytoma. **EXTREME CAUTION:** CHF, regional

G

vascular disease. **CAUTIONS:** Elderly, bronchial asthma, peptic ulcer. **PREGNANCY/LACTATION:** Not known whether drug crosses placenta or is distributed in breast milk. **Pregnancy Category B.**

INTERACTIONS

DRUG INTERACTIONS: Tricyclic antidepressants, MAO inhibitors, phenothiazines, sympathomimetics may decrease antihypertensive effect. **ALTERED LAB VALUES:** None significant.

SIDE EFFECTS

FREQUENT: Orthostasis (dizziness, syncope, weakness, feeling of faintness), diarrhea/constipation, increased bowel movements, dyspepsia, dry mouth, anorexia, drowsiness, fatigue, retrograde ejaculation, leg cramps, peripheral edema, nasal stuffiness, cough, palpitation, SOB, paresthesia, headache. **OCCASIONAL:** Impotence, visual disturbances. **RARE:** Fainting, sleep disturbances, depression.

ADVERSE REACTIONS/TOXIC EFFECTS

None significant.

NURSING IMPLICATIONS

BASELINE ASSESSMENT:

Obtain B/P immediately before each dose, in addition to regular monitoring (be alert to B/P fluctuations). Therapy should be discontinued 2-3 days before elective surgery. Advise anesthesiologist of drug therapy if emergency surgery is necessary.

INTERVENTION/EVALUATION:

Monitor pattern of daily bowel activity and stool consistency. If excessive reduction in B/P occurs, place pt in supine position w/legs elevated. Assess for peripheral edema of hands, feet (usually, first area of low extremity swelling is behind medial malleolus in ambulatory, sacral area in bedridden). Monitor both erect and supine B/P.

PATIENT/FAMILY TEACHING:

To reduce hypotensive effect, rise slowly from lying to sitting position and permit legs to dangle from bed momentarily before standing. Avoid sudden or prolonged standing, exercise, hot environment or hot shower, alcohol ingestion, particularly in morning (may aggravate orthostatic hypotension). If dizziness or weakness occurs, sit or lie down immediately. If nausea occurs, cola, unsalted crackers, or dry toast may relieve effect. Sugarless gum, sips of tepid water may relieve dry mouth.

guanfacine

gwan´fah-seen
(Tenex)

CLASSIFICATION

Antihypertensive

PHARMACOKINETICS

	ONSET	PEAK	DURATION
PO	—	1-4 hrs	—

Rapid, completely absorbed from GI tract. Widely distributed. Protein binding: 70%. Metabolized in liver. Primarily excreted in urine. Half-life: 10-30 hrs.

ACTION

Stimulates central alpha$_2$-adrenergic receptors. Decreases sympathetic outflow to heart, kidneys, peripheral vasculature. Decreases systolic, diastolic B/P. Chronic use decreases peripheral vascular resistance.

USES

Management of hypertension alone or in combination w/other antihypertensives, especially thiazide-type diuretics.

PO ADMINISTRATION

1. Give w/o regard to food.
2. Tablets may be crushed.
3. Administer at bedtime (minimizes daytime drowsiness).

INDICATIONS/DOSAGE/ROUTES

Hypertension:
PO: Adults, elderly: Initially, 1 mg/day. Increase by 1 mg/day at intervals of 3-4 wk up to 3 mg/day in single or divided doses.

PRECAUTIONS

CONTRAINDICATIONS: None significant. **CAUTIONS:** Impaired renal function. **PREGNANCY/LACTATION:** Not known whether drug crosses placenta or is distributed in breast milk. Not recommended in treatment of acute hypertension associated w/preeclampsia. **Pregnancy Category B.**

INTERACTIONS

DRUG INTERACTIONS: Beta-adrenergic blockers, hypotension producing medications may increase antihypertensive effect. **ALTERED LAB VALUES:** May increase growth hormone concentration. May decrease urinary catecholamine, VMA excretion.

SIDE EFFECTS

FREQUENT: Dry mouth, dizziness, headache, fatigue, somnolence. **OCCASIONAL:** Asthenia (loss of strength, energy). **RARE:** GI distress, leg cramps, dermatitis, bradycardia.

ADVERSE REACTIONS/TOXIC EFFECTS

Overdosage may produce severe drowsiness, bradycardia.

NURSING IMPLICATIONS

BASELINE ASSESSMENT:

Obtain B/P and pulse immediately before each dose. Withhold medication and notify physician if systolic B/P <90 mm Hg and/or pulse rate <60/min.

INTERVENTION/EVALUATION:

Monitor B/P, pulse. Sedative effect, drowsiness may require assistance w/ambulation, esp. during early therapy. If excessive B/P reduction occurs, place pt in supine position w/legs elevated.

PATIENT/FAMILY TEACHING:

Sugarless gum or sips of tepid water may help relieve dry mouth. Avoid tasks that require alertness, motor skills until drug response is established. Side effects usually diminish w/continued therapy. Tolerance to alcohol or other CNS depressants may be reduced. Do not abruptly withdraw medication after long-term use. Therapeutic effect may take 1 wk; peak effect noted in 1-3 mo.

halcinonide

hal-sin′oh-nide
(Halog)

H

CANADIAN AVAILABILITY:
Halog

(See Classifications section under Corticosteroids: topical)

halobetasol

halo-bet´ah-sol
(Ultravate)
(See Classifications section under Corticosteroids: topical)

haloperidol

hal-oh-pear´ih-dawl
(Haldol)

CANADIAN AVAILABILITY:
Apo-Haloperidol, Haldol, Novo-peridol, Peridol

CLASSIFICATION

Antipsychotic

PHARMACOKINETICS

Readily absorbed from GI tract. Protein binding: 92%. Extensively metabolized in liver. Primarily excreted in urine. Half-life: *oral:* 12-37 hrs; *IM:* 17-25 hrs, *IV:* 10-19 hrs.

ACTION

Competitively blocks postsynaptic dopamine receptors, increases turnover of brain dopamine producing tranquilizing effect. Has anticholinergic, alpha-adrenergic blocking activity.

USES

Management of psychotic disorders, control of tics, vocal utterances in Tourette's syndrome. Used in management of severe behavioral problems in children, short-term treatment of hyperactivity in children.

STORAGE/HANDLING

Store all preparations at room temperature. Discard if precipitate forms, discoloration occurs.

PO/IM ADMINISTRATION

PO:

1. Give w/o regard to meals.
2. Scored tablets may be crushed.

IM:

Parenteral administration: Pt must remain recumbent for 30-60 min in head-low position w/legs raised to minimize hypotensive effect.

1. Prepare IM injection using 21-gauge needle.
2. Do not exceed a maximum volume of 3 ml per IM injection site.
3. Inject slow, deep IM into upper outer quadrant of gluteus maximus.

INDICATIONS/DOSAGE/ROUTES

NOTE: Increase dosage gradually to optimum response, then decrease to lowest effective level for maintenance. Replace parenteral therapy w/oral therapy as soon as possible.

Moderate symptoms:
PO: Adults, elderly: Initially, 0.5-2 mg 2-3 times/day; may titrate up to 100 mg/day. **Maintenance:** Lowest effective dose.

Severe symptoms:
PO: Adults, elderly: Initially, 3-5 mg 2-3 times/day; may titrate up to 100 mg/day. **Maintenance:** Lowest effective dose.

Usual parenteral dosage:
IM: Adults, elderly: 2-5 mg; may repeat at 1-8 hr intervals. Give oral dose 12-24 hrs after last parenteral dose administered.

Usual elderly dosage (nonpsychotic):
PO: Elderly: Initially, 0.25-0.5 mg 1-2 times/day. May increase by 0.25-0.5 mg q4-7days. **Maximum:** 50 mg/day.

Usual pediatric dosage:
PO: Children (3-12 yrs): Initially, 0.5 mg/day. May increase by 0.5 mg q5-7 days. Total daily dose given in 2-3 doses/day. **Psychotic disorders:** 0.05-0.15 mg/kg/day. **Nonpsychiatric disorders, Tourette's disorder:** 0.05-0.075 mg/kg/day.

PRECAUTIONS

CONTRAINDICATIONS: Coma, alcohol ingestion, Parkinson's disease, thyrotoxicosis. **CAUTIONS:** Impaired respiratory/hepatic/cardiovascular function, alcohol withdrawal, history of seizures, urinary retention, glaucoma, prostatic hypertrophy, elderly. **PREGNANCY/LACTATION:** Crosses placenta; distributed in breast milk. **Pregnancy Category C.**

INTERACTIONS

DRUG INTERACTIONS: Alcohol, CNS depressants may increase CNS depression. Epinephrine may block alpha-adrenergic effects. Extrapyramidal symptom (EPS) producing medications may increase EPS. Lithium may increase neurologic toxicity. **ALTERED LAB VALUES:** None significant.

SIDE EFFECTS

OCCASIONAL: Orthostatic hypotension, mild, transient leukopenia, dry mouth, blurred vision, lethargy, constipation or diarrhea, peripheral edema, urinary retention, nausea.

ADVERSE REACTIONS/TOXIC EFFECTS

Extrapyramidal symptoms appear to be dose related and may be noted in first few days of therapy. Marked drowsiness and lethargy, excessive salivation, fixed stare may be mild to severe in intensity. Less frequently seen are severe akathisia (motor restlessness), and acute dystonias: torticollis (neck muscle spasm), opisthotonos (rigidity of back muscles), and oculogyric crisis (rolling back of eyes). Tardive dyskinesia (protrusion of tongue, puffing of cheeks, chewing/puckering of the mouth) may occur during long-term administration or following drug discontinuance, and may be irreversible. Risk is greater in female geriatric pts. Abrupt withdrawal following long-term therapy may provoke transient dyskinesia signs.

NURSING IMPLICATIONS

BASELINE ASSESSMENT:

Assess behavior, appearance, emotional status, response to environment, speech pattern, thought content.

INTERVENTION/EVALUATION:

Supervise suicidal-risk pt closely during early therapy (as depression lessens, energy level improves, causing increased suicide potential). Monitor B/P for hypotension. Assess for peripheral edema behind medial malleolus (sacral area in bedridden pts). Assess stool consistency and frequency. Monitor for rigidity, tremor, masklike facial expression, fine tongue movement. Assess for therapeutic response (interest in surroundings, improvement in self-care, increased ability to concentrate, relaxed facial expression).

PATIENT/FAMILY TEACHING:

Full therapeutic effect may take up to 6 wks. Do not abruptly withdraw from long-term drug therapy. Report visual disturbances. Sugarless gum or sips of tepid water may relieve dry mouth. Drowsiness generally subsides during continued therapy. Avoid tasks that require alertness, motor skills until response to drug is established. Avoid alcohol.

haloprogin

ha-low-proe´jin
(Halotex)

CANADIAN AVAILABILITY:
Halotex

CLASSIFICATION

Antifungal

USES

Treatment of tinea pedis, tinea cruris, tinea corporis, tinea manuum, tinea versicolor.

INDICATIONS/DOSAGE/ROUTES

Usual dosage:
TOPICAL: Adults, elderly: 2 times/day for 2-4 wks.

PRECAUTIONS

CONTRAINDICATIONS: Hypersensitivity to haloprogin or ingredients of preparation. **PREGNANCY/LACTATION:** Unknown if drug is excreted in breast milk. **Pregnancy Category B.**

INTERACTIONS

DRUG INTERACTIONS: None significant. **ALTERED LAB VALUES:** None significant.

SIDE EFFECTS

FREQUENT: Transient stinging. **OCCASIONAL:** Localized burning, itching, stinging, blistering.

ADVERSE REACTIONS/TOXIC EFFECTS

None significant.

NURSING IMPLICATIONS

BASELINE ASSESSMENT:

Question for history of hypersensitivity to haloprogin, ingredients of preparation.

INTERVENTION/EVALUATION:

Assess for therapeutic response or local increased irritation: burning, itching, stinging, blistering.

PATIENT/FAMILY TEACHING:

Rub well into affected areas. Complete full course of therapy (may take several weeks). Do not use occlusive covering or use other preparations w/o consulting physician. Avoid contact w/eyes. Keep areas clean, dry; wear light clothing to promote ventilation. Separate personal items, linens. Notify physician of increased irritation.

heparin sodium

hep´ah-rin
(Liquaemin)

CANADIAN AVAILABILITY:
Hepalean

CLASSIFICATION

Anticoagulant

PHARMACOKINETICS

Well absorbed after SubQ administration. Protein binding: high. Metabolized in liver, removed from circulation by uptake by reticuloendothelial system. Primarily excreted in urine. Half-life: 1-6 hrs.

ACTION

Potentiates inhibitory action of antithrombin III on several coagulation factors. Inhibits actions of thrombin, prevents conversion of fibrinogen to fibrin, and prevents formation of stable fibrin clot.

USES

Prophylaxis, treatment of venous thrombosis, pulmonary embolism, peripheral arterial embolism, atrial fibrillation w/embolism. Prevention of thromboembolus in cardiac and vascular surgery, dialysis procedures, blood transfusions, and blood sampling for laboratory purposes. Adjunct in treatment of coronary occlusion w/acute MI. Maintain patency of indwelling intravascular devices. Diagnoses and treatment of acute/chronic consumptive coagulopathies (e.g., DIC). Prevents cerebral thrombosis in progressive strokes.

STORAGE/HANDLING

Store parenteral form at room temperature.

SubQ/IV ADMINISTRATION

NOTE: Do *not* give by IM injection (pain, hematoma, ulceration, erythema).

SubQ: Note: Used in low dose therapy.

1. After withdrawal of heparin from vial, change needle before injection (prevents leakage along needle track).
2. Inject above iliac crest or in abdominal fat layer. Do not inject within 2 inches of umbilicus, or any scar tissue.
3. Withdraw needle rapidly, apply prolonged pressure at injection site. Do not massage.
4. Rotate injection sites.

IV: Note: Used in full dose therapy. Intermittent IV produces higher incidence of bleeding abnormalities. Continuous IV preferred.

1. Dilute IV infusion in isotonic sterile saline, 5% dextrose in water, or lactated Ringer's.
2. Invert container at least 6 times (ensures mixing, prevents pooling of medication).
3. Use constant-rate IV infusion pump or microdrip.

INDICATIONS/DOSAGE/ROUTES

NOTE: Dosage expressed in USP units. Dosage requirements highly individualized.

SubQ: Adults, elderly: 5,000 U IV injection and 10,000-20,000 U SubQ, followed by 8,000-10,000 U q8h or 15,000-20,000 U q12h.

Prophylaxis of postoperative thrombosis:

SubQ: Adults, elderly: 5,000 U given 2 hrs before surgery, then q8-12h after surgery for 5-7 days or when pt is ambulatory.

Full dose-therapy:

CONTINUOUS IV: Adults, elderly: 5,000 U IV injection to start, followed by 20,000-40,000 U IV infusion given over 24 hrs. **Children:** 50 U/kg IV to start, followed by 20,000 U/m^2 continuous IV infusion per 24 hrs.

INTERMITTENT IV: Adults, elderly: 10,000 U to start, followed by 5,000-10,000 U q4-6h. **Children:** 100

U/kg to start, followed by 50-100 U/kg q4h.

Maintaining patency of indwelling intravascular devices:

IV: Adults, elderly: 10-100 U injected into diaphragm of device after each use, designated interval, or as necessary.

PRECAUTIONS

CONTRAINDICATIONS: Bleeding abnormalities, vitamin K insufficiency, chronic alcoholism, severe hepatic/renal disease, salicylate therapy, severe hypertension, pregnancy, hypersensitivity to heparin, ergot alkaloids, lidocaine; peripheral artery disease, coronary insufficiency, angina, sepsis, thrombocytopenia, brain/spinal cord surgery, spinal anesthesia, eye surgery, oral anticoagulants. **CAUTIONS:** Severe hypertension, peripheral vascular disease, indwelling catheters, those >60 yrs, factors increasing risk of hemorrhage, diabetes, mild hepatic/renal disease. **PREGNANCY/LACTATION:** Use w/ caution, particularly during last trimester, immediate postpartum period (increased risk of maternal hemorrhage). Does not cross placenta; not distributed in breast milk. **Pregnancy Category C.**

INTERACTIONS

DRUG INTERACTIONS: Anticoagulants, platelet aggregation inhibitors, thrombolytics may increase risk of bleeding. Antithyroid medications, cefoperazone, cefotetan, valproic acid may cause hypoprothrombinemia. Probenecid may increase effect. **ALTERED LAB VALUES:** May increase free fatty acids, SGOT (AST), SGPT (ALT). May decrease triglycerides, cholesterol.

SIDE EFFECTS

OCCASIONAL: Itching, burning, particularly on soles of feet (due to vasospastic reaction). **RARE:** Pain, cyanosis of extremity 6-10 days after initial therapy, lasts 4-6 hrs; hypersensitivity reaction (chills, fever, pruritus, urticaria, asthma, rhinitis, lacrimation, headache).

ADVERSE REACTIONS/TOXIC EFFECTS

Bleeding complications ranging from local ecchymoses to major hemorrhage occur more frequently in high dose therapy, intermittent IV infusion, and in women >60 yrs. *Antidote:* Protamine sulfate 1-1.5 mg for q 100 U heparin SubQ if overdosage occurred before 30 min, 0.5-0.75 mg for q 100 U heparin SubQ if overdosage occurred within 30-60 min, 0.25-0.375 mg for q 100 U heparin SubQ if 2 hrs have elapsed since overdosage, 25-50 mg if heparin given by IV infusion.

NURSING IMPLICATIONS

BASELINE ASSESSMENT:

Cross-check dose w/co-worker. Determine activated partial thromboplastin time (APTT) before administration and 24 hrs after initiation of therapy, then 24-48 hrs for first week of therapy or until maintenance dose is established. Follow with APTT determinations 1-2 times weekly for 3-4 wks. Long-term therapy: 1-2 times month.

INTERVENTION/EVALUATION:

Monitor APTT (therapeutic dosage at 1.5-2.5 times normal) diligently. Assess hematocrit, platelet count, urine/stool culture for occult blood, SGOT (AST), SGPT (ALT), regardless of route of administration. Assess for decrease in B/P, increase in pulse rate, complaint of abdominal or back pain, severe headache (may be evidence of hemorrhage). Question for increase in amount of discharge during menses. Check peripheral pulses; skin for bruises, petechiae. Check for excessive bleeding from minor cuts, scratches. Assess gums for erythema, gingival bleeding. Assess urine output for hematuria. Avoid IM injections of other medications because of potential for hematomas. When converting to coumadin therapy, monitor PT results (will be 10-20% higher while heparin is given concurrently).

PATIENT/FAMILY TEACHING:

Use electric razor, soft toothbrush to prevent bleeding. Report any sign of red or dark urine, black or red stool, coffee-ground vomitus, red-speckled mucus from cough. Do not use any over-the-counter medication w/o physician approval (may interfere w/platelet aggregation). Wear/carry identification that notes anticoagulant therapy. Inform dentist, other physicians of heparin therapy.

hetastarch

het´ah-starch

(Hespan)

CLASSIFICATION

Plasma volume expander

PHARMACOKINETICS

Smaller molecules (<50,000 molecular weight) rapidly excreted by kidneys; larger molecules (>50,000 molecular weight) slowly degraded to smaller-sized molecules, then excreted. Half-life: 17 days.

ACTION

Increases circulating blood volume by exerting osmotic pull on tissue fluids; reduces hemoconcentration and blood viscosity.

USES

Fluid replacement and plasma volume expansion in treatment of shock due to hemorrhage, burns, surgery, sepsis, trauma, leukapheresis.

STORAGE/HANDLING

Store solutions at room temperature. Solution should appear clear, pale yellow to amber. Do not use if discolored (deep turbid brown) or if precipitate forms.

IV ADMINISTRATION

1. Administer only by IV infusion.
2. Do not add drugs or mix w/ other IV fluids.
3. In acute hemorrhagic shock, administer at rate approaching 1.2 Gm/kg (20 ml/kg) per hour. Use slower rates for burns, septic shock.
4. Monitor central venous pressure (CVP) when given by rapid infusion. If there is a precipitous rise in CVP, immediately discontinue drug (overexpansion of blood volume).

INDICATIONS/DOSAGE/ROUTES

Plasma volume expansion:
IV: Adults, elderly: 500-1,000 ml/day up to 1,500 ml/day (20 mg/kg) at a rate up to 20 ml/kg/hr in hemorrhagic shock (slower rates for burns or septic shock).

Leukapheresis:
IV: Adults, elderly: 250-700 ml infused at constant rate, usually 1:8 to venous whole blood.

PRECAUTIONS

CONTRAINDICATIONS: Severe bleeding disorders, severe CHF, oliguria, anuria. **CAUTIONS:** Thrombocytopenia, elderly or very young, pulmonary edema, CHF, impaired renal function, hepatic disease, those on sodium restriction. **PREGNANCY/LACTATION:** Do not use in pregnancy unless benefits outweigh risk to fetus. **Pregnancy Category C.**

INTERACTIONS

DRUG INTERACTIONS: None significant. **ALTERED LAB VALUES:** May prolong prothrombin time (PT), partial thromboplastin time (PTT), bleeding, and clotting times; decrease hematocrit.

SIDE EFFECTS

RARE: Allergic reaction resulting in vomiting, mild temperature elevation, chills, itching; submaxillary and parotid gland enlargement, peripheral edema of lower extremities, mild flulike symptoms: headache, muscle aches.

ADVERSE REACTIONS/TOXIC EFFECTS

Fluid overload (headache, weakness, blurred vision, behavioral changes, incoordination, isolated muscle twitching) and pulmonary edema (rapid breathing, rales, wheezing, coughing, increased B/P, distended neck veins) may occur. Anaphylactoid reaction may be observed as periorbital edema, urticaria, wheezing.

NURSING IMPLICATIONS

INTERVENTION/EVALUATION:

Monitor for fluid overload (peripheral and/or pulmonary edema, impending CHF symptoms). Assess lung sounds for wheezing, rales. During leukapheresis, monitor CBC, leukocyte and platelet counts, differential, hemoglobin, hematocrit, PT, PTT, I&O. Monitor central venous B/P (detects overexpansion of blood volume). Monitor urine output closely (increase in output generally occurs in oliguric pts after administration). Assess for periorbital edema, itching, wheezing, urticaria (allergic reaction). Monitor for oliguria, anuria, any change in output ratio. Monitor for bleeding from surgical or trauma sites.

homatropine hydrobromide

home-ah´trow-peen
(Isopto Homatropine, Homatrine)

CANADIAN AVAILABILITY:
Homatropine, Isopto Homatropine

CLASSIFICATION

Cycloplegic/mydriatic

PHARMACOKINETICS

Mydriatic effect: Peak occurs in 40-60 min; recovery in 1-3 days. *Cycloplegic effect:* Peak occurs in 30-60 min; recovery in 1-3 days.

ACTION

Blocks response of acetylcholine stimulation to sphincter muscle of iris and accommodative muscle of ciliary body. Produces mydriasis (dilated pupils) and paralysis of accommodation (cycloplegia).

USES

Cycloplegic refraction and dilation of pupil in inflammatory conditions of iris and uveal tract. Optical aid in some cases of axial lens opacities. Preop and postop conditions if mydriasis required.

OPHTHALMIC ADMINISTRATION

1. Place finger on lower eyelid and pull out until pocket is formed between eye and lower lid.
2. Hold dropper above pocket and place prescribed number of drops into pocket. Close eye gently.
3. Apply digital pressure to lacrimal sac for 1-2 min (minimizes drainage into nose and throat, reducing risk of systemic effects).
4. Remove excess solution around eye w/tissue.

INDICATIONS/DOSAGE/ROUTES

Refraction:
OPHTHALMIC: Adults, elderly: 1-2 drops into eye; repeat in 5-10 min if necessary.

Inflammation:
OPHTHALMIC: Adults, elderly: 1-2 drops into eye q3-4h.

PRECAUTIONS

CONTRAINDICATIONS: Narrow-angle glaucoma, severe ulcerative colitis, toxic megacolon, obstructive disease of GI tract, paralytic ileus, intestinal atony, bladder neck obstruction due to prostatic hypertrophy, myasthenia gravis in those not treated w/neostigmine, tachycardia secondary to cardiac insufficiency or thyrotoxicosis, cardiospasm, unstable cardiovascular status in acute hemorrhage. **EXTREME CAUTION:** Autonomic neuropathy, known or suspected GI infections, diarrhea, mild to moderate ulcerative colitis. **CAUTIONS:** Hyperthyroidism, hepatic or renal disease, hypertension, tachyarrhythmias, CHF, coronary artery disease, gastric ulcer, esophageal reflux or hiatal hernia associated w/reflux esophagitis, infants, elderly. **PREGNANCY LACTATION:** Unknown if drug crosses placenta or is distributed in breast milk. **Pregnancy Category C.**

INTERACTIONS

DRUG INTERACTIONS: Acetylcholine, medications w/anticholinergic properties may increase anticholinergic effects. May decrease effects of carbachol, physostigmine, pilocarpine. **ALTERED LAB VALUES:** None significant.

SIDE EFFECTS

FREQUENT: Dry mouth (sometimes severe), decreased sweating, constipation. **OCCASIONAL:** Blurred vision, bloated feeling, urinary hesitancy, drowsiness (w/high dosage), headache, sensitivity to light, photophobia, loss of taste, nervousness, flushing, insomnia, impotence, mental confusion/excitement (particularly in elderly, children). **RARE:** Dizziness, faintness.

ADVERSE REACTIONS/TOXIC EFFECTS

Overdosage may produce temporary paralysis of ciliary muscle, pupillary dilation, tachycardia, palpitation, hot, dry, flushed skin, absence of bowel sounds, hyperthermia, increased respiratory rate, ECG abnormalities, nausea, vomiting, rash over face, upper trunk, CNS stimulation, psychosis (agitation, restlessness, rambling speech, visual hallucination, paranoid behavior, delusions), followed by depression.

NURSING IMPLICATIONS

Baseline Assessment:

Before giving medication, instruct pt to void (reduces risk of urinary retention).

Intervention/Evaluation:

Monitor daily bowel activity and stool consistency. Assess for urinary retention. Monitor changes in B/P, temperature. Assess skin turgor, mucous membranes to evaluate hydration status (encourage adequate fluid intake), bowel sounds for peristalsis. Be alert for fever (increased risk of hyperthermia).

Patient/Family Teaching:

Do not become overheated during exercise in hot weather (may result in heat stroke). Avoid hot baths, saunas. Avoid tasks that require alertness, motor skills until response to drug is established. Sugarless gum, sips of tepid water may relieve dry mouth. Do not take antacids or medicine for diarrhea within 1 hr of taking this medication (decreased effectiveness).

hydralazine hydrochloride

hy-dral´ah-zeen

(Apresoline)

FIXED-COMBINATION(S):
W/hydrochlorothiazide, a diuretic (Apresodex, Apresoline-Esidrex, Apresazide, Hydralazine PLUS, Hydrazide); w/reserpine, an antihypertensive (Serpasil-Apresoline); w/hydrochlorothiazide and reserpine (Cherapas, Ser-Ap-Es, Serathide).

CANADIAN AVAILABILITY:
Apresoline, Novohylazin

CLASSIFICATION

Antihypertensive

PHARMACOKINETICS

	ONSET	PEAK	DURATION
PO	10-20 min	0.5-2 hrs	2-4 hrs

Well absorbed from GI tract. Widely distributed. Protein binding: 87%. Metabolized in liver to active metabolite. Primarily excreted in urine. Half-life: 3-7 hrs (increased in decreased renal function).

ACTION

Reduces B/P by direct relaxation of vascular smooth muscle (greater effect on arterioles). Produces decreased peripheral vascular resistance, increased heart rate, cardiac output. Decreases afterload (increases CO, decreases systemic resistance).

USES

Management of moderate/severe hypertension.

STORAGE/HANDLING

Store oral form at room temperature.

PO ADMINISTRATION

1. Best given w/food or regularly spaced meals.
2. Tablets may be crushed.

INDICATIONS/DOSAGE/ROUTES

Hypertension:
PO: Adults: Initially, 10 mg 4

times/day for 2-4 days. Increase to 25 mg 4 times/day for remainder of first week. Increase second week and subsequent weeks to 50 mg 4 times/day. **Elderly:** Initially, 10 mg 2-3 times/day. May increase by 10-25 mg/day q2-5days. **Children:** Initially, 0.75 mg/kg in 4 divided doses (maximum 25 mg). May be increased over 1-4 wks up to 7.5 mg/kg/day or 200 mg/day.

PRECAUTIONS

CONTRAINDICATIONS: Coronary artery disease, rheumatic heart disease, lupus erythematosus. **CAUTIONS:** Impaired renal function, cerebrovascular disease. **PREGNANCY/LACTATION:** Drug crosses placenta; unknown if drug is distributed in breast milk. Thrombocytopenia, leukopenia, petechial bleeding, hematomas have occurred in newborns (resolved within 1-3 wks). **Pregnancy Category C.**

INTERACTIONS

DRUG INTERACTIONS: Diuretics, other hypotensives may increase hypotensive effect. **ALTERED LAB VALUES:** May produce positive direct Coomb's test.

SIDE EFFECTS

FREQUENT: Transient headache, palpitations, tachycardia should disappear in 7-10 days. **OCCASIONAL:** Postural hypotension, edema and/or weight gain (drug causes sodium and water retention), flushing, lacrimation, nasal congestion. High doses may produce GI disturbances (nausea, anorexia, diarrhea) and lupus erythematosis-like reaction (fever, facial rash, muscle and joint aches, splenomegaly).

ADVERSE REACTIONS/TOXIC EFFECTS

Severe orthostatic hypotension, generalized skin flushing, severe headache, myocardial ischemia, cardiac arrhythmias may develop. Profound shock may occur in cases of severe overdosage.

NURSING IMPLICATIONS

BASELINE ASSESSMENT:

Obtain B/P, pulse immediately before each dose administration, in addition to regular monitoring (be alert to fluctuations). Keep tissues readily available at pt's bedside for lacrimation, nasal congestion.

INTERVENTION/EVALUATION:

Assess for peripheral edema of hands, feet (usually, first area of low extremity swelling is behind medial malleolus in ambulatory, sacral area in bedridden). Monitor temperature for fever (lupuslike reaction). Monitor pattern of daily bowel activity and stool consistency.

PATIENT/FAMILY TEACHING:

To reduce hypotensive effect, rise slowly from lying to sitting position and permit legs to dangle from bed momentarily before standing. Unsalted crackers, dry toast may relieve nausea. Report muscle and joint aches, fever (lupuslike reaction).

hydrochlorothiazide

high-drow-chlor-oh-thigh´ah-zide

(HydroDIURIL, Esidrix, Oretic)

FIXED COMBINATION(S): W/methyldopa, an antihypertensive (Aldoril); w/propranolol, a beta blocker (Inderide); w/hydralazine, a vasodilator (Apresazide); w/captopril, an ACE inhibitor (Capozide); w/enalapril, an ACE inhibitor (Vaseretic); w/metoprolol, a beta blocker (Lopressor HCT); w/timolol, a beta blocker (Timolide); w/labetolol, an alpha-beta blocker (Normozide); w/potassium sparing diuretics (amiloride [Moduretic]) (spironolactone [Aldactazide]) (triamterene [Dyazide, Maxzide]).

CANADIAN AVAILABILITY: Apo-Hydro, Diuchlor H, Hydrodiuril, Neo-Codema

CLASSIFICATION

Diuretic: Thiazide

PHARMACOKINETICS

	ONSET	PEAK	DURATION
PO (diuretic)	2 hrs	4-6 hrs	6-12 hrs

Variably absorbed from GI tract. Primarily excreted unchanged in liver. Half-life: 5.6-14.8 hrs.

ACTION

Diuretic: Inhibits sodium, water reabsorption in early distal tubule. Increases delivery of sodium, water to site of potassium secretion promoting sodium reabsorption, increasing potassium excretion. Increases aldosterone secretion due to decreased plasma volume. *Antihypertensive:* Reduces plasma, extracellular fluid volume. Decreases PVR by direct effect on blood vessels.

USES

Adjunctive therapy in edema associated w/CHF, hepatic cirrhosis, corticoid or estrogen therapy, renal impairment. In treatment of hypertension, may be used alone or w/other antihypertensive agents.

PO ADMINISTRATION

May give w/food or milk if GI upset occurs, preferably w/breakfast (may prevent nocturia).

INDICATIONS/DOSAGE/ROUTES

Edema:
PO: Adults: Initially, 25-200 mg in 1-3 divided doses. **Maintenance:** 25-100 mg/day. **Maximum:** 200 mg/day.

Hypertension:
PO: Adults: Initially, 12.5-25 mg/day. Gradually increase up to 50 mg/day. **Maintenance:** 25-50 mg/day.

Usual elderly dosage:
PO: Elderly: 12.5-25 mg/day.

Usual dosage for children:
PO: Children, 2-12 yrs: 37.5-100 mg/day. **Children <2 yrs:** 12.5-37.5 mg/day.

PRECAUTIONS

CONTRAINDICATIONS: History of hypersensitivity to sulfonamides or thiazide diuretics, renal decompensation, anuria. **CAUTIONS:** Severe renal disease, impaired hepatic function, diabetes mellitus, elderly/debilitated, thyroid disorders. **PREGNANCY/LACTATION:** Crosses placenta; small amount distributed in breast milk—nursing not advised. **Pregnancy Category B.**

INTERACTIONS

DRUG INTERACTIONS: Cholestyramine, colestipol may decrease absorption, effects. May increase digoxin toxicity (due to hypokalemia). May increase lithium toxicity.

ALTERED LAB VALUES: May increase bilirubin, serum calcium, LDL, cholesterol, triglycerides, creatinine, glucose, uric acid. May decrease urinary calcium, magnesium, potassium, sodium.

SIDE EFFECTS

EXPECTED: Increase in urine frequency/volume. **FREQUENT:** Potassium depletion. **OCCASIONAL:** Postural hypotension, headache, GI disturbances, photosensitivity reaction.

ADVERSE REACTIONS/TOXIC EFFECTS

Vigorous diuresis may lead to profound water loss and electrolyte depletion, resulting in hypokalemia, hyponatremia, dehydration. Acute hypotensive episodes may occur. Hyperglycemia may be noted during prolonged therapy. GI upset, pancreatitis, dizziness, paresthesias, headache, blood dyscrasias, pulmonary edema, allergic pneumonitis, dermatologic reactions occur rarely. Overdosage can lead to lethargy, coma w/o changes in electrolytes or hydration.

NURSING IMPLICATIONS

BASELINE ASSESSMENT:

Check vital signs, especially B/P for hypotension prior to administration. Assess baseline electrolytes, particularly check for low potassium. Evaluate edema, skin turgor, mucous membranes for hydration status. Assess muscle strength, mental status. Note skin temperature, moisture. Obtain baseline weight. Initiate I&O.

INTERVENTION/EVALUATION:

Continue to monitor B/P, vital signs, electrolytes, I&O, weight. Note extent of diuresis. Watch for changes from initial assessment (hypokalemia may result in weakness, tremor, muscle cramps, nausea, vomiting, change in mental status, tachycardia; hyponatremia may result in confusion, thirst, cold/clammy skin). Be esp. alert for potassium depletion in pts taking digoxin (cardiac arrhythmias). Potassium supplements are frequently ordered. Check for constipation (may occur w/exercise diuresis).

PATIENT/FAMILY TEACHING:

Expect increased frequency and volume of urination. To reduce hypotensive effect, rise slowly from lying to sitting position and permit legs to dangle momentarily before standing. Eat foods high in potassium such as whole grains (cereals), legumes, meat, bananas, apricots, orange juice, potatoes (white, sweet), raisins. Protect skin from sun/ultraviolet rays (photosensitivity may occur).

hydrocodone bitartrate

high-drough-koe´doan

FIXED-COMBINATION(S): W/acetaminophen (Anexsia, Lortab, Vicodin); w/aspirin (Lortab ASA); w/chlorpheniramine, an antihistamine (Tussionex); w/phenylpropanolamine, a sympathomimetic (Hycomine)

CANADIAN AVAILABILITY: Hycodan, Robidone

CLASSIFICATION

Opioid: Analgesic **(Schedule III)**

PHARMACOKINETICS

	ONSET	PEAK	DURATION
PO	—	—	4-6 hrs

Well absorbed from GI tract. Metabolized in liver. Primarily excreted in urine. Half-life: 3.8 hrs (increased in elderly).

ACTION

Binds w/opioid receptors within CNS, altering processes affecting pain perception, emotional response to pain.

USES

Relief of moderate to moderately severe pain, nonproductive cough.

PO ADMINISTRATION

1. Give w/o regard to meals.
2. Tablets may be crushed.

INDICATIONS/DOSAGE/ROUTES

Analgesia:
PO: Adults, children >12 yrs: 5-10 mg q4-6h. **Elderly:** 2.5-5 mg q4-6h.

Antitussive:
PO: Adults: 5-10 mg q4-6h as needed. **Maximum:** 15 mg/dose. **Children:** 0.6 mg/kg/day in 3-4 divided doses at intervals of no less than 4 hrs. **Maximum single dose in children 2-12 yrs:** 5 mg. **Maximum single dose in children <2 yrs:** 1.25 mg.

Extended-release:
PO: Adults: 10 mg q12h. **Children 6-12 yrs:** 5 mg q12h.

PRECAUTIONS

CONTRAINDICATIONS: None significant. **EXTREME CAUTION:** CNS depression, anoxia, hypercapnia, respiratory depression, seizures, acute alcoholism, shock, untreated myxedema, respiratory dysfunction. **CAUTIONS:** Increased intracranial pressure, impaired hepatic function, acute abdominal conditions, hypothyroidism, prostatic hypertrophy, Addison's disease, urethral stricture, COPD. **PREGNANCY/LACTATION:** Readily crosses placenta; distributed in breast milk. May prolong labor if administered in latent phase of first stage of labor, or before cervical dilation of 4-5 cm has occurred. Respiratory depression may occur in neonate if mother received opiates during labor. Regular use of opiates during pregnancy may produce withdrawal symptoms (irritability, excessive crying, tremors, hyperactive reflexes, fever, vomiting, diarrhea, yawning, sneezing, seizures) in the neonate. **Pregnancy Category C.**

INTERACTIONS

DRUG INTERACTIONS: Alcohol, CNS depressants may increase CNS, respiratory depression, hypotension. MAO inhibitors, may produce severe, fatal reaction (reduce dose to 1/4 usual dose). **ALTERED LAB VALUES:** May increase amylase, lipase plasma concentrations.

SIDE EFFECTS

NOTE: Effects are dependent on dosage amount but occur infrequently w/oral antitussives. Ambulatory pts and those not in severe pain may experience dizziness, nausea, vomiting, hypotension more frequently than those who are in supine position or having severe pain. **FREQUENT:** Suppressed breathing depth. **OCCASIONAL:** Sweating, flushing, feeling of facial and neck warmth, lightheadedness, mental clouding, dizziness, sedation, hypotension, nausea, vomiting, euphoria/dysphoria, constipation (drug delays digestion), urinary retention.

ADVERSE REACTIONS/TOXIC EFFECTS

Overdosage results in respiratory depression, skeletal muscle flaccidity, cold, clammy skin, cyanosis, extreme somnolence progressing to convulsions, stupor, coma. Tolerance to analgesic effect, physical dependence may occur w/repeated use. Prolonged duration of action, cumulative effect may occur in those w/impaired hepatic, renal function.

NURSING IMPLICATIONS

BASELINE ASSESSMENT:

Obtain vital signs before giving medication. If respirations are 12/min or lower (20/min or lower in children), w/hold medication, contact physician. *Analgesic:* Assess onset, type, location, and duration of pain. Effect of medication is reduced if full pain recurs before next dose. *Antitussive:* Assess type, severity, frequency of cough, and productions.

INTERVENTION/EVALUATION:

Increase fluid intake and environmental humidity to improve viscosity of lung secretions. Palpate bladder for urinary retention. Monitor pattern of daily bowel activity and stool consistency. Initiate deep breathing and coughing exercises, particularly in those w/impaired pulmonary function. Assess for clinical improvement and record onset of relief of pain or cough.

PATIENT/FAMILY TEACHING:

Change positions slowly to avoid orthostatic hypotension. Avoid tasks that require alertness, motor skills until response to drug is established. Tolerance/dependence may occur w/prolonged use of high doses.

H

hydrocortisone

high-droe-core´tah-sewn

(Cortef, Cort-Dome, Cortenema, Hydrocortone, Hytone)

hydrocortisone acetate

(Cortaid, Corticaine)

hydrocortisone butyrate

(Locoid)

hydrocortisone cypionate

(Cortef Suspension)

hydrocortisone sodium phosphate

(Hydrocortone Phosphate)

hydrocortisone sodium succinate

(A-hydroCort, Solu-Cortef)

hydrocortisone valerate

(WestCort)

FIXED-COMBINATION(S):

W/Neomycin, an antibiotic, (Neo-Cort-Dome); w/Bacitracin, Neomycin, Polymyxin B, anti-infectives, (Cortisporin); hydrocortisone acetate w/Neomycin, an antibiotic, (Neo-Cortef)

CANADIAN AVAILABILITY: Cortamed, Cortaid, Cortef, Cortenema, Corticreme, SoluCortef, Westcort

CLASSIFICATION

PHARMACOTHERAPEUTIC: Adrenocorticosteroid

CLINICAL: Glucocorticoid

PHARMACOKINETICS

Well absorbed from GI tract, after IM administration. Widely distributed. Protein binding: high. Metabolized in liver. Half-life: *plasma:* 1.5-2 hrs; *biologic:* 8-12 hrs.

ACTION

Decreases/prevents tissue response to inflammatory process. Inhibits accumulation of inflammatory cells at inflammation sites, phagocytosis, lysosomal enzyme release and synthesis and/or release of mediators of inflammation. Prevents/suppresses cell-mediated immune reactions.

USES

Substitution therapy in deficiency states (acute/chronic adrenal insufficiency, congenital adrenal hyperplasia, adrenal insufficiency secondary to pituitary insufficiency); nonendocrine disorders (arthritis, rheumatic carditis, allergic, collagen, intestinal tract, liver, ocular, renal, skin diseases, bronchial asthma, cerebral edema, malignancies). Rectal: Adjunctive therapy in treatment of ulcerative colitis.

STORAGE/HANDLING

Store parenteral forms at room temperature. *Hydrocortisone sodium succinate:* After reconstitution, use solution within 72 hrs. Use immediately if further diluted w/ 5% dextrose, 0.9% NaCl, or other compatible diluent.

PO/IM/IV/TOPICAL/OPHTHALMIC/OTIC ADMINISTRATION

PO:

1. Give w/milk or food (decreases GI upset).
2. Give single dose before 9 AM, give multiple doses at evenly spaced intervals.

TOPICAL:

1. Gently cleanse area prior to application.
2. Use occlusive dressings only as ordered.
3. Apply sparingly and rub into area thoroughly.

IM/IV:

1. Once reconstituted, solution stable for 72 hrs at room temperature.
2. May further dilute w/5% dextrose or 0.9% NaCl.

RECTAL:

1. Shake homogeneous suspension well.
2. Instruct pt to lie on left side w/left leg extended, right leg flexed.
3. Gently insert applicator tip into rectum, pointed slightly toward naval (umbilicus).
4. Aim nozzle to back, then slowly instill medication.

INDICATIONS/DOSAGE/ROUTES

Hydrocortisone:

PO: Adults, elderly: 20-240 mg/day.

IM: Adults, elderly: ⅓-½ oral dose q12h.

Hydrocortisone sodium phosphate:
IM/IV/SubQ: Adults, elderly: 15-240 mg/day, usually ⅓-½ oral dose q12h.

Hydrocortisone sodium succinate:
IM/IV: Adults, elderly: Initially, 100-500 mg/day.

Hydrocortisone acetate:
INTRA-ARTICULAR, INTRALESIONAL, SOFT TISSUE: Adults, elderly: 5-50 mg.

Usual rectal dosage:
RECTAL: Adults, elderly: 100 mg at bedtime for 21 nights or until clinical and proctologic remission occurs. (May require 2-3 mo therapy.)
CORTIFOAM: Adults, elderly: 1 applicator 1-2 times/day for 2-3 wks, then every second day thereafter.

Usual topical dosage:
TOPICAL: Adults, elderly: Apply sparingly 2-4 times/day.

PRECAUTIONS

CONTRAINDICATIONS: Hypersensitivity to any corticosteroid or sulfite, systemic fungal infection, peptic ulcers (except life-threatening situations). Avoid live virus vaccine such as smallpox. *Topical:* Marked circulation impairment. Do not instill ocular solution when topical corticosteroids are being used on eyelids or surrounding skin. **CAUTIONS:** Thromboembolic disorders, history of tuberculosis (may reactivate disease), hypothyroidism, cirrhosis, nonspecific ulcerative colitis, CHF, hypertension, psychosis, renal insufficiency, seizure disorders. Prolonged therapy should be discontinued slowly. *Topical:* Do not apply to extensive areas. **PREGNANCY/LACTATION:** Crosses placenta, distributed in breast milk. May produce cleft palate if used chronically during first trimester. Nursing contraindicated. **Pregnancy Category C.**

INTERACTIONS

DRUG INTERACTIONS: Amphotericin may increase hypokalemia. May decrease effect of oral hypoglycemics, insulin, diuretics, potassium supplements. May increase digoxin toxicity (due to hypokalemia). Hepatic enzyme inducers may decrease effect. Live virus vaccines may potentiate virus replication, increase vaccine side effects, decrease pt's antibody response to vaccine. **ALTERED LAB VALUES:** May decrease calcium, potassium, thyroxine. May increase cholesterol, lipids, glucose, sodium, amylase.

SIDE EFFECTS

NOTE: W/high dose, prolonged therapy: **FREQUENT:** Increased susceptibility to infection (signs/symptoms masked); delayed wound healing; hypokalemia; hypocalcemia; nausea, vomiting, anorexia or increased appetite, diarrhea or constipation; sodium and water retention, hypertension. **OCCASIONAL:** Hypercholesterolemia, thrombophlebitis, fat embolism, headache, vertigo, insomnia, mood swings, depression, euphoria, hyperglycemia and aggravation or induction of diabetes mellitus, hirsutism, acne, suppression of pituitary w/decreased release of corticotropin, muscle wasting, osteoporosis, menstrual difficulties or amenorrhea, ulcer development (2%), hypo/hyperpigmentation w/

parenteral, growth retardation in children. *Topical:* Itching, redness, irritation. **RARE:** Increased blood coagulability, sterile abscess, or atrophy at site w/parenteral, symptoms of vitamin A or C deficiency, posterior subcapsular cataracts (esp. in children), tachycardia, frequency or urgency of urination, seizures, psychosis. *Topical:* Allergic contact dermatitis, purpura. Systemic absorption more likely w/occlusive dressings or extensive application in young children.

ADVERSE REACTIONS/TOXIC EFFECTS

Anaphylaxis w/parenteral administration, pathologic and vertebral compression fractures. Sudden discontinuance may be fatal. Rarely, intralesional injection around face, head may produce blindness.

NURSING IMPLICATIONS

BASELINE ASSESSMENT:

Question for hypersensitivity to any corticosteroids, sulfite. Obtain baselines for height, weight, B/P, glucose, cholesterol, electrolytes. Check results of initial tests, e.g. TB skin test, X-rays, EKG.

INTERVENTION/EVALUATION:

Monitor I&O, daily weight. Assess for edema. Check lab results for blood coagulability and clinical evidence of thromboembolus, thrombophlebitis. Evaluate food tolerance and bowel activity; report hyperacidity promptly. Check B/P, vital signs at least 2 times/day. Be alert to infection: sore throat, fever, or vague symptoms. Monitor electrolytes. Watch for hypocalcemia (muscle twitching, cramps, positive Trousseau's or Chvostek's signs) or hypokalemia (weakness and muscle cramps, numbness/tingling esp. lower extremities, nausea and vomiting, irritability, EKG changes). Assess emotional status, ability to sleep. Provide assistance w/ambulation. Retention enema of hydrocortisone (Cortenema) may be ordered to reduce GI inflammation.

PATIENT/FAMILY TEACHING:

Take w/food or milk. Carry identification of drug and dose, physician's name and phone number. Do not change dose/schedule or stop taking drug, must taper off gradually under medical supervision. Notify physician of fever, sore throat, muscle aches, sudden weight gain/swelling. W/dietician give instructions for prescribed diet (usually sodium restricted w/ high vitamin D, protein, potassium). Maintain careful personal hygiene, avoid exposure to disease or trauma. Severe stress (serious infection, surgery, or trauma) may require increased dosage. Do not take aspirin or any other medication w/o consulting physician. Follow-up visits, lab tests are necessary; children must be assessed for growth retardation. Inform dentist or other physicians of hydrocortisone therapy now or within past 12 mos. Caution against overuse of joints injected for symptomatic relief. *Topical.* Apply after shower or bath for best absorption. Do not cover unless physician orders; do not use tight diapers, plastic pants, or coverings. Avoid contact w/eyes. Do not expose treated area to sunlight.

hydromorphone hydrochloride

high-dro-more´phone
(Dilaudid)

FIXED-COMBINATION(S): W/guaifenesin, an expectorant (Dilaudid Cough Syrup)

CANADIAN AVAILABILITY: Dilaudid

CLASSIFICATION

Opioid: Analgesic **(Schedule II)**

PHARMACOKINETICS

	ONSET	PEAK	DURATION
PO	30 min	90-120 min	4 hrs
SubQ	15 min	30-90 min	4 hrs
IM	15 min	30-60 min	4-5 hrs
IV	10-15 min	15-30 min	2-3 hrs
Rectal	15-30 min	—	—

Well absorbed from GI tract, after IM administration. Widely distributed. Metabolized in liver. Excreted in urine. Half-life: 1-3 hrs.

ACTION

Binds w/opioid receptors within CNS, altering processes affecting pain perception, emotional response to pain.

USES

Relief of moderate to severe pain, persistent nonproductive cough.

STORAGE/HANDLING

Store oral/parenteral form at room temperature. Slight yellow discoloration of parenteral form does not indicate loss of potency. Refrigerate suppositories.

PO/IM/IV/RECTAL ADMINISTRATION

PO: 1. Give w/o regard to meals.
2. Tablets may be crushed.

SubQ/IM:

1. Use short 30-gauge needle for SubQ injection.
2. Administer slowly, rotating injection sites.
3. Pts w/circulatory impairment experience higher risk of overdosage because of delayed absorption of repeated administration.

IV: Note: High concentration injection (10 mg/ml) should only be used in those tolerant to opiate agonists, currently receiving high doses of another opiate agonist for severe, chronic pain due to cancer.

1. Administer very slowly (over 2-3 min).
2. Rapid IV increases risk of severe adverse reactions (chest wall rigidity, apnea, peripheral circulatory collapse, anaphylactoid effects, cardiac arrest).

RECTAL:

1. Moisten suppository w/cold water before inserting well up into rectum.

INDICATIONS/DOSAGE/ROUTES

Analgesia:
PO/SubQ/IM/IV: Adults, elderly: 2 mg q4-6h, as needed. Severe pain may require up to 4 mg q4-6h.
RECTAL: Adults, elderly: 3 mg q6-8h.

Antitussive:
PO: Adults, children >12 yrs, elderly: 1 mg q3-4h. **Children 6-12 yrs:** 0.5 mg q3-4h.

PRECAUTIONS

CONTRAINDICATIONS: None significant. **EXTREME CAUTION:** CNS depression, anoxia, hypercapnia, respiratory depression, seizures, acute alcoholism, shock, untreated myxedema, respiratory dysfunction. **CAUTIONS:** Increased intracranial pressure, impaired hepatic function, acute abdominal conditions, hypothyroidism, prostatic hypertrophy, Addison's disease, urethral stricture, COPD. **PREGNANCY/LACTATION:** Readily crosses placenta; unknown if distributed in breast milk. May prolong labor if administered in latent phase of first stage of labor, or before cervical dilation of 4-5 cm has occurred. Respiratory depression may occur in neonate if mother receives opiates during labor. Regular use of opiates during pregnancy may produce withdrawal symptoms in the neonate (irritability, excessive crying, tremors, hyperactive reflexes, fever, vomiting, diarrhea, yawning, sneezing, seizures). **Pregnancy Category C.**

INTERACTIONS

DRUG INTERACTIONS: Alcohol, CNS depressants may increase CNS, respiratory depression, hypotension. MAO inhibitors may produce severe, fatal reaction (reduce dose to 1/4 usual dose). **ALTERED LAB VALUES:** May increase amylase, lipase plasma concentrations.

SIDE EFFECTS

NOTE: Effects are dependent on dosage amount, route of administration but occur infrequently w/ oral antitussives. Ambulatory pts and those not in severe pain may experience dizziness, nausea, vomiting, hypotension more frequently than those in supine position or having severe pain. **FREQUENT:** Sedation, suppressed breathing depth. **OCCASIONAL:** Lightheadedness, mental clouding, dizziness, sedation, hypotension, nausea, vomiting, euphoria/dysphoria, constipation (drug delays digestion), sweating, flushing, feeling of facial and neck warmth, urinary retention.

ADVERSE REACTIONS/TOXIC EFFECTS

Overdosage results in respiratory depression, skeletal muscle flaccidity, cold, clammy skin, cyanosis, extreme somnolence progressing to convulsions, stupor, coma. Tolerance to analgesic effect, physical dependence may occur w/repeated use. Prolonged duration of action, cumulative effect may occur in those w/impaired hepatic, renal function.

NURSING IMPLICATIONS

BASELINE ASSESSMENT:

Obtain vital signs before giving medication. If respirations are 12/min or lower (20/min or lower in children), withhold medication, contact physician. *Analgesic:* Assess onset, type, location, and duration of pain. Effect of medication is reduced if full pain recurs before next dose. *Antitussive:* Assess type, severity, frequency of cough and productions.

INTERVENTION/EVALUATION:

Monitor B/P, pulse, respirations. Assess cough, lung sounds. Increase fluid intake and environmental humidity to improve viscosity of lung secretions. To prevent pain cycles, instruct pt to request pain medication as soon as discomfort begins. Check for constipation (esp. in long-term use) and increase fiber, fluids, and exercise as appropriate. Initiate deep breathing and coughing exercises, particularly in those w/impaired pulmonary function. Assess for clinical improvement and record onset of relief of pain or cough.

PATIENT/FAMILY TEACHING:

Discomfort may occur w/injection. Change positions slowly to avoid orthostatic hypotension. Avoid tasks that require alertness, motor skills until response to drug is established. Tolerance/dependence may occur w/prolonged use of high doses. Avoid alcohol.

hydroxychloroquine sulfate

hi-drocks-ee-klor′oh-kwin
(Plaquenil Sulfate)

CANADIAN AVAILABILITY:
Plaquenil

CLASSIFICATION

Antimalarial, antirheumatic

PHARMACOKINETICS

Variably absorbed from GI tract. Widely distributed. Protein binding: 45%. Slowly excreted in urine. Minimal removal by hemodialysis. Half-life: 1.9-5.5 hrs.

ACTION

Concentrates in parasite acid vesicles, increases pH (inhibits parasite growth). May interfere w/parasite protein synthesis. Antirheumatic action unknown, but may involve suppressing formation of antigens responsible for hypersensitivity reactions.

USES

Treatment of falciparum malaria (terminates acute attacks and cures nonresistant strains), suppression of acute attacks and prolongation of interval between treatment/relapse in vivax, ovale, malariae malaria. Treatment of discoid or systematic lupus erythematosus, acute and chronic rheumatoid arthritis.

H

ADMINISTRATION

Administer w/meals to reduce GI upset.

INDICATIONS/DOSAGE/ROUTES

NOTE: 200 mg hydroxychloroquine = 155 mg base.

Suppression of malaria:
PO: Adults: 310 mg base weekly on same day each week. **Children:** 5 mg base/kg/wk. Begin 2 wks prior to exposure; continue 6-8 wks after leaving endemic area or if therapy is not begun prior to exposure.
PO: Adults: 620 mg base. **Children:** 10 mg base/kg given in 2 divided doses 6 hrs apart.

Treatment of malaria (acute attack): Dose (mg base)

DOSE	TIMES	ADULTS	CHILDREN
Initial	Day 1	620 mg	10 mg/kg
2nd	6 hrs later	310 mg	5 mg/kg
3rd	Day 2	310 mg	5 mg/kg
4th	Day 3	310 mg	5 mg/kg

Rheumatoid arthritis:
PO: Adults: Initially, 400-600 mg (310-465 mg base) daily for 5-10 days; gradually increase dose to optimum response level. **Maintenance (usually within 4-12 wks):** Decrease dose by 50%, continue at level of 200-400 mg/day. Maximum effect may not be seen for several months.

Lupus erythematosus:
PO: Adults: Initially, 400 mg 1-2 times/day for several weeks or months. **Maintenance:** 200-400 mg/day.

PRECAUTIONS

CONTRAINDICATIONS: Hypersensitivity to 4-aminoquinolones, retinal, or visual field changes, long-term therapy for children, psoriasis, porphyria. After weighing risk/benefit ratio, physician may still elect to use drug, esp. w/ plasmodial forms. **CAUTIONS:** Alcoholism, hepatic disease, G-6-PD deficiency. Children are esp. susceptible to hydroxychloroquine fatalities. **PREGNANCY/LACTATION:** Unknown if drug crosses placenta; small amount excreted in breast milk. If possible, avoid use in pregnancy. **Pregnancy Category C.**

INTERACTIONS

DRUG INTERACTIONS: May increase concentration of penicillamine, increase risk of hematologic/renal or severe skin reaction. **ALTERED LAB VALUES:** None significant.

SIDE EFFECTS

FREQUENT: Mild transient headache, anorexia, nausea, vomiting. **OCCASIONAL:** Visual disturbances (blurring and difficulty focusing); nervousness; fatigue; pruritus (esp. of palms, soles, scalp); bleaching of hair; irritability, personality changes, diarrhea, skin eruptions. **RARE:** Stomatitis, exfoliative dermatitis, reduced hearing (nerve deafness).

ADVERSE REACTIONS/TOXIC EFFECTS

Ocular toxicity (esp. retinopathy, which may progress even after drug is discontinued). Prolonged therapy: peripheral neuritis, neuromyopathy, hypotension, ECG changes, agranulocytosis, aplastic anemia, thrombocytopenia, convulsions, psychosis. Overdosage: headache, vomiting, visual disturbance, drowsiness, convulsions, hypokalemia followed by cardiovascular collapse, death.

NURSING IMPLICATIONS

BASELINE ASSESSMENT:

Question for hypersensitivity to hydroxychloroquine sulfate or chloroquine. Evaluate CBC, hepatic function results.

INTERVENTION/EVALUATION:

Monitor and report any visual disturbances promptly. Evaluate for GI distress: give dose w/food, (for malaria); discuss w/physician dividing the dose into separate days during week. Monitor hepatic function tests and check for fatigue, jaundice, other signs of hepatic effects. Assess skin and buccal mucosa; inquire about pruritus. Check vital signs. Be alert to signs/symptoms of overdosage (esp. w/children). Monitor CBC results for adverse hematologic effects. Report reduced hearing immediately. W/ prolonged therapy, test for muscle weakness.

PATIENT/FAMILY TEACHING:

Continue drug for full length of treatment. In long-term therapy therapeutic response may not be evident for up to 6 mo. Immediately notify physician of *any* new symptom of visual difficulties, muscular weakness, decreased hearing, tinnitus. Do not take any other medication w/o consulting physician. Periodic lab and visual tests are important part of therapy. Keep out of reach of children (small amount can cause serious effects, death).

hydroxyurea

high-drocks-ee-your´e-ah
(Hydrea)

CANADIAN AVAILABILITY: Hydrea

CLASSIFICATION

Antineoplastic

PHARMACOKINETICS

Well absorbed from GI tract. Crosses blood-brain barrier. Metabolized in liver. Primarily excreted in urine; partially removed in lungs as CO_2. Half-life: 3-4 hrs.

ACTION

Cell cycle-specific for S-phase. May be involved w/interference of DNA synthesis.

USES

Treatment of melanoma, resistant chronic myelocytic leukemia, recurrent, metastatic, or inoperable ovarian carcinoma. Also used in combination w/radiation therapy for local control of primary squamous cell carcinoma of head and neck, excluding lip.

PO ADMINISTRATION

NOTE: May be carcinogenic, mutagenic, or teratogenic. Handle w/ extreme care during administration.

If unable to swallow, dissolve contents of capsule in water immediately before administration.

INDICATIONS/DOSAGE/ROUTES

NOTE: Dosage individualized based on clinical response, tolerance to adverse effects. When used in combination therapy, consult specific protocols for optimum dosage, sequence of drug administration. Dosage based on actual or ideal body weight, whichever is less. Therapy interrupted when platelets fall below 100,000/mm^3 or leukocytes fall below 2,500/mm^3. Resume when counts rise towards normal.

Solid tumors, carcinoma of head and neck (with irradiation):
PO: Adults: 60-80 mg/kg (2-3 Gm/m^2) as single dose every third day, or 20-30 mg/kg as single daily dose begun at least 7 days prior to irradiation initiation.

Resistant chronic myelocytic leukemia:
PO: Adults: 20-30 mg/kg as single daily dose or 2 divided doses.

PRECAUTIONS

CONTRAINDICATIONS: WBC less than 2,500/mm^3 or platelet count $<$100,000/mm^3. **CAUTIONS:** Previous irradiation therapy, other cytoxic drugs, impaired renal, hepatic function. **PREGNANCY/LACTATION:** If possible, avoid use during pregnancy, especially first trimester. Breast feeding not recommended. **Pregnancy Category C.**

INTERACTIONS

DRUG INTERACTIONS: May decrease effect of antigout medications. Bone marrow depressants may increase bone marrow depression. Live virus vaccines may potentiate virus replication, increase vaccine side effects, decrease pt's antibody response to vaccine. **ALTERED LAB VALUES:** May increase BUN, creatinine, uric acid.

SIDE EFFECTS

FREQUENT: Nausea, vomiting, anorexia, constipation/diarrhea. **OCCASIONAL:** Mild, reversible rash, facial flushing, pruritus, fever, chills, malaise. **RARE:** Alopecia, headache, drowsiness, dizziness, disorientation.

ADVERSE REACTIONS/TOXIC EFFECTS

Bone marrow depression manifested as hematologic toxicity (leukopenia, and to lesser extent, thrombocytopenia, anemia).

NURSING IMPLICATIONS

BASELINE ASSESSMENT:

Obtain bone marrow studies, liver, kidney function tests before therapy begins, periodically thereafter. Obtain Hgb, WBC, platelet count weekly during therapy. Those w/marked renal impairment may develop visual, auditory hallucinations, marked hematologic toxicity.

INTERVENTION/EVALUATION:

Assess pattern of daily bowel activity and stool consistency. Monitor for hematologic toxicity (fever, sore throat, signs of local infection, easy bruising, or unusual bleeding from any site), symptoms of anemia (excessive tiredness, weakness). Assess skin for rash, erythema.

PATIENT/FAMILY TEACHING:

Alopecia is reversible, but new hair growth may have different color or texture. Do not have immunizations w/o physician's approval (drug lowers body's resistance). Avoid contact w/those who have recently received live virus vaccine. Promptly report fever, sore throat, signs of local infection, easy bruising, or unusual bleeding from any site. Contact physician if nausea/vomiting continues at home.

hydroxyzine hydrochloride

high-drox´ih-zeen

(Atarax, Vistaril)

hydroxyzine pamoate

(Vistaril)

CANADIAN AVAILABILITY: Apo-Hydroxyzine, Atarax, Novo-hydroxyzin

CLASSIFICATION

Antihistamine

PHARMACOKINETICS

	ONSET	PEAK	DURATION
PO	15-30 min	—	—

Well absorbed from GI tract, after IM administration. Metabolized in liver. Primarily excreted in urine. Half-life: 20-25 hrs (increased in elderly).

ACTION

Prevents, antagonizes most histamine effects (e.g., urticaria, pruritus). Anticholinergic effects cause drying of nasal mucosa. Suppresses activity in subcortical area of CNS. Diminishes vestibular stimulation and depresses labyrinthine function. May act on CTZ in medulla.

USES

Relief of anxiety, tension; pruritus caused by allergic conditions, preop and postop sedation, control of muscle spasm, nausea and vomiting.

STORAGE/HANDLING

Store oral solution/suspension, parenteral form at room temperature.

PO/IM ADMINISTRATION

PO:

1. Shake oral suspension well.
2. Scored tablets may be crushed.
3. Do not crush or break capsule.

IM: Note: Significant tissue damage, thrombosis, gangrene may occur if injection is given SubQ, intra-arterial, or IV injection.

1. IM may be given undiluted.
2. Use Z-track technique of injection to prevent SubQ infiltration.
3. Inject deep IM into gluteus maximus or midlateral thigh in adults, midlateral thigh in children.

INDICATIONS/DOSAGE/ROUTES

Anxiety, tension:
PO: Adults, elderly: 25-100 mg 3-4 times/day. **Children >6 yrs:** 50-100 mg/day in divided doses. **Children <6 yrs:** 50 mg/day in divided doses.
IM: Adults, elderly: 25-100 mg q4-6h, as needed. **Children:** 0.5 mg/kg.

Nausea, vomiting:
IM: Adults, elderly: 25-100 mg. **Children:** 1.1 mg/kg.

Pruritus:
PO: Adults, elderly: 25 mg 3-4 times/day. **Children >6 yrs:** 50-100/day in divided doses. **Children <6 yrs:** 50 mg/day in divided doses.

Agitation due to alcohol withdrawal:
IM: Adults, elderly: 50-100 mg. May be repeated q4-6h, as needed.

PRECAUTIONS

CONTRAINDICATIONS: None significant. **CAUTIONS:** None significant. **PREGNANCY/LACTATION:** Unknown if hydroxyzine crosses placenta or is distributed in breast milk. **Pregnancy Category C.**

INTERACTIONS

DRUG INTERACTIONS: Alcohol, CNS depressants may increase CNS depressant effects. MAO inhibitors may increase anticholinergic, CNS depressant effects. **ALTERED LAB VALUES:** May cause false positives w/17-hydroxy corticosteroid determinations.

SIDE EFFECTS

Side effects are generally mild and transient. **FREQUENT:** Drowsiness, dry mouth, marked discomfort w/IM injection. **OCCASIONAL:** Dizziness, ataxia (muscular incoordination), weakness, slurred speech, headache, agitation, increased anxiety. **RARE:** Paradoxical CNS hyperactivity/nervousness in children, excitement/restlessness in elderly/debilitated pts (generally noted during first 2 wks of therapy, particularly noted in presence of uncontrolled pain).

ADVERSE REACTIONS/TOXIC EFFECTS

Hypersensitivity reaction (wheezing, dyspnea, tightness of chest).

NURSING IMPLICATIONS

BASELINE ASSESSMENT:

Anxiety: Offer emotional support to anxious pt. Assess motor responses (agitation, trembling, tension) and autonomic responses (cold, clammy hands, sweating). *Antiemetic:* Assess for dehydration (poor skin turgor, dry mucous membranes, longitudinal furrows in tongue).

INTERVENTION/EVALUATION:

For those on long-term therapy, liver/renal function tests, blood counts should be performed periodically. Monitor lung sounds for signs of hypersensitivity reaction. Monitor serum electrolytes in those w/severe vomiting. Assess for paradoxical reaction, particularly during early therapy. Assist w/ambulation if drowsiness, lightheadedness occur.

PATIENT/FAMILY TEACHING:

Marked discomfort may occur w/IM injection. Sugarless gum, sips of tepid water may relieve dry mouth. Drowsiness usually diminishes w/continued therapy. Avoid tasks that require alertness, motor skills until response to drug is established.

hyoscyamine hydrobromide

high-oh-sigh´ah-meen

hyoscyamine sulfate

(Anaspaz, Levsin, Levsinex, Neoquess, Cystospaz)

FIXED-COMBINATION(S):

W/phenobarbital, a sedative-hypnotic (Levsinex w/PB, Anaspaz PB)

CANADIAN AVAILABILITY:
Buscopan, Levsin

CLASSIFICATION

Anticholinergic

PHARMACOKINETICS

Well absorbed from GI tract. Widely distributed. Protein binding: 50%. Metabolized in liver. Primarily excreted in urine. Half-life: 3.5 hrs.

ACTION

Inhibits action of acetylcholine on structures innervated by postganglionic sites: smooth, cardiac muscle, SA, AV nodes, exocrine glands. Larger doses may decrease motility, secretory activity of GI system, tone of ureter, urinary bladder.

USES

Adjunct in treatment of peptic ulcer disease; GI hypermotility (i.e., irritable bowel syndrome). Treatment of neurogenic bowel syndrome. Drying agent in acute rhinitis. Aid in controlling gastric secretion, visceral spasm, hypermotility in spastic colitis, spastic bladder, pylorospasm, associated abdominal cramps. Reduce duodenal motility to facilitate diagnostic radiologic procedure. Preop to reduce salivary, tracheobronchial, pharyngeal secretions. Reduces volume, acidity of gastric secretions.

PO/SubQ/IM/IV ADMINISTRATION

PO:

1. May give w/o regard to meals.

2. Tablets may be crushed, chewed.

3. Extended-release capsule should be swallowed whole.

INDICATIONS/DOSAGE/ROUTES

Usual oral dose:
PO: Adults, elderly: 0.125-0.25 mg 3-4 times/day. **Children:** Based on weight q4h as needed.

Usual parenteral dosage:
IM/IV/SubQ: Adults, elderly: 0.25-0.5 mg 2-4 times/day.

Duodenography:
IV: Adults, elderly: 0.25-0.5 mg 10 min prior to procedure.

Preop:
IM: Adults, elderly: 0.5 mg (0.005 mg/kg) 30-60 min prior to induction of anesthesia or administration of preop medications.

PRECAUTIONS

CONTRAINDICATIONS: Narrow-angle glaucoma, severe ulcerative colitis, toxic megacolon, obstructive disease of GI tract, paralytic ileus, intestinal atony, bladder neck obstruction due to prostatic hypertrophy, myasthenia gravis in those not treated w/neostigmine, tachycardia secondary to cardiac insufficiency or thyrotoxicosis, cardiospasm, unstable cardiovascular status in acute hemorrhage. **EXTREME CAUTION:** Autonomic neuropathy, known or suspected GI infections, diarrhea, mild to moderate ulcerative colitis, bronchial asthma. **CAUTIONS:** Hyperthyroidism, hepatic or renal disease, hypertension, tachyarrhythmias, CHF, coronary artery disease, gastric ulcer, esophageal reflux or hiatal hernia associated w/reflux esophagitis, infants, elderly, those w/COPD. **PREGNANCY LACTATION:** Crosses placenta; distributed in breast milk. Parenteral form near term may produce tachycardia in fetus. **Pregnancy Category C.**

INTERACTIONS

DRUG INTERACTIONS: Antacids, antidiarrheals may decrease absorption. Anticholinergics may increase effects. May decrease absorption of ketoconazole. May increase severity GI lesions with potassium chloride (wax matrix). **ALTERED LAB VALUES:** None significant.

SIDE EFFECTS

FREQUENT: Dry mouth (sometimes severe), decreased sweating, constipation. **OCCASIONAL:** Blurred vision, bloated feeling, urinary hesitancy, drowsiness (w/high dosage), headache, intolerance to light, loss of taste, nervousness, flushing, insomnia, impotence, mental confusion/excitement (particularly in elderly, children). Parenteral form may produce temporary lightheadedness, local irritation. **RARE:** Dizziness, faintness.

ADVERSE REACTIONS/TOXIC EFFECTS

Overdosage may produce temporary paralysis of ciliary muscle, pupillary dilation, tachycardia, palpitation, hot/dry/flushed skin, absence of bowel sounds, hyperthermia, increased respiratory rate, EKG abnormalities, nausea, vomiting, rash over face/upper trunk, CNS stimulation, psychosis (agitation, restlessness, rambling speech, visual hallucination, paranoid behavior, delusions), followed by depression.

NURSING IMPLICATIONS

BASELINE ASSESSMENT:

Before giving medication, instruct pt to void (reduces risk of urinary retention).

INTERVENTION/EVALUATION:

Monitor daily bowel activity and stool consistency. Palpate bladder for urinary retention. Monitor changes in B/P, temperature. Assess skin turgor, mucous membranes to evaluate hydration status (encourage adequate fluid intake), bowel sounds for peristalsis. Be alert for fever (increased risk of hyperthermia).

PATIENT/FAMILY TEACHING:

Do not become overheated during exercise in hot weather (may result in heat stroke). Avoid hot baths, saunas. Avoid tasks that require alertness, motor skills until response to drug is established. Sugarless gum, sips of tepid water may relieve dry mouth. Do not take antacids or medicine for diarrhea within 1 hr of taking this medication (decreased effectiveness).

ibuprofen

eye-byew-pro´fen

(Advil, Motrin, Nuprin, Rufen, Trendar)

CANADIAN AVAILABILITY:

Actiprofen, Advil, Amersol, Motrin, Novoprofen

CLASSIFICATION

Nonsteroidal anti-inflammatory

PHARMACOKINETICS

	ONSET	PEAK	DURATION
PO (analgesic)	0.5 hrs	—	4-6 hrs
PO (anti-rheumatic)	2 days	1-2 wks	—

Rapidly absorbed from GI tract. Protein binding: 99%. Metabolized in liver. Primarily excreted in urine. Half-life: 2-4 hrs.

ACTION

Inhibits prostaglandin synthesis. Inhibits action of cyclooxygenase, decreases formation of prostaglandin, thromboxane precursors from arachidonic acid.

USES

Symptomatic treatment of acute/chronic rheumatoid arthritis and osteoarthritis; reduces fever. Relief of mild to moderate pain, primary dysmenorrhea. Temporary relief of minor aches/pain associated w/common cold, headache, toothache, muscular aches, backaches, menstrual cramps.

PO ADMINISTRATION

1. Do not crush or break enteric-coated form.
2. May give w/food, milk, or antacids if GI distress occurs.

INDICATIONS/DOSAGE/ROUTES

NOTE: Do not exceed 3.2 Gm/day.

Acute/chronic rheumatoid arthritis, osteoarthritis:
PO: Adults, elderly: 300-800 mg 3-4 times/day.

Mild to moderate pain, primary dysmenorrhea:
PO: Adults, elderly: 400 mg q4-6h.

Fever, minor aches/pain:
PO: Adults, elderly: 200-400 mg q4-6h. **Maximum:** 1.2 Gm/day. **Children:** 5-10 mg/kg/dose. **Maximum:** 40 mg/kg/day.

Juvenile arthritis:
PO: Children: 30-40 mg/kg/day in 3-4 divided doses.

PRECAUTIONS

CONTRAINDICATIONS: Active peptic ulcer, GI ulceration, chronic inflammation of GI tract, GI bleeding disorders, history of hypersensitivity to aspirin or nonsteroidal anti-inflammatory agent. **CAUTIONS:** Impaired renal/hepatic function, history of GI tract disease, predisposition to fluid retention. **PREGNANCY/LACTATION:** Unknown if drug crosses placenta or is distributed in breast milk. Avoid use during 3rd trimester (may adversely affect fetal cardiovascular system: premature closure of ductus arteriosus). **Pregnancy Category C.**

INTERACTIONS

DRUG INTERACTIONS: May increase effects of oral anticoagulants, heparin, thrombolytics. May decrease effect of antihypertensives, diuretics. Salicylates, aspirin may increase risk of GI side effects, bleeding. Bone marrow depressants may increase risk of hematologic reactions. May increase concentration, toxicity of lithium. May increase methotrexate toxicity. Probenecid may increase concentration. **ALTERED LAB VALUES:** May prolong bleeding time. May alter blood glucose. May increase BUN, creatinine, potassium, liver function tests. May decrease Ccr, Hgb, Hct.

SIDE EFFECTS

FREQUENT: Dyspepsia (heartburn, nausea, epigastric distress), dizziness, rash/dermatitis. **OCCASIONAL:** Diarrhea/constipation, abdominal cramps/distention, flatulence, pruritus, tinnitus, peripheral edema/fluid retention. **RARE:** Blurred and/or diminished vision.

ADVERSE REACTIONS/TOXIC EFFECTS

Acute overdosage may result in metabolic acidosis. Peptic ulcer, GI bleeding, gastritis, severe hepatic reaction (cholestasis, jaundice) occur rarely. Nephrotoxicity (dysuria, hematuria, proteinuria, nephrotic syndrome) and severe hypersensitivity reaction (particularly those w/systemic lupus erythematosus, other collagen diseases) occur rarely.

NURSING IMPLICATIONS

BASELINE ASSESSMENT:

Assess onset, type, location, and duration of pain or inflammation. Inspect appearance of affected joints for immobility, deformities, and skin condition.

INTERVENTION/EVALUATION:

Monitor for evidence of nausea, dyspepsia. Monitor pattern of daily bowel activity and stool consistency. Check behind medial malleolus for fluid retention (usually first area noted). Assess skin for evidence of rash. Assist w/ambulation if dizziness occurs. Evaluate for therapeutic response: relief of pain, stiffness, swelling, increase in joint mobility, reduced joint tenderness, improved grip strength.

PATIENT/FAMILY TEACHING:

Avoid aspirin, alcohol during therapy (increases risk of GI bleeding). If GI upset occurs, take w/food, milk, or antacids. Report blurred vision, ringing/roaring in ears. Avoid tasks that require alertness until response to drug is established. Do not crush or chew enteric-coated tablet.

idarubicin hydrochloride

eye-dah-roo´bi-sin
(Idamycin)

CANADIAN AVAILABILITY:
Idamycin

CLASSIFICATION

Antineoplastic

PHARMACOKINETICS

Widely distributed. Protein binding: 94-97%. Rapidly metabolized in liver to active metabolite. Primarily eliminated via biliary excretion. Not removed by hemodialysis. Half-life: 4-46 hrs; metabolite: 8-92 hrs.

ACTION

Intercalates DNA (inhibits DNA synthesis), inhibits nucleic acid synthesis; interacts with enzyme topoisomerase II (an enzyme promoting DNA strand supercoiling).

USES

Treatment of acute myeloid leukemia (AML) in adults.

STORAGE/HANDLING

Reconstituted solution stable for 72 hrs (3 days) at room temperature or 168 hrs (7 days) if refrigerated. Discard unused solution.

IV ADMINISTRATION

NOTE: Give by free-flowing IV infusion (*never* SubQ or IM). Gloves, gowns, eye goggles recommended during preparation and administration of medication. If powder or solution come in contact with skin, wash thoroughly. Avoid small veins, swollen or edematous extremities, and areas overlying joints, tendons.

1. Reconstitute each 10 mg vial with 10 ml 0.9% NaCl injection (5 ml/5 mg vial) to provide a concentration of 1 mg/ml.
2. Administer into tubing of freely running IV infusion of 5% dextrose or 0.9% NaCl, preferably via butterfly needle, *slowly* (>10-15 min).
3. Extravasation produces immediate pain, severe local tissue damage. Terminate infusion immediately. Apply cold compresses for ½ hr immediately, then ½ hr 4 times/day for 3 days. Keep extremity elevated.

INDICATIONS/DOSAGE/ROUTES

NOTE: Dosage individualized based on clinical response, tolerance to adverse effects. When used in combination therapy, consult specific protocols for optimum dosage, sequence of drug administration.

Usual dose:
IV: Adults: 12 mg/m^2/day for 3 days (combined with Ara-C).

Dosage in hepatic/renal impairment:
Dosage may be decreased in pts with liver/renal dysfunction.

PRECAUTIONS

CONTRAINDICATIONS: None significant. **EXTREME CAUTION:** Preexisting myelosuppression, cardiac disease, impaired hepatic/renal function. **PREGNANCY/LACTATION:** If possible, avoid use during pregnancy (may be embryotoxic). Unknown if drug is distributed in breast milk (advise to discontinue nursing before drug initiation). **Pregnancy Category D.**

INTERACTIONS

DRUG INTERACTIONS: May decrease effect of antigout medications. Bone marrow depressants may increase bone marrow depression. Live virus vaccines may potentiate virus replication, increase vaccine side effects, decrease pt's antibody response to vaccine. **ALTERED LAB VALUES:** May increase uric acid, SGOT (AST), SGPT (ALT), alkaline phosphatase, bilirubin. May cause ECG changes.

SIDE EFFECTS

FREQUENT: Complete alopecia (scalp, axillary, pubic hair), nausea, vomiting, abdominal pain (suggestive of stomatitis), diarrhea, esophagitis (especially if drug given daily on several successive days). **OCCASIONAL:** Anorexia, hyperpigmentation of nailbeds, phalangeal and dermal creases. **RARE:** Fever, chills, conjunctivitis, lacrimation.

ADVERSE REACTIONS/TOXIC EFFECTS

Bone marrow depression manifested as hematologic toxicity (principally leukopenia, and to lesser extent anemia, thrombocytopenia). Generally occurs within 10-15 days, returns to normal levels by third week. Cardiotoxicity noted as either acute, transient abnormal EKG findings and/or cardiomyopathy manifested as CHF.

NURSING IMPLICATIONS

BASELINE ASSESSMENT:

Determine baseline renal and hepatic function, CBC results. Obtain EKG before therapy. Antiemetic before and during therapy may prevent, relieve nausea.

INTERVENTION/EVALUATION:

Severe myelosuppression of idarubicin requires frequent CBC assessment and close observation of pt: thrombocytopenia (easy bruising, unusual bleeding to frank hemorrhage), leukemia (fever, sore throat, signs of infection), and anemia (excessive fatigue, weakness, dyspnea). Avoid IM injections, rectal temperatures, and other trauma that may precipitate bleeding. Check infusion site frequently for extravasation (causes severe local necrosis). Assess for potentially fatal CHF dyspnea, rales, edema) and life threatening arrhythmias.

PATIENT/FAMILY TEACHING:

Total body alopecia is frequent but reversible. Assist w/ways to cope w/hair loss. New hair growth resumes 2-3 mo after last therapy dose and may have different color, texture. Maintain fastidious oral hygiene. Do not have immunizations without physician's approval (drug lowers body's resistance). Avoid crowds, those w/infections. Teach pt and family the early signs of bleeding and infection.

idoxuridine

eye-dox-yoor´ih-deen
(Stoxil, Herplex Liquifilm)

CANADIAN AVAILABILITY: Herplex, Stoxil

CLASSIFICATION

Antiviral

PHARMACOKINETICS

Rapidly inactivated by deaminases or necleotidases.

ACTION

Incorporated into DNA causing increased rate of mutation and errors in protein formation w/inhibition of viral replication.

USES

Treatment of herpes simplex keratitis.

OPHTHALMIC ADMINISTRATION

1. Place finger on lower eyelid and pull out until a pocket is formed between eye and lower lid. Hold dropper above pocket and place correct number of drops (¼-½ inch ointment) into pocket. Close eye gently. *Solution:* Apply digital pressure to lacrimal sac for 1-2 min (minimizes drainage into nose and throat, reducing risk of systemic effects). *Ointment:* Close eye for 1-2 min, rolling eyeball (increases contact area of drug to eye). Remove excess solution or ointment around eye w/tissue.

INDICATIONS/DOSAGE/ROUTES

Usual ophthalmic dosage:

OPHTHALMIC: Adults, elderly: *Solution:* Instill 1 drop into each infected eye q1h during day and q2h at night. After improvement noted (loss of staining w/fluorescein) reduce to 1 drop q2h during day and q4h during night. Continue 3-5 days after healing appears complete OR 1 drop every min × 5 min. Repeat q4h. *Ointment:* 5 instillations/day q4h (last dose at bedtime). Continue 3-5 days after complete healing.

PRECAUTIONS

CONTRAINDICATIONS: Hypersensitivity to idoxuridine or any component in preparation; long-term use; deep ulcerations. **PREGNANCY/LACTATION:** Potentially carcinogenic. Unknown if drug crosses placenta or distributed in breast milk. **Pregnancy Category C.**

INTERACTIONS

DRUG INTERACTIONS: None significant. **ALTERED LAB VALUES:** None significant.

SIDE EFFECTS

OCCASIONAL: Irritation, redness, mild edema of eyelids and cornea, pain, itching, photophobia. **RARE:** Allergic reactions.

ADVERSE REACTIONS/TOXIC EFFECTS

Squamous cell carcinoma at application site has been reported.

NURSING IMPLICATIONS

BASELINE ASSESSMENT:

Question for hypersensitivity to idoxuridine or components of preparation.

INTERVENTION/EVALUATION:

Evaluate for therapeutic results or onset of redness, itching, pain, edema.

PATIENT/FAMILY TEACHING:

Temporary visual haze may occur after administration (assure proper administration). Refrigerate, do not freeze. Use only under care of physician; do not share medication or personal items. Dosage schedule must be strictly followed. Do not stop medication or increase frequency of doses w/o checking w/physician (continue for 5-7 days after appears completely healed). Contact physician if no improvement after 7-8 days of treatment or for onset of: redness, itching, swelling, pain. Wear sunglasses to reduce sensitivity to light. Do not use *any* other products, including makeup, on the eye w/o advice of physician.

ifosfamide

eye-fos´fah-mid
(Ifex)

CANADIAN AVAILABILITY:
Ifex

CLASSIFICATION

Antineoplastic

PHARMACOKINETICS

Metabolized in liver to active metabolite. Crosses blood-brain barrier (limited). Primarily excreted in urine. Half-life: 15 hrs.

ACTION

Converted to active metabolite, bind w/intracellular structures. Action primarily due to cross-linking strands of DNA, RNA, inhibiting protein synthesis.

USES

Third-line chemotherapy of germ cell testicular carcinoma (used in combination w/agents that protect against hemorrhagic cystitis).

STORAGE/HANDLING

NOTE: May be carcinogenic, mutagenic, or teratogenic. Handle w/extreme care during preparation/administration.

Store vial at room temperature. After reconstitution w/bacteriostatic water for injection, solution stable for 1 wk at room temperature; stable for 3 wks if refrigerated (further diluted solution stable for 6 wks, refrigerated). Solutions prepared w/other diluents should be used within 6 hrs.

IV ADMINISTRATION

1. Reconstitute 1 Gm vial w/20 ml sterile water for injection or bacteriostatic water for injection to provide concentration of 50 mg/ml. Shake to dissolve.
2. Further dilute w/5% dextrose or 0.9% NaCl to provide concentration of 0.6-20 mg/ml.
3. Infuse over 30 min minimum.
4. Give w/at least 2,000 ml oral or IV fluid (prevents bladder toxicity).
5. Give w/protector against hemorrhagic cystitis (e.g., mesna).

INDICATIONS/DOSAGE/ROUTES

NOTE: Dosage individualized based on clinical response, tolerance to adverse effects. When used in combination therapy, consult specific protocols for optimum dosage, sequence of drug administration.

Germ cell testicular carcinoma:
IV: Adults: 1.2 Gm/m^2/day for 5 consecutive days. Repeat q3wks or after recovery from hematologic toxicity. Administer w/mesna.

PRECAUTIONS

CONTRAINDICATIONS: Severely depressed bone marrow function. **CAUTIONS:** Impaired renal, liver function, compromised bone marrow function. **PREGNANCY/LACTATION:** If possible, avoid

I

use during pregnancy, especially first trimester. May cause fetal damage. Drug is distributed in breast milk. Breast feeding not recommended. **Pregnancy Category D.**

INTERACTIONS

DRUG INTERACTIONS: Bone marrow depressants may increase bone marrow depression. Live virus vaccines may potentiate virus replication, increase vaccine side effects, decrease pt's antibody response to vaccine. **ALTERED LAB VALUES:** May increase BUN, creatinine, uric acid, SGOT (AST), SGPT (ALT), LDH, bilirubin. May decrease Ccr.

SIDE EFFECTS

FREQUENT: Alopecia, nausea, vomiting. **OCCASIONAL:** Infection. **RARE:** Anorexia, diarrhea/constipation, fatigue, hypo/hypertension, FUO.

ADVERSE REACTIONS/TOXIC EFFECTS

Hemorrhagic cystitis (occurs frequently), severe myelosuppression, CNS toxicity (confusion, hallucinations, somnolence, coma) may require discontinuation of therapy.

NURSING IMPLICATIONS

BASELINE ASSESSMENT:

Obtain urinalysis before each dose. If hematuria occurs (>10 RBCs per field), withhold therapy until resolution occurs. Obtain WBC, platelet count, Hgb before each dose.

INTERVENTION/EVALUATION:

Monitor hematologic studies, urinalysis diligently. Assess for fever, sore throat, signs of local infection, easy bruising, unusual bleeding from any site, symptoms of anemia (excessive tiredness, weakness).

PATIENT/FAMILY TEACHING:

Maintain copious daily fluid intake (protects against cystitis). Therapy may interfere w/wound healing. Do not have immunizations w/o physician's approval (drug lowers body's resistance). Avoid contact w/those who have recently received live virus vaccine. Contact physician if nausea/vomiting continues at home.

imiglucerase (Cerezyme)
See supplement

imipenem/cilastatin sodium

im-ih´peh-nem/sill-as-tah´tin
(Primaxin)

CANADIAN AVAILABILITY:
Primaxin

CLASSIFICATION

Antibiotic

PHARMACOKINETICS

Readily absorbed after IM administration. Widely distributed. Protein binding: 20%. Metabolized in kidney. Primarily excreted in urine. Removed by hemodialysis. Half-life: 1 hr (increase in decreased renal function).

ACTION

Imipenem: Bactericidal. Binds to bacterial membranes, inhibiting bacterial cell wall synthesis. *Cilastatin:* Prevents renal metabolism of imipenem.

USES

Treatment of respiratory tract, skin/skin structure, gynecologic, bone/joint, intra-abdominal, complicated/uncomplicated urinary tract infections, endocarditis, polymicrobic infections, septicemia; serious nosocomial infections.

STORAGE/HANDLING

Solution appears colorless to yellow, discard if solution turns brown. IV infusion (piggyback) stable for 4 hrs at room temperature, 24 hrs if refrigerated. Discard if precipitate forms.

IM/IV ADMINISTRATION

IM:

1. Prepare w/1% lidocaine w/o epinephrine; 500 mg vial w/2 ml, 750 mg vial w/3 ml lidocaine HCl.
2. Administer suspension within 1 hr of preparation.
3. Do not mix w/any other medications.
4. Inject deep in large muscle; aspirate to decrease risk of injection into a blood vessel.

IV:

1. Give by intermittent IV infusion (piggyback). Do not give IV push.
2. Dilute each 250 mg or 500 mg vial w/100 ml 5% dextrose; 0.9% NaCl, or other compatible IV fluid. Infuse >20-30 min (1 Gm dose >40-60 min).
3. Use large veins to reduce risk of phlebitis; alternate sites.
4. Observe pt during first 30 min of infusion to observe for possible hypersensitivity reaction.

INDICATIONS/DOSAGE/ROUTES

NOTE: Space doses evenly around the clock.

Uncomplicated urinary tract infections:
IV: Adults, elderly: 250 mg q6h.

Complicated urinary tract infections:
IV: Adults, elderly: 500 mg q6h.

Mild infections:
IV: Adults, elderly: 250-500 mg q6h.

Moderate infections:
IV: Adults, elderly: 500 mg q6-8h.

Severe, life-threatening infections:
IV: Adults, elderly: 500 mg q6h.

Dosage in renal impairment:
Dose and/or frequency is modified based on creatinine clearance and/or severity of infection.

CREATININE CLEARANCE	DOSAGE
31-70 ml/min	500 mg q8h
21-30 ml/min	500 mg q12h
0-20 ml/min	250 mg q12h

Usual Intramuscular Dosage

NOTE: Do not use for severe or life-threatening infections.

Mild to moderate lower respiratory tract, skin/skin structure, gynecologic infections:
IM: Adults, elderly: 500-750 mg q12h.

Mild to moderate intra-abdominal infections:
IM: Adults, elderly: 750 mg q12h.

PRECAUTIONS

CONTRAINDICATIONS: Hypersensitivity to imipenem/cilastatin sodium, other beta lactams. Not for children under 12 yrs of age. IM: Hypersensitivity to any local anesthetics of amide-type; pts w/severe shock or heart block (due to use of lidocaine diluent). **CAU-**

TIONS: Hypersensitivity to penicillins, cephalosporins, other allergens; renal dysfunction, CNS disorders, particularly w/history of seizures. **PREGNANCY/LACTATION:** Crosses placenta; distributed in cord blood, amniotic fluid, breast milk. **Pregnancy Category C.**

INTERACTIONS

DRUG INTERACTIONS: None significant. **ALTERED LAB VALUES:** May increase SGOT (AST), SGPT (ALT), alkaline phosphatase, LDH, bilirubin, BUN, creatinine. May decrease Hgb, Hct.

SIDE EFFECTS

FREQUENT: Phlebitis, thrombophlebitis, pain at IV or IM site, nausea, vomiting, diarrhea. **OCCASIONAL:** Confusion, headache, seizures, rash, urticaria, pruritus, fever, hypotension. **RARE:** Tachycardia, palpitations, heartburn, abdominal pain, transient hearing loss, tinnitus, oliguria or polyuria, increased potassium/decreased sodium, increased BUN.

ADVERSE REACTIONS/TOXIC EFFECTS

Antibiotic-associated colitis, other superinfections may occur. Anaphylactic reactions in those receiving beta lactams have occurred.

NURSING IMPLICATIONS

BASELINE ASSESSMENT:

Question pt for history of allergies, particularly to imipenem/cilastatin sodium, other beta lactams, penicillins, cephalosporins. Inquire about history of seizures. Obtain culture and sensitivity tests before giving first dose (therapy may begin before results are known).

INTERVENTION/EVALUATION:

Evaluate for phlebitis (heat, pain, red streaking over vein), pain at IV injection site. Assess for GI discomfort, nausea, vomiting. Determine pattern of bowel activity and stool consistency. Assess skin for rash. Monitor I&O, renal function tests. Check mental status, be alert to tremors and possible seizures. Assess temperature, B/P twice daily, more often if necessary. Assess for hearing loss, tinnitus. Monitor electrolytes, esp. potassium.

PATIENT/FAMILY TEACHING:

Continue therapy for full length of treatment. Doses should be evenly spaced. Do not take any other medication unless approved by physician. Notify physician in event of tremors, seizures, rash, diarrhea, or other new symptom.

imipramine hydrochloride

ih-mip´prah-meen

(Janimine, Tofranil)

Imipramine pamoate

(Tofranil-PM)

CANADIAN AVAILABILITY:
Api-Imipramine, Impril, Novopramine, Tofranil

CLASSIFICATION

Antidepressant: Tricyclic

PHARMACOKINETICS

Rapidly, well absorbed from GI tract. Widely distributed. Protein binding: 89-95%. Metabolized in liver, undergoing first-pass effect. Primarily excreted in urine. Half-life: 11-25 hrs.

ACTION

Increases synaptic concentration of norepinephrine and/or serotonin (inhibits re-uptake by presynaptic membrane). Antienuretic effect due to anticholinergic action.

USES

Treatment of various forms of depression, often in conjunction w/ psychotherapy. Treatment of nocturnal enuresis in children >6 yrs.

STORAGE/HANDLING

Parenteral form takes on yellow or reddish hue when exposed to light. Slight discoloration does not affect potency but marked discoloration is associated w/potency loss.

PO/IM ADMINISTRATION

PO:

1. Give w/food or milk if GI distress occurs.
2. Do not crush or break film-coated tablets.

IM:

1. Give by IM only if oral administration is not feasible.
2. Crystals may form in injection. Redissolve by immersing ampoule in hot water for 1 min.
3. Give deep IM slowly.

INDICATIONS/DOSAGE/ROUTES

Depression:

PO: Adults: Initially, 75-100 mg daily. Dosage may be gradually increased to 300 mg daily for hospitalized pts, 200 mg for outpatients, then reduce dosage to effective maintenance level (50-150 mg daily). **Elderly:** Initially, 10-25 mg/day at bedtime. May increase by 10-25 mg q3-7days. **Range:** 50-150 mg. **Adolescents:** 30-40 mg daily in divided doses to maximum of 100 mg/day.

IM: Adults: Do not exceed 100 mg/day, administered in divided doses.

Childhood enuresis:

PO: Children >6 yrs: 25 mg 1 hr before bedtime.

PRECAUTIONS

CONTRAINDICATIONS: Acute recovery period following MI, within 14 days of MAO inhibitor ingestion. **CAUTIONS:** Prostatic hypertrophy, history of urinary retention or obstruction, glaucoma, diabetes mellitus, history of seizures, hyperthyroidism, cardiac/hepatic/renal disease, schizophrenia, increased intraocular pressure, hiatal hernia. **PREGNANCY/LACTATION:** Crosses placenta; distributed in breast milk. **Pregnancy Category C.**

INTERACTIONS

DRUG INTERACTIONS: Alcohol, CNS depressants may increase CNS, respiratory depression, hypotensive effects. Antithyroid agents may increase risk of agranulocytosis. Phenothiazines may increase sedative, anticholinergic effects. Cimetidine may increase concentration, toxicity. May decrease effects of clonidine, guanadrel. May increase cardiac effects w/sympathomimetics. May increase risk of hypertensive crisis, hyperpyretic, convulsions w/ MAO inhibitors. Phenytoin may decrease concentrations. **ALTERED LAB VALUES:** May alter ECG readings, glucose.

SIDE EFFECTS

FREQUENT: Drowsiness, fatigue,

dry mouth, blurred vision, constipation, delayed micturition, postural hypotension, excessive sweating, disturbed concentration, increased appetite, urinary retention. **OCCASIONAL:** GI disturbances (nausea, metallic taste sensation). **RARE:** Paradoxical reaction (agitation, restlessness, nightmares, insomnia), extrapyramidal symptoms (particularly fine hand tremor).

ADVERSE REACTIONS/TOXIC EFFECTS

High dosage may produce cardiovascular effects (severe postural hypotension, dizziness, tachycardia, palpitations, arrhythmias) and seizures. May also result in altered temperature regulation (hyperpyrexia or hypothermia). Abrupt withdrawal from prolonged therapy may produce headache, malaise, nausea, vomiting, vivid dreams.

NURSING IMPLICATIONS

BASELINE ASSESSMENT:

For those on long-term therapy, liver/renal function tests, blood counts should be performed periodically.

INTERVENTION/EVALUATION:

Supervise suicidal-risk pt closely during early therapy (as depression lessens, energy level improves, causing increased suicide potential). Assess appearance, behavior, speech pattern, level of interest, mood. Monitor pattern of daily bowel activity and stool consistency. Monitor B/P, pulse for hypotension, arrhythmias. Assess for urinary retention by bladder palpation.

PATIENT/FAMILY TEACHING:

Change positions slowly to avoid hypotensive effect. Tolerance to postural hypotension, sedative, and anticholinergic effects usually develop during early therapy. Therapeutic effect may be noted within 2-5 days, maximum effect within 2-3 wks. Photosensitivity to sun may occur. Dry mouth may be relieved by sugarless gum, or sips of tepid water. Report visual disturbances. Do not abruptly discontinue medication. Avoid tasks that require alertness, motor skills until response to drug is established. Avoid alcohol.

immune globulin IM (IGIM, gamma globulin, ISG)

(Gamastan, Gammar)

immune globulin IV (IGIV)

(Gamimune N, Gammagard, Gammar-IV, Iveegam, Sandoglobulin, Venoglobulin-I)

CANADIAN AVAILABILITY:
Gamastan, Gamimume N, Iveegam

CLASSIFICATION

Immune serum

PHARMACOKINETICS

Evenly distributed between intravascular and extravascular space. Half-life: 21-23 days.

ACTION

Provides passive immunity against infection by increasing antibody titer and antigen-antibody reaction potential. Induces rapid increase in platelet counts. Has anti-inflammatory effect.

USES

IGIM: Provides passive immunity to those exposed to hepatitis A virus, hepatitis B virus, or hepatitis B surface antigen (HBsAg); prevents or modifies symptoms of measles (rubeola) in susceptible individuals exposed <6 days previously; provides replacement therapy in prophylactic management of infections with those with IgG or other antibody deficiency diseases. *IGIV:* Maintenance treatment in those unable to produce sufficient amounts of IgG antibodies; treatment of idiopathic thrombocytopenic purpura (ITP); prevent bacterial infections in those with hypogammaglobulinemia and/or recurrent bacterial infections associated with B-cell chronic lymphocytic leukemia (CLL).

STORAGE/HANDLING

Refrigerate IM vials; refer to individual IV preparations for storage requirements, stability after reconstitution. Reconstitute only with diluent provided by manufacturer. Discard partially used or turbid preparations.

IM/IV ADMINISTRATION

NOTE: Do not mix with other medications. Do not perform skin testing prior to administration.

IM:

1. Inject into deltoid muscle or anterolateral aspect of thigh.
2. Use upper outer quadrant of gluteal muscle only for large volumes or multiple injections (when dose >10 ml).

IV:

1. For IV infusion only.
2. After reconstituted, administer via separate tubing.
3. Avoid mixing with other medication/IV infusion fluids.
4. Rate of infusion varies with product used.
5. Monitor vital signs and B/P diligently during and immediately following IV administration (precipitous fall in B/P may produce picture of anaphylactic reaction). Stop infusion immediately. Epinephrine should be readily available.

I

INDICATIONS/DOSAGE/ROUTES

Hepatitis A infection:
IM: Adults, elderly, children: (after exposure): 0.02 ml/kg as single dose as soon as possible after exposure; (before exposure): 0.02 ml/kg as single dose; 0.06 ml/kg if exposure >3 mo, repeat every 4-6 mo.

Non-A, non-B hepatitis:
IM: Adults, elderly, children: 0.06 ml/kg as single dose as soon as possible after exposure.

Measles (after exposure):
IM: Adults, children: 0.25 ml/kg as single dose within 6 days of exposure; 0.5 ml/kg if pt suspected of having leukemia, lymphoma, generalized malignancy, or immunodeficiency disorder, receiving steroids, or other immunosuppression therapy.

Immunodeficiency diseases:
IM: Adults, elderly, children: Initially, 1.2 ml/kg. **Maintenance:** 0.6 ml/kg (at least 100 mg/kg) q2-4wks. **Maximum single dose:** 30-50 ml (adults); 20-30 ml (infants, small children).

Primary immunodeficiency diseases:
IV INFUSION: Adults, elderly, children: *(Gamimune N):* 100-200

mg/kg or 2-4 ml/kg once monthly; may increase to 400 mg/kg or 8 ml/kg once monthly or more frequently. *(Gammagard):* 200-400 mg/kg once monthly. **Minimum:** 100 mg/kg once monthly. *(Gammar-IV):* 100-200 mg/kg q3-4wks. Loading dose 200 mg/kg may be given at more frequent intervals until therapeutic concentration attained. *(Iveegam):* 200 mg/kg once monthly. *(Sandoglobulin):* 200 mg/kg once monthly, may increase to 300 mg/kg once monthly or at more frequent intervals. *(Venoglobulin-I):* 200 mg/kg once monthly, may increase to 300-400 mg/kg once monthly or at more frequent intervals.

Idiopathic thrombocytopenic purpura (ITP):
IV INFUSION: Adults, elderly, children: *(Gamimune-N, Sandoglobulin):* Initially, 400 mg/kg/day for 2-5 days depending on platelet count/clinical response. *(Gammagard):* 1 Gm/kg as single dose; may give up to 3 doses on alternate days. *(Venoglobulin-I):* Initially, 500 mg/kg/day for 2-7 days; then, if necessary, 500-2,000 mg/kg q2wks or less to maintain platelets $>30,000/m^3$ in children or $>20,000/m^3$ in adults.

Hypogammaglobulinemia and/or recurrent bacterial infections in B-cell CLL:
IV INFUSION: Adults, elderly, children: *(Gammagard):* 400 mg/kg q3-4wks.

PRECAUTIONS

CONTRAINDICATIONS: History of allergic response to gamma globulin or anti-immunoglobulin A (IgA) antibodies, allergic response to thimerosal, those with isolated immunoglobulin A (IgA) deficiency. IM also contraindicated in those who have severe thrombocytopenia and any coagulation disorder. **CAUTIONS:** Prior systemic allergic reactions following administration of human immunoglobulin preparations. **PREGNANCY/LACTATION:** Unknown if drug crosses placenta, or is distributed in breast milk. **Pregnancy Category C.**

INTERACTIONS

DRUG INTERACTIONS: Live virus vaccines may potentiate virus replication, increase vaccine side effects, decrease pt's antibody response to vaccine. **ALTERED LAB VALUES:** None significant.

SIDE EFFECTS

FREQUENT: Localized tenderness at IM injection site with pain and muscle stiffness. **OCCASIONAL:** Urticaria, angioedema. **RARE:** Chills, fever, lethargy, chest tightness, nausea, vomiting.

ADVERSE REACTIONS/TOXIC EFFECTS

Anaphylactic reactions occur rarely but increased incidence when given large IM doses or in those receiving repeated injections of immune globulin. Epinephrine should be readily available.

NURSING IMPLICATIONS

BASELINE ASSESSMENT:

Inquire about history of exposure to disease for both pt and family as appropriate. Have epinephrine readily available.

INTERVENTION/EVALUATION:

Control rate of IV infusion carefully; too rapid infusion increases risk of precipitous fall in B/P and signs of anaphylaxis (facial flushing, chest tightness, chills, fever, nausea, vomiting, diaphoresis). Assess pt closely during infusion, esp. 1st hour, monitor vital signs continuously. Stop infusion temporarily if above signs noted. For treatment of ITP, monitor platelets.

PATIENT/FAMILY TEACHING:

Explain rationale for therapy. Rapid response, lasts 1-3 mo. Local pain or muscle tenderness may occur at IM injection site.

indapamide

in-dap'ah-myd
(Lozol)

CANADIAN AVAILABILITY:
Lozide

CLASSIFICATION

Diuretic: Thiazide

PHARMACOKINETICS

	ONSET	PEAK	DURATION
PO (diuretic)	1-2 hrs	<2 hrs	Up to 36 hrs

Completely absorbed from GI tract. Protein binding: 71-79%. Metabolized in liver. Primarily excreted in urine. Half-life: 14-18 hrs.

ACTION

Inhibits reabsorption of water, electrolytes primarily at cortical diluting segment of distal tubule. Reduces peripheral vascular resistance.

USES

Treatment of hypertension and edema associated w/CHF. May be used alone or w/antihypertensive agents.

PO ADMINISTRATION

1. Give w/food or milk if GI upset occurs, preferably w/breakfast (may prevent nocturia).
2. Do not crush or break tablets.

INDICATIONS/DOSAGE/ROUTES

Edema:
PO: Adults: initially, 2.5 mg/day, may increase to 5 mg/day in 1 wk.

Hypertension:
PO: Adults: Initially, 1.25 mg, may increase to 2.5 mg/day in 4 wks or 5 mg/day after additional 4 wks.

Usual elderly dosage:
PO: Elderly: Initially 1.25 mg/day or every other day. May increase up to 5 mg/day.

PRECAUTIONS

CONTRAINDICATIONS: History of hypersensitivity to sulfonamides or thiazide diuretics, renal decompensation, anuria. **CAUTIONS:** Severe renal disease, impaired hepatic function, diabetes mellitus, elderly/debilitated, thyroid disorders. **PREGNANCY/LACTATION:** Crosses placenta; small amount distributed in breast milk; nursing not advised. **Pregnancy Category B.**

INTERACTIONS

DRUG INTERACTIONS: May increase risk of digoxin toxicity (due to hypokalemia). May decrease clearance, increase toxicity of lithium. **ALTERED LAB VALUES:** May increase plasma renin activity. May decrease calcium, protein-bound iodine, potassium, sodium.

SIDE EFFECTS

EXPECTED: Increase in urine frequency/volume. **FREQUENT:** Potassium depletion. **OCCA-**

SIONAL: Postural hypotension, headache, GI/CNS disturbances.

ADVERSE REACTIONS/TOXIC EFFECTS

Vigorous diuresis may lead to profound water loss and electrolyte depletion, resulting in hypokalemia, hyponatremia, dehydration. Acute hypotensive episodes may occur. Hyperglycemia may be noted during prolonged therapy. GI upset, pancreatitis, dizziness, paresthesias, headache, blood dyscrasias, pulmonary edema, allergic pneumonitis, dermatologic reactions occur rarely. Overdosage can lead to lethargy, coma w/o changes in electrolytes or hydration.

NURSING IMPLICATIONS

BASELINE ASSESSMENT:

Check vital signs, especially B/P for hypotension prior to administration. Assess baseline electrolytes, particularly check for low potassium. Assess edema, skin turgor, mucous membranes for hydration status. Assess muscle strength, mental status. Note skin temperature, moisture. Obtain baseline weight. Initiate I&O.

INTERVENTION/EVALUATION:

Continue to monitor B/P, vital signs, electrolytes, I&O, weight. Note extent of diuresis. Watch for electrolyte disturbances (hypokalemia may result in weakness, tremor, muscle cramps, nausea, vomiting, change in mental status, tachycardia; hyponatremia may result in confusion, thirst, cold/clammy skin).

PATIENT/FAMILY TEACHING:

Expect increased frequency and volume of urination. To reduce hypotensive effect, rise slowly from lying to sitting position and permit legs to dangle momentarily before standing. Eat foods high in potassium such as whole grains (cereals), legumes, meat, bananas, apricots, orange juice, potatoes (white, sweet), raisins.

indomethacin

in-doe-meth´ah-sin

(Indocin, Indocin-SR)

indomethacin sodium trihydrate

(Indocin IV)

CANADIAN AVAILABILITY:
Apo-Indomethacin, Indocid, Novomethacin

CLASSIFICATION

Nonsteroidal anti-inflammatory

PHARMACOKINETICS

	ONSET	PEAK	DURATION
PO (analgesic)	0.5 hr	—	4-6 hrs
PO (anti-rheumatic)	7 days	1-2 wks	—

Well absorbed from GI tract. Protein binding: 99%. Metabolized in liver. Primarily excreted in urine. Half-life: 4-6 hrs (increased in neonates: 2-60 hrs).

ACTION

Inhibits prostaglandin synthesis. Inhibits action of cyclooxygenase, decreases formation of prostaglandin, thromboxane precursors from arachidonic acid. *Patent ductus:* Constriction of patent ductus arteriosus and/or increased sensitivity of premature ductus to dilating effects of prostaglandins.

USES

Treatment of active stages of rhemuatoid arthritis, osteoarthritis, ankylosing spondylitis, acute gouty arthritis, acute painful shoulder. Relief of acute bursitis and/or tendonitis of shoulder. For closure of hemodynamically significant patent ductus arteriosus of premature infants weighing 500-1,750 Gm.

STORAGE/HANDLING

Store capsules, suppositories, oral suspension at room temperature. IV solutions made w/o preservatives should be used immediately. Use IV immediately after reconstitution. IV solution appears clear; discard if cloudy or if precipitate forms. Discard unused portion.

PO/IV ADMINISTRATION

PO:

1. Give after meals or w/food or antacids.
2. Do not crush sustained-release capsules.

RECTAL:

1. If suppository is too soft, chill for 30 min in refrigerator or run cold water over foil wrapper.
2. Moisten suppository w/cold water before inserting well up into rectum.

IV:

NOTE: IV injection perferred for patent ductus arteriosus in nenoate (may give dose orally via NG tube or rectally).

1. To 1 mg vial, add 1-2 ml preservative free sterile water for injection or 0.9% NaCl injection to provide concentration of 1 mg or 0.5 mg/ml, respectively. Do not further dilute.
2. Administer over 5-10 seconds.
3. Restrict fluid intake.

INDICATIONS/DOSAGE/ROUTES

Moderate-severe rheumatoid arthritis, osteoarthritis, ankylosing spondylitis:
PO: Adults, elderly: Initially, 25 mg 2-3 times/day. Increase by 25-50 mg/wk up to 150-200 mg/day.
EXTENDED-RELEASE: Adults, elderly: Initially, 75 mg/day up to 75 mg two times/day.

Acute gouty arthritis:
PO: Adults, elderly: Initially, 100 mg, then 50 mg three times/day.

Acute painful shoulder:
PO: Adults, elderly: 75-150 mg/day in 3-4 divided doses.

Usual rectal dosage:
RECTAL: Adults, elderly: 50 mg four times/day. **Children:** Initially, 1.5-2.5 mg/kg/day, up to 4 mg/kg/day. Do not exceed 150-200 mg/day.

Patent ductus arteriosus:
NOTE: May give up to 3 doses at 12-24 hr intervals.
IV: Neonates: Initially, 0.2 mg/kg. **>7 days old:** 0.25 mg/kg for 2nd and 3rd doses. **Age 2-7 days:** 0.2 mg/kg for 2nd and 3rd doses. **<48 hrs old:** 0.1 mg/kg for second and third doses.

PRECAUTIONS

CONTRAINDICATIONS: History of allergic reaction to aspirin or other nonsteroidal anti-inflammatory agents, history of recurrent or active GI lesions. *Suppositories:* History of proctitis or recent rectal bleeding. **CAUTIONS:** Impaired renal/hepatic function, elderly,

I

volume depletion, CHF, sepsis, epilepsy, parkinsonism, psychiatric disturbances, coagulation defects. **PREGNANCY/LACTATION:** Crosses placenta; distributed in breast milk. Avoid use during third trimester (may adversely affect fetal cardiovascular system: premature closure of ductus arteriosus). **Pregnancy Category C.**

INTERACTIONS

DRUG INTERACTIONS: May increase effects of oral anticoagulants, heparin, thrombolytics. May decrease effect of antihypertensives, diuretics. Salicylates, aspirin may increase risk of GI side effects, bleeding. Bone marrow depressants may increase risk of hematologic reactions. May increase concentration, toxicity of lithium. May increase methotrexate toxicity. Probenecid may increase concentration. May increase concentration of aminoglycosides in neonates. **ALTERED LAB VALUES:** May prolong bleeding time. May alter blood glucose. May increase BUN, creatinine, potassium, liver function tests. May decrease Ccr, sodium, platelet count.

SIDE EFFECTS

FREQUENT: Headache (usually severe in morning), nausea, dyspepsia (heartburn, indigestion, epigastric pain), dizziness. **RARE:** Constipation or diarrhea, vomiting, abdominal distress, fatigue, tinnitus. Prolonged therapy may produce ocular disturbances.

ADVERSE REACTIONS/TOXIC EFFECTS

Ulceration of esophagus, stomach, duodenum, or small intestine may occur. In those w/impaired renal function, hyperkalemia along w/worsening of impairment may occur. May aggravate depression or psychiatric disturbances, epilepsy, parkinsonism. Nephrotoxicity (dysuria, hematuria, proteinuria, nephrotic syndrome) occurs rarely.

NURSING IMPLICATIONS

BASELINE ASSESSMENT:

May mask signs of infection. Do not give concurrently w/triamterene (may potentiate acute renal failure). Assess onset, type, location, and duration of pain, fever, or inflammation. Inspect appearance of affected joints for immobility, deformities, and skin condition.

INTERVENTION/EVALUATION:

Monitor for evidence of nausea, dyspepsia. Assist w/ambulation if dizziness occurs. Evaluate for therapeutic response: relief of pain, stiffness, swelling, increase in joint mobility, reduced joint tenderness, improved grip strength.

PATIENT/FAMILY TEACHING:

Avoid aspirin, alcohol during therapy (increases risk of GI bleeding). If GI upset occurs, take w/food, milk. Report headache. Avoid tasks that require alertness, motor skills until response to drug is established. Swallow capsule whole; do not crush or chew.

insulin

in′sull-in

Rapid acting:

INSULIN INJECTION

(Humulin R, Novolin R, Regular, Velosulin)

PROMPT INSULIN ZINC SUSPENSION

(Semilente)

Intermediate acting:

ISOPHANE INSULIN SUSPENSION

(Humulin N, Insulatard, Novolin N, NPH)

INSULIN ZINC SUSPENSION

(Humulin L, Lente, Novolin L)

Long acting:

PROTAMINE ZINC INSULIN SUSPENSION

(PZI)

EXTENDED INSULIN ZINC SUSPENSION

(Humulin U, Ultralente)

FIXED-COMBINATION(S): Isophane Insulin Suspension w/insulin injection: Humulin 70/30, Mixtard, Novolin 70/30.

CANADIAN AVAILABILITY: See Fixed-Combination(s).

CLASSIFICATION

Hypoglycemic

PHARMACOKINETICS

	ONSET (HRS)	PEAK (HRS)	DURATION (HRS)
Regular	0.5-1	—	6-8
Semilente	1-1.5	5-10	12-16
NPH	1-1.5	4-12	24
Lente	1-2.5	7-15	24
PZI	4-8	14-24	36
Ultralente	4-8	10-30	>36

ACTION

Hormone controls storage, metabolism of carbohydrates, protein, fats. Primarily acts in liver, muscle, adipose tissue by attaching to receptors on cellular membranes, facilitating passage of glucose, K, Mg.

USES

Treatment of insulin-dependent type I diabetes mellitus; noninsulin-dependent type II diabetes mellitus when diet/weight control therapy has failed to maintain satisfactory blood glucose levels or in event of pregnancy, surgery, trauma, infection, fever, severe renal, hepatic or endocrine dysfunction. Regular insulin used in emergency treatment of ketoacidosis, to promote passage of glucose across cell membrane in hyperalimentation, to facilitate intracellular shift of K^+ in hyperkalemia.

STORAGE/HANDLING

Store currently used insulin at room temperature (avoid extreme temperatures, direct sunlight). Store extra vials in refrigerator. Discard unused vials if not used for several weeks. No insulin should have precipitate or discoloration.

SubQ ADMINISTRATION

1. Give SubQ only. (Regular Insulin is the *only* insulin that may be given IV, IM for ketoacidosis or other specific situations).
2. Use only insulin syringes (marked in units, e.g., U40, U100) that coordinate to strength of insulin to be administered.
3. Do not give cold insulin; warm to room temperature.
4. Rotate vial gently between hands; do not shake. Regular insulin should be clear; no insulin should have precipitate or discoloration.
5. Usually administered approximately 30 min before a meal. Check blood glucose concentration before administration; dosage highly individualized.
6. When insulin is mixed, regular insulin is always drawn up first.

Insulins to be combined must be the same concentration (units per milliliter). Mixtures must be administered at once (binding can occur within 5 min).

7. SubQ injections may be given in thigh, abdomen, upper arm, buttocks, or upper back if there is adequate adipose tissue.

8. Rotation of injection sites is essential; maintain careful record.

9. For home situations, prefilled syringes are stable for 1 wk under refrigeration (this includes mixtures once they have stabilized, e.g., 15 min for NPH/Regular, 24 hrs for Lente/Regular). Prefilled syringes should be stored in vertical or oblique position to avoid plugging; plunger should be pulled back slightly and the syringe rocked to remix the solution before injection.

INDICATIONS/DOSAGE/ROUTES

Dosage for insulin is individualized/monitored.

Usual dosage guidelines:

NOTE: Adjust dosage to achieve premeal and bedtime glucose level of 80-140 mg/dl (children <5 yrs: 100-200 mg/dl).

SubQ: Adults, elderly, children: 0.5-1 unit/kg/day. **Adolescents (during growth spurt):** 0.8-1.2 units/kg/day.

PRECAUTIONS

CONTRAINDICATIONS: Hypersensitivity or insulin resistance may require change of type or species source of insulin. **PREGNANCY/LACTATION:** Insulin is drug of choice for diabetes in pregnancy; close medical supervision is needed. Following delivery, insulin needs may drop for 24-72 hrs, then rise to prepregnancy levels. Not secreted in breast milk; lactation may decrease insulin requirements. **Pregnancy Category B.**

INTERACTIONS

DRUG INTERACTIONS: Glucocorticoids, thiazide diuretics may increase blood glucose. Alcohol may increase insulin effect. Beta-adrenergic blockers may increase risk of hypo/hyperglycemia, mask signs of hypoglycemia, prolong period of hypoglycemia. **ALTERED LAB VALUES:** May decrease potassium, magnesium, phosphate concentrations.

SIDE EFFECTS

OCCASIONAL: Local redness, swelling, itching (due to improper injection technique or allergy to cleansing solution or insulin). **INFREQUENT:** Somogyi effect (rebound hyperglycemia) w/chronically excessive insulin doses. Systemic allergic reaction (rash, angioedema, anaphylaxis), lipodystrophy (depression at injection site due to breakdown of adipose tissue), lipohypertrophy (accumulation of SubQ tissue at injection site due to lack of adequate site rotation). **RARE:** Insulin resistance.

ADVERSE REACTIONS/TOXIC EFFECTS

Severe hypoglycemia (due to hyperinsulinism) may occur in overdose of insulin, decrease or delay of food intake, excessive exercise, or those w/brittle diabetes. Diabetic ketoacidosis may result from stress, illness, omission of insulin dose, or long-term poor insulin control.

NURSING IMPLICATIONS

BASELINE ASSESSMENT:

Question for allergies. Check

blood glucose level. Discuss lifestyle to determine extent of learning, emotional needs.

INTERVENTION/EVALUATION:

Monitor blood glucose and food intake; assure between meal/bedtime nourishments. Assess for hypoglycemia (refer to pharmacokinetics table for peak times/duration): cool wet skin, tremors, dizziness, headache, anxiety, tachycardia, numbness in mouth, hunger, diplopia. Check sleeping pt for restlessness or diaphoresis. Check for hyperglycemia: polyuria (excessive urine output), polyphagia (excessive food intake), polydipsia (excessive thirst), nausea and vomiting, dim vision, fatigue, deep rapid breathing. Be alert to conditions altering glucose requirements: fever, increased activity or stress, surgical procedure.

PATIENT/FAMILY TEACHING:

Prescribed diet is essential part of treatment; do not skip or delay meals. Diabetes mellitus requires life-long control. Check blood glucose/urine as ordered. Instruct signs and symptoms, treatment of hypo/hyperglycemia, proper handling, and administration of medication. Carry candy, sugar packets, other sugar supplements for immediate response to hypoglycemia. Wear/carry medical alert identification. Check w/physician when insulin demands are altered, e.g., fever, infection, trauma, stress, heavy physical activity. Avoid alcoholic beverages. Do not take other medication w/o consulting physician. Weight control, exercise, hygiene (including foot care) and not smoking are integral part of therapy. Protect skin, limit sun exposure. Avoid exposure to infections. Important to keep follow-up appointments. Select clothing, positions that do not restrict blood flow. Inform dentist, physician, or surgeon of medication before any treatment is given. Assure follow-up instruction if pt/family does not thoroughly understand diabetes management or administration techniques.

interferon alfa-2a

inn-ter-fear´on
(Roferon-A)

CANADIAN AVAILABILITY:
Roferon-A

CLASSIFICATION

Antineoplastic

PHARMACOKINETICS

Well absorbed after IM, SubQ administration. Undergoes proteolytic degradation during reabsorption in kidney. Half-life: *IM* 6-8 hrs; *IV* 3.7-8.5 hrs.

ACTION

Inhibits viral replication in virus infected cells, suppressing cell proliferation, increasing phagocytic action of macrophages; augments specific lymphocytic cytotoxicity.

USES

Treatment of hairy cell leukemia, AIDS-related Kaposi's sarcoma.

STORAGE/HANDLING

Refrigerate. Do not shake vial. Reconstituted solutions stable for 30 days if refrigerated. Solutions appear colorless. Do not use if precipitate or discoloration occurs.

SubQ/IM ADMINISTRATION

NOTE: SubQ preferred for thrombocytopenic pts, those at risk for bleeding.

Reconstitute 18 million-U vial w/ 3 ml diluent (provided by manufacturer) to provide concentration of 6 million U/ml (3 million U/0.5 ml).

INDICATIONS/DOSAGE/ROUTES

NOTE: Dosage individualized based on clinical response, tolerance to adverse effects. When used in combination therapy, consult specific protocols for optimum dosage, sequence of drug administration. If severe adverse reactions occur, modify dose or temporarily discontinue medication.

Hairy cell leukemia:
SubQ/IM: Adults: Initially, 3 million units/day for 16-24 wks. **Maintenance:** 3 million units 3 times/ wk. Do not use 36 million-U vial.

AIDS-related Kaposi's sarcoma:
SubQ/IM: Adults: Initially, 36 million U/day for 10-12 wks (may give 3 million U on day 1; 9 million U on day 2; 18 million U on day 3; then begin 36 million U/day for remainder of 10-12 wks). **Maintenance:** 36 million U/day 3 times/wk.

PRECAUTIONS

CONTRAINDICATIONS: Hypersensitivity to alpha interferon. **CAUTIONS:** Renal, hepatic impairment, seizure disorders, compromised CNS function, cardiac disease, history of cardiac abnormalities, myelosuppression. **PREGNANCY/LACTATION:** If possible, avoid use during pregnancy. Breast feeding not recommended. **Pregnancy Category C.**

INTERACTIONS

DRUG INTERACTIONS: Bone marrow depressants may have additive effect. **ALTERED LAB VALUES:** May increase SGOT (AST), SGPT (ALT), alkaline phosphatase, LDH. May decrease Hgb, Hct, leukocyte, platelet counts.

SIDE EFFECTS

FREQUENT: Flu-like symptoms (fever, fatigue, headache, aches, pains, anorexia, chills) nausea, vomiting, coughing, dyspnea, hypotension, edema, chest pain, dizziness, diarrhea, weight loss, taste change, abdominal discomfort, confusion, paresthesia, depression, visual and sleep disturbances, sweating, lethargy. **OCCASIONAL:** Partial alopecia, rash, dry throat/skin, pruritus, flatulence, constipation, hypertension, palpitations, sinusitis. **RARE:** Hot flashes, hypermotility, Raynaud's syndrome, bronchospasm, earache, ecchymosis.

ADVERSE REACTIONS/TOXIC EFFECTS

Arrhythmias, stroke, transient ischemic attacks, CHF, pulmonary edema, myocardial infarction occurs rarely.

NURSING IMPLICATIONS

INTERVENTION/EVALUATION:

Offer emotional support. Monitor all levels of clinical function (numerous side effects). Encourage ample fluid intake, particularly during early therapy.

PATIENT/FAMILY TEACHING:

Clinical response may take 1-3 mo. Flu-like symptoms tend to diminish with continued therapy. Do not have immunizations w/o physician's approval (drug lowers body's resistance). Avoid contact w/those who have recently received live virus vaccine. Contact physician if nausea/vomiting continues at home.

interferon alfa-2b

inn-ter-fear′on
(Intron-A)

CANADIAN AVAILABILITY:
Intron-A, Wellferon

CLASSIFICATION

Antineoplastic

PHARMACOKINETICS

Well absorbed after IM, SubQ administration. Undergoes proteolytic degradation during reabsorption in kidney. Half-life: 2-3 hrs.

ACTION

Inhibits viral replication in virus-infected cells, suppresses cell proliferation, increases phagocytic action of macrophages, augments specific cytotoxicity of lymphocytes.

USES

Treatment of hairy cell leukemia, condylomata acuminata (genital, venereal warts), AIDS-related Kaposi's sarcoma, chronic hepatitis non-A, non-B/C, chronic hepatitis B.

STORAGE/HANDLING

Refrigerate vial. After reconstitution, solution stable for 1 mo. Solution appears clear, colorless to light yellow.

IM/SubQ ADMINISTRATION

1. Do not give IM if platelets <50,000/m^3; give SubQ.
2. For hairy cell leukemia, reconstitute each 3 million IU vial w/ 1 ml bacteriostatic water for injection to provide concentration of 3 million IU/ml (1 ml to 5 million IU vial; 2 ml to 10 million IU vial; 5 ml to 25 million IU vial provides concentration of 5 million IU/ml).
3. For condylomata acuminata, reconstitute each 10 million IU vial w/1 ml bacteriostatic water for injection to provide concentration of 10 million IU/ml.
4. For AIDS-related Kaposi's sarcoma, reconstitute 50 million IU vial w/1 ml bacteriostatic water for injection to provide concentration of 50 million IU/ml.
5. Agitate vial gently, withdraw w/sterile syringe.

INDICATIONS/DOSAGE/ROUTES

NOTE: Dosage individualized based on clinical response, tolerance to adverse effects. When used in combination therapy, consult specific protocols for optimum dosage, sequence of drug administration.

Hairy cell leukemia:
IM/SubQ: Adults: 2 million IU/m^2 3 times/wk. If severe adverse reactions occur, modify dose or temporarily discontinue.

Condylomata acuminata:
INTRALESIONAL: Adults: 1 million IU/lesion 3 times/wk for 3 wks. Use only 10 million IU vial, reconstitute w/no more than 1 ml diluent. Use TB syringe w/25- or 26-gauge needle. Give in evening w/acetaminophen (alleviates side effects).

AIDS-related Kaposi's sarcoma:
IM/SubQ: Adults: 30 million IU/m^2 3 times/wk. Use only 50 million IU vials. If severe adverse reactions occur, modify dose or temporarily discontinue.

Chronic hepatitis non-A, non-B/C:
IM/SubQ: Adults: 3 million IU 3 times/wk for up to 6 mo.

Chronic hepatitis B:
IM/SubQ: Adults: 30-35 million IU/wk (5 million IU/day or 10 million IU 3 times/wk).

PRECAUTIONS

CONTRAINDICATIONS: Hypersensitivity to interferon alfa-2b. **CAUTIONS:** Renal, hepatic impairment, seizure disorders, compromised CNS function, cardiac diseases, history of cardiac abnormalities, myelosuppression. **PREGNANCY/LACTATION:** If possible, avoid use during pregnancy. Breast feeding not recommended. **Pregnancy Category C.**

INTERACTIONS

DRUG INTERACTIONS: Bone marrow depressants may have additive effect. **ALTERED LAB VALUES:** May increase SGOT (AST), SGPT (ALT), alkaline phosphatase, LDH, prothrombin time, partial thromboplastin time. May decrease Hgb, Hct, leukocyte, platelet counts.

SIDE EFFECTS

NOTE: Dose-related effects. **FREQUENT:** Flu-like symptoms (fever, fatigue, headache, aches, pains, anorexia, chills), rash (hairy cell leukemia, Kaposi's sarcoma only). *Kaposi's sarcoma:* All previously mentioned side effects plus depression, dyspepsia, dry mouth/thirst, alopecia, rigors. **OCCASIONAL:** Dizziness, pruritus, dry skin, dermatitis, alteration in taste. **RARE:** Confusion, leg cramps, back pain, gingivitis, flushing, tremor, nervousness, eye pain.

ADVERSE REACTIONS/TOXIC EFFECTS

Hypersensitivity reaction occurs rarely. Severe adverse reactions of flu-like symptoms appear dose-related.

NURSING IMPLICATIONS

INTERVENTION/EVALUATION:

Offer emotional support. Monitor all levels of clinical function (numerous side effects). Encourage ample fluid intake, particularly during early therapy.

PATIENT/FAMILY TEACHING:

Clinical response occurs in 1-3 mo. Flu-like symptoms tend to diminish w/continued therapy. Some symptoms may be alleviated or minimized by bedtime doses. Do not have immunizations w/o physician's approval (drug lowers body's resistance). Avoid contact w/those who have recently received live virus vaccine.

interferon alfa-n3

inn-ter-fear´on
(Alferon N)

CLASSIFICATION

Antineoplastic

PHARMACOKINETICS

Well absorbed after IM, SubQ administration. Undergoes proteolytic degradation during reabsorption in kidney. Half-life: 6-8 hrs.

ACTION

Inhibits viral replication in virus-infected cells, suppresses cell proliferation, increases phagocytic action of macrophages, augments specific cytotoxicity of lymphocytes.

USES

Treatment of refractory or recurring condylomata acuminata (genital, venereal warts).

STORAGE/HANDLING

Refrigerate vial. Do not freeze or shake.

INTRALESIONAL ADMINISTRATION

Inject into base of each wart w/ 30-gauge needle.

INDICATIONS/DOSAGE/ROUTES

Condylomata acuminata:
INTRALESIONAL: Adults >18 yrs: 0.05 ml (250,000 IU) per wart 2 times/wk up to 8 wks. **Maximum dose/treatment session:** 0.5 ml (2.5 million IU). Do not repeat for 3 mo after initial 8 wks unless warts enlarge or new warts appear.

PRECAUTIONS

CONTRAINDICATIONS: Hypersensitivity to interferon alfa, previous history of anaphylactic reaction to mouse immunoglobulin (IgG), egg protein, or neomycin. **CAUTIONS:** Unstable angina, uncontrolled CHF, severe pulmonary disease, diabetes mellitus w/ketoacidosis, thrombophlebitis, pulmonary embolism, hemophilia, severe myelosuppression, seizure disorders. **PREGNANCY/LACTATION:** If possible, avoid use during pregnancy. Breast feeding not recommended. **Pregnancy Category C.**

INTERACTIONS

DRUG INTERACTIONS: Bone marrow depressants may have additive effect. **ALTERED LAB VALUES:** May increase SGOT (AST), SGPT (ALT), alkaline phosphatase, LDH. May decrease Hgb, Hct, leukocyte, platelet counts.

SIDE EFFECTS

FREQUENT: Flu-like symptoms (fever, fatigue, headache, aches, pains, anorexia, chills). **OCCASIONAL:** Dizziness, pruritus, dry skin, dermatitis, alteration in taste. **RARE:** Confusion, leg cramps, back pain, gingivitis, flushing, tremor, nervousness, eye pain.

ADVERSE REACTIONS/TOXIC EFFECTS

Hypersensitivity reaction occurs rarely. Severe adverse reactions of flu-like symptoms appear dose-related.

NURSING IMPLICATIONS

INTERVENTION/EVALUATION:

Offer emotional support. Monitor all levels of clinical function (numerous side effects). Encourage ample fluid intake, particularly during early therapy.

PATIENT/FAMILY TEACHING:

Clinical response occurs in 1-3 mo. Flu-like symptoms tend to diminish w/continued therapy. Some symptoms may be alleviated or minimized by bedtime doses. Do not have immunizations w/o physician's approval (drug lowers body's resistance). Avoid contact w/those who have recently received live virus vaccine.

interferon beta 1b

in-tear-fair'on
(Betaseron)

CLASSIFICATION

Interferon

PHARMACOKINETICS

Half-life: 8 minutes to 4.3 hrs.

ACTION

Possesses antiviral and immunoregulatory activities. Action mediated through its interactions w/ specific cell receptors found on surface of human cells.

USES

Reduces frequency of clinical exacerbations w/pts w/relapsing-remitting multiple sclerosis (recurrent attacks of neurologic dysfunction).

STORAGE/HANDLING

Refrigerate vials. After reconstitution, stable for 3 hrs if refrigerated. Use within 3 hrs of reconstitution. Discard if discolored, contains a precipitate.

SubQ ADMINISTRATION

1. Reconstitute 0.3 mg (9.6 million IU) vial w/1.2 ml diluent (supplied by manufacturer) to provide concentration of 0.25 mg/ml (8 million U/ml).
2. Gently swirl to dissolve medication; do not shake.
3. Discard if discolored, contains particulate matter.
4. Withdraw 1 ml solution and inject SubQ into arms, abdomen, hips, or thighs using 27-gauge needle.
5. Discard unused portion (contains no preservative).

INDICATIONS/DOSAGE/ROUTES

Relapsing-remitting multiple sclerosis:
SubQ: Adults: 0.25 mg (8 million IU) every other day.

PRECAUTIONS

CONTRAINDICATIONS: Hypersensitivity to interferon, albumin. **CAUTIONS:** Chronic progressive multiple sclerosis, children <18 yrs of age. **PREGNANCY/LACTATION:** Unknown whether distributed in breast milk. **Pregnancy Category C.**

INTERACTIONS

DRUG INTERACTIONS: None significant. **ALTERED LAB VALUES:** May increase SGOT (AST), SGPT (ALT), bilirubin, alkaline phosphatase, BUN, calcium, glucose. May decrease Hgb, platelets, WBCs, neutrophils.

SIDE EFFECTS

FREQUENT: Injection site reaction, headache, fever, flu-like symptoms, pain, asthenia, chills, abdominal pain, sinusitis, myalgia, myasthenia, diarrhea, constipation, vomiting, conjunctivitis, dysmenorrhea, menstrual disorders, malaise, migraine, mental symptoms, sweating. **OCCASIONAL:** Edema, pelvic pain, palpitations, hypertension, dyspnea, abnormal vision, cystitis, breast pain.

ADVERSE REACTIONS/TOXIC EFFECTS

None significant.

NURSING IMPLICATIONS

BASELINE ASSESSMENT:

Obtain Hgb, CBC and differential, platelet count, blood chemistries including liver function tests. Assess home situation for support of therapy.

INTERVENTION/EVALUATION:

Periodically monitor lab results and reevaluate injection technique. Assess for depression and suicidal ideation.

PATIENT/FAMILY TEACHING:

Do not change schedule or dosage w/o consultation w/physician. Instruct on correct reconstitution of product and administration, including aseptic technique. Provide puncture resistant container for used needles, syringes, and explain proper disposal. Explain that injection site reactions may occur. These do not require discontinuation of therapy, but note type and extent carefully. Depression or suicidal ideation must be reported immediately. Inform physician of flu-like symptoms (occur commonly but decrease over time). Wear sunscreens, protective clothing if exposed to ultraviolet light or sunlight until tolerance known. Interferon beta 1b has abortifacient potential.

interferon gamma-1b

inter-fear´on
(Actimmune)

CLASSIFICATION

Biologic response modifier

PHARMACOKINETICS

Slowly absorbed following SubQ administration. Metabolic fate unknown.

ACTION

Induces activation of macrophages in blood monocytes to phagocytes (necessary in cellular immune response to intracellular and extracellular pathogens). Enhances phagocytic function, antimicrobial activity of monocytes.

USES

Reduces frequency, severity of serious infections due to chronic granulomatous disease.

STORAGE/HANDLING

Refrigerate vials. Do not freeze. Do not keep at room temperature >12 hrs, discard if left out longer. Vials are single dose; discard unused portion. Clear, colorless solution. Do not use if discolored, precipitate formed.

SubQ ADMINISTRATION

NOTE: Avoid excessive agitation of vial; do not shake.
SubQ: When given 3 times/week (Monday, Wednesday, Friday), give in left deltoid, right deltoid, and anterior thigh.

INDICATIONS/DOSAGE/ROUTES

Chronic granulomatous disease:
SubQ: Adults, children >1 yr: 50 mcg/m^2 (1.5 million U/m^2) in pts with body surface area (BSA) >0.5 m^2; 1.5 mcg/kg/dose in pts with BSA ≤0.5 m^2.

PRECAUTIONS

CONTRAINDICATIONS: Hypersensitivity to *Escherichia coli* products. **CAUTIONS:** Seizure disorders, compromised CNS function, preexisting cardiac disease (including ischemia, CHF, arrhythmia), myelosuppression. **PREGNANCY/LACTATION:** Unknown if drug crosses placenta or is distributed in breast milk. **Pregnancy Category C.**

INTERACTIONS

DRUG INTERACTIONS: Bone marrow depressants may increase bone marrow depression. **AL-**

I

TERED LAB VALUES: May increase SGOT (AST), SGPT (ALT), alkaline phosphatase, LDH, cortisol, triglyceride concentrations. May decrease leukocyte counts.

SIDE EFFECTS

FREQUENT: Fever, headache, rash, chills, fatigue, diarrhea. **OCCASIONAL:** Nausea, vomiting, muscle aches. **RARE:** Anorexia, hypersensitivity reaction.

ADVERSE REACTIONS/TOXIC EFFECTS

May exacerbate preexisting CNS, cardiac abnormalities demonstrated as decreased mental status, gait disturbance, dizziness.

NURSING IMPLICATIONS

Baseline Assessment:

CBC, differential and platelet counts, blood chemistries, urinalysis, renal and liver function tests should be performed prior to initial therapy and at 3 mo intervals during course of treatment.

Intervention/Evaluation:

Monitor for "flu-like" symptoms (fever, chills, fatigue, muscle aches). Assess for evidence of hypersensitivity reaction. Check for gait disturbance, dizziness. Assist with walking if these symptoms appear.

Patient/Family Teaching:

Flu-like symptoms fever, chills, fatigue, muscle aches, are generally mild, and tend to disappear as treatment continues. Symptoms may be minimized by bedtime administration. Avoid tasks that require alertness, motor skills until response to drug is established. If home use prescribed, instruct in proper technique of administration, care in proper disposal of needles, syringes. Vial should remain refrigerated.

iodinated glycerol

eye-oh´din-ay-ted gligh´sir-all
(Iophen, Organidin)

NOTE: Iodinated glycerol replaced by guaifenesin (reformulated by manufacturer).

FIXED-COMBINATION(S):
W/codeine, an opiate agonist (Tussi-Organidin); w/dextromethorphan, a nonnarcotic antitussive (Tussi-Organidin DM); w/theophylline, a bronchodilator (Theo-Organidin)

CANADIAN AVAILABILITY:
Organidin

CLASSIFICATION

Expectorant, antitussive

PHARMACOKINETICS

Readily absorbed from GI tract. Primarily concentrated in respiratory tract. Primarily excreted in urine.

ACTION

Increases respiratory tract secretions (decreases viscosity of mucus).

USES

Symptomatic relief of cough in presence of mucus in respiratory tract due to bronchial asthma, bronchitis, emphysema.

PO ADMINISTRATION

1. Give w/o regard to meals.
2. Scored tablets may be crushed.

INDICATIONS/DOSAGE/ROUTES

Expectorant:
PO: Adults, elderly: 60 mg 4 times/day. **Children >12 yrs:** 30 mg 4 times day.

PRECAUTIONS

CONTRAINDICATIONS: History of hypersensitivity to iodides, pregnancy, nursing women, neonates. **CAUTIONS:** Evidence or history of thyroid disease. **PREGNANCY/LACTATION:** Unknown if drug crosses placenta or is distributed in breast milk. Drug should be discontinued if pregnancy occurs. **Pregnancy Category X.**

INTERACTIONS

DRUG INTERACTIONS: May increase hypothyroid effect of lithium, other antithyroid medications. **ALTERED LAB VALUES:** May alter thyroid function test results.

SIDE EFFECTS

RARE: Dizziness, headache, rash.

ADVERSE REACTIONS/TOXIC EFFECTS

Excessive dosage may produce nausea, vomiting.

NURSING IMPLICATIONS

BASELINE ASSESSMENT:

Assess type, severity, frequency of cough, and productions. Increase fluid intake and environmental humidity to lower viscosity of lung secretions.

INTERVENTION/EVALUATION:

Initiate deep breathing and coughing exercises, particularly in those w/impaired pulmonary function. Assess for clinical improvement and record onset of relief of cough.

PATIENT/FAMILY TEACHING:

Avoid tasks that require alertness, motor skills until response to drug is established. Do not take during pregnancy.

ipecac syrup

ip´eh-kak

CANADIAN AVAILABILITY:
PMS Ipecac Syrup

CLASSIFICATION

Antidote

PHARMACOKINETICS

	ONSET	PEAK	DURATION
PO	<30 min	—	—

After administration, vomiting occurs within 20-30 min.

ACTION

Acts centrally by stimulating medullary chemoreceptor trigger zone and locally by irritating gastric mucosa, producing emesis.

USES

Induces vomiting in early treatment of unabsorbed oral poisons, drug overdosage.

STORAGE/HANDLING

Store syrup at room temperature.

PO ADMINISTRATION

1. Before administering, instruct pt to sit upright before drinking syrup (enhances emetic effect).
2. Do not confuse ipecac fluid extract w/ipecac syrup (fluid extract is 14 times more potent and may cause death if given inadvertently at syrup dosage).

3. Emetic action may be facilitated if 200-300 ml water or clear liquid is given immediately following ipecac.

INDICATIONS/DOSAGE/ROUTES

NOTE: If vomiting has not occurred within 20 min after first dose, repeat w/15 ml. If vomiting has not occurred within 30 min after last dose, initiate gastric lavage, activated charcoal.

Emetic:
PO: Adults, elderly, children >12 yrs: 15-30 ml; follow w/3-4 glasses water immediately following administration. **Children 1-12 yrs:** 15 ml; follow w/1-2 glasses water. **Children 6 mo-1 yr:** 5-10 ml; follow w/1 glass water. If vomiting has not occurred within 30 min, repeat initial dosage.

PRECAUTIONS

CONTRAINDICATIONS: Ingestion of petroleum distillates (paint thinner, gasoline, kerosene), alkali (lye), acids, strychnine. **CAUTIONS:** Impaired cardiac function, pathologic blood vessel disease. **PREGNANCY/LACTATION:** Unknown if drug crosses placenta or is distributed in breast milk. **Pregnancy Category C.**

INTERACTIONS

DRUG INTERACTIONS: Antiemetics may decrease effect. Avoid carbonated beverages (causes stomach distention), milk or milk products (decreases effectiveness). **ALTERED LAB VALUES:** None significant.

SIDE EFFECTS

EXPECTED RESPONSE: Nausea, vomiting. After vomiting, diarrhea and mild CNS symptoms commonly occur.

ADVERSE REACTIONS/TOXIC EFFECTS

Cardiotoxicity may occur if ipecac syrup is not vomited (noted as hypotension, tachycardia, precordial chest pain, pulmonary congestion, dyspnea, ventricular tachycardia and fibrillation, cardiac arrest).

NURSING IMPLICATIONS

BASELINE ASSESSMENT:

Do not administer to semiconscious, unconscious, or convulsing pt. Gastric lavage, activated charcoal is necessary if vomiting does not occur within 30 min of second dosage to avoid drug toxicity (bloody stools, vomitus, abdominal pain, hypotension, dyspnea, shock, cardiac disturbances, seizures, coma). Maintain pt in upright position to enhance emetic effect.

INTERVENTION/EVALUATION:

Closely monitor vital signs, EKG during and after drug is administered. Watch for changes from initial assessment. Check for reversal of poisoning or overdosage symptoms. Monitor daily bowel activity and stool consistency (watery, loose, soft, semisolid, solid) and record time of evacuation. Assess for dehydration in excessive vomiting: poor skin turgor, dry mucous membranes, longitudinal furrows in tongue.

ipratropium bromide

ih-prah-trow´pea-um
(Atrovent)

FIXED-COMBINATION(S):
W/albuterol, a bronchodilator (Combivent)

CANADIAN AVAILABILITY:
Atrovent

CLASSIFICATION

Bronchodilator

PHARMACOKINETICS

	ONSET	PEAK	DURATION
Inhalation	<15 min	1-2 hrs	3-4 hrs

Minimal systemic absorption. Metabolized in liver (systemic absorption). Primarily eliminated in feces. Half-life: 1.5-4 hrs.

ACTION

Competitively inhibits cholinergic receptors on bronchial smooth muscle (blocks action of acetylcholine). Local effect occurring throughout airways.

USES

Relief of bronchospasm due to chronic obstructive airway disease, bronchitis, bronchial asthma. Not to be used for immediate bronchospasm relief. *Nasal spray:* rhinorrhea.

INHALATION ADMINISTRATION

1. Shake container well, exhale completely then holding mouthpiece 1 inch away from lips; inhale and hold breath as long as possible before exhaling.
2. Wait 1-10 min before inhaling second dose (allows for deeper bronchial penetration).
3. Rinse mouth w/water immediately after inhalation (prevents mouth/throat dryness).

INDICATIONS/DOSAGE/ROUTES

Bronchospasm:
INHALATION: Adults, elderly: 2 inhalations 4 times/day. Wait 1-10 min before administering second inhalation. **Maximum:** 12 inhalations/24 hrs.
NEBULIZATION: Adults, elderly: 500 mcg 3-4 times/day.

PRECAUTIONS

CONTRAINDICATIONS: History of hypersensitivity to atropine. **CAUTIONS:** Narrow-angle glaucoma, prostatic hypertrophy, bladder neck obstruction. **PREGNANCY/LACTATION:** Unknown if distributed in breast milk. **Pregnancy Category B.**

INTERACTIONS

DRUG INTERACTIONS: Avoid mixing w/cromolyn inhalation solution (forms precipitate). **ALTERED LAB VALUES:** None significant.

SIDE EFFECTS

OCCASIONAL: Dry mouth/throat, cough, headache, nausea. **RARE:** Blurred vision, palpitations, rash, insomnia.

ADVERSE REACTIONS/TOXIC EFFECTS

Worsening of narrow-angle glaucoma, acute eye pain, hypotension occur rarely.

NURSING IMPLICATIONS

BASELINE ASSESSMENT:

Offer emotional support (high incidence of anxiety due to difficulty in breathing and sympathomimetic response to drug).

INTERVENTION/EVALUATION:

Monitor rate, depth, rhythm, type of respiration; quality and rate of pulse. Assess lung sounds for rhonchi, wheezing, rales. Monitor arterial blood gases. Observe lips, fingernails for blue or dusky color in light-skinned pts; gray in dark-skinned pts. Observe for clavicular retractions, hand tremor. Evaluate for clinical improvement (quieter, slower respirations, relaxed facial expression, cessation of clavicular retractions).

PATIENT/FAMILY TEACHING:

Increase fluid intake (decreases lung secretion viscosity). Do not take more than 2 inhalations at any one time (excessive use may produce paradoxical bronchoconstriction, or a decreased bronchodilating effect). Rinsing mouth with water immediately after inhalation may prevent mouth/throat dryness. Avoid excessive use of caffeine derivatives (chocolate, coffee, tea, cola, cocoa).

iron dextran

iron dex´tran
(Infed)

CANADIAN AVAILABILITY:
Imferon

CLASSIFICATION

Hematinic

PHARMACOKINETICS

Readily absorbed after IM administration. Major portion of absorption occurs within 72 hrs; remainder within 3-4 wks. Iron is bound to protein to form hemosiderin, ferritin, or transferrin. No physiologic system of elimination. Small amounts lost daily in shedding of skin, hair, and nails, and in feces, urine, and perspiration. Half-life: 5-20 hrs.

ACTION

Essential component of formation of hemoglobin, replenishes hemoglobin and depleted iron stores. Necessary for effective erythropoiesis and oxygen transport capacity of blood. Serves as cofactor of several essential enzymes.

USES

Treatment of established iron deficiency anemia. Use only when oral administration is not feasible or when rapid replenishment of iron is warranted.

STORAGE/HANDLING

Store at room temperature. Dark brown, slightly viscous liquid.

IM/IV ADMINISTRATION

NOTE: Test doses are generally given before the full dosage; stay w/pt for several minutes after injection due to potential for anaphylactic reaction and keep epinephrine and resuscitative equipment available.

IM:

1. Draw up medication w/one needle, use new needle for injection (minimizes skin staining).
2. Administer deep IM in upper outer quadrant of buttock only.
3. Use Z-tract technique (displacement of SubQ tissue lateral to injection site before inserting needle) to minimize skin staining.

IV:

1. May give undiluted or diluted in normal saline for infusion.
2. Do not exceed IV administration rate of 50 mg/min (1 ml/min). A too-rapid IV rate may produce chest pain, shock, hypotension, tachycardia, flushing.
3. Pt must remain recumbent 30-45 min following IV administration (avoid postural hypotension).

INDICATIONS/DOSAGE/ROUTES

NOTE: Discontinue oral iron form before administering iron dextran.

Dosage expressed in terms of milligrams of elemental iron. Dosage individualized based on degree of anemia; pt weight, presence of any bleeding. Use periodic hematologic determinations as guide to therapy.

Iron deficiency anemia (no blood loss):
IM/IV: Adults, elderly: Mg iron = 0.66 × weight (kg) × (100 − Hgb <Gm/dl>/14.8)

Replacement secondary to blood loss:
IM/IV: Adults, elderly: Replacement iron (mg) = blood loss (ml) × hematocrit

PRECAUTIONS

CONTRAINDICATIONS: All anemias except iron deficiency anemia (eliminates pernicious, aplastic, normocytic, refractory). **EXTREME CAUTION:** Serious liver impairment. **CAUTIONS:** History of allergies, bronchial asthma, rheumatoid arthritis. **PREGNANCY/LACTATION:** May cross placenta in some form (unknown); trace distributed in breast milk. **Pregnancy Category B.**

INTERACTIONS

DRUG INTERACTIONS: None significant. **ALTERED LAB VALUES:** May increase bilirubin. May decrease calcium. May prolong partial thromboplastin time when blood sample mixed w/anticoagulant citrate dextrose solution (does not occur w/anticoagulant sodium citrate solution).

SIDE EFFECTS

FREQUENT: Pain, inflammation, staining of skin at IM injection site. **OCCASIONAL:** Nausea, vomiting, abdominal pain, diarrhea, metallic taste. W/IV administration: phlebitis at injection site; exacerbation of joint pain and swelling w/rheumatoid arthritis; delayed reactions (1-2 days after injection) of moderately high fever, chills, backache, headache, myalgia, nausea, vomiting, dizziness. Flushing and hypotension may occur w/too-rapid IV injection. **RARE:** Abscess at IM site, chest pain, tachycardia, leukocytosis, lymphadenopathy.

ADVERSE REACTIONS/TOXIC EFFECTS

Anaphylaxis has occurred during the first few minutes after injection, causing death on rare occasions.

NURSING IMPLICATIONS

BASELINE ASSESSMENT:

Do not give concurrently w/oral iron form (excessive iron may produce excessive iron storage [hemosiderosis]). Be alert to those w/rheumatoid arthritis or iron deficiency anemia (acute exacerbation of joint pain and swelling may occur). Inguinal lymphadenopathy may occur w/IM injection. Assess for adequate muscle mass before injecting medication.

INTERVENTION/EVALUATION:

Monitor IM site for abscess formation, necrosis, atrophy, swelling, brownish color to skin. Question pt regarding soreness, pain, inflammation at or near IM injection site. Check IV site for phlebitis. Monitor serum ferritin levels.

PATIENT/FAMILY TEACHING:

Pain and brown staining may occur at injection site. Oral iron should not be taken when receiving iron injections. Stools frequently become black w/iron therapy; this is harmless unless accompanied by red streaking, sticky consistency of stool, abdominal pain or cramping that should be reported to physician. Oral hygiene, hard candy or gum may reduce metallic taste. Notify physician immediately if fever, back pain, headache occur.

isoetharine hydrochloride

eye-sew-eth´ah-reen

(Bronkosol, Dey-Dose)

isoetharine mesylate

(Bronkometer)

CLASSIFICATION

Bronchodilator

PHARMACOKINETICS

	ONSET	PEAK	DURATION
Aerosol	1-6 min	5-15 min	1-4 hrs
Nebulization	1-6 min	5-15 min	1-4 hrs
IPPB	1-6 min	5-15 min	1-4 hrs

Inhaled medication rapidly absorbed from respiratory tract. Metabolized in GI tract, lungs, liver; excreted in urine.

ACTION

Stimulates beta$_2$-adrenergic receptors in lungs (relaxes bronchial smooth muscle by increasing cAMP). Relieves bronchospasm; reduces airway resistance.

USES

Relief of acute bronchial asthma, bronchospasm associated w/ chronic bronchitis, emphysema.

STORAGE/HANDLING

Store at room temperature. Do not use if solution is pink to brown, contains a precipitate, or becomes cloudy.

PO ADMINISTRATION

METERED DOSE AEROSOL (i. mesylate):

1. Shake container well, exhale completely then holding mouthpiece 1 inch away from lips, inhale and hold breath as long as possible before exhaling.
2. Wait 1-10 min before inhaling 2nd dose (allows for deeper bronchial penetration).
3. Rinse mouth w/water immediately after inhalation (prevents mouth/throat dryness).

NEBULIZATION, IPPB (i. hydrochloride):

1. Dilute 0.5 or 1% solution with sterile water, sterile purified water, or 0.45 or 0.9% NaCl solution at 1:3 ratio (0.125, 0.2, or 0.25% may be given undiluted).
2. Adjust oxygen flow rate at 4-6 L/min over 120 min.
3. For IPPB, adjust at 15 L/min at cycling pressure of 15 cm water (allowing for adjustment of flow rate, cycling pressure, further dilution).

INDICATIONS/DOSAGE/ROUTES

HAND-BULB NEBULIZER:
Adults, elderly: 4 inhalations (range: 3-7 inhalations) undiluted. May be repeated up to 5 times/day.
METERED DOSE INHALATION: Adults, elderly: 1-2 inhalations q4h. Wait 1 min before administering 2nd inhalation.
IPPB, OXYGEN AEROLIZATION: Adults, el-

derly: 0.5-1 ml of a 0.5% or 0.5 ml of a 1% solution diluted 1:3.

PRECAUTIONS

CONTRAINDICATIONS: History of hypersensitivity to sympathomimetics. **CAUTIONS:** Hypertension, cardiovascular disease, hyperthyroidism, diabetes mellitus. **PREGNANCY/LACTATION:** Unknown if drug crosses placenta or is distributed in breast milk. May inhibit uterine contractility. **Pregnancy Category C.**

INTERACTIONS

DRUG INTERACTIONS: May decrease effects of beta-blockers. Digoxin may increase risk of arrhythmias. **ALTERED LAB VALUES:** May decrease serum potassium levels.

SIDE EFFECTS

OCCASIONAL: Tremor, nausea, nervousness, palpitations, tachycardia, peripheral vasodilation, dryness of mouth, throat.

ADVERSE REACTIONS/TOXIC EFFECTS

Excessive sympathomimetic stimulation may cause palpitations, extrasystoles, tachycardia, chest pain, slight increase in B/P followed by a substantial decrease, chills, sweating, and blanching of skin. Too-frequent or excessive use may lead to loss of bronchodilating effectiveness and/or severe, paradoxical bronchoconstriction.

NURSING IMPLICATIONS

BASELINE ASSESSMENT:

Offer emotional support (high incidence of anxiety due to difficulty in breathing and sympathomimetic response to drug).

INTERVENTION/EVALUATION:

Monitor rate, depth, rhythm, type of respiration; quality and rate of pulse. Assess lung sounds for rhonchi, wheezing, rales. Monitor arterial blood gases. Observe lips, fingernails for blue or dusky color in light-skinned pts; gray in dark-skinned pts. Observe for clavicular retractions, hand tremor. Evaluate for clinical improvement (quieter, slower respirations, relaxed facial expression, cessation of clavicular retractions).

PATIENT/FAMILY TEACHING:

Increase fluid intake (decreases lung secretion viscosity). Do not take more than 2 inhalations at any one time (excessive use may produce paradoxical bronchoconstriction, or a decreased bronchodilating effect). Rinsing mouth with water immediately after inhalation may prevent mouth/throat dryness. Avoid excessive use of caffeine derivatives (chocolate, coffee, tea, cola, cocoa).

isoflurophate

eye-soh-floor´oh-fate
(Floropryl)

CLASSIFICATION

Anticholinesterase agent

PHARMACOKINETICS

	ONSET	PEAK	DURATION
Ophthalmic (miosis)	5-10 min	15-30 min	1-4 wks

Maximal decrease in intraocular pressure seen w/in 24 hrs, persists for 1 wk.

ACTION

Prolongs effect of acetylcholine by inactivating cholinesterase causing constriction of iris sphincter muscle (miosis) and ciliary muscle. Lowers resistance to outflow of aqueous humor.

USES

Treatment of open-angle glaucoma and conditions obstructing aqueous outflow (e.g., synechial formation) that are responsive to miotic therapy; following iridectomy; in accommodative esotropia (convergent strabismus).

OPHTHALMIC ADMINISTRATION

1. For topical ophthalmic use only.
2. Administer at bedtime to reduce side effects.
3. Pt should be supine, looking up.
4. Gently pull lower lid down to form pouch and apply ointment.
5. Do not touch tip of tube to lids or any surface.
6. Instruct pt to close eye for 1-2 min and roll the eyeball in all directions.
7. Remove any excess ointment around eye w/tissue. Wash hands immediately to remove medication.
8. Do not rinse tip of tube or permit contact w/tears; cover tightly.

INDICATIONS/DOSAGE/ROUTES

Glaucoma:
OPHTHALMIC: Adults, elderly: ¼ inch strip q8-72h.

Accommodative esotropia:
OPHTHALMIC: Adults, elderly: *Diagnosis:* <½ inch strip every hr for 2 wks. If eyes become straightened, an accommodative factor is demonstrated. *Treatment:* <½ inch strip to both eyes every hr for 2 wks, then reduce to ½ inch every 2-7 days for 2 mo. If improvement not maintained w/dose interval of at least 48 hrs, discontinue therapy.

PRECAUTIONS

CONTRAINDICATIONS: Hypersensitivity to cholinesterase inhibitors or any component of the preparation; active uveal inflammation; angle-closure (narrow-angle) glaucoma; glaucoma associated w/iridocyclitis. **CAUTIONS:** Bronchial asthma, gastrointestinal disturbances, peptic ulcer, bradycardia, hypotension, recent myocardial infarction, epilepsy, parkinsonism, and other disorders that may respond adversely to vagotonic effects. **PREGNANCY/LACTATION:** Contraindicated in women who are or may become pregnant due to potential hazard to fetus. Discontinue nursing during isoflurophate therapy. **Pregnancy Category X.**

INTERACTIONS

DRUG INTERACTIONS: Anticholinergics, antimyasthenics, cholinesterase inhibitors may increase toxicity. **ALTERED LAB VALUES:** None significant.

SIDE EFFECTS

FREQUENT: Stinging, burning, tearing, painful ciliary or accommodative spasm, blurred vision or myopia, poor vision in dim light. **OCCASIONAL:** Iris cysts (more frequent in children), increased visibility of floaters, headache, browache, photophobia, ocular pain, hypersensitivity reactions (including allergic conjunctivitis, dermatitis or keratitis), potential hemorrhage during ocular surgery. **RARE:** Lens opacities, paradoxical increase in intraocular pressure, acute fibrinous iritis.

ADVERSE REACTIONS/TOXIC EFFECTS

Systemic toxicity may occur; retinal detachment.

NURSING IMPLICATIONS

INTERVENTION/EVALUATION:

Be alert for systemic toxicity: severe nausea, vomiting, diarrhea, frequent urination, excessive salivation, bradycardia (may trigger asthma attack in asthmatics). Assess vision acuity and provide assistance w/ambulation as needed.

PATIENT/FAMILY TEACHING:

Close observation is necessary for first 24 hrs. Teach proper administration. Do not use more often than directed due to risk of overdosage. Do not drive or engage in activities requiring visual acuity when vision is impaired; side effects often subside after the first few days of therapy. Avoid night driving, activities requiring visual acuity in dim light. Avoid insecticides, pesticides; inhalation or absorption through skin may add to systemic effects of isoflurophate. Report promptly any systemic effects (see Nursing Implications) or ocular problems. Inform dentist or physician of isoflurophate therapy.

isoniazid

eye-soe-nye´a-zid

(INH, Laniazid, Nydrazid)

FIXED-COMBINATION(S):

W/rifampin, an antitubercular (Rifamate); w/pyrazinamide and rifampin, antituberculars (Rifater).

CANADIAN AVAILABILITY:

Isotamine, PMS Isoniazid

CLASSIFICATION

Antitubercular

PHARMACOKINETICS

Readily absorbed from GI tract. Widely distributed (including CSF). Protein binding: 0-10%. Metabolized in liver. Primarily excreted in urine. Removed by hemodialysis. Half-life: 0.5-5 hrs.

ACTION

Inhibits mycolic acid synthesis that causes disruption of bacterial cell wall and loss of acid-fast properties in susceptible mycobacteria. Active only during cell division. Bactericidal.

USES

Drug of choice in tuberculosis prophylaxis. Used in combination w/one or more other antitubercular agents for treatment of all forms of active tuberculosis.

PO ADMINISTRATION

1. Give 1 hr before or 2 hrs after meals (may give w/food to decrease GI upset, but will delay absorption).
2. Administer at least 1 hr before antacids, esp. those containing aluminum.

INDICATIONS/DOSAGE/ROUTES

Tuberculosis (treatment):

PO/IM: Adults, elderly: 5 mg/kg/day (maximum 300 mg/day) as single dose. **Children:** 10-20 mg/kg/day (maximum 300 mg/day) as single dose.

Tuberculosis (prevention):

PO/IM: Adults, elderly: 300 mg/day as single dose. **Children:** 10 mg/kg/day (maximum 300 mg/day) as single dose.

PRECAUTIONS

CONTRAINDICATIONS: Acute liver disease, history of hypersensitivity reactions or hepatic injury w/previous isonizid therapy. **CAUTIONS:** Chronic liver disease or alcoholism, severe renal impairment. May be cross-sensitive w/ nicotinic acid or other chemically related medications. **PREGNANCY/LACTATION:** Prophylaxis usually postponed until after delivery. Crosses placenta; distributed in breast milk. **Pregnancy Category C.**

INTERACTIONS

DRUG INTERACTIONS: Alcohol may increase hepatotoxicity, metabolism. May increase toxicity of carbamazepine, phenytoin. May decrease ketoconazole concentrations. Disulfiram may increase CNS effects. Hepatotoxic medications may increase hepatotoxicity. **ALTERED LAB VALUES:** May increase SGOT (AST), SGPT (ALT), bilirubin.

SIDE EFFECTS

FREQUENT: Peripheral neuritis (esp. in alcoholics, diabetics, malnourished). Irritation at injection site w/IM administration. **OCCASIONAL:** Nausea, vomiting, dry mouth, hepatitis (esp. in those over age 35), pyridoxine deficiency, dizziness, hyperglycemia. **RARE:** Hypersensitivity reactions w/fever, skin eruptions, vasculitis; optic neuritis, memory impairment, seizures, gynecomastia, agranulocytosis, hemolytic anemia, rheumatic syndrome, lupus erythematosus-like syndrome.

ADVERSE REACTIONS/TOXIC EFFECTS

Neurotoxicity, hepatotoxicity.

NURSING IMPLICATIONS

BASELINE ASSESSMENT:

Question for history of hypersensitivity reactions or hepatic injury from isoniazid, sensitivity to nicotinic acid or chemically related medications. Assure collection of specimens for culture, sensitivity. Evaluate initial hepatic function results.

INTERVENTION/EVALUATION:

Monitor hepatic function test results and assess for hepatitis: anorexia, nausea, vomiting, weakness, fatigue, dark urine, jaundice (hold INH and inform physician promptly). Check for tingling, numbness, or burning of extremities (those esp. at risk for neuropathy may be given pyridoxine prophylactically: malnourished, elderly, diabetics, those w/chronic liver disease, including alcoholics). Be alert for fever, skin eruptions (hypersensitivity reaction). Report vision difficulties at once. Evaluate mental status. Check for dizziness, assist w/ambulation as needed. Monitor CBC results and blood sugar.

PATIENT/FAMILY TEACHING:

Do not skip doses; continue taking isonizid for full length of therapy (6 to 24 mo). Office visits, vision and lab tests are important part of treatment. Take preferably 1 hr before or 2 hrs after meals (w/food if GI upset). Avoid alcohol during treatment. Do not take any other medications w/o consulting physician, including antacids; must take isoniazid at least 1 hr before antacid. Avoid tuna, skipjack, sauerkraut, aged cheeses, smoked fish (provide list of tyramine-containing foods) that may cause reaction such as red/itching skin, pounding heartbeat, lightheadedness, hot or clammy feeling, headache; contact physician. Be certain not experiencing vision difficulty, dizziness, or other impairment before driving, using machinery. Notify physician of any new symptom, immediately for vision difficulties, nausea/vomiting, dark urine, yellowing of skin/eyes, fatigue, numbness or tingling of hands or feet.

isoproterenol hydrochloride

eye-sew-pro-tear´en-all

(Isuprel, Dey-Dose)

isoproterenol sulfate

(Medihaler-Iso)

FIXED-COMBINATION(S):
W/phenylephrine, a vasoconstrictor (Duo-Medihaler)

CANADIAN AVAILABILITY:
Isuprel, Medihaler-Iso

CLASSIFICATION

Cardiac stimulant, bronchodilator

PHARMACOKINETICS

	ONSET	PEAK	DURATION
Inhalation	2-5 min	—	0.5-2 hrs
Sublingual	15-30 min	—	1-2 hrs
SubQ, IM	Prompt	—	1-2 hrs
IV	Immediate	—	Length of infusion

Rapidly absorbed after inhalation/parenteral administration. Metabolized in liver. Primarily excreted in urine. Half-life: 2.5-5 minutes.

ACTION

Stimulates $beta_2$-adrenergic receptors in lungs (relaxes bronchial smooth muscle by increasing cAMP). Relieves bronchospasm; reduces airway resistance. Stimulates $beta_1$-adrenergic receptors (increases myocardial contractility, stroke volume, cardiac output).

USES

Treatment of carotid sinus hypersensitivity, Adams-Stokes syndrome, ventricular arrhythmias due to AV nodal block, reversible bronchospasm, diagnosis of coronary artery disease; adjunct in treatment of shock.

STORAGE/HANDLING

Do not use if solution is pink to brown, contains a precipitate, or appears cloudy.

PO/INHALATION/IV ADMINISTRATION

SUBLINGUAL:

1. Dissolve sublingual tablet under tongue (do not chew or swallow tablet).
2. Do not swallow saliva until tablet is dissolved.

INHALATION:

1. Shake container well, exhale completely then holding mouthpiece 1 inch away from lips, inhale and hold breath as long as possible before exhaling.
2. Wait 1-10 min before inhaling second dose (allows for deeper bronchial penetration).
3. Rinse mouth w/water immediately after inhalation (prevents mouth/throat dryness).

IV:

NOTE: May also be given SubQ, IM, intracardiac.

1. For IV injection, dilute 0.2 mg (1 ml) of 1:5,000 solution to a volume of 10 ml 0.9% NaCl injection or 5% dextrose injection.

2. Administer IV injection at rate of 1 ml/min, regulated by EKG monitoring.

3. For IV infusion, dilute 0.2 mg-2 mg (1-10 ml) of 1:5,000 solution in 500 ml of 5% dextrose in water to provide a solution of 0.4-4 mcg/ml.

4. Rate of IV infusion determined by pt's heart rate, central venous pressure, systemic B/P, and urine flow measurements.

5. Use microdrip (60 drops/ml) or infusion pump to administer drug.

6. If EKG changes occur, heart rate exceeds 110 beats/min, or premature beats occur, reduction in rate of infusion or temporarily stopping infusion should be considered.

INDICATIONS/DOSAGE/ROUTES

Arrhythmias:

IV BOLUS: Adults, elderly: Initially, 0.02-0.06 mg (1-3 ml of diluted solution). Subsequent dose range: 0.01-0.2 mg (0.5-10 ml of diluted solution).

IV INFUSION: Adults, elderly: Initially, 5 mcg/min (1.25 ml/min of diluted solution). Subsequent dose range: 2-20 mcg/min. **Children:** 2.5 mcg/min or 0.1 mcg/kg per min.

IM/SubQ: Adults, elderly: 0.2 mg, then 0.02-1 mg, as needed.

Mild arrhythmias:

SUBLINGUAL: Adults, elderly: 10-30 mg 4-6 times/day.

Complete heart block following closure of ventricular septal defects:

IV: Adults, elderly: 0.04-0.06 mg (2-3 ml of diluted solution). **Infants:** 0.01-0.03 (0.5-1.5 ml of diluted solution).

Shock:

IV INFUSION: Adults, elderly: Rate of 0.5-5 mcg/min (0.25-2.5 ml of 1:500,000 dilution); rate of infusion based on clinical response (heart rate, central venous pressure, systemic B/P, urine flow measurements).

Bronchospasm:

METERED DOSE INHALATION: Adults, elderly, children >6 yrs: 1-2 inhalations 4-6 times/day at no less than 3-4 hr intervals. Wait 1-5 min before administering second inhalation.

IPPB: Adults, elderly: 2 ml (0.125%) or 2.5 ml (0.1%) up to 5 times/day. Flow rate adjusted to administer dose over 15-20 min IPPB: 10-20 min via nebulization. **Children:** 2 ml (0.0625%) or 2.5 ml (0.05%) up to 5 times/day.

NEBULIZATION SOLUTION: Adults, elderly, children: 6-12 inhalations (0.025%). Repeat at 5-15 min intervals (maximum 3 treatments). **Maximum:** 8 treatments/ 24 hrs.

SUBLINGUAL: Adults, elderly: 10-20 mg q6-8h. **Children >6 yrs:** 5-10 mg q6-8h.

IV INFUSION: Adults, elderly: 0.01-0.02 mg (0.5-1 ml of a diluted solution). **Children:** 1/10-1/2 adult dose.

PRECAUTIONS

CONTRAINDICATIONS: Tachycardia due to digitalis toxicity, preexisting arrhythmias, angina, precordial distress. **CAUTIONS:** Hypersensitivity to sulfite, elderly/ debilitated, hypertension, cardiovascular disease, impaired renal function, hyperthyroidism, diabetes mellitus, prostatic hypertrophy, glaucoma. **PREGNANCY/LAC-**

TATION: Unknown if drug crosses placenta or is distributed in breast milk. May inhibit uterine contractility. **Pregnancy Category C.**

INTERACTIONS

DRUG INTERACTIONS: Tricyclic antidepressants may increase cardiovascular effects. May decrease effects of beta-blockers. Digoxin may increase risk of arrhythmias. **ALTERED LAB VALUES:** May decrease serum potassium levels.

SIDE EFFECTS

OCCASIONAL: Restlessness, nervousness, insomnia, anxiety. **RARE:** Nausea, sweating, flushing of face, headache, weakness.

ADVERSE REACTIONS/TOXIC EFFECTS

Excessive sympathomimetic stimulation may cause palpitations, extrasystoles, tachycardia, chest pain, slight increase in B/P followed by a substantial decrease, chills, sweating, and blanching of skin. Ventricular arrhythmias may occur if heart rate is above 130 beats/min. When used for bronchospasm, too-frequent or excessive use may lead to loss of bronchodilating effectiveness and/or severe, paradoxical bronchoconstriction. Parotid gland swelling may occur w/prolonged use.

NURSING IMPLICATIONS

BASELINE ASSESSMENT:

Be alert to anginal pain or precordial distress, pulse rate exceeding 110 beats/min.

INTERVENTION/EVALUATION:

Cardiac stimulant: Monitor EKG, blood P_{CO_2} or bicarbonate and blood pH, central venous pressure, pulse, systemic B/P, urine output. *Bronchospasm:* Monitor rate, depth, rhythm, type of respiration; quality and rate of pulse. Assess lung sounds for rhonchi, wheezing, rales. Monitor arterial blood gases. Observe lips, fingernails for blue or dusky color in light-skinned pts; grey in dark-skinned pts. Observe for clavicular retractions, hand tremor. Evaluate for clinical improvement (quieter, slower respirations, relaxed facial expression, cessation of clavicular retractions).

PATIENT/FAMILY TEACHING:

Bronchospasm: Increase fluid intake (decreases lung secretion viscosity). Do not take more than 2 inhalations at any one time (excessive use may produce paradoxical bronchoconstriction, or a decreased bronchodilating effect).

Rinsing mouth with water immediately after inhalation may prevent mouth/throat dryness. Saliva may turn pink after sublingual administration. Due to acidity of drug, frequent sublingual use may damage teeth. Avoid excessive use of caffeine derivatives (chocolate, coffee, tea, cola, cocoa).

isosorbide dinitrate

eye-sew-sore´bide

(Dilatrate, Isordil, Sorbitrate)

isosorbide mononitrate

(Imdur, ISMO, Monoket)

CANADIAN AVAILABILITY: Apo-ISDN, Coronex, Novosorbide

CLASSIFICATION

Nitrate

PHARMACOKINETICS

	ONSET	PEAK	DURATION
Chewable	5-20 min	15-60 min	1-4 hrs
Sublingual	5-20 min	15-60 min	1-4 hrs
Extended release	up to 4 hrs	—	6-8 hrs
Tablets, capsules	20-40 min	45-120 min	4-6 hrs
Mononitrate	30-60 min	—	—

Poorly absorbed from GI tract; well absorbed after sublingual administration. Protein binding: 60%. Metabolized in liver (undergoes first-pass effect). Primarily excreted in urine. Half-life: *oral:* 4 hrs, *sublingual:* 1 hr. *Mononitrate:* Not subjected to first-pass metabolism in liver.

ACTION

Decreases myocardial O_2 demand. Reduces left ventricular preload and afterload. Dilates coronary arteries; improves collateral blood flow to ischemic areas within myocardium.

USES

Relief of acute angina; prophylaxis prior to event well-known to cause angina. Chronic prophylaxis of angina. *Mononitrate:* Prevents angina pectoris due to coronary artery disease.

PO/SUBLINGUAL ADMINISTRATION

PO:

1. Best if taken on an empty stomach.
2. Oral tablets may be crushed.
3. Do not crush or break sublingual or extended-release form.
4. Do not crush chewable form before administering.

SUBLINGUAL:

1. Do not crush/chew sublingual tablets.
2. Dissolve tablets under tongue, do not swallow.

INDICATIONS/DOSAGE/ROUTES

Acute angina, prophylactic management in situations likely to provoke attack:
SUBLINGUAL/CHEWABLE:
Adults, elderly: Initially, 2.5-5 mg. Repeat at 5-10 min intervals. No more than 3 doses in 15-30 min period.

Acute prophylactic management of angina:
SUBLINGUAL/CHEWABLE:
Adults, elderly: 5-10 mg q2-3h.

Long-term prophylaxis of angina:
PO: Adults, elderly: Initially, 5-20 mg 3-4 times/day. **Maintenance:** 10-40 mg q6h. Consider 2-3 times/day, last dose no later than 7 PM to minimize intolerance.
MONONITRATE: Adults, elderly: 20 mg 2 times/day, 7 hrs apart. First dose upon awakening in morning.
EXTENDED RELEASE: Adults, elderly: Initially, 40 mg. **Maintenance:** 40-80 mg q6-12h. Consider 1-2 times/day, last dose at 2 PM to minimize intolerance.
IMDUR: 60-120 mg/day as single dose.

PRECAUTIONS

CONTRAINDICATIONS: Hypersensitivity to nitrates, severe anemia, closed-angle glaucoma, postural hypotension, head trauma, increased intracranial pressure. *Extended release:* GI hypermotility/malabsorption, severe anemia. **CAUTIONS:** Acute MI, hepatic/renal disease, glaucoma (contraindicated in closed-angle glaucoma), blood volume depletion from diuretic therapy, systolic B/P below 90 mm Hg. **PREGNANCY/ LACTATION:** Unknown if drug crosses placenta or is distributed in breast milk. **Pregnancy Category C.**

INTERACTIONS

DRUG INTERACTIONS: Alcohol, antihypertensives, vasodilators may increase risk of orthostatic hypotension. **ALTERED LAB VALUES:** May increase urine catecholamines, urine VMA.

SIDE EFFECTS

FREQUENT: Headache (may be severe) occurs mostly in early therapy, diminishes rapidly in intensity, usually disappears during continued treatment; transient flushing of face and neck, dizziness (especially if pt is standing immobile or is in a warm environment), weakness, postural hypotension. *Sublingual:* Burning, tingling sensation at oral point of dissolution. **OCCASIONAL:** GI upset.

ADVERSE REACTIONS/TOXIC EFFECTS

Drug should be discontinued if blurred vision, dry mouth occur. Severe postural hypotension manifested by fainting, pulselessness, cold/clammy skin, profuse sweating. Tolerance may occur w/repeated, prolonged therapy (minor tolerance w/intermittent use of sublingual tablets). Tolerance may not occur w/extended-release form. High dose tends to produce severe headache.

NURSING IMPLICATIONS

BASELINE ASSESSMENT:

Record onset, type (sharp, dull, squeezing), radiation, location, intensity and duration of anginal pain, and precipitating factors (exertion, emotional stress). If headache occurs during management therapy, administer medication w/meals.

INTERVENTION/EVALUATION:

Assist w/ambulation if lightheadedness, dizziness occurs. Assess for facial/neck flushing. Monitor B/P for hypotension.

PATIENT/FAMILY TEACHING:

Rise slowly from lying to sitting position and dangle legs momentarily before standing. Take oral form on empty stomach (however, if headache occurs during management therapy, take medication w/meals). Dissolve sublingual tablet under tongue, do not swallow. Take at first signal of angina. If not relieved within 5 min, dissolve second tablet under tongue. Repeat if no relief in another 5 min. If pain continues, contact physician. Expel from mouth any remaining sublingual tablet after pain is completely relieved. Place transmucosal tablets under upper lip or buccal pouch (between cheek and gum); do not chew or swallow tablet. Do not change from one brand of drug to another. Avoid alcohol (intensifies hypotensive effect). If alcohol is ingested soon after taking nitroglycerin, possible acute hypotensive episode (marked drop in B/P, vertigo, pallor) may occur.

isotretinoin

eye-soe-tret´ih-noyn
(Accutane)

CANADIAN AVAILABILITY:
Accutane

CLASSIFICATION

Acne aid

PHARMACOKINETICS

Rapidly absorbed from GI tract. Protein binding: 99.9%. Metabolized in liver. Excreted in urine; via biliary system. Half-life: 10-20 hrs.

ACTION

Reduces sebaceous gland size; inhibits its activity. Has antikeratinizing, anti-inflammatory effects.

USES

Treatment of severe, recalcitrant cystic acne that is unresponsive to conventional acne therapies.

PO ADMINISTRATION

1. Administer whole; do not crush.
2. Give w/food to facilitate absorption.

INDICATIONS/DOSAGE/ROUTES

Recalcitrant cystic acne:
PO: Adults: Initially, 0.5-2 mg/kg/day divided in 2 doses for 15-20 wks. May repeat after at least 2 mo off therapy.

PRECAUTIONS

CONTRAINDICATIONS: Hypersensitivity to isotretinoin or parabens (component of capsules). **CAUTIONS:** Renal, hepatic dysfunction. Safety in children not established. **PREGNANCY/LACTATION:** Contraindicated in females who are or may become pregnant while undergoing treatment. Extremely high risk of major deformities in infant if pregnancy occurs while taking any amount of isotretinoin, even for short periods. Pt must be capable of understanding and carrying out instructions and of complying w/mandatory contraception. Excretion in milk unknown; due to potential for serious adverse effects, not recommended during nursing. **Pregnancy Category X.**

INTERACTIONS

DRUG INTERACTIONS: Etretinate, tretinoin, vitamin A may increase toxic effects. Tetracycline may increase potential of pseudotumor cerebri. **ALTERED LAB VALUES:** May increase triglycerides, cholesterol, SGPT (ALT), SGOT (AST), alkaline phosphatase, LDH, sedimentation rate, fasting blood glucose, uric acid; may decrease HDL.

SIDE EFFECTS

FREQUENT: Cheilitis (90% of pts); skin/mucous membrane dryness (up to 80%) including dry skin, fragility of skin, pruritus, epistaxis, dry nose and mouth; conjunctivitis (40%); hypertriglyceridemia (25%); nausea, vomiting, abdominal pain (20%). **OCCASIONAL:** Musculoskeletal symptoms (16%) including bone or joint pain, arthralgia, generalized muscle aches; photosensitivity (5-10%). Some pts have problems w/control of blood glucose. **RARE:** Decreased night vision, corneal opacities, hepatitis, depression.

ADVERSE REACTIONS/TOXIC EFFECTS

Inflammatory bowel disease and pseudotumor cerebri (benign intracranial hypertension) have been temporarily associated w/isotretinoin therapy.

NURSING IMPLICATIONS

BASELINE ASSESSMENT:

Question for hypersensitivity to isotretinoin or parabens. Assess baselines for blood lipids and glucose.

INTERVENTION/EVALUATION:

Assess acne for decreased cysts. Evaluate skin and mucous membranes for excessive dryness. Monitor blood glucose, lipids.

PATIENT/FAMILY TEACHING:

A transient exacerbation of acne may occur during initial period. May have decreased tolerance to contact lenses during and after therapy. Topical acne agents should not be used w/o physician approval. Do not take vitamin supplements w/vitamin A because of additive effects. Notify physician immediately of onset of abdominal pain, severe diarrhea, rectal bleeding (possible inflammatory bowel disease), or headache, nausea and vomiting, visual disturbances (possible pseudotumor cerebri). Decreased night vision may occur suddenly; take caution w/night driving. Minimize or eliminate alcohol consumption (may potentiate serum triglyceride elevation). Avoid prolonged exposure to sunlight; use sunscreens, protective clothing until sunlight or ultraviolet light tolerance established. Do not donate blood during or for 1 mo after treatment. *Women:* Explain the serious risk to fetus if pregnancy occurs (both oral and written warnings are given, w/pt acknowledging in writing that she understands the warnings and consents to treatment). Must have a negative serum pregnancy test within 2 wks prior to starting therapy; therapy will begin on the second or third day of the next normal menstrual period. Effective contraception (using 2 reliable forms of contraception simultaneously) must be used for at least 1 mo before, during, and for at least 1 mo after therapy w/isotretinoin.

isradipine

is-rad´ih-peen
(DynaCirc, DynaCirc CR)

CLASSIFICATION

Calcium channel blocker

PHARMACOKINETICS

	ONSET	PEAK	DURATION
PO	2-3 hrs	—	—

Well absorbed from GI tract. Protein binding: 95%. Metabolized in liver (undergoes first-pass effect). Primarily excreted in urine. Half-life: 8 hrs.

ACTION

Potent peripheral vasodilator; does not depress SA, AV nodes. Reflex increased heart rate masks negative inotropic effect.

USES

Management of hypertension. May be used alone or w/thiazide-type diuretics.

PO ADMINISTRATION

Do not crush or break capsule.

INDICATIONS/DOSAGE/ROUTES

Hypertension:
PO: Adults, elderly: Initially, 2.5 mg 2 times/day. May increase by 5 mg q2-4wks. **Maximum:** 20 mg/day. *DynaCirc CR:* 5-20 mg/day as single dose.

PRECAUTIONS

CONTRAINDICATIONS: Sick sinus syndrome/second- or third-degree AV block (except in presence of pacemaker). **CAUTIONS:** Impaired renal/hepatic function, CHF. **PREGNANCY/LACTATION:** Unknown if drug crosses placenta or is distributed in breast milk. **Pregnancy Category C.**

INTERACTIONS

DRUG INTERACTIONS: Beta-blockers may have additive effect. **ALTERED LAB VALUES:** None significant.

SIDE EFFECTS

FREQUENT: Headache, peripheral edema, dizziness/lightheadedness. **OCCASIONAL:** Palpitations, facial flushing. **RARE:** Nausea, vomiting, diarrhea, rash, dyspepsia, cough.

ADVERSE REACTIONS/TOXIC EFFECTS

CHF. Overdosage produces nausea, drowsiness, confusion, slurred speech.

NURSING IMPLICATIONS

BASELINE ASSESSMENT:

Assess baseline renal/liver function tests. Assess B/P, apical pulse immediately before drug is administered (if pulse is 60/min or below, or systolic B/P is below 90 mm Hg, withhold medication, contact physician).

INTERVENTION/EVALUATION:

Assist w/ambulation if lightheadedness, dizziness occurs. Assess for peripheral edema behind medial malleolus (sacral area in bedridden pts). Monitor pulse rate for bradycardia. Assess skin for flushing. Monitor liver enzyme tests.

PATIENT/FAMILY TEACHING:

Do not abruptly discontinue medication. Compliance w/therapy regimen is essential to control hypertension. To avoid hypotensive effect, rise slowly from lying to sitting position, wait momentarily before standing. Avoid tasks that require alertness, motor skills until response to drug is established. Contact physician/nurse if irregular heart beat, shortness of breath, pronounced dizziness, or nausea occurs.

itraconazole

eye-tra-con'ah-zoll
(Sporanex)

CLASSIFICATION

Antifungal

PHARMACOKINETICS

Moderately absorbed from GI tract (increased w/food). Widely distributed (primarily in liver, kidney, fatty tissue). Protein binding: >99%. Metabolized in liver to active metabolite. Primarily excreted in urine. Not removed by hemodialysis. Half-life: 21 hrs; metabolite: 12 hrs.

ACTION

Inhibits cytochrome P-450 dependent synthesis of ergosterol (vital component of fungal cell membranes). Alters membrane function. May directly damage membrane phospholipids.

USES

Treatment of blastomycosis (pulmonary, extrapulmonary), histoplasmosis, aspergillosis.

PO ADMINISTRATION

Take w/food (increases absorption).

INDICATIONS/DOSAGE/ROUTES

NOTE: Doses >200 mg given in 2 divided doses.

Blastomycosis, histoplasmosis:
PO: Adults, elderly: Initially, 200 mg/day w/food. May increase in 100 mg increments. **Maximum:** 400 mg/day.

Aspergillosis:
PO: Adults, elderly: 200-400 mg/day.

Life-threatening infection:
PO: Adults, elderly: Initially, 200 mg 3 times/day for 3 days as loading dose.

PRECAUTIONS

CONTRAINDICATIONS: Co-administration of terfenadine. Hypersensitivity to itraconazole, fluconazole, ketoconazole, miconazole. **CAUTIONS:** Hepatitis, HIV-infected pts, pts w/achlorhydria, hypochlorhydria (decreases absorption), impaired liver function. **PREGNANCY/LACTATION:** Distributed in breast milk. **Pregnancy Category C.**

INTERACTIONS

DRUG INTERACTIONS: May increase cyclosporine, digoxin concentrations. May increase terfenadine, astemizole concentration, increasing risk of cardiac dysrhythmias. May increase effect of oral anticoagulants. Phenytoin, rifampin may decrease concentrations. Antacids, H_2 antagonists, didanosine may decrease absorption. **ALTERED LAB VALUES:** May increase SGOT (AST), SGPT (ALT), alkaline phosphatase, LDH, bilirubin. May decrease potassium.

SIDE EFFECTS

OCCASIONAL: Skin rash, abdominal pain, nausea, vomiting, diarrhea, constipation, anorexia, headache. **RARE:** Hepatitis (loss of appetite, stomach pain, unusual tiredness/weakness, yellow eyes/skin, dark urine).

ADVERSE REACTIONS/TOXIC EFFECTS

None significant.

NURSING IMPLICATIONS

BASELINE ASSESSMENT:

Obtain specimens for fungal cultures and other lab studies before first dose. Therapy may begin before results are known. Determine baseline temperature, liver function tests. Assess allergies.

INTERVENTION/EVALUATION:

Assess for signs and symptoms of liver dysfunction and monitor hepatic enzyme test results in pts w/pre-existing liver dysfunction. Check temperature.

PATIENT/FAMILY TEACHING:

Take w/food. Therapy will continue for at least 3 months and until lab tests and clinical presentation indicate infection is controlled. Report the following at once: unusual fatigue, yellow skin, dark urine, pale stool, anorexia/nausea/vomiting.

kanamycin sulfate

can-ah-my´sin
(Kantrex)

CLASSIFICATION

Antibiotic: Aminoglycoside

PHARMACOKINETICS

Rapid, complete absorption after IM administration. Widely distributed (does not cross blood-brain barrier, low concentrations in CSF). Protein binding: 10%. Excreted unchanged in urine. Removed by hemodialysis. Half-life: 2-4 hrs (increased in decreased renal function, neonates; decreased in cystic fibrosis, burn or febrile pts).

ACTION

Irreversibly binds to protein on 30S subunit of bacterial ribosome, interfering in protein synthesis of susceptible microorganisms.

USES

Treatment of skin/skin structure, bone, joint, respiratory tract, intra-abdominal and complicated urinary tract infections; wound and surgical site irrigation, burns, septicemia, hepatic encephalopathy. Adjunctive therapy for tuberculosis; before operation for intestinal antisepsis.

STORAGE/HANDLING

Store parenteral form, capsules at room temperature. Solutions appear clear, colorless to pale yellow. Darkening of solution does not indicate loss of potency. Intermittent IV infusion (piggyback) stable for 24 hrs at room temperature. Discard if precipitate forms.

PO/IM/IV ADMINISTRATION

NOTE: Coordinate peak and trough lab draws w/administration times.

PO:

1. Give w/o regard to meals.
2. If GI upset occurs, give w/ food or milk.

IM:

1. To minimize discomfort, give deep IM slowly. Less painful to inject into gluteus maximus rather than lateral aspect of thigh.

IV:

1. Dilute each 500 mg w/100-200 ml 5% dextrose, 0.9% NaCl, or other compatible IV fluid. Amount of diluent for infants, children depends on individual needs.
2. Administer IV infusion (piggyback) over 30-60 min.
3. Alternating IV sites, use large veins to reduce risk of phlebitis.

INDICATIONS/DOSAGE/ROUTES

Space doses evenly around the clock.

Mild to moderate infections:
IM/IV: Adults, children: 15 mg/kg/day in divided doses q8-12h (IM doses may be given q6h). **Elderly:** 5-7.5 mg/kg/dose q12-24h.

Hepatic encephalopathy (adjunctive treatment):
PO: Adults, elderly: 8-12 Gm/day in 4 divided doses.

Preop intestinal antisepsis:
PO: Adults, elderly: 1 Gm every hour for 4 doses, then 1 Gm q6h for up to 3 days.

INTRAPERITONEAL INSTILLATIONS: Adults: 500 mg dissolved in 20 ml sterile water, instilled via catheter into wound.

IRRIGATION: Adults: 0.25% solution to irrigate pleural space, ventricular or abscess cavities, wounds, or surgical sites.

INHALATION: Adults: 250 mg diluted w/3 ml 0.9% NaCl and nebulized 2-4 times/day.

Dosage in renal impairment:

Dose and/or frequency is modified based on degree of renal impairment, serum concentration of drug.

PRECAUTIONS

CONTRAINDICATIONS: Hypersensitivity to kanamycin, other aminoglycosides (cross-sensitivity). Oral administration contraindicated in intestinal obstruction. **CAUTIONS:** Elderly, neonates (due to renal insufficiency or immaturity); neuromuscular disorders (potential for respiratory depression), prior hearing loss, vertigo, renal impairment. Not for long-term therapy due to associated toxicities. Cumulative effects may occur when given via more than one route. **PREGNANCY/LACTATION:** Readily crosses placenta; distributed in breast milk. May cause fetal nephrotoxicity. **Pregnancy Category C.**

INTERACTIONS

DRUG INTERACTIONS: Other aminoglycosides, nephrotoxic, ototoxic medications may increase toxicity. May increase effects of neuromuscular blocking agents. **ALTERED LAB VALUES:** May increase BUN, SGPT (ALT), SGOT (AST), bilirubin, creatinine, LDH concentrations; may decrease serum calcium, magnesium, potassium, sodium concentrations.

SIDE EFFECTS

FREQUENT: *Oral:* Nausea, vomiting, diarrhea. **OCCASIONAL:** *IM:* Pain, irritation at injection site. *IV:* Phlebitis; hypersensitivity reactions: rash, fever, urticaria, pruritus. **RARE:** Headache.

ADVERSE REACTIONS/TOXIC EFFECTS

Nephrotoxicity (evidenced by increased BUN and serum creatinine, decreased creatinine clearance) may be reversible if drug stopped at first sign of symptoms; irreversible otoxicity (tinnitus, dizziness, ringing/roaring in ears, reduced hearing) and neurotoxicity (headache, dizziness, lethargy, tremors, visual disturbances) occur occasionally. Risk is greater w/higher dosages, prolonged therapy. Superinfections, particularly w/fungi, may result from bacterial imbalance. Severe respiratory depression, anaphylaxis occur rarely.

NURSING IMPLICATIONS

BASELINE ASSESSMENT:

Dehydration must be treated before aminoglycoside therapy. Establish pt's baseline hearing acuity before beginning therapy. Question for history of allergies, especially to aminoglycosides. Obtain specimens for culture, sensitivity before giving first dose (therapy may begin before results are known). Maintain adequate hydration.

INTERVENTION/EVALUATION:

Monitor I&O (maintain hydration), urinalysis (casts, RBCs, WBCs, decrease in specific gravity). Monitor results of peak/trough blood tests. Be alert to ototoxic and neurotoxic symptoms (see Adverse Reactions/Toxic Effects). Check IM injection site for pain, induration. Evaluate IV site for phlebitis (heat, pain, red streaking over vein). Assess for rash. Be alert to respiratory depression. Assess for superinfection, particularly genital/anal pruritus, changes of oral mucosa, diarrhea.

PATIENT/FAMILY TEACHING:

Continue antibiotic for full length of treatment. Space doses evenly. Discomfort may occur w/IM injection. Notify physician in event of headache, shortness of breath, dizziness, hearing or urinary problem even after therapy is completed. Do not take other medication w/o consulting physician. Lab tests are an essential part of therapy.

kaolin/pectin

kay´oh-lyn
(Kaopectate, Kapectolin)

FIXED-COMBINATION(S):
W/atropine, hyoscyamine, scopolamine, belladonna alkaloids, opium (Donnagel PG, Kapectolin PG); w/opium (Parepectolin)

CANADIAN AVAILABILITY:
Donnagel-MB, Kao-Con, Kaopectate

CLASSIFICATION

CLINICAL: Antidiarrheal

PHARMACOKINETICS

Not absorbed orally. Up to 90% of pectin decomposed in GI tract.

ACTION

Adsorbent, protectant (adsorbs bacteria, toxins, reduces water loss).

USES

Symptomatic treatment of mild to moderate acute diarrhea.

PO ADMINISTRATION

Shake suspension well before administration.

INDICATIONS/DOSAGE/ROUTES

Antidiarrheal:
PO: Adults, elderly: 60-120 ml after each loose bowel movement. **Children >12 yrs:** 60 ml after each loose bowel movement; **6-12 yrs:** 30-60 ml after each loose bowel movement; **3-6 yrs:** 15-30 ml after each loose bowel movement.

PRECAUTIONS

CONTRAINDICATIONS: None significant. **CAUTIONS:** None significant. **PREGNANCY/LACTATION:** Unknown if drug crosses placenta or is distributed in breast milk. **Pregnancy Category C.**

INTERACTIONS

DRUG INTERACTIONS: May decrease absorption of digoxin. **ALTERED LAB VALUES:** None significant.

SIDE EFFECTS

RARE: Constipation.

ADVERSE REACTIONS/TOXIC EFFECTS

None significant.

NURSING IMPLICATIONS

INTERVENTION/EVALUATION:

Encourage adequate fluid intake. Assess bowel sounds for peristalsis. Assess stools for frequency and consistency (watery, loose, soft, semisolid, solid).

PATIENT/FAMILY TEACHING:

Do not use for more than 2 days or w/high fever. Not for children under 3 years of age w/o physician direction.

ketamine hydrochloride

ket´ah´meen
(Ketalar)

CANADIAN AVAILABILITY:
Ketalar

CLASSIFICATION

Rapid-acting general anesthetic

PHARMACOKINETICS

	ONSET	PEAK	DURATION
IV	30 sec	—	5-10 min
IM	3-4 min	—	12-25 min

Rapidly absorbed, distributed. Metabolized in liver. Primarily excreted in urine. Half-life: 2-3 hrs.

ACTION

Blocks afferent impulses associated w/emotional component of pain perception. Suppresses spinal cord activity, interacts w/CNS transmitter systems.

USES

Sole anesthetic for procedures not requiring skeletal muscle relaxation; induction of anesthesia prior to administering other general anesthetics; supplement low potency anesthetics.

IV ADMINISTRATION

IV:

1. For IV use, dilute 100 mg/ml w/equal volume sterile water for injection, 0.9% NaCl, or 5% dextrose.
2. Administer slowly over 60 sec (too-rapid IV may produce marked severe hypotension, respiratory depression, irregular muscular movements).
3. For IV infusion, add 10 ml (50 mg/ml) or 5 ml (100 mg/ml) to 250-500 ml 0.9% NaCl or 5% dextrose to provide a concentration of 1-2 mg/ml.
4. Observe for signs of intra-arterial injection (pain, discolored skin patches, white/blue color to hand, delayed onset of drug action).
5. Inadvertent intra-arterial injection may result in arterial spasm w/severe pain, thrombosis, gangrene.

INDICATIONS/DOSAGE/ROUTES

NOTE: Do not use alone; individualize dosage.

Induction:
IV: Adults: Initially, 1-4.5 mg/kg to produce 5-10 min surgical anesthesia.
IV INFUSION: Adults: 1-2 mg/kg infused at rate of 0.5 mg/kg/min.
IM: Adults: 6.5-13 mg/kg to produce 12-25 min surgical anesthesia.

Maintenance:
IM/IV: Adults: ½ the 100% induction dose repeated as needed for maintenance anesthesia.

PRECAUTIONS

CONTRAINDICATIONS: Those in whom significant increase in B/P would be hazardous, psychiatric disorders (schizophrenia, acute psychoses, known intolerance to drug). **CAUTIONS:** Hypertension, cardiac decompensation, chronic alcoholism, acute alcohol intoxication, debilitated, impaired respiratory, circulatory, renal, hepatic, endocrine function. **PREGNANCY/LACTATION:** Crosses placenta; unknown if distributed in breast milk. **Pregnancy Category C.**

K

INTERACTIONS

DRUG INTERACTIONS: Antihypertensives, CNS depressants may increase risk of hypotension or respiratory depression. **ALTERED LAB VALUES:** May increase IOP.

SIDE EFFECTS

FREQUENT: Increase in B/P, pulse. Emergence reaction occurs commonly (least in those <15 yrs, >65 yrs) resulting in dream-like state, vivid imagery, hallucination, delirium, occasionally w/confusion, excitement, irrational behavior. Duration: Few hours to 24 hrs after operation. **OCCASIONAL:** Local pain at injection site. **RARE:** Rash.

ADVERSE REACTIONS/TOXIC EFFECTS

Continuous or repeated intermittent infusion may result in extreme somnolence, respiratory/circulatory depression. A too-rapid IV may produce marked severe hypotension, respiratory depression, irregular muscular movements. Acute allergic reaction (erythema, pruritus, urticaria, rhinitis, dyspnea, hypotension, restlessness, anxiety, abdominal pain) may occur.

NURSING IMPLICATIONS

BASELINE ASSESSMENT:

Resuscitative equipment, endotracheal tube, suction, oxygen must be available. Obtain vital signs before administration.

INTERVENTION/EVALUATION:

Monitor vital signs every 3-5 min during and after administration until recovery is achieved. Assess for emergence reaction (hypnotic/barbiturate may be needed). Keep verbal, tactile, visual stimulation at minimum during recovery.

PATIENT/FAMILY TEACHING:

Do not drive or operate machinery for 24 hrs after anesthesia.

ketoconazole

keet-oh-con´ah-zol
(Nizoral)

CANADIAN AVAILABILITY: Nizoral

CLASSIFICATION

Antifungal

PHARMACOKINETICS

Oral: Readily absorbed from GI tract. Widely distributed. Protein binding: 99%. Metabolized in liver. Primarily excreted via biliary elimination. Half-life: 8 hrs. *Topical:* Minimal systemic absorption.

ACTION

Fungistatic. Inhibits ergosterol synthesis. Damages fungal cell membrane, altering permeability (causes loss of essential intracellular elements).

USES

Treatment of histoplasmosis, blastomycosis, candidiasis, chronic mucocutaneous candidiasis, coccidioidomycosis, paracoccidioidomycosis, chromomycosis, seborrheic dermatitis, tineas (ringworm): corporis, capitis, manus, cruris, pedis, unguium (onychomycosis), oral thrush, candiduria. Shampoo: Reduce scaling due to dandruff.

PO ADMINISTRATION

1. Give w/food to minimize GI irritation.
2. Tablets may be crushed.
3. Ketoconazole requires acidity; give antacids, anticholinergics, H_2 blockers *at least* 2 hrs after dosing.

INDICATIONS/DOSAGE/ROUTES

Mild to moderate infections:
PO: Adults, elderly: 200 mg/day. **Children >2 yrs:** 3.3-6.6 mg/kg/day as single dose.

Severe infections:
PO: Adults, elderly: 400 mg/day.

Cutaneous fungal infections:
TOPICAL: Adults, elderly: Apply 1-2 times/day for 2-4 wks.

Dandruff:
SHAMPOO: Adults, elderly: 2 times/wk for 4 wks, allowing at least 3 days between each shampoo. Intermittent use to maintain control.

PRECAUTIONS

CONTRAINDICATIONS: Hypersensitivity to ketoconazole, children <2 yrs. **CAUTIONS:** Hepatic impairment. **PREGNANCY/LACTATION:** Unknown if crosses placenta; probably distributed in breast milk. **Pregnancy Category C.**

INTERACTIONS

DRUG INTERACTIONS: Alcohol, hepatotoxic medications may increase hepatotoxicity. Antacids, anticholinergics, H_2 antagonists, omeprazole may decrease absorption (allow 2 hr interval). May increase concentration, toxicity of cyclosporine. Isoniazid, rifampin may decrease concentration. May increase concentration terfenadine causing cardiotoxicity. **ALTERED LAB VALUES:** May increase SGOT (AST), SGPT (ALT), alkaline phosphatase, bilirubin. May decrease corticosteroid, testosterone concentrations.

SIDE EFFECTS

FREQUENT: Nausea, vomiting, pruritus. **OCCASIONAL:** Abdominal pain, diarrhea or constipation, GI bleeding, rash, urticaria, photophobia, headache, dizziness, gynecomastia, fever, chills, abnormal dreams, somnolence, impotence, arthralgia, adrenocortical insufficiency. **RARE:** Topical application may cause itching, burning, irritation.

ADVERSE REACTIONS/TOXIC EFFECTS

Hematologic toxicity occurs occasionally (thrombocytopenia, hemolytic anemia, leukopenia). Hepatotoxicity may occur within first week to several months of therapy. Anaphylaxis occurs rarely.

NURSING IMPLICATIONS

BASELINE ASSESSMENT:

Question for history of allergies, especially to ketoconazole (sulfite when using topical cream). Confirm that a culture or histologic test was done for accurate diagnosis; therapy may begin before results known.

INTERVENTION/EVALUATION:

Monitor hepatic function tests; be alert for hepatotoxicity: dark urine, pale stools, fatigue, anorexia/nausea/vomiting (unrelieved by giving medication w/food). Determine pattern of bowel activity, stool consistency, check for blood in stool. Assess mental status (dizziness, somnolence) and provide assistance as needed.

Evaluate skin for rash, urticaria, itching. Check sleep pattern. *Topical:* Check for local burning, itching, irritation.

PATIENT/FAMILY TEACHING:

Prolonged therapy (weeks or months) is usually necessary. Do not miss a dose; continue therapy as long as directed. Avoid alcohol (due to potential liver problem). Wear sunglasses and avoid bright light in event of photophobia. Do not drive car, machinery if dizziness, drowsiness occur. Take any antacids/anti-ulcer medications at least 2 hrs after ketoconazole. Notify physician of dark urine, pale stool, yellow skin/eyes, increased irritation in topical use, or onset of other new symptom. Consult physician before taking any other medication. GI distress: take tablets w/food. *Topical:* Rub well into affected areas. Avoid contact w/ eyes. Keep skin clean, dry; wear light clothing for ventilation. Separate personal items in direct contact w/affected area. Do not use other preparations or occlusive covering w/o consulting physician. *Shampoo:* Apply shampoo to wet hair to produce enough lather to wash hair and scalp. Leave in place about 1 min, then rinse. Apply shampoo and lather a second time, leaving on scalp 3 min, then rinse again thoroughly. Initially use twice weekly for 4 wks w/at least 3 days between shampooing; frequency then will be determined by response.

ketoprofen

key-toe-pro´fen

(Orudis, Oruvail)

CANADIAN AVAILABILITY:

Apo-Keto, Orudis, Rhodis

CLASSIFICATION

Nonsteroidal anti-inflammatory

PHARMACOKINETICS

Rapid, complete absorption from GI tract. Protein binding: 99%. Primarily metabolized in liver, excreted in urine. Removed by hemodialysis. Half-life: 1.5-4 hrs.

ACTION

Inhibits prostaglandin synthesis. Inhibits action of cyclooxygenase; decreases formation of prostaglandin, thromboxane precursors from arachidonic acid.

USES

Symptomatic treatment of acute and chronic rheumatoid arthritis and osteoarthritis. Relief of mild to moderate pain, primary dysmenorrhea.

PO ADMINISTRATION

May give w/food, milk, or full glass (8 ounces) water (minimizes potential GI distress).

INDICATIONS/DOSAGE/ROUTES

NOTE: Do not exceed 300 mg/ day. Oruvail not recommended as initial therapy in pts who are small, >75 yrs of age, or renally impaired.

Acute and chronic rheumatoid arthritis, osteoarthritis:

PO: Adults: Initially, 75 mg three times/day or 50 mg four times/day. **Elderly:** Initially, 25-50 mg 3-4 times/day. **Maintenance:** 150-300 mg/day in 3-4 divided doses. *Oruvail:* 200 mg/day.

Mild to moderate pain, dysmenorrhea:

PO: Adults: 25-50 mg q6-8h.

PRECAUTIONS

CONTRAINDICATIONS: Active peptic ulcer, GI ulceration, chronic inflammation of GI tract, GI bleeding disorders, history of hypersensitivity to aspirin or nonsteroidal anti-inflammatory agents. **CAUTIONS:** Impaired renal/hepatic function, history of GI tract disease, predisposition to fluid retention. **PREGNANCY/LACTATION:** Unknown if drug is distributed in breast milk. Avoid use during third trimester (may adversely affect fetal cardiovascular system: premature closure of ductus arteriosus). **Pregnancy Category B.**

INTERACTIONS

DRUG INTERACTIONS: May increase effects of oral anticoagulants, heparin, thrombolytics. May decrease effect of antihypertensives, diuretics. Salicylates, aspirin may increase risk of GI side effects, bleeding. Bone marrow depressants may increase risk of hematologic reactions. May increase concentration, toxicity of lithium. May increase methotrexate toxicity. Probenecid may increase concentration. **ALTERED LAB VALUES:** May prolong bleeding time. May increase alkaline phosphatase, LDH, liver function tests. May decrease sodium, Hgb, Hct.

SIDE EFFECTS

FREQUENT: Dyspepsia (heartburn, indigestion, epigastric pain). **OCCASIONAL:** Nausea, diarrhea/constipation, flatulence, headache, dizziness, peripheral edema/fluid retention. **RARE:** Anorexia, vomiting, visual disturbances.

ADVERSE REACTIONS/TOXIC EFFECTS

Peptic ulcer, GI bleeding, gastritis, severe hepatic reaction (cholestasis, jaundice) occur rarely. Nephrotoxicity (dysuria, hematuria, proteinuria, nephrotic syndrome) and severe hypersensitivity reaction (bronchospasm, angiofacial edema) occur rarely.

NURSING IMPLICATIONS

BASELINE ASSESSMENT:

Assess onset, type, location, and duration of pain or inflammation. Inspect appearance of affected joints for immobility, deformities, skin condition.

INTERVENTION/EVALUATION:

Monitor for evidence of dyspepsia. Assist w/ambulation if dizziness occurs. Monitor pattern of daily bowel activity and stool consistency. Check behind medial malleolus for fluid retention (usually first area noted). Evaluate for therapeutic response: relief of pain, stiffness, swelling, increase in joint mobility, reduced joint tenderness, improved grip strength.

PATIENT/FAMILY TEACHING:

Avoid aspirin, alcohol during therapy (increases risk of GI bleeding). If GI upset occurs, take w/food, milk. Avoid tasks that require alertness, motor skills until response to drug is established. Swallow capsule whole, do not crush or chew.

ketorolac tromethamine

key-tore´oh-lack
(Toradol, Acular)

CLASSIFICATION

Nonsteroidal anti-inflammatory

K

PHARMACOKINETICS

	ONSET	PEAK	DURATION
IM	10 min	1-2 hrs	4-6 hrs
IV	10 min	1-2 hrs	4-6 hrs

Readily absorbed from GI tract, after IM administration. Protein binding: 99%. Partially metabolized primarily in kidneys. Primarily excreted in urine. Half-life: 3.8-6.3 hrs (increased in decreased renal function, elderly).

ACTION

Inhibits prostaglandin synthesis. Inhibits action of cyclooxygenase; decreases formation of prostaglandin, thromboxane precursors from arachidonic acid. Reduces prostaglandin levels in aqueous humor.

USES

Short-term relief of pain. *Ophthalmic:* Relief of ocular itching due to seasonal allergic conjunctivitis.

STORAGE/HANDLING

Store oral, parenteral form at room temperature.

PO/IM/IV/OPHTHALMIC ADMINISTRATION

PO: May give with food, milk or antacids if GI distress occurs.
IM: Give slowly, deeply into muscle.
IV: Give over at least 15 sec.
OPHTHALMIC:
1. Place finger on lower eyelid and pull out until pocket is formed between eye and lower lid. Hold dropper above pocket and place prescribed number of drops in pocket.
2. Close eye gently. Apply digital pressure to lacrimal sac for 1-2 min (minimized drainage into nose and throat, reducing risk of systemic effects).
3. Remove excess solution w/ tissue.

INDICATIONS/DOSAGE/ROUTES

NOTE: Combined duration of IM/IV and oral not to exceed 5 days. May give as single dose, regular, or as needed schedule.

Analgesic (multiple dosing):
PO: Adults, elderly: 10 mg q4-6h. **Maximum:** 40 mg/24 hrs.
IV/IM: Adults <65 yrs: 30 mg q6h. **Maximum:** 120 mg/24 hrs. **>65 yrs, renally impaired, <50 kg:** 15 mg q6h. **Maximum:** 60 mg/24 hrs.

Analgesic (single dose):
IM: Adults <65 yrs: 60 mg; **>65 yrs, renally impaired, <50 kg:** 30 mg.
IV: Adults <65 yrs: 30 mg; **>65 yrs, renally impaired, <50 kg:** 15 mg.

Usual ophthalmic dosage:
OPHTHALMIC: Adults, elderly: 1 drop 4 times/day.

PRECAUTIONS

CONTRAINDICATIONS: Active peptic ulcer, GI ulceration, chronic inflammation of GI tract, GI bleeding disorders, history of hypersensitivity to aspirin or nonsteroidal anti-inflammatory agent. **CAUTIONS:** Impaired renal/hepatic function, history of GI tract disease, predisposition to fluid retention. **PREGNANCY/LACTATION:** Unknown if drug is excreted in breast milk. Avoid use during third trimester (may adversely affect fetal cardiovascular system: premature closure of ductus arteriosus). **Pregnancy Category C.**

INTERACTIONS

DRUG INTERACTIONS: May increase effects of oral anticoagulants, heparin, thrombolytics. Salicylates, aspirin may increase risk of GI side effects, bleeding. May increase concentration, toxicity of lithium. May increase methotrexate toxicity. Probenecid may increase concentration **ALTERED LAB VALUES:** May prolong bleeding time. May increase liver function tests.

SIDE EFFECTS

NOTE: Age increases possibility of side effects.
FREQUENT: Diarrhea/constipation, indigestion, nausea, maculopapular rash, dermatitis, dizziness, headache. *Ophthalmic:* Transient stinging and burning. **OCCASIONAL:** Anorexia, GI cramps, flatulence. *Ophthalmic:* Ocular irritation, allergic reactions, superficial ocular infection, keratitis.

ADVERSE REACTIONS/TOXIC EFFECTS

GI bleeding, peptic ulcer occur infrequently. Nephrotoxicity (glomerular nephritis, interstitial nephritis, and nephrotic syndrome) may occur in those with preexisting impaired renal function. Acute hypersensitivity reaction (fever, chills, joint pain) occurs rarely.

NURSING IMPLICATIONS

Baseline Assessment:

Assess onset, type, location, and duration of pain.

Intervention/Evaluation:

Assist with ambulation if dizziness occurs. Monitor stool frequency, consistency. Assess for evidence of rash. Evaluate for therapeutic response: relief of pain, stiffness, swelling, increase in joint mobility, reduced joint tenderness, improved grip strength. Be alert to signs of bleeding (may also occur w/ophthalmic due to systemic absorption).

Patient/Family Teaching:

Avoid aspirin, alcohol during therapy w/oral or ophthalmic ketorolac (increases tendency to bleed). If GI upset occurs, take with food, milk. Avoid tasks that require alertness, motor skills until response to drug is established. *Ophthalmic:* Transient stinging and burning may occur upon instillation. Do not wear soft contact lenses (causes redness and burning).

L

labetolol hydrochloride

lah-bet´ah-lol
(Normodyne)

FIXED-COMBINATION(S):
W/hydrochlorothiazide, a diuretic (Normozide).

CANADIAN AVAILABILITY:
Trandate

CLASSIFICATION

Beta-adrenergic blocker

PHARMACOKINETICS

	ONSET	PEAK	DURATION
PO	0.5-2 hrs	2-4 hrs	8-12 hrs
IV	2-5 min	5-15 min	2-4 hrs

Completely absorbed from GI tract. Undergoes first-pass metabolism. Protein binding: 50%. Metabolized in liver. Primarily excreted in urine. Half-life: oral: 6-8 hrs, IV: 5.5 hrs.

ACTION

Selectively blocks $beta_1$-adrenergic receptors, slowing sinus heart rate, decreasing cardiac output, decreasing B/P (exact mechanism unknown but may block peripheral adrenergic receptors, decrease sympathetic outflow from CNS, or decrease renin release from kidney). Large dose may block $beta_2$-adrenergic receptors, increasing airway resistance. Alpha blockage causes vasodilation, decreased peripheral vascular resistance, postural hypotension.

USES

Management of mild, moderate, severe hypertension. May be used alone or in combination w/other antihypertensives.

STORAGE/HANDLING

Store oral, parenteral form at room temperature. After dilution, IV solution is stable for 24 hours. Solution appears clear, colorless to light yellow. Discard if precipitate forms or discoloration occurs.

PO/IV ADMINISTRATION

PO:

1. May give w/o regard to food.
2. Tablets may be crushed.

IV:

NOTE: Pt must be in supine position for IV administration and for 3 hrs after receiving medication (substantial drop in B/P on standing should be expected).

1. For IV injection, give over 2 min at 10 min intervals.
2. For IV infusion, dilute 200 mg in 160 ml 5% dextrose, 0.9% NaCl, or other compatible IV fluid to provide concentration of 1 mg/ml.
3. Administer at rate of 2 mg/min (2 ml/min) initially. Rate is adjusted according to B/P.
4. Monitor B/P immediately before, and every 5-10 min during IV administration (maximum effect occurs within 5 min).

INDICATIONS/DOSAGE/ROUTES

Hypertension:

PO: Adults: Initially, 100 mg 2 times/day adjusted in increments of 100 mg 2 times/day every 2-3 days. **Maintenance:** 200-400 mg 2 times/day. **Maximum:** 2.4 Gm/day.

Usual elderly dosage:

PO: Elderly: Initially, 100 mg 1-2 times/day. May increase as needed.

Severe hypertension, hypertensive emergency:

IV: Adults: Initially, 20 mg. Additional doses of 20-80 mg may be given at 10 min intervals, up to total dose of 300 mg.

IV INFUSION: Adults: Initially, 2 mg/min up to total dose of 300 mg.

PO: Adults: (After IV therapy): Initially, 200 mg; then, 200-400 mg in 6-12 hrs. Increase dose at 1-day intervals to desired level.

PRECAUTIONS

CONTRAINDICATIONS: Bronchial asthma, uncontrolled CHF, second- or third-degree heart block, severe bradycardia, cardiogenic shock. **CAUTIONS:** Drug-controlled CHF, nonallergic bronchospastic disease (chronic bronchitis, emphysema), impaired hepatic, cardiac function, pheochromocytoma, diabetes mellitus. **PREGNANCY/LACTATION:** Drug crosses placenta; small amount distributed in breast milk. **Pregnancy Category C.**

INTERACTIONS

DRUG INTERACTIONS: Diuretics, other hypotensives may increase hypotensive effect; sympathomimetics, xanthines may mutually inhibit effects; may mask symptoms of hypoglycemia, prolong hypoglycemic effect of insulin, oral hypoglycemics. MAO inhibitors may produce hypertension. **ALTERED LAB VALUES:** May increase ANA titer, SGOT (AST), SGPT (ALT), alkaline phosphatase, LDH, bilirubin, BUN, creatinine, potassium uric acid, lipoproteins, triglycerides.

SIDE EFFECTS

FREQUENT: Dizziness, nausea, fatigue. Orthostatic hypotension likely to occur if recumbent pt is tilted upward or assumes standing position within 3 hrs following IV administration (hypotension occurs rarely w/oral administration). **OCCASIONAL:** Dyspepsia (heartburn, indigestion, epigastric discomfort), nasal congestion. **RARE:** Headache, vertigo, wheezing.

ADVERSE REACTIONS/TOXIC EFFECTS

May precipitate or aggravate CHF (due to decreased myocardial stimulation). Abrupt withdrawal may precipitate ischemic heart disease, producing sweating, palpitations, headache, tremulousness. Beta blockers may mask signs, symptoms of acute hypoglycemia (tachycardia, B/P changes) in diabetic pts.

NURSING IMPLICATIONS

BASELINE ASSESSMENT:

Assess baseline renal/liver function tests. Assess B/P, apical pulse immediately before drug is administered (if pulse is 60/min or below, or systolic B/P is below 90 mm Hg, withhold medication, contact physician).

INTERVENTION/EVALUATION:

Monitor B/P for hypotension, respiration for shortness of breath. Assess pulse for strength/weakness, irregular rate, bradycardia. Monitor EKG for cardiac arrhythmias. Monitor stool frequency and consistency. Assist w/ambulation if dizziness occurs. Assess for evidence of CHF: dyspnea (particularly on exertion or lying down), night cough, peripheral edema, distended neck veins. Monitor I&O (increase in weight, decrease in urine output may indicate CHF). Assess for nausea, diaphoresis, headache, fatigue.

PATIENT/FAMILY TEACHING:

Do not discontinue drug except upon advice of physician (abrupt discontinuation may precipitate heart failure). Transient scalp tingling may occur, esp. when drug is initiated. Compliance w/therapy regimen is essential to control hypertension, arrhythmias. Avoid tasks that require alertness, motor skills until response to drug is established. Report shortness of breath, excessive fatigue, weight gain, prolonged dizziness or headache. Do not use nasal decongestants, over-the-counter cold preparations (stimulants) w/o physician approval. Outpatients should monitor B/P, pulse before taking medication. Restrict salt, alcohol intake.

lactulose

lack´tyoo-lows
(Chronulac)

CANADIAN AVAILABILITY:
Chronulac, Lactulax

CLASSIFICATION

Laxative: Osmotic

PHARMACOKINETICS

	ONSET	PEAK	DURATION
PO	24-48 hrs	—	—
Rectal	30-60 min	—	—

Poorly absorbed from GI tract. Acts in colon.

ACTION

Decrease blood ammonia concentration. Retains ammonia in colon. Laxative effect expels ammonia from colon. *Laxative:* Produces osmotic effect in colon. Accumulation of fluid causes distention, promotes increased peristalsis, bowel evacuation.

USES

Prevention/treatment of portal systemic encephalopathy (including hepatic pre-coma, coma); treatment of constipation.

STORAGE/HANDLING

Store solution at room temperature. Solution appears pale yellow to yellow, sweet, viscous liquid. Cloudiness, darkened solutions do not indicate potency loss.

PO/RECTAL ADMINISTRATION

PO:

1. Drink water, juice, or milk w/each dose (aids stool softening, increases palatability).

RECTALLY:

1. Lubricate anus w/petroleum jelly before enema insertion.
2. Insert carefully (prevents damage to rectal wall) w/nozzle toward navel.
3. Squeeze container until entire dose expelled.
4. Retain until definite lower abdominal cramping felt.

INDICATIONS/DOSAGE/ROUTES

Constipation:
PO: Adults, elderly: 15-30 ml/day up to 60 ml/day.

Portal-systemic encephalopathy:
PO: Adults, elderly: Initially, 30-45 ml every hour. Then, 30-45 ml 3-4 times/day. Adjust dose every 1-2 days to produce 2-3 soft stools/day. **Children:** 40-90 ml/day in divided doses. **Infants:** 2.5-10 ml/day in divided doses.

Usual rectal dosage (as retention enema):
RECTAL: Adults, elderly: 300 ml w/700 ml water or saline; retain 30-60 min; repeat every 4-6 hrs. (If evacuation occurs too promptly, repeat immediately.)

PRECAUTIONS

CONTRAINDICATIONS: Those on galactose-free diet, abdominal pain, nausea, vomiting, appendicitis. **CAUTIONS:** Diabetes mellitus. **PREGNANCY/LACTATION:** Unknown if drug crosses placenta or is distributed in breast milk. **Pregnancy Category C.**

INTERACTIONS

DRUG INTERACTIONS: May decrease transient time of concurrently administered oral medication, decreasing absorption. **ALTERED LAB VALUES:** May decrease potassium concentration.

SIDE EFFECTS

FREQUENT: Some degree of abdominal discomfort, mild cramps, griping. **OCCASIONAL:** Nausea.

ADVERSE REACTIONS/TOXIC EFFECTS

Diarrhea indicates overdosage. Long-term use may result in laxative dependence, chronic constipation, loss of normal bowel function.

NURSING IMPLICATIONS

INTERVENTION/EVALUATION:

Encourage adequate fluid intake. Assess bowel sounds for peristalsis. Monitor daily bowel activity and stool consistency (watery, loose, soft, semisolid, solid) and record time of evacuation. Assess for abdominal disturbances. Monitor serum electrolytes in those exposed to prolonged, frequent, or excessive use of medication.

PATIENT/FAMILY TEACHING:

Evacuation occurs in 24-48 hrs of initial dose. Institute measures to promote defecation: increase fluid intake, exercise, high-fiber diet. Cola, unsalted crackers, dry toast may relieve nausea.

---

lamotrigine (Lamictal)
See supplement

---

lansoprazole (Prevacid)
See supplement

---

leucovorin calcium (folinic acid, citrovorum factor)

lou´koe-vear´in
(Wellcovorin)

CANADIAN AVAILABILITY:
Lederle, Leucovorin

CLASSIFICATION

Folic acid antagonist

PHARMACOKINETICS

Readily absorbed from GI tract. Widely distributed. Primarily concentrated in liver. Metabolized in liver, intestinal mucosa to active metabolite. Primarily excreted in urine. Half-life: 6.2 hrs.

ACTION

Competes w/methotrexate for same transport processes into cells (limits methotrexate action on normal cells). Allows purine, DNA, RNA, protein synthesis.

USES

Antidote (diminishes toxicity, counteracts effect of unintentional overdose of folic acid antagonists [e.g., methotrexate]); prevention/treatment of undesired hematopoietic effects of folic acid antagonists (e.g., rescue w/high dose methotrexate therapy); treatment of megaloblastic anemias due to folic acid deficiency. Palliative treatment of advanced colorectal cancer (in combination w/5-fluorouracil).

STORAGE/HANDLING

Store tablets/vials for parenteral use at room temperature. Injection is clear, yellowish solution.

IM/IV ADMINISTRATION

PO:

1. Scored tablets may be crushed.

IV:

1. Reconstitute each 50 mg vial w/5 ml sterile water for injection or bacteriostatic water for injection containing benzyl alcohol to provide concentration of 10 mg/ml. Due to benzyl alcohol in 1 mg ampoule and in bacteriostatic water, reconstitute doses >10 mg/m^2 w/sterile water.

2. Use immediately if reconstituted w/sterile water; stable for 7 days if reconstituted w/bacteriostatic water for injection.

3. Further dilute w/5% dextrose or 0.9% NaCl.

4. Do not exceed 160 mg/min if given by IV infusion (because of calcium content).

INDICATIONS/DOSAGE/ROUTES

Antidote, prevention/treatment of hematopoietic effects of folic acid antagonists:
NOTE: For rescue therapy in cancer chemotherapy, refer to specific protocol being used for optimal dosage and sequence of leucovorin administration.
CONVENTIONAL RESCUE DOSAGE: 10 mg/m² parenterally one time then q6h orally until serum methotrexate $<10^{-8}$M. If 24 hr serum creatinine increased by 50% or more over baseline or methotrexate $>5 \times 10^{-6}$M or 48 hr level $>9 \times 10^{7}$M increase to 100 mg/m² IV q3h until methotrexate level $<10^{-8}$M.

Megaloblastic anemia:
IM: Adults: Up to 1 mg/day.

Advanced colorectal cancer:
IV: Adults: 200 mg/m² over minimum of 3 min (follow w/5-fluorouracil 370 mg/m² by IV injection) or 20 mg/m² (follow w/5-fluorouracil 425 mg/m²). Repeat daily for 5 days; repeat cycle at 4 wk intervals for 2 cycles; then, at 4-5 wk intervals. **Note:** Do not start next cycle until pt recovered from prior treatment course (until WBC are 4,000/mm³ and platelets are 130,000/mm³).

PRECAUTIONS

CONTRAINDICATIONS: Pernicious anemia, other megalobastic anemias secondary to vitamin B_{12} deficiency. **CAUTIONS:** History of allergies, bronchial asthma. *W/5-fluorouracil:* Pts w/GI toxicities (more common/severe). **PREGNANCY/LACTATION:** Unknown if drug crosses placenta or is distributed in breast milk. **Pregnancy Category C.**

INTERACTIONS

DRUG INTERACTIONS: May decrease effect of anticonvulsants. May increase effect, toxicity of 5-fluorouracil. **ALTERED LAB VALUES:** None significant.

SIDE EFFECTS

FREQUENT: W/5-fluorouracil: Diarrhea, stomatitis, nausea, vomiting, lethargy/malaise/fatigue, alopecia, anorexia. **OCCASIONAL:** Urticaria, dermatitis.

ADVERSE REACTIONS/TOXIC EFFECTS

Excessive dosage may negate chemotherapeutic effect of folic acid antagonists. Anaphylaxis occurs rarely. Diarrhea may cause rapid clinical deterioration and death.

NURSING IMPLICATIONS

BASELINE ASSESSMENT:

Give as soon as possible, preferably within 1 hr, for treatment of accidental overdosage of folic acid antagonists.

INTERVENTION/EVALUATION:

Monitor for vomiting—may need to change from oral to parenteral therapy. Observe elderly and debilitated closely because of risk of severe toxicities. Assess CBC, differential, platelet count (also electrolytes and liver function tests for combination w/5-fluorouracil).

PATIENT/FAMILY TEACHING:

Explain purpose of medication

in treatment of cancer. Report allergic reaction, vomiting.

leuprolide acetate

leu´pro-lied
(Lupron, Lupron Depot Ped)

CANADIAN AVAILABILITY:
Lupron

CLASSIFICATION

Antineoplastic

PHARMACOKINETICS

Rapid, well absorbed after SubQ administration. Slow absorption after IM administration. Half-life: 3-4 hrs.

ACTION

Initial or intermittent administration stimulates release of luteinizing hormone (LH) and follicle-stimulating hormone (FSH) from anterior pituitary, increasing testosterone levels within 1 wk. Continuous daily administration suppresses secretion of gonadotropin-releasing hormone, producing fall in testosterone level within 2-4 wks.

USES

Treatment of advanced prostatic carcinoma, endometriosis, central precocious puberty, uterine fibroid tumors.

STORAGE/HANDLING

NOTE: May be carcinogenic, mutagenic, or teratogenic. Handle w/ extreme care during preparation/ administration.

Injection appears clear, colorless. Refrigerate. Store opened vial at room temperature. Discard if precipitate forms or solution appears discolored. Depot vials: Store at room temperature. Reconstitute only w/diluent provided, use immediately. Do not use needles <22-gauge.

SubQ ADMINISTRATION

Use syringes provided by manufacturer (0.5 ml low-dose insulin syringe may be used as alternative).

INDICATIONS/DOSAGE/ROUTES

Prostatic carcinoma:
SubQ: Adults, elderly: 1 mg daily.
IM: Adults, elderly: Depot: 7.5 mg q28-33days.

Endometriosis:
IM: Adults: Depot: 3.75 mg monthly.

Central precocious puberty:
SubQ: Children: Initially, 50 mcg/ kg/day; if down regulation not achieved, titrate upward by 10 mcg/kg/day.
IM: Children: Initially, 0.3 mg/kg/ 4 wks (minimum: 7.5 mg); if down regulation not achieved, titrate upward in 3.75 mg increments q4wks.

PRECAUTIONS

CONTRAINDICATIONS: None significant. **EXTREME CAUTION:** Patients w/life-threatening disease when rapid symptomatic relief is necessary. **CAUTIONS:** Hypersensitivity to benzyl alcohol. **PREGNANCY/LACTATION:** *Depot:* Contraindicated in pregnancy. May cause spontaneous abortion. **Pregnancy Category X.**

INTERACTIONS

DRUG INTERACTIONS: None significant. **ALTERED LAB VALUES:** May increase serum acid phosphatase. Initially increases testosterone then decreases testosterone concentration.

SIDE EFFECTS

FREQUENT: Hot flashes (ranging from mild flushing to sweating), peripheral edema, impotence, decreased libido during therapy. **OCCASIONAL:** Irritation at injection site, dizziness, headache, paresthesia, erythema, ecchymosis, blurred vision, lethargy, insomnia, irritability, arrhythmias, nausea, constipation/diarrhea, rash, itching.

ADVERSE REACTIONS/TOXIC EFFECTS

Occasionally, a worsening of signs/symptoms of prostatic carcinoma occurs 1-2 wks after initial dosing (subsides during continued therapy). Increased bone pain and less frequently dysuria or hematuria, weakness or paresthesia of lower extremities may be noted.

NURSING IMPLICATIONS

Baseline Assessment:

Question for possibility of pregnancy before initiating therapy (Pregnancy Category X). Obtain serum testosterone, prostatic acid phosphatase (PAP) levels periodically during therapy. Serum testosterone and PAP levels should increase during first week of therapy. Testosterone level then should decrease to baseline level or less within 2 wks, PAP level within 4 wks.

Intervention/Evaluation:

Monitor closely for signs/symptoms of worsening of disease.

Patient/Family Teaching:

Hot flashes tend to decrease during continued therapy. A temporary exacerbation of signs/symptoms of disease may occur during first few weeks of therapy.

levamisole hydrochloride

lev-am´ih-sole
(Ergamisol)

CANADIAN AVAILABILITY:
Ergamisol

CLASSIFICATION

Antineoplastic

PHARMACOKINETICS

Rapidly absorbed from GI tract. Metabolized in liver. Primarily excreted in urine. Half-life: 3-4 hrs.

ACTION

Immunorestorative agent. Causes T-cell activation, proliferation; augments monocyte and macrophage activity; increases neutrophil mobility, adherence, chemotaxis.

USES

Adjunctive treatment with concurrent use of fluorouracil after surgical resection in those with Duke's stage C colon cancer.

INDICATIONS/DOSAGE/ROUTES

Colon cancer:
PO: Adults, elderly: Initially, 50 mg q8h for 3 days (begin 7-30 days postop); repeat 50 mg q8h for 3 days every 2 wks for 1 yr.

PRECAUTIONS

CONTRAINDICATIONS: None significant. **PREGNANCY/LACTATION:** Unknown if drug crosses placenta or is distributed in breast milk. **Pregnancy Category C.**

INTERACTIONS

DRUG INTERACTIONS: Bone marrow depressants may increase

bone marrow depression. **ALTERED LAB VALUES:** None significant.

SIDE EFFECTS

FREQUENT: Anorexia, diarrhea, fatigue, minimal alopecia, fever, dry skin, fissuring, scaling, erythema, mild to moderate nausea, mild sensory peripheral neuropathy, mild anemia. **OCCASIONAL:** Moderate to severe sensory peripheral neuropathy, moderate to severe anemia. **RARE:** Severe nausea and vomiting, anorexia, fatigue, rash, alopecia.

ADVERSE REACTIONS/TOXIC EFFECTS

Earliest sign of toxicity (4-8 days after beginning therapy) is stomatitis (dry mouth, burning sensation, mucosal erythema, ulceration at inner margin of lips). Most common dermatologic toxicity is pruritic rash (generally appears on extremities, less frequently on trunk). Leukopenia generally occurs within 9-14 days after drug administration (may occur as late as 25th day). Thrombocytopenia occasionally occurs within 7-17 days after administration. Hematologic toxicity may also manifest itself as agranulocytosis, evidenced as fever, chills.

NURSING IMPLICATIONS

BASELINE ASSESSMENT:

Give emotional support to pt and family. Perform neurologic function tests prior to chemotherapy. Check blood counts prior to each course of therapy, monthly or as clinically indicated. Drug should be discontinued if intractable vomiting, diarrhea, stomatitis, GI bleeding occurs.

INTERVENTION/EVALUATION:

Monitor for hematologic toxicity (fever, sore throat, signs of local infection, easy bruising, unusual bleeding), symptoms of anemia (excessive tiredness, weakness). Measure all vomitus (general guideline requiring immediate notification of physician: 750 ml/8 hrs, urinary output less than 100 ml/hr). Monitor for rapidly falling WBC and/or intractable diarrhea, GI bleeding (bright red or tarry stool). Assess oral mucosa for mucosal erythema, ulceration at inner margin of lips, sore throat, difficulty swallowing (stomatitis). Assess skin for rash. Assess pattern of daily bowel activity and stool consistency. Be alert to symptoms of chills, fever (may be evidence of agranulocytosis).

PATIENT/FAMILY TEACHING:

Exposure to sunlight may intensify skin reaction. Maintain fastidious oral hygiene. Do not have immunizations without physician's approval (drug lowers body's resistance). Avoid contact with those who have recently received live virus vaccine. Promptly report fever, sore throat, signs of local infection, easy bruising, unusual bleeding from any site. Avoid alcohol (disulfiram-effect may occur [facial flushing, throbbing headache, extreme nausea, copious vomiting, diaphoresis, marked uneasiness]). Contact physician/nurse if chills, fever occur.

levobunolol hydrochloride

lev-oh-beau′no-lol

(Betagan Liquifilm)

CANADIAN AVAILABILITY:
Betagan

CLASSIFICATION

Beta-adrenergic blocker

PHARMACOKINETICS

	ONSET	PEAK	DURATION
Eye drops	<60 min	2-6 hrs	12-24 hrs

Systemic absorption may occur. Maximal effect of decreased intraocular pressure within 2-3 wks of 2 times/day drug instillation.

ACTION

Reduces elevated/normal intraocular pressure. Reduces aqueous humor production.

USES

Reduces intraocular pressure in management of chronic open-angle glaucoma, ocular hypertension.

STORAGE/HANDLING

Store ophthalmic solution at room temperature.

OPHTHALMIC ADMINISTRATION

1. Place finger on lower eyelid and pull out until pocket is formed between eye and lower lid.
2. Hold dropper above pocket and place prescribed number of drops into pocket. Instruct pt to close eyes gently so medication will not be squeezed out of sac.
3. Apply gentle finger pressure to the lacrimal sac at inner canthus for 1 min following instillation (lessens risk of systemic absorption).

INDICATIONS/DOSAGE/ROUTES

Glaucoma:
EYE DROPS: Adults, elderly: Initially, 1 drop 1-2 times/day. If further decrease in intraocular pressure occurs, add other ocular hypotensive to regimen.

PRECAUTIONS

CONTRAINDICATIONS: History of/or bronchial asthma, COPD, sinus bradycardia, overt cardiac failure, cardiogenic shock, second-degree and third-degree AV block. **CAUTIONS:** Chronic bronchitis, emphysema, diabetes mellitus, cerebrovascular insufficiency, thyroid deficiency. **PREGNANCY/LACTATION:** Unknown if drug crosses placenta or is distributed in breast milk. May produce bradycardia, apnea, hypoglycemia, hypothermia during delivery, small-birth weight infants. **Pregnancy Category C.**

INTERACTIONS

DRUG INTERACTIONS: May be additive w/dipivefrin, epinephrine ophthalmics. May increase effects of systemic beta-adrenergic blockers. **ALTERED LAB VALUES:** None significant.

SIDE EFFECTS

Generally well tolerated, w/ mild and transient side effects. **FREQUENT:** Eye irritation (burning, stinging), conjunctivitis. **RARE:** Ataxia, dizziness, lethargy.

ADVERSE REACTIONS/TOXIC EFFECTS

Overdosage may produce bradycardia, hypotension, bronchospasm, acute cardiac failure.

NURSING IMPLICATIONS

BASELINE ASSESSMENT:

Assess B/P, apical pulse.

INTERVENTION/EVALUATION:

Assess pulse for strength/weakness, irregular rate, bradycardia.

PATIENT/FAMILY TEACHING:

Do not abruptly discontinue medication. Compliance w/therapy regimen is essential to control glaucoma. Monitor B/P, pulse before taking medication. Ocular stinging/discomfort commonly occurs.

levocabastine hydrochloride

lev-oh-cah-bass'teen
(Livostin)

CLASSIFICATION

Antiallergic

PHARMACOKINETICS

	ONSET	PEAK	DURATION
Ophthalmic	—	—	2 hrs

Minimal systemic absorption.

ACTION

Selective H_1 receptor antagonist. Blocks histamine-associated symptoms of allergic conjunctivitis.

USES

Temporary relief of signs and symptoms of seasonal allergic conjunctivitis.

STORAGE/HANDLING

Store at room temperature, protect from freezing. Discard if suspension is discolored. Keep tightly closed.

OPHTHALMIC ADMINISTRATION

1. Instruct pt to lie down or tilt head backward and look up.
2. Shake suspension well.
3. Gently pull lower lid down to form pouch and instill medication.
4. Do not touch tip of applicator to any surface.
5. When lower lid is released, have pt keep eye open w/o blinking for at least 30 sec.
6. Apply gentle finger pressure to lacrimal sac (bridge of the nose, inside corner of the eye) for 1-2 min.
7. Remove excess solution around eye w/tissue.
8. Tell pt not to close eyes tightly or blink more often than necessary.
9. Never rinse dropper.

INDICATIONS/DOSAGE/ROUTES

Allergic conjunctivitis:
OPHTHALMIC: Adults, elderly, children >12 yrs: 1 drop 4 times/day, for up to 2 wks.

PRECAUTIONS

CONTRAINDICATIONS: Hypersensitivity. Wearing soft contact lenses (product contains benzalkonium chloride). **CAUTIONS:** For ophthalmic use only. Not for injection. Safety in children <12 years not known. **PREGNANCY/LACTATION:** Excreted in breast milk. **Pregnancy Category C.**

INTERACTIONS

DRUG INTERACTIONS: None significant. **ALTERED LAB VALUES:** None significant.

SIDE EFFECTS

FREQUENT: Transient stinging, burning, discomfort, headache. **OCCASIONAL:** Dry mouth, fatigue, eye dryness, lacrimation/discharge, eyelid edema. **RARE:** Rash, erythema, nausea, dyspnea.

ADVERSE REACTIONS/TOXIC EFFECTS

None significant.

NURSING IMPLICATIONS

BASELINE ASSESSMENT:

Assess for hypersensitivity to any component of suspension. Evaluate ocular signs and symptoms.

PATIENT/FAMILY TEACHING:

Shake well before using. Do not use if suspension is discolored. Teach correct procedure for administration of drops. Do not wear soft contact lenses during therapy. For ophthalmic use only. May experience mild transitory burning, stinging upon instillation. Therapy may last up to 2 wks. If disorder does not improve or new symptoms develop, notify physician.

levorphanol tartrate

lev-orphan´ole
(Levo-Dromoran)

CANADIAN AVAILABILITY:
Levo-Dromoran

CLASSIFICATION

Opioid: Analgesic

PHARMACOKINETICS

	ONSET	PEAK	DURATION
PO	30-45 min	60-120 min	4 hrs (analgesic) 4-6 hrs (antitussive)
IM	10-30 min	30-60 min	4 hrs
SubQ	10-30 min	—	2.5-4 hrs

Well absorbed from GI tract, after IM, SubQ administration. Protein binding: moderate. Metabolized in liver. Primarily excreted in urine. Half-life: 11 hrs.

ACTION

Binds w/opioid receptors within CNS, altering processes affecting pain perception, emotional response to pain.

USES

Relief of moderate to severe pain. Used preoperatively to produce sedation, and as adjunct w/ nitrous oxide/oxygen anesthesia.

STORAGE/HANDLING

Store oral, parenteral forms at room temperature.

PO/SubQ/IV ADMINISTRATION

PO:

1. May be given w/o regard to meals.
2. Tablets may be crushed.

SubQ:

1. Pt should be in recumbent position before administering.
2. Those w/circulatory impairment may experience overdosage due to delayed absorption of repeated SubQ administration.

IV:

1. Always administer very slowly (over 2-3 min).
2. Rapid IV increases risk of severe adverse reactions (chest wall rigidity, apnea, peripheral circulatory collapse, anaphylactoid effect, cardiac arrest).

INDICATIONS/DOSAGE/ROUTES

NOTE: Reduce initial dosage in those w/hypothyroidism, Addison's disease, renal insufficiency, elderly/debilitated, those on concurrent CNS depressants.

PO/SubQ: Adults, elderly: 2 mg. May be increased to 3 mg, if needed.

IV: Adults: Optimum dosage not established.

PRECAUTIONS

CONTRAINDICATIONS: None significant. **EXTREME CAUTION:** CNS depression, anoxia, hypercapnia, respiratory depression, seizures, acute alcoholism, shock, untreated myxedema, respiratory dysfunction. **CAUTIONS:** Increased intracranial pressure, impaired hepatic function, acute abdominal conditions, hypothyroidism, prostatic hypertrophy, Addison's disease, urethral stricture, COPD. **PREGNANCY/LACTATION:** Readily crosses placenta; unknown if distributed in breast milk. Respiratory depression may occur in neonate if mother received opiates during labor. Regular use of opiates during pregnancy may produce withdrawal symptoms in neonate (irritability, excessive crying, tremors, hyperactive reflexes, fever, vomiting, diarrhea, yawning, sneezing, seizures). **Pregnancy Category C.**

INTERACTIONS

DRUG INTERACTIONS: Alcohol, CNS depressants may increase CNS, respiratory depression, hypotension. MAO inhibitors may produce severe, fatal reaction (reduce dose to 1/4 usual dose). **ALTERED LAB VALUES:** May increase amylase, lipase plasma concentrations.

SIDE EFFECTS

NOTE: Effects are dependent on dosage amount, route of administration. Ambulatory pts and those not in severe pain may experience dizziness, nausea, vomiting, hypotension more frequently than those in supine position or having severe pain.

FREQUENT: Suppressed breathing depth. **OCCASIONAL:** Lightheadedness, mental clouding, dizziness, sedation, hypotension, nausea, vomiting, euphoria/dysphoria, constipation (drug delays digestion), sweating, flushing, feeling of facial, neck warmth, urinary retention.

ADVERSE REACTIONS/TOXIC EFFECTS

Overdosage results in respiratory depression, skeletal muscle flaccidity, cold, clammy skin, cyanosis, extreme somnolence progressing to convulsions, stupor, coma. Tolerance to analgesic effect, physical dependence may occur w/repeated use.

NURSING IMPLICATIONS

BASELINE ASSESSMENT:

Pt should be in a recumbent position before drug is administered by parenteral route. Assess onset, type, location, and duration of pain. Obtain vital signs before giving medication. If respirations are 12/min or lower (20/min or lower in children), withhold medication, contact physician.

INTERVENTION/EVALUATION:

Monitor vital signs after parenteral administration for decreased B/P, a change in rate or quality of pulse, decreased respirations. Assess for adequate voiding, possible constipation. Initiate deep breathing and coughing exercises, particularly in those w/impaired pulmonary function. Assess therapeutic response and contact physician if pain relief is inadequate.

PATIENT/FAMILY TEACHING:

Promptly report recurrence of pain (effect of medication is reduced if full pain recurs before next dose). Discomfort may occur w/injection. Change positions slowly to avoid orthostatic hypotension. Avoid tasks that require alertness, motor skills until response to drug is established. Tolerance/dependence may occur w/prolonged use of high doses. Avoid alcohol.

levothyroxine

lee-voe-thye-rox'een

(Levothroid, Levoxyl, Synthroid)

FIXED-COMBINATION(S):
W/liothyronine, T_3 (Thyrolar)

CANADIAN AVAILABILITY:
Eltroxin, Synthroid

CLASSIFICATION

Thyroid

PHARMACOKINETICS

Variably, incomplete absorption from GI tract. Widely distributed. Protein binding: >99%. Deiodinated in peripheral tissues, minimal metabolism in liver. Eliminated by biliary excretion. Half-life: 6-7 days.

ACTION

Involved in normal metabolism, growth and development (esp. CNS of infants). Possesses catabolic and anabolic effects. Increases basal metabolic rate, enhances gluconeogenesis, stimulates protein synthesis.

USES

Replacement in decreased or absent thyroid function (partial or complete absence of gland, primary atrophy, functional deficiency, effects of surgery, radiation or antithyroid agents, pituitary or hypothalamic hypothyroidism); management of simple (nontoxic) goiter and chronic lymphocytic thyroiditis; treatment of thyrotoxicosis (w/antithyroid drugs) to prevent goitrogenesis and hypothyroidism. Management of thyroid cancer. Diagnostic in thyroid suppression tests.

PO/IM/IV ADMINISTRATION

Do not interchange brands since there have been problems w/bioequivalence between manufacturers.

PO:

1. Give at same time each day to maintain hormone levels.
2. Administer before breakfast to prevent insomnia.
3. Tablets may be crushed.

IV:

1. Reconstitute 200 mcg or 500 mcg vial w/5 ml 0.9% NaCl to provide a concentration of 40 or 100 mcg/ml, respectively; shake until clear.
2. Do not use or mix w/other IV solutions.
3. Use immediately and discard unused portions.

INDICATIONS/DOSAGE/ROUTES

NOTE: Begin therapy w/small doses, gradually increase.

Hypothyroidism:
PO: Adults, elderly: Initially, 0.05 mg/day. Increase by 0.025 mg q2-3wks. **Maintenance:** 0.1-0.2 mg/day.

Myxedema coma or stupor (medical emergency):
IV: Adults, elderly: Initially, 0.4 mg. Follow w/daily supplements of

0.1-0.2 mg. **Maintenance:** 0.05-0.1 mg/day.

Thyroid suppression therapy:
PO: Adults, elderly: 2.6 mcg/kg/day for 7-10 days.

TSH suppression in thyroid cancer, nodules, euthroid goiters:
PO: Adults, elderly: Use larger doses than that used for replacement therapy.

Congenital hypothyroidism:
PO: Children >12 yrs: >0.15 mg/day; **Children 6-12 yrs:** 0.1-0.15 mg/day; **Children 1-5 yrs:** 0.075-0.1 mg/day; **Children 6-12 mo:** 0.05-0.075 mg/day; **Infants 0-6 mo:** 0.025-0.05 mg/day.

Usual parenteral dosage:
IV: Adults, elderly: ½ previously established oral dosage.

PRECAUTIONS

CONTRAINDICATIONS: Thyrotoxicosis and myocardial infarction uncomplicated by hypothyroidism, hypersensitivity to any component (w/tablets: tartrazine, allergy to aspirin, lactose intolerance), treatment of obesity. **CAUTIONS:** Elderly, angina pectoris, hypertension or other cardiovascular disease. **PREGNANCY/LACTATION:** Drug does not cross placenta; minimal excretion in breast milk. **Pregnancy Category A.**

INTERACTIONS

DRUG INTERACTIONS: May alter effect of oral anticoagulants. Cholestyramine, colestipol may decrease absorption. Sympathomimetics may increase effects, coronary insufficiency. **ALTERED LAB VALUES:** None significant.

SIDE EFFECTS

OCCASIONAL: Children may have reversible hair loss upon initiation. **RARE:** Dry skin, GI intolerance.

ADVERSE REACTIONS/TOXIC EFFECTS

Excessive dosage produces signs/symptoms of hyperthyroidism: weight loss, palpitations, increased appetite, tremors, nervousness, tachycardia, increased B/P, headache, insomnia, menstrual irregularities. Cardiac arrhythmias occur rarely.

NURSING IMPLICATIONS

BASELINE ASSESSMENT:

Question for hypersensitivity to tartrazine, aspirin, lactose. Obtain baseline weight, vital signs. Check results of thyroid function tests. Signs and symptoms of diabetes mellitus, diabetes insipidus, adrenal insufficiency, hypopituitarism may become intensified. Treat w/adrenocortical steroids prior to thyroid therapy in coexisting hypothyroidism and hypoadrenalism.

INTERVENTION/EVALUATION:

Monitor pulse for rate, rhythm (report pulse of 100 or marked increase). Assess for tremors, nervousness. Check appetite and sleep pattern.

PATIENT/FAMILY TEACHING:

Do not discontinue; replacement for hypothyroidism is lifelong. Follow-up office visits and thyroid function tests are essential. Take medication at the same time each day, preferably in morning. Monitor pulse, report marked increase, pulse of 100 or above, change of rhythm. Do not change brands. Take other medications only on advice of physician. Notify physician promptly of chest pain, weight loss, nervousness or tremors, insomnia. Children may have reversible hair loss or increased aggressiveness during the first few months of therapy. Full therapeutic effect may take 1-3 wks.

lidocaine hydrochloride

lie´doe-cane
(LidoPen, Xylocaine)

FIXED-COMBINATION(S): W/epinephrine, a sympathomimetic (Lidocaine with Epinephrine, Xylocaine with Epinephrine)

CANADIAN AVAILABILITY: Xylocard

CLASSIFICATION

Antiarrhythmic, anesthetic

PHARMACOKINETICS

	ONSET	PEAK	DURATION
IV	30-90 sec	—	10-20 min
Local anesthetic	2.5 min	—	30-60 min

Completely absorbed after IM administration. Widely distributed. Protein binding: 60-80%. Metabolized in liver. Primarily excreted in urine. Half-life: 1-2 hrs.

ACTION

Anesthetic: Inhibits conduction of nerve impulses causing temporary loss of feeling and sensation. *Antiarrhythmic:* Decreases depolarization, automaticity, excitability of ventricle during diastole by direct action.

USES

Antiarrhythmic: Rapid control of acute ventricular arrhythmias following myocardial infarction, cardiac catheterization, cardiac surgery, digitalis-induced ventricular arrhythmias. *Local anesthetic:* Infiltration or nerve block for dental or surgical procedures, childbirth. *Topical anesthetic:* Local skin disorders (minor burns, insect bites, prickly heat, skin manifestations of chickenpox, abrasions). Mucous membranes (local anesthesia of oral, nasal, and laryngeal mucous membranes, respiratory or urinary tracts; relieve discomfort of pruritus ani, hemorrhoids, pruritus vulvae).

IM/IV/INFILTRATION-NERVE BLOCK/TOPICAL ADMINISTRATION

NOTE: Resuscitative equipment and drugs (including oxygen) must always be readily available when administering lidocaine by any route.

IM:

1. Use 10% (100 mg/ml); clearly identify lidocaine that is *for IM use.*
2. Give in deltoid muscle (blood level is significantly higher than if injection is given in gluteus muscle or lateral thigh).

IV:

NOTE: Use only lidocaine without preservative, clearly marked *for IV use.*

1. For direct IV, use 1% (10 mg/ml) or 2% (20 mg/ml).
2. Administer for direct IV at rate of 25-50 mg/min.
3. For IV infusion, prepare solution by adding 1 Gm to 1 liter 5% dextrose to provide concentration of 1 mg/ml (0.1%).
4. Commercially available preparations of 0.2%, 0.4%, and 0.8% may be used for IV infusion.

5. Administer for IV infusion at rate of 1-4 mg/min (1-4 ml); use volume control IV set.

6. Monitor EKG constantly during infusion.

7. Terminate IV infusion when cardiac rhythm is stable or toxic effects occur.

8. Monitor pt response during IV administration.

9. If excessive cardiac depression (arrhythmias; prolongation of PR interval, QRS complex) occurs, discontinue medication immediately, institute supportive measures.

10. Unused lidocaine without preservative must be discarded.

INFILTRATION/NERVE BLOCK

NOTE: Only clinicians skilled in administration of anesthetics may give lidocaine for local anesthesia.

1. For spinal or epidural anesthesia, only solutions without preservatives are to be used.

2. B/P, pulse, respirations, and pts state of consciousness should be monitored throughout regional anesthesia due to potential for cardiovascular or CNS toxicity.

3. Consult standard textbooks for positioning and general care of pts undergoing regional anesthesia.

TOPICAL

1. Not for ophthalmic use.

2. For skin disorders, apply directly to affected area or put on gauze or bandage which is then applied to the skin.

3. For mucous membrane use, apply to desired area using manufacturer's insert.

4. Administer the lowest dose possible that still provides anesthesia.

INDICATIONS/DOSAGE/ROUTES

Ventricular arrhythmias:
IM: Adults, elderly: 300 mg (or 4.3 mg/kg). May repeat in 60-90 min.
IV: Adults, elderly: Initially, 50-100 mg (1 mg/kg) IV bolus at rate of 25-50 mg/min. May repeat in 5 min. Give no more than 200-300 mg in 1 hr. **Maintenance:** 20-50 mcg/kg/min (1-4 mg/min) as IV infusion. **Children, infants:** Initially, 0.5-1 mg/kg IV bolus, may repeat but total dose not to exceed 3-5 mg/kg. **Maintenance:** 10-50 mcg/kg/min as IV infusion.

Usual local anesthetic dosage:
NOTE: Do not use any preparation containing preservatives for spinal or epidural anesthesia.
INFILTRATION: 0.5 or 1% solution.
EPIDURAL (INCLUDING CAUDAL): 1 or 2% solution.
PERIPHERAL NERVE BLOCK: 1 or 1.5% solution.
SYMPATHETIC NERVE BLOCK: 1% solution.
SPINAL ANESTHESIA: 1.5 or 5% solution (with dextrose).

Usual topical dosage:
TOPICAL: Adults, elderly: Apply to affected areas as needed.

PRECAUTIONS

CONTRAINDICATIONS: Hypersensitivity to amide-type local anesthetics, Adams-Stokes syndrome, supraventricular arrhythmias, Wolff-Parkinson-White syndrome. Spinal anesthesia contraindicated in septicemia. **CAUTIONS:** Dosage should be reduced for elderly, debilitated, acutely ill; safety in children not established. Severe renal/hepatic disease, hypovolemia, CHF, shock, heart block, marked hypoxia, severe respiratory depression, bradycardia, incomplete heart block. Anesthetic solutions containing epinephrine should be used with caution in peripheral or hypertensive vascular disease, and during or following potent general anesthesia. Sulfite sensitivity or asthma for some local and topical anesthetic preparations. Tartrazine or aspirin sensitivity with some topical preparations. **PREGNANCY/LACTATION:** Crosses placenta; distributed in breast milk. **Pregnancy Category B.**

INTERACTIONS

DRUG INTERACTIONS: May increase cardiac effects w/other antiarrhythmics. Anticonvulsants may increase cardiac depressant effects. Beta-adrenergic blockers may increase risk of toxicity. **ALTERED LAB VALUES:** IM lidocaine may increase CPK level (used in diagnostic test for presence of acute MI).

SIDE EFFECTS

CNS effects generally dose related and of short duration. **OCCASIONAL:** *IM:* pain at injection site. *Topical:* Burning, stinging, tenderness. **RARE:** Generally with high dose: drowsiness, dizziness, disorientation, lightheadedness, tremors, apprehension, euphoria, sensation of heat/cold/numbness, blurred/double vision, ringing/roaring in ears (tinnitus), nausea.

ADVERSE REACTIONS/TOXIC EFFECTS

Although serious adverse reactions to lidocaine are uncommon, high dosage by any route may produce cardiovascular depression: bradycardia, somnolence, hypotension, arrhythmias, heart block, cardiovascular collapse, cardiac arrest. Potential for malignant hyperthermia. CNS toxicity may occur, esp. with regional anesthesia use, progressing rapidly from mild side effects to tremors, convulsions, vomiting, respiratory depression, arrest. Methemoglobinemia (evidenced by cyanosis) has occurred following topical application of lidocaine for teething discomfort and laryngeal anesthetic spray. Overuse of oral lidocaine has caused seizures in children. Allergic reactions are rare.

NURSING IMPLICATIONS

BASELINE ASSESSMENT:

Question for hypersensitivity to lidocaine, amide anesthetics or components of preparation. Obtain baseline B/P, pulse, respirations, and EKG, electrolytes.

INTERVENTION/EVALUATION:

Monitor EKG, vital signs closely during and after drug is administered for cardiac performance. If EKG shows arrhythmias, prolongation of PR interval or QRS complex, inform physician immediately. Assess pulse for irregularity, strength/weakness, bradycardia. Assess B/P for evidence of hypotension. Monitor I&O, electrolyte serum level. Monitor for therapeutic serum level (1.5-6 mcg/ml). For lidocaine given by all routes, monitor vital signs and pt state of consciousness. Drowsiness should be considered a warning sign of high blood levels of lidocaine.

PATIENT/FAMILY TEACHING:

Explain action of lidocaine. Report drowsiness or CNS effects promptly (see Adverse Reactions/Toxic Effects). *Local anesthesia:* Assure that pt understands loss of feeling, sensation and need for protection until anesthetic wears off (e.g., no ambulation, including special positions for some regional anesthesia; not chewing gum, eating, or drinking following administration to oral area, etc.). *Topical anesthesia:* Use only as directed; too-frequent use may cause overdosage. Do not eat, drink, or chew gum for 1 hr following application (swallowing reflex may be impaired increasing risk of aspiration; numbness of tongue or buccal mucosa may lead to biting trauma).

liothyronine

lye-oh-thye´roe-neen
(Cytomel)

FIXED-COMBINATION(S):
W/levothyroxine, T_4 (Thyrolar)

CANADIAN AVAILABILITY:
Cytomel

CLASSIFICATION

Thyroid

PHARMACOKINETICS

Almost complete absorption from GI tract. Widely distributed. Protein binding: >99%. Deiodinated in peripheral tissues, minimal metabolism in liver. Eliminated by biliary excretion. Half-life: 1 day.

ACTION

Involved in normal metabolism, growth and development (esp. CNS of infants). Possesses catabolic and anabolic effects. Increases basal metabolic rate, enhances gluconeogenesis, stimulates protein synthesis.

USES

Oral: Replacement in decreased or absent thyroid function (partial or complete absence of gland, primary atrophy, functional deficiency, effects of surgery, radiation or antithyroid agents, pituitary or hypothalamic hypothyroidism). Management of simple (nontoxic) goiter; diagnostically in T_3 suppression test (differentiates hyperthyroidism from euthroidism). *IV:* Myxedema coma, precoma.

STORAGE/HANDLING

Refrigerate parenteral dosage form; store oral tablets at room temperature.

PO/IV ADMINISTRATION

PO:

1. Give at the same time each day to maintain hormone levels.
2. Administer before breakfast to prevent insomnia.
3. When transferred *from* another thyroid preparation, the other thyroid agent should be discontinued first, begin liothyronine at low dose.
4. When transferring *to* another thyroid preparation, continue liothyronine for several days to prevent relapse (rapid action, short duration).

IV:

1. Do not administer IM or SubQ.
2. Switch to oral as soon as pt stabilized clinically. Initiate oral therapy at low dose increasing gradually according to pt response.

INDICATIONS/DOSAGE/ROUTES

Hypothyroidism:
PO: Adults: Initially, 25 mcg/day. Increase by 12.5-25 mcg q1-2wks. **Elderly:** Initially, 5 mcg/day. May increase by 5 mcg/day q1-2wks. **Maintenance:** 25-75 mcg/day.

Myxedema:
PO: Adults, elderly: Initially, 5 mcg/day. Increase by 5-10 mcg q1-2wks (after 25 mcg/day reached, may increase by 12.5 mcg increments). **Maintenance:** 50-100 mcg/day.

Nontoxic goiter:
PO: Adults, elderly: Initially, 5 mcg/day. Increase by 5-10 mcg/day q1-2wks. When 25 mcg/day obtained, may increase by 12.5-25 mcg/day q1-2wks. **Maintenance:** 75 mcg/day.

Congenital hypothyroidism:
PO: Children: Initially, 5 mcg/day. Increase by 5 mcg/day q3-4days. **Maintenance: (Infants):** 20 mcg/day. **(1 yr):** 50 mcg/day. **(>3 yrs):** Full adult dosage.

T_3 suppression test:
PO: Adults, elderly: 75-100 mcg/day for 7 days, then repeat I^{131} thyroid uptake test.

Myxedema coma, precoma:
NOTE: Initial and subsequent dosage based on pts clinical status, response. Administer IV dose at least 4 hrs but no longer than 12 hrs apart.
IV: Adults, elderly: Initially, 25-50 mcg (10-20 mcg in pts w/cardiovascular disease). Total dose at least 65 mcg/day.

PRECAUTIONS

CONTRAINDICATIONS: Thyrotoxicosis and MI uncomplicated by hypothyroidism, treatment of obesity. **CAUTIONS:** Elderly, angina pectoris, hypertension, or other cardiovascular disease. **PREGNANCY/LACTATION:** Drug does not cross placenta, minimal excretion in breast milk. **Pregnancy Category A.**

INTERACTIONS

DRUG INTERACTIONS: May alter effect of oral anticoagulants. Cholestyramine, colestipol may decrease absorption. Sympathomimetics may increase effects, coronary insufficiency. **ALTERED LAB VALUES:** None significant.

SIDE EFFECTS

OCCASIONAL: Children may have reversible hair loss upon initiation. **RARE:** Dry skin, GI intolerance.

ADVERSE REACTIONS/TOXIC EFFECTS

Excessive dosage produces signs/symptoms of hyperthyroidism: weight loss, palpitations, increased appetite, tremors, nervousness, tachycardia, increased B/P, headache, insomnia, menstrual irregularities. Cardiac arrythmias occur rarely.

NURSING IMPLICATIONS

BASELINE ASSESSMENT:

Question for hypersensitivity to tartrazine, aspirin. Obtain baseline weight, vital signs. Check results of thyroid function tests. Signs and symptoms of diabetes mellitus, diabetes insipidus, adrenal insufficiency, hypopituitarism may become intensified. Treat w/adrenocortical steroids prior to thyroid therapy in coexisting hypothyroidism and hypoadrenalism.

INTERVENTION/EVALUATION:

Monitor pulse for rate, rhythm (report pulse ≥ 100 or marked increase). Assess for tremors, nervousness. Check appetite and sleep pattern.

PATIENT/FAMILY TEACHING:

Do not discontinue; replacement

for hypothyroidism is lifelong. Follow-up office visits and thyroid function tests are essential. Take medication at the same time each day, preferably in morning. Teach pt or family to take pulse correctly, report marked increase, pulse of 100 or above, change of rhythm. Do not change brands (not equivalent). Take other medications only on advice of physician. Notify physician promptly of chest pain, weight loss, nervousness or tremors, insomnia. Children may have reversible hair loss or increased aggressiveness during first few months of therapy.

lisinopril

lih-sin′oh-prill
(Prinivil, Zestril)

FIXED-COMBINATION(S):
W/hydrochlorothiazide, a diuretic (Prinzide, Zestoretic)

CANADIAN AVAILABILITY:
Prinivil, Zestril

CLASSIFICATION

Angiotensin converting enzyme (ACE) inhibitor

PHARMACOKINETICS

	ONSET	PEAK	DURATION
PO	1 hr	6 hrs	24 hrs

Incompletely absorbed from GI tract. Protein binding: none. Primarily excreted unchanged in urine. Removed by hemodialysis. Half-life: 12 hrs (increase in decreased renal function).

ACTION

Suppresses renin-angiotensin-aldosterone system (prevents conversion of angiotensin I to angiotensin II, a potent vasoconstrictor; may also inhibit angiotensin II at local vascular and renal sites). Decreases plasma angiotensin II, increases plasma renin activity, decreases aldosterone secretion. Reduces peripheral arterial resistance. *Vasodilator:* Decreases peripheral vascular resistance (afterload), PCWP (preload), pulmonary vascular resistance.

USES

Treatment of hypertension. Used alone or in combination w/ other antihypertensives. Adjunctive therapy in management of heart failure.

PO ADMINISTRATION

1. May give w/o regard to food.
2. Tablets may be crushed.

INDICATIONS/DOSAGE/ROUTES

Hypertension (used alone):
PO: Adults: Initially, 10 mg/day. **Maintenance:** 20-40 mg/day as single dose. **Maximum:** 80 mg/day.

Hypertension (combination therapy):
NOTE: Discontinue diuretic 2-3 days prior to initiating lisinopril therapy.
PO: Adults: Initially, 5 mg/day titrated to pt's needs.

Heart failure:
PO: Adults: Initially, 5 mg/day (2.5 mg/day in pts w/hyponatremia). **Range:** 5-20 mg/day.

Usual elderly dosage:
PO: Elderly: Initially, 2.5-5 mg/day. May increase by 2.5-5 mg/day at 1-2 wk intervals. **Maximum:** 40 mg/day.

Dosage in renal impairment:

Titrate to pt's needs after giving the following initial dose:

CREATININE CLEARANCE	INITIAL DOSE
>30 ml/min	10 mg
10-30 ml/min	5 mg
<10 ml/min	2.5 mg

PRECAUTIONS

CONTRAINDICATIONS: MI, coronary insufficiency, angina, evidence of coronary artery disease, hypersensitivity to phentolamine, history of angioedema w/previous treatment w/ACEIs. **CAUTIONS:** Renal impairment, those w/sodium depletion or on diuretic therapy, dialysis, hypovolemia, coronary or cerebrovascular insufficiency. **PREGNANCY/LACTATION:** Crosses placenta; unknown if distributed in breast milk. **Pregnancy Category C:** First trimester. **Pregnancy Category D:** Second and third trimesters. Has caused fetal/neonatal mortality, morbidity.

INTERACTIONS

DRUG INTERACTIONS: Alcohol, diuretics, hypotensive agents may increase effects. NSAIDs may decrease effect. Potassium sparing diuretics, potassium supplements may cause hyperkalemia. May increase lithium concentration, toxicity. **ALTERED LAB VALUES:** May increase potassium, SGOT (AST), SGPT (ALT), alkaline phosphatase, bilirubin, BUN, creatinine. May decrease sodium. May cause positive ANA titer.

SIDE EFFECTS

FREQUENT: Dizziness, headache. **OCCASIONAL:** Diarrhea, nausea, hypotension, fatigue. **RARE:** Chest pain, vomiting.

ADVERSE REACTIONS/TOXIC EFFECTS

Excessive hypotension ("first-dose syncope") may occur in those w/CHF, severely salt/volume depleted. Angioedema (swelling of face/lips), hyperkalemia occur rarely. Agranulocytosis, neutropenia may be noted in those w/impaired renal function or collagen vascular disease (systemic lupus erythematosus, scleroderma). Nephrotic syndrome may be noted in those w/history of renal disease.

NURSING IMPLICATIONS

BASELINE ASSESSMENT:

Obtain B/P and apical pulse immediately before each dose, in addition to regular monitoring (be alert to fluctuations). If excessive reduction in B/P occurs, place pt in supine position, feet slightly elevated. Renal function tests should be performed before therapy begins. In those w/renal impairment, autoimmune disease, or taking drugs that affect leukocytes or immune response, CBC and differential count should be performed before therapy begins and q2wks for 3 mo, then periodically thereafter.

INTERVENTION/EVALUATION:

Assess for edema; check lungs for rales. Monitor I&O; weigh daily. Assess stools for frequency and consistency; prevent constipation. Assist w/ambulation if dizziness occurs.

PATIENT/FAMILY TEACHING:

To reduce hypotensive effect, rise slowly from lying to sitting position and permit legs to dangle from bed momentarily before standing. Full therapeutic effect may take 2-4 wks. Report any sign of infection (sore throat, fever), swelling of hands or feet or face, chest pain, difficulty breathing or swallowing. Skipping doses or voluntarily discontinuing drug may produce severe, rebound hypertension. Do not take cold preparations, nasal decongestants. Restrict sodium and alcohol as ordered.

lithium carbonate

lith´ee-um

(Eskalith, Lithane, Lithobid)

lithium citrate

(Cibalith-S)

CANADIAN AVAILABILITY: Carbolith, Duralith, Lithane, Lithizine

CLASSIFICATION

Antimanic

PHARMACOKINETICS

Rapid, complete absorption from GI tract. Protein binding: none. Primarily excreted unchanged in urine. Half-life: 18-24 hrs (increased in elderly).

ACTION

Alters ion transport at cellular sites in body tissue. Cations necessary in synthesis, storage, release, reuptake of neurotransmitters involved in producing antimanic, antidepressant effects.

USES

Prophylaxis, treatment of acute mania, manic phase of bipolar disorder (manic-depressive illness).

STORAGE/HANDLING

Store all forms at room temperature.

PO ADMINISTRATION

1. Preferable to administer w/ meals or milk.
2. Do not crush, chew, or break extended-release or film-coated tablets.

INDICATIONS/DOSAGE/ROUTES

NOTE: During acute phase, therapeutic serum lithium concentration of 1-1.4 mEq/L is required. Desired level during long-term control: 0.5-1.3 mEq/L.

Acute manic phase:
PO: Adults: Initially, 1.8 Gm (or 20-30 mg/kg) lithium carbonate or 30 ml lithium citrate/day, in 2-3 divided doses. **Elderly:** 600-900 mg/day.

Long-term control:
PO: Adults: 900 mg-1.2 Gm lithium carbonate or 15-20 ml lithium citrate, daily, in 2-4 divided doses.

Usual elderly dosage:
PO: Elderly: Initially, 300 mg 2 times/day. May increase by 300 mg/day at weekly intervals. **Maintenance:** 900-1200 mg/day.

PRECAUTIONS

CONTRAINDICATIONS: Severe cardiovascular disease, severe renal disease, severe dehydration/sodium depletion, debilitated patients. **CAUTIONS:** Cardiovascular disease, thyroid disease, elderly. **PREGNANCY/LACTATION:** Freely crosses placenta; distributed in breast milk. **Pregnancy Category D.**

INTERACTIONS

DRUG INTERACTIONS: May increase effects of antithyroid med-

L

ication, iodinated glycerol, potassium iodide. NSAIDs may increase concentration, toxicity. May decrease absorption of phenothiazines. Phenothiazines may increase intracellular concentration, increase renal excretion, extrapyramidal symptoms (EPS), delirium, mask early signs of lithium toxicity. Diuretics may increase concentration, toxicity. Haloperidol may increase EPS, neurologic toxicity. Molindone may increase risk of neurotoxic symptoms. **ALTERED LAB VALUES:** May increase blood glucose, calcium, immunoreactive parathyroid hormone.

SIDE EFFECTS

HIGH INCIDENCE: Polyuria (increased urination), polydipsia (excessive thirst) due to reversible diabetes insipidus. **FREQUENT:** Dry mouth, lethargy, fatigue, muscle weakness, headache, GI disturbances (mild nausea, anorexia, diarrhea, abdominal bloating), fine hand tremor, and inability to concentrate. **RARE:** Muscle hyperirritability (hyperactive reflexes, twitching), vertigo, hypothyroidism.

ADVERSE REACTIONS/TOXIC EFFECTS

Serum lithium concentration of 1.5-2.0 mEq/L may produce vomiting, diarrhea, drowsiness, incoordination, coarse hand tremor, muscle twitching, ECG T-wave depression, mental confusion. Serum lithium concentration of 2.0-2.5 mEq/L may result in ataxia, giddiness, tinnitus, blurred vision, clonic movements, severe hypotension. Acute toxicity characterized by seizures, oliguria, circulatory failure, coma, death.

NURSING IMPLICATIONS

BASELINE ASSESSMENT:

Serum lithium levels should be tested every 3-4 days during initial phase of therapy, every 1-2 mo thereafter, and weekly if there is no improvement of disorder or adverse effects occur.

INTERVENTION/EVALUATION:

Lithium serum testing should be performed as close as possible to 12th hour after last dose. Besides serum lithium concentration levels, clinical assessment of therapeutic effect or tolerance to drug effect are necessary for correct dosing level management. Assess behavior, appearance, emotional status, response to environment, speech pattern, thought content. Monitor serum lithium concentrations, differential count, urinalysis, creatinine clearance. Assess for increased urine output, persistent thirst. Report polyuria, prolonged vomiting, diarrhea, fever to physician (may need to temporarily reduce or discontinue dosage). Monitor for signs of lithium toxicity. Supervise suicidal-risk pt closely during early therapy (as depression lessens, energy level improves, and suicide potential increases). Assess for therapeutic response (interest in surroundings, improvement in self-care, increased ability to concentrate, relaxed facial expression).

PATIENT/FAMILY TEACHING:

Take as directed; do not discontinue except on physician's advice. Do not engage in activities requiring alert response until effects of drug are known. Thirst, frequent urination may occur. A fluid intake of 2-3 quarts liquid per day and maintenance of a normal salt intake are necessary during initial phase of treatment to avoid dehydration. Thereafter, 1-1.5 L fluid intake daily is necessary. GI disturbances generally disappear during continued therapy. Thyroid function tests should be performed every 6-12 mo in elderly pts (increased incidence of goiter, hypothyroidism). Therapeutic improvement noted in 1-3 wks. Avoid alcohol and over-the-counter drugs. Consult physician regarding contraception.

Iodoxamide tromethamine

low-dox'ah-myd

(Alomide)

CLASSIFICATION

Antiallergic

PHARMACOKINETICS

Minimal systemic absorption. Primarily excreted in urine. Half-life: 8.5 hrs.

ACTION

Mast cell stabilizer. Inhibits Type I immediate hypersensitivity reaction. Inhibits increase in cutaneous vascular permeability, prevents antigen-stimulated histamine release and may prevent calcium influx into mast cells.

USES

Treatment of vernal keratoconjunctivitis, conjunctivitis, and keratitis.

STORAGE/HANDLING

Keep at room temperature; protect from freezing. Do not use if discolored. Keep tightly closed.

OPHTHALMIC ADMINISTRATION

1. Instruct pt to lie down or tilt head backward and look up.
2. Gently pull lower lid down to form pouch and instill medication.
3. Do not touch tip of applicator to any surface.
4. When lower lid is released, have pt keep eye open w/o blinking for at least 30 sec.
5. Apply gentle finger pressure to lacrimal sac (bridge of the nose, inside corner of the eye) for 1-2 min.
6. Remove excess solution around eye w/tissue.
7. Tell pt not to close eyes tightly or blink more often than necessary.
8. Never rinse dropper.

INDICATIONS/DOSAGE/ROUTES

Usual ophthalmic dosage:
OPHTHALMIC: Adults, elderly, children >2 yrs: 1-2 drops 4 times/day, for up to 3 mo.

PRECAUTIONS

CONTRAINDICATIONS: Hypersensitivity. Wearing soft contact lenses (product contains benzalkonium chloride). **CAUTIONS:** For ophthalmic use only. Not for injection. Safety in children <2 yrs not known. **PREGNANCY/LACTATION:** Unknown if excreted in breast milk. **Pregnancy Category B.**

INTERACTIONS

DRUG INTERACTIONS: None significant. **ALTERED LAB VALUES:** None significant.

SIDE EFFECTS

FREQUENT Transient stinging, burning, instillation discomfort. **OCCASIONAL:** Ocular itching, blurred vision, dry eye, tearing/

discharge/foreign body sensation, headache. **RARE:** Scales on lid/lash, ocular swelling, sticky sensation, dizziness, somnolence, nausea, sneezing, dry nose, rash.

ADVERSE REACTIONS/TOXIC EFFECTS

None significant.

NURSING IMPLICATIONS

BASELINE ASSESSMENT:

Assess for hypersensitivity to any component of suspension. Evaluate ocular signs and symptoms.

PATIENT/FAMILY TEACHING:

Teach correct procedure for administration of drops. Do not wear soft contact lenses during therapy. For ophthalmic use only. May experience mild transitory burning, stinging upon instillation; inform physician if continues. Therapy may last up to 3 mo. If disorder does not improve or new symptoms develop, notify physician.

lomefloxacin hydrochloride

low-meh-flocks´ah-sin
(Maxaquin)

CLASSIFICATION

Anti-infective: Quinolone

PHARMACOKINETICS

Well absorbed from GI tract. Widely distributed. Protein binding: 20-40%. Metabolized in liver. Primarily excreted in urine. Minimal removal by hemodialysis. Half-life: 4-6 hrs (increased in decreased renal function, elderly).

ACTION

Inhibits DNA-gyrase in susceptible microorganisms, interfering w/bacterial DNA replication and repair. Bactericidal.

USES

Treatment of infections of urinary tract, lower respiratory tract, postop prophylaxis in pts undergoing transurethral procedures.

PO ADMINISTRATION

1. May be given w/o regard to meals (preferred dosing time: 2 hrs after meals).
2. Do not administer antacids (aluminum, magnesium) within 2 hrs of lomefloxacin.
3. Encourage cranberry juice, citrus fruits (to acidify urine).

INDICATIONS/DOSAGE/ROUTES

Urinary tract infections:
PO: Adults, elderly: 400 mg/day for 10-14 days.

Lower respiratory tract infections:
PO: Adults, elderly: 400 mg/day for 10 days.

Postop prophylaxis:
PO: Adults, elderly: 400 mg 2-6 hrs prior to surgery.

Dosage in renal impairment:
The dose and/or frequency is modified in pts based on severity of renal impairment.

CREATININE CLEARANCE	DOSAGE
>40 ml/min	No change
10-40 ml/min	400 mg initially, then 200 mg/day for 10-14 days

PRECAUTIONS

CONTRAINDICATIONS: Hyper-

sensitivity to lomefloxacin, quinolones, any component of the preparation. **CAUTIONS:** Renal impairment, CNS disorders, seizures, those taking theophylline or caffeine. **PREGNANCY/LACTATION:** Unknown if distributed in breast milk. If possible, do not use during pregnancy/lactation (risk of arthropathy to fetus/infant). **Pregnancy Category C.**

INTERACTIONS

DRUG INTERACTIONS: Antacids, iron prep, sucralfate may decrease absorption. Decreases clearance, may increase concentration, toxicity of theophylline. May increase effects of oral anticoagulants. **ALTERED LAB VALUES:** May increase SGOT (AST), SGPT (ALT), alkaline phosphatase, LDH, serum bilirubin, BUN, serum creatinine concentration.

SIDE EFFECTS

FREQUENT: Nausea, diarrhea, headache, dizziness, photosensitivity.

ADVERSE REACTIONS/TOXIC EFFECTS

Superinfection (bacterial or fungal overgrowth of nonsusceptible organisms), photosensitivity reaction.

NURSING IMPLICATIONS

BASELINE ASSESSMENT:

Question for history of hypersensitivity to lomefloxacin, quinolones, any component of preparation. Obtain specimen for diagnostic tests before giving first dose (therapy may begin before results are known).

INTERVENTION/EVALUATION:

Evaluate food tolerance. Determine pattern of bowel activity; be alert to blood in feces. Check for dizziness, headache. Monitor B/P at least twice daily. Assess for chest, joint pain.

PATIENT/FAMILY TEACHING:

Do not skip dose; take full course of therapy. Take w/8 ounces water; drink several glasses of water between meals. Eat/drink high sources of ascorbic acid to prevent crystalluria (cranberry juice, citrus fruits). Do not take antacids (reduces/destroys effectiveness). Avoid sunlight/ultraviolet exposure; wear sunscreen, protective clothing if photosensitivity develops. Notify nurse/physician if new symptoms occur.

lomustine

low-mus´steen
(CeeNU)

CANADIAN AVAILABILITY:
CeeNu

CLASSIFICATION

Antineoplastic

PHARMACOKINETICS

Rapid, well absorbed from GI tract. Widely distributed. Crosses blood-brain barrier. Protein binding: 50%. Metabolized in liver to active metabolite. Primarily excreted in urine. Half-life: 16-48 hrs.

ACTION

Cell cycle-phase nonspecific. Interferes w/DNA, RNA function. Inhibits DNA synthesis.

USES

Treatment of primary and metastatic brain tumors, disseminated Hodgkin's disease.

PO ADMINISTRATION

NOTE: May be carcinogenic, mutagenic, or teratogenic. Handle w/ extreme care during administration.

Give on empty stomach (reduces potential for nausea).

INDICATIONS/DOSAGE/ROUTES

NOTE: Dosage is individualized based on clinical response and tolerance to adverse effects. When used in combination therapy, consult specific protocols for optimum dosage, sequence of drug administration.

Usual dosage:
PO: Adults, elderly, children: 100-130 mg/m^2 as single dose. Repeat dose at intervals of at least 6 wks but not until circulating blood elements have returned to acceptable levels. Adjust dose based on hematologic response to previous dose.

PRECAUTIONS

CONTRAINDICATIONS: Previous hypersensitivity to drug. **CAUTIONS:** Depressed platelet, leukocyte, erythrocyte counts. **PREGNANCY/LACTATION:** If possible, avoid use during pregnancy, especially first trimester. May cause fetal harm. Unknown if distributed in breast milk. Breast feeding not recommended. **Pregnancy Category D.**

INTERACTIONS

DRUG INTERACTIONS: Bone marrow depressants may increase bone marrow depression. Live virus vaccines may potentiate virus replication, increase vaccine side effects, decrease pt's antibody response to vaccine. **ALTERED LAB VALUES:** May increase liver function tests.

SIDE EFFECTS

FREQUENT: Nausea, vomiting occur 45 min-6 hrs after dosing, lasts 12-24 hrs. Anorexia often follows for 2-3 days. **OCCASIONAL:** Hair thinning, stomatitis.

ADVERSE REACTIONS/TOXIC EFFECTS

Bone marrow depression manifested as hematologic toxicity (principally leukopenia, mild anemia, thrombocytopenia). Leukopenia occurs at about 6 wks, thrombocytopenia at about 4 wks, and persists for 1-2 wks. Refractory anemia, thrombocytopenia occur commonly if therapy continued longer than 1 yr. Hepatotoxicity occurs infrequently. Large cumulative doses may result in renal damage.

NURSING IMPLICATIONS

BASELINE ASSESSMENT:

Manufacturer recommends weekly blood counts; experts recommend first blood count obtained 2-3 wks after initial therapy, subsequent blood counts indicated by prior toxicity. Antiemetics can reduce duration, frequency of nausea, vomiting.

INTERVENTION/EVALUATION:

Monitor hematologic status, liver function tests. Monitor for stomatitis (burning/erythema of oral mucosa at inner margin of lips, sore throat, difficulty swallowing). Monitor for hematologic toxicity (fever, sore throat, signs of local infection, easy bruising, unusual bleeding from any site), symptoms of anemia (excessively tired, weak).

PATIENT/FAMILY TEACHING:

Nausea, vomiting abates generally in <1 day. Fasting prior to therapy can reduce frequency/duration of GI effects. Maintain fastidious oral hygiene. Do not have immunizations w/o physician's approval (drug lowers body's resistance). Avoid crowds and those w/known illness. Promptly report fever, sore throat, signs of local infection, easy bruising or unusual bleeding from any site, swelling of legs and feet, yellow skin. Contact physician if nausea/vomiting continues at home. Avoid alcohol and over-the-counter medications. Contraception is recommended during therapy.

loperamide hydrochloride

low-pear´ah-myd

(Imodium, Imodium A-D)

CANADIAN AVAILABILITY:
Imodium

CLASSIFICATION

CLINICAL: Antidiarrheal

PHARMACOKINETICS

Poorly absorbed from GI tract. Protein binding: 97%. Metabolized in liver. Eliminated in feces, excreted in urine. Half-life: 9.1-14.4 hrs.

ACTION

Slows intestinal motility (direct effect on intestinal wall muscles); prolongs transit time of intestinal contents (reduces fecal volume, diminishes loss of fluid/electrolytes, increases viscosity, bulk).

USES

Controls, provides symptomatic relief of acute nonspecific diarrhea; chronic diarrhea associated w/inflammatory bowel disease; traveler's diarrhea. Reduces volume of discharge from ileostomy.

INDICATIONS/DOSAGE/ROUTES

Acute diarrhea (capsules):
PO: Adults, elderly: Initially, 4 mg, then 2 mg after each unformed stool. **Maximum:** 16 mg/day. **Children, 8-12 yrs, >30 kg:** Initially, 2 mg 3 times/day for 24 hrs. **5-8 yrs, 20-30 kg:** Initially, 2 mg 2 times/day for 24 hrs. **2-5 yrs, 13-20 kg:** Initially, 1 mg 3 times/day for 24 hrs. **Maintenance:** 1 mg/10 kg only after loose stool.

Chronic diarrhea:
PO: Adults, elderly: Initially 4 mg, then 2 mg after each unformed stool until diarrhea is controlled.

Traveler's diarrhea:
PO: Adults, elderly: Initially, 4 mg, then 2 mg after each loose bowel movement (LBM). **Maximum:** 8 mg/day for 2 days. **Children 9-11 yrs:** Initially 2 mg, then 1 mg after each LBM. **Maximum:** 6 mg/day for 2 days. **Children 6-8 yrs:** Initially, 1 mg, then 1 mg after each LBM. **Maximum:** 4 mg/day for 2 days.

PRECAUTIONS

CONTRAINDICATIONS: Those who must avoid constipation, diarrhea associated w/pseudomembranous enterocolitis due to broad-spectrum antibiotics or w/organisms that invade intestinal mucosa (*Escherichia coli,* shigella, salmonella), acute ulcerative colitis (may produce toxic megacolon). **CAU-**

TIONS: Those w/fluid/electrolyte depletion, hepatic impairment. **PREGNANCY/LACTATION:** Unknown if drug crosses placenta or is distributed in breast milk. **Pregnancy Category B.**

INTERACTIONS

DRUG INTERACTIONS: Opioid (narcotic) analgesics may increase risk of constipation. **ALTERED LAB VALUES:** None significant.

SIDE EFFECTS

INFREQUENT: Dry mouth, drowsiness, abdominal discomfort. **RARE:** Hypersensitivity reaction (including rash).

ADVERSE REACTIONS/TOXIC EFFECTS

Toxicity results in constipation, GI irritation including nausea, vomiting, CNS depression. Treatment: Activated charcoal.

NURSING IMPLICATIONS

BASELINE ASSESSMENT:

Do not administer in presence of bloody diarrhea or temperature >101°F.

INTERVENTION/EVALUATION:

Encourage adequate fluid intake. Assess bowel sounds for peristalsis. Monitor stool frequency and consistency (watery, loose, soft, semisolid, solid). Withhold drug and notify physician promptly in event of abdominal pain, distention, or fever.

PATIENT/FAMILY TEACHING:

Do not exceed prescribed dose. Avoid tasks that require alertness, motor skills until response to drug is established. Notify physician if diarrhea does not stop within 3 days, if abdominal distention or pain occurs, or if fever develops.

loracarbef

laur-ah-car'bef

(Lorabid)

CLASSIFICATION

Antibiotic: Cephalosporin

PHARMACOKINETICS

Well absorbed from GI tract. Widely distributed. Protein binding: 25%. Primarily excreted unchanged in urine. Removed by hemodialysis. Half-life: 1 hr (increased in decreased renal function).

ACTION

Bactericidal. Binds to bacterial membranes. Inhibits cell wall synthesis.

USES

Treatment of bronchitis, otitis media, pharyngitis, pneumonia, sinusitis, skin and soft tissue infections, urinary tract infections (uncomplicated cystitis, pyelonephritis).

STORAGE/HANDLING

After reconstitution, powder for suspension may be kept at room temperature for 14 days. Discard unused portion after 14 days.

PO ADMINISTRATION

1. Give 1 hr before or 2 hrs after meal.
2. Shake oral suspension well before using.

INDICATIONS/DOSAGE/ROUTES

Bronchitis:
PO: Adults, elderly, children >12 yrs: 200-400 mg q12h for 7 days.

Pharyngitis:
PO: Adults, elderly, children >12 yrs: 200 mg q12h for 10 days. **Children <12 yrs:** 7.5 mg/kg q12h for 10 days.

Pneumonia:
PO: Adults, elderly, children >12 yrs: 400 mg q12h for 14 days.

Sinusitis:
PO: Adults, elderly, children >12 yrs: 400 mg q12h for 10 days.

Skin, soft tissue infections:
PO: Adults, elderly, children >12 yrs: 200 mg q12h for 7 days. **Children <12 yrs:** 7.5 mg/kg q12h for 7 days.

Urinary tract infections:
PO: Adults, elderly, children >12 yrs: 200-400 mg q12h for 7-14 days.

Otitis media:
PO: Children: 15 mg/kg q12h for 10 days.

PRECAUTIONS

CONTRAINDICATIONS: History of hypersensitivity to cephalosporins, anaphylactic reaction to penicillins. **CAUTIONS:** Renal impairment. **PREGNANCY/LACTATION:** Unknown whether distributed in breast milk. **Pregnancy Category B.**

INTERACTIONS

DRUG INTERACTIONS: Probenecid increases serum concentrations, half-life of loracarbef. **ALTERED LAB VALUES:** May increase SGOT (AST), SGPT (ALT), alkaline phosphatase, BUN, creatinine. May decrease leukocytes, platelets.

SIDE EFFECTS

FREQUENT: Abdominal pain, anorexia, nausea, vomiting, diarrhea. **OCCASIONAL:** Skin rash, itching. **RARE:** Dizziness, headache, vaginitis.

ADVERSE REACTIONS/TOXIC EFFECTS

Antibiotic-associated colitis, other superinfections may result from altered bacterial balance. Hypersensitivity reactions (ranging from rash, urticaria, fever to anaphylaxis) occur in less than 5%, generally those w/history of allergies, especially penicillin.

NURSING IMPLICATIONS

BASELINE ASSESSMENT:

Question history of allergies, particularly cephalosporins, penicillins. Obtain culture and sensitivity test before giving first dose (therapy may begin before results are known).

INTERVENTION/EVALUATION:

Assess for nausea, vomiting. Check stool frequency and consistency. Assess skin for rash (diaper area in children). Monitor I&O, urinalysis, renal function reports for nephrotoxicity. Be alert for superinfection: genital/anal pruritus, moniliasis, abdominal pain, sore mouth or tongue, moderate to severe diarrhea.

PATIENT/FAMILY TEACHING:

Continue antibiotic therapy for full length of treatment. Doses should be evenly spaced, given at least 1 hr before or 2 hrs after a meal. Notify physician in event of diarrhea, rash, or onset of other new symptoms.

loratadine

lor-ah'tah-deen
(Claritin)

FIXED-COMBINATION(S):
W/pseudoephedrine, a sympathomimetic (Claritin-D)

CANADIAN AVAILABILITY:
Claritin

CLASSIFICATION

Antihistamine

PHARMACOKINETICS

	ONSET	PEAK	DURATION
PO	1-3 hrs	8-12 hrs	24 hrs

Rapidly, almost completely absorbed from GI tract. Distributed mainly in liver, lungs, GI tract, bile. Protein binding: 99%. Metabolized in liver to active metabolite (undergoes extensive first-pass metabolism). Excreted in urine, eliminated in feces. Half-life: 3-20 hrs; metabolite: 28 hrs (increased in elderly, liver disease).

ACTION

Long-acting w/selective peripheral histamine H_1 receptor antagonist action. Prevents, antagonizes most histamine effects (e.g., urticaria, pruritus). Has no significant anticholinergic effects.

USES

Relief of nasal and nonnasal symptoms of seasonal allergic rhinitis (hay fever).

PO ADMINISTRATION

Preferably give on an empty stomach (food delays absorption).

INDICATIONS/DOSAGE/ROUTES

Allergic rhinitis:
PO: Adults, elderly, children >12 yrs: 10 mg once daily. **Hepatic function impairment:** 10 mg every other day.

PRECAUTIONS

CONTRAINDICATIONS: Hypersensitivity to loratadine or any ingredient. **CAUTIONS:** Pts w/liver impairment. Safety in children <12 yrs not known. **PREGNANCY/LACTATION:** Excreted in breast milk. **Pregnancy Category B.**

INTERACTIONS

DRUG INTERACTIONS: Alcohol, CNS depressants may increase CNS depression. Ketoconazole, erythromycin may increase concentrations resulting in cardiotoxic effects. **ALTERED LAB VALUES:** May suppress wheal and flare reactions to antigen skin testing, unless antihistamines are discontinued 4 days before testing.

SIDE EFFECTS

FREQUENT: Headache, somnolence, fatigue, dry mouth. **OCCASIONAL:** Conjunctivitis, blurred vision, eye pain, malaise, fever, aggravated allergy, increased sweating.

ADVERSE REACTIONS/TOXIC EFFECTS

Somnolence, tachycardia, headache. General symptomatic and supportive measures should be instituted.

NURSING IMPLICATIONS

BASELINE ASSESSMENT:

Assess lung sound, rhinitis, urticaria, or other symptoms.

INTERVENTION/EVALUATION:

For upper respiratory allergies, increase fluids to maintain thin secretions and offset thirst, loss of fluids from increased sweating. Monitor symptoms for therapeutic response.

PATIENT/FAMILY TEACHING:

Take loratadine on an empty stomach. Does not cause drowsiness; however, if blurred vision or eye pain occur, do not drive or perform activities requiring visual acuity. Avoid alcohol during antihistamine therapy.

lorazepam

lor-az´ah-pam
(Alzapam, Ativan)

CANADIAN AVAILABILITY:
Apo-Lorazepam, Ativan, Novolorazepam

CLASSIFICATION

Antianxiety

PHARMACOKINETICS

	ONSET	PEAK	DURATION
IM	15-30 min	—	12-24 hrs
IV	1-5 min	—	12-24 hrs

Well absorbed after oral, IM administration. Widely distributed. Protein binding: 85%. Metabolized in liver. Primarily excreted in urine. Half-life: 10-20 hrs.

ACTION

Enhances action of inhibitory neurotransmitter gamma-aminobutyric acid (GABA). Depressant effects occur at all levels of CNS. Enhances presynaptic inhibition, suppresses spread of seizure activity. Inhibits spinal polysynaptic pathways. Directly depresses motor nerve, muscle function.

USES

Management of anxiety disorders associated w/depressive symptoms. Parenteral form used preoperatively to provide sedation, relieve anxiety, and produce anterograde amnesia.

STORAGE/HANDLING

Refrigerate parenteral form. Do not use if precipitate forms or solution appears discolored. Avoid freezing.

PO/IM/IV ADMINISTRATION

PO:

1. Give w/food.
2. Tablets may be crushed.

IM:

1. Give deep IM into large muscle mass.

IV:

1. Dilute w/equal volume of sterile water for injection, 0.9% NaCl injection, or 5% dextrose injection.
2. To dilute prefilled syringe, remove air from half-filled syringe, aspirate equal volume of diluent, pull plunger back slightly to allow for mixing, and gently invert syringe several times (do not shake vigorously).
3. Give by direct IV injection or into tubing of free-flowing IV infusion (0.9% NaCl, 5% dextrose) at rate of infusion not to exceed 2 mg/min.
4. Direct IV injection should be made w/repeated aspiration to ensure prevention of intra-arterial administration (produces arteriospasm; may result in gangrene).

INDICATIONS/DOSAGE/ROUTES

Anxiety:
PO: Adults: 1-2 mg daily in 2-3 evenly divided doses. **Elderly:** Initially, 0.5-1 mg/day. May increase gradually.

Insomnia due to anxiety:

PO: Adults: 2-4 mg at bedtime. **Elderly:** 0.5-1 mg at bedtime.

Preop:

IM: Adults, elderly: 0.05 mg/kg given 2 hrs before procedure. Do not exceed 4 mg.

IV: Adults, elderly: 0.044 mg/kg (up to 2 mg total) 15-20 min before surgery.

PRECAUTIONS

CONTRAINDICATIONS: Acute narrow-angle glaucoma, acute alcohol intoxication. **CAUTIONS:** Impaired kidney/liver function. **PREGNANCY/LACTATION:** May cross placenta; may be distributed in breast milk. May increase risk of fetal abnormalities if administered during 1st trimester of pregnancy. Chronic ingestion during pregnancy may produce fetal toxicity, withdrawal symptoms, CNS depression in neonates. **Pregnancy Category D.**

INTERACTIONS

DRUG INTERACTIONS: Alcohol, CNS depressants may increase CNS depressant effect. **ALTERED LAB VALUES:** None significant.

SIDE EFFECTS

FREQUENT: Drowsiness, dizziness, incoordination. Morning drowsiness may occur initially. **OCCASIONAL:** Blurred vision, slurred speech, hypotension, headache. **RARE:** Paradoxical CNS restlessness, excitement in elderly/debilitated (generally noted during first 2 wks of therapy, particularly noted in presence of uncontrolled pain).

ADVERSE REACTIONS/TOXIC EFFECTS

Abrupt or too-rapid withdrawal may result in pronounced restlessness, irritability, insomnia, hand tremors, abdominal/muscle cramps, sweating, vomiting, seizures. Overdosage results in somnolence, confusion, diminished reflexes, coma.

NURSING IMPLICATIONS

BASELINE ASSESSMENT:

Offer emotional support to anxious pt. Pt must remain recumbent for up to 8 hrs (individualized) after parenteral administration to reduce hypotensive effect. Assess motor responses (agitation, trembling, tension) and autonomic responses (cold, clammy hands, sweating).

INTERVENTION/EVALUATION:

For those on long-term therapy, liver/renal function tests, blood counts should be performed periodically. Assess for paradoxical reaction, particularly during early therapy. Assist w/ambulation if drowsiness, lightheadedness occur. Evaluate for therapeutic response: a calm facial expression, decreased restlessness and/or insomnia.

PATIENT/FAMILY TEACHING:

Drowsiness usually disappears during continued therapy. If dizziness occurs, change positions slowly from recumbent to sitting position before standing. Avoid tasks that require alertness, motor skills until response to drug is established. Smoking reduces drug effectiveness. Do not abruptly withdraw medication after long-term therapy. Do not use alcohol or CNS depressants. Contraception is recommended for long-term therapy. Notify physician at once if pregnancy is suspected.

losartan (Cozaar)
See supplement

lovastatin

low-vah-stah´tin
(Mevacor)

CANADIAN AVAILABILITY:
Mevacor

CLASSIFICATION

Antihyperlipoproteinemic

PHARMACOKINETICS

Incompletely absorbed from GI tract (increased on empty stomach). Protein binding: >95%. Hydrolyzed in liver to active metabolite. Primarily eliminated in feces. Half-life: 3 hrs.

ACTION

Inhibits HMG-CoA preventing conversion of HMG-CoA to mevalonate (early step in cholesterol synthesis). Decrease LDL, cholesterol, VLDL, plasma triglycerides; increases HDL concentration slightly.

USES

Adjunct to diet therapy to decrease elevated total and LDL cholesterol concentrations in those w/ primary hypercholesterolemia (types IIa and IIb) and in those w/ combined hypercholesterolemia, hypertriglyceridemia. May slow progression and promote regression of atherosclerosis.

PO ADMINISTRATION

Give w/meals.

INDICATIONS/DOSAGE/ROUTES

Hyperlipoproteinemia:
PO: Adults, elderly: Initially, 20-40 mg/day w/evening meal. Increase at 4 wk intervals up to maximum of 80 mg/day. **Maintenance:** 20-80 mg/day in single or divided doses.

PRECAUTIONS

CONTRAINDICATIONS: Hypersensitivity to lovostatin, active liver disease, unexplained serum transaminases. **CAUTIONS:** Anticoagulant therapy, history of liver disease, substantial alcohol consumption. Withholding/discontinuing lovostatin may be necessary when pt is at risk for renal failure (secondary to rhabdomyolysis); major surgery, severe acute infection, trauma, hypotension, severe metabolic, endocrine or electrolyte disorders, or uncontrolled seizures. **PREGNANCY/LACTATION:** Contraindicated in pregnancy (suppression of cholesterol biosynthesis may cause fetal toxicity) and lactation. Unknown if drug is distributed in breast milk. **Pregnancy Category X.**

INTERACTIONS

DRUG INTERACTIONS: Increased risk of rhabdomyolysis, acute renal failure w/cyclosporine, erythromycin, gemfibrozil, niacin, other immunosuppressants. **ALTERED LAB VALUES:** May increase creatinine kinase, serum transaminase concentrations.

SIDE EFFECTS

Generally well tolerated. Side effects usually mild and transient. **FREQUENT:** Nausea, dyspepsia, diarrhea and/or constipation, flatulence, abdominal pain, headache, rash, pruritus. **OCCASIONAL:** Heartburn, myalgia, muscle cramping, blurred vision, insomnia, malaise, dizziness. **RARE:** Dysgeusia (distorted sense of taste), myopathy (myalgia and/or muscle weakness w/markedly elevated CK concentrations).

ADVERSE REACTIONS/TOXIC EFFECTS

Potential for malignancy, cataracts.

NURSING IMPLICATIONS

BASELINE ASSESSMENT:

Question for possibility of pregnancy before initiating therapy (Pregnancy Category X). Question history of hypersensitivity to lovostatin. Assess baseline lab results: cholesterol, triglycerides, liver function tests.

INTERVENTION/EVALUATION:

Evaluate food tolerance. Determine pattern of bowel activity. Check for headache, dizziness, blurred vision. Assess for rash, pruritus. Monitor cholesterol and triglyceride lab results for therapeutic response. Be alert for malaise, muscle cramping or weakness. Monitor temperature at least twice a day.

PATIENT/FAMILY TEACHING:

Take w/meals. Follow special diet (important part of treatment). Periodic lab tests are essential part of therapy. Do not take other medications w/o physician's knowledge. Do not stop medication w/o consulting physician. Report promptly any muscle pain or weakness, especially if accompanied by fever or malaise. Do not drive or perform activities that require alert response if dizziness occurs.

loxapine hydrochloride

lox´ah-peen

(Loxitane)

loxapine succinate

(Loxitane)

CANADIAN AVAILABILITY:
Loxapac

CLASSIFICATION

Antipsychotic

PHARMACOKINETICS

	ONSET	PEAK	DURATION
PO (sedation)	20-30 min	1.5-3 hrs	12 hrs
IM (sedation)	15-30 min	—	12 hrs

Well absorbed after oral, IM administration. Metabolized in liver to active metabolite. Primarily excreted in urine. Half-life: 12-19 hrs.

ACTION

Blocks dopamine at postsynaptic receptor sites in brain. Has strong alpha blocking, anticholinergic effects.

USES

Symptomatic management of psychotic disorders.

STORAGE/HANDLING

Store oral, parenteral form at room temperature. Yellow discoloration of solutions does not affect potency, but discard if markedly discolored.

PO/IM ADMINISTRATION

NOTE: Give by oral or IM route.

PO:

1. Give w/o regard to meals.
2. Dilute oral concentrate w/ orange or grapefruit juice.

IM:

1. Inject slow, deep IM into up-

per outer quadrant of gluteus maximus.

INDICATIONS/DOSAGE/ROUTES

PO: Adults: 10 mg 2 times/day. Increase dosage rapidly during first week to 50 mg, if needed. **Usual therapeutic, maintenance range:** 60-100 mg daily in 2-4 divided doses. **Maximum daily dose:** 250 mg.
IM: Adults: 12.5-50 mg q4-6h.

Usual elderly dosage (nonpsychotic):
PO: Elderly: Initially, 5-10 mg 1-2 times/day. May increase by 5-10 mg q4-7days.
IM: Elderly: 12.5-25 mg q48h. May increase by 12.5 mg up to 50 mg.

PRECAUTIONS

CONTRAINDICATIONS: Severe CNS depression, comatose states. **EXTREME CAUTION:** History of seizures. **CAUTION:** Cardiovascular disorders, glaucoma, history of urinary retention, prostatic hypertrophy. **PREGNANCY/LACTATION:** Crosses placenta; distributed in breast milk. **Pregnancy Category C**

INTERACTIONS

DRUG INTERACTIONS: Alcohol, CNS depressants may increase CNS depression. Antacids, antidiarrheals may decrease absorption. Extrapyramidal symptom (EPS) producing medications may increase risk of EPS. **ALTERED LAB VALUES:** None significant.

SIDE EFFECTS

FREQUENT: Transient drowsiness, dry mouth, constipation, blurred vision, nasal congestion. **OCCASIONAL:** Diarrhea, peripheral edema, urinary retention, nausea, mild/transient postural hypotension, tachycardia.

ADVERSE REACTIONS/TOXIC EFFECTS

Extrapyramidal symptoms frequently noted are akathisia (motor restlessness, anxiety). Less frequently noted are akinesia (rigidity, tremor, salivation, mask-like facial expression, reduced voluntary movements). Infrequently noted are dystonias: torticollis (neck muscle spasm), opisthotonos (rigidity of back muscles), and oculogyric crisis (rolling back of eyes). Tardive dyskinesia (protrusion of tongue, puffing of cheeks, chewing/puckering of mouth) occurs rarely but may be irreversible. Risk is greater in female elderly pts. Grand-mal seizures may occur in epileptic pts (risk higher w/IM administration).

NURSING IMPLICATIONS

BASELINE ASSESSMENT:

Assess behavior, appearance, emotional status, response to environment, speech pattern, thought content.

INTERVENTION/EVALUATION:

Supervise suicidal-risk pt closely during early therapy (as depression lessens, energy level improves, and suicide potential increases). Monitor B/P for hypotension. Assess for peripheral edema behind medial malleolus (sacral area in bedridden pts). Assess stool consistency and frequency. Monitor for rigidity, tremor, mask-like facial expression (especially in those receiving IM injection). Assess for therapeutic response (interest in surroundings, improvement in self-care, increased ability to concentrate, relaxed facial expression).

PATIENT/FAMILY TEACHING:

Full therapeutic effect may take up to 6 wks. Report visual disturbances. Sugarless gum or sips of tepid water may relieve dry mouth. Drowsiness generally subsides during continued therapy. Avoid tasks that require alertness, motor skills until response to drug is established. Avoid alcohol, CNS depressants, over-the-counter medications. Describe signs and symptoms of extrapyramidal involvement and tardive dyskinesia for pt to report immediately.

lypressin

lye-press´in

(Diapid)

CLASSIFICATION

Antidiuretic

PHARMACOKINETICS

	ONSET	PEAK	DURATION
Intranasal	Rapid	0.5-2 hrs	3-8 hrs

Rapidly absorbed from nasal mucosa. Metabolized in liver, kidney. Primarily excreted in urine. Half-life: 15 minutes.

ACTION

Increases water reabsorption by increasing cellular permeability of collecting ducts. Increases urine osmolality w/decreased urine output.

USES

Prevention or control of polydipsia, polyuria, dehydration of neurogenic diabetes insipidus (caused by insufficient ADH). Esp. useful in diabetes insipidus refractory to other forms of treatment or pts allergic to preparations of animal origin.

INTRANASAL ADMINISTRATION

1. W/pt vertical and head up, bottle should be held upright and nozzle placed into nostril.
2. Pt should be instructed *not* to inhale.
3. A bedtime dose helps prevent nocturia.
4. If more than 2 sprays q4-6h needed, increase frequency, not number of sprays.

INDICATIONS/DOSAGE/ROUTES

NOTE: 1-2 sprays into one or both nostrils whenever increased urinary frequency or significant thirst develops.

Diabetes insipidus:
INTRANASAL: Adults, elderly, children: 1-2 sprays 4 times/day. Additional dose given at HS to control nocturia.

PRECAUTIONS

CONTRAINDICATIONS: None known. **CAUTIONS:** Hypertension, coronary artery disease. Pts w/known sensitivity to vasopressin should be tested prior to administration of lypressin. Effectiveness decreased in pts w/nasal congestion, allergic rhinitis, or upper respiratory infections. **PREGNANCY/LACTATION: Pregnancy Category C.**

INTERACTIONS

DRUG INTERACTIONS: May increase effects w/carbamazepine, chlorpropamide, clofibrate. May decrease effects w/demeclocycline, lithium, norepinephrine. **AL-**

TERED LAB VALUES: None significant.

SIDE EFFECTS

OCCASIONAL: Rhinorrhea, nasal congestion, irritation of nasal passages, headache, dizziness, increased bowel movements, abdominal cramps, conjunctivitis. **RARE:** Heartburn secondary to excessive administration dripping into pharynx.

ADVERSE REACTIONS/TOXIC EFFECTS

Overdosage has caused marked, but transient fluid retention. Coronary vasoconstriction, hypertension have occurred w/ large doses.

NURSING IMPLICATIONS

BASELINE ASSESSMENT:

Question previous sensitivity w/ vasopressin. Establish baselines for B/P, pulse, electrolytes, weight, urine specific gravity.

INTERVENTION/EVALUATION:

Monitor I&O; weigh daily if water retention suspected. Check B/P and pulse 2 times/day. Monitor electrolytes, urine specific gravity. Report side effects to physician for dose reduction. Hold medication and report promptly water retention or chest pain.

PATIENT/FAMILY TEACHING:

Teach proper administration of medication, importance of I&O. Report swelling of hands or feet, chest pain, shortness of breath, nasal discomfort, or other symptom promptly.

mafenide acetate

ma´fe-nide
(Sulfamylon)

CANADIAN AVAILABILITY: Sulfamylon

CLASSIFICATION

Burn preparation

PHARMACOKINETICS

Absorbed through devascularized areas into systemic circulation. Rapidly metabolized. Primarily excreted in urine.

ACTION

Bacteriostatic. Decreases number of bacteria in avascular tissue of second and third degree burns. Promotes spontaneous healing of deep partial-thickness burns.

USES

Adjunctive therapy for second- and third-degree burns to prevent infection, septicemia; protection against conversion from partial to full thickness wounds (infection causes extended tissue destruction).

TOPICAL ADMINISTRATION

1. Apply to cleansed, debrided burns using sterile glove.
2. Keep burn areas covered w/ mafenide cream at all times; reapply to any areas where removed (e.g., w/pt activity).
3. Dressings usually not required; if ordered (e.g., when eschar begins to separate), apply thin layer.

INDICATIONS/DOSAGE/ROUTES

Usual topical dosage:
TOPICAL: Adults, elderly: Apply 1-2 times/day.

PRECAUTIONS

CONTRAINDICATIONS: Hypersensitivity to mafenide or sulfite. **CAUTIONS:** Impaired renal function that increases risk of metabolic acidosis. Cross-sensitivity to sulfonamides not certain. **PREGNANCY/LACTATION:** Unknown if distributed in breast milk. Safety during lactation unknown; potential for serious adverse effects to neonate. Not recommended during pregnancy unless burn area is >20% of body surface; contraindicated at or near term. **Pregnancy Category C.**

INTERACTIONS

DRUG INTERACTIONS: None significant. **ALTERED LAB VALUES:** None significant.

SIDE EFFECTS

Difficult to distinguish side effects and effects of severe burn. **FREQUENT:** Pain, burning upon application. **OCCASIONAL:** Allergic reaction (usually 10-14 days after initiation of mafenide): itching, rash, facial edema, swelling; unexplained syndrome of marked hyperventilation w/respiratory alkalosis. **RARE:** Delay in eschar separation, excoriation of new skin.

ADVERSE REACTIONS/TOXIC EFFECTS

Hemolytic anemia, porphyria, bone marrow depression, superinfections (esp. w/fungi), metabolic acidosis occur rarely.

NURSING IMPLICATIONS

BASELINE ASSESSMENT:

Question for hypersensitivity to mafenide, sulfite (more frequent in asthmatics). Evaluate arterial blood gases (ABGs) for acid/base balance, renal function tests and CBCs for baseline.

INTERVENTION/EVALUATION:

Be alert to fluid balance and renal function: monitor I&O, renal function tests, urinary pH and promptly report changes. Watch for signs/symptoms of metabolic acidosis: Kussmaul's respirations, nausea, vomiting, diarrhea, headache, tremors, weakness and cardiac arrhythmias (due to associated hyperkalemia), sensorium changes, decreased P_{CO_2}, blood pH, and HCO_3. Monitor vital signs, evaluate ABG results. Assess burns, surrounding skin areas for allergic reaction or superinfection: rash, excoriation, swelling, itching, increased pain, purulent exudate. Monitor hematologic tests.

PATIENT/FAMILY TEACHING:

Application may cause temporary pain or burning; burn areas must be completely covered by cream. Therapy must not be interrupted (attempts will be made to reduce adverse reaction before considering discontinuance of drug).

magaldrate (hydroxymagnesium aluminate)

mag´ul-drate
(Lowsium, Riopan)

FIXED-COMBINATION(S):
W/simethicone, an antiflatulent (Lowsium Plus, Riopan Plus)

CANADIAN AVAILABILITY:
Riopan

CLASSIFICATION

Antacid

PHARMACOKINETICS

Minimal absorption from GI tract. Onset of action based on solubility in stomach and reaction w/ hydrochloric acid. Duration of action based primarily on gastric emptying time (20 min when given before meals, up to 3 hrs when given after meals).

ACTION

Neutralizes existing gastric acid (no effect on output). Reduces acid concentration within lumen of esophagus (increases pH, decreases pepsin activity).

USES

Symptomatic relief of upset stomach associated w/hyperacidity (heartburn, acid indigestion, sour stomach) associated w/gastric, duodenal ulcers. Symptomatic treatment of gastroesophageal reflux disease. Prophylactic treatment of GI bleeding secondary to gastritis and stress ulceration.

PO ADMINISTRATION

1. Have pt chew tablets thoroughly before swallowing (follow w/glass of water or milk).
2. Shake well before administering suspension.

INDICATIONS/DOSAGE/ROUTES

Antacid:

PO: Adults, elderly: 5-10 ml between meals and at bedtime.

PRECAUTIONS

CONTRAINDICATIONS: Fecal impaction, renal failure. **CAUTIONS:** Impaired renal function, gastric outlet obstruction, elderly, dehydration, fluid restriction, intestinal obstruction, GI bleeding, diarrhea. **PREGNANCY/LACTATION:** May be distributed in breast milk. **Pregnancy Category C.**

INTERACTIONS

DRUG INTERACTIONS: May decrease excretion of quinidine, anticholinergics. May decrease effects of methenamine. May increase salicylate excretion. May decrease absorption of quinolones, iron preparations, isoniazid, ketoconazole, tetracyclines. **ALTERED LAB VALUES:** May increase gastrin, systemic/urinary pH. May decrease serum phosphate.

M

SIDE EFFECTS

None significant.

ADVERSE REACTIONS/TOXIC EFFECTS

Hypermagnesemia evidenced by hypotension, nausea, vomiting, EKG changes, respiratory/mental depression.

NURSING IMPLICATIONS

BASELINE ASSESSMENT:

Do not give other oral medication within 1-2 hrs of antacid administration.

INTERVENTION/EVALUATION:

Assess pattern of daily bowel activity and stool consistency. Monitor serum phosphate levels. Assess for relief of gastric distress.

PATIENT/FAMILY TEACHING:

Chew tablets thoroughly before swallowing (may be followed by water or milk). Maintain adequate fluid intake.

magnesium

magnesium chloride

(Slow-Mag)

magnesium citrate

(Citrate of Magnesia, Citroma, Citro-Nesia)

magnesium hydroxide

(MOM)

magnesium oxide

(Mag-Ox 400, Maox)

magnesium protein complex

(Mg-PLUS)

magnesium sulfate

(Epsom salt, Magnesium Sulfate injection)

FIXED-COMBINATION(S): W/aluminum, an antacid (Aludrox, Delcid, Gaviscon, Maalox); w/ aluminum and simethicone, an antiflatulent (Di-Gel, Gelusil, Maalox Plus, Mylanta, Silain-Gel); w/ aluminum and calcium, antacid (Camalox); w/mineral oil, a lubricant laxative (Haley's MO)

CANADIAN AVAILABILITY: Citro-Mag, Phillips' Magnesia Tablets

CLASSIFICATION

Antacid, anticonvulsant, electrolyte, laxative

PHARMACOKINETICS

Antacid, laxative: Minimal absorption through intestine. Absorbed dose primarily excreted in urine. *Systemic:* Widely distributed. Primarily excreted in urine.

ACTION

Antacid: Acts in stomach to neutralize gastric acid, increase pH. *Laxative:* Osmotic effect primarily in small intestine. Draws water into intestinal lumen, produces distention, promotes peristalsis, bowel evacuation. *Systemic:* Found primarily in intracellular fluids. Essential for activity of enzymes, nerve conduction, and muscle contraction. Prevents/controls convulsions by blocking neuromuscular transmission, decreasing amount of acetylcholine released at motor end plate.

USES

Antacid: Symptomatic relief of upset stomach associated w/hyperacidity (heartburn, acid indigestion, sour stomach), gastric, duodenal ulcers. Symptomatic treatment of GERD. Prophylactic treatment of GI bleeding secondary to gastritis and stress ulceration. *Laxative:* Evacuation of colon for rectal and bowel examination, elective colon surgery. Accelerates excretion of various parasites, poisonous substances (except acid or alkali) from GI tract. *Systemic:* Dietary supplement, replacement therapy. Nutritional adjunct in hyperalimentation. *Anticonvulsant:* Immediate control of life-threatening seizures in treatment of severe toxemia of pregnancy, seizures associated w/acute nephritis in children.

STORAGE/HANDLING

Store oral, parenteral forms at room temperature. Refrigerate citrate of magnesia (retains potency, palatability).

PO/IM/IV ADMINISTRATION

PO (ANTACID):

1. Suspensions to be shaken well before use.
2. Chew chewable tablets thoroughly before swallowing and follow w/full glass of water.

PO (LAXATIVE):

1. Drink full glass of liquid (8 oz) w/each dose (prevents dehydration).
2. Flavor improved by following w/fruit juice or citrus carbonated beverage.

IM:

1. For adults, elderly use 250 mg/ml (25%) or 500 mg/ml (50%) magnesium sulfate concentration.
2. For infants, children do not exceed 200 mg/ml (20%).

IV:

1. For IV infusion, do not exceed magnesium sulfate concentration 200 mg/ml (20%).
2. Do not exceed IV infusion rate of 150 mg/min.

INDICATIONS/DOSAGE/ROUTES

NOTE: 1 Gm = 8.12 mEq as magnesium sulfate.

ANTACID:

Magnesium hydroxide:
PO: Adults, elderly, children >12 yrs: 5-15 ml or 0.65-1.3 Gm 4 times/day.

Magnesium oxide:
PO: Adults, elderly: 400-840 mg/day.

LAXATIVE:

Citrate of magnesia:
PO: Adults, elderly: 240 ml as needed. **Children:** 1/2 adult dose, repeat as needed.

Magnesium hydroxide:
PO: Adults, elderly: 30-60 ml/day w/liquids. **Children ≥2 yrs:** 5-30 ml (dependent on age).

Magnesium sulfate:
PO: Adults, elderly: 10-15 Gm in glass of water. **Children:** 5-10 Gm in glass of water.

DIETARY SUPPLEMENT:

PO: Adults, elderly: 54-483 mg/day (refer to individual products).

MILD DEFICIENCY:

IM: Adults, elderly: 1 Gm q6h for 4 doses.

SEVERE DEFICIENCY:

IM: Adults, elderly: Up to 250 mg/kg (2 mEq/kg) within 4 hr period.
IV INFUSION: Adults, elderly: 1-5 Gm (8-40 mEq).

HYPERALIMENTATION:

IV: Adults, elderly: 1-3 Gm (8-24 mEq)/day. **Children:** 0.25-1.25 Gm (2-10 mEq)/day.

ANTICONVULSANT:

IM: Adults: 4-5 Gm (32-40 mEq) of 50% solution q4h as needed. **Children:** 20-40 mg/kg of 20% solution, may repeat as needed.
IV: Adults: 4 Gm (32 mEq) of 10-20% solution (do not exceed rate of 1.5 ml/min of 10% solution).
IV INFUSION: Adults: 4-5 Gm (32-40 mEq)/250 ml 5% dextrose or 0.9% NaCl (do not exceed rate of 3 ml/min).

PRECAUTIONS

CONTRAINDICATIONS: *Antacids:* Severe renal impairment, appendicitis or symptoms of appendicitis, ileostomy, intestinal obstruction. *Laxative:* Appendicitis, undiagnosed rectal bleeding, CHF, intestinal obstruction, hyper-

M

sensitivity, colostomy, ileostomy. *Systemic:* Heart block, myocardial damage, renal failure. **CAUTIONS:** Safety in children <6 yrs not known. *Antacids:* Undiagnosed gastrointestinal or rectal bleeding, ulcerative colitis, colostomy, diverticulitis, chronic diarrhea. *Laxative:* Diabetes mellitus or pts on low salt diet (some products contain sugar, sodium). *Systemic:* Severe renal impairment. **PREGNANCY/LACTATION:** *Antacid:* Unknown whether distributed in breast milk. **Pregnancy Category C.** *Parenteral:* Readily crosses placenta; distributed in breast milk for 24 hrs after magnesium therapy is discontinued. Continuous IV infusion increases risk of magnesium toxicity in neonate. IV administration should not be used 2 hrs preceding delivery. **Pregnancy Category A.**

INTERACTIONS

DRUG INTERACTIONS: *Antacids:* May decrease absorption of ketoconazole, tetracyclines. May decrease effect of methenamine. *Antacids, laxatives:* May decrease effects of oral anticoagulants, digoxin, phenothiazines. May form nonabsorbable complex w/tetracyclines. *Systemic:* Calcium may neutralize effects. CNS depression producing medications may increase CNS depression. May cause changes in cardiac conduction/heart block w/digoxin. **ALTERED LAB VALUES:** *Antacid:* May increase gastrin, pH. *Laxative:* May decrease potassium. *Systemic:* None significant.

SIDE EFFECTS

FREQUENT: *Antacid:* Chalky taste, diarrhea, laxative effect. **OCCASIONAL:** *Antacid:* Nausea, vomiting, stomach cramps. *Antacid, laxative:* Prolonged use or large dose w/renal impairment may cause increased magnesium (dizziness, irregular heartbeat, mental changes, tiredness, weakness). *Laxative:* Cramping, diarrhea, increased thirst, gas. *Systemic:* Reduced respiratory rate, decreased reflexes, flushing, hypotension, decreased heart rate.

ADVERSE REACTIONS/TOXIC EFFECTS

Antacid, laxative: None significant. *Systemic:* May produce prolonged PQ interval, widening of QRS intervals. May cause loss of deep-tendon reflexes, heart block, respiratory paralysis and cardiac arrest. *Antidote:* 10-20 ml 10% calcium gluconate (5-10 mEq of calcium).

NURSING IMPLICATIONS

BASELINE ASSESSMENT:

Assess if pt is sensitive to magnesium. *Antacid:* Assess gastrointestinal pain (duration, location, time of occurrence, relief w/food or caused by food or alcohol, constant or sporadic, worsened when lying down or bending over). *Laxative:* Assess color, amount, consistency of stool. Assess bowel habits (usual pattern), bowel sound for peristalsis. Assess pt for any abdominal pain, weight loss, nausea, vomiting, history of recent abdominal surgery. *Systemic:* Assess renal function, magnesium level.

INTERVENTION/EVALUATION:

Antacid: Assess for relief of gastric distress. Monitor renal function (esp. if dosing is long term or frequent). *Laxative:* Monitor stools for diarrhea or constipation. Maintain adequate fluid intake. *Systemic:* Monitor renal function, magnesium levels, EKG for cardiac function.

Test patellar reflex or knee jerk reflexes before giving repeat parenteral doses (used as indication of CNS depression, suppressed reflex may be sign of impending respiratory arrest). Patellar reflex must be present, respiratory rate >16/min before each parenteral dose. Provide seizure precautions).

PATIENT/FAMILY TEACHING:

Antacid: Give at least 2 hrs apart from other medication. Do not take >2 wks unless directed by physician. For peptic ulcer take 1 and 3 hrs after meals and at bedtime for 4-6 wks. Chew tablets thoroughly followed w/glass of water; shake suspensions well. Repeat dosing/large doses may have laxative effect. *Laxative:* Drink full glass (8 oz) liquid to aid stool softening. Use only for short term. Teach other methods of bowel regulation (diet, exercise, increased fluid intake). Do not use if abdominal pain, vomiting, nausea are present. Inform pt of normal bowel movement range; 3 per day to 3 per wk. *Systemic:* Inform physician of any signs of hypermagnesemia (confusion, irregular heartbeat, cramping, unusual tiredness or weakness, lightheadedness, or dizziness).

mannitol

man´ih-tole

(Osmitrol)

CANADIAN AVAILABILITY:
Osmitrol

CLASSIFICATION

Osmotic diuretic

PHARMACOKINETICS

Remains in extracellular fluid. Primarily excreted in urine. Half-life: 100 minutes. Onset diuresis occurs in 1-3 hrs, decreases intraocular pressure in 0.5-1 hr, duration lasts 4-6 hrs. Decreases cerebral spinal fluid pressure in 15 min, duration lasts 3-8 hrs.

ACTION

Increases osmolality. Increases flow of water into interstitial fluid and plasma, enhances excretion of water, inhibits renal tubular reabsorption of sodium, chloride, enhances flow of water from eye into plasma.

USES

Prevention, treatment of oliguric phase of acute renal failure (before evidence of permanent renal failure). Reduces increased intracranial pressure because of cerebral edema, edema of injured spinal cord, intraocular pressure because of acute glaucoma. Promotes urinary excretion of toxic substances (aspirin, bromides, imipramine, barbiturates).

STORAGE/HANDLING

Store at room temperature. Crystallization can occur. Do not use if crystals remain after warming procedure (see IV Administration).

IV ADMINISTRATION

NOTE: Assess IV site for patency before each dose. Extravasation noted w/pain, thrombosis.

1. Rate of administration should be titrated to promote urinary output of 30-50 ml/hr.
2. If crystals are noted in solution, warm bottle in hot water and shake vigorously at intervals. Cool to

body temperature before administration.

3. Use filter for infusion of 20% or more concentration.

4. Do not add KCl or NaCl to mannitol 20% or greater. Do not add to whole blood for transfusion.

INDICATIONS/DOSAGE/ROUTES

NOTE: Dosage based on pt's condition/fluid requirements, urinary output, concentration and rate of administration.

Test dose for marked oliguria/suspected inadequate renal function:
IV: Adults, elderly: 0.2 Gm/kg or 12.5 Gm w/15-20% solution. Infuse over 3-5 min to produce urinary output of 30-50 ml in 2-3 hrs. Test dose may be repeated once.

Oliguria/acute renal failure prevention:
IV: Adults, elderly: 50-100 Gm of a concentrated solution followed by 5-10% solution.

Treatment of oliguria:
IV: Adults, elderly: 100 Gm w/15-20% solution infused over 90 min to a few hrs.

Intracranial/intraocular pressure:
IV: Adults, elderly: 1.5-2 Gm/kg administered as a 15-20-25% solution, infused over 30-60 min. Rebound increase of intracranial pressure may occur 12 hrs after use. For preop use, administer 1-1½ hrs before surgery.

Treatment of drug intoxications:
IV: Adults, elderly: Loading dose of 25 Gm followed by dosage titrated to maintain urinary output of 100-500 ml/hr. For barbiturates, 0.5 Gm/kg w/5-10% solutions titrated to urine output. Dosage and treatment based on fluid balance, urine pH, urine volume.

PRECAUTIONS

CONTRAINDICATIONS: Increasing oliguria or anuria, CHF, pulmonary edema, organic CNS disease, severe dehydration, fluid overload, active intracranial bleeding (except during craniotomy), severe electrolyte depletion. **CAUTIONS:** Impaired renal, hepatic function. **PREGNANCY/LACTATION:** Unknown whether drug crosses placenta or is distributed in breast milk. **Pregnancy Category C.**

INTERACTIONS

DRUG INTERACTIONS: May increase digoxin toxicity (due to hypokalemia). **ALTERED LAB VALUES:** May decrease phosphate, potassium, sodium.

SIDE EFFECTS

FREQUENT: Dry mouth, thirst. **OCCASIONAL:** Blurred vision, urinary retention, headache, arm pain, backache, nausea, vomiting, urticaria (hives), dizziness, hypotension, hypertension, tachycardia, fever, angina-like chest pain.

ADVERSE REACTIONS/TOXIC EFFECTS

Fluid and electrolyte imbalance may occur because of rapid administration of large doses or inadequate urinary output resulting in overexpansion of extracellular fluid. Circulatory overload may produce pulmonary edema, CHF. Excessive diuresis may produce hypokalemia, hyponatremia. Fluid loss in excess of electrolyte excretion may produce hypernatremia, hyperkalemia.

NURSING IMPLICATIONS

BASELINE ASSESSMENT:

Check B/P, pulse before giving medication. Baseline electrolyte, renal and hepatic function, BUN may be ordered. Assess skin turgor, mucous membranes, mental status, muscle strength. Obtain baseline weight. Initiate I&O. For acute situations, a Foley catheter may assist in measuring hourly outputs.

INTERVENTION/EVALUATION:

Monitor urinary output to ascertain therapeutic response. Monitor electrolyte, BUN, renal, hepatic reports. Assess vital signs, skin turgor, mucous membranes. Weigh daily. Signs of hyponatremia include confusion, drowsiness, thirst or dry mouth, cold/clammy skin. Signs of hypokalemia include changes in muscle strength, tremors, muscle cramps, changes in mental status, cardiac arrhythmias. Signs of hyperkalemia include colic, diarrhea, muscle twitching followed by weakness or paralysis, arrhythmias.

PATIENT/FAMILY TEACHING:

Expect increased frequency and volume of urination.

maprotiline hydrochloride

mah-pro´tih-leen

(Ludiomil)

CANADIAN AVAILABILITY:
Ludiomil

CLASSIFICATION

Antidepressant

PHARMACOKINETICS

Slowly, completely absorbed from GI tract. Widely distributed. Protein binding: 88%. Metabolized in liver to active metabolites. Primarily excreted in urine. Half-life: 27-58 hrs; metabolite: 60-90 hrs.

ACTION

Blocks reuptake of norepinephrine by presynaptic neuronal membranes. May change beta-adrenergic receptor sensitivity and enhance response to alpha adrenergic, serotonergic stimulation. Has moderate anticholinergic activity.

USES

Relief of depressive-affective (mood) disorders, including depressive neurosis, major depression. Also used for depression phase of bipolar disorder (manic-depressive illness).

PO ADMINISTRATION

1. Give w/food or milk if GI distress occurs.
2. Do not crush or break enteric-coated tablets.
3. Scored tablets may be crushed.

INDICATIONS/DOSAGE/ROUTES

Mild to moderate depression:
PO: Adults: 75 mg/day to start, in 1-4 divided doses. **Elderly:** 50-75 mg/day. In 2 wks, increase dosage gradually in 25 mg increments until therapeutic response is achieved. Reduce to lowest effective maintenance level.

Severe depression:
PO: Adults: 100-150 mg/day in 1-4 divided doses. May increase

gradually to maximum 225 mg/day.

Usual elderly dosage:
PO: Elderly: Initially, 25 mg at bedtime. May increase by 25 mg q3-7days. **Maintenance:** 50-75 mg/day.

PRECAUTIONS

CONTRAINDICATIONS: Acute recovery period following MI, within 14 days of MAO inhibitor ingestion. **CAUTIONS:** Prostatic hypertrophy, history of urinary retention or obstruction, glaucoma, diabetes mellitus, history of seizures, hyperthyroidism, cardiac/hepatic/renal disease, schizophrenia, increased intraocular pressure, hiatal hernia. **PREGNANCY/LACTATION:** Crosses placenta; distributed in breast milk. **Pregnancy Category C.**

INTERACTIONS

DRUG INTERACTIONS: Alcohol, CNS depressants may increase effect. MAO inhibitors may increase risk of hypertensive crisis, severe convulsions. Sympathomimetics may increase cardiovascular effects (arrhythmias, tachycardia, severe hypertension). **ALTERED LAB VALUES:** None significant.

SIDE EFFECTS

FREQUENT: Drowsiness, fatigue, dry mouth, blurred vision, constipation, delayed micturition, postural hypotension, excessive sweating, disturbed concentration, increased appetite, urinary retention. **OCCASIONAL:** GI disturbances (nausea, GI distress, metallic taste sensation). **RARE:** Paradoxical reaction (agitation, restlessness, nightmares, insomnia), extrapyramidal symptoms (particularly fine hand tremor).

ADVERSE REACTIONS/TOXIC EFFECTS

Higher incidence of seizures than w/tricyclic antidepressants (esp. in those w/no previous history of seizures). High dosage may produce cardiovascular effects (severe postural hypotension, dizziness, tachycardia, palpitations, arrhythmias) and seizures. May also result in altered temperature regulation (hyperpyrexia or hypothermia). Abrupt withdrawal from prolonged therapy may produce headache, malaise, nausea, vomiting, vivid dreams.

NURSING IMPLICATIONS

BASELINE ASSESSMENT:

For those on long-term therapy, liver/renal function tests, blood counts should be performed periodically.

INTERVENTION/EVALUATION:

Supervise suicidal-risk pt closely during early therapy (as depression lessens, energy level improves, increasing suicide potential. Assess appearance, behavior, speech pattern, level of interest, mood. Monitor bowel activity; avoid constipation. Monitor B/P, pulse for hypotension, arrhythmias. Assess for urinary retention.

PATIENT/FAMILY TEACHING:

Change positions slowly to avoid hypotensive effect. Tolerance to postural hypotension, sedative and anticholinergic effects usually develops during early therapy. Therapeutic effect may be noted within 3-7 days, maximum effect within 2-3 wks. Wear protective clothing, use sunscreen to protect skin from ultraviolet or sunlight. Dry mouth may be relieved by sugarless gum or sips of tepid water. Report visual disturbances. Do not abruptly discontinue medication. Avoid tasks that require alertness, motor skills until response to drug is established.

masoprocol

mass-oh-pro′call
(Actinex)

CLASSIFICATION

Topical

PHARMACOKINETICS

Minimal absorption systemically (<2%).

ACTION

Produces antiproliferative activity against keratinocytes.

USES

Topical treatment for actinic (solar) keratoses.

TOPICAL ADMINISTRATION

1. Wash and dry affected area before application.
2. Apply directly to desired area, massaging gently (avoid eyes and mucus membranes of nose/mouth).
3. Avoid occlusive dressing.
4. If applied w/fingers, wash hands immediately w/soap and water after use.

INDICATIONS/DOSAGE/ROUTES

Actinic (solar) keratoses:
TOPICAL: Adults, elderly: Apply to area topically as needed. Do not cover surface (minimizes irritation). Repeat each morning and evening for 28 days.

PRECAUTIONS

CONTRAINDICATIONS: Hypersensitivity to masoprocol or other components of preparation. **CAUTIONS:** Sulfite sensitivity. For external use only. Avoid occlusive dressings. Safety in children not established. **PREGNANCY/LACTATION:** Unknown whether excreted in breast milk. **Pregnancy Category B.**

INTERACTIONS

DRUG INTERACTIONS: None significant. **ALTERED LAB VALUES:** None significant.

SIDE EFFECTS

FREQUENT: Erythema, flaking, itching, dryness, edema, burning sensation, soreness. **OCCASIONAL:** Rash, skin irritation, crusting, bleeding, tingling sensation. **RARE:** Blistering, eczema, excoriation, fissuring, skin roughness, wrinkling.

ADVERSE REACTIONS/TOXIC EFFECTS

Allergic contact dermatitis, represents sensitization. Discontinue medication, contact physician.

NURSING IMPLICATIONS

BASELINE ASSESSMENT:

Question for hypersensitivity to masoprocol or other components of preparation.

INTERVENTION/EVALUATION:

Assess for irritation.

PATIENT/FAMILY TEACHING:

Use only as directed. For external use only. Take special care to avoid eyes, nose, mouth. If contact w/eyes occurs, rinse promptly and thoroughly w/water. If applied w/ fingers, wash hands immediately after application. Do not use occlusive coverings. Do not use other skin products or makeup during therapy w/o advice of physician. May stain clothing, fabrics. Does not cause photosensitivity, but avoid undue sun exposure because of keratoses. May have transient local burning after application. Contact physician if oozing, blistering, or other severe reaction occurs.

mebendazole

meh-ben´dah-zole
(Vermox)

CANADIAN AVAILABILITY: Vermox

CLASSIFICATION

Anthelmintic

PHARMACOKINETICS

Poorly absorbed from GI tract (absorption increases w/food). Highest concentration in liver. Protein bonding: 90-95%. Metabolized in liver. Primarily eliminated in feces. Half-life: 2.5-9 hrs (increased in decreased renal function).

ACTION

Vermicidal. Degrades parasite cytoplasmic microtubules, irreversibly blocks glucose uptake in helminths and larvae (depletes glycogen, decreases ATP, causes helminth death).

USES

Treatment of trichuriasis (whipworm), enterobiasis (pinworm), ascariasis (roundworm), hookworm caused by *Ancylostoma duodenale* or *Necator americanus*. Effective in mixed helminthic infections due to broad spectrum of activity.

PO ADMINISTRATION

1. No special fasting is required.
2. Tablet may be crushed, chewed, swallowed, or mixed w/food.
3. For high dosage, best if taken w/food.

INDICATIONS/DOSAGE/ROUTES

Trichuriasis, ascariasis, hookworm:

PO: Adults, elderly, children >2 yrs: 1 tablet in morning and at bedtime for 3 days.

Enterobiasis:

PO: Adults, elderly, children >2 yrs: 1 tablet one time.

PRECAUTIONS

CONTRAINDICATIONS: None significant. **CAUTIONS:** None significant. **PREGNANCY/LACTATION:** Unknown whether drug crosses placenta or is distributed in breast milk. **Pregnancy Category C.**

INTERACTIONS

DRUG INTERACTIONS: Carbamazepine may decrease concentrations. **ALTERED LAB VALUES:** May increase SGOT (AST), SGPT (ALT), alkaline phosphatase, BUN. May decrease Hgb.

SIDE EFFECTS

OCCASIONAL: Nausea, vomiting, headache, dizziness. Transient abdominal pain, diarrhea w/massive infection and expulsion of helminths. **RARE:** Fever.

ADVERSE REACTIONS/TOXIC EFFECTS

High dosage may produce reversible myelosuppression (granulocytopenia, leukopenia, neutropenia).

NURSING IMPLICATIONS

BASELINE ASSESSMENT:

Question for history of hypersensitivity to mebendazole. Obtain specimens to confirm diagnosis: (1) stool must be collected in clean, dry bedpan or container (parasites may be destroyed by urine, water, or medications) and (2) pinworm specimens obtained early in morning by applying transparent tape to tongue blade and pressing sticky side of tape to perianal area (female pinworms usually deposit eggs in this area during night).

INTERVENTION/EVALUATION:

Encourage intake of fruits, vegetables, fluids to avoid constipation (parasites expelled by normal peristalsis). Collect stool or perianal specimens as required to confirm cure. Monitor CBCs w/high dosage. Assess food tolerance. Provide assistance w/ambulation if dizzy.

PATIENT/FAMILY TEACHING:

Complete full course of therapy; may need to repeat. Wash hands thoroughly after toileting, before eating. Keep hands away from mouth, fingernails short. Disinfect toilet facilities daily. Due to high transmission of pinworm infections, all family members should be treated simultaneously; infected person should sleep alone, shower frequently. Do not shake bedding; change and launder underclothing, pajamas, bedding, towels and wash clothes daily. W/hookworm, avoid walking barefoot (larval entry into system). Continue iron supplements as long as ordered (may be 6 mo after treatment) for anemia associated w/whipworm, hookworm. Notify physician if symptoms do not improve in a few days, or if they become worse. Follow-up w/office visits, stool collection are important parts of therapy. Don't drive, use machinery if dizzy.

mechlorethamine hydrochloride

meh-klor-eth´ah-meen
(Mustargen)

CANADIAN AVAILABILITY:
Mustargen

CLASSIFICATION

Antineoplastic

PHARMACOKINETICS

Incompletely absorbed after intracavitary administration. Rapidly deactivated in fluids/tissues. Primarily excreted in urine.

ACTION

Cell cycle-phase nonspecifc. Primarily crosslinks strands of DNA, RNA. Inhibits protein synthesis.

USES

Treatment of advanced Hodgkin's disease, lymphosarcoma, mycosis fungoides, bronchogenic carcinoma, chronic myelocytic and lymphocytic leukemia, polycythemia vera, malignant effusions (pericardial, peritoneal, pleural) by intracavitary administration.

STORAGE/HANDLING

NOTE: May be carcinogenic, mutagenic, or teratogenic. Handle w/

extreme care during preparation/administration.

Prepare solution immediately before use. Use only clear, colorless solutions. Discard if change in color occurs, precipitate forms, or water droplets are noted inside vial prior to reconstitution.

IV ADMINISTRATION

NOTE: Give by IV injection. Avoid high concentration, prolonged local contact w/drug. Wear gloves when preparing solution. Avoid inhalation of dust or vapors, contact w/skin, mucous membranes. If eye contact occurs, immediately institute copious irrigation w/0.9% NaCl or ophthalmic irrigating solution. If skin contact occurs, wash affected part immediately w/copious amounts of water for 15 min, followed by 2% sodium thiosulfate solution.

1. Reconstitute each 10 mg vial w/10 ml sterile water for injection or 0.9% NaCl injection to provide concentration of 1 mg/ml.
2. Shake vial several times w/needle still in rubber stopper (minimizes risk of skin contact) to ensure complete dissolution.
3. Withdraw dose from vial using one sterile needle; use second sterile needle for injection.
4. Give desired dose over a few min directly into suitable vein or tubing of running IV infusion.
5. Flush vein and/or tubing for 2-5 min after administration to remove any remaining drug from tubing.
6. Extravasation produces painful inflammation, induration (may last 4-6 wks). Sloughing may occur. If extravasation occurs, infiltrate the area promptly w/isotonic sodium thiosulfate and apply cold compresses for 6-12 hrs. Vein irritation produces dark bluish-grey hyperpigmentation.

INDICATIONS/DOSAGE/ROUTES

NOTE: Dosage individualized based on clinical response, tolerance to adverse effects. When used in combination therapy, consult specific protocols for optimum dosage, sequence of drug administration. Dosage based on ideal body weight.

Usual dosage:
IV: Adults: 0.4 mg/kg per course as single dose, or 0.1-0.2 mg/kg/day in 2-4 divided doses. Repeat q3-6wks.

Advanced Hodgkin's disease:
IV: Adults: MOPP Regimen: 6 mg/m^2 on days 1 and 8 of 28-day cycle.

PRECAUTIONS

CONTRAINDICATIONS: Acute phase of herpes zoster infection, those w/foci of acute/chronic pustule inflammation, presence of known infectious disease. **EXTREME CAUTION:** Leukopenia, thrombocytopenia, anemia due to infiltration of bone marrow w/malignant cells. **PREGNANCY/LACTATION:** If possible, avoid use during pregnancy, esp. first trimester. Breast feeding not recommended. **Pregnancy Category D.**

INTERACTIONS

DRUG INTERACTIONS: May decrease effect of antigout medications. Bone marrow depressants may increase bone marrow depression. Live virus vaccines may potentiate virus replication, increase vaccine side effects, decrease pt's antibody response to vaccine. **ALTERED LAB VALUES:** May increase uric acid.

SIDE EFFECTS

FREQUENT: Nausea, vomiting occurs within 1-3 hrs after therapy; vomiting usually stops within 8 hrs but nausea may persist for 24 hrs. Lymphocytopenia occurs within 24 hrs of first dose; anorexia, diarrhea, dehydration secondary to vomiting. **OCCASIONAL:** Weakness, headache, drowsiness, lightheadedness, maculopapular rash. **INFREQUENT:** Alopecia. **RARE:** Tinnitus, fever, metallic taste sensation.

ADVERSE REACTIONS/TOXIC EFFECTS

Severe bone marrow depression manifested as hematologic toxicity (severe leukopenia, anemia, thrombocytopenia, bleeding) may occur, particularly when dose exceeds 0.4 mg/kg for single course. Leukopenia occurs within 6-8 days and persists for 10-21 days, recovery within 2 wks. Risk of neurotoxicity (seizures, paresthesia, vertigo) increases w/age and in those who also receive procarbazine or cyclophosphamide.

NURSING IMPLICATIONS

BASELINE ASSESSMENT:

Check CBC and establish baseline for myelosuppressive action of drug. Antiemetics may be effective in preventing, treating nausea, vomiting.

INTERVENTION/EVALUATION:

Assess for severe thrombocytopenia (bleeding from gums, tarry stool, petechiae, small subcutaneous hemorrhages). Monitor I&O; assess for dehydration. Check stools for frequency, consistency. Monitor Hgb, Hct, WBC, differential, platelet count, serum uric acid level. Monitor for hematologic toxicity (fever, sore throat, signs of local infection, easy bruising, unusual bleeding from any site), symptoms of anemia (excessive tiredness, weakness). Avoid IM injections, rectal temperatures, other traumas that may induce bleeding.

PATIENT/FAMILY TEACHING:

Do not have immunizations w/o physician's approval (drug lowers body's resistance). Avoid crowds and those w/infections. Promptly report fever, sore throat, signs of local infection, easy bruising or unusual bleeding from any site. Contact physician if nausea/vomiting continues at home. Do not take alcohol or any medication (including over-the-counter drugs) w/o consulting physician. Contraception should be used.

meclizine

mek´lih-zeen
(Antivert, Bonine)

CANADIAN AVAILABILITY:
Bonamine

CLASSIFICATION

Antiemetic, antivertigo

PHARMACOKINETICS

	ONSET	PEAK	DURATION
PO	30-60 min	—	12-24 hrs

Well absorbed from GI tract. Widely distributed. Metabolized in liver. Primarily excreted in urine. Half-life: 6 hrs.

ACTION

Central anticholinergic activity. Diminishes vestibular stimulation, depresses labyrinth function, may affect medullary CTZ.

USES

Prevention and treatment of nausea, vomiting, vertigo due to motion sickness. Treatment of vertigo associated with diseases affecting vestibular system.

PO ADMINISTRATION

1. Give w/o regard to meals.
2. Scored tablets may be crushed.
3. Do not crush or break capsule form.

INDICATIONS/DOSAGE/ROUTES

Motion sickness:

PO: Adults, elderly, children >12 yrs: 25-50 mg 1 hr before exposure to motion. Repeat q24h as needed.

Vertigo:

PO: Adults, elderly, children >12 yrs: 25-100 mg/day in divided doses as needed.

PRECAUTIONS

CONTRAINDICATIONS: None significant. **CAUTIONS:** Narrow-angle glaucoma, prostatic hypertrophy, pyloroduodenal or bladder neck obstruction, asthma, COPD, increased intraocular pressure, cardiovascular disease, hyperthyroidism, hypertension, seizure disorders. **PREGNANCY/LACTATION:** Unknown whether drug crosses placenta or is distributed in breast milk (may produce irritability in nursing infants). **Pregnancy Category B.**

INTERACTIONS

DRUG INTERACTIONS: Alcohol, CNS depression producing medications may increase CNS depressant effect. **ALTERED LAB VALUES:** May suppress wheal, flare reactions to antigen skin testing, unless meclizine discontinued 4 days before testing.

SIDE EFFECTS

NOTE: Elderly (>60 yrs) tend to develop mental confusion, disorientation, agitation, psychotic-like symptoms. **FREQUENT:** Drowsiness, dizziness, muscular weakness, dry mouth/nose/throat/lips, urinary retention, thickening of bronchial secretions. Sedation, dizziness, hypotension more likely noted in elderly. **OCCASIONAL:** Epigastric distress, flushing, visual disturbances, hearing disturbances, paresthesia, sweating, chills.

ADVERSE REACTIONS/TOXIC EFFECTS

Children may experience dominant paradoxical reaction (restlessness, insomnia, euphoria, nervousness, tremors). Overdosage in children may result in hallucinations, convulsions, death. Hypersensitivity reaction (eczema, pruritus, rash, cardiac disturbances, photosensitivity) may occur. Overdosage may vary from CNS depression (sedation, apnea, cardiovascular collapse, death) to severe paradoxical reaction (hallucinations, tremor, seizures).

NURSING IMPLICATIONS

BASELINE ASSESSMENT:

Drug may mask signs of ototoxicity when given concurrently with medications that may produce ototoxicity.

INTERVENTION/EVALUATION:

Monitor B/P, esp. in elderly (increased risk of hypotension). Monitor children closely for paradoxical reaction. Monitor serum electrolytes in those with severe vomiting. Assess skin turgor, mucous membranes to evaluate hydration status.

PATIENT/FAMILY TEACHING:

Tolerance to sedative effect may occur. Avoid tasks that require alertness, motor skills until response to drug is established. Dry mouth, drowsiness, dizziness may be an expected response of drug. Avoid alcoholic beverages during therapy. Sugarless gum, sips of tepid water may relieve dry mouth. Coffee or tea may help reduce drowsiness.

meclofenamate sodium

meh-klow-fen´ah-mate

(Meclodium, Meclomen)

CLASSIFICATION

Nonsteroidal anti-inflammatory

PHARMACOKINETICS

	ONSET	PEAK	DURATION
Antirheumatic	Several days	—	2-3 wks

Rapidly absorbed from GI tract. Protein binding: 99%. Metabolized in liver. Primarily excreted in urine. Half-life: 2 hrs.

ACTION

Inhibits prostaglandin synthesis. Inhibits action of cyclooxygenase, decreases formation of prostaglandin, thromboxane precursors from arachidonic acid.

USES

Symptomatic treatment of acute and/or chronic rheumatoid arthritis, osteoarthritis, control of mild to moderate pain.

PO ADMINISTRATION

Give with food, milk, or 8 oz water (minimizes potential GI distress).

INDICATIONS/DOSAGE/ROUTES

NOTE: Do not exceed 400 mg/day.

Rheumatoid arthritis, osteoarthritis:
PO: Adults, elderly: Initially, 200-300 mg/day in 3-4 divided doses.

Mild to moderate pain:
PO: Adults, elderly: 50 mg q4-6h as needed.

PRECAUTIONS

CONTRAINDICATIONS: Active peptic ulcer, GI ulceration, chronic inflammation of GI tract, GI bleeding disorders, history of hypersensitivity to aspirin or NSAIDs. **CAUTIONS:** Impaired renal/hepatic function, history of GI tract disease, predisposition to fluid retention. **PREGNANCY/LACTATION:** Breast feeding not recommended. Avoid use during third trimester (may adversely affect fetal cardiovascular system: premature closure of ductus arteriosus). **Pregnancy Category C.**

INTERACTIONS

DRUG INTERACTIONS: May increase effects of oral anticoagulants, heparin, thrombolytics. May decrease effect of antihypertensives, diuretics. Salicylates, aspirin may increase risk of GI side effects, bleeding. Bone marrow depressants may increase risk of hematologic reactions. May increase concentration, toxicity of lithium. May increase methotrexate toxicity. Probenecid may increase concentration. **ALTERED LAB VALUES:** May increase serum transaminase activity, BUN, creatinine, potassium, alkaline phosphatase, LDH. May decrease creatinine clearance.

SIDE EFFECTS

FREQUENT: Diarrhea, nausea, rash/dermatitis. **OCCASIONAL:** Headache, dyspepsia (heartburn, indigestion, epigastric pain), flatulence, dizziness, peripheral edema. **RARE:** Anorexia, vomiting, stomatitis, visual disturbances.

ADVERSE REACTIONS/TOXIC EFFECTS

Peptic ulcer, GI bleeding, gastritis, severe hepatic reaction (cholestasis, jaundice) occur rarely. Nephrotoxicity (dysuria, hematuria, proteinuria, nephrotic syndrome) and severe hypersensitivity reaction (fever, chills, bronchospasm) occur rarely.

NURSING IMPLICATIONS

BASELINE ASSESSMENT:

Assess onset, type, location and duration of pain or inflammation. Inspect appearance of affected joints for immobility, deformities, and skin condition.

INTERVENTION/EVALUATION:

Assist with ambulation if dizziness occurs. Monitor pattern of daily bowel activity and stool consistency. Assess skin for evidence of rash. Check behind medial malleolus for fluid retention (usually first area noted). Evaluate for therapeutic response: relief of pain, stiffness, swelling, increase in joint mobility, reduced joint tenderness, improved grip strength.

PATIENT/FAMILY TEACHING:

Anti-inflammatory effect noted in 2-3 wks. Avoid aspirin, alcohol during therapy (increases risk of GI bleeding). If GI upset occurs, take with food, milk. Avoid tasks that require alertness, motor skills until response to drug is established.

medroxyprogesterone acetate

meh-drocks-ee-pro-jest´er-own
(Amen, Curretab, Depo-Provera, Provera)

FIXED-COMBINATION(S): W/conjugated estrogens (Premphase, Prempro)

CANADIAN AVAILABILITY: Depo-Provera, Provera

CLASSIFICATION

Progestin, antineoplastic

PHARMACOKINETICS

Slow absorption after IM administration. Metabolized in liver. Primarily excreted in urine.

ACTION

Transforms endometrium from proliferative to secretory (in an estrogen-primed endometrium); inhibits secretion of pituitary gonadotropins, preventing follicular maturation and ovulation. Stimulates growth of mammary alveolar tissue; relaxes uterine smooth muscle.

USES

Oral: Prevention of endometrial hyperplasia (concurrently given with estrogen to women with intact uterus), treatment of secondary amenorrhea, abnormal uterine bleeding. *IM:* Adjunctive therapy, palliative treatment of inoperable, recurrent, metastatic endometrial carcinoma, renal carcinoma; prevention of pregnancy.

PO/IM ADMINISTRATION

PO:

1. Give w/o regard to meals.

IM:

1. Shake vial immediately before administering (ensures complete suspension).
2. Rarely, a residual lump, change in skin color, or sterile abscess occurs at injection site.

INDICATIONS/DOSAGE/ROUTES

Endometrial hyperplasia:
PO: Adults: 2-10 mg/day for 14 days.

Secondary amenorrhea:
PO: Adults: 5-10 mg/day for 5-10 days (begin at any time during menstrual cycle).

Abnormal uterine bleeding:
PO: Adults: 5-10 mg/day for 5-10 days (begin on calculated day 16 or day 21 of menstrual cycle).

Endometrial, renal carcinoma:
IM: Adults, elderly: Initially, 400-1000 mg, repeat at 1 wk intervals. If improvement occurs, disease stabilized, begin maintenance w/ as little as 400 mg/mo.

Pregnancy prevention:
IM: Adults: 150 mg q3mo.

PRECAUTIONS

CONTRAINDICATIONS: History of or active thrombotic disorders (cerebral apoplexy, thrombophlebitis, thromboembolic disorders), hypersensitivity to progestins, severe liver dysfunction, estrogen-dependent neoplasia, undiagnosed abnormal genital bleeding, missed abortion, use as pregnancy test, undiagnosed vaginal bleeding, carcinoma of breast, known or suspected pregnancy. **CAUTIONS:** Those w/conditions aggravated by fluid retention (asthma, seizures, migraine, cardiac or renal dysfunction), diabetes, history of mental depression. **PREGNANCY/LACTATION:** Avoid use during pregnancy, esp. first 4 mo (congenital heart, limb reduction defects may occur). Distributed in breast milk. **Pregnancy Category X.**

INTERACTIONS

DRUG INTERACTIONS: May interfere w/effects of bromocriptine. **ALTERED LAB VALUES:** May increase alkaline phosphatase, LDL. May decrease HDL.

SIDE EFFECTS

FREQUENT: Transient menstrual abnormalities (spotting, change in menstrual flow or cervical secretions, amenorrhea) at initiation of therapy. **OCCASIONAL:** Edema, weight change, breast tenderness, nervousness, insomnia, fatigue, dizziness. **RARE:** Alopecia, mental depression, dermatologic changes, headache, fever, nausea.

ADVERSE REACTIONS/TOXIC EFFECTS

Thrombophlebitis, pulmonary or cerebral embolism, retinal thrombosis occur rarely.

NURSING IMPLICATIONS

BASELINE ASSESSMENT:

Question for hypersensitivity to progestins, possibility of pregnancy before initiating therapy (Pregnancy Category X). Obtain baseline weight, blood glucose, B/P.

INTERVENTION/EVALUATION:

Check weight daily; report weekly gain of 5 lb or more. Check B/P periodically. Assess skin for rash, hives. Report immediately the development of chest pain, sudden shortness of breath, sudden decrease in vision, migraine headache, pain (esp. w/swelling, warmth, and redness) in calves, numbness of an arm or leg (thrombotic disorders). Monitor I&O in those with renal carcinoma or those experiencing weight gain. Note medroxyprogesterone therapy on pathology specimens.

PATIENT/FAMILY TEACHING:

Importance of medical supervision. Do not take other medications without physician approval. Use sunscreens, protective clothing to protect from sunlight or ultraviolet light until tolerance determined. Notify physician of abnormal vaginal bleeding or other symptoms. Teach how to perform Homans' test and the signs and symptoms of blood clots (report these to physician immediately). Teach self-breast exam. Stop taking medication and contact physician at once if pregnancy is suspected.

medrysone

med'rih-sohn
(HMS Liquifilm)

CANADIAN AVAILABILITY:
HMS

CLASSIFICATION

Corticosteroid, ophthalmic

PHARMACOKINETICS

Absorbed into conjunctival sac, systemically absorbed.

ACTION

Causes vasoconstriction and inhibits edema, fibrin deposition and migration of leukocytes and phagocytes in the inflammatory response to mechanical, chemical, or immunologic agents.

USES

Symptomatic relief of inflammatory conditions of the conjunctiva, cornea, lid, and anterior segment of the globe (e.g., allergic conjunctivitis, superficial punctate keratitis, herpes zoster keratitis and cyclitis). Also used to help prevent fibrosis, scarring and potential visual impairment caused by chemical, radiation, or thermal burns or penetration of foreign bodies.

OPHTHALMIC ADMINISTRATION

1. For topical ophthalmic use only.
2. Position pt w/head tilted back, looking up.
3. Gently pull lower lid down to form pouch and instill drops.
4. Do not touch tip of applicator to lids or any surface.
5. When lower lid is released, have pt keep eye open w/o blinking for at least 30 sec.
6. Apply gentle finger pressure to lacrimal sac (bridge of the nose, inside corner of the eye) for 1-2 min after administration of solution.
7. Remove excess solution around eye with a tissue. Wash hands immediately to remove medication.

INDICATIONS/DOSAGE/ROUTES

Usual ophthalmic dosage:
OPHTHALMIC: Adults, elderly:

Instill 1 drop into conjunctival sac q4h; may increase to 1 drop q1-2h for severe cases. Gradually taper dosage when discontinuing medication.

PRECAUTIONS

CONTRAINDICATIONS: Hypersensitivity to any component of preparation, acute superficial herpes simplex keratitis, fungal diseases of ocular structure. In pts w/vaccinia, varicella, or most other viral diseases of the cornea and conjunctiva; ocular tuberculosis. Not for use in iritis or uveitis. **CAUTIONS:** Safety and efficacy in children not established. **PREGNANCY/LACTATION:** Safety during pregnancy, lactation not established. **Pregnancy Category C.**

INTERACTIONS

DRUG INTERACTIONS: None significant. **ALTERED LAB VALUES:** None significant.

SIDE EFFECTS

OCCASIONAL: Transient stinging, burning on instillation. High doses may slow corneal healing. **RARE:** Filtering blebs after cataract surgery; hypersensitivity.

ADVERSE REACTIONS/TOXIC EFFECTS

Systemic reactions occur rarely with extensive use.

NURSING IMPLICATIONS

BASELINE ASSESSMENT:

Question for hypersensitivity to any components of preparation.

INTERVENTION/EVALUATION:

Assess for therapeutic response, superinfection, delayed healing or irritation.

PATIENT/FAMILY TEACHING:

Explain possible burning or stinging upon application. Visual acuity may be decreased after administration; avoid driving or operating machinery if vision decreases. Do not discontinue use w/o consulting physician. Notify physician if no improvement in 7-8 days, if condition worsens, or if pain, itching or swelling of eye occurs. Sensitivity to bright light may occur; wear sunglasses to minimize discomfort.

megestrol acetate

meh-jes´troll
(Megace)

CANADIAN AVAILABILITY:
Megace

CLASSIFICATION

Antineoplastic

PHARMACOKINETICS

Well absorbed from GI tract. Metabolized in liver; excreted in urine.

ACTION

Suppresses release of luteinizing hormone from anterior pituitary by inhibiting pituitary function.

USES

Palliative management of recurrent, inoperable, or metastatic endometrial or breast carcinoma. Treatment of anorexia, cachexia, or unexplained significant weight loss in pts w/AIDS.

INDICATIONS/DOSAGE/ROUTES

Palliative treatment of advanced breast cancer:
PO: Adults, elderly: 160 mg/day in 4 equally divided doses.

Palliative treatment of advanced endometrial carcinoma:
PO: Adults, elderly: 40-320 mg/day in divided doses. **Maximum:** 800 mg/day.

Anorexia, cachexia, weight loss:
PO: Adults, elderly: 800 mg (20 ml)/day.

PRECAUTIONS

CONTRAINDICATIONS: None significant. **CAUTIONS:** History of thrombophlebitis. **PREGNANCY/LACTATION:** If possible, avoid use during pregnancy, esp. first 4 mo. Breast feeding not recommended. **Pregnancy Category X.**

INTERACTIONS

DRUG INTERACTIONS: None significant. **ALTERED LAB VALUES:** May increase serum glucose levels.

SIDE EFFECTS

FREQUENT: Weight gain secondary to increased appetite. **OCCASIONAL:** Nausea, breakthrough bleeding, backache, headache, breast tenderness, carpal tunnel syndrome. **RARE:** Feeling of coldness.

ADVERSE REACTIONS/TOXIC EFFECTS

Thrombophlebitis, pulmonary embolism occur rarely.

NURSING IMPLICATIONS

BASELINE ASSESSMENT:

Question for possibility of pregnancy before initiating therapy (Pregnancy Category X). Provide support to pt, family, recognizing this drug is palliative, not curative.

PATIENT/FAMILY TEACHING:

Alopecia is reversible, but new hair growth may have different color or texture. Importance of contraception. Notify physician if headache, nausea, breast tenderness, or other symptom persists.

melphalan

melf′ah-lan
(Alkeran)

CANADIAN AVAILABILITY:
Alkeran

CLASSIFICATION

Antineoplastic

PHARMACOKINETICS

Variably, incompletely absorbed from GI tract. Protein binding: <30%. Deactivated in body fluids, tissues. Excreted in urine, eliminated in feces. Half-life: 90 minutes.

ACTION

Cell cycle-phase nonspecific. Primarily crosslinks strands of DNA, RNA. Inhibits protein synthesis.

USES

Treatment of multiple myeloma, nonresectable epithelial carcinoma of ovary.

STORAGE/HANDLING

Store vials at room temperature. Protect from light. After reconstitution, use immediately; do not refrigerate.

IV ADMINISTRATION

NOTE: Use caution, wear gloves when preparing/handling solution. Skin reactions may occur. If contacted w/skin, wash thoroughly w/ soap and water.

1. Reconstitute 50 mg vial w/10 ml sterile diluent to provide concentration of 5 mg/ml.
2. Immediately after reconstitution, further dilute w/0.9% NaCl injection to concentration ≤0.45 mg/ml.
3. Administer over minimum of 15 min.
4. Complete administration within 60 min of reconstitution.

INDICATIONS/DOSAGE/ROUTES

NOTE: May be carcinogenic, mutagenic, or teratogenic. Handle w/ extreme care during administration. Dosage individualized based on clinical response, tolerance to adverse effects. When used in combination therapy, consult specific protocols for optimum dosage, sequence of drug administration. Leukocyte count usually maintained between 3,000-4,000/mm^3.

Ovarian carcinoma:
PO: Adults, elderly: 0.2 mg/kg/day for 5 successive days. Repeat at 4-6 wk intervals.

Multiple myeloma:
PO: Adults, elderly: Initially, 6 mg/day as single dose for 2-3 wks. Discontinue drug for up to 4 wks. **Maintenance:** 2 mg/day when leukocytes, platelets increase.

Usual parenteral dosage:
IV: Adults, elderly: 16 mg/m^2 q2wks × 4 doses, then q4wks.

PRECAUTIONS

CONTRAINDICATIONS: Known hypersensitivity to drug, resistance to previous therapy w/drug. **EXTREME CAUTION:** Compromised bone marrow reserve from previous irradiation or chemotherapy, bone marrow function recovery from previous cytotoxic therapy. **PREGNANCY/LACTATION:** If possible, avoid use during pregnancy, esp. first trimester. May cause fetal harm. Unknown whether drug crosses placenta or distributed in breast milk. Breast feeding not recommended. **Pregnancy Category D.**

INTERACTIONS

DRUG INTERACTIONS: May decrease effect of antigout medications. Bone marrow depressants may increase bone marrow depression. Live virus vaccines may potentiate virus replication, increase vaccine side effects, decrease pt's antibody response to vaccine. **ALTERED LAB VALUES:** May increase uric acid.

SIDE EFFECTS

FREQUENT: Severe nausea, vomiting (large dose). **OCCASIONAL:** Diarrhea, stomatitis, mild nausea, vomiting (usual dose), rash, itching, temporary alopecia.

ADVERSE REACTIONS/TOXIC EFFECTS

Bone marrow depression manifested as hematologic toxicity (principally leukopenia, thrombocytopenia, and to lesser extent, anemia, pancytopenia, agranulocytosis). Leukopenia may occur as early as 5 days. WBC, platelet counts return to normal levels during fifth wk, but leukopenia or thrombocytopenia may last more than 6 wks after discontinuing drug. Hyperuricemia noted by hematuria, crystalluria, flank pain.

NURSING IMPLICATIONS

BASELINE ASSESSMENT:

Obtain blood counts weekly. Dosage may be decreased or discontinued if WBC falls below 3,000/mm^3 or platelet count falls below 100,000/mm^3. Antiemetics may be effective in preventing, treating nausea, vomiting.

INTERVENTION/EVALUATION:

Monitor Hgb, Hct, WBC, differential, platelet count, urinalysis, serum uric acid level. Monitor for stomatitis (burning/erythema of oral mucosa at inner margin of lips, sore throat, difficulty swallowing, oral ulceration). Monitor for hematologic toxicity (fever, sore throat, signs of local infection, easy bruising, unusual bleeding from any site), symptoms of anemia (excessive tiredness, weakness), signs of hyperuricemia (hematuria, flank pain). Avoid IM injections, rectal temperatures, other traumas that may induce bleeding.

PATIENT/FAMILY TEACHING:

Increase fluid intake (may protect against hyperuricemia). Maintain fastidious oral hygiene. Alopecia is reversible, but new hair growth may have different color or texture. Do not have immunizations w/o physician's approval (drug lowers body's resistance). Avoid crowds and those w/infections. Promptly report fever, sore throat, signs of local infection, easy bruising or unusual bleeding from any site, yellow discoloration of eyes or skin, black, tarry stools. Contact physician if nausea/vomiting continues at home. Contraceptives are recommended during therapy.

menotropins

men-oh-troe´pins

(Humegon, Pergonal)

CANADIAN AVAILABILITY:
Pergonal

CLASSIFICATION

Gonadotropin

PHARMACOKINETICS

Well absorbed after IM administration. Excreted in urine. Half-life: *FSH:* 70 hrs, *LH:* 4 hrs.

ACTION

Gonadotropic agent w/follicle-stimulating hormone (FSH) and luteinizing hormone (LH) actions. Promotes ovarian follicular growth and maturation in women; stimulates spermatogenesis in men.

USES

Treatment of infertility: in conjunction w/chorionic gonadotropin (HCG) to stimulate ovulation and pregnancy in women w/secondary ovarian dysfunction and to stimulate spermatogenesis in men w/primary or secondary hypogonadotropic hypogonadism.

STORAGE/HANDLING

Powder for reconstitution may be refrigerated or kept at room temperature.

IM ADMINISTRATION

1. Reconstitute w/1-2 ml 0.9% NaCl injection.
2. Administer immediately after reconstitution; discard unused portion.
3. Give IM only.

INDICATIONS/DOSAGE/ROUTES

Induction ovulation/pregnancy:
IM: Adults: Initially, 75 IU FSH/75 IU LH per day for 9-12 days. Follow w/10,000 IU HCG 1 day after last dose menotropin. May repeat at least 2 courses before increasing dose to 150 IU FSH/150 IU LH if evidence of ovulation, but no pregnancy.
NOTE: Omit HCG if hyperstimulation syndrome likely to occur (total estrogen excretion >100 mcg/24 hrs or estradiol excretion >50 mcg/24 hrs) or ovaries abnormally enlarged on last day of menotropin therapy.

Stimulation of spermatogenesis:
NOTE: Pretreat w/HCG alone (5,000 IU 3 times/wk) until normal serum testosterone level and masculinization. May take 4-6 mo.
IM: Adults: Initially, 75 IU FSH/75 IU LH 3 times/wk and HCG 2,000 IU 2 times/wk for at least 4 mo. If no response, may increase dose to 150 IU FSH/150 IU LH w/same HCG dose.

PRECAUTIONS

CONTRAINDICATIONS: Prior hypersensitivity to menotropins; primary ovarian failure; thyroid or adrenal dysfunction; organic intracranial lesion (e.g., pituitary tumor); ovarian cysts or enlargement not due to polycystic ovary syndrome; abnormal vaginal bleeding of undetermined origin; men w/normal urinary gonadotropin concentrations, primary testicular failure or infertility problems other than hypogonadotropic hypogonadism. **PREGNANCY/LACTATION:** Excretion in breast milk unknown. **Pregnancy Category X.**

INTERACTIONS

DRUG INTERACTIONS: None significant. **ALTERED LAB VALUES:** None significant.

SIDE EFFECTS

OCCASIONAL: Pain, rash, swelling, irritation at injection site; mild to moderate ovarian enlargement w/abdominal distention and pain; gynecomastia in males. **RARE:** Fever and flu-like symptoms, nausea, vomiting, diarrhea.

ADVERSE REACTIONS/TOXIC EFFECTS

Risk of atelectasis and acute respiratory distress syndrome, intravascular thrombosis and embolism, ovarian hyperstimulation syndrome (OHSS), high incidence (20%) of multiple births (premature deliveries and neonatal prematurity), ruptured ovarian cysts.

M

NURSING IMPLICATIONS

BASELINE ASSESSMENT:

Question for prior allergic reaction to drug.

INTERVENTION/EVALUATION:

Monitor carefully for OHSS; early signs include weight gain, severe pelvic pain, nausea, vomiting progressing to ascites, dyspnea; report immediately. (Ascitic, pleural, or pericardial fluids should not be removed unless absolutely necessary because of potential injury to the ovary. Pelvic examination should be avoided due to potential rupture of an ovarian cyst.)

PATIENT/FAMILY TEACHING:

Importance of close physician supervision during treatment. Promptly report abdominal pain/distention, vaginal bleeding or signs of edema (weigh 2-3 times/week; report >5 lb/wk gain or swelling of fingers or feet). In anovulation treatment, proper method of taking/recording daily basal temperature; advise intercourse daily beginning the day preceding HCG treatment. Intercourse should be discontinued w/ significant ovarian enlargement. Possibility of multiple births.

meperidine hydrochloride

meh-pear´ih-deen
(Demerol)

CANADIAN AVAILABILITY:
Demerol

CLASSIFICATION

PHARMACOTHERAPEUTIC: Opiate agonist **(Schedule II)**

CLINICAL: Narcotic analgesic

PHARMACOKINETICS

	ONSET	PEAK	DURATION
PO	15 min	60 min	2-4 hrs
SubQ	10-15 min	30-50 min	2-4 hrs
IM	10-15 min	30-50 min	2-4 hrs
IV	1 min	5-7 min	2-4 hrs

Variably absorbed from GI tract, well absorbed after IM administration. Widely distributed. Protein binding: 65-75%. Metabolized in liver to active metabolite. Primarily excreted in urine. Half-life: 2.4-4 hrs (increased in elderly).

ACTION

Binds w/opioid receptors within CNS, altering processes affecting pain perception, emotional response to pain.

USES

Relief of moderate to severe pain, preop sedation, obstetrical support, anesthesia adjunct.

STORAGE/HANDLING

Store oral, parenteral form at room temperature. Do not use if solution appears cloudy or contains a precipitate.

PO/SubQ/IM/IV ADMINISTRATION

PO:

1. May give w/o regard to meals.
2. Dilute syrup in ½ glass H_2O (prevents anesthetic effect on mucous membranes).

SubQ/IM:

NOTE: IM preferred over SubQ route (SubQ produces pain, local irritation, induration).

1. Administer slowly.
2. Those with circulatory impairment experience higher risk of overdosage due to delayed absorbtion of repeated administration.

IV:

NOTE: Give by slow IV injection or IV infusion. Physically incompatible with amobarbital, aminophylline, ephedrine, heparin, hydrocortisone, methicillin, methylprednisolone, morphine, nitrofurantoin, oxytetracycline, pentobarbital, phenobarbital, secobarbital, sodium bicarbonate, sodium iodide, tetracycline, thiamylal, thiopental, solutions containing potassium iodide, aminosalicylic acid, salicylamide.

1. Dilute in 5% dextrose and lactated Ringer's, dextrose-saline combination, 2.5%, 5%, or 10% dextrose in water, Ringer's, lactated Ringer's, 0.45% or 0.9% NaCl, or ⅙

molar sodium lactate diluent for IV injection or infusion.

2. IV dosage must always be administered very slowly, over 2-3 min.

3. Rapid IV increases risk of severe adverse reactions (chest wall rigidity, apnea, peripheral circulatory collapse, anaphylactoid effects, cardiac arrest).

INDICATIONS/DOSAGE/ROUTES

Pain:
PO/SubQ/IM: Adults: 50-150 mg q3-4h. **Children:** 1.1-1.8 mg/kg q3-4h. Do not exceed single pediatric dose 100 mg.
IV: Adults: 15-35 mg/hr.

Usual elderly dosage:
PO: Elderly: 50 mg q4h as needed.
IM: Elderly: 25 mg q4h as needed.

Preop:
PO/SubQ/IM: Adults: 50-100 mg given as single dose 30-90 min before induction of anesthesia. **Children:** 1-2 mg/kg 30-90 min before anesthesia.

Labor:
IM: Adults: 50-100 mg when labor pains are regular. Repeat at 1-3 hr intervals.

PRECAUTIONS

CONTRAINDICATIONS: Those receiving MAO inhibitors in past 14 days, diarrhea due to poisoning, delivery of premature infant. **EXTREME CAUTION:** Impaired renal, hepatic function, elderly/debilitated, supraventricular tachycardia, cor pulmonale, history of seizures, acute abdominal conditions, increased intracranial pressure, respiratory abnormalities. **PREGNANCY/LACTATION:** Crosses placenta; distributed in breast milk. Respiratory depression may occur in neonate if mother received opiates during labor. Regular use of opiates during pregnancy may produce withdrawal symptoms in neonate (irritability, excessive crying, tremors, hyperactive reflexes, fever, vomiting, diarrhea, yawning, sneezing, seizures). **Pregnancy Category C.**

INTERACTIONS

DRUG INTERACTIONS: Alcohol, CNS depressants may increase CNS, respiratory depression, hypotension. MAO inhibitors may produce severe, fatal reaction (reduce dose to 1/4 usual dose). **ALTERED LAB VALUES:** May increase amylase, lipase.

M

NOTE: Effects are dependent on dosage amount, route of administration. Ambulatory pts and those not in severe pain may experience dizziness, nausea, vomiting more frequently than those in supine position or having severe pain. **FREQUENT:** Sedation, decreased respirations, nausea, vomiting, lightheadedness, dizziness, sweating. **OCCASIONAL:** Euphoria/dysphoria, urinary retention.

ADVERSE REACTIONS/TOXIC EFFECTS

Overdosage results in respiratory depression, skeletal muscle flaccidity, cold, clammy skin, cyanosis, extreme somnolence progressing to convulsions, stupor, coma. Antidote: 0.4 mg naloxone (Narcan). Tolerance to analgesic effect, physical dependence may occur with repeated use.

NURSING IMPLICATIONS

BASELINE ASSESSMENT:

Pt should be in recumbent position before drug is administered by parenteral route. Assess onset, type, location, duration of pain. Obtain vital signs before giving medication. If respirations are 12/min or lower (20/min or lower in children), withhold medication, contact physician. Effect of medication is reduced if full pain recurs before next dose.

INTERVENTION/EVALUATION:

Monitor vital signs 15-30 min after SubQ/IM dose, 5-10 min after IV dose (monitor for decreased B/P, change in rate/quality of pulse). Monitor stools; avoid constipation. Check for adequate voiding. Initiate deep breathing and coughing exercises, particularly in those with impaired pulmonary function.

PATIENT/FAMILY TEACHING:

Medication should be taken before pain fully returns, within ordered intervals. Discomfort may occur with injection. Change positions slowly to avoid orthostatic hypotension. Avoid tasks that require alertness, motor skills until response to drug is established. Increase fluids, bulk to prevent constipation. Tolerance/dependence may occur with prolonged use of high doses. Avoid alcohol and other CNS depressants.

mepivacaine hydrochloride

meh-piv′ah-cane

(Carbocaine, Polocaine)

FIXED-COMBINATION(S):

W/levonordefrin, a vasoconstrictor (Isocaine)

CANADIAN AVAILABILITY:

Carbocaine, Isocaine, Polocaine

(See Classifications section under Anesthetics: local)

mercaptopurine

mur-cap-toe-pure′een

(Purinethol)

CANADIAN AVAILABILITY:

Purinethol

CLASSIFICATION

Antineoplastic

PHARMACOKINETICS

Variably, incompletely absorbed from GI tract. Crosses blood-brain barrier. Protein binding: 20%. Metabolized in liver. Primarily excreted in urine. Removed by hemodialysis. Half-life: 45 min.

ACTION

Cell cycle-specific for S phase of cell division. After activation in tissue, inhibits DNA, RNA synthesis.

USES

Treatment of acute lymphatic (lymphocytic, lymphoblastic) leukemia, acute myelogenous leukemia, acute myelomonocytic leukemia.

INDICATIONS/DOSAGE/ROUTES

NOTE: May be carcinogenic, mutagenic, or teratogenic. Handle w/ extreme care during administration. Dosage individualized based on clinical response, tolerance to adverse effects. When used in combination therapy, consult specific protocols for optimum dosage, sequence of drug administration. Reduce dose in those w/renal impairment.

Induction remission:
PO: Adults, elderly, children: 2.5 mg/kg/day as single dose (100-200 mg in average adults, 50 mg in average children). Increase dose up to 5 mg/kg/day after 4 wks if no improvement and no toxicity.

Maintenance:
PO: Adults, elderly, children: 1.5-2.5 mg/kg/day as single dose.

PRECAUTIONS

CONTRAINDICATIONS: Previous therapy resistance to drug. **EXTREME CAUTION:** Preexisting liver disease. **CAUTIONS:** Impaired liver function. **PREGNANCY/LACTATION:** If possible, avoid use during pregnancy, esp. first trimester. May cause fetal harm. Unknown if distributed in breast milk. Breast feeding not recommended. **Pregnancy Category D.**

INTERACTIONS

DRUG INTERACTIONS: May decrease effect of antigout medications. Bone marrow depressants may increase bone marrow depression. Hepatotoxic medications may increase risk of hepatotoxicity. Immunosuppressants may increase risk of infection, develop neoplasms. Live virus vaccines may potentiate virus replication, increase vaccine side effects, decrease pt's antibody response to vaccine. **ALTERED LAB VALUES:** May increase uric acid.

SIDE EFFECTS

OCCASIONAL: Nausea, vomiting, diarrhea, anorexia, abdominal discomfort, fever, headache, excessive weakness. **RARE:** Oral lesions, hyperpigmentation, rash, alopecia.

ADVERSE REACTIONS/TOXIC EFFECTS

Hepatotoxicity manifested by jaundice, ascites, cholestasis, elevated hepatic enzyme concentrations, severe fibrosis, necrosis, and bone marrow depression manifested as hematologic toxicity (principally leukopenia, anemia, thrombocytopenia, and to lesser extent, pancytopenia, agranulocytosis). Hyperuricemia results in hematuria, crystalluria, and flank pain.

M

NURSING IMPLICATIONS

BASELINE ASSESSMENT:

Risk of hepatic injury increases when dosage exceeds 2.5 mg/kg/day. Hematology tests should be performed weekly. Therapy may be discontinued if large or rapid decrease in WBC or abnormal bone marrow depression occurs, and resumed when WBC or platelet count increases, or remains constant for 2-3 days. Liver function tests should be performed weekly during initial therapy, monthly thereafter.

INTERVENTION/EVALUATION:

Monitor hepatic function tests, hemoglobin/hematocrit, WBC, differential, platelet count, urinalysis. Monitor for hematologic toxicity (fever, sore throat, signs of local infection, easy bruising, unusual bleeding from any site), symptoms of anemia (excessive tiredness, weakness), signs of hyperuricemia (hematuria, flank pain). Avoid IM injections, rectal temperatures or other traumas that may induce bleeding.

PATIENT/FAMILY TEACHING:

Increase fluid intake (may protect against hyperuricemia). Do not have immunizations w/o physician's approval (drug lowers body's resistance). Avoid crowds and those w/infection. Promptly report fever, sore throat, signs of local infection, easy bruising, unusual bleeding from any site, yellow skin or eyes, dark urine, pale stools. Contact physician if nausea/vomiting continues at home. Do not take alcohol or medications w/o consulting physician. Contraception should be practiced during therapy.

mesalamine (5-aminosalicylic acid, 5-ASA)

mess-ale´ah-meen
(Asacol, Pentasa, Rowasa)

CANADIAN AVAILABILITY:
Salofalk

CLASSIFICATION

Anti-inflammatory agent

PHARMACOKINETICS

Poorly absorbed from colon. Moderately absorbed from GI tract. Metabolized in liver to active metabolite. Unabsorbed portion eliminated in feces; absorbed portion excreted in urine. Half-life: 0.5-1.5 hrs; metabolite: 5-10 hrs.

ACTION

Blocks prostaglandin synthesis in colon. Produces local inhibitory effect on arachidonic acid metabolite production (increase in pt's w/chronic inflammatory bowel disease).

USES

Treatment of active mild to moderate distal ulcerative colitis, proctosigmoiditis or proctitis.

STORAGE/HANDLING

Store rectal suspension, suppository, oral forms at room temperature.

PO/RECTAL ADMINISTRATION

PO:

1. Have pt swallow whole; do not break outer coating of tablet.
2. May take w/o regard to food.

RECTAL:

1. Shake bottle well.
2. Instruct pt to lie on left side with lower leg extended, upper leg flexed forward.
3. Knee-chest position may also be used.
4. Insert applicator tip into rectum, pointing toward umbilicus.
5. Squeeze bottle steadily until contents are emptied.

INDICATIONS/DOSAGE/ROUTES

Ulcerative colitis, proctosigmoiditis, proctitis:
RECTAL: Adults, elderly: (suppository) 500 mg 2 times/day. Retain 1-3 hrs. (suspension) 4 Gm (60 ml) daily, preferably at bedtime.
PO: Adults, elderly: *(Asacol):* 800 mg 3 times/day for 6 wks; *(Pentasa):* 1 Gm 4 times/day for 8 wks.

PRECAUTIONS

CONTRAINDICATIONS: None significant. **CAUTIONS:** Preexisting renal disease, sulfasalazine sensitivity. **PREGNANCY/LAC-**

TATION: Unknown whether drug crosses placenta or is distributed in breast milk. **Pregnancy Category B.**

INTERACTIONS

DRUG INTERACTIONS: None significant. **ALTERED LAB VALUES:** May increase SGOT (AST), SGPT (ALT), alkaline phosphatase, BUN, serum creatinine.

SIDE EFFECTS

NOTE: Generally well tolerated, with only mild and transient effects. **OCCASIONAL:** Flatulence, nausea, fatigue. **RARE:** Dizziness, bloating, back pain, hair loss.

ADVERSE REACTIONS/TOXIC EFFECTS

Sulfite sensitivity in susceptible pts noted as cramping, headache, diarrhea, fever, rash, hives, itching, wheezing. Discontinue drug immediately.

NURSING IMPLICATIONS

INTERVENTION/EVALUATION:

Encourage adequate fluid intake. Assess bowel sounds for peristalsis. Monitor daily bowel activity and stool consistency (watery, loose, soft, semi-solid, solid) and record time of evacuation. Assess for abdominal disturbances. Assess skin for rash, hives. Discontinue medication if rash, fever, cramping, or diarrhea occurs.

PATIENT/FAMILY TEACHING:

Avoid tasks that require alertness, motor skills until response to drug is established.

mesna

mess´nah
(Mesnex)

CANADIAN AVAILABILITY:
Uromitexan

CLASSIFICATION

Antidote

PHARMACOKINETICS

Rapidly metabolized after IV administration to mesna disulfide, which is reduced to mesna in kidney. Excreted in urine. Half-life: 0.36 hrs.

ACTION

Reduced to free thiol compound, mesna, which reacts with urotoxic ifosfamide metabolites (detoxification). Inhibits ifosfamide induced hemorrhagic cystitis.

USES

Decreased incidence of ifosfamide-induced hemorrhagic cystitis.

STORAGE/HANDLING

Store parenteral form at room temperature. After dilution, stable for 24 hrs at room temperature (recommended use within 6 hrs). Discard unused medication.

IV ADMINISTRATION

1. Dilute each 100 mg with 5% dextrose or 0.9% NaCl to provide concentration of 20 mg/ml.
2. Administer direct IV injection.

INDICATIONS/DOSAGE/ROUTES

Hemorrhagic cystitis:
IV: Adults, elderly: 20% of ifosfamide dose at time of ifosfamide administration and 4 and 8 hrs after each dose of ifosfamide. Total dose: 60% of ifosfamide dosage.

PRECAUTIONS

CONTRAINDICATIONS: None significant. **CAUTIONS:** None significant. **PREGNANCY/LACTA-**

TION: Unknown whether drug crosses placenta or is distributed in breast milk. **Pregnancy Category B.**

INTERACTIONS

DRUG INTERACTIONS: None significant. **ALTERED LAB VALUES:** May produce false positive test for urinary ketones.

SIDE EFFECTS

FREQUENT: Bad taste in mouth, soft stools. Large doses: Diarrhea, limb pain, headache, fatigue, nausea, hypotension, allergic reaction.

ADVERSE REACTIONS/TOXIC EFFECTS

Occasionally, hematuria develops.

NURSING IMPLICATIONS

Baseline Assessment:

Each dose must be administered with ifosfamide.

Intervention/Evaluation:

Assess morning urine specimen for hematuria. If such occurs, dosage reduction or discontinuation may be necessary. Monitor daily bowel activity and stool consistency (watery, loose, soft, semisolid, solid) and record time of evacuation. Monitor B/P for hypotension.

Patient/Family Teaching:

Inform physician/nurse if headache, limb pain, or nausea occurs.

mesoridazine besylate

mess-oh-rid´ah-zeen

(Serentil)

CANADIAN AVAILABILITY: Serentil

CLASSIFICATION

Antipsychotic

PHARMACOKINETICS

Variably absorbed from GI tract. Protein binding: >90%. Metabolized in liver to some active metabolites. Primarily excreted in urine. Half-life: 20-40 hrs.

ACTION

Blocks postsynaptic dopaminergic receptors in brain. Possesses strong alpha-adrenergic blocking, anticholinergic effects.

USES

Symptomatic management of psychotic disorders, treatment of hyperactivity, uncooperativeness associated w/mental deficiency, chronic brain syndrome; as adjunctive treatment of alcohol dependence, management of anxiety/tension associated w/neurosis.

STORAGE/HANDLING

Store oral, parenteral form at room temperature. Yellow discoloration of solution does not affect potency, but discard if markedly discolored or if precipitate forms.

PO/IM ADMINISTRATION

PO:

1. Dilute oral solution w/water, orange, grape juice.

IM:

NOTE: Pt must remain recumbent for 30-60 min in head-low position w/legs raised, to minimize hypotensive effect.

1. Inject slow, deep IM into upper outer quadrant of gluteus maximus. If irritation occurs, further injections may be diluted w/0.9% NaCl or 2% procaine hydrochloride.

2. Massage IM injection site to reduce discomfort.

INDICATIONS/DOSAGE/ROUTES

NOTE: Increase dosage gradually to optimum response, then decrease to lowest effective level for maintenance. Replace parenteral therapy w/oral therapy as soon as possible.

Usual parenteral dosage:
IM: Adults, children >12 yrs: 25 mg given as single dose. May repeat in 30-60 min, if needed. **Maximum dose:** 200 mg/day.

Psychotic disorders:
PO: Adults, children >12 yrs: Initially, 50 mg 3 times/day. **Maintenance:** 100-400 mg/day.

Hyperactivity:
PO: Adults, children >12 yrs: 25 mg 3 times/day. **Maintenance:** 75-300 mg/day.

Alcohol dependence:
PO: Adults, children >12 yrs: 25 mg twice/day. **Maintenance:** 50-200 mg/day.

Anxiety/tension:
PO: Adults, children >12 yrs: 10 mg 3 times/day. **Maintenance:** 30-150 mg/day.

Usual elderly dosage (nonpsychotic):
PO: Elderly: Initially, 10 mg 1-2 times/day. May increase by 10-25 mg/day every 7-10 days. **Maximum:** 250 mg/day.

PRECAUTIONS

CONTRAINDICATIONS: Severe CNS depression, comatose states, severe cardiovascular disease, bone marrow depression, subcortical brain damage. **CAUTIONS:** Impaired respiratory/hepatic/renal/cardiac function, alcohol withdrawal, history of seizures, urinary retention, glaucoma, prostatic hypertrophy. **PREGNANCY/LACTATION:** Crosses placenta, distributed in breast milk. **Pregnancy Category C.**

INTERACTIONS

DRUG INTERACTIONS: Alcohol, CNS depressants may increase CNS, respiratory depression, hypotensive effects. Tricyclic antidepressants, MAO inhibitors may increase sedative, anticholinergic effects. Antithyroid agents may increase risk of agranulocytosis. Extrapyramidal symptoms (EPS) may increase w/EPS producing medications. Hypotensives may increase hypotension. May decrease levodopa effects. Lithium may decrease absorption, produce adverse neurologic effects.

SIDE EFFECTS

FREQUENT: Hypotension, dizziness and fainting occur frequently after first injection, occasionally after subsequent injections, and rarely w/oral dosage. **OCCASIONAL:** Drowsiness during early therapy, dry mouth, blurred vision, lethargy, constipation or diarrhea, nasal congestion, peripheral edema, urinary retention. **RARE:** Ocular changes, skin pigmentation (those on high doses for prolonged periods).

ADVERSE REACTIONS/TOXIC EFFECTS

Extrapyramidal symptoms appear dose-related (particularly high dosage), and is divided into three categories: akathisia (inability to sit still, tapping of feet, urge to move around), parkinsonian symptoms (mask-like face, tremors, shuffling gait, hypersalivation), and acute dystonias: torticollis (neck muscle spasm), opisthotonos (rigidity of back muscles), and oculogyric crisis (rolling back of eyes). Dystonic reaction may also produce profuse sweating, pallor. Tardive dyskinesia (protrusion of tongue, puffing of cheeks, chewing/puckering of the mouth) occurs rarely (may be irreversible). Abrupt withdrawal following long-term therapy may precipitate nausea, vomiting, gastritis, dizziness, tremors. Blood dyscrasias, particularly agranulocytosis, mild leukopenia (sore mouth/gums/throat) may occur. May lower seizure threshold.

NURSING IMPLICATIONS

BASELINE ASSESSMENT:

Avoid skin contact w/solution (contact dermatitis). Assess behavior, appearance, emotional status, response to environment, speech pattern, thought content.

INTERVENTION/EVALUATION:

Monitor B/P for hypotension. Assess for extrapyramidal symptoms. Monitor WBC, differential count for blood dyscrasias. Monitor for fine tongue movement (may be early sign of tardive dyskinesia). Supervise suicidal-risk pt closely during early therapy (as depression lessens, energy level improves, increasing suicide potential). Assess for therapeutic response (interest in surroundings, improvement in self-care, increased ability to concentrate, relaxed facial expression).

PATIENT/FAMILY TEACHING:

Full therapeutic effect may take up to 6 wks. Urine may become pink, reddish brown. Do not abruptly withdraw from long-term drug therapy. Report visual disturbances. Sugarless gum or sips of tepid water may relieve dry mouth. Drowsiness generally subsides during continued therapy. Avoid tasks that require alertness, motor skills until response to drug is established. Do not use alcohol or other CNS depressants. Use sunscreen, protective clothing for possible photosensitivity.

metaproterenol sulfate

met-ah-pro-tair′in-all
(Alupent, Metaprel)

CANADIAN AVAILABILITY:
Alupent

CLASSIFICATION

Bronchodilator

PHARMACOKINETICS

	ONSET	PEAK	DURATION
Aerosol	1 min	1 hr	4 hrs
PO	15 min	1 hr	4 hrs
Nebulization	5-30 min	1 hr	3-4 hrs

Partially absorbed from GI tract, minimal after inhalation. Metabolized in liver. Primarily excreted in urine.

ACTION

Stimulates $beta_2$-adrenergic receptors in lungs (relaxes bronchial smooth muscle by increasing cAMP). Relieves bronchospasm, reduces airway resistance.

USES

Relief of reversible bronchospasm due to bronchial asthma, bronchitis, emphysema.

STORAGE/HANDLING

Do not use solution for nebulization if brown in color or contains a precipitate.

PO/INHALATION ADMINISTRATION

AEROSOL:

1. Shake container well, exhale completely, then holding mouthpiece 1 inch away from lips, inhale and hold breath as long as possible before exhaling.
2. Wait 1-10 min before inhaling second dose (allows for deeper bronchial penetration).
3. Rinse mouth w/water immediately after inhalation (prevents mouth/throat dryness).

PO:

1. Give w/o regard to meals.
2. Tablets may be crushed.

NEBULIZATION:

1. Administer undiluted solution in hand nebulizer .

IPPB: Dilute in 2.5 ml saline solution.

INDICATIONS/DOSAGE/ROUTES

Bronchospasm:
Metered-dose inhalation: Adults, elderly, children >12 yrs: 2-3 inhalations as single dose. Wait 2 min before administering second dose. Do not repeat for 3-4 hrs. **Maximum:** 12 inhalations/day.
PO: Adults, children >9 yrs or weigh >60 lb: 20 mg 3-4 times/day. **Children 6-9 yrs or weigh <60 lb:** 10 mg 3-4 times/day.
Nebulization: Adults, elderly, children >12 yrs: 10 inhalations (range 5-15 inhalations) of undiluted 5% solution, up to 3-4 times/day.
IPPB: Adults, elderly: 0.3 ml 3-4 times/day. May repeat no more often than q4h.

Usual elderly dosage:
PO: Elderly: Initially, 10 mg 3-4 times/day. May increase up to 20 mg 3-4 times/day.

PRECAUTIONS

CONTRAINDICATIONS: Preexisting arrhythmias. **CAUTIONS:** Impaired cardiac function, diabetes mellitus, hypertension, hyperthyroidism. **PREGNANCY/LACTATION:** Unknown whether drug crosses placenta or is distributed in breast milk. May inhibit uterine contractility. **Pregnancy Category C.**

INTERACTIONS

DRUG INTERACTIONS: Tricyclic antidepressants may increase cardiovascular effects. MAO inhibitors may increase risk of hypertensive crises. May decrease effects of beta-blockers. Digoxin, sympathomimetics may increase risk of arrhythmias. **ALTERED LAB VALUES:** May decrease serum potassium levels.

SIDE EFFECTS

FREQUENT: Shakiness, restlessness, palpitations, and mild, transient nausea if taken on an empty stomach. Drying or irritation of oropharynx with inhalation therapy. **OCCASIONAL:** Muscle cramping in extremities.

ADVERSE REACTIONS/TOXIC EFFECTS

Excessive sympathomimetic stimulation may cause palpitations, extrasystoles, tachycardia, chest pain, slight increase in B/P followed by a substantial decrease, chills, sweating, and blanching of skin. Too-frequent or excessive use may lead to loss of bronchodilating effectiveness and/or severe, paradoxical bronchoconstriction.

NURSING IMPLICATIONS

BASELINE ASSESSMENT:

Offer emotional support (high incidence of anxiety because of difficulty in breathing and sympathomimetic response to drug).

INTERVENTION/EVALUATION:

Monitor rate, depth, rhythm, type of respiration; quality and rate of pulse. Assess lung sounds for rhonchi, wheezing, rales. Monitor arterial blood gases. Observe lips, fingernails for blue or dusky color in light-skinned pts; gray in dark-skinned pts. Observe for clavicular retractions, hand tremor. Evaluate for clinical improvement (quieter, slower respirations, relaxed facial expression, cessation of clavicular retractions).

PATIENT/FAMILY TEACHING:

Increase fluid intake (decreases lung secretion viscosity). Do not take more than 2 inhalations at any one time (excessive use may produce paradoxical bronchoconstriction, or a decreased bronchodilating effect). Rinsing mouth w/water immediately after inhalation may prevent mouth/throat dryness. Avoid excessive use of caffeine derivatives (chocolate, coffee, tea, cola, cocoa).

metaraminol bitartrate

met-ah-ram′in-all

(Aramine)

CLASSIFICATION

Sympathomimetic

PHARMACOKINETICS

	ONSET	PEAK	DURATION
SubQ	5-20 min	—	1 hr
IM	10 min	—	1 hr
IV	1-2 min	—	20 min

Well absorbed after IM administration. Metabolized in liver. Excreted in urine, eliminated in feces via biliary system.

ACTION

Directly stimulates alpha-adrenergic receptors (produces vasoconstriction), indirectly releases norepinephrine from its storage sites. Stimulates $beta_1$-adrenergic receptors (produces cardiac stimulation).

USES

Treatment of hypotension caused by spinal anesthesia and produces vasoconstriction, cardiac stimulation in hypotensive states caused by hemorrhage, drug reactions, surgical complications, or shock resulting from trauma or tumor.

STORAGE/HANDLING

Store at room temperature. Use within 24 hrs after mixing with infusion diluent.

IM/IV ADMINISTRATION

NOTE: Hypovolemia should be corrected before therapy begins. Avoid SubQ, if possible (may result in local tissue injury).

IM:

1. Inject deeply into large muscle mass.

IV INFUSION:

1. **Adult:** Add 15-100 mg metaraminol to 500 ml 5% dextrose or 0.9% NaCl. **Children:** Add 1 mg metaraminol to 25 ml diluent.
2. Administer in large veins of antecubital fossa or thigh (do not use veins in ankle or dorsum of hand).
3. Rate of infusion should be adjusted according to pt B/P.
4. Systolic B/P should be maintained at 80-100 mm Hg in previously normotensive pts, 30-40 mm Hg below the normal B/P in previously hypertensive pts.
5. When discontinuing IV, slow infusion rate gradually.
6. Therapy should not be reinstated unless B/P falls to 70-80 mm Hg.
7. If extravasation occurs, immediately infiltrate liberally with 10-15 ml sterile saline containing 5-10 mg phentolamine mesylate.

INDICATIONS/DOSAGE/ROUTES

Hypotension:
IV INFUSUION: Adults, elderly: 15-100 mg in 250-500 ml D5W or NaCl. Infuse to maintain B/P at desired level.

Shock:
IV: Adults, elderly: 0.5-5 mg IV push, then IV infusion as noted above.

PRECAUTIONS

CONTRAINDICATIONS: Mesenteric/peripheral vascular thrombosis, profound hypoxia. **CAUTIONS:** Severe cardiac disease, hypertensive and hypothyroid pts, diabetes mellitus, cirrhosis, digitalized pts, pts on MAO inhibitors. **PREGNANCY/LACTATION:** Unknown whether drug crosses placenta or is distributed in breast milk. Fetal anoxia may occur because of uterine contractility. **Pregnancy Category C.**

M

INTERACTIONS

DRUG INTERACTIONS: Tricyclic antidepressants, maprotiline may increase cardiovascular effects. May decrease effects of beta-blockers. Ergonovine, methergine, oxytocin may increase vasoconstriction. Digoxin, sympathomimetics may increase risk of arrhythmias. MAO inhibitors may prolong, intensify cardiac stimulation, vasopressor effects. **ALTERED LAB VALUES:** None significant.

SIDE EFFECTS

OCCASIONAL: Anxiety, weakness, dizziness, flushing, pallor, sweating, headache. Hypovolemic pts may experience reduced urine flow, peripheral vasoconstriction.

ADVERSE REACTIONS/TOXIC EFFECTS

Overdosage may produce palpitation, bradycardia, cardiac arrhythmias. Extravasation may produce tissue necrosis and sloughing. Prolonged therapy may result in plasma volume depletion. Hypotension may recur if plasma volume is not maintained.

NURSING IMPLICATIONS

BASELINE ASSESSMENT:

Obtain B/P, pulse, respirations before administering drug. Never leave pt alone during IV infusion.

INTERVENTION/EVALUATION:

Monitor B/P q2min until stabilized, q5min during infusion. Monitor IV infusion site closely for free flow. Assess for extravasation characterized by blanching of skin over vein, coolness (results from local vasoconstriction). Assess color and temperature of IV site extremity for pallor, cyanosis, mottling. Assess nailbed capillary refill. Monitor I&O diligently (drug produces reduced renal profusion). Assess B/P (be alert to severe B/P drop).

metformin (Glucophage)
See supplement

methadone hydrochloride

meth´ah-doan
(Dolophine)

CLASSIFICATION

Opioid analgesic **(Schedule II)**

PHARMACOKINETICS

	ONSET	PEAK	DURATION
PO	30-60 min	0.5-1 hr	4-6 hrs
SubQ	10-15 min	—	4-6 hrs
IM	10-15 min	—	4-6 hrs

Well absorbed after IM injection. Protein binding: 80-85%. Metabolized in liver. Primarily excreted in urine. Half-life: 15-25 hrs.

ACTION

Binds w/opioid receptors within CNS, altering processes affecting pain perception, emotional response to pain.

USES

Relief of severe pain, detoxification and temporary maintenance treatment of narcotic abstinence syndrome.

STORAGE/HANDLING

Store oral, parenteral form at room temperature. Do not use if solution appears cloudy or contains a precipitate.

PO/SubQ/IM ADMINISTRATION

PO:

1. May give w/o regard to meals.
2. Dilute syrup in ½ glass H_2O (prevents anesthetic effect on mucous membranes).

SubQ/IM:

NOTE: IM preferred over SubQ route (SubQ produces pain, local irritation, induration).

1. Administer slowly.
2. Those w/circulating impairment experience higher risk of overdosage because of delayed absorption of repeated administration.

INDICATIONS/DOSAGE/ROUTES

Pain:
PO/SubQ/IM: Adults: 2.5-10 mg q3-4h as necessary. **Elderly:** 2.5 mg q8-12h.

Detoxification:
NOTE: Refer to local FDA-approved methadone programs.
PO: Adults: 15-40 mg/day until suppression of withdrawal symptoms. **Maintenance:** 20-100 mg/day.

PRECAUTIONS

CONTRAINDICATIONS: Hyper-

sensitivity to narcotics, diarrhea due to poisoning, delivery of premature infant, during labor. **EXTREME CAUTION:** Impaired renal, hepatic function, elderly/debilitated, supraventricular tachycardia, cor pulmonale, history of seizures, acute abdominal conditions, increased intracranial pressure, respiratory abnormalities. **PREGNANCY/LACTATION:** Crosses placenta; distributed in breast milk. Respiratory depression may occur in neonate if mother received opiates during labor. Regular use of opiates during pregnancy may produce withdrawal symptoms in neonate (irritability, excessive crying, tremors, hyperactive reflexes, fever, vomiting, diarrhea, yawning, sneezing, seizures). **Pregnancy Category C.**

INTERACTIONS

DRUG INTERACTIONS: Alcohol, CNS depressants may increase CNS, respiratory depression, hypotension. MAO inhibitors may produce severe, fatal reaction (reduce dose to 1/4 usual dose). Effects may be decreased w/buprenorphine. **ALTERED LAB VALUES:** May increase amylase, lipase.

SIDE EFFECTS

NOTE: Effects are dependent on dosage amount, route of administration. Ambulatory pts and those not in severe pain may experience dizziness, nausea, vomiting more frequently than those in supine position or having severe pain. **FREQUENT:** Sedation, decreased respirations, nausea, vomiting/constipation, lightheadedness, dizziness, sweating. **OCCASIONAL:** Euphoria/dysphoria, urinary retention.

ADVERSE REACTIONS/TOXIC EFFECTS

Overdosage results in respiratory depression, skeletal muscle flaccidity, cold, clammy skin, cyanosis, extreme somnolence progressing to convulsions, stupor, coma. *Antidote:* 0.4 mg naloxone (Narcan). Tolerance to analgesic effect, physical dependence may occur w/repeated use.

NURSING IMPLICATIONS

BASELINE ASSESSMENT:

Pt should be in recumbent position before drug is administered by parenteral route. Assess onset, type, location, duration of pain. Obtain vital signs before giving medication. If respirations are 12/min or lower (20/min or lower in children), withhold medication, contact physician. Effect of medication is reduced if full pain recurs before next dose.

INTERVENTION/EVALUATION:

Monitor vital signs 15-30 min after SubQ/IM dose, 5-10 min after IV dose (monitor for decreased B/P and/or respirations, change in rate or quality of pulse). Oral medication is one-half as potent as parenteral. Assess for adequate voiding. Monitor stools; avoid constipation with increased fluids, bulky foods, and exercise. Initiate deep breathing and coughing exercises, particularly in those w/impaired pulmonary function. Assess for clinical improvement and record onset of relief of pain. Provide support to pt in detoxification program; monitor for withdrawal symptoms.

PATIENT/FAMILY TEACHING:

Discomfort may occur with injection. Change positions slowly to avoid orthostatic hypotension. Avoid tasks that require alertness, motor skills until response to drug is established. Tolerance/dependence may occur w/prolonged use of high doses. Do not take alcohol or other CNS depressants.

methazolamide

meth-ah-zole´ah-myd
(Neptazane)

CANADIAN AVAILABILITY: Neptazane

CLASSIFICATION

Carbonic anhydrase inhibitor

PHARMACOKINETICS

	ONSET	PEAK	DURATION
PO	2-4 hrs	6-8 hrs	10-18 hrs

Slowly, completely absorbed from GI tract. Widely distributed. Protein binding: moderate. Partially metabolized in liver. Primarily excreted in urine. Half-life: 14 hrs.

ACTION

Reduces formation of hydrogen and bicarbonate ions from carbon dioxide and water by inhibiting, in proximal renal tubule, the enzyme carbonic anhydrase, thereby promoting renal excretion along with potassium, bicarbonate, water. Reduces aqueous humor formation. Reduces intraocular pressure.

USES

Treatment of open-angle (noncongestive, chronic simple) glaucoma. Used prior to surgery in correction of acute angle-closure (obstructive, narrow-angle glaucoma).

PO ADMINISTRATION

1. Scored tablet may be crushed.
2. May give w/food if GI upset occurs.

INDICATIONS/DOSAGE/ROUTES

Glaucoma:
PO: Adults, elderly: 50-100 mg 2-3 times/day.

PRECAUTIONS

CONTRAINDICATIONS: Hypersensitivity to sulfonamides, severe renal disease, adrenal insufficiency, hypochloremic acidosis. **CAUTIONS:** History of hypercalcemia, diabetes mellitus, gout, digitalized patients, obstructive pulmonary disease. **PREGNANCY/LACTATION:** Unknown whether drug crosses placenta or is distributed in breast milk. May produce skeletal anomalies, embryocidal effects at high doses. **Pregnancy Category C.**

INTERACTIONS

DRUG INTERACTIONS: May increase excretion of lithium; decrease excretion of quinidine, procainamide, methenamine. May increase digoxin toxicity due to hypokalemia. **ALTERED LAB VALUES:** May increase ammonia, bilirubin, glucose, chloride, uric acid, calcium; may decrease bicarbonate, potassium.

SIDE EFFECTS

OCCASIONAL: Paresthesia in extremities/lips/mouth/anus, anorexia, polyuria, drowsiness, confusion. **RARE:** Nausea, vomiting, diarrhea, altered taste or smell, excessive thirst, headache, malaise, irritability, sedation, dizziness.

ADVERSE REACTIONS/TOXIC EFFECTS

Long-term therapy may result in acidotic state. Bone marrow depression may be manifested as aplastic anemia, thrombocytopenia or thrombocytopenic purpura, leukopenia, agranulocytosis, hemolytic anemia. Renal effects may include dysuria, crystalluria, renal colic/calculi.

NURSING IMPLICATIONS

BASELINE ASSESSMENT:

Assess peripheral vision, acuity. Assess affected pupil for dilation, response to light.

INTERVENTION/EVALUATION:

Monitor I&O, BUN, electrolytes (particularly serum potassium). Monitor pattern of daily bowel activity and stool consistency. Observe for signs of infection (fever, sore throat, unusual bleeding/bruising, fatigue) due to bone marrow depression. Monitor for acidosis (headache, lethargy progressing to drowsiness, CNS depression, Kussmaul respiration).

PATIENT/FAMILY TEACHING:

Report presence of tingling or tremor in hands or feet, unusual bleeding/bruising, unexplained fever, sore throat, flank pain. Avoid tasks that require alertness, motor skills until response to drug is established.

methenamine hippurate

meth-en´ah-meen

(Hiprex, Urex)

methenamine mandelate

(Mandelamine, Mandelets)

FIXED-COMBINATION(S):
W/hyoscyamine, an antispasmodic (Urisedamine); w/belladonna alkaloids, an anticholinergic/antispasmodic, and salicylate, an analgesic (Urised).

CANADIAN AVAILABILITY:
Hip-Rex, Mandelamine

CLASSIFICATION

Anti-infective

PHARMACOKINETICS

Readily absorbed from GI tract. Widely distributed. Metabolized in liver. Primarily excreted in urine. Half-life: 4.3 hrs.

ACTION

In acid medium (urine), methenamine is hydrolyzed to formaldehyde, a nonspecific antibacterial agent (usually bactericidal).

USES

Prophylaxis or suppression of recurrent urinary tract infections.

PO ADMINISTRATION

1. Administer after meals, bedtime.
2. Restrict alkalinizing foods, e.g., milk products, medication.
3. Drink sufficient fluids.
4. Do not crush enteric coated tablets, swallow whole.

INDICATIONS/DOSAGE/ROUTES

Prophylaxis and suppression of urinary tract infections:
PO: Adults, elderly: (Mandelate): 1 Gm 4 times/day. (Hippurate): 1 Gm 2 times/day. **Children, 6-12**

M

yrs: (Mandelate): 500 mg 4 times/day. (Hippurate): 500 mg-1 Gm 2 times/day. **Children <6 yrs:** (Mandelate): 18.4 mg/kg 4 times/day. (Hippurate): None.

PRECAUTIONS

CONTRAINDICATIONS: Hypersensitivity to methenamine, renal insufficiency, severe hepatic impairment, dehydration. Not for use alone in acute infections. **CAUTIONS:** Elderly, debilitated due to potential for lipid pneumonia w/oral suspension of methenamine mandelate (oil base). Tartrazine sensitivity when administering methenamine hippurate (frequently in those sensitive to aspirin). Do not use in those w/renal and/or severe liver impairment. **PREGNANCY/LACTATION:** Crosses placenta, distributed in breast milk. **Pregnancy Category C.**

INTERACTIONS

DRUG INTERACTIONS: Urinary alkalizers (e.g., antacids), thiazide diuretics may decrease effect. **ALTERED LAB VALUES:** May falsely increase 17-hydroxycorticosteroids. May falsely decrease 5-HIAA.

SIDE EFFECTS

FREQUENT: Anorexia, nausea, vomiting, abdominal cramps, diarrhea. **RARE:** Headache, generalized edema, dyspnea, hypersensitivity reaction: rash, pruritus, urticaria. Bladder irritation, frequency, hematuria, dysuria, crystalluria have occurred w/high dosages.

ADVERSE REACTIONS/TOXIC EFFECTS

Lipid pneumonia occurs rarely.

NURSING IMPLICATIONS

BASELINE ASSESSMENT:

Question for history of hypersensitivity to methenamine, tartrazine, or aspirin. Obtain specimens for diagnostic tests before giving first dose (therapy may begin before results are known).

INTERVENTION/EVALUATION:

Evaluate food tolerance. Determine pattern of bowel activity. Assess skin for rash, urticaria; inquire about pruritus. Be alert to frequent or painful micturition, hematuria. Monitor I&O, culture and sensitivity results.

PATIENT/FAMILY TEACHING:

Take after meals and at bedtime. Avoid large intake of milk products. Do not take other medications, esp. antacids w/o checking w/physician. Drink adequate fluids at and between meals. Take full course of therapy. Notify physician in event of rash, painful or difficult urination, GI upset.

methicillin sodium

meth´ih-sill-in
(Staphcillin)

CLASSIFICATION

Antibiotic: Penicillin

PHARMACOKINETICS

Widely distributed. Protein binding: 40%. Partially metabolized in liver. Primarily excreted in urine. Half-life: 0.4-0.8 hrs (increased in decreased renal function).

ACTION

Bactericidal. Binds to bacterial membranes. Inhibits cell wall synthesis.

USES

Treatment of respiratory tract, skin/skin structure infections, osteomyelitis, meningitis, endocarditis, perioperatively esp. cardiovascular, orthopedic procedures. Predominantly treatment of infections caused by penicillinase-producing staphylococci.

STORAGE/HANDLING

Solution for IM injection is stable for 24 hrs at room temperature, 96 hrs if refrigerated; IV infusion (piggyback) is stable for 8 hrs at room temperature. Discard if precipitate forms.

IM/IV ADMINISTRATION

NOTE: Space doses evenly around the clock for full effectiveness.

IM:

1. Reconstitute 500 mg vial w/ 1.5 ml sterile water for injection or 0.9% NaCl injection to provide concentration of 500 mg/ml.
2. Inject IM deeply into gluteus maximus.
3. Administer IM injection slowly.

IV:

1. For IV injection, further dilute w/20-25 ml sterile water for injection or 0.9% NaCl injection; administer at rate of 10 ml/min.
2. For intermittent IV infusion (piggyback), further dilute w/50-100 ml 5% dextrose, 0.9% NaCl or other compatible IV fluid; infuse over 20-30 min.
3. Alternating IV sites, use large veins to reduce risk of phlebitis.
4. Because of potential for hypersensitivity/anaphylaxis, start initial dose at few drops per minute, increase slowly to ordered rate; stay w/pt first 10-15 min, then check q10min.

INDICATIONS/DOSAGE/ROUTES

Usual adult dosage:
IM/IV: Adults, elderly: 1-2 Gm q4-6h.

Usual pediatric dosage:
IM/IV: Children >1 mo: 100-300 mg/kg/day in divided doses q4-6h.

Usual dosage (neonates):
IM/IV: Neonates 0-7 days, <2 kg: 50-100 mg/kg/day in divided doses q12h. **Neonates 7-28 days, <2 kg or 0-7 days, >2 kg:** 75-150 mg/kg/day in divided doses q8h. **Neonates 7-28 days, >2 kg:** 100-200 mg/kg/day in divided doses q6h.

PRECAUTIONS

CONTRAINDICATIONS: Hypersensitivity to any penicillin. **CAUTIONS:** Renal impairment, history of allergies, particularly cephalosporins. **PREGNANCY/LACTATION:** Readily crosses placenta, appears in cord blood, amniotic fluid. Distributed in breast milk in low concentrations. May lead to allergic sensitization, diarrhea, candidiasis, skin rash in infant. **Pregnancy Category B.**

INTERACTIONS

DRUG INTERACTIONS: Probenecid may increase concentration, toxicity risk. **ALTERED LAB VALUES:** May increase SGOT (AST). May cause positive Coombs' test.

SIDE EFFECTS

FREQUENT: Mild hypersensitivity reaction (fever, rash, pruritus), nausea, vomiting, diarrhea more common w/oral therapy. **OCCASIONAL:** Phlebitis, thrombophlebitis (more common in elderly). **RARE:** Sterile abscess at IM injection site.

ADVERSE REACTIONS/TOXIC EFFECTS

Superinfections, potentially fatal antibiotic-associated colitis may result from bacterial imbalance. Neurotoxicity w/IV methicillin. Adverse hematologic effects, severe hypersensitivity reactions, rarely anaphylaxis. Acute interstitial nephritis occurs occasionally.

NURSING IMPLICATIONS

BASELINE ASSESSMENT:

Question history of allergies, esp. penicillins, cephalosporins. Obtain specimen for culture and sensitivity before giving first dose (therapy may begin before results are known).

INTERVENTION/EVALUATION:

Hold medication and promptly report rash (possible hypersensitivity) or diarrhea (w/fever, abdominal pain, mucous and blood in stool may indicate antibiotic-associated colitis). Assess food tolerance. Evaluate IV site for phlebitis (heat, pain, red streaking over vein). Monitor I&O; check for hematuria. Assess IM injection sites for pain, induration. Be alert for superinfection: increased fever, onset sore throat, nausea, vomiting, diarrhea, ulceration or changes of oral mucosa, anal/genital pruritus. Check hematology reports (esp. WBCs), periodic renal or hepatic reports in prolonged therapy.

PATIENT/FAMILY TEACHING:

Space doses evenly. Continue antibiotic for full length of treatment. Discomfort may occur w/IM injection. Notify physician in event of diarrhea, rash, blood in urine, or other new symptom.

methimazole

meth-im´ah-zole
(Tapazole)

CANADIAN AVAILABILITY: Tapazole

CLASSIFICATION

Antithyroid

PHARMACOKINETICS

Readily absorbed from GI tract (food may alter absorption). Primarily concentrated in thyroid gland. Protein binding: minimal. Metabolized in liver. Primarily excreted in urine. Minimally removed by hemodialysis. Half-life: 5-6 hrs.

ACTION

Inhibits thyroid hormone synthesis. Diverts iodine from thyroid hormone synthesis.

USES

Palliative treatment of hyperthyroidism; adjunct to ameliorate hyperthyroidism in preparation for surgical treatment or radioactive iodine therapy.

PO ADMINISTRATION

Space doses evenly, usually at 8 hr intervals.

INDICATIONS/DOSAGE/ROUTES

Hyperthyroidism:
PO: Adults, elderly: Initially: 15-60 mg/day. **Maintenance:** 5-15

mg/day. **Children:** Initially, 0.4 mg/kg/day. **Maintenance:** ½ initial dose.

PRECAUTIONS

CONTRAINDICATIONS: Hypersensitivity to the drug. **CAUTIONS:** Pts >40 yrs or in combination w/ other agranulocytosis inducing drugs. **PREGNANCY/LACTATION:** Readily crosses placenta, distributed in breast milk. Contraindicated in nursing mothers (can induce goiter, cretinism in neonate). **Pregnancy Category D.**

INTERACTIONS

DRUG INTERACTIONS: Amiodarone, iodinated glycerol, iodine, potassium iodide may decrease response. May decrease effect of oral anticoagulants. May increase concentration of digoxin (as pt becomes euthyroid). May decrease thyroid uptake of I^{131}. **ALTERED LAB VALUES:** May increase SGOT (AST), SGPT (ALT), alkaline phosphatase, LDH, bilirubin, prothrombin time. May decrease prothrombin level.

SIDE EFFECTS

FREQUENT: Urticaria, rash, pruritus, nausea, vomiting, skin pigmentation, hair loss, headache, paresthesia. **OCCASIONAL:** Drowsiness, lymphadenopathy, vertigo. **RARE:** Periarteritis, fever, lupus-like syndrome.

ADVERSE REACTIONS/TOXIC EFFECTS

Agranulocytosis (which may occur as long as 4 mo after therapy), pancytopenia and fatal hepatitis have occurred.

NURSING IMPLICATIONS

BASELINE ASSESSMENT:

Question for hypersensitivity. Obtain baseline weight, pulse.

INTERVENTION/EVALUATION:

Monitor pulse and weight daily. Assess food tolerance. Check for skin eruptions, itching, swollen lymph glands. Be alert to hepatitis: nausea, vomiting, drowsiness, jaundice. Monitor hematology results for bone marrow suppression; check for signs of infection or bleeding.

PATIENT/FAMILY TEACHING:

Do not exceed ordered dose; follow-up w/physician is essential. Space evenly around the clock. Take resting pulse (teach pt/family) daily to monitor therapeutic results and report as directed. Do not take other medications w/o approval of physician. Seafood and iodine products may be restricted. Report illness, unusual bleeding or bruising immediately. Inform physician of sudden or continuous weight gain, cold intolerance or depression.

M

methocarbamol

meth-oh-car´bah-moll
(Robaxin)

FIXED-COMBINATION(S): W/aspirin, a salicylate (Robaxisal)

CANADIAN AVAILABILITY: Robaxin

CLASSIFICATION

Skeletal muscle relaxant

PHARMACOKINETICS

	ONSET	PEAK	DURATION
PO	30 min	—	—
IV	Immediate	—	—

Rapid, completely absorbed from GI tract. Metabolized in liver. Excreted in urine. Half-life: 0.9-2.2 hrs.

ACTION

Muscle relaxant related to CNS depressant effects (sedation). Blocks interneuronal activity in descending reticular formation and spinal cord.

USES

Adjunctive therapy for relief of discomfort associated with mild to moderate painful musculoskeletal conditions.

STORAGE/HANDLING

Store oral, parenteral form at room temperature. After dilution, do not refrigerate (may precipitate). Solution stable for 6 days after dilution with 5% dextrose or 0.9% NaCl.

PO/IM/IV ADMINISTRATION

PO:

1. Give w/o regard to meals.
2. Tablets may be crushed.

IM:

1. Do not give >5 ml into each gluteal region.

IV:

1. For direct IV, give undiluted at rate of 3 ml/min (300 mg/min).
2. For infusion, dilute each 1 Gm methocarbamol with 250 ml of 0.9% NaCl or 5% dextrose.
3. Pt must remain recumbent 10-15 min following administration.
4. A too-rapid IV rate may produce hypotension, syncope, bradycardia.
5. Extravasation (stinging, swelling, coolness, little or no blood return) may result in thrombophlebitis, tissue sloughing.

INDICATIONS/DOSAGE/ROUTES

Musculoskeletal conditions:

PO: Adults: Initially, 1500 mg 4 times/day for first 2-3 days. **Elderly:** Initially, 500 mg 4 times/day. **Maintenance:** 4-4.5 Gm/day in 3-6 divided doses.

IM/IV: Adults: 1 Gm up to 3 times/day for 3 consecutive days. May repeat after a 2-day drug-free interval.

PRECAUTIONS

CONTRAINDICATIONS: *Parenteral:* Impaired renal function. **CAUTIONS:** Myasthenia gravis pts receiving concurrent anticholinesterase agents. **PREGNANCY/LACTATION:** Unknown whether drug crosses placenta or is distributed in breast milk. **Pregnancy Category C.**

INTERACTIONS

DRUG INTERACTIONS: CNS depressing medications may have additive effect. **ALTERED LAB VALUES:** May falsely elevate 5-HIAA, VMA.

SIDE EFFECTS

FREQUENT: Drowsiness, dizziness, lightheadedness. *Parenteral:* Metallic taste, GI upset, flushing, hypotension. **OCCASIONAL:** Blurred vision, headache, fever, nausea. **RARE:** Hypersensitivity reaction (rash, hives, itching, nasal congestion).

ADVERSE REACTIONS/TOXIC EFFECTS

Overdosage results in CNS depression.

NURSING IMPLICATIONS

BASELINE ASSESSMENT:

Record onset, type, location, and duration of muscular spasm. Check for immobility, stiffness, swelling.

INTERVENTION/EVALUATION:

Assist with ambulation at all times. Assess for evidence of extravasation (stinging, swelling, coolness, little or no blood return). Evaluate for therapeutic response: decreased intensity of skeletal muscle pain, improved mobility, decrease in stiffness, swelling.

PATIENT/FAMILY TEACHING:

Drowsiness usually diminishes w/continued therapy. Discomfort may occur w/IM injection. Urine may darken to brown, black, or green. Avoid tasks that require alertness, motor skills until response to drug is established. Avoid alcohol or other depressants while taking medication. Avoid sudden changes in posture.

methohexital sodium

meth-oh-hex′ih-tall

(Brevital)

CANADIAN AVAILABILITY:
Brietal

(See Classifications section under Anesthetics: general)

methotrexate sodium

meth-oh-trex′ate

(Folex, Mexate, Rheumatrex)

CANADIAN AVAILABILITY:
Methotrexate

CLASSIFICATION

Antineoplastic, antiarthritic, antipsoriatic

PHARMACOKINETICS

Variably absorbed from GI tract. Widely distributed. Protein binding: 50% Metabolized in liver, intracellularly. Primarily excreted in urine. Half-life: 3-10 hrs (high doses: 8-15 hrs).

ACTION

Cell cycle-specific for S phase of cell division. Irreversibly binds w/dihydrofolate reductase preventing reduction to tetrahydrofolate. Inhibits DNA, RNA, protein synthesis. Has mild immunosuppressant activty.

USES

Treatment of trophoblastic neoplasms (gestational choriocarcinoma, chorioadenoma destruens, hydatidiform mole), acute leukemias, breast cancer, epidermoid cancers of head and neck, lung cancer, advanced stages of lymphosarcoma, mycosis fungoides, meningeal leukemia, severe psoriasis, rheumatoid arthritis.

STORAGE/HANDLING

NOTE: May be carcinogenic, mutagenic, or teratogenic. Handle w/ extreme care during preparation/ administration.

Solutions w/o preservatives should be prepared immediately before use.

IM/IV ADMINISTRATION

NOTE: May give IM, IV, intra-arterially, intrathecally. Wear gloves when preparing solution. If powder or solution come in contact w/

skin, wash immediately, thoroughly w/soap, water.

1. Reconstitute vial w/2-10 ml sterile water for injection or 0.9% NaCl injection.

2. May further dilute w/5% dextrose or 0.9% NaCl.

3. For intrathecal use, dilute w/ preservative-free 0.9% NaCl to provide a 1 mg/ml concentration.

INDICATIONS/DOSAGE/ROUTES

NOTE: Dosage individualized based on clinical response, tolerance to adverse effects. When used in combination therapy, consult specific protocols for optimum dosage, sequence of drug administration.

Trophoblastic neoplasms, choriocarcinoma:
PO/IM: Adults: 15-30 mg/day for 5 days. Repeat 3-5 times w/rest periods of 1-2 wks between courses.

Leukemia:
PO: Adults, children: (Combined w/prednisone): *Induction:* 3.3 mg/ m^2/day produces remission within 4-6 wks.
PO/IM: Adults, children: Maintenance: 30 mg/m^2/wk in divided doses 2 times/wk.
IV: Adults, children: Maintenance: 2.5 mg/kg every 14 days.

Meningeal leukemia:
INTRATHECAL: Adults, children >2 yrs: 12 mg/m^2 every 2-5 days until CSF normal, then give one additional dose. **Children 2 yrs:** 10 mg/m^2. **Children 1-2 yrs:** 8 mg/m^2. **Children <1 yr:** 6 mg/ m^2.

Burkitt's lymphoma, stage I or II:
PO: Adults: 10-25 mg/day for 4-8 days. Repeat in 7-10 days.

Stage III lymphosarcoma:
PO: Adults: 0.625-2.5 mg/kg/day.

Osteosarcoma:
IV INFUSION: Adults: (Combination therapy): Initially, 12 Gm/m^2 over 4 hrs. May increase to 15 Gm/ m^2 w/subsequent treatments. Give w/leucovorin 15 mg orally q6h for 10 doses, begin 24 hrs after start of methotrexate (MTX) infusion. Give IM/IV if pt vomiting/unable to tolerate oral medication. Dosage may vary based upon serum (MTX) levels, impairment of liver function. **NOTE:** Delay MTX therapy w/leucovorin rescue until recovery if WBCs <1500/mm^3, neutrophil count <200/mm^3, platelet count <75,000/mm^3, serum bilirubin >1.2 mg/dl, SGPT (ALT) level >450 U. If mucositis present, until evidence of healing. If persistent pleural effusion, drain prior to infusion. Serum creatinine must be normal, creatinine clearance >60 ml/min before initiation of therapy. Pt must be well hydrated.

Mycosis fungoides:
PO: Adults: 2.5-10 mg/day.
IM: Adults: 50 mg once/wk or 25 mg 2 times/wk.

Psoriasis:
IM/IV: Adults: 5-10 mg 1 wk prior to initiation of therapy to detect idiosyncratic reaction.
PO: Adults: *Divided doses:* 2.5-5 mg q12h for 3 doses or q8h for 4 doses each wk. Increase dose by 2.5 mg/wk. Do not exceed 25-30 mg/wk. **Daily dose:** 2.5 mg/day for 5 days. Rest 2 days. Repeat. **Maximum daily dose:** 6.25 mg.
PO/IM/IV: Adults: *Weekly single dose:* 10-25 mg/wk up to 50 mg/ wk

Rheumatoid arthritis:
PO: Adults: Initially: 7.5 mg/wk as single dose or 2.5 mg q12h × 3

doses. Adjust dose gradually to achieve optimal response, usually not >20 mg/wk.

Usual elderly dose (rheumatoid arthritis/psoriasis):

PO: Elderly: Initially, 5 mg/wk as single or divided doses. May increase up to 7.5 mg/wk. **Maximum:** 20 mg/wk.

PRECAUTIONS

CONTRAINDICATIONS: Impaired renal function. *Psoriasis:* Poor nutritional status, severe renal/hepatic disease, preexisting blood dyscrasias. **EXTREME CAUTION:** Infection, peptic ulcer, ulcerative colitis, very young, elderly, debilitated, preexisting liver damage, impaired hepatic function, preexisting bone marrow depression. **CAUTIONS:** Impaired renal, hepatic function, peptic ulcer, ulcerative colitis. **PREGNANCY/LACTATION:** Avoid pregnancy during MTX therapy and minimum 3 mo after therapy in males or at least 1 ovulatory cycle after therapy in females. May cause fetal death, congenital anomalies. Drug is distributed in breast milk. Breast feeding not recommended. **Pregnancy Category D.** In pregnant psoriatic and rheumatoid arthritic pt: **Pregnancy Category X.**

INTERACTIONS

DRUG INTERACTIONS: Parenteral acyclovir may increase neurotoxicity. Alcohol, hepatotoxic medications may increase hepatotoxicity. NSAIDs may increase toxicity. Asparaginase may decrease effects of methotrexate. Bone marrow depressants may increase bone marrow depression. Probenecid, salicylates may increase concentration, toxicity. Live virus vaccines may potentiate virus replication, increase vaccine side effects, decrease pt's antibody response to vaccine. **ALTERED LAB VALUES:** May increase uric acid, SGOT (AST).

SIDE EFFECTS

FREQUENT: Anorexia, nausea, vomiting, diarrhea; in psoriatic pts, burning, erythema of psoriatic site for 1-2 days after each dose. **OCCASIONAL:** Malaise, excessive fatigue, headache, drowsiness, dizziness, blurred vision, alopecia.

ADVERSE REACTIONS/TOXIC EFFECTS

High potential for various, severe toxicity. GI toxicity may produce oral ulcers of mouth, gingivitis, glossitis, pharyngitis, stomatitis, enteritis, hematemesis. Hepatotoxicity occurs more frequently w/frequent, small doses than w/large, intermittent doses. Pulmonary toxicity characterized as interstitial pneumonitis. Hematologic toxicity resulting from marked bone marrow depression may be manifested as leukopenia, thrombocytopenia, anemia, hemorrhage (may develop rapidly). Skin toxicity produces rash, pruritus, urticaria, pigmentation, photosensitivity, petechiae, ecchymosis, pustules. Severe nephropathy produces azotemia, hematuria, renal failure.

NURSING IMPLICATIONS

BASELINE ASSESSMENT:

Question for possibility of pregnancy before initiating therapy (Pregnancy Category X). Obtain all functional tests before therapy and repeat throughout therapy. Antiemetics may prevent nausea, vomiting.

INTERVENTION/EVALUATION:

Monitor hepatic and renal function tests, Hgb, Hct, WBC, differential, platelet count, urinalysis, chest radiographs, serum uric acid level. Monitor for hematologic toxicity (fever, sore throat, signs of local infection, easy bruising, unusual bleeding from any site), symptoms of anemia (excessive tiredness, weakness). Assess skin for evidence of dermatologic toxicity. Keep pt well hydrated, urine alkaline. Avoid IM injections, rectal temperatures, traumas that induce bleeding. Apply 5 full mins. of pressure to IV sites.

PATIENT/FAMILY TEACHING:

Maintain fastidious oral hygiene. Do not have immunizations w/o physician's approval (drug lowers body's resistance). Avoid crowds, those w/infection. Avoid alcohol, salicylates. Avoid sunlamp and sunlight exposure. Use contraceptive measures during therapy and for 3 mos. (males) or one ovular cycle (females) after therapy. Promptly report fever, sore throat, signs of local infection, easy bruising, unusual bleeding from any site. Alopecia is reversible, but new hair growth may have different color or texture. Contact physician if nausea/vomiting continues at home.

methylcellulose

meth-ill-cell´you-los

(Citrucel, Cologel)

CLASSIFICATION

Laxative: Bulk-forming

PHARMACOKINETICS

	ONSET	PEAK	DURATION
PO	12-24 hrs	—	—

Full effect may not be evident for 2-3 days. Acts in small/large intestine.

ACTION

Dissolves, swells in water (provides increased bulk, moisture content in stool, increasing peristalsis, bowel motility).

USES

Prophylaxis in those who should not strain during defecation. Facilitates defecation in those w/diminished colonic motor response.

PO ADMINISTRATION

1. Instruct pt to drink 6-8 glasses of water/day (aids stool softening).
2. Not to be swallowed in dry form; mix w/at least 1 full glass (8 oz) liquid.

INDICATIONS/DOSAGE/ROUTES

Laxative:

PO: Adults, elderly: 1 tbsp (15 ml) in 8 oz water 1-3 times/day. **Children 6-12 yrs:** 1 tsp (5 ml) in 4 oz water 3-4 times/day.

PRECAUTIONS

CONTRAINDICATIONS: Abdominal pain, nausea, vomiting, symptoms of appendicitis, partial bowel obstruction, dysphagia. **CAUTIONS:** None significant. **PREGNANCY/LACTATION:** Safe for use in pregnancy. **Pregnancy Category C.**

INTERACTIONS

DRUG INTERACTIONS: May interfere w/effects of potassium-sparing diuretics, potassium supplements. May decrease effect of oral anticoagulants, digoxin, salicylates by decreasing absorption. **ALTERED LAB VALUES:** May increase glucose. May decrease potassium.

SIDE EFFECTS

RARE: Some degree of abdominal discomfort, nausea, mild cramps, griping, faintness.

ADVERSE REACTIONS/TOXIC EFFECTS

Esophageal or bowel obstruction may occur if administered with insufficient liquid (less than 250 ml or 1 full glass).

NURSING IMPLICATIONS

INTERVENTION/EVALUATION:

Encourage adequate fluid intake. Assess bowel sounds for peristalsis. Monitor daily bowel activity and stool consistency (watery, loose, soft, semi-solid, solid) and record time of evacuation. Monitor serum electrolytes in those exposed to prolonged, frequent, or excessive use of medication.

PATIENT/FAMILY TEACHING:

Institute measures to promote defecation: increase fluid intake, exercise, high-fiber diet.

methyldopa

meth-ill-doe´pah

(Aldomet)

methyldopate hydrochloride

FIXED-COMBINATION(S): W/hydrochlorothiazide, a diuretic (Aldoril); w/chlorothiazide, a diuretic (Aldoclor).

CANADIAN AVAILABILITY: Aldomet, Apo-Methyldopa, Dopamet, Novomedopa

CLASSIFICATION

Antihypertensive

PHARMACOKINETICS

	ONSET	PEAK	DURATION
PO	—	4-6 hrs	—
IV	—	4-6 hrs	10-16 hrs

Variably absorbed from GI tract. Protein binding: <20%. Metabolized in liver. Primarily excreted in urine. Removed by hemodialysis. Half-life: 1.7 hrs (increased in decreased renal function).

ACTION

Stimulates central inhibitory alpha-adrenergic receptors (lowers arterial pressure, reduces plasma renin activity).

USES

Management of moderate to severe hypertension.

STORAGE/HANDLING

Store tablets at room temperature. IV solution is stable for 24 hrs at room temperature.

PO/IV ADMINISTRATION

PO:

1. May give w/o regard to food. If GI upset occurs, give w/food.
2. Tablets may be crushed.

M

IV:

1. Give by IV infusion (piggyback). Avoid SubQ, IM (unpredictable absorption).
2. For IV infusion, dilute 250 or 500 mg vial w/50 or 100 ml 5% dextrose.
3. Infuse slowly over 30-60 min.

INDICATIONS/DOSAGE/ROUTES

Hypertension:
PO: Adults: Initially, 250 mg 2-3 times/day for 2 days. Adjust dosage at intervals of 2 days (minimum). **Elderly:** Initially, 125 mg 1-2 times/day. May increase by 125 mg q2-3days. **Maintenance:** 500 mg to 2 Gm/day in 2-4 divided doses. **Children:** Initially, 10 mg/kg/day in 2-4 divided doses. Adjust dose at intervals of 2 days (minimum). **Maximum:** 65 mg/kg/day or 3 Gm/day, whichever is less.
IV: Adults: 250-500 mg q6h up to 1 Gm q6h. **Children:** 20-40 mg/kg/day in divided doses q6h. **Maximum:** 65 mg/kg/day or 3 Gm/day, whichever is less.

PRECAUTIONS

CONTRAINDICATIONS: Acute hepatitis, active cirrhosis. **CAUTIONS:** Impaired hepatic function. **PREGNANCY/LACTATION:** Crosses placenta; distributed in breast milk. Reduction of neonate systolic B/P (4-5 mm Hg) has occurred for 2-3 days after delivery; tremors reported. **Pregnancy Category B.**

INTERACTIONS

DRUG INTERACTIONS: Tricyclic antidepressants, NSAIDs may decrease effect. Hypotensive-producing medications may increase effect. May increase risk of toxicity of lithium. May cause hyperexcitability w/MAO inhibitors. Sympathomimetics may decrease effects. **ALTERED LAB VALUES:** May increase SGOT (AST), SGPT (ALT), alkaline phosphatase, bilirubin, BUN, creatinine, potassium, sodium, prolactin, uric acid. May produce false positive Coombs' test, prolong prothrombin time.

SIDE EFFECTS

FREQUENT: Transient drowsiness, headache, weakness during initial therapy. W/increased dose: postural hypotension, dry mouth. **OCCASIONAL:** Edema, weight gain.

ADVERSE REACTIONS/TOXIC EFFECTS

Hepatotoxicity (abnormal liver function tests, jaundice, hepatitis), hemolytic anemia, unexplained fever and flu-like symptoms: discontinue medication, contact physician.

NURSING IMPLICATIONS

BASELINE ASSESSMENT:

Obtain baseline B/P, pulse, weight.

INTERVENTION/EVALUATION:

Monitor B/P, pulse closely q30min until stabilized. Monitor weight daily during initial therapy. Monitor liver function tests. Assess for peripheral edema of hands, feet (usually, first area of low extremity swelling is behind medial malleolus in ambulatory, sacral area in bedridden).

PATIENT/FAMILY TEACHING:

Urine may darken in color. To reduce hypotensive effect, rise slowly from lying to sitting position and permit legs to dangle from bed momentarily before standing. Avoid sudden or prolonged standing, exercise, hot environment or hot shower, alcohol ingestion, particularly in morning (may aggravate orthostatic hypotension). Full therapeutic effect of oral administration may take 2-3 days. Drowsiness usually disappears during continued therapy. Sugarless gum, sips of tepid water may relieve dry mouth.

methylergonovine

meth-ill-er-goe-noe´veen
(Methergine)

CLASSIFICATION

Oxytocic

PHARMACOKINETICS

	ONSET	PEAK	DURATION
PO	5-10 min	—	—
IM	2-5 min	—	—
IV	Immediate	—	3 hrs

Rapidly absorbed from GI tract, after IM administration. Distributed rapidly to plasma, extracellular fluid, tissues. Metabolized in liver (undergoes first-pass effect). Primarily excreted in urine.

ACTION

Directly stimulates uterine muscle (increases force, frequency of contractions). Induces cervical contractions. Stimulates alpha-adrenergic, serotonin receptors producing arterial vasoconstriction. Causes vasospasm of coronary arteries.

USES

To prevent and treat postpartum, postabortion hemorrhage due to atony or involution. (Not for induction or augmentation of labor).

PO/IM/IV ADMINISTRATION

1. Initial dose may be given parenterally, followed by oral regimen.
2. IV use in life-threatening emergencies only; dilute to volume of 5 ml w/0.9% NaCl injection and give over at least 1 min, carefully monitoring B/P.

INDICATIONS/DOSAGE/ROUTES

Usual parenteral dosage:
IM/IV: Adults: Initially, 0.2 mg. May repeat no more often than q2-4h for no more than 5 doses total.

Usual oral dosage:
PO: Adults: 0.2 mg 3-4 times/day for maximum of 7 days.

PRECAUTIONS

CONTRAINDICATIONS: Hypersensitivity to ergot, hypertension, pregnancy, toxemia, untreated hypocalcemia. **CAUTIONS:** Renal or hepatic impairment, coronary artery disease, occlusive peripheral vascular disease, sepsis. **PREGNANCY/LACTATION:** Contraindicated during pregnancy. Small amounts in breast milk. **Pregnancy Category C.**

INTERACTIONS

DRUG INTERACTIONS: Vasoconstrictors, vasopressors may increase effect. **ALTERED LAB VALUES:** May decrease prolactin concentration.

SIDE EFFECTS

OCCASIONAL: Nausea, vomiting, esp. w/IV administration. **RARE:** Dizziness, diaphoresis, tinnitus, foul taste, palpitations, temporary chest pain, headache, pruritus; pale/cold hands or feet; pain in arms, legs, lower back; weakness in legs.

M

ADVERSE REACTIONS/TOXIC EFFECTS

Severe hypertensive episodes may result in cerebrovascular accident, serious arrhythmias, seizures; hypertensive effects more frequent w/pt susceptibility, rapid IV administration, concurrent regional anesthesia or vasoconstrictors. Peripheral ischemia may lead to gangrene.

NURSING IMPLICATIONS

BASELINE ASSESSMENT:

Question for hypersensitivity to any ergot derivatives. Determine calcium, B/P and pulse baselines. Assess bleeding prior to administration.

INTERVENTION/EVALUATION:

Monitor uterine tone, bleeding, B/P and pulse every 15 min until stable (about 1-2 hrs). Assess extremities for color, warmth, movement, pain. Report chest pain promptly. Provide support w/ambulation if dizziness occurs.

PATIENT/FAMILY TEACHING:

Avoid smoking because of added vasoconstriction. Report increased cramping, bleeding, or foul-smelling lochia. Pale, cold hands or feet should be reported because may mean decreased circulation.

methylphenidate hydrochloride

methyl-fen´ihdate

(Ritalin)

CANADIAN AVAILABILITY:

Ritalin

CLASSIFICATION

CNS stimulant

PHARMACOKINETICS

	ONSET	PEAK	DURATION
PO (tablets)	—	—	3-6 hrs
PO (extended-release)	—	—	8 hrs

Slowly, incompletely absorbed from GI tract. Metabolized in liver. Excreted in urine, eliminated in feces via biliary system. Half-life: 2-4 hrs.

ACTION

Blocks reuptake mechanisms of dopaminergic neurons. Decreases motor restlessness, enhances ability to pay attention. Increases motor activity, mental alertness; diminishes sense of fatigue, enhances spirit, produces mild euphoria.

USES

Adjunct to treatment of attention deficit disorder with moderate to severe distractability, short attention spans, hyperactivity, emotional impulsivity in children >6 yrs. Management of narcolepsy in adults.

PO ADMINISTRATION

1. Do not give drug in afternoon or evening (prevents insomnia).
2. Do not crush or break sustained-release capsules.
3. Tablets may be crushed.
4. Give dose 30-45 min before meals.

INDICATIONS/DOSAGE/ROUTES

NOTE: Do not use extended-release for initial therapy.

Attention deficit disorder:
PO: Children >6 yrs: Initially, 5 mg before breakfast and lunch. May increase dosage by 5-10 mg/day at weekly intervals. **Maximum:** 60 mg/day. Therapy usually discontinued when adolescence reached.

Narcolepsy:
PO: Adults, elderly: 10 mg 2-3 times/day. **Range:** 10-60 mg/day.

PRECAUTIONS

CONTRAINDICATIONS: History of marked anxiety, tension, agitation; glaucoma, those with motor tics, family history of Tourette's disorder. **CAUTIONS:** History of seizures, hypertension, history of drug dependence. **PREGNANCY/LACTATION:** Unknown whether drug crosses placenta or is distributed in breast milk. **Pregnancy Category C.**

INTERACTIONS

DRUG INTERACTIONS: CNS stimulants may have additive effect. MAO inhibitors may increase effects. **ALTERED LAB VALUES:** None significant.

SIDE EFFECTS

FREQUENT: Nervousness, insomnia, anorexia. **OCCASIONAL:** Headache, nausea, dizziness, drowsiness, dry throat, abdominal discomfort. **RARE:** Gingival bleeding, easy bruising.

ADVERSE REACTIONS/TOXIC EFFECTS

Prolonged administration to children w/attention deficit disorder may produce a temporary suppression of normal weight gain pattern. Overdose may produce tachycardia, palpitations, cardiac irregularities, chest pain, psychotic episode, seizures, coma. Hypersensitivity reactions, blood dyscrasias occur rarely.

NURSING IMPLICATIONS

INTERVENTION/EVALUATION:

CBC, differential, and platelet count should be performed routinely during therapy. If paradoxical return of attention deficit occurs, dosage should be reduced or discontinued.

PATIENT/FAMILY TEACHING:

Avoid tasks that require alertness, motor skills until response to drug is established. Dry mouth may be relieved by sugarless gum or sips of tepid water.

methylprednisolone

meth-ill-pred-niss′oh-lone
(Medrol)

methylprednisolone acetate

(Depo-Medrol, Duralone)

methylprednisolone sodium succinate

(Solu-Medrol, A-Methapred)

FIXED-COMBINATIONS: Methylprednisolone acetate w/Neomycin, an anti-infective (Neo-Medrol)

CANADIAN AVAILABILITY: Medrol, Depo-Medrol, Solu-Medrol

CLASSIFICATION

Corticosteroid

PHARMACOKINETICS

Well absorbed from GI tract, after IM administration. Widely distributed. Protein binding: high. Metabolized in liver. Excreted in urine. Half-life: >3.5 hrs.

ACTION

Decreases/prevents tissue response to inflammatory process. Inhibits accumulation inflammatory cells at inflammation sites, phagocytosis, lysosomal enzyme release and synthesis and/or release of mediators of inflammation. Prevents/suppresses cell-mediated immune reactions.

USES

Substitution therapy of deficiency states: acute/chronic adrenal insufficiency, congenital adrenal hyperplasia, adrenal insufficiency secondary to pituitary insufficiency. Nonendocrine disorders: arthritis, rheumatic carditis, allergic, collagen, intestinal tract, liver, ocular, renal, and skin diseases, bronchial asthma, cerebral edema, malignancies.

PO/IM/IV/TOPICAL ADMINISTRATION

PO:

1. Give w/food or milk.
2. Single doses given prior to 9 AM; multiple doses at evenly spaced intervals.

IM:

1. Methylprednisolone acetate should not be further diluted.
2. Methylprednisolone sodium succinate should be reconstituted w/bacteriostatic water.
3. Give deep IM in gluteus maximus.

IV:

1. For infusion, add to 5% dextrose, 0.9% NaCl or 5% dextrose in 0.9% NaCl.
2. Do *not* give methylprednisolone acetate IV.

TOPICAL:

1. Gently cleanse area prior to application.
2. Use occlusive dressings only as ordered.
3. Apply sparingly and rub into area thoroughly.

INDICATIONS/DOSAGE/ROUTES

NOTE: Individualize dose based on disease, pt, and response.

ORAL METHYLPREDNISOLONE:

PO: Adults, elderly: Initially, 4-48 mg/day.

METHYLPREDNISOLONE SODIUM SUCCINATE:

IV: Adults, elderly: (High dose): 30 mg/kg over at least 30 min. Repeat q4-6h for 48-72 hrs.
IV: Adults, elderly: Initially, 10-40 mg q4-6h, may give subsequent doses IM. **Children, infants:** Not less than 0.5 mg/kg/day.

METHYLPREDNISOLONE ACETATE:

Adrenogenital syndrome:
IM: Adults, elderly: 40 mg q2wks.

Rheumatoid arthritis:
IM: Adults: 40-120 mg/wk.

Dermatologic lesions:
IM: Adults, elderly: 40-120 mg/wk for 1-4 wks.

Asthma, allergic rhinitis:
IM: Adults, elderly: 80-120 mg/wk.

Usual topical dosage:
TOPICAL: Adults, elderly: 2-4 times/day.

PRECAUTIONS

CONTRAINDICATIONS: Hypersensitivity to any corticosteroid, systemic fungal infection, peptic ulcers (except life-threatening situations). Avoid immunizations, smallpox vaccination. *Topical:* marked circulation impairment. **CAUTIONS:** History of tuberculosis (may reactivate disease), hypothyroidism, cirrhosis, nonspecific ulcerative colitis, CHF, hypertension, psychosis, renal insufficiency. Prolonged therapy should be discontinued slowly. **PREGNANCY/LACTATION:** Drug crosses placenta, distributed in breast milk. May cause cleft palate (chronic use first trimester). Nursing contraindicated. **Pregnancy Category C.**

INTERACTIONS

DRUG INTERACTIONS: Amphotericin may increase hypokalemia. May decrease effect of oral hypoglycemics, insulin, diuretics, potassium supplements. May increase digoxin toxicity (due to hypokalemia). Hepatic enzyme inducers may decrease effect. Live virus vaccines may potentiate virus replication, increase vaccine side effects, decrease pt's antibody response to vaccine. **ALTERED LAB VALUES:** May decrease calcium, potassium, thyroxine. May increase cholesterol, lipids, glucose, sodium, amylase.

SIDE EFFECTS

FREQUENT: Increased appetite, exaggerated sense of well-being, abdominal distention, weight gain, insomnia, mood swings. *High dose, prolonged therapy:* Increased susceptibility to infection (signs/symptoms masked); slow wound healing; hypokalemia, hypocalcemia, GI distress. **OCCASIONAL:** Headache, vertigo. **RARE:** Increased blood coagulability, tachycardia, frequency or urgency of urination, psychosis. *Topical:* Redness, itching, irritation.

ADVERSE REACTIONS/TOXIC EFFECTS

Long-term therapy: Muscle wasting (esp. arms, legs), osteoporosis, spontaneous fractures, amenorrhea, cataracts, glaucoma, peptic ulcer, CHF. *Abrupt withdrawal following long-term therapy:* Anorexia, nausea, fever, headache, joint pain, rebound inflammation, fatigue, weakness, lethargy, dizziness, orthostatic hypotension.

NURSING IMPLICATIONS

BASELINE ASSESSMENT:

Question for hypersensitivity to any of the corticosteroids, components. Obtain baselines for height, weight, B/P, glucose, electrolytes. Check results of initial tests, e.g., TB skin test, x-rays, EKG.

INTERVENTION/EVALUATION:

Monitor I&O, daily weight; assess for edema. Evaluate food tolerance and bowel activity; report hyperacidity promptly. Check B/P, TPR at least 2 times/day. Be alert to infection: sore throat, fever or vague symptoms. Monitor electrolytes. Watch for hypocalcemia (muscle twitching, cramps, positive Trousseau's or Chvostek's signs) or hypokalemia (weakness and muscle cramps, numbness/tingling [esp. lower extremities], nausea and vomiting, irritability, EKG changes). Assess emotional status, ability to sleep. Check lab results for blood coagulability and clinical evidence of thromboembolism. Provide assistance w/ambulation.

PATIENT/FAMILY TEACHING:

Take w/food or milk. Carry identification of drug and dose, physician name and phone number. Do not change dose/schedule or stop taking drug, must taper off gradually under medical supervision. Notify physician of fever, sore throat, muscle aches, sudden weight gain/swelling. W/dietician give instructions for prescribed diet (usually sodium restricted w/high vitamin D, protein and potassium). Maintain careful personal hygiene, avoid exposure to disease or trauma. Severe stress (serious infection, surgery or trauma) may require increased dosage. Do not take any other medication w/o consulting physician. Follow-up visits, lab tests are necessary; children must be assessed for growth retardation. Inform dentist or other physicians of methylprednisolone therapy now or within past 12 mo. Caution against overuse of joints injected for symptomatic relief. Retention enema of methylprednisolone (Medrol Enpak) may be ordered to soothe GI inflammation. *Topical:* Apply after shower or bath for best absorption. Do not cover unless physician orders; do not use tight diapers, plastic pants, or coverings. Avoid contact w/eyes. Do not expose treated area to sunlight.

methysergide maleate

meth-i-sir′guide
(Sansert)

CANADIAN AVAILABILITY:
Sansert

CLASSIFICATION

Antimigraine

PHARMACOKINETICS

Rapidly absorbed from GI tract. Widely distributed. Metabolized in liver to active metabolite. Primarily excreted in urine. Half-life: 10 hrs.

ACTION

Directly stimulates smooth muscle leading to vasoconstriction. May have antiserotonin effect.

USES

Prevents or aborts vascular headaches (e.g., migraine, cluster headaches).

PO ADMINISTRATION

Give w/meals to avoid GI upset.

INDICATIONS/DOSAGE/ROUTES

Vascular headaches:
PO: Adults: 4-8 mg/day in divided doses. Do not give continuously >6 mo w/o 3-4 wk drug-free interval between courses of therapy. Discontinue gradually over 2-3 wks (avoids rebound headaches).

PRECAUTIONS

CONTRAINDICATIONS: Hypersensitivity to ergot alkaloids, peripheral vascular disease (thromboangiitis obliterans, leutic arteritis, severe arteriosclerosis. Raynaud's disease), phlebitis or cellulitis of lower limbs, pulmonary disease, collagen diseases, fibrotic disease, impaired renal or hepatic function, severe pruritus, valvular heart disease, coronary artery disease, severe hypertension, debilitated, malnutrition. **CAUTIONS:** None significant. **PREGNANCY/LACTATION:** Contraindicated in pregnancy (produces uterine stimulant action, resulting in possible fetal death or retarded fetal growth, increases vasoconstriction of placental vascular bed). Drug distributed in breast milk. May produce diarrhea, vomiting in neonate. May inhibit lactation. **Pregnancy Category X.**

INTERACTIONS

DRUG INTERACTIONS: Ergot alkaloids, systemic vasoconstrictors (e.g., norepinephrine) may increase vasoconstrictor effect. **ALTERED LAB VALUES:** May increase BUN.

SIDE EFFECTS

FREQUENT: Nausea, vomiting, diarrhea/constipation, heartburn (may be alleviated if given w/ meals); peripheral edema, facial flushing, lightheadedness, insomnia, feeling of dissociation.

ADVERSE REACTIONS/TOXIC EFFECTS

Prolonged administration or excessive dosage may produce ergotamine poisoning: nausea, vomiting, weakness of legs, pain in limb muscles, numbness and tingling of fingers/toes, precordial pain, tachycardia or bradycardia, hyper/hypotension. Localized edema, itching due to vasoconstriction of peripheral arteries and arterioles. Feet and hands will become cold, pale, numb. Muscle pain occurs when walking and later, even at rest. Gangrene may occur. Occasionally, confusion, depression, drowsiness, convulsions may appear.

NURSING IMPLICATIONS

BASELINE ASSESSMENT:

Question pt regarding history of peripheral vascular disease, renal or hepatic impairment, or possibility of pregnancy. Contact physician with findings before administering drug. Question pt regarding onset, location and duration of migraine, and possible precipitating symptoms.

INTERVENTION/EVALUATION:

Monitor closely for evidence of ergotamine overdosage as result of prolonged administration or excessive dosage (see Adverse Reactions/Toxic Effects). Contact physician if any signs and symptoms of ergotamine poisoning presents itself.

PATIENT/FAMILY TEACHING:

Initiate therapy at first sign of migraine attack. Inform physician/nurse if need to progressively increase dose in order to relieve vascular headaches or if irregular heartbeat, nausea, vomiting, numbness or tingling of fingers or toes or if pain or weakness of extremities is noted. Use of nonhormonal contraception.

metipranolol hydrochloride

met-ih-pran´oh-lol

(OptiPranolol)

CLASSIFICATION

Beta-adrenergic blocker

PHARMACOKINETICS

	ONSET	PEAK	DURATION
Eye drops	<0.5 hr	2 hrs	12-24 hrs

Systemic absorption may occur.

M

ACTION

Decreases intraocular pressure by reducing aqueous humor production. May increase aqueous humor outflow.

USES

Reduces intraocular pressure, including those w/chronic open-angle glaucoma, ocular hypertension.

STORAGE/HANDLING

Store ophthalmic solution at room temperature.

OPHTHALMIC ADMINISTRATION

1. Place finger on lower eyelid and pull out until pocket is formed between eye and lower lid.
2. Hold dropper above pocket and place prescribed number of drops into pocket.
3. Instruct pt to close eyes gently so medication will not be squeezed out of sac. Apply gentle finger pressure to the lacrimal sac at inner canthus for 1 min following installation (lessens risk of systemic absorption).

INDICATIONS/DOSAGE/ROUTES

Glaucoma:
EYE DROPS: Adults, elderly: 1 drop 2 times/day alone or in combination w/other agents.

PRECAUTIONS

CONTRAINDICATIONS: History of/or bronchial asthma, COPD, sinus bradycardia, overt cardiac failure, cardiogenic shock, second- and third-degree AV block. **CAUTIONS:** Chronic bronchitis, emphysema, diabetes mellitus, cerebrovascular insufficiency, thyroid deficiency. **PREGNANCY/LACTATION:** Unknown whether drug crosses placenta or is distributed in breast milk. May produce bradycardia, apnea, hypoglycemia, hypothermia during delivery, small birth weight infants. **Pregnancy Category C.**

INTERACTIONS

DRUG INTERACTIONS: Diuretics, other hypotensives may increase hypotensive effect. Dipivefrin, epinephrine may have additive effects. **ALTERED LAB VALUES:** None significant.

SIDE EFFECTS

Generally well tolerated, w/ mild and transient side effects. **FREQUENT:** Eye irritation (burning, stinging), conjunctivitis. **RARE:** Ataxia, dizziness, lethargy.

ADVERSE REACTIONS/TOXIC EFFECTS

Overdosage may produce bradycardia, hypotension, bronchospasm, acute cardiac failure.

NURSING IMPLICATIONS

BASELINE ASSESSMENT:

Assess B/P, apical pulse immediately before drug is administered (if pulse is 60/min or below, or systolic B/P is below 90 mm Hg, withhold medication, contact physician).

INTERVENTION/EVALUATION:

Assess pulse for strength/weakness, irregular rate, bradycardia.

PATIENT/FAMILY TEACHING:

Do not abruptly discontinue medication. Compliance w/therapy regimen is essential to control glaucoma. Monitor B/P, pulse before taking medication. Ocular stinging/discomfort commonly occurs.

metoclopramide

meh-tah-klo´prah-myd
(Reglan)

CANADIAN AVAILABILITY:
Apo-Metoclop, Emex, Maxeran, Reglan

CLASSIFICATION

GI stimulant, antiemetic

PHARMACOKINETICS

Well absorbed from GI tract. Protein binding: 30%. Metabolized in liver. Primarily excreted in urine. Half-life: 4-6 hrs.

ACTION

Inhibits gastric smooth muscle relaxation, accelerates intestinal transit and gastric emptying. Decreases reflux into esophagus. Raises threshold of activity in CTZ.

USES

To facilitate small bowel intubation, stimulate gastric emptying, intestinal transit. Relieves symptoms of acute, recurrent gastroparesis (nausea, vomiting, persistent fullness after meals). Prevents nausea, vomiting associated w/ cancer chemotherapy. Treatment of heartburn, delayed gastric emptying secondary to reflux esophagitis.

STORAGE/HANDLING

Store tablets, syrup at room temperature. After reconstitution, IV infusion (piggyback) is stable for 48 hrs.

PO/IV ADMINISTRATION

PO:

1. Give 30 min before meals and at bedtime.
2. Tablets may be crushed.

IV:

1. For IV infusion (piggyback), may dilute w/5% dextrose or 0.9% NaCl.
2. Infuse >15 min.
3. May give slow IV push at rate of 10 mg over 1-2 min.
4. A too-rapid IV injection may produce intense feeling of anxiety or restlessness, followed by drowsiness.

INDICATIONS/DOSAGE/ROUTES

NOTE: May give PO, IM, direct IV, IV infusion.

Diabetic gastroparesis:
PO/IV: Adults: 10 mg 4 times/day for 2-8 wks.
PO: Elderly: Initially, 5 mg 30 min before meals and at bedtime. May increase to 10 mg for 2-8 wks.
IV: Elderly: 5 mg over 1-2 min. May increase to 10 mg.

Symptomatic gastroesophageal reflux:
PO: Adults: 10-15 mg up to 4 times/day; single doses up to 20 mg, as needed. **Elderly:** Initially, 5 mg 4 times/day. May increase to 10 mg.

Prevent cancer chemotherapy-induced nausea and vomiting:
IV: Adults, elderly, children: 1-2 mg/kg 30 min prior to chemotherapy; repeat q2h for 2 doses, then q3h, as needed.

To facilitate small bowel intubation (single dose):
IV: Adults, elderly: 10 mg. **Children 6-14 yrs:** 2.5-5 mg. **Children <6 yrs:** 0.1 mg/kg.

PRECAUTIONS

CONTRAINDICATIONS: Pheochromocytoma, history of seizure disorders, concurrent use of medications likely to produce extra-

M

pyramidal reactions, GI obstruction or perforation, GI hemorrhage. **CAUTIONS:** Impaired renal function, CHF, cirrhosis. **PREGNANCY/LACTATION:** Crosses placenta; distributed in breast milk. **Pregnancy Category B.**

INTERACTIONS

DRUG INTERACTIONS: Alcohol may increase CNS depressant effect. CNS depressants may increase sedative effect. **ALTERED LAB VALUES:** May increase aldosterone, prolactin concentrations.

SIDE EFFECTS

NOTE: Doses of 2 mg/kg or higher or length of therapy may result in a greater incidence of side effects. **FREQUENT:** Restlessness/drowsiness, fatigue, insomnia, dizziness, headache. **OCCASIONAL:** Constipation/diarrhea, periorbital edema, rash, urticaria. **RARE:** Galactorrhea, gynecomastia, menstrual disorders.

ADVERSE REACTIONS/TOXIC EFFECTS

Extrapyramidal reactions occur most frequently in children and young adults (age 18-30) receiving high doses (2 mg/kg) during cancer chemotherapy, and is usually limited to akathisia (motor restlessness), involuntary limb movement, and facial grimacing.

NURSING IMPLICATIONS

BASELINE ASSESSMENT:

Antiemetic: Assess for dehydration (poor skin turgor, dry mucous membranes, longitudinal furrows in tongue).

INTERVENTION/EVALUATION:

Monitor for anxiety, restlessness, extrapyramidal symptoms during IV administration. Monitor pattern of daily bowel activity and stool consistency. Assess for periorbital edema. Assess skin for rash, hives. Evaluate for therapeutic response from gastroparesis (nausea, vomiting, persistent fullness after meals).

PATIENT/FAMILY TEACHING:

Avoid tasks that require alertness, motor skills until drug response is established. Report involuntary eye, facial, or limb movement. Avoid alcohol.

metolazone

met-oh´lah-zone
(Diulo, Mykrox, Zaroxolyn)

CANADIAN AVAILABILITY:
Zaroxolyn

CLASSIFICATION

Diuretic: Thiazide

PHARMACOKINETICS

	ONSET	PEAK	DURATION
PO (diuretic)	1 hr	2 hrs	12-24 hrs

Incompletely absorbed from GI tract. Protein binding: 95%. Primarily excreted unchanged in urine. Half-life: 14 hrs.

ACTION

Diuretic: Blocks reabsorption of sodium, potassium, chloride at distal convoluted tubule, promoting delivery of sodium to potassium side, increasing potassium excretion (Na-K exchange). *Antihypertensive:* Reduces plasma, extracellular fluid volume. Decreases peripheral vascular resistance by direct effect on blood vessels.

USES

Diulo, Zaroxolyn: Treatment of mild to moderate essential hypertension, edema of renal disease, edema due to CHF; *Micrsox:* Treatment of mild to moderate hypertension.

PO ADMINISTRATION

May give w/food or milk if GI upset occurs, preferably w/breakfast (may prevent nocturia).

INDICATIONS/DOSAGE/ROUTES

DIULO, ZAROXOLYN:

Edema due to CHF:
PO: Adults: 5-10 mg once daily in morning. Reduce dose to lowest maintenance level when dry weight is achieved (nonedematous state).

Edema due to renal disease:
PO: Adults: 5-20 mg once daily in morning. Reduce dose to lowest maintenance level when dry weight is achieved (nonedematous state).

Hypertension:
PO: Adults: 2.5-5 mg once daily in morning.

Usual elderly dosage (Diulo, Zaroxolyn):
PO: Elderly: Initially, 2.5 mg/day or every other day.

MYKROX:

Hypertension:
PO: Adults: 0.5 mg once daily in morning. Dose may be increased to 1 mg once daily if B/P response is insufficient.

PRECAUTIONS

CONTRAINDICATIONS: History of hypersensitivity to sulfonamides or thiazide diuretics, renal decompensation, anuria, hepatic coma or precoma. **CAUTIONS:** Severe renal disease, impaired hepatic function, diabetes mellitus, elderly/debilitated, thyroid disorders. **PREGNANCY/LACTATION:** Crosses placenta; small amount distributed in breast milk—nursing not advised. **Pregnancy Category B.**

INTERACTIONS

DRUG INTERACTIONS: Cholestyramine, colestipol may decrease absorption, effects. May increase digoxin toxicity (due to hypokalemia). May increase lithium toxicity. **ALTERED LAB VALUES:** May increase bilirubin, serum calcium, LDL, cholesterol, triglycerides, creatinine, glucose, uric acid. May decrease urinary calcium, magnesium, potassium, sodium.

M

SIDE EFFECTS

EXPECTED: Increase in urine frequency/volume. **FREQUENT:** Potassium depletion. **OCCASIONAL:** Postural hypotension, headache, abdominal bloating, palpitations, chills.

ADVERSE REACTIONS/TOXIC EFFECTS

Vigorous diuresis may lead to profound water loss and electrolyte depletion, resulting in hypokalemia, hyponatremia, dehydration. Acute hypotensive episodes may occur. Hyperglycemia may be noted during prolonged therapy. GI upset, pancreatitis, dizziness, paresthesias, headache, blood dyscrasias, pulmonary edema, allergic pneumonitis, dermatologic reactions occur rarely. Overdosage can lead to lethargy, coma w/o changes in electrolytes or hydration.

NURSING IMPLICATIONS

Baseline Assessment:

Check vital signs, especially B/P for hypotension prior to administration. Assess baseline electrolytes, particularly check for low potassium. Assess edema, skin turgor, mucous membranes for hydration status. Assess muscle strength, mental status. Note skin temperature, moisture. Obtain baseline weight. Initiate I&O.

Intervention/Evaluation:

Continue to monitor B/P, vital signs, electrolytes, I&O, weight. Note extent of diuresis. Watch for electrolyte disturbances (hypokalemia may result in weakness, tremor, muscle cramps, nausea, vomiting, change in mental status, tachycardia; hyponatremia may result in confusion, thirst, cold/clammy skin).

Patient/Family Teaching:

Expect increased frequency and volume of urination. To reduce hypotensive effect, rise slowly from lying to sitting position and permit legs to dangle momentarily before standing. Eat foods high in potassium such as whole grains (cereals), legumes, meat, bananas, apricots, oranges juice, potatoes (white, sweet), raisins.

metoprolol tartrate

meh-toe´pro-lol

(Lopressor, Toprol XL)

FIXED-COMBINATION(S):

W/hydrochlorothiazide, a diuretic (Lopressor HCT)

CANADIAN AVAILABILITY:

Apo-Metoprolol, Betaloc, Lopressor, Novometoprol

CLASSIFICATION

Beta-adrenergic blocker

PHARMACOKINETICS

	ONSET	PEAK	DURATION
PO	10-15 min	—	6 hrs
IV	—	20 min	5-8 hrs

Well absorbed from GI tract. Widely distributed. Protein binding: 12%. Metabolized in liver (undergoes significant first-pass metabolism). Primarily excreted in urine. Half-life: 3-7 hrs.

ACTION

Selectively blocks $beta_1$-adrenergic receptors, slowing sinus heart rate, decreasing cardiac output, decreasing B/P (exact mechanism unknown but may block peripheral adrenergic receptors, decrease sympathetic outflow from CNS or decrease renin release from kidney). Large dose may block $beta_2$-adrenergic receptors, increasing airway resistance. Decreases myocardial ischemia severity by decreasing oxygen requirements.

USES

Management of mild to moderate hypertension. Used alone or in combination with diuretics, especially thiazide-type. Management of chronic stable angina pectoris. Reduces cardiovascular mortality in those with definite or suspected acute MI. *Extended release:* Management of hypertension, long-term treatment of angina pectoris.

STORAGE/HANDLING

Store parenteral form at room temperature.

PO/IV ADMINISTRATION

PO:

1. Tablets may be crushed; do not crush or break extended-release tablets.
2. Give at same time each day.
3. May be given w/or immediately after meals (enhances absorption).

IV:

1. Administer IV injection rapidly.
2. Monitor EKG during administration.

INDICATIONS/DOSAGE/ROUTES

Hypertension, angina pectoris:
PO: Adults: Initially, 100 mg/day as single or divided dose. Increase at weekly (or longer) intervals. **Maintenance:** 100-450 mg/day.

Usual elderly dosage:
PO: Elderly: Initially, 25 mg/day. **Range:** 25-300 mg/day.

Usual dosage for extended-release tablets:
PO: Adults: *Hypertension:* 50-100 mg/day as single dose. May increase at least at weekly intervals until optimum B/P attained. *Angina:* Initially, 100 mg/day as single dose. May increase at least weekly intervals until optimum clinical response achieved.

Myocardial infarction (early treatment):
IV: Adults: 5 mg q2min for 3 doses, followed by 50 mg orally q6h for 48 hrs. Begin oral dose 15 min after last IV dose. Alternatively, in those who do not tolerate full IV dose, give 25-50 mg orally q6h, 15 min after last IV dose.

Myocardial infarction (late treatment, maintenance):
PO: Adults: 100 mg 2 times/day for at least 3 mo.

PRECAUTIONS

CONTRAINDICATIONS: Overt cardiac failure, cardiogenic shock, heart block greater than first degree, sinus bradycardia. *MI:* Heart rate <45 beats/min, systolic B/P <100 mm Hg. **CAUTIONS:** Bronchospastic disease, impaired renal function, peripheral vascular disease, hyperthyroidism, diabetes, inadequate cardiac function. **PREGNANCY/LACTATION:** Crosses placenta; distributed in breast milk. Avoid use during first trimester. May produce bradycardia, apnea, hypoglycemia, hypothermia during delivery, small birth weight infants. **Pregnancy Category C.**

INTERACTIONS

DRUG INTERACTIONS: Diuretics, other hypotensives may increase hypotensive effect; sympathomimetics, xanthines may mutually inhibit effects; may mask symptoms of hypoglycemia, prolong hypoglycemic effect of insulin, oral hypoglycemics; NSAIDs may decrease antihypertensive effect; cimetidine may increase concentration. **ALTERED LAB VALUES:** May increase ANA titer, SGOT (AST), SGPT (ALT), alkaline phosphatase, LDH, bilirubin, BUN, creatinine, potassium, uric acid, lipoproteins, triglycerides.

SIDE EFFECTS

Generally well tolerated, w/ transient and mild side effects. **FREQUENT:** Dizziness, tiredness. **OCCASIONAL:** Depression, pruritus, rash, shortness of breath, bradycardia. **RARE:** Increased dreaming, insomnia, diarrhea, heartburn, nausea, cold extremities, hypotension, palpitations, impotence, edema.

ADVERSE REACTIONS/TOXIC EFFECTS

Excessive dosage may produce profound bradycardia, hypotension, bronchospasm. Abrupt withdrawal may result in sweating, palpitations, headache, tremulousness, exacerbation of angina, MI, ventricular arrhythmias. May precipitate CHF, MI in those with cardiac disease, thyroid storm in those with thyrotoxicosis, peripheral ischemia in those w/existing peripheral vascular disease. Hypoglycemia may occur in previously controlled diabetics.

NURSING IMPLICATIONS

BASELINE ASSESSMENT:

Assess baseline renal/liver function tests. Assess B/P, apical pulse immediately before drug is administered (if pulse is 60/min or below, or systolic B/P is below 90 mm Hg, withhold medication, contact physician). *Antianginal:* Record onset, type (sharp, dull, squeezing), radiation, location, intensity and duration of anginal pain, and precipitating factors (exertion, emotional stress).

INTERVENTION/EVALUATION:

Measure B/P near end of dosing interval (determines if B/P is controlled throughout day). Monitor B/P for hypotension, respiration for shortness of breath. Assess pulse for strength/weakness, irregular rate, bradycardia. Assist w/ambulation if dizziness occurs. Check skin for evidence of rash. Assess for evidence of CHF: dyspnea (particularly on exertion or lying down), night cough, peripheral edema, distended neck veins. Monitor I&O (increase in weight, decrease in urine output may indicate CHF). Therapeutic response to hypertension noted in 1-2 wks.

PATIENT/FAMILY TEACHING:

Do not abruptly discontinue medication. Compliance w/therapy regimen is essential to control hypertension, arrhythmias. If a dose is missed, take next scheduled dose (do not double dose). To avoid hypotensive effect, rise slowly from lying to sitting position, wait momentarily before standing. Avoid tasks that require alertness, motor skills until response to drug is established. Report excessive fatigue, dizziness. Do not use nasal decongestants, over-the-counter cold preparations (stimulants) w/o physician approval. Outpatients should monitor B/P, pulse before taking medication. Restrict salt, alcohol intake.

metronidazole hydrochloride

meh-trow-nye′dah-zoll
(Flagyl, MetroGel, Protostat, Satric)

CANADIAN AVAILABILITY:
Apo-Metronidazole, Flagyl, Neo-Metric, Novonidazol

CLASSIFICATION

Antibacterial, antiprotozoal

PHARMACOKINETICS

Well absorbed from GI tract,

minimal absorption after topical application. Widely distributed, crosses blood-brain barrier. Protein binding: <20%. Metabolized in liver to active metabolite. Primarily excreted in urine; partially eliminated in feces. Removed by hemodialysis. Half-life: 8 hrs (increased in alcoholic liver disease, neonates).

ACTION

Taken up by cells in susceptible microorganisms. Reduced to unidentified polar products, disrupting DNA and inhibiting nucleic acid synthesis producing bactericidal, amebicidal, trichomonacidal effects. Produces anti-inflammatory, immunosuppressive effects when applied topically.

USES

Treatment of anaerobic infections (skin/skin structure, CNS, lower respiratory tract, bone and joints, intra-abdominal, gynecologic, endocarditis, septicemia). Treatment of trichomoniasis, amebiasis, perioperatively for contaminated/potentially contaminated intra-abdominal surgery, antibiotic-associated pseudomembranous colitis. Topical application replaces oral therapy in treatment of acne rosacea. Also used in treatment of grade III, IV decubitus ulcers w/anaerobic infection. Treatment of bacterial vaginosis.

PO/IV ADMINISTRATION

PO:

1. May give w/o regard to meals. Give w/food to decrease GI irritation.

IV:

1. Infuse >30-60 min. Do not give bolus.
2. Avoid prolonged use of indwelling catheters.

INDICATIONS/DOSAGE/ROUTES

Anaerobic bacterial infections:
IV: Adults, elderly: Initially, 1 Gm, then 500 mg q6-8h.
PO: Adults, elderly: 500 mg q6-8h. **Maximum:** 4 Gm/24 hrs.

Antibiotic-associated pseudomembranous colitis:
PO: Adults, elderly: 750 mg to 2 Gm/day in 3-4 divided doses for 7-14 days.

Trichomoniasis:
PO: Adults: 2 Gm as single or in 2 divided doses × 1 day or 250 mg three times/day × 7 days. **Children:** 15 mg/kg in 3 divided doses × 7-10 days. **Infants:** 10-30 mg/kg/day × 5-8 days.

Bacterial vaginosis:
INTRAVAGINALLY: Adults: One applicatorful 2 times/day for 5 days.

Amebiasis:
PO: Adults, elderly: 500-750 mg 3 times/day for 5-10 days. **Children:** 35-50 mg/kg/day in 3 divided doses for 5 days.

Perioperative prophylaxis:
IV: Adults, elderly: 1 Gm 1 hr before surgery and 500 mg 6 and 12 hrs after initial dose.

Rosacea:
TOPICAL: Adults: Thin application 2 times/day to affected area.

PRECAUTIONS

CONTRAINDICATIONS: Hypersensitivity to metronidazole or

other nitroimidazole derivatives (also parabens w/topical application). **CAUTIONS:** Blood dyscrasias, severe hepatic dysfunction, CNS disease, predisposition to edema, concurrent corticosteroid therapy. Safety and efficacy of topical administration in those <21 yrs of age not established. **PREGNANCY/LACTATION:** Readily crosses placenta; distributed in breast milk. Contraindicated during first trimester in those w/ trichomoniasis. Topical use during pregnancy or lactation discouraged. **Pregnancy Category B.**

INTERACTIONS

DRUG INTERACTIONS: Alcohol may cause disulfiram-type reaction. May increase effect of oral anticoagulants. May increase toxicity w/disulfiram. **ALTERED LAB VALUES:** May increase SGOT (AST), SGPT (ALT), LDH.

SIDE EFFECTS

FREQUENT: Anorexia, nausea, dry mouth, metallic taste. *Vaginal:* Symptomatic cervicitis/vaginitis, abdominal cramps, uterine pain. **OCCASIONAL:** Diarrhea or constipation, vomiting, dizziness, erythematous rash, urticaria, reddish brown or dark urine. Oral metronidazole may result in furry tongue, glossitis, cystitis, dysuria. *Topical:* Transient redness, mild dryness, burning, irritation, stinging (also tearing when applied too close to eyes). *Vaginal:* Vaginal, perineal, vulvar itching, vulvar swelling. **RARE:** Mild, transient leukopenia, convulsive seizures, peripheral neuropathy (numbness, tingling, paresthesia). Thrombophlebitis w/ IV therapy. Pancreatitis and flattening of T waves on EKG readings w/oral therapy.

ADVERSE REACTIONS/TOXIC EFFECTS

Superinfection. Peripheral neuropathy (usually reversible if treatment is stopped immediately upon appearance of neurologic symptoms).

NURSING IMPLICATIONS

BASELINE ASSESSMENT:

Question for history of hypersensitivity to metronidazole or other nitroimidazole derivatives (and parabens w/topical). Obtain specimens for diagnostic tests before giving first dose (therapy may begin before results are known).

INTERVENTION/EVALUATION:

Evaluate food tolerance. Determine pattern of bowel activity. Check leukocyte counts frequently. Monitor I&O and assess for urinary problems. Be alert to neurologic symptoms: dizziness, numbness, tingling or paresthesia of extremities. Assess for rash, urticaria. Watch for onset of superinfection: ulceration or change of oral mucosa, furry tongue, vaginal discharge, genital/anal pruritus.

PATIENT/FAMILY TEACHING:

Urine may be red-brown or dark because of metabolism of drug. Avoid alcohol and alcohol-containing preparations, e.g., cough syrups, elixirs. Hard candy, gum, or ice chips may help w/dry mouth. If dizziness occurs, do not drive or use machines that require alertness. If taking metronidazole for trichomoniasis, refrain from sexual intercourse until physician advises. Report any new symptom to physician, esp. dizziness, numbness, tingling. For amebiasis, frequent stool specimen checks will be necessary. *Topical:* Avoid contact w/

eyes. May apply cosmetics after application. Metronidazole acts on redness, papules and pustules but has no effect on rhinophyma (hypertrophy of nose), telangiectasia or ocular problems (conjunctivitis, keratitis, blepharitis). Other recommendations for rosacea include avoidance of hot or spicy foods, alcohol, extremes of hot or cold temperatures, excessive sunlight.

mexiletine hydrochloride

mex-ill'eh-teen

(Mexitil)

CANADIAN AVAILABILITY: Mexitil

CLASSIFICATION

Antiarrhythmic

PHARMACOKINETICS

	ONSET	PEAK	DURATION
PO	0.5-2 hrs	2-3 hrs	—

Well absorbed from upper intestinal section of GI tract. Protein binding: 60-75%. Metabolized in liver (undergoes first-pass effect). Excreted via biliary system. Removed by hemodialysis. Half-life: 10-12 hrs (increase in liver disease, decreased renal function).

ACTION

Blocks fast sodium channels in cardiac tissue without autonomic involvement. Shortens action potential duration, decreases effective refractory period esp. in Purkinje system.

USES

Suppress symptomatic ventricular arrhythmias (PVCs, unifocal or multifocal, couplets, and ventricular tachycardia).

PO ADMINISTRATION

1. Do not crush or break capsules.
2. Give w/food or antacid to reduce GI distress.

INDICATIONS/DOSAGE/ROUTES

Usual dosage for arrhythmias:
PO: Adults, elderly: Initially, 200 mg q8h. Adjust dose by 50-100 mg at 2-3 day intervals. **Maintenance:** 200-300 mg q8h. **Maximum:** 1200 mg/day. **Note:** If 300 mg q8h or less controls arrhythmias, may give dose q12h. **Maximum:** 450 mg q12h.

Rapid control of arrhythmias:
PO: Adults, elderly: Initially, 400 mg, then 200 mg q8h.

PRECAUTIONS

CONTRAINDICATIONS: Cardiogenic shock, preexisting second- or third-degree AV block (w/o presence of pacemaker). **CAUTIONS:** Impaired myocardial function, second- or third-degree AV block (w/pacemaker), CHF, sick sinus syndrome (bradycardia-tachycardia). **PREGNANCY/LACTATION:** Unknown whether drug crosses placenta; distributed in breast milk. **Pregnancy Category B.**

INTERACTIONS

DRUG INTERACTIONS: Urinary acidifiers may increase excretion, urinary alkalizers may decrease excretion. Hepatic enzyme inducers may decrease concentrations. Metoclopramide may increase absorption. **ALTERED LAB VAL-**

UES: May cause positive ANA titers. May increase SGOT (AST).

SIDE EFFECTS

FREQUENT: GI distress (nausea, vomiting, heartburn), dizziness, lightheadedness, tremor. **OCCASIONAL:** Nervousness, change in sleep habits, headache, visual disturbances, paresthesia, diarrhea/constipation, palpitations, chest pain, rash, respiratory difficulty, edema. **RARE:** Dry mouth, weakness, fatigue, tinnitus, depression, speech difficulties.

ADVERSE REACTIONS/TOXIC EFFECTS

Has ability to worsen existing arrhythmias or produce new ones. May produce or worsen CHF.

NURSING IMPLICATIONS

INTERVENTION/EVALUATION:

Monitor EKG, vital signs closely during and after drug administration for cardiac performance. Assess pulse for irregular rate, strength/weakness. Observe for GI disturbances (high incidence). Monitor pattern of daily bowel activity and stool consistency. Assess for dizziness, syncope. Evaluate hand movement for tremor. Check for evidence of CHF (cough, dyspnea [particularly on exertion], rales at base of lungs, fatigue). Monitor fluid and electrolyte serum levels. Check for therapeutic serum level (0.5-2 mcg/ml).

PATIENT/FAMILY TEACHING:

Compliance w/therapy regimen is essential to control cardiac arrhythmias. Report shortness of breath, cough, unexplained sore throat or fever, generalized fatigue. Do not use nasal decongestants, over-the-counter cold preparations (stimulants) w/o physician approval. Restrict salt, alcohol intake.

mezlocillin sodium

mezz-low-sill′in

(Mezlin)

CLASSIFICATION

Antibiotic: Penicillin

PHARMACOKINETICS

Well absorbed after IM administration. Widely distributed. Protein binding: 30%. Primarily excreted unchanged in urine. Removed by hemodialysis. Half-life: 50-70 minutes.

ACTION

Bactericidal. Binds to bacterial membranes. Inhibits cell wall synthesis.

USES

Treatment of gynecologic, skin/skin structure, respiratory, urinary tract, bone and joint, intra-abdominal infections, septicemia, gonorrhea (w/probenecid), perioperative prophylaxis, esp. in abdominal surgery.

STORAGE/HANDLING

Solution appears clear, colorless to pale yellow; may darken slightly (does not indicate loss of potency). If precipitate forms, redissolve in warm water, agitate. IV infusion (piggyback) is stable for 24 hrs at room temperature.

IM/IV ADMINISTRATION

NOTE: Space doses evenly around the clock.

IM:

1. For IM injection, reconstitute each Gm w/3-4 ml sterile water for injection (may require vigorous agitation).
2. Inject slowly and deeply into gluteus maximus.
3. Avoid IM injections >2 Gm.

IV:

1. For IV injection, reconstitute each Gm w/10 ml sterile water for injection or 0.9% NaCl injection. Administer over 3-5 min.
2. For intermittent IV infusion (piggyback), further dilute w/50-100 ml 5% dextrose, 0.9% NaCl, or other compatible IV fluid. Infuse over 30 min.
3. Because of potential for hypersensitivity/anaphylaxis, start initial dose at few drops per min, increase slowly to ordered rate; stay w/pt first 10-15 min, then check q10min.
4. Alternating IV sites, use large veins to reduce risk of phlebitis.

INDICATIONS/DOSAGE/ROUTES

Uncomplicated UTI:
IM/IV: Adults, elderly: 1.5-2 Gm q6h.

Complicated UTI:
IM/IV: Adults, elderly: 3 Gm q6h.

Lower respiratory tract, intra-abdominal, gynecologic, skin/skin structure infections, septicemia:
IV: Adults, elderly: 4 Gm q6h or 3 Gm q4h.

Life-threatening infections:
IV: Adults, elderly: Up to 4 Gm q4h. **Maximum:** 24 Gm/day.

Acute, uncomplicated gonococcal urethritis:
IM/IV: Adults: 1-2 Gm one time w/1 Gm probenecid.

Perioperative prophylaxis:
IV: Adults, elderly: 4 Gm 30-90 min before surgery and 6 and 12 hrs after first dose.

Cesarean section:
IV: Adults: 4 Gm after umbilical cord clamped, then 4 and 8 hrs after first dose.

Usual dosage (children):
IM/IV: Children 1 mo-12 yrs: 50 mg/kg q4h.

Usual dosage (neonates):
IM/IV: Neonates 0-7 days: 75 mg/kg q8-12h. **Neonates 7-28 days:** 75 mg/kg q6-12h.

Dosage in renal impairment:
Dose and/or frequency modified on basis of creatinine clearance and/or severity of infection.

	CREATININE CLEARANCE	
	10-30 ml/min	**<10ml/min**
Uncomplicated UTI	1.5 Gm q8h	1.5 Gm q8h
Complicated UTI	1.5 Gm q6h	1.5 Gm q8h
Serious infections	3 Gm q8h	2 Gm q8h
Life-threatening infections	3 Gm q6h	2 Gm q6h

PRECAUTIONS

CONTRAINDICATIONS: Hypersensitivity to any penicillin. **CAUTIONS:** History of allergies, esp. cephalosporins. **PREGNANCY/LACTATION:** Readily crosses placenta, appears in cord blood, amniotic fluid. Distributed in breast milk in low concentrations. May lead to allergic sensitization, diarrhea, candidiasis, skin rash in infant. **Pregnancy Category B.**

M

INTERACTIONS

DRUG INTERACTIONS: Probenecid may increase concentration, toxicity risk. **ALTERED LAB VALUES:** May increase SGOT (AST), SGPT (ALT), alkaline phosphatase, bilirubin, creatinine, sodium. May cause positive Coombs' test. May decrease potassium.

SIDE EFFECTS

FREQUENT: Rash, urticaria, pain and induration at IM injection site; phlebitis, thrombophlebitis w/IV doses. **OCCASIONAL:** Nausea, vomiting, diarrhea, hypernatremia. **RARE:** Bleeding may occur w/ high IV dosage; hypokalemia, headache, fatigue, dizziness.

ADVERSE REACTIONS/TOXIC EFFECTS

Superinfections, potentially fatal antibiotic-associated colitis may result from altered bacterial balance. Seizures, neurological reactions may occur w/overdosage (most often w/renal impairment). Acute interstitial nephritis, severe hypersensitivity reactions occur rarely.

NURSING IMPLICATIONS

BASELINE ASSESSMENT:

Question for history of allergies, esp. penicillins, cephalosporins. Obtain specimen for culture and sensitivity before giving first dose (therapy may begin before results are known).

INTERVENTION/EVALUATION:

Hold medication and promptly report rash (hypersensitivity) or diarrhea (w/fever, abdominal pain, mucus and blood in stool may indicate antibiotic-associated colitis). Assess food tolerance. Evaluate IV site for phlebitis (heat, pain, red streaking over vein). Check IM injection sites for pain, induration. Monitor I&O, urinalysis, renal function tests. Assess for bleeding: overt bleeding, bruising or tissue swelling; check hematology reports. Monitor electrolytes, particularly sodium, potassium. Be alert for superinfection: increased fever, onset sore throat, diarrhea, vomiting, ulceration or other oral changes, anal/genital pruritus.

PATIENT/FAMILY TEACHING:

Continue antibiotic for full length of treatment. Space doses evenly. Discomfort may occur at IM injection site. Notify physician in event of rash, diarrhea, bleeding, bruising, other new symptom.

miconazole nitrate

mih-koh-na´zoll

(Micatin, Monistat 3, 7, Monistat-Derm)

miconazole

(Monistat IV)

CANADIAN AVAILABILITY:
Micatin, Monistat

CLASSIFICATION

Antifungal

PHARMACOKINETICS

Parenteral: Widely distributed in tissues. Protein binding: 90%. Metabolized in liver. Primarily excreted in urine. Half-life: 24 hrs. *Topical:* No systemic absorption following application to intact skin. *Intravaginally:* Small amount absorbed systemically.

ACTION

Binds w/phospholipids in fungal cell membrane to alter membrane permeability resulting in loss of cellular components.

USES

Treatment of coccidioidomycosis, paracoccidioidomycosis, cryptococcosis, petriellidiosis (allescheriosis), disseminated candidiasis, chronic mucocutaneous candidiasis. Fungal meningitis usually treated intrathecally as well as IV; urinary bladder infections w/ instillations as well as IV miconazole. *Vaginally:* Vulvovaginal candidiasis. *Topical:* Cutaneous candidiasis, tinea cruris, t. corporis, t. pedis, t. versicolor.

STORAGE/HANDLING

After reconstitution, IV solution is stable for 24 hrs at room temperature w/5% dextrose or 0.9% NaCl.

IV ADMINISTRATION

1. Dilute each 200 mg ampoule w/at least 200 ml 5% dextrose or 0.9% NaCl to provide maximum concentration of 1 mg/ml.
2. Give IV infusion (piggyback) over at least 30-60 min (rapid administration may cause arrhythmias).
3. Because of incidence of phlebitis, central venous catheters are recommended.
4. Initial treatment should be performed in hospital w/physician in attendance for first 200 mg dose.

INDICATIONS/DOSAGE/ROUTES

NOTE: IV doses may be divided over 3 IV infusions.

Coccidioidomycosis:
IV: Adults, elderly: 1.8-3.6 Gm/day for 3-20 wks or longer.

Cryptococcosis:
IV: Adults, elderly: 1.2-2.4 Gm/day for 3-12 wks or longer.

Petriellidiosis:
IV: Adults, elderly: 0.6-3.0 Gm/day for 5-20 wks or longer.

Candidiasis:
IV: Adults, elderly: 0.6-1.8 Gm/day for 1-20 wks or longer.

Paracoccidioidomycosis:
IV: Adults, elderly: 0.2-1.2 Gm/day for 2-16 wks or longer.

Usual dosage for children:
IV: Children: 20-40 mg/kg/day in 3 divided doses. (Do not exceed 15 mg/kg for any 1 infusion.)

Vulvovaginal candidiasis:
INTRAVAGINALLY: Adults, elderly: 1-200 mg suppository at bedtime for 3 days; 1-100 mg suppository or 1 applicatorful at bedtime for 7 days.

Topical fungal infections, cutaneous candidiasis:
TOPICAL: Adults, elderly: Apply liberally 2 times/day, morning and evening.

PRECAUTIONS

CONTRAINDICATIONS: Hypersensitivity to miconazole. Children <1 yr; topically, children <2 yrs. **CAUTIONS:** Hepatic insufficiency. **PREGNANCY/LACTATION:** Unknown whether drug crosses placenta or distributed in breast milk. **Pregnancy Category C.**

INTERACTIONS

DRUG INTERACTIONS: May increase effects of oral anticoagulants, oral hypoglycemics. Isoniazid, rifampin may decrease concentrations. **ALTERED LAB VALUES:** None significant.

SIDE EFFECTS

FREQUENT: Nausea, vomiting, phlebitis, pruritus, rash. **OCCASIONAL:** Fever, chills, diarrhea, drowsiness, dizziness. Vaginal and cutaneous application may cause burning, itching, and irritation. **RARE:** Headache, pelvic cramps w/vaginal administration.

ADVERSE REACTIONS/TOXIC EFFECTS

Anemia, thrombocytopenia occur rarely.

NURSING IMPLICATIONS

BASELINE ASSESSMENT:

Question for history of allergies, esp. to miconazole. Confirm that cultures or histologic tests were done. Check for/obtain orders for antiemetics, antihistamines (given before infusion to reduce nausea, vomiting).

INTERVENTION/EVALUATION:

Check for nausea, vomiting (administer medication for symptomatic relief; avoid dosing at mealtimes, slow infusion rate). Assess skin for rash. Evaluate IV site for phlebitis. Determine pattern of bowel activity, stool consistency. Assess mental status (dizziness, drowsiness), provide assistance as needed. Monitor Hgb/Hct results, be alert for bleeding, bruising. *Topical/vaginal:* Assess for burning, itching, irritation.

PATIENT/FAMILY TEACHING:

Continue full length of treatment; prolonged therapy (weeks or months) may be necessary for some conditions. Discomfort may occur at IV site. Notify physician in event of bleeding, bruising, soft tissue swelling or other new symptom. Do not ambulate w/o assistance or use any machinery if dizziness, drowsiness occur. Consult physician before taking any other medication. *Vaginal preparations:* Base interacts w/certain latex products such as contraceptive diaphragm. Ask physician about douching, sexual intercourse. *Topical:* Rub well into affected areas. Avoid getting in eyes. Do not apply any other preparations or occlusive covering w/o consulting physician. Use ointment (sparingly) or lotion in intertriginous areas. Keep areas clean, dry; wear light clothing for ventilation. Separate personal items in contact w/affected areas.

midazolam hydrochloride

my-dah´zoe-lam
(Versed)

CANADIAN AVAILABILITY: Versed

CLASSIFICATION

Sedative **(Schedule IV)**

PHARMACOKINETICS

	ONSET	PEAK	DURATION
IM	5-15 min	45 min	1-6 hrs
IV	1-5 min	—	Dose-related

Well absorbed after IM administration. Protein binding: 97%. Metabolized in liver to active metabolite. Primarily excreted in urine. Half-life: 1-5 hrs.

ACTION

Enhances action of inhibitory neurotransmitter gamma-aminobutyric acid (GABA). Depressant effects occur at all levels of CNS.

USES

IM: Preop for sedation, relief of anxiety; produces anterograde amnesia. *IV:* Sedation (w/o loss of consciousness) to relieve anxiety; produces anterograde amnesia for short diagnostic, endoscopic procedures.

STORAGE/HANDLING

Store at room temperature. Although undiluted solution should be protected from light, it is unnecessary to protect diluted solution from light.

IM/IV ADMINISTRATION

NOTE: Compatible w/5% dextrose, 0.9% NaCl, lactated Ringer's. Compatible for 30 min w/atropine, meperidine, morphine, scopolamine, low doses of opiate agonists.

IM:

1. Give deep IM into large muscle mass.

IV:

1. Oxygen, resuscitative equipment must be readily available before IV is administered.
2. Administer by slow IV injection, in incremental dosages: give each incremental dose over 2 or more min at intervals of at least 2 min.
3. Reduce IV rate in those >60 yrs, and/or debilitated, those w/ chronic disease states, and/or impaired pulmonary function.
4. A too-rapid IV rate, excessive doses, or a single large dose increases risk of respiratory depression/arrest.

INDICATIONS/DOSAGE/ROUTES

Preop:
IM: Adults >18 yrs: 70-80 mcg/kg (0.07-0.08 mg/kg) 30-60 min before surgery. **Elderly/debilitated:** Dosage should be lowered.

Conscious sedation:
IV: Adults: Initially, up to 2.5 mg. May further titrate in small increments to desired effect. Total dose rarely >5 mg. **Elderly:** Initially, up to 1.5 mg. May further titrate to desired effect. Total dose rarely >3.5 mg.

Adjunct to anesthesia:
IV: Adults: Initially, 150-350 mcg/kg. **Elderly:** Initially, 150-300 mcg/kg. Additional doses, 25% of initial dose.

M

PRECAUTIONS

CONTRAINDICATIONS: Shock, comatose pts, acute alcohol intoxication, acute narrow-angle glaucoma. **CAUTIONS:** Acute illness, severe fluid/electrolyte imbalance, impaired renal function, CHF, treated open-angle glaucoma. **PREGNANCY/LACTATION:** Crosses placenta; unknown whether drug is distributed in breast milk. **Pregnancy Category D.**

INTERACTIONS

DRUG INTERACTIONS: Alcohol, CNS depressants may increase CNS, respiratory depression, hypotensive effects. Hypotension-producing medications may increase hypotensive effects. **ALTERED LAB VALUES:** None significant.

SIDE EFFECTS

FREQUENT: Decreased respiratory rate, pain w/IM injection, tenderness at IV injection site, hiccups. **OCCASIONAL:** Nausea, vomiting, erythema, induration at IV site. **RARE:** Hypotensive episodes.

ADVERSE REACTIONS/TOXIC EFFECTS

Too much or too little dosage, improper administration, or cerebral hypoxia may result in agitation, involuntary movements, hyperactivity, combativeness. Underventilation/apnea may produce hypoxia, cardiac arrest. A too-rapid IV rate, excessive doses, or a single large dose increases risk of respiratory depression/arrest.

NURSING IMPLICATIONS

Baseline Assessment:

Resuscitative equipment, endotracheal tube, suction, oxygen must be available. Obtain vital signs before administration.

Intervention/Evaluation:

Monitor respiratory rate continuously during parenteral administration for underventilation, apnea. Monitor vital signs q3-5min during recovery period.

Patient/Family Teaching:

Discomfort may occur w/IM injection.

milrinone lactate

mill'rih-known
(Primacor)

CLASSIFICATION

Cardiotonic

PHARMACOKINETICS

	ONSET	PEAK	DURATION
IV	5-15 min	—	—

Protein binding: 70%. Metabolized in liver; excreted in urine. Half-life: 2.4 hrs.

ACTION

Inhibits phosphodiesterase activity in cardiac and vascular muscle; possesses positive inotropic effect (increases force of myocardial contraction), direct arterial vasodilation.

USES

Short-term management of congestive heart failure (CHF).

STORAGE/HANDLING

Store parenteral form at room temperature.

IV ADMINISTRATION

1. Avoid furosemide injections into tubing of milrinone IV infusion (precipitate forms immediately).
2. For IV injection (loading dose) administer slowly over 10 min.
3. For IV infusion, dilute 20 mg (20 ml) vial with 80 or 180 ml diluent (0.9% NaCl, 5% dextrose) to provide concentration of 200 or 100 mcg/ml respectively.
4. Monitor for arrhythmias, hypotension during IV therapy. Reduce or temporarily discontinue infusion until condition stabilizes.

INDICATIONS/DOSAGE/ROUTES

Congestive heart failure:
IV: Adults: Initially, give 50 mcg/kg over 10 min. Continue w/maintenance infusion rate of 0.375-0.75 mcg/kg/min based on hemodynamic and clinical response (total daily dose: 0.59-1.13 mg/kg). Re-

duce dose to 0.2-0.43 mcg/kg/min in pts w/severe renal impairment.

PRECAUTIONS

CONTRAINDICATIONS: Severe obstructive aortic or pulmonic valvular disease. **CAUTIONS:** Impaired renal, hepatic function. **PREGNANCY/LACTATION:** Unknown whether drug crosses placenta or is distributed in breast milk. **Pregnancy Category C.**

INTERACTIONS

DRUG INTERACTIONS: Produces additive inotropic effects w/ cardiac glycosides. **ALTERED LAB VALUES:** None significant.

SIDE EFFECTS

OCCASIONAL: Headache, hypotension. **RARE:** Angina, chest pain.

ADVERSE REACTIONS/TOXIC EFFECTS

Supraventricular and ventricular arrhythmias occur in 12%; nonsustained ventricular tachycardia occurs in 2%, sustained ventricular tachycardia in 1% of those treated.

NURSING IMPLICATIONS

BASELINE ASSESSMENT:

Offer emotional support (difficulty breathing may produce anxiety). Assess B/P, apical pulse rate before treatment begins and during IV therapy. Assess lung sounds, check edema.

INTERVENTION/EVALUATION:

Hemodynamic monitoring. Assess hypotension, heart rate, serum electrolytes, I&O, renal function studies. Assess lungs for rales, wheezing; check for edema. Monitor CHF symptoms.

minocycline hydrochloride

min-know-sigh′clean
(Minocin)

CANADIAN AVAILABILITY:
Minocin

CLASSIFICATION

Antibiotic: Tetracycline

PHARMACOKINETICS

Well absorbed from GI tract. Widely distributed. Protein binding: 76%. Partially inactivated in liver. Excreted in urine, eliminated in feces via biliary secretion. Minimally removed by hemodialysis. Half-life: 11-23 hrs.

ACTION

Bacteriostatic because of binding to ribosomes, inhibiting protein synthesis.

USES

Treatment of prostate, urinary tract, CNS infections (not meningitis), uncomplicated gonorrhea, inflammatory acne, brucellosis, skin granulomas, cholera, trachoma, nocardiasis, yaws, and syphilis when penicillins are contraindicated.

STORAGE/HANDLING

Store capsules, oral suspension at room temperature. IV solution stable for 24 hrs at room temperature. Use IV infusion (piggyback) immediately after reconstitution. Discard if precipitate forms.

PO/IV ADMINISTRATION

PO:

1. Give oral capsules, tablets w/ full glass of water.

IV:

NOTE: Give by intermittent IV infusion (piggyback).

1. For intermittent IV infusion (piggyback), reconstitute each 100 mg vial w/5-10 ml sterile water for injection to provide concentration of 20 or 10 mg/ml respectively.
2. Further dilute w/500-1,000 ml 5% dextrose, 0.9% NaCl, or other compatible IV fluid. Infuse over >6 hrs.
3. Alternating IV sites, use large veins to reduce risk of phlebitis.

INDICATIONS/DOSAGE/ROUTES

NOTE: Space doses evenly around the clock.

Mild to moderate to severe infections:
PO: Adults, elderly: Initially, 100-200 mg, then 100 mg q12h, or 50 mg q6h.
IV: Adults, elderly: Initially, 200 mg, then 100 mg q12h up to 400 mg/day.
PO/IV: Children >8 yrs: Initially, 4 mg/kg, then 2 mg/kg q12h.

PRECAUTIONS

CONTRAINDICATIONS: Hypersensitivity to tetracyclines, last half of pregnancy, children <8 yrs. **CAUTIONS:** Renal impairment, sun or ultraviolet exposure (severe photosensitivity reaction). **PREGNANCY/LACTATION:** Readily crosses placenta; distributed in breast milk. Avoid use in women during last half of pregnancy. May produce permanent teeth discoloration, enamel hypoplasia, inhibit fetal skeletal growth in children <8 yrs. **Pregnancy Category D.**

INTERACTIONS

DRUG INTERACTIONS: Cholestyramine, colestipol may decrease absorption. May decrease effect of oral contraceptives. Carbamazepine, phenytoin may decrease concentrations. **ALTERED LAB VALUES:** May increase SGOT (AST), SGPT (ALT), alkaline phosphatase, amylase, bilirubin concentrations.

SIDE EFFECTS

FREQUENT: Headache, dizziness, vertigo, drowsiness, fatigue, anorexia, nausea, vomiting, diarrhea, dysphagia. **OCCASIONAL:** Vaginal candidiasis, rash, urticaria, thrombophlebitis.

ADVERSE REACTIONS/TOXIC EFFECTS

Superinfection (esp. fungal), anaphylaxis, increased intracranial pressure, bulging fontanelles occur rarely in infants.

NURSING IMPLICATIONS

BASELINE ASSESSMENT:

Question for history of allergies, esp. tetracyclines, sulfite. Obtain culture and sensitivity test before giving first dose (therapy may begin before results are known).

INTERVENTION/EVALUATION:

Check IV site for phlebitis (heat, pain, red streaking over vein). Assess ability to ambulate: drowsiness, vertigo, dizziness. Determine pattern of bowel activity and stool consistency. Monitor food intake, tolerance. Assess skin for rash. Check B/P and level of consciousness for increased intracranial pressure. Be alert for superinfection: diarrhea, ulceration or changes of oral mucosa, anal/genital pruritus.

PATIENT/FAMILY TEACHING:

Continue antibiotic for full length of treatment. Space doses evenly.

Drink full glass of water w/capsules, tablets and avoid bedtime doses. Avoid tasks that require alertness, motor skills until response to drug is established. Notify physician if diarrhea, rash, other new symptom occurs. Protect skin from sun exposure. Consult physician before taking any other medication.

minoxidil

min-ox'ih-dill
(Loniten, Rogaine)

CANADIAN AVAILABILITY:
Loniten, Rogaine

CLASSIFICATION

Antihypertensive

PHARMACOKINETICS

	ONSET	PEAK	DURATION
PO	0.5 hrs	2-8 hrs	2-5 days

Well absorbed from GI tract, minimal absorption after topical application. Widely distributed. Metabolized in liver to active metabolite. Primarily excreted in urine. Removed by hemodialysis. Half-life: 4.2 hrs.

ACTION

Direct vasodilator of arterioles (decreases peripheral vascular resistance). *Topical:* Increases cutaneous blood flow, stimulates resting hair follicles, hair follicle cells.

USES

Treatment of severe symptomatic hypertension, or hypertension associated w/organ damage. Used for those who fail to respond to maximal therapeutic dosages of diuretic and two other antihypertensive agents. Treatment of alopecia androgenetica (males: baldness of vertex of scalp; females: diffuse hair loss or thinning of frontoparietal areas).

PO/TOPICAL ADMINISTRATION

PO:

1. Give w/o regard to food (w/food if GI upset occurs).
2. Tablets may be crushed.

TOPICAL:

1. Shampoo and dry hair before applying medication.
2. Wash hands immediately after application.
3. Do not use hair dryer after application (reduces effectiveness).

INDICATIONS/DOSAGE/ROUTES

Hypertension:
PO: Adults: Initially, 5 mg/day. Increase w/at least 3-day intervals to 10 mg, 20 mg, up to 40 mg/day in 1-2 doses. **Elderly:** Initially, 2.5 mg/day. May increase gradually. **Maintenance:** 10-40 mg/day. **Maximum:** 100 mg/day. **Children:** Initially, 0.2 mg/kg (5 mg maximum) daily. Gradually increase at minimum 3-day intervals of 0.1-2 mg/kg. **Maintenance:** 0.25-1 mg/kg/day in 1-2 doses. **Maximum:** 50 mg/day.

Hair regrowth:
TOPICAL: Adults: 1 ml to total affected areas of scalp 2 times/day. Total daily dose not to exceed 2 ml.

PRECAUTIONS

CONTRAINDICATIONS: Pheochromocytoma. **CAUTIONS:** Severe renal impairment, chronic CHF, coronary artery disease, recent MI (1 mo). **PREGNANCY/LACTATION:** Crosses placenta;

M

distributed in breast milk. **Pregnancy Category C.**

INTERACTIONS

DRUG INTERACTIONS: Parenteral antihypertensives may increase hypotensive effect. NSAIDs may decrease effect. **ALTERED LAB VALUES:** May increase BUN, creatinine, plasma renin activity, alkaline phosphatase, sodium. May decrease Hgb, Hct, erythrocyte count.

SIDE EFFECTS

FREQUENT: *Oral:* Edema with concurrent weight gain, hypertrichosis (elongation, thickening, increased pigmentation of fine body hair) develops in 80% of pts within 3-6 wks after beginning therapy. Occurs on face first and later extends to back, arms, legs. **OCCASIONAL:** T wave changes but usually these revert to pretreatment state with continued therapy or drug withdrawal. **RARE:** Rash, pruritus, breast tenderness in male and female, headache.

ADVERSE REACTIONS/TOXIC EFFECTS

Tachycardia and angina pectoris may occur, because of increased oxygen demands associated w/increased heart rate, cardiac output. Fluid and electrolyte imbalance, CHF may be observed (esp. if diuretic is not given concurrently). Too-rapid reduction in B/P may result in syncope, cerebral vascular accident, MI, ischemia of special sense organs (vision, hearing). Pericardial effusion and tamponade may be seen in those w/impaired renal function not on dialysis.

NURSING IMPLICATIONS

BASELINE ASSESSMENT:

Assess B/P on both arms and take pulse for 1 full min immediately before giving medication. If pulse increases 20 beats/min or more over baseline, or systolic or diastolic B/P decreases more than 20 mm Hg, withhold drug, contact physician.

INTERVENTION/EVALUATION:

Assess for peripheral edema of hands, feet (usually, first area of low extremity swelling is behind medial malleolus in ambulatory, sacral area in bedridden). Assess for signs of CHF (cough, rales at base of lungs, cool extremities, dyspnea on exertion). Monitor fluid and electrolyte serum levels. Assess for distant or muffled heart sounds by auscultation (pericardial effusion, tamponade).

PATIENT/FAMILY TEACHING:

Maximum B/P response occurs in 3-7 days. Reversible growth of fine body hair may begin 3-6 wks after treatment is initiated. When used topically for stimulation of hair growth, treatment must continue on a permanent basis—cessation of treatment will begin reversal of new hair growth.

misoprostol

mis-oh-pros´toll
(Cytotec)

CANADIAN AVAILABILITY:
Cytotec

CLASSIFICATION

Antisecretory, gastric protectant

PHARMACOKINETICS

Rapidly absorbed from GI tract. Protein binding: 85%. Rapidly deesterified to active metabolite. Primarily excreted in urine. Half-life: 20-40 min.

ACTION

Increases production of gastric mucus. Inhibits basal, nocturnal gastric acid secretion via direct action on parietal cells.

USES

Prevention of NSAID-induced gastric ulcers and in those at high risk of developing gastric ulcer or gastric ulcer complication.

PO ADMINISTRATION

Give after meals or w/meals (minimizes diarrhea).

INDICATIONS/DOSAGE/ROUTES

Prevention of NSAID-induced gastric ulcer:

PO: Adults: 200 mcg 4 times/day w/food (last dose at bedtime). Continue for duration of NSAID therapy. May reduce dosage to 100 mcg if 200 mcg dose is not tolerable. **Elderly:** 100-200 mcg 4 times/day w/food.

PRECAUTIONS

CONTRAINDICATIONS: Pregnancy, history of allergy to prostaglandins. **CAUTIONS:** Impaired renal function. **PREGNANCY/LACTATION:** Unknown whether distributed in breast milk. Produces uterine contractions, uterine bleeding, expulsion of products of conception (abortifacient property). **Pregnancy Category X.**

INTERACTIONS

DRUG INTERACTIONS: None significant. **ALTERED LAB VALUES:** None significant.

SIDE EFFECTS

FREQUENT: Diarrhea, abdominal discomfort. **OCCASIONAL:** Nausea, flatulence, dyspepsia, headache. **RARE:** Vomiting, constipation, gynecologic abnormalities (spotting, cramps, excessive bleeding).

ADVERSE REACTIONS/TOXIC EFFECTS

Overdosage may produce sedation, tremor, convulsions, dyspnea, palpitations, hypotension, bradycardia.

NURSING IMPLICATIONS

BASELINE ASSESSMENT:

Question for possibility of pregnancy before initiating therapy (Pregnancy Category X).

PATIENT/FAMILY TEACHING:

Avoid magnesium-containing antacids (minimizes potential for diarrhea). Women of childbearing potential must not be pregnant before or during medication therapy (may result in hospitalization, surgery, infertility, death).

mitomycin

my-toe-my´sin

(Mutamycin)

CANADIAN AVAILABILITY:

Mutamycin

CLASSIFICATION

Antineoplastic

PHARMACOKINETICS

Widely distributed. Does not cross blood-brain barrier. Primarily metabolized in liver and excreted in urine. Half-life: 50 min.

ACTION

Cell cycle-phase nonspecific (most active in G and S phase of cell division). Crosslinks DNA inhibiting DNA, RNA, protein synthesis.

USES

Treatment of disseminated adenocarcinoma of stomach, pancreas.

STORAGE/HANDLING

NOTE: May be carcinogenic, mutagenic, or teratogenic. Handle w/ extreme care during preparation/ administration.

Use only clear, blue-grey solutions. Concentrations of 0.5 mg/ml are stable for 7 days at room temperature or 2 wks if refrigerated. Further diluted solutions w/5% dextrose are stable for 3 hrs, 24 hrs if diluted w/0.9% NaCl.

IV ADMINISTRATION

NOTE: Give IV via IV catheter, IV infusion. Extremely irritating to vein. May produce pain on injection, w/induration, thrombophlebitis, paresthesia.

1. Reconstitute 5 mg vial w/10 ml sterile water for injection (40 ml for 20 mg vial) to provide solution containing 0.5 mg/ml.
2. Do not shake vial to dissolve. Allow vial to stand at room temperature until complete dissolution occurs.
3. Give IV through tubing of functional IV catheter or running IV infusion.
4. For IV infusion, further dilute w/50-100 ml 5% dextrose or 0.9% NaCl injection.
5. Extravasation may produce cellulitis, ulceration, tissue sloughing. Terminate immediately, inject ordered antidote. Apply ice intermittently for up to 72 hrs; keep area elevated.

INDICATIONS/DOSAGE/ROUTES

NOTE: Dosage individualized based on clinical response, tolerance to adverse effects. When used in combination therapy, consult specific protocols for optimum dosage, sequence of drug administration.

Initial dosage:
IV: Adults, elderly: 20 mg/m^2 as single dose. Repeat q6-8wks. Give additional courses only after circulating blood elements (platelets, WBC) are within acceptable levels.

PRECAUTIONS

CONTRAINDICATIONS: Platelet count less than 75,000/mm^3, WBC less than 3000/mm^3, serum creatinine greater than 1.7 mg/dl, coagulation disorders/bleeding tendencies, serious infection. **CAUTIONS:** Impaired renal function, pulmonary disorders. **PREGNANCY/LACTATION:** If possible, avoid use during pregnancy, esp. first trimester. Breast feeding not recommended. **Pregnancy Category C.**

INTERACTIONS

DRUG INTERACTIONS: Bone marrow depressants may increase bone marrow depression. Live virus vaccines may potentiate virus replication, increase vaccine side effects, decrease pt's antibody response to vaccine. **ALTERED**

LAB VALUES: May increase BUN, creatinine.

SIDE EFFECTS

FREQUENT: Nausea, vomiting within 1-2 hrs after IV administration. Vomiting subsides rapidly; nausea may persist 2-3 days, fever, anorexia, prolonged malaise w/ weakness, weight loss. **OCCASIONAL:** Alopecia, mouth ulcers, pruritus.

ADVERSE REACTIONS/TOXIC EFFECTS

Marked bone marrow depression results in hematologic toxicity manifested as leukopenia, thrombocytopenia, and to lesser extent, anemia (generally occurs within 2-4 wks after initial therapy). Renal toxicity may be evidenced by rise in BUN and/or serum creatinine. Pulmonary toxicity manifested as dyspnea, cough, hemoptysis, pneumonia. Long-term therapy may produce hemolytic-uremic syndrome (HUS), characterized by hemolytic anemia, thrombocytopenia, renal failure, hypertension.

NURSING IMPLICATIONS

BASELINE ASSESSMENT:

Obtain WBC, platelet, differential, prothrombin, bleeding time, Hgb before and periodically during therapy. Antiemetics before and during therapy may alleviate nausea/vomiting.

INTERVENTION/EVALUATION:

Monitor hematologic status, BUN, serum creatinine, kidney function studies. Assess IV site for phlebitis, extravasation. Monitor for hematologic toxicity (fever, sore throat, signs of local infection, easy bruising, unusual bleeding from any site), symptoms of anemia (excessive tiredness, weakness). Assess for renal toxicity (foul odor, rise in BUN, serum creatinine).

PATIENT/FAMILY TEACHING:

Maintain fastidious oral hygiene. Immediately report any stinging, burning at injection site. Do not have immunizations w/o physician's approval (drug lowers body's resistance). Avoid contact w/those who have recently received live virus vaccine. Promptly report fever, sore throat, signs of local infection, easy bruising, unusual bleeding from any site, burning on urination, increased frequency. Alopecia is reversible, but new hair growth may have different color or texture. Contact physician if nausea/vomiting continues at home.

mitotane

my´tow-tain

(Lysodren)

CANADIAN AVAILABILITY: Lysodren

CLASSIFICATION

Antineoplastic

PHARMACOKINETICS

Partially absorbed from GI tract. Widely distributed. Metabolized in liver/kidney. Primarily excreted in urine. Half-life: 18-159 days.

ACTION

Selectively inhibit adrenocortical function, functional and nonfunctional adrenocortical neoplasms by direct cytoxic effect.

USES

Treatment of inoperable functional and nonfunctional adenocortical carcinomas.

INDICATIONS/DOSAGE/ROUTES

NOTE: May be carcinogenic, mutagenic, or teratogenic. Handle w/ extreme care during administration.

Adenocortical carcinomas:
PO: Adults: Initially, 2-6 Gm/day in 3-4 divided doses. Increase by 2-4 Gm/day q3-7days, up to 9-10 Gm/day. **Range:** 2-16 Gm/day.

PRECAUTIONS

CONTRAINDICATIONS: Known hypersensitivity to drug. **CAUTIONS:** Hepatic disease. **PREGNANCY/LACTATION:** If possible, avoid use during pregnancy, esp. first trimester. Breast feeding not recommended. **Pregnancy Category C.**

INTERACTIONS

DRUG INTERACTIONS: CNS depressants may increase CNS depression. **ALTERED LAB VALUES:** May decrease plasma cortisol, urinary 17-OH, PBI, uric acid.

SIDE EFFECTS

FREQUENT: Anorexia, nausea, vomiting, diarrhea, lethargy, somnolence, adrenocortical insufficiency, dizziness, vertigo, maculopapular rash, hypouricemia. **OCCASIONAL:** Blurred or double vision, retinopathy, decreased hearing, excess salivation, urine abnormalities (hematuria, cystitis, albuminuria), hypertension, orthostatic hypotension, flushing, wheezing, shortness of breath, generalized aching, fever.

ADVERSE REACTIONS/TOXIC EFFECTS

Brain damage, functional impairment may occur w/long-term, high dosage therapy.

NURSING IMPLICATIONS

BASELINE ASSESSMENT:

Therapy should be discontinued immediately following shock, trauma (drug produces adrenal suppression). Steroid-replacement therapy generally necessary during therapy.

INTERVENTION/EVALUATION:

Monitor uric acid serum levels, hepatic function studies, urine tests. Perform neurologic and behavioral assessments periodically in those receiving prolonged therapy (over 2 yrs). Assess pattern of daily bowel activity and stool consistency. Assess skin for maculopapular rash.

PATIENT/FAMILY TEACHING:

Immediately report injury, infection, other illnesses. Do not have immunizations w/o physician's approval (drug lowers body resistance). Increase fluid intake (may protect against urine abnormalities). Contact physician if nausea/vomiting continues at home. Do not drive or perform tasks requiring alert response if dizziness, drowsiness occur. Contraception is recommended during therapy.

mitoxantrone

my-toe-zan´trone
(Novantrone)

CANADIAN AVAILABILITY:
Novantrone

CLASSIFICATION

Antineoplastic

PHARMACOKINETICS

Widely distributed. Protein binding: 78%. Metabolized in liver. Primarily eliminated in feces via biliary system. Half-life: 2.3-13 days.

ACTION

Cell cycle-phase nonspecific. Most active in late S phase of cell division. Binds to DNA. Inhibits DNA, RNA synthesis.

USES

Treatment of acute, nonlymphocytic leukemia (monocytic, myelogenous, promyelocytic).

IV ADMINISTRATION

NOTE: May be carcinogenic, mutagenic, or teratogenic. Handle w/ extreme care during preparation/ administration. Give by IV injection, IV infusion. Must dilute before administration.

1. Dilute w/at least 50 ml 5% dextrose or 0.9% NaCl. Infuse into freely running IV over at least 3 min.
2. Do not mix w/heparin in same IV solution (precipitate forms).

INDICATIONS/DOSAGE/ROUTES

NOTE: Dosage individualized based on clinical response, tolerance to adverse effects. When used in combination therapy, consult specific protocols for optimum dosage, sequence of drug administration.

Usual dosage:
IV: Adults: Combined w/cytosine: *Induction:* 12 mg/m^2/day on days 1-3. *Second course (for incomplete response):* 12 mg/m^2/day on days 1 and 2.

PRECAUTIONS

CONTRAINDICATIONS: None significant. **CAUTIONS:** None significant. **PREGNANCY/LACTATION:** If possible, avoid use during pregnancy, esp. first trimester. May cause fetal harm. Breast feeding not recommended. **Pregnancy Category D.**

INTERACTIONS

DRUG INTERACTIONS: May decrease effect of antigout medications. Bone marrow depressants may increase bone marrow depression. Live virus vaccines may potentiate virus replication, increase vaccine side effects, decrease pt's antibody response to vaccine. **ALTERED LAB VALUES:** May increase SGOT (AST), SGPT (ALT), bilirubin, uric acid.

SIDE EFFECTS

FREQUENT: Nausea, vomiting, diarrhea, cough, headache, inflammation of mucous membranes, abdominal discomfort, fever, alopecia. **OCCASIONAL:** Easy bruising, fungal infection, conjunctivitis, urinary tract infection. **RARE:** Arrhythmias.

ADVERSE REACTIONS/TOXIC EFFECTS

Bone marrow suppression may be severe, resulting in GI bleeding, sepsis, pneumonia. Renal failure, seizures, jaundice, CHF may occur.

NURSING IMPLICATIONS

BASELINE ASSESSMENT:

Establish baseline for CBC, temperature, rate and quality of pulse, lung status.

INTERVENTION/EVALUATION:

Monitor lung sounds for pulmonary toxicity (dyspnea, fine lung rales). Monitor hematologic status, pulmonary function studies, hepatic and renal function tests. Monitor for stomatitis (burning/erythema of oral mucosa at inner margin of lips) fever, sore throat, signs of local infection, easy bruising or unusual bleeding from any site.

PATIENT/FAMILY TEACHING:

Urine will appear blue/green 24 hrs after administration. Blue tint to sclera may also appear. Maintain adequate daily fluid intake (may protect against renal impairment). Do not have immunizations w/o physician's approval (drug lowers body's resistance). Avoid contact w/those who have recently received live virus vaccine. Contact physician if nausea/vomiting continues at home.

mivacurium chloride

miv'ah-cure-ee-um
(Mivacron)

(See Classifications section under Neuromuscular blocking agents)

molindone hydrochloride

mole-in'doan
(Moban)

CLASSIFICATION

Antipsychotic

PHARMACOKINETICS

	ONSET	PEAK	DURATION
PO	—	—	36 hrs

Rapidly absorbed from GI tract. Widely distributed. Protein binding: 90-99%. Metabolized in liver to active metabolite. Primarily excreted in urine.

ACTION

Decreases dopamine activity. Occupies dopamine receptors in reticular activating, limbic systems in brain.

USES

Symptomatic management of schizophrenic disorders.

PO ADMINISTRATION

1. Give w/o regard to meals.
2. Give oral concentrate alone or mix w/water, milk, fruit juice, or carbonated beverages.

INDICATIONS/DOSAGE/ROUTES

Management of schizophrenia:
PO: Adults: Initially, 50-75 mg/day in 3-4 divided doses. Increase to 100 mg/day in 3-4 days, if needed.

Maintenance (mild symptoms):
PO: Adults: 5-15 mg 3-4 times/day.

Maintenance (moderate symptoms):
PO: Adults: 10-25 mg 3-4 times/day.

Maintenance (severe symptoms):
PO: Adults: Up to 225 mg may be needed.

Usual elderly dosage (nonpsychotic):
PO: Elderly: Initially, 5-10 mg 1-2 times/day. May increase by 5-10

mg every 4-7 days. **Maximum:** 112 mg/day.

PRECAUTIONS

CONTRAINDICATIONS: Severe CNS depression, comatose states. **CAUTIONS:** Severe cardiovascular disorders, history of seizures. **PREGNANCY/LACTATION:** Unknown whether drug crosses placenta or is distributed in breast milk. **Pregnancy Category C.**

INTERACTIONS

DRUG INTERACTIONS: Alcohol, CNS depression producing medications may prolong CNS effects. Anticholinergics, antihistamines, MAO inhibitors, maprotiline, tricyclic antidepressants may increase anticholinergic, sedative effects. Extrapyramidal symptoms (EPS) may increase in severity, frequency w/EPS producing medications. May cause neurotoxic symptoms w/lithium. **ALTERED LAB VALUES:** May alter BUN, RBCs, glucose values. May increase prolactin concentration, WBCs.

SIDE EFFECTS

FREQUENT: Transient drowsiness, dry mouth, constipation, blurred vision, nasal congestion. **OCCASIONAL:** Diarrhea, peripheral edema, rash, urinary retention, nausea, mild/transient postural hypotension, tachycardia. **RARE:** Skin pigmentation, ocular changes.

ADVERSE REACTIONS/TOXIC EFFECTS

Frequently noted extrapyramidal symptom is akathisia (motor restlessness, anxiety). Occurring less frequently is akinesia (rigidity, tremor, salivation, mask-like facial expression, reduced voluntary movements). Infrequently noted are dystonias: torticollis (neck muscle spasm), opisthotonos (rigidity of back muscles), and oculogyric crisis (rolling back of eyes). Tardive dyskinesia (protrusion of tongue, puffing of cheeks, chewing/puckering of mouth) occurs rarely but may be irreversible. Risk is greater in female geriatric pts. Potentially fatal neuroleptic malignant syndrome (NMS) requires immediate discontinuation of the drug.

NURSING IMPLICATIONS

Baseline Assessment:

Assess behavior, appearance, emotional status, response to environment, speech pattern, thought content.

Intervention/Evaluation:

Supervise suicidal-risk pt closely during early therapy (as depression lessens, energy level improves, increasing suicide potential). Monitor B/P for hypotension. Assess for peripheral edema behind medial malleolus (sacral area in bedridden pts). Monitor stools; avoid constipation. Assess for extrapyramidal symptoms (see above), hyperthermia, altered mental status or level of consciousness, and autonomic instability (NMS); evaluate for evidence of tardive dyskinesia. Assess for therapeutic response (interest in surroundings, improvement in self-care, increased ability to concentrate, relaxed facial expression).

Patient/Family Teaching:

Full therapeutic effects may take up to 6 wks. Report visual disturbances. Sugarless gum or sips of tepid water may relieve dry mouth. Drowsiness generally subsides during continued therapy. Avoid tasks that require alertness, motor skills until response to drug is established. Avoid alcohol and CNS depressants.

mometasone

moe-met´ah-sone

(Elocon)

(See Classifications section under Corticosteroids: topical)

moricizine hydrochloride

mor-ih-see´zeen

(Ethmozine)

CLASSIFICATION

Antiarrhythmic

PHARMACOKINETICS

	ONSET	PEAK	DURATION
PO	—	2-4 hrs	—

Well absorbed from GI tract. Undergoes significant first-pass metabolism. Protein binding: 95%. Metabolized in liver (induces own metabolism). Primarily eliminated in feces via biliary system. Minimal removal by hemodialysis. Half-life: 1.5-3.5 hrs.

ACTION

Inhibits sodium current across myocardial cell membranes. Has potent local anesthetic activity and membrane stabilizing effects. Slows AV, Purkinje conduction, decreases action potential duration, effective refractory period.

USES

Treatment of documented, life-threatening ventricular arrhythmias (e.g., sustained ventricular tachycardia).

PO ADMINISTRATION

1. May be given w/o regard to food but give w/food if GI upset occurs.
2. Monitor EKG for cardiac changes, particularly, increase in PR and QRS intervals. Notify physician of any significant interval changes.

INDICATIONS/DOSAGE/ROUTES

Usual dosage for arrhythmias:
PO: Adults, elderly: 200-300 mg q8h; may increase by 150 mg/day at 3-day intervals until desired effect achieved.

Dosage in hepatic/renal impairment:
Initially, 600 mg or less/day.

PRECAUTIONS

CONTRAINDICATIONS: Preexisting second- or third-degree AV block or right-bundle-branch block associated w/left hemiblock (bifascicular block), w/o pacemaker; cardiogenic shock. **CAUTIONS:** CHF, electrolyte imbalance, sick sinus syndrome (bradycardia-tachycardia), impaired hepatic/renal function. **PREGNANCY/LACTATION:** Unknown if drug crosses placenta; distributed in breast milk. **Pregnancy Category B.**

INTERACTIONS

DRUG INTERACTIONS: Cimetidine may increase concentrations; moricizine may decrease theophylline concentrations. **ALTERED LAB VALUES:** May cause EKG changes (prolong PR, QT intervals).

SIDE EFFECTS

FREQUENT: Dizziness, nausea, heachache, fatigue, dyspnea. **OCCASIONAL:** Nervousness, paresthesia, sleep disturbances, dyspepsia, vomiting, diarrhea. **RARE:** Urinary retention/frequency, sweating, dry mouth, swelling of lips/tongue, periorbital edema, impotence, decreased libido, generalized body aches.

ADVERSE REACTIONS/TOXIC EFFECTS

Has ability to worsen existing arrhythmias or produce new ones. Jaundice w/hepatitis occurs rarely. Overdosage produces emesis, lethargy, syncope, hypotension, conduction disturbances, exacerbation of CHF, MI, sinus arrest.

NURSING IMPLICATIONS

BASELINE ASSESSMENT:

Correct electrolyte imbalance before administering medication.

INTERVENTION/EVALUATION:

Monitor EKG for cardiac changes, particularly, increase in PR and QRS intervals. Notify physician of any significant interval changes. Assess pulse for strength/weakness, irregular rate. Question for headache, GI upset, dizziness, nausea. Monitor fluid and electrolyte serum levels. Monitor pattern of daily bowel activity and stool consistency. Assess for dizziness, unsteadiness. Monitor liver enzymes results.

PATIENT/FAMILY TEACHING:

Do not abruptly discontinue medication. Compliance w/therapy regimen is essential to control arrhythmias.

morphine sulfate

(Astramorph, Duramorph, MS Contin, MSIR, RMS, Roxanol)

CANADIAN AVAILABILITY: Epimorph, Morphitec, M.O.S., MS Contin, Roxanol

CLASSIFICATION

Opioid: Analgesic **(Schedule II)**

M

PHARMACOKINETICS

	ONSET	PEAK	DURATION
PO	Variable	60-120 min	4-5 hrs
Extended release	—	60-120 min	8-12 hrs
SubQ	5-30 min	50-90 min	4-5 hrs
IM	5-30 min	30-60 min	3-7 hrs
IV	Rapid	20 min	4-5 hrs
Rectal	20-60 min	—	4-5 hrs
Epidural	15-60 min	—	16-24 hrs
Intrathecal	15-60 min	—	16-24 hrs

Variably absorbed from GI tract. Readily absorbed after SubQ, IM administration. Widely distributed. Protein binding: low. Metabolized in liver. Primarily excreted in urine. Half-life: 2-3 hrs.

ACTION

Binds w/opioid receptors within CNS, altering processes affecting pain perception, emotional response to pain. Decreases intestinal motility by local, central actions.

USES

Relief of severe, acute, chronic pain, preop sedation, anesthesia supplement, analgesia during labor. Drug of choice for pain due to myocardial infarction, dyspnea from pulmonary edema not resulting from chemical respiratory irritant.

STORAGE/HANDLING

Store suppositories, parenteral, oral form at room temperature. Discard unused portion from pt-controlled IV infusion.

PO/SubQ/IM/IV/RECTAL ADMINISTRATION

NOTE: Give by IM injection if repeated doses necessary (repeated SubQ may produce local tissue irritation, induration). May also be given slow IV injection or IV infusion. Incompatible w/aminophylline, amobarbital, chlorothiazide, phenytoin, heparin, meperidine, methicillin, nitrofurantoin, pentobarbital, phenobarbital, sodium bicarbonate, sodium iodide, thiopental.

PO:

1. Mix liquid form w/fruit juice to improve taste.
2. Do not crush or break extended-release capsule.

SubQ/IM:

1. Administer slowly, rotating injection sites.
2. Pts with circulatory impairment experience higher risk of overdosage because of delayed absorption of repeated administration.

IV:

1. For IV injection, dilute 2.5-15 mg morphine in 4-5 ml sterile water for injection.
2. Always administer very slowly, over 4-5 min. Rapid IV increases risk of severe adverse reactions (apnea, chest wall rigidity, peripheral circulatory collapse, cardiac arrest, anaphylactoid effects).
3. For multiple IV injections, may give pt-controlled analgesia, using pt-controlled infusion device.
4. For continuous IV infusion, dilute to concentration of 0.1-1 mg/ml in 5% dextrose and give through controlled infusion device.

RECTAL:

1. If suppository is too soft, chill for 30 min in refrigerator or run cold water over foil wrapper.
2. Moisten suppository w/cold water before inserting well up into rectum.

INDICATIONS/DOSAGE/ROUTES

NOTE: Reduce dosage in elderly/debilitated, those on concurrent CNS depressants.

Pain:
PO: Adults, elderly: 10-30 mg q4h. **Extended-release:** 30 mg q8-12h.
RECTAL: Adults, elderly: 10-30 mg q4h.
SubQ/IM: Adults, elderly: 10 mg q4h, as needed. **Usual dosage range:** 5-20 mg q4h. **Children:** 0.1-0.2 mg/kg SubQ per dose. Give q4h, as needed. Do not exceed single dose of 15 mg.
IV INJECTION: Adults, elderly: 4-10 mg, given very slowly.

Severe, chronic pain associated w/cancer:
IV INFUSION: Adults, elderly: 0.8-10 mg/hr. Increase to effective dosage level, as needed. **Maintenance:** 0.8-80 mg/hr. **Children**

(Maintenance): 0.025-2.6 mg/kg/hr.

EPIDURAL: Adults, elderly: Initially, 5 mg. If pain relief not obtained in 1 hr, may give additional doses in increments of 1-2 mg at sufficient intervals. **Maximum total daily dose:** 10 mg.

CONTINUOUS EPIDURAL INFUSION: Adults, elderly: Initially, 2-4 mg/day. May be increased by 1-2 mg/day if needed.

INTRATHECAL: Adults, elderly: 0.2-1 mg.

SubQ: Children: Usual maintenance level: 0.025-1.79 mg/kg/hr.

Myocardial infarction pain:
SubQ/IM/IV: Adults, elderly: 8-15 mg. Give additional smaller doses q3-4h.

Analgesia during labor:
SubQ/IM: Adults: 10 mg.

PRECAUTIONS

CONTRAINDICATIONS: Postop biliary tract surgery, surgical anastomosis. **EXTREME CAUTION:** CNS depression, anoxia, hypercapnia, respiratory depression, seizures, acute alcoholism, shock, untreated myxedema, respiratory dysfunction. **CAUTIONS:** Toxic psychoses, increased intracranial pressure, impaired hepatic function, acute abdominal conditions, hypothyroidism, prostatic hypertrophy, Addison's disease, urethral stricture, COPD. **PREGNANCY/LACTATION:** Crosses placenta; distributed in breast milk. May prolong labor if administered in latent phase of first stage of labor, or before cervical dilation of 4-5 cm has occurred. Respiratory depression may occur in neonate if mother received opiates during labor. Regular use of opiates during pregnancy may produce withdrawal symptoms in neonate (irritability, excessive crying, tremors, hyperactive reflexes, fever, vomiting, diarrhea, yawning, sneezing, seizures). **Pregnancy Category C.**

INTERACTIONS

DRUG INTERACTIONS: Alcohol, CNS depressants may increase CNS, respiratory depression, hypotension. MAO inhibitors may produce severe, fatal reaction (reduce dose to 1/4 usual dose). **ALTERED LAB VALUES:** May increase amylase, lipase.

SIDE EFFECTS

NOTE: Effects dependent on dosage amount, route of administration. Ambulatory pts, those not in severe pain may experience dizziness, nausea, vomiting, hypotension more frequently than those in supine position or who have severe pain.

FREQUENT: Suppressed breathing depth. **OCCASIONAL:** Lightheadedness, mental clouding, dizziness, sedation, hypotension, nausea, vomiting, euphoria/dysphoria, constipation (drug delays digestion), sweating, flushing, feeling of facial and neck warmth, urinary retention.

ADVERSE REACTIONS/TOXIC EFFECTS

Overdosage results in respiratory depression, skeletal muscle flaccidity, cold, clammy skin, cyanosis, extreme somnolence progressing to convulsions, stupor, coma. Tolerance to analgesic effect, physical dependence may occur w/repeated use. Prolonged duration of action, cumulative effect may occur in those w/impaired hepatic, renal function.

NURSING IMPLICATIONS

BASELINE ASSESSMENT:

Pt should be in a recumbent position before drug is given by parenteral route. Assess onset, type, location and duration of pain. Obtain vital signs before giving medication. If respirations are 12/min or lower (20/min or lower in children), withhold medication, contact physician. Effect of medication is reduced if full pain recurs before next dose.

INTERVENTION/EVALUATION:

Monitor vital signs 5-10 min after IV administration, 15-30 min after SubQ or IM. Be alert for decreased respirations or B/P. Check for adequate voiding; palpate bladder if output questionable. Monitor stools; avoid constipation. Initiate deep breathing and coughing exercises, particularly in those w/impaired pulmonary function. Assess for clinical improvement and record onset of pain relief. Consult physician if pain relief is not adequate.

PATIENT/FAMILY TEACHING:

Discomfort may occur w/injection. Change positions slowly to avoid orthostatic hypotension. Avoid tasks that require alertness, motor skills until response to drug is established. Avoid alcohol and CNS depressants. Tolerance/dependence may occur with prolonged use of high doses.

mupirocin

mew pee-ro-sin

(Bactroban)

CANADIAN AVAILABILITY:
Bactroban

CLASSIFICATION

Topical antibacterial

PHARMACOKINETICS

Metabolized in skin to inactive metabolite. Transport to skin surface; removed by normal skin desquamation.

ACTION

Bacteriostatic. Inhibits bacterial protein, RNA synthesis. Less effective on DNA synthesis.

USES

Topical treatment of impetigo.

TOPICAL ADMINISTRATION

1. Gown and gloves are to be worn until 24 hrs after therapy is effective. Disease is spread by direct contact w/moist discharges.
2. Apply small amount to affected areas.
3. Cover affected areas w/gauze dressing if desired.

INDICATIONS/DOSAGE/ROUTES

Usual topical dosage:
TOPICAL: Adults, elderly, children: Apply 3 times/day (may cover w/gauze).

PRECAUTIONS

CONTRAINDICATIONS: Hypersensitivity to any of the components. **CAUTIONS:** Impaired renal function. **PREGNANCY LACTATION:** Not known whether present in breast milk; temporarily discontinue nursing while using mupirocin. **Pregnancy Category B.**

INTERACTIONS

DRUG INTERACTIONS: None significant. **ALTERED LAB VALUES:** None significant.

SIDE EFFECTS

INFREQUENT: Burning, stinging, pain (1.5% of pts); itching (1%). **RARE:** Erythema, rash, dry skin, swelling, nausea, increased exudate (<1%).

ADVERSE REACTIONS/TOXIC EFFECTS

Superinfection may result in bacterial or fungal infections, esp. w/prolonged or repeated therapy.

NURSING IMPLICATIONS

BASELINE ASSESSMENT:

Question for hypersensitivity to components. Assess skin for type and extent of lesions.

INTERVENTION/EVALUATION:

Keep neonates or pts w/poor hygiene isolated. Wear gloves and gown if necessary when contact w/discharges is likely; continue until 24 hrs after therapy is effective. Cleanse/dispose of articles soiled with discharge according to institutional guidelines. In event of skin reaction, stop applications, cleanse area gently and notify physician.

PATIENT/FAMILY TEACHING:

For external use only. Avoid contact w/eyes. Explain precautions to avoid spread of infection; teach how to apply medication. If skin reaction, irritation develops, notify physician. If there is no improvement in 3-5 days pt should be reevaluated.

muromonab-CD3

meur-oh-mon´ab

(Orthoclone, OKT3)

CANADIAN AVAILABILITY:

Orthoclone

CLASSIFICATION

Immunosuppressant

ACTION

Antibody (purified IgG2 immune globulin) to T3 (CD3) antigen of human T cells which acts as an immunosuppressant. Reverses graft rejection by blocking T cell function which has major role in acute renal rejections. Reacts w/and blocks function of molecule CD3 in human T cell membrane.

USES

Treatment of acute allograft rejection in renal transplant pts, steroid-resistant acute allograft rejection in cardiac, hepatic transplant pts.

STORAGE/HANDLING

Refrigerate ampoule. Do not shake ampoule before using. Fine translucent particles may develop; does not affect potency.

IV ADMINISTRATION

IV:

1. Administer direct IV over <1 min.
2. Give methylprednisolone 1 mg/kg before and 100 mg hydrocortisone 30 min after dose (decreases adverse reaction to first dose).
3. Draw solution into syringe through 0.22 micron filter. Discard filter; use needle for IV administration.

INDICATIONS/DOSAGE/ROUTES

Prevention of allograft rejection:
IV: Adults, elderly: 5 mg/day for 10-14 days. Begin when acute renal rejection is diagnosed.

PRECAUTIONS

CONTRAINDICATIONS: History of hypersensitivity to muromonab-CD3 or any murine origin product, those in fluid overload evidenced by chest x-ray or >3% weight gain within the wk before initial treatment. **CAUTIONS:** Impaired hepatic, renal, cardiac function. **PREGNANCY/LACTATION:** Unknown whether drug crosses placenta or is distributed in breast milk. Avoid nursing. **Pregnancy Category C.**

INTERACTIONS

DRUG INTERACTIONS: Other immunosuppressants may increase risk of infection or development of lymphoproliferative disorders. Live virus vaccines may potentiate virus replication, increase vaccine side effects, decrease pt's antibody response to vaccine. **ALTERED LAB VALUES:** None significant.

SIDE EFFECTS

FREQUENT: First-dose reaction: Fever, chills, dyspnea, malaise occurs 30 min to 6 hrs after first dose (reaction markedly reduced w/ subsequent dosing after first 2 days of treatment). **OCCASIONAL:** Chest pain, nausea, vomiting, diarrhea, tremor.

ADVERSE REACTIONS/TOXIC EFFECTS

Cytokine release syndrome (CRS) may range from flu-like illness to life threatening shock-like reaction. Occasionally fatal hypersensitivity reactions. Severe pulmonary edema occurs in <2% of those treated w/muromonab-CD3. Infection (due to immunosuppression) generally occurs within 45 days after initial treatment; cytomegalovirus occurs in 19%, herpes simplex in 27%. Severe and life-threatening infection occurs in <4.8%.

NURSING IMPLICATIONS

BASELINE ASSESSMENT:

Chest x-ray must be taken within 24 hrs of initiation of therapy and be clear of fluid. Weight should be ≤3% above minimum weight the wk before treatment begins (pulmonary edema occurs where fluid overload was present before treatment). Have resuscitative drugs and equipment immediately available.

INTERVENTION/EVALUATION:

Monitor WBC, differential, platelet count, renal and hepatic function tests, and immunologic tests (plasma levels or quantitative T lymphocyte surface phenotyping) before and during therapy. If fever exceeds 100° F, antipyretics should be instituted. Monitor for fluid overload by chest x-ray and weight gain of >3% over weight before treatment began. Assess lung sounds for evidence of fluid overload. Monitor I&O. Assess stool frequency and consistency.

PATIENT/FAMILY TEACHING:

Inform pt of first-dose reaction prior to treatment, headache, tremor may occur as a response to medication. Avoid crowds, those w/infections. Do not receive immunizations.

nabumetone

nah-byew′meh-tone

(Relafen)

CLASSIFICATION

Nonsteroidal anti-inflammatory

PHARMACOKINETICS

Readily absorbed from GI tract. Widely distributed. Protein binding: >90%. Metabolized in liver to active metabolite. Primarily excreted in urine. Half-life: 22-30 hrs.

ACTION

Inhibits prostaglandin synthesis. Inhibits action of cyclooxygenase, decreases formation of prostaglandin, thromboxane precursors from arachidonic acid.

USES

Acute and chronic treatment of osteoarthritis, rheumatoid arthritis.

PO ADMINISTRATION

1. Give w/food, milk, or antacids if GI distress occurs.
2. Do not crush; swallow whole.

INDICATIONS/DOSAGE/ROUTES

Rheumatoid arthritis, osteoarthritis:

PO: Adults, elderly: Initially, 1,000 mg as single dose or in 2 divided doses. May increase up to 2,000 mg/day as single or in 2 divided doses.

PRECAUTIONS

CONTRAINDICATIONS: Active peptic ulcer, GI ulceration, chronic inflammation of GI tract, GI bleeding disorders, history of hypersensitivity to aspirin or NSAIDs, history of significantly impaired renal function. **CAUTIONS:** Impaired renal/hepatic function, history of GI tract disease, predisposition to fluid retention. **PREGNANCY/LACTATION:** Distributed in low concentration in breast milk. Avoid use during last trimester (may adversely affect fetal cardiovascular system: premature closing of ductus arteriosus). **Pregnancy Category C.**

INTERACTIONS

DRUG INTERACTIONS: May increase effects of oral anticoagulants, heparin, thrombolytics. May decrease effect of antihypertensives, diuretics. Salicylates, aspirin may increase risk of GI side effects, bleeding. Bone marrow depressants may increase risk of hematologic reactions. May increase concentration, toxicity of lithium. May increase methotrexate toxicity. Probenecid may increase concentration. **ALTERED LAB VALUES:** May increase serum transaminase activity. May decrease uric acid.

SIDE EFFECTS

FREQUENT: Headache, somnolence/drowsiness, dyspepsia (heartburn, indigestion, epigastric pain), nausea, vomiting, constipation. **OCCASIONAL:** Dizziness, pruritus, nervousness, asthenia (loss of strength), diarrhea, abdominal cramps, flatulence, tinnitus, blurred vision, peripheral edema/fluid retention.

ADVERSE REACTIONS/TOXIC EFFECTS

Overdose may result in acute hypotension, tachycardia. Peptic ulcer, GI bleeding, nephrotoxicity (dysuria, cystitis, hematuria, proteinuria, nephrotic syndrome), gastritis, severe hepatic reaction (cholestasis, jaundice), severe hypersensitivity reaction (bronchospasm, angiofacial edema) occur rarely.

NURSING IMPLICATIONS

BASELINE ASSESSMENT:

Assess onset, type, location, and duration of pain or inflammation. Inspect appearance of affected joints for immobility, deformities, and skin condition.

INTERVENTION/EVALUATION:

Assist w/ambulation if somnolence/drowsiness/dizziness occurs. Monitor for evidence of dyspepsia. Monitor pattern of daily bowel activity and stool consistency. Check behind medial malleolus for fluid retention (usually first area noted). Evaluate for therapeutic response: relief of pain, stiffness, swelling, increase in joint mobility, reduced joint tenderness, improved grip strength.

PATIENT/FAMILY TEACHING:

Swallow capsule whole, do not crush or chew. Avoid tasks that require alertness, motor skills until response to drug is established. If GI upset occurs, take w/food, milk. Avoid aspirin, alcohol during therapy (increases risk of GI bleeding). Report headache, GI distress, visual disturbances, edema.

nadolol

nay-doe´lol
(Corgard)

FIXED-COMBINATION(S):
W/bendroflumethiazide, a diuretic (Corzide)

CANADIAN AVAILABILITY:
Corgard, Syn-Nadolol

CLASSIFICATION

Beta-adrenergic blocker

PHARMACOKINETICS

	ONSET	PEAK	DURATION
PO	—	—	24 hrs

Partially absorbed from GI tract. Protein binding: 30%. Primarily excreted unchanged in urine. Moderately removed by hemodialysis. Half-life: 20-24 hrs (increased in decreased renal function).

ACTION

Nonselective beta blocker. Blocks $beta_1$-adrenergic receptors, slowing sinus heart rate, decreasing cardiac output, decreasing B/P (exact mechanism unknown but may block peripheral adrenergic receptors, decrease sympathetic outflow from CNS or decrease renin release from kidney). Blocks $beta_2$-adrenergic receptors, increasing airway resistance. Decreases myocardial ischemia severity by decreasing oxygen requirements.

USES

Management of mild to moderate hypertension. Used alone or in combination w/diuretics, esp. thiazide-type. Management of chronic stable angina pectoris.

PO ADMINISTRATION

1. May be given w/o regard to meals.
2. Tablets may be crushed.

INDICATIONS/DOSAGE/ROUTES

Hypertension:
PO: Adults: Initially, 40 mg/day. Increase by 40-80 mg/day at 7 day intervals. **Maintenance:** 40-80 mg/day up to 240-320 mg/day.

Angina pectoris:
PO: Adults: Initially, 40 mg/day. Increase by 40-80 mg/day at 3-7 day intervals. **Maintenance:** 40-80 mg/day up to 160-240 mg/day.

Usual elderly dosage:
PO: Elderly: Initially, 20 mg/day for angina/hypertension.

Dosage in renal impairment:
Dose is modified based on creatinine clearance.

CREATININE CLEARANCE	DOSAGE INTERVAL
>50 ml/min	q24h
31-50 ml/min	q24-36h
10-30 ml/min	q24-48h
<10 ml/min	q40-60h

PRECAUTIONS

CONTRAINDICATIONS: Bronchial asthma, COPD, uncontrolled cardiac failure, sinus bradycardia, heart block greater than first degree, cardiogenic shock, CHF unless secondary to tachyarrhythmias, those on MAO inhibitors. **CAUTIONS:** Inadequate cardiac function, impaired renal/hepatic function, diabetes mellitus, hyperthyroidism. **PREGNANCY/LACTATION:** Crosses placenta; distributed in breast milk. Avoid use during first trimester. May produce bradycardia, apnea, hypoglycemia, hypothermia during delivery, small birth weight infants. **Pregnancy Category C.**

INTERACTIONS

DRUG INTERACTIONS: Diuretics, other hypotensives may increase hypotensive effect; sympathomimetics, xanthines may mutually inhibit effects; may mask symptoms of hypoglycemia, prolong hypoglycemic effect of insulin, oral hypoglycemics; NSAIDs may decrease antihypertensive effect; cimetidine may increase concentration. **ALTERED LAB VALUES:** May increase ANA titer, SGOT (AST), SGPT (ALT), alkaline phosphatase, LDH, bilirubin, BUN, creatinine, potassium, uric acid, lipoproteins, triglycerides.

SIDE EFFECTS

Generally well tolerated, w/ transient and mild side effects. **OCCASIONAL:** Bradycardia, peripheral vascular insufficiency (usually Raynaud's type), dizziness, fatigue. **RARE:** Sedation, change in behavior, hypotension, GI upset, rhythm/conduction disturbances.

ADVERSE REACTIONS/TOXIC EFFECTS

Excessive dosage may produce profound bradycardia, hypotension. Abrupt withdrawal may result in sweating, palpitations, headache, tremulousness, exacerbation of angina, MI, ventricular arrhythmias. May precipitate CHF, MI in those w/cardiac disease, thyroid storm in those w/thyrotoxicosis, peripheral ischemia in those w/ existing peripheral vascular disease. Hypoglycemia may occur in previously controlled diabetics.

NURSING IMPLICATIONS

BASELINE ASSESSMENT:

Assess baseline renal/liver function tests. Assess B/P, apical pulse immediately before drug is administered (if pulse is 60/min or below, or systolic B/P is below 90 mm Hg, withhold medication, contact physician). *Antianginal:* Record onset, type (sharp, dull, squeezing), radiation, location, intensity, and duration of anginal pain, and precipitating factors (exertion, emotional stress).

INTERVENTION/EVALUATION:

Monitor B/P for hypotension, respiration for shortness of breath. Assess pulse for strength/weakness, irregular rate, bradycardia. Assess fingers for color, numbness (Raynaud's). Assist w/ambulation if dizziness occurs. Assess for evidence of CHF: Dyspnea (particularly on exertion or lying down), night cough, peripheral edema, distended neck veins. Monitor I&O (increase in weight, decrease in urine output may indicate CHF).

PATIENT/FAMILY TEACHING:

Do not abruptly discontinue medication. Compliance w/therapy regimen is essential to control hypertension, arrhythmias. To avoid hypotensive effect, rise slowly from lying to sitting position, wait momentarily before standing. Avoid tasks that require alertness, motor skills until response to drug is established. Report excessive fatigue, dizziness. Do not use nasal decongestants, over-the-counter cold preparations (stimulants) w/o physician approval. Outpatients should monitor B/P, pulse before taking medication. Restrict salt, alcohol intake.

nafarelin acetate

naf-ah-rell´in
(Synarel)

CLASSIFICATION

Gonadotropin inhibitor

PHARMACOKINETICS

Well absorbed after intranasal administration. Primarily eliminated in feces. Half-life: 3 hrs.

ACTION

Initially stimulates the release of the pituitary gonadotropins, luteinizing hormone and follicle-stimulating hormone, resulting in temporary increase of ovarian steroidogenesis. Continued dosing abolishes the stimulatory effect on the pituitary gland, and, after about 4 wks, leads to decreased secretion of gonadal steroids.

USES

Management of endometriosis, including pain relief and reduction of endometriotic lesions. Treatment of central precocious puberty.

INTRANASAL ADMINISTRATION

1. Use metered spray pump to administer correct dose.
2. When dose is given 2 times/day, alternate nostrils.
3. When a topical nasal decongestant is necessary, do not use until at least 30 min after nafarelin dose.

INDICATIONS/DOSAGE/ROUTES

Endometriosis:
NOTE: Initiate treatment between days 2 and 4 of menstrual cycle. Duration of therapy is 6 mo.
INTRANASAL: Adults: 400 mcg/day. 200 mcg (1 spray) into 1 nostril in morning, 1 spray into other nostril in evening. For pts w/persistent regular menstruation after months of treatment, increase dose to 800 mcg/day (1 spray into each nostril in morning and evening).

Central precocious puberty:
INTRANASAL: Children: 1600 mcg/day. 400 mcg (2 sprays into each nostril in morning and evening; total 8 sprays).

PRECAUTIONS

CONTRAINDICATIONS: Hypersensitivity to nafarelin, other agonist analogs and components of the preparation; undiagnosed abnormal vaginal bleeding. **CAUTIONS:** History of osteoporosis, chronic alcohol or tobacco use, intercurrent rhinitis. **PREGNANCY/LACTATION:** Contraindicated during pregnancy or breast feeding. **Pregnancy Category X.**

INTERACTIONS

DRUG INTERACTIONS: None significant. **ALTERED LAB VALUES:** None significant.

SIDE EFFECTS

FREQUENT: Acne, decreased breast size, flushing, sweating, headaches, nervousness, emotional lability, fatigue, decreased bone density. Nasal irritation in 10% of pts. **OCCASIONAL:** Vaginitis (itching, dryness, burning, vaginal bleeding). **RARE:** Hypersensitivity.

ADVERSE REACTIONS/TOXIC EFFECTS

None significant.

NURSING IMPLICATIONS

BASELINE ASSESSMENT:

Question for hypersensitivity to any agonist analog, ingredients. Inquire about menstrual cycle; therapy should begin between days 2 and 4 of cycle.

INTERVENTION/EVALUATION:

Check for pain relief as result of therapy. Inquire about menstrual cessation and other decreased estrogen effects.

PATIENT/FAMILY TEACHING:

Pt should use nonhormonal contraceptive during therapy. Do not take drug, check w/physician if pregnancy is suspected (risk to fetus). Importance of full length of therapy, regular visits to physician's office. Notify physician if regular menstruation continues (menstruation should stop w/therapy).

nafcillin sodium

naph´sill-in

(Nafcil, Nallpen, Unipen)

CANADIAN AVAILABILITY: Unipen

CLASSIFICATION

Antibiotic: Penicillin

PHARMACOKINETICS

Poorly absorbed from GI tract (food decreases absorption). Protein binding: 87-90%. Metabolized in liver. Primarily excreted in urine. Not removed by hemodialysis. Half-life: 0.5-1 hr (increase in decreased renal function, neonates).

ACTION

Bactericidal. Binds to bacterial membranes. Inhibits cell wall synthesis.

USES

Treatment of respiratory tract, skin/skin structure infections, osteomyelitis, endocarditis, meningitis; perioperatively, esp. in cardiovascular, orthopedic procedures. Predominantly treatment of infections caused by penicillinase-producing staphylococci.

STORAGE/HANDLING

Store capsules, tablets at room temperature. *Oral solution:* After reconstitution, stable for 7 days if refrigerated. *IV infusion (piggyback):* Stable for 24 hrs at room temperature, 96 hrs if refrigerated. Discard if precipitate forms.

PO/IM/IV ADMINISTRATION

NOTE: Space doses evenly around the clock.

PO:

1. Give 1 hr before or 2 hrs after food/beverages.

IM:

1. Reconstitute each 500 mg w/ 1.7 ml sterile water for injection or 0.9% NaCl injection to provide concentration of 250 mg/ml.
2. Inject IM into large muscle mass.

IV:

1. For IV injection, further dilute each vial w/15-30 ml sterile water for injection or 0.9% NaCl injection. Administer over 5-10 min.
2. For intermittent IV infusion (piggyback), further dilute with 50-100 ml 5% dextrose, 0.9% NaCl or other compatible IV fluid. Infuse over 30-60 min.
3. Because of potential for hypersensitivity/anaphylaxis, start initial dose at few drops per min, increase slowly to ordered rate; stay w/pt first 10-15 min, then check q10min.
4. Limit IV therapy to <48 hrs, if possible. Alternating IV sites, use large veins to reduce risk of phlebitis.
5. Stop infusion if pt complains of pain.

INDICATIONS/DOSAGE/ROUTES

Usual dosage:
IV: Adults, elderly: 3-6 Gm/24 hrs in divided doses.
IM: Adults, elderly: 500 mg q4-6h.
PO: Adults, elderly: 250 mg to 1 Gm q4-6 h.

Usual pediatric dosage:
IM/IV: Children: 25 mg/kg 2 times/day.
PO: Children: 25-50 mg/kg/day in 4 divided doses.

Usual neonate dosage:
IM/IV: Neonates <7 days: 50 mg/kg/day in 2-3 divided doses. **>7 days:** 75 mg/kg/day in 4 divided doses.

PRECAUTIONS

CONTRAINDICATIONS: Hypersensitivity to any penicillin. **CAUTIONS:** History of allergies, particularly cephalosporins. **PREGNANCY/LACTATION:** Readily crosses placenta, appears in cord blood, amniotic fluid. Distributed in breast milk in low concentrations. May lead to allergic sensitization, diarrhea, candidiasis, skin rash in infant. **Pregnancy Category B.**

INTERACTIONS

DRUG INTERACTIONS: Probenecid may increase concentration, toxicity risk. **ALTERED LAB VALUES:** May cause positive Coombs' test.

SIDE EFFECTS

FREQUENT: Mild hypersensitivity reaction (fever, rash, pruritus), GI effects (nausea, vomiting, diarrhea) more frequent w/oral administration. **OCCASIONAL:** Hypokalemia w/high IV doses, phlebitis, thrombophlebitis (more common in elderly). **RARE:** Extravasation w/IV administration.

ADVERSE REACTIONS/TOXIC EFFECTS

Superinfections, potentially fatal antibiotic-associated colitis may result from altered bacterial balance. Hematologic effects (esp. involving platelets, WBCs), severe hypersensitivity reactions, rarely anaphylaxis.

NURSING IMPLICATIONS

BASELINE ASSESSMENT:

Question for history of allergies, esp. penicillins, cephalosporins. Obtain specimen for culture and sensitivity before giving first dose (therapy may begin before results are known).

INTERVENTION/EVALUATION:

Hold medication and promptly report rash (possible hypersensitivity) or diarrhea (w/fever, abdominal pain, mucus and blood in stool may indicate antibiotic-associated colitis). Assess food tolerance. Evaluate IV site frequently for phlebitis (heat, pain, red streaking over vein) and infiltration (potential extravasation). Check IM injection sites for pain, induration. Monitor potassium. Be alert for superinfection: Increased fever, onset sore throat, vomiting, diarrhea, ulceration/changes of oral mucosa, anal/genital pruritus. Check hematology reports (esp. WBCs), periodic renal or hepatic reports in prolonged therapy.

PATIENT/FAMILY TEACHING:

Continue antibiotic for full length of treatment. Doses should be evenly spaced. Discomfort may occur w/IM injection. Report IV discomfort immediately. Notify physician in event of diarrhea, rash, other new symptom.

naftifine hydrochloride

naf´tih-feen
(Naftin)

CLASSIFICATION

Antifungal

PHARMACOKINETICS

Minimal absorption after topical administration. Excreted in urine, eliminated in feces. Half-life: 2-3 days.

ACTION

Interferes with sterol biosynthesis through inhibition of the enzyme squalene monoxygenase, resulting in decreased ergosterol, accumulation of squalene in cells. Fungistatic against Candida; fungicidal against most dermatophytes and Candida in high concentrations.

USES

Treatment of tinea cruris, t. corporis.

INDICATIONS/DOSAGE/ROUTES

Usual topical dosage:
TOPICAL: Adults, elderly: 2 times/day; continue 1-2 wks after manifestations subside.

PRECAUTIONS

CONTRAINDICATIONS: Hypersensitivity to naftifine or any component in formulation. Safety in children <12 yrs not established. **PREGNANCY/LACTATION:** Unknown whether distributed in breast milk. **Pregnancy Category B.**

INTERACTIONS

DRUG INTERACTIONS: None significant. **ALTERED LAB VALUES:** None significant.

SIDE EFFECTS

OCCASIONAL: Local burning, stinging, itching, dryness, redness.

ADVERSE REACTIONS/TOXIC EFFECTS

None significant.

NURSING IMPLICATIONS

BASELINE ASSESSMENT:

Question for history of hypersensitivity to naftifine/components of formulation. Confirm that diagnosis has been made by microscopic exam or culture of infected tissue.

INTERVENTION/EVALUATION:

Check for therapeutic response or local irritation (burning, stinging, itching, redness, dryness).

PATIENT/FAMILY TEACHING:

Rub well into affected, surrounding areas. Complete full course of therapy; continue at least 1-2 wks after symptoms gone (may take several wks). Do not use occlusive covering or use other preparations w/o consulting physician. Avoid contact w/eyes, nose, mouth, mucous membranes. Keep areas clean, dry; wear light clothing to promote ventilation. Separate personal items, linens. Notify physician of increased irritation.

nalbuphine hydrochloride

nail-byew′phin
(Nubain)

CANADIAN AVAILABILITY:
Nubain

CLASSIFICATION

Opioid analgesic

PHARMACOKINETICS

	ONSET	PEAK	DURATION
SubQ	<15 min	—	3-6 hrs
IM	<15 min	—	3-6 hrs
IV	2-3 min	30 min	3-6 hrs

Well absorbed after IM, SubQ administration. Metabolized in liver. Primarily eliminated in feces via biliary secretion. Half-life: 3.5-5 hrs.

ACTION

Binds w/opioid receptors within CNS, altering processes affecting pain perception, emotional response to pain. May displace opioid agonists and competitively inhibit their action (may precipitate withdrawal symptoms).

USES

Relief of moderate to severe pain, preop sedation, obstetrical analgesia, adjunct to anesthesia.

STORAGE/HANDLING

Store parenteral form at room temperature.

SubQ/IM/IV ADMINISTRATION

IM:

Rotate IM injection sites and record.

IV:

For IV injection, administer each 10 mg >3-5 min.

INDICATIONS/DOSAGE/ROUTES

NOTE: Dosage based on severity of pain, physical condition of pt, concurrent use of other medications.

Analgesia:
SubQ/IM/IV: Adults, elderly: 10 mg q3-6 h, as necessary. Do not exceed maximum single dose of 20 mg, maximum daily dose of 160 mg. In pts chronically receiving narcotic analgesics of similar duration of action, give 25% of usual dosage.

Supplement to anesthesia:
IV: Adults, elderly: Induction: 0.3-3 mg/kg over 10-15 min. **Maintenance:** 0.25-0.5 mg/kg as necessary.

PRECAUTIONS

CONTRAINDICATIONS: Respirations <12/min. **CAUTIONS:** Impaired hepatic/renal function, elderly, debilitated, head injury, increased intracranial pressure, MI w/nausea, vomiting, respiratory disease, hypertension, before biliary tract surgery (produces spasm of sphincter of Oddi). **PREGNANCY/LACTATION:** Readily crosses placenta; distributed in breast milk (breast feeding not recommended). **Pregnancy Category C.**

INTERACTIONS

DRUG INTERACTIONS: Alcohol, CNS depressants may increase CNS, respiratory depression, hypotension. MAO inhibitors may produce severe, fatal reaction (reduce dose to 1/4 usual dose). Effects may be decreased w/buprenorphine. **ALTERED LAB VALUES:** May increase amylase, lipase.

SIDE EFFECTS

FREQUENT: Sedation, decreased respirations. **OCCASIONAL:** Sweaty palms, clammy skin, nausea, dizziness, dry mouth, headache. **RARE:** Restlessness, crying, euphoria, vomiting, bitter taste, urinary urgency, skin burning/itching, blurred vision.

ADVERSE REACTIONS/TOXIC EFFECTS

Abrupt withdrawal after prolonged use may produce symptoms of narcotic withdrawal (abdominal cramping, rhinorrhea, lacrimation, anxiety, increased temperature, piloerection [goosebumps]). Overdose results in severe respiratory depression, skeletal muscle flaccidity, cyanosis, extreme somnolence progressing to convulsions, stupor, coma. Tolerance to analgesic effect, physical dependence may occur w/chronic use.

N

NURSING IMPLICATIONS

Baseline Assessment:

Raise bedrails. Obtain vital signs before giving medication. If respirations are 12/min or lower (20/min or lower in children), withhold medication, contact physician. Assess onset, type, location, and duration of pain. Effect of medication is reduced if full pain recurs before next dose. Low abuse potential.

Intervention/Evaluation:

Increase fluid intake and environmental humidity to improve viscosity of lung secretions. Monitor for change in respirations, B/P, change in rate or quality of pulse. Monitor pattern of daily bowel activity and stool consistency. Initiate deep breathing and coughing exercises, particularly in those w/impaired pulmonary function. Change pt's position q2-4h. Assess for clinical improvement and record onset of relief of pain. Consult physician if pain relief is not adequate.

PATIENT/FAMILY TEACHING:

Change positions slowly to avoid dizziness. Avoid tasks that require alertness, motor skills until response to drug is established. Note effects of abrupt withdrawal following long-term use. Avoid alcohol and CNS depressants.

nalidixic acid

nal-ih-dix′ik
(NegGram)

CANADIAN AVAILABILITY:
NegGram

CLASSIFICATION

Anti-infective

PHARMACOKINETICS

Rapid, completely absorbed from GI tract (antacids may delay absorption). Widely distributed. Protein binding: 93%; metabolite: 63%. Metabolized in liver to active metabolite. Primarily excreted in urine. Half-life: 6-7 hrs (increased in decreased renal function, elderly).

ACTION

Interferes w/DNA polymerization. Inhibits bacterial DNA synthesis.

USES

Treatment of acute, chronic urinary tract infections.

PO ADMINISTRATION

1. May give w/o regard to meals. Give w/food if GI upset occurs.
2. Tablets may be crushed.

INDICATIONS/DOSAGE/ROUTES

Urinary tract infections:
PO: Adults, elderly: Initially, 1 Gm 4 times/day for 7-14 days. **Maintenance:** 500 mg 4 times/day. **Children >3 mo:** 55 mg/kg/day in 4 divided doses. **Maintenance:** 33 mg/kg/day in 4 divided doses.

PRECAUTIONS

CONTRAINDICATIONS: Hypersensitivity to nalidixic acid, history of convulsive disorders. Do not give to infants <3 mo of age. **CAUTIONS:** Hepatic dysfunction, respiratory insufficiency, epilepsy, severe renal failure, prepubertal children (cartilage erosion has occurred in animals). **PREGNANCY/LACTATION:** Crosses placenta; distributed in breast milk. Safety in the first trimester has not been established; use during the last 2 trimesters has not been associated w/adverse effects on mother or child. At the first sign of labor, nalidixic acid should be discontinued to prevent potentially significant nalidixic acid blood levels in neonate. **Pregnancy Category B.**

INTERACTIONS

DRUG INTERACTIONS: May enhance effects of oral anticoagulants. **ALTERED LAB VALUES:** None significant.

SIDE EFFECTS

FREQUENT: Nausea, vomiting, rash, urticaria. **OCCASIONAL:** Diarrhea, abdominal pain, photosensitivity, pruritus, headache, vertigo, malaise, confusion. **RARE:** Paresthesia, photophobia, blurred vision.

ADVERSE REACTIONS/TOXIC EFFECTS

Convulsions, psychosis, hepatotoxicity (jaundice, increased SGOT (AST), SGPT (ALT), serum bilirubin) occur rarely.

NURSING IMPLICATIONS

BASELINE ASSESSMENT:

Question for history of convulsive disorders, hypersensitivity to nalidixic acid. Obtain specimens for diagnostic tests before giving first dose (therapy may begin before results are known).

INTERVENTION/EVALUATION:

Monitor I&O, culture and sensitivity results. Evaluate food tolerance. Determine pattern of bowel activity. Assess skin for rash, urticaria. Check B/P at least 2 times/day; evaluate mental status. Assess for visual effects.

PATIENT/FAMILY TEACHING:

Take 1 hr before meals. If GI upset occurs, take after meals. Continue for full length of therapy and do not omit a dose. Maintain adequate fluids. Protect against phototoxicity: avoid sun and ultraviolet light, wear sunscreens and protective clothing. Notify nurse/physician in event of headache, blurred vision, rash or other symptom.

naloxone hydrochloride

nay-lox´own
(Narcan)

CANADIAN AVAILABILITY:
Narcan

CLASSIFICATION

Opioid antagonist

PHARMACOKINETICS

	ONSET	PEAK	DURATION
IV	1-2 min	—	1-4 hrs
IM	2-5 min	—	1-4 hrs
SubQ	2-5 min	—	1-4 hrs

Well absorbed after IM, SubQ administration. Metabolized in liver. Primariy excreted in urine. Half-life: 60-100 min.

ACTION

Displaces opioid analgesics from receptors. Competitively inhibits opioid analgesic action effects.

USES

Reversal of narcotic-induced respiratory depression, diagnostic tool in suspected acute narcotic overdosage, treatment of asphyxia neonatorum.

STORAGE/HANDLING

Store parenteral form at room temperature. Use mixture within 24 hrs; discard unused solution.

IM/IV ADMINISTRATION

IM:

1. Give in upper, outer quadrant of buttock.

IV:

1. May dilute 1 mg/ml with 50 ml sterile water for injection to provide a concentration of 0.02 mg/ml.
2. The 0.4 mg/ml and 1 mg/ml for injection used for adults, the 0.02 mg/ml concentration used for neonates.
3. For continuous IV infusion, dilute each 2 mg of naloxone with 500 ml of 5% dextrose in water or 0.9%

NaCl, producing solution containing 0.004 mg/ml.

INDICATIONS/DOSAGE/ROUTES

Respiratory depression:
SubQ/IM/IV: Adults, elderly: 0.1-0.2 mg at 2-3min intervals until adequate alertness and ventilation are achieved. **Children:** 0.005-0.01 mg q2-3min. Repeated doses may be required at 1-2 hr intervals.

Narcotic overdosage:
IV: Adults, elderly: Initially, 0.4-2 mg. May repeat at 2-3 min intervals until desired response is obtained.

Asphyxia neonatorum:
IV: Neonates: 0.01 mg/kg injected into umbilical vein. Repeat at 2-3 min intervals until desired response is obtained.

PRECAUTIONS

CONTRAINDICATIONS: Respiratory depression due to nonopiate drugs. **CAUTIONS:** Opiate-dependent pt, cardiovascular disorders. **PREGNANCY/LACTATION:** Unknown whether drug crosses placenta or is distributed in breast milk. **Pregnancy Category B.**

INTERACTIONS

DRUG INTERACTIONS: Reverses analgesic/side effects, may precipitate withdrawal symptoms of butorphanol, nalbuphine, pentazocine, opioid agonist analgesics. **ALTERED LAB VALUES:** None significant.

SIDE EFFECTS

None significant (little or no pharmacologic effect in absence of narcotics).

ADVERSE REACTIONS/TOXIC EFFECTS

Too-rapid reversal of narcotic depression may result in nausea, vomiting, tremulousness, sweating, increased B/P, tachycardia. Excessive dosage in postop pts may produce significant reversal of analgesia, excitement, tremulousness. Hypotension or hypertension, ventricular tachycardia and fibrillation, pulmonary edema may occur in those w/cardiovascular disease.

NURSING IMPLICATIONS

BASELINE ASSESSMENT:

Maintain clear airway. Obtain weight of children to calculate drug dosage.

INTERVENTION/EVALUATION:

Monitor vital signs esp rate, depth, and rhythm of respiration during and frequently after administration. Carefully observe pt after satisfactory response (duration of opiate may exceed duration of naloxone resulting in recurrence of respiratory depression). Assess for increased pain w/reversal of opiate.

---

naltrexone (Revia)
See supplement

---

nandrolone decanoate

nan´-droe-lon
(Anabolin LA, Deca-Durabolin, Hybolin Decanoate, Neo-Durabolic)

nandrolone phenpropionate

(Androlone, Durabolin, Nandrobolic)

CANADIAN AVAILABILITY:
Durabolin

CLASSIFICATION

Anabolic steroid

ACTION

Reverses catabolic processes, negative nitrogen balance (promotes protein anabolism, stimulates appetite). Increases, stimulates production of erythropoietin.

USES

Nandrolone decanoate: Management of anemia of renal insufficiency. *Nandrolone phenpropionate:* Treatment of metastatic breast cancer in women.

IM ADMINISTRATION

Inject IM deeply, preferably into the gluteal muscle.

INDICATIONS/DOSAGE/ROUTES

Nandrolone decanoate:
IM: Adults (Female): 50-100 mg/wk. **Adults (Male):** 100-200 mg/wk. **Children (2-13 yrs):** 25-50 mg q3-4wks.

Nandrolone phenpropionate:
IM: Adults: 50-100 mg/wk.

PRECAUTIONS

CONTRAINDICATIONS: Hypersensitivity to anabolic steroids; nephrosis; severe hepatic impairment; infancy; pituitary insufficiency; hypercalcemia. Male pts w/prostate or breast carcinoma, benign prostatic hypertrophy. **CAUTIONS:** Cardiac, renal, or hepatic impairment; young children, elderly, diabetic pts, history of myocardial infarction or coronary artery disease. **PREGNANCY/LACTATION:** Not recommended during nursing because of potential for serious effects on infant. **Pregnancy Category X.**

INTERACTIONS

DRUG INTERACTIONS: May increase effects of oral anticoagulants, salicylates. May increase hepatotoxicity w/hepatotoxic medications. **ALTERED LAB VALUES:** May increase SGOT (AST), SGPT (ALT), alkaline phosphatase, bilirubin, calcium, chloride, potassium, sodium, creatine, LDL, prothrombin time. May decrease HDL, serum lipids, 17 ketosteroid concentrations.

SIDE EFFECTS

FREQUENT: Acne, oily skin, nausea, vomiting, abdominal fullness. **OCCASIONAL:** Fluid retention, sore tongue. *Females:* Hirsutism, menstrual irregularities, hoarseness or deepening of voice, enlarged clitoris. *Prepubertal males:* Phallic enlargement, increased frequency of erections, virilism. *Postpubertal males:* Gynecomastia, oligospermia, chronic priapism, bladder irritability (change in libido and impotence w/prolonged, high dose therapy). **RARE:** Mental depression, ongoing headache.

ADVERSE REACTIONS/TOXIC EFFECTS

Peliosis hepatitis (liver/splenic tissue is replaced with blood-filled cysts) and hepatic tumors (benign or malignant) may be life threatening.

NURSING IMPLICATIONS

BASELINE ASSESSMENT:

Question for hypersensitivity to anabolic steroids. Establish baseline weight, B/P, blood glucose, hemoglobin, and hematocrit. Check liver function test results, electrolytes and cholesterol if ordered. Wrist x-rays may be ordered to determine bone maturation in children.

INTERVENTION/EVALUATION:

Weigh daily and report weekly gain of >5 lbs; evaluate for edema. Monitor I&O. Check B/P at least 2 times/day. Assess electrolytes, blood glucose, hemoglobin and hematocrit, liver function test results. W/breast cancer, check for hypercalcemia (lethargy, muscle weakness, confusion, irritability). Assure adequate intake of iron, protein, calories. Assess for virilization.

PATIENT/FAMILY TEACHING:

Regular visits to physician and monitoring tests are necessary. Do not take any other medications w/o consulting physician. Teach diet high in iron, protein, calories. Food may be tolerated better in small, frequent feedings. Weigh daily, report >5 lb gain/week. Notify physician if nausea, vomiting, acne or ankle swelling occurs; dark urine, light stools, yellowing of skin or eyes (liver dysfunction) should be reported at once. Female pts: Promptly report hoarseness, deepening of voice, menstrual irregularities (symptoms may not be reversible even when drug discontinued at once). Teach prepubertal and postpubertal males which symptoms to report (see Side Effects).

naphazoline

naf-az´oh-leen
(Albalon, Estivin, Naphcon, Vasocon)

FIXED-COMBINATION(S):
W/pheniramine maleate, an antihistamine (Naphcon-A)

CANADIAN AVAILABILITY:
Albalon, Naphcon, Vasocon

CLASSIFICATION

Sympathomimetic, decongestant

ACTION

Directly acts on alpha-adrenergic receptors in arterioles of conjunctiva causing vasoconstriction, decreasing congestion.

USES

Ophthalmic: Relief of itching, congestion and minor irritation; to control hyperemia in pts with superficial corneal vascularity. Occasionally may be used during some ocular diagnostic procedures. *Intranasal:* Relief of nasal congestion due to common cold, acute or chronic rhinitis, hay fever or other allergies.

STORAGE/HANDLING

Do not store in aluminum containers (degraded by aluminum). Do not use if cloudy or discolored solution.

OPHTHALMIC/INTRANASAL ADMINISTRATION

OPHTHALMIC:

1. Follow manufacturer's directions regarding contact lenses.
2. Tilt pt's head back; place solution in conjunctival sac.
3. Have pt close eyes; press gently on lacrimal sac for 1 min.
4. Take care not to touch any area w/the applicator.
5. Remove excess solution by gently blotting w/tissue.

INTRANASAL:

NOTE: Applicator should not touch any surface; rinse tip of dispenser or dropper w/hot water following use. Use for only 1 person.

Drops:

1. Position pt in lateral, head-low position or reclining w/head tilted as far back as possible.
2. Apply drops to one nostril and maintain position for 5 min. Then apply drops to second nostril and maintain position for 5 min.

Spray:

1. Administer spray into each nostril w/pt's head erect so that excess solution is not released.
2. After 2-3 min, have pt blow nose thoroughly.

INDICATIONS/DOSAGE/ROUTES

Usual nasal dosage:
INTRANASAL: Adults, elderly, children >12 yrs: 2 drops/sprays (0.05%) in each nostril q3-6h. **Children <12 yrs:** 1-2 drops/sprays (0.025%) in each nostril q3-6h.

Usual ophthalmic dosage:
OPHTHALMIC: Adults, elderly: 1-2 drops q3-4h for 3-4 days.

PRECAUTIONS

CONTRAINDICATIONS: Hypersensitivity to naphazoline or any component of the preparation; narrow-angle glaucoma or those w/a narrow angle who do not have glaucoma; before peripheral iridectomy; eyes capable of angle closure. **CAUTIONS:** Hypertension, diabetes, hyperthyroidism, heart disease, hypertensive cardiovascular disease, coronary artery disease, cerebral arteriosclerosis, long-standing bronchial asthma. Consider precautions for individual components. **PREGNANCY/LACTATION:** Safety during pregnancy and lactation not established. **Pregnancy Category C.**

INTERACTIONS

DRUG INTERACTIONS: Tricyclic antidepressants, maprotiline may increase effect. **ALTERED LAB VALUES:** None significant.

SIDE EFFECTS

FREQUENT: Stinging, burning of nasal mucosa. **OCCASIONAL:** Mild CNS stimulation (restlessness, nervousness, tremors, headache, insomnia), particularly in those hypersensitive to sympathomimetics (generally, elderly pts).

ADVERSE REACTIONS/TOXIC EFFECTS

Large doses may produce tachycardia, palpitations, lightheadedness, nausea, vomiting. Overdosage in pts >60 yrs: hallucinations, CNS depression, seizures.

NURSING IMPLICATIONS

BASELINE ASSESSMENT:

Question for hypersensitivity to naphazoline or any component of preparation.

PATIENT/FAMILY TEACHING:

Teach correct application (see Ophthalmic/Intranasal Administration). Do not use beyond 72 hrs w/o consulting a physician. Use caution w/activities that require visual acuity. Discontinue and consult physician if the following occur: Vision changes, headache, eye pain, floating spots, pain w/light exposure, acute eye redness. Too frequent use may result in rebound effect.

naproxen

nah-prox´en
(EC-Naprosyn, Naprosyn)

naproxen sodium

(Aleve, Anaprox)

CANADIAN AVAILABILITY: Anaprox, Apo-Naproxen, Naprosyn, Naxen, Novonaprox, Synflex

CLASSIFICATION

Nonsteroidal anti-inflammatory

PHARMACOKINETICS

	ONSET	PEAK	DURATION
PO: (analgesic)	<1 hr	—	Up to 7 hrs
PO: (antirheumatic)	Up to 14 days	2-4 wks	—

Completely absorbed from GI tract. Protein binding: >99%. Metabolized in liver. Primarily excreted in urine. Half-life: 13 hrs.

ACTION

Inhibits prostaglandin synthesis. Inhibits action of cyclooxygenase, decreases formation of prostaglandin, thromboxane precursors from arachidonic acid.

USES

Treatment of acute or long-term mild to moderate pain, primary dysmenorrhea, mild to moderately severe pain, rheumatoid arthritis, juvenile rheumatoid arthritis, osteoarthritis, ankylosing spondylitis, acute gouty arthritis, bursitis, tendonitis.

PO ADMINISTRATION

1. Do not crush or break enteric-coated form.
2. May give with food, milk, or antacids if GI distress occurs.

INDICATIONS/DOSAGE/ROUTES

NOTE: Each 275 or 550 mg tablet of naproxen sodium equals 250 or 500 mg naproxen, respectively.

Rheumatoid arthritis, osteoarthritis, ankylosing spondylitis:
PO: Adults, elderly: 250-500 mg (275-550 mg) 2 times/day or 250 mg (275 mg) in morning and 500 mg (550 mg) in evening.

Juvenile rheumatoid arthritis (naproxen only):
PO: Children: 10 mg/kg/day in 2 divided doses.

Acute gouty arthritis:
PO: Adults, elderly: Initially, 750 (825) mg, then 250 (275) mg q8h until attack subsides.

Mild to moderate pain, dysmenorrhea, bursitis, tendonitis:
PO: Adults, elderly: Initially, 500 (550) mg, then 250 (275) mg q6-8h as needed. Total daily dose not to exceed 1.25 (1.375) Gm.

PRECAUTIONS

CONTRAINDICATIONS: GI ulceration, chronic inflammation of GI tract, bleeding disorders, history of hypersensitivity to aspirin or NSAIDs. **CAUTIONS:** Impaired renal/hepatic function, history of GI tract disease, predisposition to fluid retention. **PREGNANCY/LACTATION:** Crosses placenta; distributed in breast milk. Avoid use during third trimester (may adversely affect fetal cardiovascular system: Premature closing of ductus arteriosus). **Pregnancy Category B.**

INTERACTIONS

DRUG INTERACTIONS: May increase effects of oral anticoagulants, heparin, thrombolytics. May decrease effect of antihypertensives, diuretics. Salicylates, aspirin may increase risk of GI side effects, bleeding. Bone marrow depressants may increase risk of hematologic reactions. May increase concentration, toxicity of lithium, May increase methotrexate toxicity. Probenecid may increase concentration. **ALTERED LAB VALUES:** May prolong bleeding time, alter blood glucose levels. May increase liver function tests. May decrease sodium, uric acid.

SIDE EFFECTS

FREQUENT: Headache, dyspepsia (heartburn, epigastric distress), nausea, dizziness, somnolence/drowsiness, constipation, pruritus, rash, ecchymoses, tinnitus, peripheral edema/fluid retention. **OCCASIONAL:** Diarrhea, stomatitis, flatulence, sweating, and purpura (purple patches on skin, mucous membranes).

ADVERSE REACTIONS/TOXIC EFFECTS

Peptic ulcer, GI bleeding, gastritis, severe hepatic reaction (cholestasis, jaundice) occur rarely. Nephrotoxicity (dysuria, hematuria, proteinuria, nephrotic syndrome) and severe hypersensitivity reaction (fever, chills, bronchospasm) occur rarely.

NURSING IMPLICATIONS

BASELINE ASSESSMENT:

Assess onset, type, location, and duration of pain or inflammation. Inspect appearance of affected joints for immobility, deformities, and skin condition.

INTERVENTION/EVALUATION:

Assist w/ambulation if dizziness occurs. Monitor pattern of daily bowel activity and stool consistency. Check behind medial malleolus for fluid retention (usually first area noted). Evaluate for therapeutic response: Relief of pain, stiffness, swelling, increase in joint mobility, reduced joint tenderness, improved grip strength.

PATIENT/FAMILY TEACHING:

Avoid tasks that require alertness, motor skills until response to drug is established. If GI upset occurs, take w/food, milk. Avoid aspirin, alcohol during therapy (increases risk of GI bleeding). Report headache, rash. Scored tablets may be broken or crushed; swallow enteric-coated form whole.

natamycin

na-ta-mye´sin

(Natacyn)

CLASSIFICATION

Antifungal

PHARMACOKINETICS

Minimal systemic absorption. Topical application produces effective concentrations in corneal stroma, but not in intraocular fluid.

ACTION

Binds to sterols in fungal cell membrane, altering membrane permeability and permitting loss of potassium and other essential components from fungal cell. Fungicidal.

USES

Fungal blepharitis, conjunctivitis, keratitis due to susceptible organisms.

OPHTHALMIC ADMINISTRATION

1. Shake vial well before use.
2. Place finger on lower eyelid and pull out until pocket is formed between eye and lower lid.
3. Hold dropper above pocket and place prescribed number of drops into pocket.
4. Close eye gently.
5. Apply digital pressure to lacrimal sac for 1-2 min (minimizes drainage into nose and throat, reducing risk of systemic effects).
6. Remove excess solution around eye w/tissue.

INDICATIONS/DOSAGE/ROUTES

Fungal keratitis:
OPHTHALMIC: Adults, elderly: 1 drop into conjunctival sac at 1-2 hr intervals; decrease to 1 drop at 3-4 hr intervals after 3-4 days. Continue therapy 14-21 days or until resolution of active fungal keratitis.

Fungal blepharitis and conjunctivitis:
OPHTHALMIC: Adults, elderly: 1 drop q4-6h.

PRECAUTIONS

CONTRAINDICATIONS: Hypersensitivity to natamycin or any component of preparation. **PREGNANCY/LACTATION: Pregnancy Category C.**

INTERACTIONS

DRUG INTERACTIONS: None significant. **ALTERED LAB VALUES:** None significant.

SIDE EFFECTS

RARE: Allergic reaction: Hyperemia, conjunctival chemosis (edema).

ADVERSE REACTIONS/TOXIC EFFECTS

None significant.

NURSING IMPLICATIONS

BASELINE ASSESSMENT:

Question for hypersensitivity to natamycin, components of suspension. Assure specimens have been obtained (therapy may begin before results are known).

INTERVENTION/EVALUATION:

Evaluate for therapeutic response or increased irritation, edema.

PATIENT/FAMILY TEACHING:

Follow dosage schedule carefully (teach proper administration). If no improvement in 7-10 days, contact physician. Continue as directed, usually 14-21 days to assure infection healed. Report any increased irritation or vision problems promptly. Do not use any other product, including makeup, except on advice of physician.

nedocromil sodium

ned-oh-crow'mul
(Tilade)

CANADIAN AVAILABILITY: Tilade

CLASSIFICATION

Anti-inflammatory

PHARMACOKINETICS

	ONSET	PEAK	DURATION
Inhalation	30 min	—	—

Minimal absorption from GI tract after inhalation. Protein binding: 89%. Distributed to plasma. Primarily excreted unchanged in urine or via biliary system. Half-life: 1.5-3.3 hrs.

ACTION

Prevents activation, release of

mediators of inflammation (e.g., histamine, leukotrienes, mast cells, eosinophils, monocytes). Prevents both early and late asthmatic responses.

USES

Maintenance therapy for preventing airway inflammation, bronchoconstriction in pts w/mild to moderate bronchial asthma.

INHALATION ADMINISTRATION

1. Shake container well, then remove cap from mouthpiece.
2. Position mouthpiece to bottom, tilt head back.
3. Breathe out through mouth to functional volume.
4. Place mouthpiece in mouth or hold 1-2 inches away from open mouth.
5. Activate inhaler while breathing in slowly and deeply.
6. Hold breath 5-10 sec (or as long as possible).
7. Remove inhaler from mouth and breath out slowly.
8. Wait 1-10 min before second inhalation.

INDICATIONS/DOSAGE/ROUTES

Asthma:
ORAL INHALATION: Adults, elderly, children >12 yrs: Two inhalations (4 mg) 4 times/day. May decrease to 3 times/day then 2 times/day as control of asthma occurs. **Maximum:** 16 mg/24 hrs.

PRECAUTIONS

CONTRAINDICATIONS: Hypersensitivity to nedocromil. **CAUTIONS:** Safety in children <12 yrs. Not for reversing acute bronchospasm. **PREGNANCY/LACTATION:** Unknown whether drug crosses placenta or is distributed in breast milk. **Pregnancy Category B.**

INTERACTIONS

DRUG INTERACTIONS: None significant. **ALTERED LAB VALUES:** None significant.

SIDE EFFECTS

Generally well tolerated. **FREQUENT:** Unpleasant taste. **OCCASIONAL:** Increased wheezing, chest tightness, difficult breathing, cough, headache, nausea, throat irritation, sleepiness, vomiting.

ADVERSE REACTIONS/TOXIC EFFECTS

None significant.

NURSING IMPLICATIONS

BASELINE ASSESSMENT:

Assess sensitivity to nedocromil. Offer emotional support.

INTERVENTION/EVALUATION:

Evaluate therapeutic response: reduced dependence on antihistamine, less frequent/less severe asthmatic attacks.

PATIENT/FAMILY TEACHING:

Increase fluid intake (decreases lung secretion viscosity). Must be administered at regular intervals (even when symptom-free) to achieve optimal results of therapy. Proper inhalation technique is essential (illustrated pt information leaflet accompanies medication). Do not increase or decrease dosage w/o consulting physician. Unpleasant taste after inhalation may be relieved by rinsing mouth w/water immediately, using sugarless hard candy or gum.

---

nefazodone (Serzone)
See supplement

neomycin sulfate

ne-oh-my´sin
(Mycifradin, Myciguent)

FIXED-COMBINATION(S):
W/polymyxin B, an anti-infective (Neosporin, Neosporin G.U. Irrigant); w/polymyxin B and bacitracin, an antibiotic (Mycitracin, Neosporin, Neo-Polycin); w/polymyxin B and hydrocortisone, a steroid (Cortisporin); w/gramicidin, an anti-infective (Spectrocin)

CANADIAN AVAILABILITY:
Mycifradin, Myciguent

CLASSIFICATION

Antibiotic: Aminoglycoside

PHARMACOKINETICS

Minimal absorption from GI tract, after ophthalmic, topical administration. Primarily eliminated unchanged in feces. Half-life: 2-3 hrs.

ACTION

Binds to specific receptor protein on 30S subunit of bacterial ribosomes, inhibits protein synthesis. Suppresses bacterial growth in bowel by decreasing ammonia production in intestine (inhibits bacteria from ammonia synthesis).

USES

Irrigation of wounds, surgical sites, bladder; preop use for intestinal antisepsis; diarrhea due to enteropathogenic *Escherichia coli,* adjunctive therapy for hepatic encephalopathy. *Ophthalmic:* Ointment/solution for superficial eye infections. *Otic:* Otitis externa only. *Topical:* Prevention or treatment of superficial skin infections. Not for long-term therapy because of associated toxicities.

PO/OPHTHALMIC/OTIC ADMINISTRATION

NOTE: Given orally, as retention enema, bladder irrigation, ophthalmic, otic, or topical. Neomycin frequently combined w/corticosteroids, anesthetics, other anti-infectives when applied in topical form.

PO:

1. Give w/o regard to meals.
2. If GI upset occurs, give w/ food or milk.
3. Tablets may be crushed.

OPHTHALMIC:

1. Place finger on lower eyelid and pull out until a pocket is formed between eye and lower lid.
2. Hold dropper above pocket and place correct number of drops (¼-½ inch ointment) into pocket.
3. Close eye gently.
4. *Solution:* Apply digital pressure to lacrimal sac for 1-2 min (minimizes drainage into nose and throat, reducing risk of systemic effects). *Ointment:* Close eye for 1-2 min, rolling eyeball (increases contact area of drug to eye).
5. Remove excess solution or ointment around eye w/tissue.

OTIC:

1. Apply into clean, dry ear canal.

INDICATIONS/DOSAGE/ROUTES

Hepatic encephalopathy, adjunctive therapy:
PO: Adults, elderly: 4-12 Gm/day in 4 divided doses.

Preop intestinal antisepsis:
PO: Adults, elderly: 1 Gm every hr for 4 doses; then 1 Gm q4h for balance of 24 hrs, or 1 Gm at 1, 2, and 11 PM on day before surgery (w/erythromycin).

Continuous bladder irrigation:
Adults, elderly: 1 ml of urogenital concentrate (contains 200,000 U polymyxin B and 57 mg neomycin) added to 1,000 ml 0.9% NaCl given over 24 hrs for up to 10 days (may increase to 2,000 ml/day).

Usual ophthalmic dosage:
OINTMENT: Adults, elderly, children: Thin strip to conjunctiva q3-4h.
LIQUID: Adults, elderly, children: 1 drop to conjunctiva q3-4h.

Usual otic dosage:
OTIC: Adults, elderly: 4 drops q6-8h. **Children:** 3 drops q6-8h.

Usual topical dosage:
TOPICAL: Adults, elderly, children: Applied gently 1-3 times/day up to 5 times/day.
NOTE: Apply no more than once daily in pts w/>20% burns.

PRECAUTIONS

CONTRAINDICATIONS: Hypersensitivity to neomycin, other aminoglycosides (cross-sensitivity). Oral administration contraindicated in intestinal obstruction. **CAUTIONS:** Elderly, infants w/renal insufficiency/immaturity; neuromuscular disorders (potential for respiratory depression), prior hearing loss, vertigo, renal impairment. **PREGNANCY/LACTATION:** Unknown whether drug crosses placenta or is distributed in breast milk. **Pregnancy Category C.**

INTERACTIONS

DRUG INTERACTIONS: If significant systemic absorption occurs, may increase nephrotoxicity, ototoxicity w/aminoglycosides, other nephrotoxic, ototoxic medications. **ALTERED LAB VALUES:** None significant.

SIDE EFFECTS

FREQUENT: Nausea, vomiting, diarrhea. **OCCASIONAL:** Hypersensitivity reactions: Rash, fever, urticaria, pruritus. *Ophthalmic:* Itching, burning, redness. *Topical:* Urticaria, rash, burning, redness. **RARE:** Headache, muscular weakness.

ADVERSE REACTIONS/TOXIC EFFECTS

Nephrotoxicity (evidenced by increased BUN and serum creatinine, decreased creatinine clearance) may be reversible if drug stopped at first sign of symptoms; irreversible ototoxicity (tinnitus, dizziness, ringing/roaring in ears, reduced hearing) and neurotoxicity (headache, dizziness, lethargy, tremors, visual disturbances) occur occasionally. Risk is greater with higher dosages, prolonged therapy, or if preparation applied directly to mucosa (particularly extensive areas). Severe respiratory depression, anaphylaxis occur rarely. Superinfections, particularly w/fungi, may result from bacterial imbalance following administration via any route.

NURSING IMPLICATIONS

BASELINE ASSESSMENT:

Dehydration must be treated before aminoglycoside therapy. Establish pt's baseline hearing acuity before beginning therapy. Cumulative effects may occur when given via more than 1 route. Question for history of allergies, esp. aminoglycosides. Obtain specimens for culture, sensitivity before giving first dose (therapy may begin before results are known).

INTERVENTION/EVALUATION:

Monitor I&O (maintain hydration), urinalysis (casts, RBCs, WBCs, decrease in specific gravity). Monitor results of peak/trough blood tests. Be alert to ototoxic and neurotoxic symptoms (see Adverse Reactions/Toxic Effects). Assess for rash (*ophthalmic*—assess for redness, burning, itching, tearing; *topical*—assess for redness, itching). Be alert for superinfection particularly genital/anal pruritus, changes of oral mucosa, diarrhea. When treating pts w/ neuromuscular disorders, assess respiratory response carefully.

PATIENT/FAMILY TEACHING:

Continue antibiotic for full length of treatment. Space doses evenly. Notify physician in event of hearing, visual, balance, urinary problems, even after therapy is completed. Do not take other medication w/o consulting physician. Lab tests are an essential part of therapy. *Ophthalmic:* Blurred vision or tearing may occur briefly after application. Contact physician if tearing, redness, irritation continue. *Topical:* Cleanse area gently before application; report redness, itching.

neostigmine bromide

knee-oh-stig´meen

(Prostigmin [oral])

neostigmine methylsulfate

(Prostigmin [parenteral])

CANADIAN AVAILABILITY:
Prostigmin

CLASSIFICATION

Anticholinesterase agent

PHARMACOKINETICS

	ONSET	PEAK	DURATION
PO	2-4 hrs	—	—
IM	10-30 min	20-30 min	2.5-4 hrs

Poorly absorbed from GI tract. Rapid absorption following IM administration. Protein binding: 15-25%. Metabolized in liver, plasma. Primarily excreted in urine. Half-life: 24-79 min.

ACTION

Prevents destruction of acetylcholine by anticholinesterase. Effects include: increased secretions, salivation, miosis, bradycardia, increased intestinal, skeletal muscle tone.

USES

Improvement of muscle strength in control of myasthenia gravis, to diagnose myasthenia gravis, prevention/treatment of postop distention and urinary retention, as antidote for reversal of effects of nondepolarizing neuromuscular blocking agents after surgery.

STORAGE/HANDLING

Store parenteral, oral form at room temperature.

PO/SubQ/IM/IV ADMINISTRATION

PO:

1. For those w/difficulty chewing, give dose 30-45 min before meals, preferably w/milk (drug produces fewer cholinergic effects if taken w/milk or food).

SubQ/IM/IV:

NOTE: May be given undiluted. Do not add to IV solutions.

1. When given as curariform block antidote following surgery (unless tachycardia is present), give 0.6-1.2 mg atropine concurrently w/neostigmine to prevent bradycardia.

2. If bradycardia is present, increase pulse rate to 80/min w/ atropine before administering neostigmine.

3. Administer IV very slowly (0.5 mg or less over 1 min).

INDICATIONS/DOSAGE/ROUTES

NOTE: Dosage, frequency of administration dependent on daily clinical pt response (remissions, exacerbations, physical and emotional stress).

Myasthenia gravis:
PO: Adults, elderly: Initially, 15-30 mg 3-4 times/day. Increase dose gradually until therapeutic response achieved. **Usual maintenance dose:** 150 mg/day w/ range of 15-375 mg. **Children:** Initially, 2 mg/kg/day divided q3-4h. **Neonatal:** 1-4 mg q2-3h.
SubQ/IM/IV: Adults: 0.5-2.5 mg as needed. **Neonatal:** 0.1-0.2 mg SubQ or 0.03 mg/kg IM q2-4h.

Diagnosis of myasthenia gravis:
NOTE: Discontinue all anticholinesterase therapy at least 8 hrs before testing. Give 0.011 mg/kg atropine sulfate IV w/, or IM 30 min before administering neostigmine (prevents adverse effects).
IM: Adults, elderly: 0.022 mg/kg. If cholinergic reaction occurs, discontinue tests and administer 0.4-0.6 mg or more atropine sulfate IV. **Children:** 0.025-0.04 mg/kg IM preceded by atropine sulfate 0.011 mg/kg SubQ.

Prevention of postop urinary retention:
SubQ/IM: Adults, elderly: 0.25 mg q4-6h for 2-3 days.

Postop distention, urinary retention:
SubQ/IM: Adults, elderly: 0.5-1 mg. Catheterize if voiding does not occur within 1 hr. After voiding, continue 0.5 mg q3h for 5 injections.

Reversal of neuromuscular blockade:
IV: Adults, elderly: 0.5-2.5 mg given slowly.

PRECAUTIONS

CONTRAINDICATIONS: Concurrent use of high doses of halothane, cyclopropane, mechanical GI or GU obstruction, peritonitis, doubtful bowel viability. **CAUTIONS:** Bronchial asthma, bradycardia, epilepsy, coronary occlusion, vagotonia, hyperthyroidism, cardiac arrhythmias, peptic ulcer. **PREGNANCY/LACTATION:** Transient muscular weakness occurs in 10-20% of neonates born to mothers treated w/drug therapy for myasthenia gravis during pregnancy. May produce uterine irritability, induce premature labor if administered IV near term. **Pregnancy Category C.**

INTERACTIONS

DRUG INTERACTIONS: Anticholinergics reverse/prevent effects. Cholinesterase inhibitors may increase toxicity. Antagonizes neuromuscular blocking agents. Quinidine, procainamide may antagonize action. **ALTERED LAB VALUES:** None significant.

SIDE EFFECTS

COMMON: Miosis, increased GI and skeletal muscle tone, reduced pulse rate, constriction of bronchi and ureters, salivary and sweat gland secretion. **OCCASIONAL:** Skin rash, transient arrhythmias when given concurrently w/atropine sulfate to reverse effects of neuromuscular blockade after surgery; slight, temporary decrease in diastolic B/P with mild reflex tachycardia; short periods of atrial fibrillation in hyperthyroid pts. Hypertensive pts may react w/ marked fall in B/P.

ADVERSE REACTIONS/TOXIC EFFECTS

Overdose produces a cholinergic reaction manifested as abdominal discomfort/cramping, nausea, vomiting, diarrhea, flushing, feeling of warmth/heat about face, excessive salivation and sweating, lacrimation, pallor, bradycardia/tachycardia, hypotension, urinary urgency, blurred vision, bronchospasm, pupillary contraction, involuntary muscular contraction visible under the skin (fasciculation).

Overdose may also produce *cholinergic crisis,* manifested by increasingly severe muscle weakness, (appears first in muscles involving chewing, swallowing, followed by muscular weakness of shoulder girdle and upper extremities), respiratory muscle paralysis followed by pelvic girdle and leg muscle paralysis. Requires a withdrawal of all cholinergic drugs and immediate use of 0.6-1.2 mg atropine sulfate IV for adults, 0.01 mg/kg in infants, children under 12 yrs.

Myasthenic crisis (due to underdose) also produces extreme muscle weakness but requires a *more* intensive drug therapy program (differentiation between the 2 crises is imperative for accurate treatment). Weakness beginning 1 hr after drug administration suggests overdosage; weakness occurring 3 hrs or more after administration suggests underdosage or resistance to anticholinesterase drugs. Extremely high doses may produce CNS stimulation followed by CNS depression.

NURSING IMPLICATIONS

BASELINE ASSESSMENT:

Larger doses should be given at time of greatest fatigue. Assess muscle strength before testing for diagnosis of myasthenia gravis, as well as after drug administration. Avoid large doses in those w/ megacolon or reduced GI motility. Have tissues readily available at pt's bedside.

INTERVENTION/EVALUATION:

Monitor vital capacity during myasthenia gravis testing, or if dosage is increased. Distinguish carefully between cholinergic crisis and myasthenic crisis (see Adverse Reactions/Toxic Effects). Monitor for therapeutic response to medication (increased muscle strength, decreased fatigue, improved chewing, swallowing functions).

PATIENT/FAMILY TEACHING:

Report nausea, vomiting, diarrhea, sweating, increased salivary secretions, irregular heartbeat, muscle weakness, severe abdominal pain, or difficulty in breathing.

netilmicin sulfate

neh-till-my'sin

(Netromycin)

CANADIAN AVAILABILITY: Netromycin

CLASSIFICATION

Antibiotic: Aminoglycoside

PHARMACOKINETICS

Rapid, complete absorption after IM administration. Widely distributed (does not cross blood-brain barrier, low concentrations in CSF). Protein binding: 10%. Excreted unchanged in urine. Removed by hemodialysis. Half-life: 2-4 hrs (increased in decreased renal function, neonates; decreased in cystic fibrosis, burn or febrile pts).

ACTION

Irreversibly binds to protein in 30S subunit of bacterial ribosome, interfering in protein synthesis of susceptible microorganisms.

USES

Skin/skin structure, bone, joint, lower respiratory tract, intra-abdominal, complicated urinary tract infections; burns, septicemia.

STORAGE/HANDLING

Store parenteral form at room temperature. Solutions appear clear, colorless to pale yellow. May be discolored by light, air (does not affect potency). Intermittent IV infusion (piggyback) stable for 72 hrs at room temperature, or refrigerated. Discard if precipitate forms.

IM/IV ADMINISTRATION

NOTE: Coordinate peak and trough lab draws w/administration times.

IM:

1. To minimize discomfort, give deep IM slowly. Less painful if injected into gluteus maximus rather than lateral aspect of thigh.

IV:

1. Dilute with 50-200 ml 5% dextrose, 0.9% NaCl or other compatible IV fluid.
2. Infuse over 30-60 min for adults, older children, and over 60-120 min for infants, young children.
3. Alternating IV sites, use large veins to reduce risk of phlebitis.

INDICATIONS/DOSAGE/ROUTES

NOTE: Space doses evenly around the clock. Dosage based on ideal body weight. Peak, trough serum concentrations determined periodically to maintain desired serum concentrations (minimizes risk of toxicity). *Recommended peak level:* 6-12 mcg/ml; *trough level:* 0.5-2 mcg/ml.

Complicated urinary tract infections:
IM/IV: Adults, elderly: 3-4 mg/kg/day in divided doses q12h.

Septicemia, skin/skin structure, intra-abdominal, lower respiratory infections:
IM/IV: Adults, elderly: 4-6.5 mg/kg/day in divided doses q8-12h. **Children >6 wks:** 5.5-8 mg/kg/day in divided doses q8-12h. **Neonates:** 4-6.5 mg/kg/day in divided doses q12h.

Dosage in renal impairment:
Dose and/or frequency is modified based on degree of renal impairment, serum concentration of drug. After loading dose of 1.3-2.2 mg/kg, maintenance doses, intervals are based on serum creatinine or creatinine clearance.

PRECAUTIONS

CONTRAINDICATIONS: Hypersensitivity to netilmicin, other aminoglycosides (cross-sensitivity). Sulfite sensitivity may result in anaphylaxis, esp. in asthmatics. **CAUTIONS:** Elderly, neonates w/ renal insufficiency/immaturity; neuromuscular disorders (potential for respiratory depression), prior hearing loss, vertigo, renal impairment. **PREGNANCY/LACTATION:** Readily crosses placenta; distributed in breast milk. May produce fetal nephrotoxicity. **Pregnancy Category D.**

INTERACTIONS

DRUG INTERACTIONS: Other aminoglycosides, nephrotoxic, ototoxic producing medications may increase toxicity. May increase effects of neuromuscular blocking agents. **ALTERED LAB VALUES:** May increase BUN, SGPT (ALT), SGOT (AST), bilirubin, creatinine, LDH concentrations; may decrease serum calcium, magnesium, potassium, sodium concentrations.

SIDE EFFECTS

OCCASIONAL: Pain, induration at IM injection site; phlebitis, thrombophlebitis w/IV administration; hypersensitivity reactions: Rash, fever, urticaria, pruritus. **RARE:** Headache.

ADVERSE REACTIONS/TOXIC EFFECTS

Nephrotoxicity (evidenced by increased BUN and serum creatinine, decreased creatinine clearance) may be reversible if drug stopped at first sign of symptoms; irreversible ototoxicity (tinnitus, dizziness, ringing/roaring in ears, reduced hearing) and neurotoxicity (headache, dizziness, lethargy, tremors, visual disturbances) occur occasionally. Risk is greater w/ higher dosages, prolonged therapy. Superinfections, particularly w/fungi, may result from bacterial imbalance.

NURSING IMPLICATIONS

BASELINE ASSESSMENT:

Dehydration must be treated before aminoglycoside therapy. Establish pt's baseline hearing acuity before beginning therapy. Question for history of allergies, esp. aminoglycosides, sulfite. Obtain specimens for culture, sensitivity before giving first dose (therapy may begin before results are known).

INTERVENTION/EVALUATION:

Monitor I&O (maintain hydration), urinalysis (casts, RBCs, WBCs, decrease in specific gravity). Monitor results of peak/trough blood tests. Be alert to ototoxic and neurotoxic symptoms (see Adverse Reactions/Toxic Effects). Check IM injection site for pain, induration. Evaluate IV site for phlebitis (heat, pain, red streaking over vein). Assess for rash. Assess for superinfection particularly genital/anal pruritus, changes of oral mucosa, diarrhea.

PATIENT/FAMILY TEACHING:

Continue antibiotic for full length of treatment. Space doses evenly. Discomfort may occur with IM injection. Notify physician in event of headache, shortness of breath, dizziness, hearing, urinary problem even after therapy is completed. Do not take other medication w/o consulting physician. Lab tests are an essential part of therapy.

niacin, nicotinic acid

(Nicobid, Nico-400, Nicotinex)

CANADIAN AVAILABILITY:
Tri-B3

CLASSIFICATION

Antihyperlipoproteinemic

PHARMACOKINETICS

Readily absorbed from GI tract. Widely distributed. Metabolized in liver. Primarily excreted in urine. Half-life: 45 minutes.

ACTION

Lowers serum cholesterol and triglycerides (decreases LDL, VLDL, increases HDL). Inhibits free fatty acid release in fat tissue, decreases rate of VLDL, LDL synthesis in liver, increases lipoprotein lipase activity. Component of coenzymes which are necessary for lipid metabolism, tissue respiration, and glycogenolysis.

USES

Adjunct to diet therapy to decrease elevated serum cholesterol and triglycerides concentrations (elevated LDL, VLDL in treatment of Type II, III, IV or V hyperlipoproteinemia). Prevention and treatment of vitamin B_3 deficiency states (i.e., pellegra).

PO ADMINISTRATION

Preferably given w/or after meals (decreases GI upset).

INDICATIONS/DOSAGE/ROUTES

Hyperlipoproteinemia:
PO: Adults, elderly: Initially, 100 mg 3 times/day. Increase by 300 mg/day at 4-7 day intervals. **Maintenance:** 1-2 Gm 3 times/day. **Maximum:** 8 Gm/day.

Nutritional supplement:
PO: Adults, elderly: 10-20 mg/day.

PRECAUTIONS

CONTRAINDICATIONS: Hypersensitivity to niacin or tartrazine (frequently seen in pts sensitive to aspirin), active peptic ulcer, severe hypotension, hepatic dysfunction, arterial hemorrhaging. **CAUTIONS:** Diabetes mellitus, gallbladder disease, gout, history of jaundice or liver disease. **PREGNANCY/LACTATION:** Not recommended for use during pregnancy/lactation. Distributed in breast milk. **Pregnancy Category C.**

INTERACTIONS

DRUG INTERACTIONS: Lovastatin, pravastatin, simvastatin may increase risk of rhabdomyolysis and acute renal failure. **ALTERED LAB VALUES:** May increase uric acid.

SIDE EFFECTS

FREQUENT: Flushing (esp. of face, neck) occurring within 20 min of administration and lasting for 30-60 min, GI upset, pruritus. **OCCASIONAL:** Dizziness, hypotension, headache, blurred vision, burning or tingling of skin, flatulence, nausea, vomiting, diarrhea. **RARE:** Hyperglycemia, glycosuria, rash, hyperpigmentation, dry skin.

ADVERSE REACTIONS/TOXIC EFFECTS

Cardiac arrhythmias, particularly in those w/CHD occur rarely.

NURSING IMPLICATIONS

BASELINE ASSESSMENT:

Question for history of hypersensitivity to niacin, tartrazine or aspirin. Assess baselines: Cholesterol, triglyceride, blood glucose, liver function tests.

INTERVENTION/EVALUATION:

Evaluate flushing and degree of discomfort. Check for headache, dizziness, blurred vision. Monitor B/P at least 2 times/day. Assess food tolerance. Determine pattern of bowel activity. Monitor liver function test results, cholesterol and triglyceride. Check blood glucose levels carefully in those on insulin or oral antihyperglycemics. Assess skin for rash, dryness.

PATIENT/FAMILY TEACHING:

Take w/meals to decrease GI upset. Follow special diet (important part of treatment). Do not alter dosage. Consult physician before taking other medication. In event of new symptoms, notify physician. If dizziness occurs, avoid sudden posture changes and activities that require steady/alert response. Flushing may decrease w/continued therapy; however, discuss considerable discomfort w/physician.

nicardipine hydrochloride

nigh-car′dih-peen

(Cardene, Cardene SR)

CANADIAN AVAILABILITY:
Cardene

CLASSIFICATION

Calcium channel blocker

PHARMACOKINETICS

	ONSET	PEAK	DURATION
PO	—	1-2 hrs	8 hrs

Rapidly, completely absorbed from GI tract. Undergoes first-pass metabolism in liver. Protein binding: 95%. Metabolized in liver. Primarily excreted in urine. Half-life: 8.6 hrs.

ACTION

Potent peripheral vasodilator; does not depress SA, AV nodes. Increased heart rate masks negative inotropic effect.

USES

Oral: Treatment of chronic stable (effort associated) angina or essential hypertension. *Sustained release:* Treatment of essential hypertension. *Parenteral:* Short-term treatment of hypertension when oral therapy not feasible or desirable.

STORAGE/HANDLING

Store oral, parenteral forms at room temperature. Diluted IV solution is stable for 24 hrs at room temperature.

PO/IV ADMINISTRATION

PO:

1. Do not crush or break oral, sustained-release capsules.
2. May take w/o regard to food.

IV:

1. Dilute each 25 mg ampoule w/240 ml 5% dextrose, 0.9% NaCl or other compatible IV to provide a concentration of 1 mg/10 ml.
2. Change IV site q12h if administered peripherally.

INDICATIONS/DOSAGE/ROUTES

Chronic stable angina:
PO: Adults, elderly: Initially, 20 mg 3 times/day. **Range:** 20-40 mg 3 times/day.

Essential hypertension:
PO: Adults, elderly: Initially, 20 mg 3 times/day. **Range:** 20-40 mg 3 times/day.
SUSTAINED RELEASE: Adults, elderly: Initially, 30 mg 2 times/day. **Range:** 30-60 mg 2 times/day.

Dosage in liver impairment:
Initially, 20 mg 2 times/day then titrate.

Dosage in renal impairment:
Initially, 20 mg q8h (30 mg 2 times/day sustained release) then titrate.

Usual parenteral dosage:
Substitute for oral nicardipine:
IV: Adults, elderly: 0.5 mg/hr (20 mg q8h); 1.2 mg/hr (30 mg q8h); 2.2 mg/hr (40 mg q8h).

Drug-free pt:
IV: Adults, elderly: *(Gradual B/P decrease):* Initially, 5 mg/hr. May increase by 2.5 mg/hr q15min. *(Rapid B/P decrease):* Initially, 5 mg/hr. May increase by 2.5 mg/hr q5min. **Maximum:** 15 mg/hr until desired B/P attained.
NOTE: After B/P goal achieved, decrease rate to 3 mg/hr.

Changing to oral antihypertensive therapy:
Begin 1 hr after IV discontinued; for nicardipine, give first dose 1 hr before discontinuing IV.

PRECAUTIONS

CONTRAINDICATIONS: Severe hypotension, advanced aortic stenosis. **CAUTIONS:** Impaired renal, hepatic function. **PREGNANCY/LACTATION:** Unknown whether distributed in breast milk. **Pregnancy Category C.**

INTERACTIONS

DRUG INTERACTIONS: Beta-blockers may have additive effect. May increase digoxin concentration. Procainamide, quinidine may increase risk of QT interval prolongation. Hypokalemia producing agents may increase risk of arrhythmias. **ALTERED LAB VALUES:** None significant.

SIDE EFFECTS

FREQUENT: Peripheral edema, dizziness, lightheadedness (hypotensive effect), headache, asthenia (loss of strength, weakness), facial flushing. **OCCASIONAL:** Palpitations, tachycardia, nausea, dyspepsia, dry mouth. **RARE:** Dermatitis/rash, tachycardia, drowsiness.

ADVERSE REACTIONS/TOXIC EFFECTS

Rapid ventricular rate in atrial flutter/fibrillation, marked hypotension, CHF.

NURSING IMPLICATIONS

BASELINE ASSESSMENT:

Concurrent therapy of sublingual nitroglycerin may be used for relief of anginal pain. Record onset, type (sharp, dull, squeezing), radiation, location, intensity, and duration of anginal pain, and precipitating factors (exertion, emotional stress).

INTERVENTION/EVALUATION:

Monitor B/P during and after IV infusion. Assist w/ambulation if dizziness occurs. Assess for peripheral edema behind medial malleolus (sacral area in bedridden pts). Assess skin for facial flushing, dermatitis, rash. Question for asthenia, headache. Monitor liver enzyme results. Assess EKG, pulse for tachycardia, palpitations.

PATIENT/FAMILY TEACHING:

Do not abruptly discontinue medication. Compliance w/therapy regimen is essential to control anginal pain. To avoid hypotensive effect, rise slowly from lying to sitting position, wait momentarily before standing. Avoid tasks that require alertness, motor skills until response to drug is established. Contact physician/nurse if irregular heart beat, shortness of breath, pronounced dizziness or nausea occurs.

nicotine polacrilex

nick´oh-teen
(Nicorette)

nicotine transdermal system

(Habitrol, Nicoderm, Nicotrol ProStep)

CANADIAN AVAILABILITY:
Habitrol, Nicoderm, Nicorette

CLASSIFICATION

Smoking deterrent

PHARMACOKINETICS

Not absorbed from GI tract. Absorption increased from buccal mucosa, well absorbed after topical administration. Metabolized in liver. Primarily excreted in urine. Half-life: 1-2 hrs.

ACTION

Nicotine, a cholinergic-receptor agonist, produces autonomic effects by binding to acetylcholine receptors. Produces both stimulating and depressant effects on peripheral and central nervous systems; respiratory stimulant; produces emesis; low amounts increase heart rate, B/P; high doses may decrease B/P; may increase motor activity of GI smooth muscle. Nicotine produces psychological and physical dependence.

USES

An alternative, less potent form of nicotine (w/o tar, carbon monoxide, carcinogenic substances of tobacco) used as part of a smoking cessation program.

TRANSDERMAL/GUM ADMINISTRATION

TRANSDERMAL:

1. Apply promptly upon removal from protective pouch (prevents evaporation loss of nicotine). Use only intact pouch.
2. Apply only once/day to hairless, clean, dry skin on upper body or outer arm.
3. Replace daily at different sites; do not use same site within 7 days; do not use same patch >24 hrs.
4. Wash hands after applying patch. Wash w/water alone (soap may increase nicotine absorption).
5. Discard used patch by folding patch in half sticky side together, placing in pouch of new patch and throwing away in such a way as to prevent child/pet accessibility.

GUM:

1. Do not swallow.

2. Chew 1 piece whenever urge to smoke present.

3. Chew slowly/intermittently for 30 min.

4. Chew until distinctive nicotine taste (peppery) or slight tingling in mouth perceived then stop; when tingling almost gone (about 1 min) repeat chewing procedure. (This allows constant slow buccal absorption).

5. Too-rapid chewing may cause excessive release of nicotine resulting in adverse effects similar to oversmoking (e.g., nausea, throat irritation).

INDICATIONS/DOSAGE/ROUTES

Smoking deterrent:

NOTE: Individualize dose; stop smoking immediately.

TRANSDERMAL: Adults, elderly: (Habitrol/Nicoderm): 21 mg/day for 6 wks; then 14 mg/day for 2 wks; then 7 mg/day for 2 wks. (ProStep): 22 mg/day for 4-8 wks; then 11 mg/day for 2-4 wks.

GUM: Adults, elderly: Usually, 10-12 pieces/day. **Maximum:** 30 pieces/day.

PRECAUTIONS

CONTRAINDICATIONS: During immediate post-MI period, life-threatening arrhythmias, severe or worsening angina, active temporomandibular joint disease. **CAUTIONS:** Hyperthyroidism, pheochromocytoma, insulin-dependent diabetes mellitus, severe renal impairment, eczematous dermatitis, oral or pharyngeal inflammation, esophagitis, peptic ulcer (delays healing in peptic ulcer disease). **PREGNANCY/LACTATION:** Passes freely into breast milk. Use of cigarettes or nicotine gum associated w/decrease in fetal breathing movements. **Pregnancy Category X:** Nicotine polacrilex; **Pregnancy Category D:** Transdermal nicotine.

INTERACTIONS

DRUG INTERACTIONS: Smoking cessation may increase effects of beta-adrenergic blockers, bronchodilators (e.g., theophylline), insulin, propoxyphene. **ALTERED LAB VALUES:** None significant.

SIDE EFFECTS

Nicotine polacrilex: **FREQUENT:** Mouth or throat soreness, nausea, hiccoughs. **OCCASIONAL:** Belching, generalized GI upset. **RARE:** Excessive salivation. *Transdermal nicotine:* **FREQUENT:** Erythema, pruritus or burning at application site, headache. **OCCASIONAL:** Muscle aches, dizziness, back pain, diarrhea or constipation, insomnia, vivid dreams, cough, rash. **RARE:** Dry mouth, impaired concentration, sinusitis, sweating.

N

ADVERSE REACTIONS/TOXIC EFFECTS

Overdose produces palpitations, tachyarrhythmias, convulsions, depression, confusion, profuse diaphoresis, hypotension, rapid/weak pulse, difficulty breathing. Lethal dose, adults: 40-60 mg. Death results from respiratory paralysis.

NURSING IMPLICATIONS

BASELINE ASSESSMENT:

Screen, evaluate those w/coronary heart disease (history of MI, angina pectoris), serious cardiac arrhythmias, Buerger's disease, Prinzmetal's variant angina.

INTERVENTION/EVALUATION:

If increase in cardiovascular symptoms occur, discontinue use.

Assess all symptoms carefully w/ regard to method of medication (see Side Effects)

PATIENT/FAMILY TEACHING:

Give instruction sheet to pt; review proper application and disposal of transdermal system. Gradually withdraw or stop nicotine gum usage <3 mo, transdermal nicotine after 4-8 wks of use, progressively decreasing dose q2-4wks. Do not eat or drink anything during or immediately before nicotine gum use (reduces salivary pH). Use contraceptive measures during therapy.

nifedipine

nye-fed´ih-peen

(Adalat, Procardia)

CANADIAN AVAILABILITY:
Adalat, Apo-Nifed, Novonifedin

CLASSIFICATION

Calcium channel blocker

PHARMACOKINETICS

Rapidly, completely absorbed from GI tract. Undergoes first-pass metabolism in liver. Protein binding: 92-98%. Metabolized in liver. Primarily excreted in urine. Half-life: 2-5 hrs.

ACTION

Potent peripheral vasodilator; does not depress SA, AV nodes. Reflex increased heart rate masks negative inotropic effect.

USES

Treatment of angina due to coronary artery spasm (Prinzmetal's variant angina), chronic stable angina (effort-associated angina). *Extended release:* Treatment of essential hypertension.

PO/SUBLINGUAL ADMINISTRATION

PO:

1. Do not crush or break film-coated tablet or sustained-release capsule.
2. May give w/o regard to meals.

SUBLINGUAL:

1. Capsule must be punctured, chewed and/or squeezed to express liquid into mouth.

INDICATIONS/DOSAGE/ROUTES

NOTE: May give 10-20 mg sublingually as needed for acute attacks of angina.

Prinzmetal's variant angina, chronic stable angina:
PO: Adults, elderly: Initially, 10 mg 3 times/day. Increase at 7-14 day intervals. **Maintenance:** 10 mg 3 times/day up to 30 mg 4 times/day.
EXTENDED RELEASE: Adults, elderly: Initially, 30-60 mg/day. **Maintenance:** Up to 120 mg/day.

Hypertension:
EXTENDED RELEASE: Adults, elderly: Initially, 30-60 mg/day. **Maintenance:** Up to 120 mg/day.

PRECAUTIONS

CONTRAINDICATIONS: Sick sinus syndrome/second- or third-degree AV block (except in presence of pacemaker). **CAUTIONS:** Impaired renal/hepatic function, aortic stenosis. **PREGNANCY/LACTATION:** Insignificant amount distributed in breast milk. **Pregnancy Category C.**

INTERACTIONS

DRUG INTERACTIONS: Beta-blockers may have additive effect. May increase digoxin concentration. Procainamide, quinidine may increase risk of QT interval prolongation. Hypokalemia producing agents may increase risk of arrhythmias. **ALTERED LAB VALUES:** May cause positive ANA, Direct Coombs' test.

SIDE EFFECTS

FREQUENT: Giddiness, dizziness, lightheadedness, peripheral edema, headache, flushing, weakness, nausea. **OCCASIONAL:** Transient hypotension, heartburn, muscle cramps, nasal congestion, cough, wheezing, sore throat, palpitations, nervousness, mood changes. **RARE:** Increase in frequency, intensity, duration of angina during initial therapy.

ADVERSE REACTIONS/TOXIC EFFECTS

May precipitate CHF, MI in those w/cardiac disease, peripheral ischemia. Overdose produces nausea, drowsiness, confusion, slurred speech.

NURSING IMPLICATIONS

Baseline Assessment:

Concurrent therapy of sublingual nitroglycerin may be used for relief of anginal pain. Record onset, type (sharp, dull, squeezing), radiation, location, intensity, and duration of anginal pain, and precipitating factors (exertion, emotional stress). Check B/P for hypotension, pulse for bradycardia immediately before giving medication.

Intervention/Evaluation:

Observe for giddiness (common effect). Assist w/ambulation if lightheadedness, dizziness occur. Assess for peripheral edema behind medial malleolus (sacral area in bedridden pts). Monitor pulse rate for bradycardia. Assess skin for flushing. Monitor liver enzyme tests.

Patient/Family Teaching:

Rise slowly from lying to sitting position and permit legs to dangle from bed momentarily before standing to reduce hypotensive effect. Contact physician/nurse if irregular heart beat, shortness of breath, pronounced dizziness, or nausea occur.

N

nimodipine

nih-moad´ih-peen

(Nimotop)

CANADIAN AVAILABILITY: Nimotop

CLASSIFICATION

Calcium channel blocker

PHARMACOKINETICS

Rapidly absorbed from GI tract. Protein binding: >95%. Metabolized in liver. Excreted in urine, eliminated in feces. Half-life: (terminal) 8-9 hrs.

ACTION

Inhibits movement of calcium ions across cellular membranes in vascular smooth muscle. Greatest effect on cerebral arteries.

USES

Improvement of neurologic deficits due to spasm following subarachnoid hemorrhage from ruptured congenital intracranial aneurysms in pts in good neurologic condition.

PO ADMINISTRATION

1. If pt unable to swallow, place hole in both ends of capsule with 18-gauge needle to extract contents into syringe.
2. Empty into nasogastric tube; wash tube w/30 ml normal saline.

INDICATIONS/DOSAGE/ROUTES

Subarachnoid hemorrhage:
PO: Adults, elderly: 60 mg q4h for 21 days. Begin within 96 hrs of subarachnoid hemorrhage.

PRECAUTIONS

CONTRAINDICATIONS: Sick sinus syndrome/second- or third-degree AV block (except in presence of pacemaker). **CAUTIONS:** Impaired renal/hepatic function. **PREGNANCY/LACTATION:** Unknown whether drug crosses placenta or distributed in breast milk. **Pregnancy Category C.**

INTERACTIONS

DRUG INTERACTIONS: None significant. **ALTERED LAB VALUES:** None significant.

SIDE EFFECTS

OCCASIONAL: Diarrhea, dyspepsia, hypotension, headache, dermatitis/rash. **RARE:** Peripheral edema, mental depression, psychosis, constipation, facial flushing, muscle cramps.

ADVERSE REACTIONS/TOXIC EFFECTS

CHF. Overdose produces nausea, drowsiness, confusion, slurred speech.

NURSING IMPLICATIONS

BASELINE ASSESSMENT:

Assess level of consciousness, neurologic response, initially and throughout therapy. Monitor baseline liver function tests. Assess B/P, apical pulse immediately before drug is administered (if pulse is 60/min or below, or systolic B/P is below 90 mm Hg, withhold medication, contact physician).

INTERVENTION/EVALUATION:

Monitor pulse rate for bradycardia. Assess skin for dermatitis, rash, flushing. Monitor daily bowel activity and stool consistency. Assess for headache.

PATIENT/FAMILY TEACHING:

To avoid hypotensive effect, rise slowly from lying to sitting position, wait momentarily before standing. Avoid tasks that require alertness, motor skills until response to drug is established. Contact physician/nurse if irregular heart beat, shortness of breath, pronounced dizziness, or nausea occurs.

nitrofurantoin sodium

ny-tro-feur-an´twon
(Furadantin, Furalan, Macrodantin)

CANADIAN AVAILABILITY:
Apo-Nitrofurantoin, Macrodantin, Nephronex

CLASSIFICATION

Anti-bacterial

PHARMACOKINETICS

Microcrystalline: rapid, completely absorbed; macrocrystalline: more slowly absorbed. Food increases absorption. Primarily concentrated in urine, kidneys. Protein binding: 60%. Metabolized in most body tissues. Primarily excreted in urine. Half-life: 20-60 min.

ACTION

Bactericidal. Inactivates or alters bacterial ribosomal proteins.

USES

Treatment of urinary tract infections, initial and chronic.

PO ADMINISTRATION

Give w/food, milk to enhance absorption, reduce GI upset.

INDICATIONS/DOSAGE/ROUTES

Initial or recurrent urinary tract infection (UTI):

PO: Adults, elderly: 50-100 mg 4 times/day. **Maximum:** 400 mg/day. **Children >1 mo:** 5-7 mg/kg in 4 divided doses.

Long-term prophylaxis therapy of UTI:

PO: Adults, elderly: 50-100 mg as single evening dose. **Children:** 1-2 mg/kg in 1-2 divided doses.

PRECAUTIONS

CONTRAINDICATIONS: Hypersensitivity to nitrofurantoin, infants <1 mo of age because of hemolytic anemia, anuria, oliguria, substantial renal impairment (creatinine clearance <40 ml/min). **CAUTIONS:** Renal impairment, diabetes mellitus, electrolyte imbalance, anemia, vitamin B deficiency, debilitated (greater risk of peripheral neuropathy), glucose 6-phosphate dehydrogenase (G-6-PD) deficiency (greater risk of hemolytic anemia). **PREGNANCY/LACTATION:** Readily crosses placenta; distributed in breast milk. Contraindicated at term and during lactation when infant suspected of having G-6-PD deficiency. **Pregnancy Category C.**

INTERACTIONS

DRUG INTERACTIONS: Hemolytics may increase risk of toxicity. Neurotoxic medications may increase risk of neurotoxicity. Probenecid may increase concentration, toxicity. **ALTERED LAB VALUES:** None significant.

SIDE EFFECTS

FREQUENT: Anorexia, nausea, vomiting. **OCCASIONAL:** Abdominal pain, diarrhea, rash, pruritus, urticaria, hypertension, headache, dizziness, drowsiness. **RARE:** Photosensitivity, transient alopecia, asthmatic attacks in those w/history of asthma.

ADVERSE REACTIONS/TOXIC EFFECTS

Superinfection, hepatotoxicity, peripheral neuropathy (may be irreversible), Stevens-Johnson syndrome, permanent pulmonary function impairment (rarely respiratory failure, death), anaphylaxis occur rarely.

NURSING IMPLICATIONS

BASELINE ASSESSMENT:

Question for history of asthma, hypersensitivity to nitrofurantoin. Obtain urine specimens for culture and sensitivity before giving first dose (therapy may begin before results are known). Evaluate lab test results for renal and hepatic baselines.

INTERVENTION/EVALUATION:

Monitor I&O, renal function results. Evaluate food tolerance. Determine pattern of bowel activity. Assess skin for rash, urticaria. Be alert for numbness or tingling, esp. of lower extremities (may signal onset of peripheral neuropathy). Watch for signs of hepatoxicity: Fever, rash, arthralgia, hepatomegaly. Check B/P at least 2 times/day. Perform respiratory assessment: Auscultate lungs, check for cough, chest pain, difficulty breathing.

PATIENT/FAMILY TEACHING:

Urine may become dark yellow or brown. Take with food or milk for best results and to reduce GI upset. Complete full course of therapy. Avoid sun and ultraviolet light; use sunscreens, wear protective clothing. Notify physician if cough, fever, chest pain, difficult breathing, numbness/tingling of fingers or toes occur. Rare occurrence of alopecia is transient.

nitroglycerin intravenous

nigh-trow-glih´sir-in

(Nitro-Bid, Nitrostat, Tridil)

nitroglycerin sublingual

(Nitrostat)

nitroglycerin sustained release

(Nitro-Bid, Nitroglyn)

nitroglycerin topical

(Nitro-Bid, Nitrol)

nitroglycerin transdermal

(Minitran, Nitro-Dur, Transderm-Nitro, Nitrodisc)

nitroglycerin translingual

(Nitrolingual)

nitroglycerin transmucosal

(Nitrogard)

CANADIAN AVAILABILITY:
Nitro-Bid, Nitrogard SR, Nitrol, Nitrolingual, Nitrong SR, Nitrostat

CLASSIFICATION

Nitrate

PHARMACOKINETICS

	ONSET	PEAK	DURATION
Sublingual	2-5 min	4-8 min	30-60 min
Transmucosal tablet	2-5 min	4-10 min	3-5 hrs
Extended release	20-45 min	—	3-8 hrs
Topical	15-60 min	0.5-2 hrs	3-8 hrs
Patch	30-60 min	1-3 hrs	8-12 hrs
IV	1-2 min	—	3-5 min

Well absorbed after oral, sublingual, topical administration. Undergoes extensive first-pass metabolism. Metabolized in liver, enzymes in bloodstream. Primarily excreted in urine. Half-life: 1-4 min.

ACTION

Decreases myocardial oxygen demand. Reduces left ventricular preload and afterload. Dilates coronary arteries, improves collateral blood flow to ischemic areas within myocardium. *Intravenous:* Produces peripheral vasodilation.

USES

Lingual/sublingual/buccal dose used for acute relief of angina pectoris. Extended-release, topical forms used for prophylaxis, long-term angina management. IV form used in treatment of CHF associated w/acute MI.

STORAGE/HANDLING

Store tablets/capsules at room temperature. Keep sublingual tablets in original container.

PO/TOPICAL/IV ADMINISTRATION

PO:

1. Do not chew extended-release form.
2. Do not shake oral aerosol canister before lingual spraying.

SUBLINGUAL:

1. Do not swallow; dissolve under the tongue.
2. Administer while seated.
3. Slight burning sensation under tongue may be lessened by placing tablet in buccal pouch.

TOPICAL:

1. Spread thin layer on clean/dry/hairless skin of upper arm or body (not below knee or elbow), using applicator or dose-measuring papers. Do not use fingers; do not rub or massage into skin.

TRANSDERMAL:

1. Apply patch on clean/dry/hairless skin of upper arm or body (not below knee or elbow).

IV:

1. Dilute in given amount of 5% dextrose in water or 0.9% NaCl.
2. Use microdrop or infusion pump.

INDICATIONS/DOSAGE/ROUTES

Acute angina, acute prophylaxis:

LINGUAL SPRAY: Adults, elderly: 1 spray onto or under tongue q3-5min until relief is noted (no more than 3 sprays in 15 min period).

SUBLINGUAL: Adults, elderly: Single dose (0.15-0.6 mg) q5min until relief is noted (no more than 3 doses in 15 min period). Use prophylactically 5-10 min before activities that may cause an acute attack.

Long-term prophylaxis of angina:

PO (EXTENDED-RELEASE): Adults, elderly: Initially, 2.5 mg 3-4 times/day. Increase by 2.5 mg 2-4 times/day at intervals of several days or wks.

TOPICAL: Adults, elderly: Initially, ½ inch q8h. Increase by ½ inch w/each application. **Range:** 1-2 inches q8h up to 4-5 inches q4h.

TRANSDERMAL PATCH: Adults, elderly: Initially, 0.2-0.4 mg/hr. **Maintenance:** 0.4-0.8 mg/hr. Consider patch on 12-14 hrs, patch off 10-12 hrs (prevents tolerance).

Usual parenteral dosage:

IV: Adults, elderly: Initially, 5 mcg/min via infusion pump. Increase in 5 mcg/min increments at 3-5 min intervals until B/P response is noted or until dosage reaches maximum of 20 mcg/min. Dosage may be further titrated according to pt, therapeutic response.

PRECAUTIONS

CONTRAINDICATIONS: Hypersensitivity to nitrates, severe anemia, closed-angle glaucoma, postural hypotension, head trauma, increased intracranial pressure. *Sublingual:* Early MI. *Transdermal:* Allergy to adhesives. *Extended release:* GI hypermotility/malabsorption, severe anemia. *IV:* Uncorrected hypovolemia, hypotension, inadequate cerebral circulation, constrictive pericarditis, pericardial tamponade. **CAUTIONS:** Acute MI, hepatic/renal disease, glaucoma (contraindicated in closed-angle glaucoma), blood volume depletion from diuretic therapy, systolic B/P below 90 mm Hg. **PREGNANCY/LACTATION:** Unknown whether drug crosses placenta or is distributed in breast milk. **Pregnancy Category C.**

INTERACTIONS

DRUG INTERACTIONS: Alcohol, antihypertensives, vasodilators may increase risk of orthostatic hypotension. **ALTERED LAB VALUES:** May increase methemoglobin, urine catecholamines, urine VMA.

SIDE EFFECTS

FREQUENT: Headache (may be severe) occurs mostly in early therapy, diminishes rapidly in intensity, usually disappears during continued treatment; transient flushing of face and neck, dizziness (esp. if pt is standing immobile or is in a warm environment), weakness, postural hypotension. *Sublingual:* Burning, tingling sensation at oral point of dissolution. *Ointment:* Erythema, pruritus. **OCCASIONAL:** GI upset. *Transdermal:* Contact dermatitis.

ADVERSE REACTIONS/TOXIC EFFECTS

Drug should be discontinued if blurred vision, dry mouth occur. Severe postural hypotension manifested by fainting, pulselessness, cold/clammy skin, profuse sweating. Tolerance may occur w/repeated, prolonged therapy (minor tolerance w/intermittent use of sublingual tablets). High dose tends to produce severe headache.

NURSING IMPLICATIONS

BASELINE ASSESSMENT:

Record onset, type (sharp, dull, squeezing), radiation, location, intensity and duration of anginal pain, and precipitating factors (exertion, emotional stress). Assess B/P and apical pulse before administration and periodically after dose. Pt must have continuous EKG monitoring for IV administration.

INTERVENTION/EVALUATION:

Assist w/ambulation if lighheadedness, dizziness occur. Assess for facial/neck flushing. Cardioverter/defibrillator must not be discharged through paddle electrode overlying nitroglycerin system (may cause burns to pt or damage to paddle via arcing).

PATIENT/FAMILY TEACHING:

Rise slowly from lying to sitting position and dangle legs momentarily before standing. Take oral form on empty stomach (however, if headache occurs during therapy, take medication w/meals). Use inhalants only when lying down. Dissolve sublingual tablet under tongue, do not swallow. Take at first sign of angina. If not relieved within 5 min, dissolve second tablet under tongue. Repeat if no relief in another 5 min. If pain continues, contact physician or go immediately to emergency room. Do not change brands. Keep container away from heat, moisture. Do not inhale lingual aerosol but spray onto or under tongue (avoid swallowing after spray is administered). Expel from mouth any remaining lingual/sublingual/intrabuccal tablet after pain is completely relieved. Place transmucosal tablets under upper lip or buccal pouch (between cheek and gum); do not chew or swallow tablet. Avoid alcohol (intensifies hypotensive effect). If alcohol is ingested soon after taking nitroglycerin, possible acute hypotensive episode (marked drop in B/P, vertigo, pallor) may occur.

nitroprusside sodium

nigh´troe-pruss-eyd
(Nipride, Nitropress)

CANADIAN AVAILABILITY:
Nipride

CLASSIFICATION

CLINICAL: Antihypertensive

PHARMACOKINETICS

	ONSET	PEAK	DURATION
IV	1-2 min	Dependent on infusion rate	Dissipates rapidly after stopping IV

Reacts w/hemoglobin in erythrocytes producing cyanmethemoglobin, cyanide ions. Primarily excreted in urine. Half-life: 2 min.

ACTION

Direct vasodilating action on arterial, venous smooth muscle. Decreases peripheral vascular resistance, preload, afterload, improves cardiac output. Dilates coronary arteries, decreases oxygen consumption, relieves persistent chest pain.

USES

Immediate reduction of B/P in hypertensive crisis. Produces controlled hypotension in surgical procedures to reduce bleeding.

STORAGE/HANDLING

Protect solution from light. Solution should appear very faint brown in color. Use only freshly prepared solution. Once prepared, do not keep or use longer than 24 hrs. Deterioration evidenced by color change from brown to blue, green, or dark red. Discard unused portion.

IV ADMINISTRATION

1. Give by IV infusion only.
2. Reconstitute 50 mg vial with 2-3 ml 5% dextrose or sterile water for injection w/o preservative.
3. Further dilute w/250-1,000 ml of 5% dextrose to provide concentration of 200 mcg–50 mcg/ml, respectively.
4. Wrap infusion bottle in aluminum foil immediately after mixing.
5. Administer using IV infusion pump or microdrip (60 gtt/ml).
6. Be alert for extravasation (produces severe pain, sloughing).

INDICATIONS/DOSAGE/ROUTES

Usual parenteral dosage:
IV: Adults, elderly, children: Initially, 0.3 mcg/kg/min. **Range:** 0.5-10 mcg/kg/min. Do not exceed 10 mcg/kg/min (risk of precipitous drop in B/P).

PRECAUTIONS

CONTRAINDICATIONS: Compensatory hypertension (arteriovenous shunt or coarctation of aorta), inadequate cerebral circulation, moribund pts. **CAUTIONS:** Severe hepatic, renal impairment, hypothyroidism, hyponatremia, elderly. Except at low concentrations or brief use, may cause increased quantities of cyanide ion (may be toxic, lethal). **PREGNANCY/LACTATION:** Unknown whether drug crosses placenta or is distributed in breast milk. **Pregnancy Category C.**

INTERACTIONS

DRUG INTERACTIONS: Dobutamine may increase cardiac output, decrease pulmonary wedge pressure. Hypotensive producing medications may increase hypotensive effect. **ALTERED LAB VALUES:** None significant.

SIDE EFFECTS

None significant.

ADVERSE REACTIONS/TOXIC EFFECTS

A too-rapid IV rate reduces B/P too quickly. Nausea, retching, diaphoresis (sweating), apprehension, headache, restlessness, muscle twitching, dizziness, palpitation, retrosternal pain, and abdominal pain may occur. Symptoms disappear rapidly if rate of administration is slowed or temporarily discontinued. Overdosage produces metabolic acidosis, tolerance to therapeutic effect.

NURSING IMPLICATIONS

BASELINE ASSESSMENT:

Pt must have continuous EKG monitoring and B/P monitoring (using either continually reinflated sphygmomanometer or an intra-arterial pressure sensor). Check w/physician for desired B/P level (B/P is normally maintained about 30-40% below pretreatment levels). Medication should be discontinued if therapeutic response is not achieved within 10 min following IV infusion at 10 mcg/kg/min.

INTERVENTION/EVALUATION:

Assess IV site for extravasation. Monitor rate of infusion frequently. Monitor blood acid-base balance, electrolytes, laboratory results, I&O. Assess for metabolic acidosis (weakness, disorientation, headache, nausea, hyperventilation, vomiting). Assess for therapeutic response to medication. Monitor B/P for potential rebound hypertension after infusion is discontinued.

nizatidine

nye-zah'tih-deen
(Axid)

CANADIAN AVAILABILITY:
Axid

CLASSIFICATION

H_2 receptor antagonist

PHARMACOKINETICS

Rapidly, well absorbed from GI tract. Protein binding: 35%. Metabolized in liver. Primarily excreted in urine. Half-life: 1-2 hrs (increased in decreased renal function).

ACTION

Inhibits histamine action at H_2 receptors of parietal cells, inhibiting basal and nocturnal gastric acid secretion.

USES

Short-term treatment of active duodenal ulcer, active benign gastric ulcer. Prevention of duodenal ulcer recurrence. Treatment of gastroesophageal reflux disease (GERD) including erosive esophagitis.

PO ADMINISTRATION

1. Give w/o regard to meals. Best given after meals or at bedtime.
2. Do not administer within 1 hr of magnesium or aluminum-containing antacids (decreases absorption).

INDICATIONS/DOSAGE/ROUTES

Active duodenal ulcer:
PO: Adults, elderly: 300 mg at bedtime or 150 mg 2 times/day.

Maintenance of healed ulcer:
PO: Adults, elderly: 150 mg at bedtime.

GERD:
PO: Adults, elderly: 150 mg 2 times/day.

Active benign gastric ulcer:
PO: Adults, elderly: 150 mg 2 times/day or 300 mg at bedtime.

Dosage in renal impairment:

CREATININE CLEARANCE	ACTIVE ULCER	MAINTENANCE THERAPY
20-50 ml/min	150 mg at bedtime	150 mg every other day
<20 ml/min	150 mg every other day	150 mg every 3 days

PRECAUTIONS

CONTRAINDICATIONS: None significant. **CAUTIONS:** Impaired renal/hepatic function. **PREGNANCY/LACTATION:** Unknown whether drug crosses placenta or is distributed in breast milk. **Pregnancy Category C.**

INTERACTIONS

DRUG INTERACTIONS: Antacids may decrease absorption (do not give within 1 hr). May decrease absorption of ketoconazole (give at least 2 hrs after). **ALTERED LAB VALUES:** Interferes w/skin tests using allergen extracts. May increase SGOT (AST), SGPT (ALT) alkaline phosphatase.

SIDE EFFECTS

OCCASIONAL: Somnolence, fatigue. **RARE:** Sweating, rash.

ADVERSE REACTIONS/TOXIC EFFECTS

Asymptomatic ventricular tachycardia, hyperuricemia (not associated w/gout), nephrolithiasis occur rarely.

NURSING IMPLICATIONS

INTERVENTION/EVALUATION:

Assess for abdominal pain, GI bleeding (overt blood in emesis or stool, tarry stools). Monitor blood tests for elevated SGOT (AST), SGPT (ALT), alkaline phosophatase (hepatocellular injury).

PATIENT/FAMILY TEACHING:

Avoid tasks that require alertness, motor skills until drug response is established. Avoid alcohol, aspirin and smoking.

norepinephrine bitartrate

nor-eh-pih-nef′rin

(Levophed)

CANADIAN AVAILABILITY: Levophed

CLASSIFICATION

Sympathomimetic

PHARMACOKINETICS

	ONSET	PEAK	DURATION
IV	Rapid	1-2 min	—

Localized in sympathetic tissue. Metabolized in liver. Primarily excreted in urine.

ACTION

Acts on beta$_1$-adrenergic receptors: stimulates myocardium, increases cardiac output; alpha-adrenergic receptors: constricts resistance and capacitance vessels, increases systemic B/P, coronary artery blood flow. Pressor effect primarily due to increased peripheral resistance.

USES

Restoration of B/P in acute hypotensive states.

STORAGE/HANDLING

Do not use if brown in color or contains precipitate.

IV ADMINISTRATION

NOTE: Blood, fluid volume depletion should be corrected before drug is administered.

1. Add 4 ml to 250 ml (16 mcg base/ml)-1,000 ml (4 mcg base/ml) of D5W.
2. Infuse through plastic catheter, using antecubital vein of arm.
3. Avoid catheter tie-in technique (encourages stasis, increases local drug concentration).
4. Closely monitor IV infusion flow rate (use microdrip or infusion pump).
5. Monitor B/P q2min during IV infusion until desired therapeutic response is achieved, then q5min during remaining IV infusion. Never leave pt unattended.
6. Maintain B/P at 80-100 mm Hg in previously normotensive pts, and 30-40 mm Hg below preexisting B/P in previously hypertensive pts.
7. Reduce IV infusion gradually. Avoid abrupt withdrawal.
8. It is imperative to check the IV site frequently for free flow and infused vein for blanching, hardness to vein, coldness, pallor to extremity.
9. If extravasation occurs, area should be infiltrated w/10-15 ml sterile saline containing 5-10 mg phentolamine (does not alter pressor effects of norepinephrine).

INDICATIONS/DOSAGE/ROUTES

Acute hypotension:

IV: Adults, elderly: Initially, administer at 8-12 mcg/min. Adjust rate of flow to establish, maintain normal B/P (40 mm Hg below preexisting systolic pressure). **Average maintenance dose:** 2-4 mcg/min. **Children:** Administer at rate of 2 mcg/min.

PRECAUTIONS

CONTRAINDICATIONS: Hypovolemic states (unless an emergency measure), mesenteric/peripheral vascular thrombosis, profound hypoxia. **CAUTIONS:** Severe cardiac disease, hypertensive and hypothyroid pts, those on MAO inhibitors. **PREGNANCY/LACTATION:** Readily crosses placenta. May produce fetal anoxia due to uterine contraction, constriction of uterine blood vessels. **Pregnancy Category D.**

INTERACTIONS

DRUG INTERACTIONS: Tricyclic antidepressants, maprotiline may increase cardiovascular effects. May decrease effect of methyldopa. May have mutually inhibitory effects w/beta-blockers. May increase risk of arrhythmias w/digoxin. Ergonovine, oxytocin may increase vasoconstriction. **ALTERED LAB VALUES:** None significant.

SIDE EFFECTS

Norepinephrine produces less pronounced and less frequent side effects than epinephrine. **OCCASIONAL:** Bradycardia, anxiety, feeling of respiratory difficulty, transient headache, awareness of slow, forceful heart beat. Hypovolemic pts may experience reduced urine flow, peripheral vasoconstriction.

ADVERSE REACTIONS/TOXIC EFFECTS

Extravasation may produce tissue necrosis, sloughing. Overdosage manifested as severe hypertension w/violent headache (may be first clinical sign of overdosage), arrhythmias, photophobia, retrosternal/pharyngeal pain, pallor, excessive sweating, vomiting. Prolonged therapy may result in plasma volume depletion. Hypotension may recur if plasma volume is not maintained.

NURSING IMPLICATIONS

BASELINE ASSESSMENT:

Assess EKG and B/P continuously (be alert to precipitous B/P drop). Never leave pt alone during IV infusion. Be alert to pt complaint of headache.

INTERVENTION/EVALUATION:

Monitor IV flow rate diligently. Assess for extravasation characterized by blanching of skin over vein, coolness (results from local vasoconstriction). Color and temperature of IV site extremity (pallor, cyanosis, mottling). Assess nailbed capillary refill. Monitor I&O; measure output hourly and report <30 cc. IV should not be reinstated unless systolic B/P falls below 70-80 mm Hg.

norfloxacin

nor-flocks´ah-sin

(Chibroxin, Noroxin)

CANADIAN AVAILABILITY: Noroxin

CLASSIFICATION

Anti-infective: Quinolone

PHARMACOKINETICS

Rapidly, incompletely absorbed from GI tract. Widely distributed. Protein binding: 10-15%. Possibly metabolized in liver. Primarily excreted in urine. Half-life: 3-4 hrs (increased in decreased renal function).

ACTION

Inhibits DNA replication and repair by interfering w/DNA-gyrase in susceptible microorganisms. Usually bactericidal.

USES

Treatment of complicated and uncomplicated urinary tract infections, uncomplicated gonococcal infections. *Ophthalmic:* Conjunctival keratitis, keratoconjunctivitis, corneal ulcers, blepharitis, blepharoconjunctivitis, acute meibomianitis, dacryocystitis.

PO/OPHTHALMIC ADMINISTRATION

PO:

1. Give 1 hr before or 2 hrs after meals, w/8 oz water.
2. Encourage additional glasses of water between meals.
3. Do not administer antacids w/ or within 2 hrs of norfloxacin dose.
4. Encourage cranberry juice, citrus fruits (to acidify urine).

OPHTHALMIC:

1. Tilt pts head back; place solution in conjunctival sac.
2. Have pt close eyes; press gently on lacrimal sac for 1 min.
3. Do not use ophthalmic solutions for injection.

INDICATIONS/DOSAGE/ROUTES

Complicated or uncomplicated urinary tract infections:
PO: Adults, elderly: 400 mg 2 times/day for 7-21 days.

Uncomplicated gonococcal infections:
PO: Adults: 800 mg as single dose.

Dosage in renal impairment:
The dose and/or frequency is modified based on degree of renal impairment.

CREATININE CLEARANCE	DOSAGE
>30 ml/min	400 mg 2 times/day
<30 ml/min	400 mg once daily

Usual ophthalmic dosage:
OPHTHALMIC: Adults, elderly: 1-2 drops 4 times/day up to 7 days. For severe infections, may give 1-2 drops q2h while awake the first day.

PRECAUTIONS

CONTRAINDICATIONS: Hypersensitivity to norfloxacin, quinolones or any component of preparation. Do not use in children <18 yrs of age—produces arthropathy. *Ophthalmic:* Epithelial herpes simplex, keratitis, vaccinia, varicella, mycobacterial infection, fungal disease of ocular structure. Do not use after uncomplicated removal of foreign body. **CAUTIONS:** Impaired renal function; any predisposition to seizures. **PREGNANCY/LACTATION:** Crosses placenta; distributed into cord blood, amniotic fluid. Unknown if distributed in breast milk. Should not be used in pregnant women. **Pregnancy Category C.**

INTERACTIONS

DRUG INTERACTIONS: Antacids, sucralfate may decrease absorption. Decrease clearance, may increase concentration, toxicity of theophylline. May increase effects of oral anticoagulants. **ALTERED LAB VALUES:** May increase SGOT (AST), SGPT (ALT), alkaline phosphatase, LDH, bilirubin, BUN, creatinine. May decrease Hct.

SIDE EFFECTS

FREQUENT: Nausea, headache, dizziness, eosinophilia. *Ophthalmic:* Bad taste in mouth. **OCCASIONAL:** *Ophthalmic:* Temporary blurring of vision, irritation, burning, stinging, itching. **RARE:** Vomiting, diarrhea, dry mouth, bitter taste, nervousness, drowsiness, insomnia, photosensitivity, tinnitus, crystalluria, rash, fever, seizures. *Ophthalmic:* Conjunctival hyperemia, photophobia, decreased vision, pain.

ADVERSE REACTIONS/TOXIC EFFECTS

Superinfection, anaphylaxis, Stevens-Johnson syndrome, arthropathy (joint disease) occur rarely.

NURSING IMPLICATIONS

BASELINE ASSESSMENT:

Question for history of hypersensitivity to norfloxacin, quinolones, any component of preparation. Obtain specimens for diagnostic tests before giving first dose (therapy may begin before results are known).

INTERVENTION/EVALUATION:

Evaluate food tolerance, taste sensation and dryness of mouth. Determine pattern of bowel activity. Assess skin for rash. Check for headache, dizziness. Monitor level of consciousness, pattern of sleep. Assess temperature at least 2 times/day. *Ophthalmic:* Check for therapeutic response, side effects (see Side Effects).

PATIENT/FAMILY TEACHING:

Take 1 hr before or 2 hrs after meals. Complete full course of therapy. Take w/8 oz of water, drink several glasses of water between meals. Eat/drink high sources of ascorbic acid, e.g., cranberry juice, citrus fruits. Do not take antacids w/or within 2 hrs of norfloxacin dose. Avoid sunlight/ultraviolet exposure, wear sun screen and protective clothing if photosensitivity develops. Avoid tasks that require alert response if dizziness/drowsiness occur. Sugarless gum or hard candy, ice chips may help dry mouth and bitter taste. Notify nurse/physician if headache, dizziness or other symptom occur. *Ophthalmic:* Report any increased burning, itching or other discomfort promptly.

nortriptyline hydrochloride

knor-trip´teh-leen

(Aventyl, Pamelor)

CANADIAN AVAILABILITY:

Aventyl

CLASSIFICATION

Antidepressant: Tricyclic

PHARMACOKINETICS

Rapid, well absorbed from GI tract. Protein binding: 92%. Metabolized in liver, undergoes first-pass metabolism. Primarily excreted in urine. Minimal removal by hemodialysis. Half-life: 18-44 hrs.

ACTION

Increases synaptic concentration of norepinephrine and/or serotonin (inhibits reuptake by presynaptic membrane).

USES

Treatment of various forms of depression, often in conjunction w/psychotherapy.

PO ADMINISTRATION

Give w/food or milk if GI distress occurs.

INDICATIONS/DOSAGE/ROUTES

PO: Adults: 75-100 mg/day in 1-4 divided doses until therapeutic response achieved. Reduce dosage gradually to effective maintenance level. **Elderly:** Initially, 10-25 mg at bedtime. May increase by 25 mg q3-7days. **Maximum:** 75 mg/day.

PRECAUTIONS

CONTRAINDICATIONS: Acute recovery period following MI, within 14 days of MAO inhibitor ingestion. **CAUTIONS:** Prostatic hypertrophy, history of urinary retention or obstruction, glaucoma, diabetes mellitus, history of seizures, hyperthyroidism, cardiac/hepatic/renal disease, schizophrenia, increased intraocular pressure, hiatal hernia. **PREGNANCY/LACTATION:** Crosses placenta; distributed in breast milk. **Pregnancy Category C.**

INTERACTIONS

DRUG INTERACTIONS: Alcohol, CNS depressants may increase CNS, respiratory depression, hypotensive effects. Antithyroid agents may increase risk of agranulocytosis. Phenothiazines may increase sedative, anticholinergic effects. Cimetidine may increase concentration, toxicity. May decrease effects of clonidine, guanadrel. May increase cardiac effects w/sympathomimetics. May increase risk of hypertensive crisis, hyperpyretic convulsions w/MAOIs. **ALTERED LAB VALUES:** May alter ECG readings, glucose.

SIDE EFFECTS

FREQUENT: Drowsiness, fatigue, dry mouth, blurred vision, constipation, delayed micturition, postural hypotension, excessive sweating, disturbed concentration, increased appetite, urinary retention. **OCCASIONAL:** GI disturbances (nausea, GI distress, metallic taste sensation). **RARE:** Paradoxical reaction (agitation, restlessness, nightmares, insomnia), extrapyramidal symptoms (particularly fine hand tremor).

ADVERSE REACTIONS/TOXIC EFFECTS

High dosage may produce cardiovascular effects (severe postural hypotension, dizziness, tachycardia, palpitations, arrhythmias) and seizures. May also result in altered temperature regulation (hyperpyrexia or hypothermia). Abrupt withdrawal from prolonged therapy may produce headache, malaise, nausea, vomiting, vivid dreams.

NURSING IMPLICATIONS

BASELINE ASSESSMENT:

For those on long-term therapy, liver/renal function tests, blood counts should be performed periodically.

INTERVENTION/EVALUATION:

Supervise suicidal-risk pt closely during early therapy (as depression lessens, energy level improves, increasing suicide potential). Assess appearance, behavior, speech pattern, level of interest, mood. Monitor stools; avoid constipation w/increased fluids, bulky foods. Monitor B/P, pulse for hypotension, arrhythmias. Assess for urinary retention including output estimate and bladder palpation if indicated.

PATIENT/FAMILY TEACHING:

Change positions slowly to avoid hypotensive effect. Tolerance to postural hypotension, sedative and anticholinergic effects usually develops during early therapy. Therapeutic effect may be noted in 2 or more wks. Photosensitivity to sun may occur. Use sunscreens, protective clothing. Dry mouth may be relieved by sugarless gum, or sips of tepid water. Report visual disturbances. Do not abruptly discontinue medication. Avoid tasks that require alertness, motor skills until response to drug is established.

nystatin

nigh-stat´in

(Mycostatin, Nilstat, O-V Statin)

FIXED-COMBINATION(S):
W/triamcinolone, a steroid (Mycolog II, Myco-Triacet II, Mykacet, Mytrex F)

CANADIAN AVAILABILITY:
Mycostatin, Nadostine, Nilstat, Nyaderm

CLASSIFICATION

Antifungal

PHARMACOKINETICS

Oral: Poorly absorbed from GI tract. Eliminated unchanged in feces. *Topical:* Not absorbed systemically from intact skin.

ACTION

Fungistatic. Binds to sterols in cell membrane increasing permeability, permitting loss of potassium, other cell components.

USES

Treatment of intestinal and oral candidiasis, cutaneous/mucocutaneous mycotic infections caused by *Candida albicans* (oral thrush, paronychia, vulvovaginal candidiasis, diaper rash, perleche).

PO ADMINISTRATION

1. Dissolve lozenges (troches) slowly/completely in mouth (optimal therapeutic effect). Do not chew or swallow lozenges whole.
2. Shake suspension well before administration.
3. Place and hold suspension in mouth or swish throughout mouth as long as possible before swallowing.

INDICATIONS/DOSAGE/ROUTES

Intestinal candidiasis:
PO: Adults, elderly: 500,000-1,000,000 U 3 times/day. **Children:** 500,000 U 4 times/day.

Oral candidiasis:
PO: Adults, elderly, children: Oral suspension: 400,000-600,000 U 4 times/day. **Infants:** 100,000-200,000 U 4 times/day.
PO: Adults, elderly, children: Troches: 200,000-400,000 U 4-5 times/day up to 14 days.

Vulvovaginal candidiasis:
INTRAVAGINALLY: Adults, elderly: 1 tablet high in vagina 1-2 times/day for 14 days.

Topical fungal infections:
TOPICAL: Adults, elderly: Apply 2-3 times/day.

PRECAUTIONS

CONTRAINDICATIONS: Hypersensitivity to nystatin or components of preparation. **PREGNANCY/LACTATION:** Unknown if distributed in breast milk. Vaginal applicators may be contraindicated, requiring manual insertion of tablets during pregnancy.) **Pregnancy Category A** (**Pregnancy Category C** for oropharyngeal use).

INTERACTIONS

DRUG INTERACTIONS: None

significant. **ALTERED LAB VALUES:** None significant.

SIDE EFFECTS

OCCASIONAL: Nausea, vomiting, diarrhea and GI distress with high dosage. **RARE:** Hypersensitivity reaction, irritation with topical use.

ADVERSE REACTIONS/TOXIC EFFECTS

None significant.

NURSING IMPLICATIONS

BASELINE ASSESSMENT:

Question for history of allergies, esp. to nystatin. Confirm that cultures or histologic tests were done for accurate diagnosis.

INTERVENTION/EVALUATION:

Evaluate food intake, tolerance. Determine pattern of bowel activity and stool consistency. Assess for increased irritation w/topical, increased vaginal discharge with vaginal application.

PATIENT/FAMILY TEACHING:

Do not miss dose; complete full length of treatment (continue vaginal use during menses). Notify physician if nausea, vomiting, diarrhea, stomach pain develop. *Vaginal:* Insert high in vagina. Check w/physician regarding douching, sexual intercourse. *Topical:* Rub well into affected areas. Must not contact eyes. Do not apply any other preparations or occlusive covering w/o consulting physician. Use cream (sparingly)/powder in intertriginous areas. Keep areas clean, dry; wear light clothing for ventilation. Separate personal items in contact w/affected areas.

octreotide acetate

ock-tree'oh-tide
(Sandostatin)

CANADIAN AVAILABILITY:
Sandostatin

CLASSIFICATION

Secretory inhibitor

PHARMACOKINETICS

	ONSET	PEAK	DURATION
SubQ	—	—	Up to 12 hrs

Rapidly, completely absorbed from injection site. Protein binding: 65%. Excreted in urine. Half-life: 1.5 hrs.

ACTION

Suppresses secretion of serotonin, gastroenteropancreatic peptides. Enhances fluid/electrolyte absorption from GI tract, prolongs intestinal transit time.

USES

Symptomatic treatment of pts w/metastatic carcinoid tumors or vasoactive intestinal peptide tumors. There is insufficient data to determine whether there is decreased size, rate of growth or development of metastases. Treatment of acromegaly.

STORAGE/HANDLING

Refrigerate ampoules. Ampoules may be kept at room temperature on day to be used. Do not use if discolored, contains particulates.

SubQ ADMINISTRATION

1. Recommended route of administration is SubQ (IV bolus has been given in emergency conditions).

2. Do not use if particulates and/or discoloration are noted.

3. Avoid multiple injections at the same site within short periods.

INDICATIONS/DOSAGE/ROUTES

NOTE: Initial dose is 50 mcg 1-2 times/day, then dose is increased based on response/tolerability of pt to medication.

Carcinoid tumors:
SubQ: Adults, elderly: 100-600 mcg/day in 2-4 divided doses during first 2 wks of therapy. **Maintenance:** 450 mcg/day (range: 50-750 mcg).

VIPomas:
SubQ: Adults, elderly: 200-300 mcg/day in 2-4 divided doses during first 2 wks of therapy (range 150-750 mcg/day). Dosage adjusted to achieve therapeutic response, usually not above 450 mcg/day.

Acromegaly:
SubQ: Adults, elderly: Initially, 50 mcg 3 times/day. Up to 100 mcg 3 times/day.

PRECAUTIONS

CONTRAINDICATIONS: Hypersensitivity to drug or any of its components. **CAUTIONS:** Insulin-dependent diabetes, renal failure. **PREGNANCY/LACTATION:** Excretion in breast milk unknown. **Pregnancy Category B.**

INTERACTIONS

DRUG INTERACTIONS: May alter glucose concentrations w/insulin, oral hypoglycemics, glucagon, growth hormone. **ALTERED LAB VALUES:** May decrease T_4 concentration.

SIDE EFFECTS

FREQUENT: Nausea, vomiting, diarrhea, abdominal pain/discomfort, pain at injection site. **OCCASIONAL:** Headache, flushing, fatigue, edema, dizziness, hyperglycemia, hypoglycemia, fat malabsorption. **RARE:** Jaundice, muscle cramping, hypertension, palpitations, shortness of breath, anxiety, Bell's palsy.

ADVERSE REACTIONS/TOXIC EFFECTS

Increased risk of cholelithiasis. Potential for hypothyroidism w/prolonged high therapy.

NURSING IMPLICATIONS

BASELINE ASSESSMENT:

Question for hypersensitivity to drug, components. Establish baseline B/P, weight, blood glucose, electrolytes.

INTERVENTION/EVALUATION:

Evaluate blood glucose levels (esp. w/diabetics), electrolytes (therapy generally reduces abnormalities). Weigh every 2-3 days, report >5 lb gain/week. Monitor B/P, pulse, respirations periodically during treatment. Be alert for decreased urinary output, swelling of ankles, fingers. Check food tolerance. Monitor stools for frequency, consistency.

PATIENT/FAMILY TEACHING:

Careful instruction on SubQ injection. Follow-up by physician and tests are essential. Report jaundice (yellow eyes or skin, dark urine, clay-colored stools), abdominal pain, edema. Therapy should provide significant improvement of symptoms.

ocular lubricant

CANADIAN AVAILABILITY:
Tears Naturale

CLASSIFICATION

Ophthalmic lubricant

ACTION

Protects and lubricates eye.

USES

Protection and lubrication of the eye in: Exposure keratitis, decreased corneal sensitivity, recurrent corneal erosions, keratitis sicca (particularly for nighttime use), after removal of a foreign body, during and following surgery.

OPHTHALMIC ADMINISTRATION

1. Do not use w/contact lenses.
2. *Ointment:* Hold tube in hand for a few min to warm ointment.
3. Avoid touching tip of tube or dropper to any surface.
4. Gently pull lower lid down to form pouch.
5. Have pt tilt head backward and look up.
6. *Ointment:* Place ordered amount of ointment in pouch w/a sweeping motion. Instruct pt to close the eye for 1-2 min and roll the eyeball around in all directions.
7. *Drops:* Instill drop(s); have pt close eye gently for 1-2 min. Apply gentle pressure w/fingers to bridge of nose (inside corner of eye).
8. Wipe away excess around eye w/a tissue.

INDICATIONS/DOSAGE/ROUTES

Usual ophthalmic dosage:
OPHTHALMIC: Adults, elderly: Small amount in conjunctival cul-de-sac.

PRECAUTIONS

CONTRAINDICATIONS: Hypersensitivity to any component of preparation. **CAUTIONS:** None. **PREGNANCY/LACTATION: Pregnancy Category Unknown.**

INTERACTIONS

DRUG INTERACTIONS: None significant. **ALTERED LAB VALUES:** None significant.

SIDE EFFECTS

FREQUENT: Temporary blurring after administration, esp. w/ointment.

ADVERSE REACTIONS/TOXIC EFFECTS

None significant.

NURSING IMPLICATIONS

PATIENT/FAMILY TEACHING:

Teach proper application. Do not use contact lenses. Temporary blurring will occur esp. w/administration of ointment. Avoid activities requiring visual acuity until blurring clears. If eye pain, change of vision, or worsening of condition occurs, or if condition is unchanged after 72 hrs, notify physician.

ofloxacin

oh-flocks´ah-sin
(Floxin, Ocuflox)

CANADIAN AVAILABILITY:
Floxin

CLASSIFICATION

Anti-infective: Quinolone

PHARMACOKINETICS

Rapid, well absorbed from GI tract. Widely distributed (penetrates CSF). Protein binding: 20-25%. Metabolized in liver. Primarily excreted in urine. Minimally removed by hemodialysis.. Half-life: 4.7-7 hrs (increased in decreased renal function, elderly, cirrhosis).

ACTION

Inhibits DNA-gyrase in susceptible microorganisms, interfering w/bacterial DNA replication and repair. Bactericidal.

USES

Treatment of infections of urinary tract, skin/skin structure, sexually transmitted diseases, lower respiratory tract, prostatitis due to *Escherichia coli. Ophthalmic:* Bacterial conjunctivitis.

STORAGE/HANDLING

Store oral, parenteral forms at room temperature. After dilution, IV stable for 72 hrs at room temperature; 14 days refrigerated. Discard unused portions.

PO/IV ADMINISTRATION

PO:

1. Do not give w/food; preferred dosing time: 1 hr before or 2 hrs after meals.
2. Do not administer antacids (aluminum, magnesium) or iron-/zinc-containing products within 2 hrs of ofloxacin.
3. Encourage cranberry juice, citrus fruits (to acidify urine).
4. Give w/8 oz water and encourage fluid intake.

IV:

1. Give only by IV infusion, avoid rapid or bolus IV administration. Must dilute the 20 mg/ml or 40 mg/ml vial.
2. Infuse over at least 60 min.
3. Must dilute each 200 mg w/50 ml 5% dextrose or 0.9% NaCl (400 mg w/100 ml) to provide concentration of 4 mg/ml.
4. Do not add or infuse other medication through same IV line at same time.

INDICATIONS/DOSAGE/ROUTES

Urinary tract infection:
PO/IV INFUSION: Adults: 200 mg q12h.

Lower respiratory tract, skin/skin structure infections:
PO/IV INFUSION: Adults: 400 mg q12h for 10 days.

Prostatitis, sexually transmitted diseases (cervicitis, urethritis):
PO: Adults: 300 mg q12h.

Prostatitis:
IV INFUSION: Adults: 300 mg q12h.

Sexually transmitted diseases:
IV INFUSION: Adults: 400 mg as single dose.

Acute, uncomplicated gonorrhea:
PO: Adults: 400 mg 1 time.

Usual elderly dosage:
PO: Elderly: 200-400 mg q12-24h for 7 days up to 6 wks.

Dosage in renal impairment:
After a normal initial dose, dosage/interval based on creatinine clearance.

CREATININE CLEARANCE	ADJUSTED DOSE	DOSAGE INTERVAL
>50 ml/min	none	12 hrs
10-50 ml/min	none	24 hrs
<10 ml/min	½	24 hrs

Bacterial conjunctivitis:
OPH: Adults, elderly: 1-2 gtts q2-4h for 2 days, then 4 times/day for 5 days.

0

PRECAUTIONS

CONTRAINDICATIONS: Syphilis, hypersensitivity to ofloxacin or any quinolones. Children <18 yrs. **CAUTIONS:** Renal impairment, CNS disorders, seizures, those taking theophylline or caffeine. May mask or delay symptoms of syphilis; serologic test for syphilis should be done at diagnosis and 3 mo after treatment. **PREGNANCY/LACTATION:** Distributed in breast milk; potentially serious adverse reactions in nursing infants. Risk of arthropathy to fetus. **Pregnancy Category C.**

INTERACTIONS

DRUG INTERACTIONS: Antacids, sucralfate may decrease absorption, effect of ofloxacin. May increase theophylline concentrations, toxicity. **ALTERED LAB VALUES:** None significant.

SIDE EFFECTS

FREQUENT: Nausea, vomiting, diarrhea, abdominal discomfort, headache, dizziness, insomnia. **OCCASIONAL:** *Oral:* Dry, painful mouth; fatigue; drowsiness; rash; pruritus; visual disturbances; fever. *Parenteral:* Phlebitis, erythema, swelling. **RARE:** Phototoxicity, constipation, depression, hearing decrease, hypertension, syncope, chest pain.

ADVERSE REACTIONS/TOXIC EFFECTS

Superinfection, severe hypersensitivity reaction occur rarely. Arthropathy (joint disease w/ swelling, pain, clubbing of fingers and toes, degeneration of stress-bearing portion of a joint) may occur if given to children <18 yrs.

NURSING IMPLICATIONS

BASELINE ASSESSMENT:

Question for history of hypersensitivity to ofloxacin or any quinolones. Obtain specimen for diagnostic tests before giving first dose (therapy may begin before results are known).

INTERVENTION/EVALUATION:

Assess skin and discontinue medication at first sign of rash or other allergic reaction. Evaluate food tolerance. Determine pattern of bowel activity, stool consistency. Assess during the night for sleeplessness, restlessness, complaint of dreaming. Check for dizziness, headache, visual difficulties, tremors; provide ambulation assistance as needed. Monitor TPR, B/P at least 2 times/day. Be alert for superinfection, e.g., genital pruritus, vaginitis, fever, sores and discomfort in mouth.

PATIENT/FAMILY TEACHING:

Do not skip dose; take full course of therapy. Take w/8 oz water; drink several glasses of water between meals. Eat/drink high sources of ascorbic acid (cranberry juice, citrus fruits). Do not take antacids (reduces/destroys effectiveness). Avoid tasks that require alertness, motor skills until response to drug is established. Avoid sunlight/ultraviolet exposure; wear sun screen, protective clothing if photosensitivity develops. Notify physician if new symptoms occur.

olsalazine sodium

CANADIAN AVAILABILITY: Dipentum

CLASSIFICATION

Anti-inflammatory agent

PHARMACOKINETICS

Minimally absorbed from GI tract (99% reaches colon). Converted to mesalamine in colon. Primarily eliminated in feces. Half-life: 0.9 hrs.

ACTION

Releases mesalamine by colonic bacterial action. Mesalamine blocks prostaglandin synthesis in colon. Produces local inhibitory effect on arachidonic acid metabolite production (increased in pts w/ chronic inflammatory bowel disease).

USES

Maintenance of remission of ulcerative colitis in those intolerant of sulfasalazine medication.

PO ADMINISTRATION

Give w/food in evenly divided doses.

INDICATIONS/DOSAGE/ROUTES

Maintenance of controlled ulcerative colitis:
PO: Adults, elderly: 1 Gm/day in 2 divided doses (preferably q12h).

PRECAUTIONS

CONTRAINDICATIONS: History of hypersensitivity to salicylates. **CAUTIONS:** Preexisting renal disease. **PREGNANCY/LACTATION:** Unknown whether drug crosses placenta or is distributed in breast milk. **Pregnancy Category C.**

INTERACTIONS

DRUG INTERACTIONS: None significant. **ALTERED LAB VALUES:** May increase SGOT (AST), SGPT (ALT).

SIDE EFFECTS

FREQUENT: Diarrhea, GI cramping. **OCCASIONAL:** Headache, nausea, dyspepsia. **RARE:** Rash, pruritus, bloating, anorexia.

ADVERSE REACTIONS/TOXIC EFFECTS

Sulfite sensitivity in susceptible pts noted as cramping, headache, diarrhea, fever, rash, hives, itching, wheezing. Discontinue drug immediately. Excessive diarrhea associated w/extreme fatigue noted rarely.

NURSING IMPLICATIONS

BASELINE ASSESSMENT:

Discontinue medication if rash, fever, cramping or diarrhea occurs.

INTERVENTION/EVALUATION:

Encourage adequate fluid intake. Assess bowel sounds for peristalsis. Monitor daily bowel activity and stool consistency (watery, loose, soft, semi-solid, solid) and record time of evacuation. Assess for abdominal disturbances. Assess skin for rash, hives.

PATIENT/FAMILY TEACHING:

Notify physician if diarrhea continues or increases, rash or pruritus occurs.

omeprazole

oh-mep´rah-zole
(Prilosec)

CANADIAN AVAILABILITY: Prilosec

CLASSIFICATION

Gastric acid pump inhibitor

PHARMACOKINETICS

Rapidly absorbed from GI tract. Primarily distributed into gastric parietal cells. Protein binding: 95%. Metabolized extensively in liver. Primarily excreted in urine. Half-life: 0.5-1 hr (increased in decreased liver function).

ACTION

Irreversibly binds to H^+/K^+ ATPase (an enzyme on surface of parietal cells). Inhibits hydrogen ion transport into gastric lumen. Inhibits basal, stimulated acid secretion.

USES

Short term treatment (4-8 wks) of severe erosive esophagitis (diagnosed by endoscopy); symptomatic gastroesophageal reflux disease (GERD) poorly responsive to other treatment. Long-term treatment of pathological hypersecretory conditions; treatment of active duodenal ulcer.

PO ADMINISTRATION

Give before meals. Do not crush or chew capsule; swallow whole.

INDICATIONS/DOSAGE/ROUTES

Severe erosive esophagitis, poorly responsive GERD, active duodenal ulcer:
PO: Adults, elderly: 20 mg/day for 4-8 wks.

Pathologic hypersecretory conditions:
PO: Adults, elderly: Initially, 60 mg/day up to 120 mg, 3 times/day.

PRECAUTIONS

CONTRAINDICATIONS: None significant. **CAUTIONS:** None significant. **PREGNANCY/LACTATION:** Unknown whether drug crosses placenta or is distributed in breast milk. **Pregnancy Category C.**

INTERACTIONS

DRUG INTERACTIONS: May increase concentration of oral anticoagulants, diazepam, phenytoin. **ALTERED LAB VALUES:** May increase SGOT (AST), SGPT (ALT), alkaline phosphatase.

SIDE EFFECTS

OCCASIONAL: Headache, diarrhea, abdominal discomfort, nausea. **RARE:** Vomiting, dizziness, rash.

ADVERSE REACTIONS/TOXIC EFFECTS

None significant.

NURSING IMPLICATIONS

INTERVENTION/EVALUATION:

Evaluate for therapeutic response, i.e., relief of GI symptoms. Question if GI discomfort, nausea, diarrhea occur.

PATIENT/FAMILY TEACHING:

Report headache.

ondansetron hydrochloride

on-dan´sah-tron
(Zofran)

CLASSIFICATION

Antiemetic

PHARMACOKINETICS

Readily absorbed from GI tract. Protein binding: 70-76%. Metabolized in liver. Primarily excreted in urine. Half-life: 4 hrs.

ACTION

Exhibits selective 5-HT_3 receptor antagonism for preventing nausea/vomiting associated w/cancer chemotherapy. Action may be central (CTZ) or peripheral (vagus nerve terminal).

USES

Prevention, treatment of nausea and vomiting due to cancer chemotherapy, including high-dose cisplatin. Prevent postop nausea, vomiting.

PO/IV ADMINISTRATION

PO:

1. May take w/o regard to food.

IV:

1. For IV infusion, dilute w/50 ml 5% dextrose or 0.9% NaCl before administration.
2. Infuse over 15 min.

STORAGE/HANDLING

Store parenteral form at room temperature. After dilution, stable at room temperature for 48 hrs.

INDICATIONS/DOSAGE/ROUTES

Nausea, vomiting: Chemotherapy

IV: Adults, elderly, children (4-18 yrs): 3 doses 0.15 mg/kg. First dose given 30 min before chemotherapy; then 4 and 8 hrs after first dose of ondansetron.

PO: Adults, elderly: 8 mg 30 min before start of chemotherapy, then 4 and 8 hrs after first dose; then, 8 mg q8h for 1-2 days after completion of chemotherapy. **Children:** 4 mg using same regimen as for adults.

Nausea, vomiting: Postop

IV: Adults, elderly: 4 mg undiluted over 2-5 min.

PRECAUTIONS

CONTRAINDICATIONS: None significant. **CAUTIONS:** None significant. **PREGNANCY/LACTATION:** Unknown whether drug crosses placenta or distributed in breast milk. **Pregnancy Category B.**

INTERACTIONS

DRUG INTERACTIONS: None significant. **ALTERED LAB VALUES:** May transiently increase SGOT (AST), SGPT (ALT), bilirubin.

SIDE EFFECTS

FREQUENT: Diarrhea, headache. **OCCASIONAL:** Constipation. **RARE:** Rash, bronchospasm, tachycardia, angina.

ADVERSE REACTIONS/TOXIC EFFECTS

Overdose may produce combination of CNS stimulation and depressant effects.

NURSING IMPLICATIONS

BASELINE ASSESSMENT:

Assess for dehydration if excessive vomiting occurs (poor skin turgor, dry mucous membranes, longitudinal furrows in tongue). Provide emotional support.

INTERVENTION/EVALUATION:

Monitor pt in environment. Assess bowel sounds for peristalsis. Provide supportive measures. Assess mental status. Monitor daily bowel activity and stool consistency (watery, loose, soft, semi-solid, solid) and record time of evacuation.

PATIENT/FAMILY TEACHING:

Relief from nausea/vomiting generally occurs shortly after drug administration. Avoid alcohol, barbiturates.

orphenadrine citrate

ore-fen´ah-dreen
(Norflex)

FIXED-COMBINATION(S): W/aspirin, nonnarcotic analgesic and caffeine, a stimulant (Norgesic)

CANADIAN AVAILABILITY: Disipal, Norflex

CLASSIFICATION

Skeletal muscle relaxant

PHARMACOKINETICS

	ONSET	PEAK	DURATION
PO	—	—	4-6 hrs

Readily absorbed from GI tract. Metabolized in liver. Primarily excreted in urine. Half-life: 14 hrs.

ACTION

Muscle relaxant related to CNS depressant effects (sedation). Blocks interneuronal activity in descending reticular formation and spinal cord. Has mild anticholinergic effects.

USES

Adjunctive therapy for relief of discomfort associated w/mild to moderate painful musculoskeletal conditions.

STORAGE/HANDLING

Store oral, parenteral form at room temperature.

PO/IM/IV ADMINISTRATION

PO:

1. Give w/o regard to meals, give w/food if epigastric distress occurs.
2. Do not crush or break sustained-release form.

IM:

1. Give deep into large mass muscle.

IV:

1. Inject over about 5 min.
2. Pt in supine position; remain there for 5-10 min after injection.

INDICATIONS/DOSAGE/ROUTES

Musculoskeletal conditions:
PO: Adults, elderly: 100 mg in morning and evening (preferably q12h).
IM/IV: Adults, elderly: 60 mg. May repeat q12h, as needed.

Combination w/aspirin and caffeine:
PO: Adults, elderly: 25-50 mg 3-4 times/day.

PRECAUTIONS

CONTRAINDICATIONS: Glaucoma, pyloric or duodenal obstruction, stenosing peptic ulcer, prostatic hypertrophy, obstruction of bladder neck, cardiospasm, myasthenia gravis, bleeding ulcer. *Fixed-combination(s):* History of hypersensitivity to aspirin or caffeine. **CAUTIONS:** Cardiac decompensation, coronary insufficiency, cardiac arrhythmias, tachycardia, sulfite sensitivity. *Fixed-combination(s)*: Coagulation abnormalities. **PREGNANCY-LACTATION:** Unknown whether drug crosses placenta or is distributed in breast milk. **Pregnancy Category C.**

INTERACTIONS

DRUG INTERACTIONS: CNS depressants may increase CNS depression **ALTERED LAB VALUES:** None significant.

SIDE EFFECTS

FREQUENT: Dry mouth. **OCCASIONAL:** Epigastric distress. *Large doses:* Blurred vision, drowsiness, dizziness, lightheadedness, constipation, urinary hesitancy or retention. **RARE:** Rash, urticaria, pruritus.

ADVERSE REACTIONS/TOXIC EFFECTS

Elderly may develop mental confusion, extreme fear, agitation, hallucinations, tachycardia, palpitations, syncope, headache. Overdose results in deep coma, seizures, shock, respiratory arrest.

NURSING IMPLICATIONS

BASELINE ASSESSMENT:

Record onset, type, location, and duration of muscular spasm. Check for immobility, stiffness, swelling. Question history of allergies, particularly aspirin, caffeine if fixed-combination is ordered.

INTERVENTION/EVALUATION:

Assist w/ambulation at all times. Assess for evidence of extravasation (stinging, swelling, coolness, little or no blood return). Palpate bladder for evidence of urinary retention. Monitor pulse rate and rhythm. Evaluate for therapeutic response: Decreased intensity of skeletal muscle pain, improved mobility, decrease in stiffness, swelling.

PATIENT/FAMILY TEACHING:

Drowsiness usually diminishes w/continued therapy. Discomfort may occur w/IM injection. Avoid tasks that require alertness, motor skills until response to drug is established. Avoid alcohol or other depressants while taking medication. Avoid sudden changes in posture.

oxacillin sodium

ox'ah-sill-in
(Bactocill, Prostaphlin)

CLASSIFICATION

Antibiotic: Penicillin

PHARMACOKINETICS

Moderately absorbed from GI tract (food decreases absorption). Widely distributed. Protein binding: 90-93%. Metabolized in liver. Primarily excreted in urine. Half-life: 0.5-0.7 hrs (increased in decreased renal function, neonates).

ACTION

Bactericidal. Binds to bacterial membranes. Inhibits cell wall synthesis.

USES

Treatment of respiratory tract, skin/skin structure infections, osteomyelitis, endocarditis, meningitis, perioperatively, esp. in cardiovascular, orthopedic procedures. Predominantly used in treatment of infections caused by penicillinase-producing staphylococci.

STORAGE/HANDLING

Store capsules at room temperature. After reconstitution, oral solution is stable for 3 days at room temperature, 14 days if refrigerated; IV infusion (piggyback) is stable for at least 6 hrs at room temperature, 8 days if refrigerated. Discard if precipitate forms.

PO/IM/IV ADMINISTRATION

NOTE: Space doses evenly around the clock.

PO:

1. Give 1 hr before or 2 hrs after food.

IM:

1. Dilute 250 mg vial w/1.4 ml (500 mg with 2.7 ml, 1 Gm w/5.7 ml, 2 Gm w/11.4 ml, or 4 Gm w/21.8 ml) sterile water for injection or 0.9% NaCl injection to provide concentration of 250 mg/1.5 ml.
2. Inject IM into large muscle mass.

IV:

1. For IV injection, dilute each 250 or 500 mg vial w/5 ml (1 Gm w/10 ml, 2 Gm w/20 ml) sterile water for injection or 0.9% NaCl injection. Administer over 10 min.
2. For intermittent IV infusion (piggyback), further dilute w/50-100 ml 5% dextrose, 0.9% NaCl or other compatible IV fluid. Infuse over 30-60 min.
3. Because of potential for hypersensitivity/anaphylaxis, start initial dose at few drops per min, increase slowly to ordered rate; stay w/pt first 10-15 min, then check q10min.
4. Alternating IV sites, use large veins to reduce risk of phlebitis.

INDICATIONS/DOSAGE/ROUTES

Mild to moderate infections of upper respiratory tract, skin/skin structure infections:
PO: Adults, elderly, children >20 kg: 500 mg q4-6h. **Children <20 kg:** 50 mg/kg/day in divided doses q6h.
IM/IV: Adults, elderly, children >40 kg: 250-500 mg q4-6h. **Children <40 kg:** 50 mg/kg/day in divided doses q6h.

Lower respiratory tract, disseminated infections, serious infections:
PO: Adults, elderly: 1 Gm q4-6h. **Children:** 100 mg/kg/day in divided doses q4-6h.
IM/IV: Adults, elderly, children >40 kg: 1 Gm q4-6h. **Maximum:** 12 Gm/day. **Children <40 kg:** 100 mg/kg/day in divided doses q4-6h. **Maximum:** 300 mg/kg/day.

Usual dosage (neonates):
IM/IV: Neonates 0-7 days: 50-75 mg/kg/day in 2-3 divided doses. **Neonates 7-28 days:** 100-150 mg/kg/day in 3-4 divided doses.

PRECAUTIONS

CONTRAINDICATIONS: Hypersensitivity to any penicillin. **CAUTIONS:** History of allergies, esp. cephalosporins. **PREGNANCY/LACTATION:** Readily crosses placenta, appears in cord blood, amniotic fluid. Distributed in breast milk in low concentrations. May lead to allergic sensitization, diarrhea, candidiasis, skin rash in infant. **Pregnancy Category B.**

INTERACTIONS

DRUG INTERACTIONS: Probenecid may increase concentration, toxicity risk. **ALTERED LAB VALUES:** May increase SGOT (AST). May cause positive Coombs' test.

SIDE EFFECTS

FREQUENT: Mild hypersensitivity reaction (fever, rash, pruritus), GI effects (nausea, vomiting, diarrhea) more frequent w/oral administration. **OCCASIONAL:** Phlebitis, thrombophlebitis (more common in elderly), hepatotoxicity w/high IV dosage.

ADVERSE REACTIONS/TOXIC EFFECTS

Superinfections, antibiotic-associated colitis may result from altered bacteria balance; hypersensitivity reaction ranging from mild to severe may occur in those allergic to penicillin.

NURSING IMPLICATIONS

BASELINE ASSESSMENT:

Question for history of allergies, esp. penicillins, cephalosporins. Obtain specimen for culture and sensitivity before giving first dose (therapy may begin before results are known).

INTERVENTION/EVALUATION:

Hold medication and promptly report rash (possible hypersensitivity) or diarrhea (w/fever, abdominal pain, blood and mucus in stool may indicate antibiotic-associated colitis). Assess food tolerance. Evaluate IV site frequently for phlebitis (heat, pain, red streaking over vein). Monitor I&O, urinalysis, renal function tests. Be alert for superinfection: Vomiting, diarrhea, black/hairy tongue, ulceration/changes of oral mucosa, anal/genital pruritus. Check hematology reports (esp. WBCs), periodic renal or hepatic reports in prolonged therapy.

PATIENT/FAMILY TEACHING:

Continue antibiotic for full length of treatment. Space doses evenly. Discomfort may occur w/IM injection. Notify physician in event of diarrhea, rash, or other new symptom.

oxaprozin

ox-ah-pro'zin

(Daypro)

CLASSIFICATION

Nonsteroidal anti-inflammatory

PHARMACOKINETICS

Well absorbed from GI tract. Widely distributed. Protein binding: >99%. Metabolized in liver. Primarily excreted in urine; partially eliminated in feces. Half-life: 42-50 hrs.

ACTION

Inhibits prostaglandin synthesis. Inhibits action of cyclooxygenase, decreases formation of prostaglandin, thromboxane precursors from arachidonic acid.

USES

Acute and chronic treatment of osteoarthritis, rheumatoid arthritis.

PO ADMINISTRATION

May give w/food, milk, or antacids if GI distress occurs.

INDICATIONS/DOSAGE/ROUTES

Osteoarthritis:

PO: Adults, elderly: 1200 mg once daily. 600 mg in pts w/low body weight, mild disease. **Maximum:** 1800 mg/day.

Rheumatoid arthritis:

PO: Adults, elderly: 1200 mg once daily. **Range:** 600-1800 mg/day.

PRECAUTIONS

CONTRAINDICATIONS: Active peptic ulcer, GI ulceration, chronic inflammation of GI tract, GI bleeding disorders, history of hypersensitivity to aspirin or nonsteroidal anti-inflammatory agent. **CAU-**

TIONS: Impaired renal/hepatic function, history of GI tract disease, predisposition to fluid retention. **PREGNANCY/LACTATION:** Unknown whether drug is excreted in breast milk. Avoid use during third trimester (may adversely affect fetal cardiovascular system: premature closure of ductus arteriosus). **Pregnancy Category C.**

INTERACTIONS

DRUG INTERACTIONS May increase effects of oral anticoagulants, heparin, thrombolytics. May decrease effect of antihypertensives, diuretics. Salicylates, aspirin may increase risk of GI side effects, bleeding. Bone marrow depressants may increase risk of hematologic reactions. May increase concentration, toxicity of lithium. May increase methotrexate toxicity. Probenecid may increase concentration. **ALTERED LAB VALUES:** May increase SGOT (AST), SGPT (ALT), serum creatinine, BUN.

SIDE EFFECTS

FREQUENT: Nausea, dyspepsia. **OCCASIONAL:** Constipation, diarrhea, rash. **RARE:** Abdominal pain/distress, anorexia, flatulence, vomiting, sedation, somnolence, sleep disturbances, tinnitus, dysuria or frequency.

ADVERSE REACTIONS/TOXIC EFFECTS

GI bleeding, coma may occur. Hypertension, acute renal failure, respiratory depression occur rarely.

NURSING IMPLICATIONS

BASELINE ASSESSMENT:

Assess onset, type, location, and duration of pain or inflammation.

INTERVENTION/EVALUATION:

Assist w/ambulation if dizziness occurs. Monitor stools; avoid constipation through high-fiber diet, appropriate exercise, and increased fluids. Check for rash. Evaluate for therapeutic response: relief of pain, stiffness, swelling, increase in joint mobility, reduced joint tenderness, improved grip strength.

PATIENT/FAMILY TEACHING:

Avoid aspirin, alcohol during therapy (increases risk of GI bleeding). Report tarry stools. If GI upset occurs, take w/food, milk. Avoid tasks that require alertness, motor skills until response to drug is established.

oxazepam

ox-az´eh-pam
(Serax)

CANADIAN AVAILABILITY:
Apo-Oxazepam, Novoxapam, Serax

CLASSIFICATION

Antianxiety: Benzodiazepine

PHARMACOKINETICS

Well absorbed from GI tract. Protein binding: 97%. Metabolized in liver. Primarily excreted in urine. Half-life: 5-15 hrs.

ACTION

Enhances action of inhibitory neurotransmitter gamma-aminobutryic acid (GABA). Depressant effects occur at all levels of CNS.

USES

Management of acute alcohol withdrawal symptoms (tremulousness, anxiety on withdrawal). Treatment of anxiety associated w/ depressive symptoms.

PO ADMINISTRATION

1. Give w/o regard to meals.
2. Capsules may be emptied and mixed w/food.

INDICATIONS/DOSAGE/ROUTES

NOTE: Use smallest effective dose in elderly, debilitated, those w/ liver disease, low serum albumin.

Mild to moderate anxiety:
PO: Adults: 10-15 mg 3-4 times/day.

Severe anxiety:
PO: Adults: 15-30 mg 3-4 times/day.

Alcohol withdrawal:
PO: Adults: 15-30 mg 3-4 times/day.

Usual elderly dosage:
PO: Elderly: Initially, 10 mg 2-3 times/day. May gradually increase up to 30-45 mg/day.

PRECAUTIONS

CONTRAINDICATIONS: Acute narrow-angle glaucoma. **CAUTIONS:** Impaired renal/hepatic function. **PREGNANCY/LACTATION:** May cross placenta; may be distributed in breast milk. Chronic ingestion during pregnancy may produce withdrawal symptoms, CNS depression in neonates. **Pregnancy Category C.**

INTERACTIONS

DRUG INTERACTIONS: Potentiated effects when used w/other CNS depressants, including alcohol. **ALTERED LAB VALUES:** None significant.

SIDE EFFECTS

FREQUENT: Mild, transient drowsiness at beginning of therapy. **OCCASIONAL:** Dizziness, headache. **RARE:** Paradoxical CNS hyperactivity/nervousness in children, excitement/restlessness in elderly/debilitated (generally noted during first 2 wks of therapy, particularly noted in presence of uncontrolled pain).

ADVERSE REACTIONS/TOXIC EFFECTS

Abrupt or too-rapid withdrawal may result in pronounced restlessness, irritability, insomnia, hand tremors, abdominal/muscle cramps, sweating, vomiting, seizures. Overdose results in somnolence, confusion, diminished reflexes, coma.

NURSING IMPLICATIONS

Baseline Assessment:

Offer emotional support to anxious pt. Assess motor responses (agitation, trembling, tension) and autonomic responses (cold, clammy hands, sweating).

Intervention/Evaluation:

For those on long-term therapy, liver/renal function tests, blood counts should be performed periodically. Assess for paradoxical reaction, particularly during early therapy. Assist w/ambulation if drowsiness, lightheadedness occur. Evaluate for therapeutic response: A calm facial expression, decreased restlessness and/or insomnia.

Patient/Family Teaching:

Drowsiness usually disappears

during continued therapy. If dizziness occurs, change positions slowly from recumbent to sitting position before standing. Avoid tasks that require alertness, motor skills until response to drug is established. Smoking reduces drug effectiveness. Do not abruptly withdraw medication after long-term therapy.

oxiconazole

ox-ee-con´ah-zole
(Oxistat)

CLASSIFICATION

Antifungal

ACTION

Inhibits ergosterol synthesis increasing permeability of fungal cell membrane, loss of essential components. Fungicidal.

USES

Treatment of *Tinea pedis, T. cruris, T. corporis.*

INDICATIONS/DOSAGE/ROUTES

Tinea pedis:
TOPICAL: Adults, elderly: 1-2 times/day for 4 wks.

Tinea corporis, cruris:
TOPICAL: Adults, elderly: 1-2 times/day for 2 wks.

PRECAUTIONS

CONTRAINDICATIONS: Hypersensitivity to oxiconazole or any ingredient in preparation. **PREGNANCY/LACTATION:** Caution during lactation, excreted in milk. **Pregnancy Category B.**

INTERACTIONS

DRUG INTERACTIONS: None significant. **ALTERED LAB VALUES:** None significant.

SIDE EFFECTS

OCCASIONAL: Itching, burning, redness, irritation. **RARE:** Fissuring, maceration.

ADVERSE REACTIONS/TOXIC EFFECTS

None significant.

NURSING IMPLICATIONS

BASELINE ASSESSMENT:

Question hypersensitivity to oxiconazole or ingredients of preparation.

INTERVENTION/EVALUATION:

Assess for therapeutic response or local irritation, burning, itching, redness, maceration, fissuring.

PATIENT/FAMILY TEACHING:

Rub well into affected, surrounding areas. Complete full course of therapy (may take several wks). For external use only; keep away from eyes. Do not use occlusive covering or use other preparations w/o consulting physician. Keep areas clean, dry; wear light clothing to promote ventilation. Separate personal items, linens. Notify physician of increased irritation.

oxybutynin chloride

oxy byoo´etih-nin
(Ditropan)

CANADIAN AVAILABILITY:
Ditropan

CLASSIFICATION

Antispasmodic

PHARMACOKINETICS

	ONSET	PEAK	DURATION
PO	0.5-1 hr	3-6 hrs	6-10 hrs

Rapid absorption from GI tract. Metabolized in liver. Primarily excreted in urine. Half-life: 1-2.3 hrs.

ACTION

Exerts antispasmodic (papaverine-like) and antimuscarinic (atropine-like) action on detrusor smooth muscle of bladder. Increases bladder capacity, diminishes frequency of uninhibited detrusor muscle contraction, delays desire to void.

USES

Relief of symptoms (urgency, incontinence, frequency, nocturia, urge incontinence) associated w/ uninhibited neurogenic bladder or reflex neurogenic bladder.

PO ADMINISTRATION

Give w/o regard to meals.

INDICATIONS/DOSAGE/ROUTES

Neurogenic bladder:
PO: Adults: 5 mg 2-3 times/day. **Maximum:** 5 mg 4 times/day. **Children >5 yrs:** 5 mg 2 times/day. **Maximum:** 5 mg 3 times/day.

Usual elderly dosage:
PO: Elderly: Initially, 2.5-5 mg/day. May increase by 2.5 mg q1-2days.

PRECAUTIONS

CONTRAINDICATIONS: Angle-closure glaucoma, GI obstruction, myasthenia gravis, paralytic ileus, megacolon, ulcerative colitis, intestinal atony, unstable cardiovascular disease. **CAUTIONS:** Impaired renal or hepatic function, elderly, autonomic neuropathy. **PREGNANCY/LACTATION:** Unknown whether drug crosses placenta or is distributed in breast milk. **Pregnancy Category B.**

INTERACTIONS

DRUG INTERACTIONS: Medication w/anticholinergic effects (e.g., antihistamines) may increase effects. **ALTERED LAB VALUES:** None significant.

SIDE EFFECTS

COMMON: Dry mouth, mydriasis, increased GI and skeletal muscle tone, reduced pulse rate, constriction of bronchi and ureters, salivary and sweat gland secretion. **OCCASIONAL:** Slight, temporary decrease in diastolic B/P w/mild reflex tachycardia, short periods of atrial fibrillation in hyperthyroid pts. Hypertensive pts may react w/ marked fall in B/P.

ADVERSE REACTIONS/TOXIC EFFECTS

Overdosage produces cholinergic reaction manifested as abdominal discomfort/cramping, nausea, vomiting, diarrhea, flushing, feeling of warmth/heat about face, excessive salivation and sweating, lacrimation, pallor, bradycardia/tachycardia, hypotension, urinary urgency, blurred vision, bronchospasm, pupillary contraction, involuntary muscular contraction visible under the skin (fasciculation).

NURSING IMPLICATIONS

INTERVENTION/EVALUATION:

Assess pulse periodically. Monitor I&O; palpate bladder for retention. Monitor stools; avoid constipation w/fluids, bulk, and exercise. Hold medication and notify physician of diarrhea at once.

PATIENT/FAMILY TEACHING:

May cause dry mouth. Avoid alcohol and sedatives. Report diarrhea promptly. Do not take medication in high environmental temperature (heat prostration may occur due to decreased sweating). Avoid tasks that require alertness, motor skills until response to drug is established.

oxycodone

ox-ih-koe´doan
(Roxicodone)

FIXED-COMBINATION(S): W/acetaminophen (Percocet, Roxicet, Tylox); w/aspirin (Percodan, Roxiprin)

CANADIAN AVAILABILITY: Supeudol

CLASSIFICATION

Opioid analgesic **(Schedule II)**

PHARMACOKINETICS

	ONSET	PEAK	DURATION
PO	10-15 min	30-60 min	3-6 hrs

Moderately absorbed from GI tract. Widely distributed. Metabolized in liver. Excreted in urine. Half-life: 2-3 hrs.

ACTION

Binds w/opioid receptors within CNS, altering processes affecting pain perception, emotional response to pain.

USES

Relief of mild to moderately severe pain.

PO ADMINISTRATION

1. Give w/o regard to meals.
2. Tablets may be crushed.

INDICATIONS/DOSAGE/ROUTES

NOTE: Reduce initial dosage in those w/hypothyroidism, concurrent CNS depressants, Addison's disease, renal insufficiency, elderly/debilitated.

Analgesia:
PO: Adults: 5 mg q6h as needed. **Elderly:** 2.5-5 mg q6h as needed.

PRECAUTIONS

CONTRAINDICATIONS: None significant. **EXTREME CAUTION:** CNS depression, anoxia, hypercapnia, respiratory depression, seizures, acute alcoholism, shock, untreated myxedema, respiratory dysfunction. **CAUTIONS:** Increased intracranial pressure, impaired hepatic function, acute abdominal conditions, hypothyroidism, prostatic hypertrophy, Addison's disease, urethral stricture, COPD. **PREGNANCY/LACTATION:** Readily crosses placenta; distributed in breast milk. Respiratory depression may occur in neonate if mother received opiates during labor. Regular use of opiates during pregnancy may produce withdrawal symptoms in neonate (irritability, excessive crying, tremors, hyperactive reflexes, fever, vomiting, diarrhea, yawning, sneezing, seizures). **Pregnancy Category C.**

INTERACTIONS

DRUG INTERACTIONS: Alcohol, CNS depressants may increase CNS, respiratory depression, hypotension. MAO inhibitors may produce severe, fatal reaction (reduce dose to 1/4 usual dose). **ALTERED LAB VALUES:** May increase amylase, lipase.

SIDE EFFECTS

NOTE: Effects are dependent on dosage amount. Ambulatory pts and those not in severe pain may experience dizziness, nausea, vomiting, hypotension more frequently than those in supine position or having severe pain.
FREQUENT: Suppressed breathing depth. **OCCASIONAL:** Lightheadedness, sweating, vivid dreaming, nightmares, hypotension, nausea, vomiting, euphoria/dysphoria, constipation (drug delays digestion), flushing, feeling of facial and neck warmth, urinary retention.

ADVERSE REACTIONS/TOXIC EFFECTS

Overdose results in respiratory depression, skeletal muscle flaccidity, cold, clammy skin, cyanosis, extreme somnolence progressing to convulsions, stupor, coma. Hepatotoxicity may occur w/overdosage of acetaminophen component. Tolerance to analgesic effect, physical dependence may occur w/repeated use.

NURSING IMPLICATIONS

BASELINE ASSESSMENT:

Assess onset, type, location, and duration of pain. Effect of medication is reduced if full pain recurs before next dose. Obtain vital signs before giving medication. If respirations are 12/min or lower (20/min or lower in children), withhold medication, contact physician.

INTERVENTION/EVALUATION:

Palpate bladder for urinary retention. Monitor pattern of daily bowel activity and stool consistency. Initiate deep breathing and coughing exercises, particularly in those w/impaired pulmonary function. Assess for clinical improvement and record onset of relief of pain.

PATIENT/FAMILY TEACHING:

Change positions slowly to avoid orthostatic hypotension. Avoid tasks that require alertness, motor skills until response to drug is established. Tolerance/dependence may occur w/prolonged use of high doses. Avoid alcohol and CNS depressants.

oxytocin

ox-ih-toe´sin
(Pitocin, Syntocinon)

CANADIAN AVAILABILITY:
Syntocinon

CLASSIFICATION

Oxytocic

PHARMACOKINETICS

	ONSET	PEAK	DURATION
IM	3-5 min	—	2-3 hrs
IV	Immediate	—	1 hr
Intranasal	Few min	—	20 min

Rapidly absorbed through nasal mucous membranes. Distributed in extracellular fluid. Protein binding: 30%. Metabolized in liver, kidney. Primarily excreted in urine.

ACTION

Stimulates contraction of uterine

smooth muscle (mimics contractions of normal, spontaneous labor). Stimulates mammary smooth muscle to enhance milk ejection from breasts.

USES

Parenteral (Antepartum): To initiate or improve uterine contraction to achieve early vaginal delivery; stimulate or reinforce labor; management of incomplete or inevitable abortion. *(Postpartum):* To produce uterine contractions during third stage of labor; control uterine bleeding. *Nasal:* To promote breast milk ejection.

IV/NASAL ADMINISTRATION

IV:

1. Requires qualified personnel, hospitalization w/availability of surgical facilities and intensive care.
2. Continuous monitoring of uterine contractions, fetal and maternal heart rates, maternal B/P, and, if possible, intrauterine pressure.
3. Dilute 10 U (1 ml) in 1,000 ml of 0.9% NaCl, lactated Ringer's or 5% dextrose injection to provide a concentration of 10 milliunits/ml solution).
4. Give by IV infusion. (Use infusion device to carefully control rate of flow.)

NASAL SPRAY:

1. W/pt in sitting position, spray in one or both nostrils.
2. Give 2-3 min before nursing or pumping breasts.

INDICATIONS/DOSAGE/ROUTES

Induction/stimulation of labor:
IV INFUSION: Adults: Initially, 1-2 milliunits/min; gradually increase in increments of 1-2 milliunits/min q15-30min (until contraction pattern similar to spontaneous labor reached). **Maximum:** Rarely >20 milliunits/min.

Incomplete/inevitable abortion:
IV INFUSION: Adults: 10 U in 500 ml (20 milliunits/ml) 5% dextrose in water or 0.9% NaCl infused at 10-20 milliunits/min.

Control postpartum bleeding:
IV INFUSION: Adults: 10-40 U (**maximum:** 40 U/1,000 ml) infused at rate of 20-40 milliunits/min after delivery of infant.
IM: Adults: 10 U after delivery of placenta.

Promote milk ejection:
NASAL: Adults: 1 spray to 1 or 2 nostrils 2-3 min before nursing or pumping breasts.

PRECAUTIONS

CONTRAINDICATIONS: Hypersensitivity to oxytocin, cephalopelvic disproportion, unfavorable fetal position or presentation, unengaged fetal head, fetal distress w/o imminent delivery, prematurity, when vaginal delivery is contraindicated (e.g., active genital herpes infection, placenta previa, cord presentation), obstetric emergencies that favor surgical intervention, grand multiparity, hypertonic or hyperactive uterus, adequate uterine activity that fails to progress. Nasal spray during pregnancy. **CAUTIONS:** Induction should be for medical, not elective reasons. **PREGNANCY/LACTATION:** Used as indicated, not expected to present risk of fetal abnormalities. Small amounts in breast milk; nursing not recommended.

INTERACTIONS

DRUG INTERACTIONS: Caudal

block anesthetics, vasopressors may increase pressor effects. Other oxytocics may cause uterine hypertonus, uterine rupture, or cervical lacerations. **ALTERED LAB VALUES:** None significant.

SIDE EFFECTS

OCCASIONAL: Tachycardia, PVCs, hypotension, nausea, vomiting. **RARE:** Hypertonicity with tearing of uterus, increased bleeding, abruptio placenta, cervical and vaginal lacerations. Fetus: Bradycardia, CNS or brain damage, trauma due to rapid propulsion, low Apgar at 5 min, retinal hemorrhage.

ADVERSE REACTIONS/TOXIC EFFECTS

Prolonged IV infusion of oxytocin w/excessive fluid volume has caused severe water intoxication w/seizures, coma, and death. Anaphylaxis that may rarely be fatal.

NURSING IMPLICATIONS

BASELINE ASSESSMENT:

Question for hypersensitivity to oxytocin. Assess baselines for TPR, B/P and fetal heart rate. Determine frequency, duration, and strength of contractions.

INTERVENTION/EVALUATION:

Monitor B/P, pulse, respirations, fetal heart rate, intrauterine pressure, contractions (duration, strength, frequency) every 15 min. Notify physician of contractions that last >1 min, occur more frequently than every 2 min, or stop. Maintain careful I&O, be alert to potential water intoxication. Check for blood loss.

PATIENT/FAMILY TEACHING:

Keep pt, family informed of labor progress. *Nasal spray:* Teach proper use.

paclitaxel

pass-leh-tax'ell

(Taxol)

CLASSIFICATION

Antineoplastic

PHARMACOKINETICS

Highly bound to plasma proteins (97%). Does not readily cross blood-brain barrier. Metabolized in liver (active metabolites); eliminated via bile. Half-life: 1.3-8.6 hrs.

ACTION

Binds to fully assembled microtubules, stabilizes microtubules, prevents depolymerization resulting in halting mitosis and cell death. May also interrupt mitosis by distorting mitotic spindles. Cell-cycle specific for G2, M phases.

USES

Treatment for metastatic ovarian cancer following failure of first-line or subsequent chemotherapy. Treatment of breast carcinoma.

STORAGE/HANDLING

Refrigerate unopened vials. Prepared solutions stable at room temperature for 24 hrs. Wear gloves during handling; if contact w/skin, wash hands thoroughly w/soap and water. If in contact w/mucous membranes, flush w/water.

IV ADMINISTRATION

1. Must dilute before administration w/0.9% NaCl, 5% dextrose to final concentration of 0.3-1.2 mg/ml.

2. Store diluted solutions in bottles or plastic bags and administer through polyethylene-lined administration sets (avoid plasticized PVC equipment or devices).

3. Administer through in-line filter not greater than 0.22 microns.

4. Monitor vital signs during infusion, especially during first hr.

5. Discontinue administration if severe hypersensitivity reaction occurs.

INDICATIONS/DOSAGE/ROUTES

NOTE: Pretreat w/corticosteroids, diphenhydramine and H_2 antagonists.

Ovarian cancer:
IV INFUSION: Adults: 175 mg/m^2 over 3 hrs q3wks.

Breast carcinoma:
IV INFUSION: Adults, elderly: 175 mg/m^2 over 3 hrs q3wks.

PRECAUTIONS

CONTRAINDICATIONS: Baseline neutropenia <1,500 cells/mm^3, hypersensitivity to drugs developed w/Cremophor EL (polyoxyethylated castor oil). **CAUTIONS:** Severe hepatic impairment, bone marrow depression. **PREGNANCY/LACTATION:** May produce fetal harm. Unknown whether distributed in breast milk. Avoid pregnancy. **Pregnancy Category D.**

INTERACTIONS

DRUG INTERACTIONS: None significant. **ALTERED LAB VALUES:** May elevate alkaline phosphatase, SGOT (AST), SGPT (ALT), bilirubin.

SIDE EFFECTS

FREQUENT: Alopecia, diarrhea, cardiac disturbances (bradycardia), abnormal EKG, peripheral neuropathy. **OCCASIONAL:** Mild to moderate nausea and vomiting, mucositis, myalgia, mild fever, taste perversion, fatigue, reactions at injection site (erythema, tenderness, hyperpigmentation).

ADVERSE REACTIONS/TOXIC EFFECTS

Severe hypersensitivity reaction (dyspnea, severe hypotension, angioedema, generalized urticaria), myelosuppression (neutropenia and leukopenia).

NURSING IMPLICATIONS

BASELINE ASSESSMENT:

Give emotional support to pt and family. Use strict asepsis and protect pt from infection. Check blood counts, particularly neutrophil, platelet count before each course of therapy, monthly, or as clinically indicated.

INTERVENTION/EVALUATION:

Monitor for hematological toxicity (fever, sore throat, signs of local infection, easy bruising, unusual bleeding), symptoms of anemia (excessive tiredness, weakness). Assess response to medication; monitor and report for diarrhea. Avoid IM injections, rectal temperatures, other traumas that may induce bleeding. Put pressure to injection sites for full 5 min.

PATIENT/FAMILY TEACHING:

Explain that alopecia is reversible, but new hair may have different color, texture. Do not have immunizations w/o physician's approval (drug lowers body's resistance). Avoid crowds, persons w/known infections. Report signs of infection at once (fever, flu-like symptoms). Contact physician if nausea/vomiting continue at-home. Teach signs of peripheral neuropathy. Avoid pregnancy during therapy.

pamidronate disodium

pam-ih-draw′nate

(Aredia)

CLASSIFICATION

Hypocalcemic

PHARMACOKINETICS

After IV administration, rapidly absorbed by bone. Slowly excreted unchanged in urine.

ACTION

Inhibits accelerated bone resorption, which is responsible for hypercalcemia in malignancy (bone formation and mineralization are not inhibited).

USES

Treatment of moderate to severe hypercalcemia associated w/ malignancy (w/o or w/bone metastases). Treatment of moderate to severe Paget's disease.

STORAGE/HANDLING

Store parenteral form at room temperature. Reconstituted vials stable for 24 hrs refrigerated; IV solution stable for 24 hrs after dilution.

IV ADMINISTRATION

1. Adequate hydration is essential in conjunction w/pamidronate therapy (avoid overhydration in pts w/potential for cardiac failure).
2. Reconstitute each 30 mg vial w/10 ml sterile water for injection to provide concentration of 3 mg/ml.
3. Allow drug to dissolve before withdrawing.
4. Further dilute w/1,000 ml sterile 0.45% or 0.9% NaCl or 5% dextrose.
5. Administer IV infusion over 24 hrs.
6. Do not mix w/Ringer's solution or other calcium-containing solutions.

INDICATIONS/DOSAGE/ROUTES

Hypercalcemia:

IV INFUSION: Adults, elderly: Moderate (corrected serum calcium 12-13.5 mg/dl): 60-90 mg over 24 hrs. Severe (corrected serum calcium >13.5 mg/dl): 90 mg over 24 hrs.

Paget's disease:

IV INFUSION: Adults, elderly: 30 mg/day for 3 days.

PRECAUTIONS

CONTRAINDICATIONS: Hypersensitivity to biphosphonates. **CAUTIONS:** Safety and efficacy in children not established. **PREGNANCY/LACTATION:** There are no adequate and well-controlled studies in pregnant women; not known whether fetal harm can occur. Excretion in breast milk unknown. **Pregnancy Category C.**

INTERACTIONS

DRUG INTERACTIONS: None significant. **ALTERED LAB VALUES:** May decrease phosphate, potassium, magnesium, calcium levels.

SIDE EFFECTS

FREQUENT: 27% of pts have temperature elevation (at least 1° C.) 24-48 hrs after administration. Drug-related redness, swelling, induration, pain at catheter site (18% of pts receiving 90 mg). Anorexia, nausea, fatigue, hypophosphatemia, hypokalemia, hypomagnesemia, hypocalcemia occur more frequently w/higher dosage. **OCCASIONAL:** Constipation, GI hemorrhage, rales, rhinitis, anemia, hypertension, tachycardia, atrial fibrillation, somnolence occur more often w/90 mg dosages.

ADVERSE REACTIONS/TOXIC EFFECTS

Cardiac failure may occur w/ overhydration accompanying pamidronate therapy.

NURSING IMPLICATIONS

Baseline Assessment:

Obtain electrolyte and CBC levels; check B/P, pulse, temperature. Assess lungs for rales, dependent parts of the body for edema.

Intervention/Evaluation:

Provide adequate hydration; avoid overhydration. Monitor I&O carefully; check lungs for rales, dependent body parts for edema. Monitor B/P, temperature, pulse. Assess catheter site for redness, swelling pain. Check electrolytes (esp. calcium and potassium) and CBC results. Monitor food intake and stool frequency. Be alert for potential GI hemorrhage w/90 mg dosage.

Patient/Family Teaching:

Explain the rationale for the therapy and how to assist in maintaining an accurate I&O.

pancreatin

pan-kree-ah´tin

(Pancreatin)

CLASSIFICATION

Digestive enzyme

ACTION

Enhances digestion of protein, carbohydrate, fat in GI tract (primarily in duodenum, upper jejunum).

USES

Pancreatic enzyme replacement/supplement when enzymes are absent or deficient (i.e., chronic pancreatitis, cystic fibrosis, ductal obstruction from pancreatic cancer, common bile duct). Treatment of steatorrhea associated w/postgastrectomy syndrome, bowel resection; reduces malabsorption.

PO ADMINISTRATION

Give before or w/meals. Tablets may be crushed. Do not crush enteric-coated tablets. Instruct pt not to chew (minimizes irritation to mouth, lips, tongue).

INDICATIONS/DOSAGE/ROUTES

Usual oral dosage:

PO: Adults, elderly: 1-3 tablets before or w/meals, snacks.

PRECAUTIONS

CONTRAINDICATIONS: Hypersensitivity to pork protein. **CAUTIONS:** None significant. **PREGNANCY/LACTATION:** Unknown whether drug crosses placenta or is distributed in breast milk. **Pregnancy Category C.**

INTERACTIONS

DRUG INTERACTIONS: Antacids may decrease effect. May decrease absorption of iron supplements. **ALTERED LAB VALUES:** May decrease bilirubin. May increase uric acid.

SIDE EFFECTS

None significant.

ADVERSE REACTIONS/TOXIC EFFECTS

Excessive dosage may produce diarrhea, GI upset, hypersensitivity reaction. Hyperuricosuria, hyperuricemia reported with extremely high doses.

NURSING IMPLICATIONS

INTERVENTION/EVALUATION:

Question for therapeutic relief from GI symptoms.

pancrelipase

pan-kree-lie´pace

(Cotazym, Ilozyme, Pancrease, Viokase)

CANADIAN AVAILABILITY: Cotazyme, Pancrease

CLASSIFICATION

Digestive enzyme

ACTION

Enhances digestion of protein, carbohydrate, fat in GI tract (primarily in duodenum, upper jejunum).

USES

Pancreatic enzyme replacement/supplement when enzymes are absent or deficient (i.e., chronic pancreatitis, cystic fibrosis, ductal obstruction from pancreatic cancer, common bile duct). Treatment of steatorrhea associated w/postgastrectomy syndrome, bowel resection; reduces malabsorption.

PO ADMINISTRATION

Give before or w/meals. Tablets may be crushed. Do not crush enteric-coated tablets. Instruct pt not to chew (minimizes irritation to mouth, lips, tongue).

INDICATIONS/DOSAGE/ROUTES

Usual oral dosage:
PO: Adults, elderly: 1-3 capsules or tablets before or w/meals, snacks. May increase up to 8 tablets/dose.

PRECAUTIONS

CONTRAINDICATIONS: Hypersensitivity to pork protein. **CAUTIONS:** None significant. **PREGNANCY/LACTATION:** Unknown whether drug crosses placenta or is distributed in breast milk. **Pregnancy Category C.**

INTERACTIONS

DRUG INTERACTIONS: Antacids may decrease effect. May decrease absorption of iron supplements. **ALTERED LAB VALUES:** May increase uric acid.

SIDE EFFECTS

None significant.

ADVERSE REACTIONS/TOXIC EFFECTS

Excessive dosage may produce nausea, cramping, and/or diarrhea. Hyperuricosuria, hyperuricemia reported with extremely high doses.

NURSING IMPLICATIONS

BASELINE ASSESSMENT:

Spilling powder on hands (Viokase) may irritate skin. Inhaling powder may irritate mucous membranes, produce bronchospasm.

INTERVENTION/EVALUATION:

Question for therapeutic relief from GI symptoms.

pancuronium bromide

pan-cure-oh´knee-um
(Pavulon)

CANADIAN AVAILABILITY:
Pavulon

(See Classifications section under Neuromuscular blockers)

paroxetine hydrochloride

pear-ox'eh-teen
(Paxil)

CLASSIFICATION

Antidepressant

PHARMACOKINETICS

Well absorbed from GI tract. Widely distributed. Highly bound to plasma proteins (95%). Metabolized in liver; excreted in urine. Half-life: 24 hrs.

ACTION

Selectively blocks uptake of neurotransmitter, serotonin, at CNS neuronal presynaptic membranes, thereby increasing availability at postsynaptic neuronal receptor sites. Resulting enhancement of synaptic activity produces antidepressant effect.

USES

Treatment of major depression.

PO ADMINISTRATION

1. Give w/food or milk if GI distress occurs.
2. Scored tablet may be crushed.
3. Best if given as single morning dose.

INDICATIONS/DOSAGE/ROUTES

NOTE: Reduce dosage in elderly, pts w/severe renal, hepatic impairment. Dose changes should occur at 1 wk intervals.

Depression:
PO: Adults: Initially, 20 mg/day, usually in morning. Dosage may be gradually increased in 10 mg/day increments to 50 mg/day. **Elderly, debilitated, those w/severe hepatic, renal impairment:** Initially, 10 mg/day. Do not exceed maximum 40 mg/day.

PRECAUTIONS

CONTRAINDICATIONS: Within 14 days of MAO inhibitor therapy. **CAUTIONS:** Severe renal, hepatic impairment. History of mania, seizures, those w/metabolic or hemodynamic disease, history of drug abuse. **PREGNANCY/LACTATION:** May impair reproductive function. Distributed in breast milk. **Pregnancy Category B.**

INTERACTIONS

DRUG INTERACTIONS: MAO inhibitors may cause serotonergic syndrome (excitement, diaphoresis, rigidity, hyperthermia, autonomic hyperactivity, coma). Cimetidine may increase concentrations; phenytoin may decrease concentrations. **ALTERED LAB VALUES:** May increase liver enzymes.

SIDE EFFECTS

FREQUENT: Nausea, somnolence, headache, dry mouth, weakness, constipation/diarrhea, dizziness, insomnia, ejaculatory disturbance, sweating, tremor. **OCCASIONAL:** Decreased appetite, nervousness, anxiety, flatulence, paresthesia, decrease in libido, abdominal discomfort, urinary frequency, yawning. **RARE:** Palpitations, vomiting, blurred vision, taste change, confusion.

ADVERSE REACTIONS/TOXIC EFFECTS

None significant.

NURSING IMPLICATIONS

BASELINE ASSESSMENT:

Assess appearance, behavior, speech pattern, level of interest, mood. Assess for history of drug abuse.

INTERVENTION/EVALUATION:

For those on long-term therapy, liver/renal function tests, blood counts should be performed periodically. Supervise suicidal-risk pt closely during early therapy (as depression lessens, energy level improves, increasing suicide potential). Assess appearance, behavior, speech pattern, level of interest, mood.

PATIENT/FAMILY TEACHING:

Therapeutic effect may be noted within 1-4 weeks. Dry mouth may be relieved by sugarless gum or sips of tepid water. Do not abruptly discontinue medication. Avoid tasks that require alertness, motor skills until response to drug is established. Inform physician if intention of pregnancy or if pregnancy occurs. Avoid alcohol.

---

pegaspargase (Oncaspar)
See supplement

---

pemoline

pem´oh-leen
(Cylert)

CANADIAN AVAILABILITY:
Cylert

CLASSIFICATION

CNS stimulant

PHARMACOKINETICS

	ONSET	PEAK	DURATION
PO (adults)	Gradual	4 hrs	8 hrs
PO (children)	Gradual	—	—

Readily absorbed from GI tract. Protein binding: 50%. Metabolized in liver. Primarily excreted in urine. Half-life: 12 hrs.

ACTION

Appears to act through dopaminergic receptor sites. In children, appears to reduce motor restlessness, increases mental alertness, provides mood elevation, reduces sense of fatigue.

USES

Treatment of attention deficit disorder in children w/moderate to severe distraction, short attention span, hyperactivity, emotional impulsiveness.

PO ADMINISTRATION

1. Do not administer in afternoon or evening (to avoid insomnia).
2. Tablets may be crushed.

INDICATIONS/DOSAGE/ROUTES

Attention deficit disorder:
PO: Children >6 yrs: Initially, 37.5 mg/day given as single dose in morning. May increase by 18.75

P

mg at weekly intervals until therapeutic response is achieved. **Range:** 56.25-75 mg/day. **Maximum:** 112.5 mg/day.

PRECAUTIONS

CONTRAINDICATIONS: Impaired hepatic function, pts w/ motor tics, family history of Tourette's disorder. **CAUTIONS:** Impaired renal function. **PREGNANCY/LACTATION:** Unknown whether drug crosses placenta or is distributed in breast milk. **Pregnancy Category B.**

INTERACTIONS

DRUG INTERACTIONS: CNS stimulating medications may increase CNS stimulation. **ALTERED LAB VALUES:** May increase SGOT (AST), SGPT (ALT), LDH.

SIDE EFFECTS

FREQUENT: Anorexia, insomnia. **OCCASIONAL:** Nausea, abdominal discomfort, diarrhea, headache, dizziness, drowsiness.

ADVERSE REACTIONS/TOXIC EFFECTS

Dyskinetic movements of tongue, lips, face, and extremities, and visual disturbances, rash have occurred. Large doses may produce extreme nervousness, tachycardia. Hepatic effects (hepatitis, jaundice) appear to be reversible when drug is discontinued. Prolonged administration to children w/attention deficit disorder may produce a temporary suppression of weight and/or height patterns.

NURSING IMPLICATIONS

BASELINE ASSESSMENT:

Liver function tests should be performed before therapy begins and periodically during therapy.

PATIENT/FAMILY TEACHING:

Therapeutic response to medication may take 3-4 wks. Insomnia, anorexia usually disappear during continued therapy. Anorexia usually accompanied by weight loss. Return to normal weight usually occurs within 3-6 mo.

penbutolol

pen-beaut´oh-lol
(Levatol)

CLASSIFICATION

Beta-adrenergic blocker

PHARMACOKINETICS

	ONSET	PEAK	DURATION
PO	—	1 hr	24 hrs

Completely absorbed from GI tract. Protein binding: 80-90%. Metabolized in liver. Primarily excreted in urine. Half-life: 5 hrs (increased in decreased renal function).

ACTION

Nonselective beta-blocker. Blocks $beta_1$-adrenergic receptors, slowing sinus heart rate, decreasing cardiac output, decreasing B/P (exact mechanism unknown but may block peripheral adrenergic receptors, decrease sympathetic outflow from CNS or decrease renin release from kidney). Blocks $beta_2$-adrenergic receptors, increasing airway resistance. Decreases myocardial ischemia severity by decreasing oxygen requirements. Has moderate intrinsic sympathomimetic activity.

USES

Treatment of mild to moderate hypertension.

PO ADMINISTRATION

1. May give w/o regard to food.
2. Tablets may be crushed.

INDICATIONS/DOSAGE/ROUTES

Hypertension:
PO: Adults: Initially, 20 mg/day as single dose. May increase to 40-80 mg/day. **Elderly:** Initially, 10 mg/day.

PRECAUTIONS

CONTRAINDICATIONS: Bronchial asthma, COPD, sinus bradycardia, heart block greater than first degree, cardiogenic shock, CHF (unless secondary to tachyarrhythmias), overt cardiac failure. **CAUTIONS:** Inadequate cardiac function, impaired renal/hepatic function, diabetes mellitus, hyperthyroidism. **PREGNANCY/LACTATION:** Crosses placenta; distributed in breast milk. Avoid use during first trimester. May produce bradycardia, apnea, hypoglycemia, hypothermia during delivery, small birth weight infants. **Pregnancy Category C.**

INTERACTIONS

DRUG INTERACTIONS: Diuretics, other hypotensives may increase hypotensive effect; sympathomimetics, xanthines may mutually inhibit effects; may mask symptoms of hypoglycemia, prolong hypoglycemic effect of insulin, oral hypoglycemics; NSAIDs may decrease anti-hypertensive effect; cimetidine may increase concentration. **ALTERED LAB VALUES:** May increase ANA titer, SGOT (AST), SGPT (ALT), alkaline phosphatase, LDH, bilirubin, BUN, creatinine, potassium, uric acid, lipoproteins, triglycerides.

SIDE EFFECTS

FREQUENT: Dizziness, fatigue, insomnia, bizarre dreams, paresthesia, visual disturbances, anxiety, peripheral edema, dyspnea, weight gain. **OCCASIONAL:** Nausea, GI distress, palpitation, coldness of extremities, syncope, tachycardia, chest pain, muscle/joint pain. **RARE:** Lethargy, hallucinations, diarrhea, vomiting, wheezing, rash, pruritus, urinary frequency, impotence.

ADVERSE REACTIONS/TOXIC EFFECTS

Abrupt withdrawal (particularly in those w/coronary artery disease) may produce angina or precipitate MI. May precipitate thyroid crisis in those w/thyrotoxicosis.

NURSING IMPLICATIONS

BASELINE ASSESSMENT:

Assess baseline renal/liver function tests. Assess B/P, apical pulse immediately before drug is administered (if pulse is 60/min or below or systolic B/P is below 90 mm Hg, withhold medication, contact physician).

INTERVENTION/EVALUATION:

Assess pulse for strength/weakness, irregular rate, bradycardia. Monitor EKG for cardiac changes. Assist w/ambulation if dizziness occurs. Assess for peripheral edema of hands, feet (usually, first area of low extremity swelling is behind medial malleolus in ambulatory, sacral area in bedridden). Monitor pattern of daily

P

bowel activity, stool consistency. Assess skin for development of rash. Monitor any unusual changes in pt.

PATIENT/FAMILY TEACHING:

Do not abruptly discontinue medication. Compliance w/therapy regimen is essential to control hypertension. If dizziness occurs, sit or lie down immediately. Full therapeutic response may not occur for up to 2 wks. Avoid tasks that require alertness, motor skills until response to drug is established. Report excessively slow pulse rate (<60 beats/min), peripheral numbness, dizziness. Do not use nasal decongestants, over-the-counter cold preparations (stimulants) w/o physician approval. Outpatients should monitor B/P, pulse before taking medication. Restrict salt, alcohol intake.

penicillamine

pen-ih-sill´ah-mine
(Cuprimine, Depen)

CANADIAN AVAILABILITY:
Cuprimine, Depen

CLASSIFICATION

Chelating agent, anti-inflammatory

PHARMACOKINETICS

Well absorbed from GI tract. Protein binding: 80%. Metabolized in liver. Primarily excreted in urine. Half-life: 1.7-3.2 hrs.

ACTION

Chelates copper, iron, mercury, lead to form complexes excreted by kidney. Combines w/cystine forming complex, thus reducing concentration of cystine to below levels for formation of cystine stones. May dissolve existing stones. *Rheumatoid arthritis:* Exact mechanism unknown. May decrease cell-mediated immune response; acts as anti-inflammatory drug; may inhibit collagen formation.

USES

Promotes excretion of copper in treatment of Wilson's disease; decreases excretion of cystine, prevents renal calculi in cystinuria associated w/nephrolithiasis; treatment of active rheumatoid arthritis not controlled w/conventional therapy.

PO ADMINISTRATION

1. Preferably, give on empty stomach (1 hr before or 2 hrs after meals) or at least 1 hr from any drug, food, or milk.
2. Take w/large amounts of water when treating cystinuria.
3. Largest single dose is 500 mg; give larger amounts in divided doses.
4. Tablets may be crushed; do not crush or break capsules.

INDICATIONS/DOSAGE/ROUTES

Wilson's disease:
NOTE: Base dosage on urinary copper excretion, serum free copper concentration that produces/maintains negative copper balance. Give w/10-40 mg sulfurated potash at each meal for 6-12 mo.
PO: Adults, elderly, children: Initially, 250 mg 4 times/day. (Some pts may start at 250 mg/day, gradually increase.) Doses of 750-1500 mg/day that produce initial 24 hr cupruresis >2 mg should be continued for 3 mo. **Maintenance:** Based on serum free copper con-

centration (<10 mcg/dl indicative of adequate maintenance). **Maximum:** 2 Gm/day.

Cystinuria:
NOTE: Give in 4 equal doses; if not feasible, give larger dose at bedtime. Dose based on urinary cystine excretion. Maintain high fluid intake.
PO: Adults, elderly: Initially, 250 mg/day. Gradually increase dose. **Maintenance:** 2 Gm/day. **Range:** 1-4 Gm/day. **Children:** 30 mg/kg/day.

Rheumatoid arthritis:
PO: Adults, elderly: Initially, 125-250 mg/day. May increase by 125-250 mg/day at 1-3 mo intervals. **Maintenance:** 500-750 mg/day. After 2-3 mo w/no improvement or toxicity, may increase by 250 mg/day at 2-3 mo intervals until remission or toxicity. **Maximum:** 1 Gm up to 1.5 Gm/day.

PRECAUTIONS

CONTRAINDICATIONS: History of penicillamine-related aplastic anemia or agranulocytosis, rheumatoid arthritis pts w/history or evidence of renal insufficiency, pregnancy, breast-feeding. **CAUTIONS:** Elderly, debilitated, impaired renal/hepatic function, penicillin allergy. **PREGNANCY/LACTATION:** Birth defects noted (pyloric stenosis, hypotonia, perforated bowel, growth retardation, vein fragility, hypertrophy of skin and subcutaneous tissues). Pregnancy, lactation contraindicated. **Pregnancy Category C.**

INTERACTIONS

DRUG INTERACTIONS: Iron supplements, antacids, food may decrease absorption. Bone marrow depressants, gold compounds, immunosuppressants may increase risk of hematologic, renal adverse effects. **ALTERED LAB VALUES:** None significant.

SIDE EFFECTS

FREQUENT: Rash (pruritic, erythematous, maculopapular, morbilliform), reduced/altered sense of taste (hypogeusia), GI disturbances (anorexia, epigastric pain, nausea, vomiting, diarrhea), oral ulcers, glossitis. **OCCASIONAL:** Proteinuria, hematuria, hot flashes, drug fever. **RARE:** Alopecia, tinnitus, pemphigoid rash (water blisters).

ADVERSE REACTIONS/TOXIC EFFECTS

Aplastic anemia, agranulocytosis, thrombocytopenia, leukopenia, myasthenia gravis, bronchiolitis, erythematous-like syndrome, evening hypoglycemia, skin friability at sites of pressure/trauma producing extravasation or white papules at venipuncture, surgical sites reported. Iron deficiency (particularly children, menstruating women) may develop.

P

NURSING IMPLICATIONS

BASELINE ASSESSMENT:

Baseline WBC, differential, hemoglobin, platelet count should be performed before therapy begins, every 2 wks thereafter for first 6 mo, then monthly during therapy. Liver function tests (GGT, SGOT, SGPT, LDH) and x-ray for renal stones should also be ordered. A 2 hr interval is necessary between iron and penicillamine therapy. In event of upcoming surgery, dosage should be reduced to 250 mg/day until wound healing is complete.

INTERVENTION/EVALUATION:

Encourage copious amounts of

water in those w/cystinuria. Monitor WBC, differential, platelet count. If WBC <3500, neutrophils <2000/mm^3, monocytes >500/mm^3, or platelet counts <100,000 or if a progressive fall in either platelet count or WBC in 3 successive determinations noted, inform physician (drug withdrawal necessary). Assess for evidence of hematuria. Monitor urinalysis for hematuria, proteinuria (if proteinuria exceeds 1 Gm/24 hrs, inform physician).

PATIENT/FAMILY TEACHING:

Promptly report any missed menstrual periods/other indications of pregnancy, fever, sore throat, chills, bruising, bleeding, difficulty breathing on exertion, unexplained cough or wheezing. Take medication 1 hr before or 2 hrs after meals or at least 1 hr from any other drug, food, or milk.

penicillin G benzathine

pen-ih-sil´lin G benz´ah-thene
(Bicillin)

FIXED COMBINATION(S):
W/penicillin G procaine, an antibiotic (Bicillin CR)

CANADIAN AVAILABILITY:
Bicillin, Megacillin

CLASSIFICATION

Antibiotic: Penicillin

PHARMACOKINETICS

Slowly absorbed after IM administration. Widely distributed. Protein binding: 60%. Metabolized in liver. Primarily excreted in urine. Moderately removed by hemodialysis. Half-life: 0.5-0.7 hrs (increase in decreased renal function).

ACTION

Bactericidal. Binds to bacterial membranes. Inhibits cell wall synthesis.

USES

Mild to moderate infections of respiratory tract, skin and skin structure, rheumatic fever prophylaxis, early syphilis, yaws, bejel, pinta. Follow-up to IM/IV therapy w/penicillin G potassium, sodium.

STORAGE/HANDLING

Refrigerate.

IM ADMINISTRATION

NOTE: Do not give IV, intra-arterially, intravascularly, or SubQ. Space doses evenly around the clock.

IM:

1. Give IM injection deeply into gluteus maximus or midlateral thigh.
2. Do not administer if blood is aspirated; draw up new dose; select another site.
3. Avoid areas of nerves, repeated IM injections into anterolateral thigh.
4. Administer IM injection slowly; stop if pt complains of severe pain.

INDICATIONS/DOSAGE/ROUTES

Usual parenteral dosage:
IM: Adults, elderly: 1.2 million U one time. **Children >27 kg:** 900,000-1.2 million U one time. **Children <27 kg, infants:** 300,000-600,000 U/kg one time. **Neonates:** 50,000 U/kg one time.

PRECAUTIONS

CONTRAINDICATIONS: Hypersensitivity to any penicillin. **CAUTIONS:** Renal impairment, history of allergies, particularly cephalosporins, aspirin (tartrazine reaction may occur in those sensitive to aspirin). **PREGNANCY/LACTATION:** Readily crosses placenta, appears in cord blood, amniotic fluid. Distributed in breast milk in low concentrations. May lead to allergic sensitization, diarrhea, candidiasis, skin rash in infant. **Pregnancy Category B.**

INTERACTIONS

DRUG INTERACTIONS: Probenecid may increase concentration, toxicity risk. **ALTERED LAB VALUES:** May cause positive Coombs' test.

SIDE EFFECTS

FREQUENT: GI reactions (nausea, vomiting, diarrhea). **OCCASIONAL:** Pain, induration at IM injection site. **RARE:** Bleeding.

ADVERSE REACTIONS/TOXIC EFFECTS

Hypersensitivity reactions occur frequently, ranging from rash, fever/chills to anaphylaxis. Nephrotoxicity may occur w/high parenteral dosages, preexisting renal disease. Superinfections, potentially fatal antibiotic-associated colitis may result from altered bacterial balance.

NURSING IMPLICATIONS

BASELINE ASSESSMENT:

Question for history of allergies, particularly penicillins, cephalosporins, aspirin. Obtain specimen for culture and sensitivity before giving first dose (therapy may begin before results are known).

INTERVENTION/EVALUATION:

Hold medication and promptly report rash (hypersensitivity) or diarrhea (w/fever, abdominal pain, mucus and blood in stool may indicate antibiotic-associated colitis). Assess for food tolerance. Check IM injection sites for induration, tenderness. Check for wheezing, respiratory difficulty due to tartrazine sensitivity. Monitor I&O, urinalysis, renal function tests for nephrotoxicity. Be alert for superinfection: Increased fever, onset sore throat, nausea, vomiting, diarrhea, ulceration or changes of oral mucosa, vaginal discharge, anal/genital pruritus. Evaluate hemoglobin levels and assess for signs of bleeding: Overt bleeding, bruising/swelling of tissue.

PATIENT/FAMILY TEACHING:

Continue antibiotic for full length of treatment. Space doses evenly. Discomfort may occur w/IM injection. Notify physician in event of rash, diarrhea, bleeding, bruising, other new symptom.

penicillin G potassium, sodium

(Pentids, Pfizerpen)

CANADIAN AVAILABILITY: Crystapen, Megacillin

CLASSIFICATION

Antibiotic: Penicillin

PHARMACOKINETICS

Poorly absorbed from GI tract. Widely distributed. Protein binding: 65%. Metabolized in liver. Primarily excreted in urine. Moderately removed by hemodialysis. Half-life: 20-50 min.

ACTION

Bactericidal. Binds to bacterial membranes. Inhibits cell wall synthesis.

USES

Treatment of infections of respiratory tract, skin and skin structure, bone and joints; septicemia, meningitis, endocarditis, pericarditis, diphtheria, Listeria, clostridium, disseminated gonococcal infections, actinomycosis, rheumatic fever prophylaxis, syphilis, necrotizing ulcerative gingivitis, anthrax, Lyme disease.

STORAGE/HANDLING

Store tablets at room temperature. Oral solution, after reconstitution, is stable for 14 days if refrigerated; IV infusion (piggyback) is stable for 24 hrs at room temperature, 7 days if refrigerated. Discard if precipitate forms.

PO/IV ADMINISTRATION

NOTE: Space doses evenly around the clock. For IM or IV injection, reconstitute vial based on individual manufacturer's directions.

PO:

1. Give 1 hr before or 2 hrs after meals.

IV:

1. After reconstitution, dilute w/ 50-100 ml 5% dextrose, 0.9% NaCl, or other compatible IV fluid. Infuse over 1-2 hrs in adults, 15-30 min in neonates, children.
2. Because of potential for hypersensitivity/anaphylaxis, start initial dose at few drops/min, increase slowly to ordered rate; stay w/pt first 10-15 min, then check q10min.
3. Alternating IV sites, use large veins to reduce risk of phlebitis.

INDICATIONS/DOSAGE/ROUTES

Usual oral dosage:
PO: Adults, elderly: 200,000-500,000 U q6-8h. **Children:** 25,000-90,000 U/day in 3-6 divided doses.

Usual parenteral dosage:
IV: Adults, elderly: 5 million U/day minimum. **Children:** 100,000-250,000 U/kg/day in divided doses q4h. **Infants:** 50,000-100,000 U/kg/day in divided doses q6-12h.

PRECAUTIONS

CONTRAINDICATIONS: Hypersensitivity to any penicillin. **CAUTIONS:** Renal impairment, history of allergy, particularly cephalosporins. **PREGNANCY/LACTATION:** Readily crosses placenta; appears in cord blood, amniotic fluid. Distributed in breast milk in low concentrations. May lead to allergic sensitization, diarrhea, candidiasis, skin rash in infant. **Pregnancy Category B.**

INTERACTIONS

DRUG INTERACTIONS: Probenecid may increase concentration, toxicity risk. Angiotensin converting enzyme inhibitors, potassium sparing diuretics, potassium supplements may increase risk of hyperkalemia. **ALTERED LAB VALUES:** May cause positive Coombs' test.

SIDE EFFECTS

FREQUENT: GI reactions (nausea, vomiting, diarrhea) especially w/ oral penicillin. **OCCASIONAL:** High IV dosage may cause electrolyte imbalance, phlebitis, thrombophlebitis. **RARE:** Bleeding.

ADVERSE REACTIONS/TOXIC EFFECTS

Hypersensitivity reactions occur frequently, ranging from rash, fever/chills to anaphylaxis. Nephrotoxicity, neurotoxicity have occurred w/high dosages, preexisting renal impairment. Superinfections, potentially fatal antibiotic-associated colitis may result from altered bacterial balance.

NURSING IMPLICATIONS

BASELINE ASSESSMENT:

Question for history of allergies, esp. penicillins, cephalosporins. Obtain specimen for culture and sensitivity before giving first dose (therapy may begin before results are known).

INTERVENTION/EVALUATION:

Hold medication and promptly report rash (hypersensitivity) or diarrhea (w/fever, abdominal pain, mucus and blood in stool may indicate antibiotic-associated colitis). Assess food tolerance. Monitor electrolytes, particularly potassium. Evaluate IV site for phlebitis (heat, pain, red streaking over vein). Check IM injection sites for induration, tenderness. Monitor I&O, urinalysis, renal function tests for nephrotoxicity. Check for superinfection: Increased fever, onset sore throat, nausea, vomiting, diarrhea, ulceration or changes of oral mucosa, vaginal discharge, anal/genital pruritus. Review hemoglobin levels and be alert for signs of bleeding: Overt bleeding, bruising or swelling of tissue.

PATIENT/FAMILY TEACHING:

Continue antibiotic for full length of treatment. Space doses evenly. Notify physician immediately in event of rash, diarrhea, bleeding, bruising, or other new symptom. Sodium content of penicillin G sodium must be considered for those on sodium-restricted diets.

penicillin G procaine

(Crystacillin, Duracillin, Pfizerpen, Wycillin)

FIXED-COMBINATION(S):
W/probenecid, a renal tubular blocking agent (Wycillin & Probenecid); w/penicillin G benzathine, an antibiotic (Bicillin-CR)

CANADIAN AVAILABILITY:
Ayercillin, Wycillin 5 Million

CLASSIFICATION

Antibiotic: Penicillin

PHARMACOKINETICS

Slowly absorbed after IM administration. Widely distributed. Protein binding: 60%. Metabolized in liver. Primarily excreted in urine. Moderately removed by hemodialysis. Half-life: 0.5-0.7 hrs (increase in decreased renal function).

ACTION

Bactericidal. Binds to bacterial membranes. Inhibits cell wall synthesis.

USES

Treatment of moderately severe infections of respiratory tract, skin, skin structure, otitis media, yaws, bejel, pinta, syphilis; prophylactically for rheumatic fever, dental procedures.

STORAGE/HANDLING

Refrigerate parenteral form.

IM ADMINISTRATION

NOTE: Do not give IV, intra-arterially, intravascularly, or SubQ. Space doses evenly around the clock.

1. Give IM injection deeply into gluteus maximus or midlateral thigh.
2. Do not administer if blood is aspirated; draw up new dose, select another site.
3. Avoid repeated IM injections into anterolateral thigh, areas w/ nerves.
4. Administer slowly.

INDICATIONS/DOSAGE/ROUTES

Moderate to severe upper respiratory tract, otitis media, tonsillitis, pharyngitis, skin/skin structure infections, uncomplicated pneumonia:
IM: Adults, elderly, children: 600,000-1,200,000 U/day. **Children <60 lbs:** 300,000 U/day.

Acute uncomplicated gonorrhea:
IM: Adults, elderly: 4.8 million U one time in divided doses (w/1 Gm probenecid 30 min before penicillin).

Syphilis:
IM: Adults, elderly: 600,000 U/day for 8 days.

Neurosyphilis:
IM: Adults, elderly: 2.4 million U/day and probenecid 500 mg 4 times/day for 10 days, follow w/ penicillin G benzathine 2.4 million U weekly × 3 wks.

Congenital syphilis:
IM: Children <70 lbs, neonates: 50,000 U/kg/day for 10-14 days.

PRECAUTIONS

CONTRAINDICATIONS: Hypersensitivity to any penicillin or procaine. **CAUTIONS:** Renal impairment, history of asthma, allergies, particularly cephalosporins. **PREGNANCY/LACTATION:** Readily crosses placenta; appears in cord blood, amniotic fluid. Distributed in breast milk in low concentrations. May lead to allergic sensitization, diarrhea, candidiasis, skin rash in infant. **Pregnancy Category B.**

INTERACTIONS

DRUG INTERACTIONS: Probenecid may increase concentration, toxicity risk. **ALTERED LAB VALUES:** May cause positive Coombs' test.

SIDE EFFECTS

FREQUENT: Mild hypersensitivity reaction (rash, fever/chills), GI reactions, particularly diarrhea. **OCCASIONAL:** Pain, induration at IM injection site. **RARE:** Bleeding.

ADVERSE REACTIONS/TOXIC EFFECTS

Severe hypersensitivity reactions, including anaphylaxis, occur frequently. Toxic reaction to procaine (confusion, combativeness, seizures) may occur when large dose is administered. Nephrotoxicity, superinfection (including potentially fatal antibiotic-associated colitis) may result from high dosage, prolonged therapy.

NURSING IMPLICATIONS

BASELINE ASSESSMENT:

Question for history of allergies, particularly penicillins, procaine, cephalosporins. Obtain specimen for culture and sensitivity before giving first dose (therapy may begin before results are known).

INTERVENTION/EVALUATION:

Hold medication and promptly

report rash (possible hypersensitivity) or diarrhea (w/fever, abdominal pain, mucus and blood in stool may indicate antibiotic-associated colitis). Assess food tolerance. Evaluate IM injection sites for induration, tenderness. Monitor I&O, urinalysis, renal function tests for nephrotoxicity. Be alert to superinfection: Increased fever, onset sore throat, nausea, vomiting, diarrhea, ulceration or changes of oral mucosa, vaginal discharge, anal/genital pruritus. Review hemoglobin levels; check for bleeding: Overt bleeding, bruising or swelling of tissue.

PATIENT/FAMILY TEACHING:

Continue antibiotic for full length of treatment. Space doses evenly. Discomfort may occur at IM injection site (less discomfort than other penicillins because of procaine). Notify physician in event of rash, diarrhea, bleeding, bruising, other new symptom.

penicillin V potassium

(Pen Vee K, V-Cillin-K, Veetids)

CANADIAN AVAILABILITY: Apo-Pen VK, Nadopen-V, Novopen VK, V-Cillin-K

CLASSIFICATION

Antibiotic: Penicillin

PHARMACOKINETICS

Moderately absorbed from GI tract. Widely distributed. Protein binding: 80%. Metabolized in liver. Primarily excreted in urine. Half-life: 1 hr (increased in decreased renal function).

ACTION

Bactericidal. Binds to bacterial membranes. Inhibits cell wall synthesis.

USES

Treatment of mild to moderate infections of respiratory tract and skin/skin structure, otitis media, necrotizing ulcerative gingivitis, prophylaxis for rheumatic fever, dental procedures.

STORAGE/HANDLING

Store tabs at room temperature. Oral solution, after reconstitution, is stable for 14 days if refrigerated.

PO ADMINISTRATION

1. Space doses evenly around the clock.
2. Give w/o regard to meals.

INDICATIONS/DOSAGE/ROUTES

Usual adult, elderly dosage:
PO: Adults, elderly: 125-500 mg 4 times/day.

Usual children's dosage:
PO: Children: 15-50 mg/kg/day in divided doses q6-8h.

PRECAUTIONS

CONTRAINDICATIONS: Hypersensitivity to any penicillin. **CAUTIONS:** Renal impairment, history of allergies, particularly cephalosporins, aspirin. **PREGNANCY/LACTATION:** Readily crosses placenta; appears in cord blood, amniotic fluid. Distributed in breast milk in low concentrations. May lead to allergic sensitization, diarrhea, candidiasis, skin rash in infant. **Pregnancy Category B.**

P

INTERACTIONS

DRUG INTERACTIONS: Probenecid may increase concentration, toxicity risk. **ALTERED LAB VALUES:** May cause positive Coombs' test.

SIDE EFFECTS

FREQUENT: Mild hypersensitivity reaction (rash, fever/chills), nausea, vomiting, diarrhea. **RARE:** Bleeding, allergic reactions.

ADVERSE REACTIONS/TOXIC EFFECTS

Severe hypersensitivity reaction, including anaphylaxis, may occur. Nephrotoxicity, superinfections (including potentially fatal antibiotic-associated colitis) may result from high dosages, prolonged therapy.

NURSING IMPLICATIONS

BASELINE ASSESSMENT:

Question for history of allergies, particularly penicillins, cephalosporins. Obtain specimen for culture and sensitivity before giving first dose (therapy may begin before results are known).

INTERVENTION/EVALUATION:

Hold medication and promptly report rash (hypersensitivity) or diarrhea (w/fever, abdominal pain, mucus and blood in stool may indicate antibiotic-associated colitis). Assess food tolerance. Monitor I&O, urinalysis, renal function tests for nephrotoxicity. Be alert for superinfection: Increased fever, onset sore throat, nausea, vomiting, diarrhea, ulceration or changes of oral mucosa, vaginal discharge, anal/genital pruritus. Review hemoglobin levels; check for bleeding: Overt bleeding, bruising or swelling of tissue.

PATIENT/FAMILY TEACHING:

Continue antibiotic for full length of treatment. Space doses evenly. Notify physician immediately in event of rash, diarrhea, bleeding, bruising, or other new symptom.

pentaerythritol tetranitrate (P.E.T.N.)

pen-tah-rith´rih-toll
(Duotrate, Peritrate)

CANADIAN AVAILABILITY:
Peritrate Forte

CLASSIFICATION

Nitrate

PHARMACOKINETICS

	ONSET	PEAK	DURATION
PO	30 min	—	5 hrs
Ext-release	30 min	—	Up to 12 hrs

Readily absorbed from GI tract. Undergoes extensive first-pass metabolism. Metabolized in liver, blood (enzymatic). Primarily excreted in urine.

ACTION

Decreases myocardial oxygen demand. Reduces left ventricular preload and afterload. Dilates coronary arteries, improves collateral blood flow to ischemic areas within myocardium.

USES

Prophylaxis, treatment of angina unassociated w/acute attacks.

PO ADMINISTRATION

1. May crush scored tablets.
2. Do not crush or break extended-release tablets or capsules.
3. Give extended-release form on empty stomach.

INDICATIONS/DOSAGE/ROUTES

Prophylaxis, treatment of angina:
PO: Adults, elderly: 10-20 mg 4 times/day. Increase up to 40 mg 4 times/day.
EXTENDED RELEASE: Adults, elderly: 30-80 mg q8-12h.

PRECAUTIONS

CONTRAINDICATIONS: Hypersensitivity to nitrates, severe anemia, closed angle glaucoma, postural hypotension, head trauma, increased intracranial pressure. **CAUTIONS:** Acute MI, hepatic/renal disease, glaucoma (contraindicated in closed angle glaucoma), blood volume depletion from diuretic therapy, systolic B/P below 90 mm Hg. **PREGNANCY/LACTATION:** Unknown whether drug crosses placenta or is distributed in breast milk. **Pregnancy Category C.**

INTERACTIONS

DRUG INTERACTIONS: Alcohol, antihypertensives, vasodilators may increase risk of orthostatic hypotension. **ALTERED LAB VALUES:** None significant.

SIDE EFFECTS

FREQUENT: Headache (may be severe) occurs mostly in early therapy, diminishes rapidly in intensity, usually disappears during continued treatment; transient flushing of face and neck, dizziness (esp. if pt is standing immobile or is in a warm environment), weakness, postural hypotension. **OCCASIONAL:** GI upset.

ADVERSE REACTIONS/TOXIC EFFECTS

Drug should be discontinued if blurred vision, dry mouth occur. Severe postural hypotension manifested by fainting, pulselessness, cold/clammy skin, profuse sweating. Tolerance may occur w/repeated, prolonged therapy (minor tolerance w/intermittent use of sublingual tablets). High dose tends to produce severe headache.

NURSING IMPLICATIONS

BASELINE ASSESSMENT:

Record onset, type (sharp, dull, squeezing), radiation, location, intensity, and duration of anginal pain and precipitating factors (exertion, emotional stress).

INTERVENTION/EVALUATION:

Assist w/ambulation if lightheadedness, dizziness occurs. Assess for facial/neck flushing. Monitor B/P for hypotension.

PATIENT/FAMILY TEACHING:

Rise slowly from lying to sitting position and dangle legs momentarily before standing. Take oral form on empty stomach. Do not change from one brand of drug to another. Avoid alcohol (intensifies hypotensive effect). If alcohol is ingested soon after taking nitroglycerin, possible acute hypotensive episode (marked drop in B/P, vertigo, pallor) may occur.

pentamidine isethionate

pen-tam´ih-deen
(NebuPent, Pentam-300)

CANADIAN AVAILABILITY:
Pentacarinat, Pneumopent

CLASSIFICATION

Anti-infective

PHARMACOKINETICS

Minimal absorption following inhalation, well absorbed after IM administration. Widely distributed. Protein binding: 69%. Primarily excreted in urine. Minimally removed by hemodialysis. Half-life: 6.5 hrs (increased in decreased renal function).

ACTION

Exact mechanism unknown. May interfere w/incorporation of nucleotides into RNA, DNA; may inhibit oxidative phosphorylation. Inhibits DNA, RNA, phospholipid, protein synthesis.

USES

Treatment of pneumonia caused by *Pneumocystis carinii* (PCP). Prevention of PCP in high-risk HIV-infected pts.

STORAGE/HANDLING

Store vials at room temperature. After reconstitution, IV solution and aerosol are stable for 48 hrs at room temperature. Use freshly prepared aerosol solution. Discard unused portion.

IM/IV/INHALATION ADMINISTRATION

NOTE: Pt must be in supine position during administration w/frequent B/P checks until stable (potential for life-threatening hypotensive reaction). Have resuscitative equipment nearby.

IM:

1. Reconstitute 300 mg vial w/3 ml sterile water for injection to provide concentration of 100 mg/ml.

IV:

1. For intermittent IV infusion (piggyback), reconstitute each vial w/3-5 ml 5% dextrose or sterile water for injection.
2. Withdraw desired dose and further dilute w/50-250 ml 5% dextrose; infuse over 60 min.
3. Do not give by IV injection or rapid IV infusion (increases potential for severe hypotension).

AEROSOL (NEBULIZER):

1. Reconstitute 300 mg vial w/6 ml sterile water for injection. Avoid saline (may cause precipitate).
2. Do not mix w/other medication in nebulizer reservoir.

INDICATIONS/DOSAGE/ROUTES

Pneumocystis carinii ***pneumonia:***
IM/IV: Adults, elderly, children: 4 mg/kg/day once daily for 14 days.

Prevention **P. carinii** ***pneumonia:***
AEROSOL (NEBULIZER):
Adults, elderly: 300 mg once q4wks via nebulizer.

PRECAUTIONS

CONTRAINDICATIONS: When PCP has been firmly established, there are no absolute contraindications. Inhalation of drug is contraindicated in those w/history of severe asthma or anaphylactic reaction to drug, by any route. **CAUTIONS:** Hyper/hypotension, hepatic/renal dysfunction, hyper/hypoglycemia, hypocalcemia, thrombocytopenia, leukopenia, anemia. **PREGNANCY/LACTATION:** Unknown whether crosses placenta or is distributed in breast milk. **Pregnancy Category C.**

INTERACTIONS

DRUG INTERACTIONS: Blood dyscrasias–producing medication, bone marrow depressants may increase abnormal hematologic effects. Didanosine may increase risk of pancreatitis. Foscarnet may increase hypocalcemia, hypomagnesemia, nephrotoxicity. Nephrotoxic medications may increase risk of nephrotoxicity. **ALTERED LAB VALUES:** May increase SGOT (AST), SGPT (ALT), alkaline phosphatase, bilirubin, BUN, creatinine. May decrease calcium, magnesium. May alter glucose levels.

SIDE EFFECTS

FREQUENT: Pain, induration, sterile abscess at IM site, elevated serum creatinine w/mild to moderate renal insufficiency. **OCCASIONAL:** Moderate to severe hypotension, ulceration/necrosis at IM site, phlebitis w/IV administration, leukopenia, thrombocytopenia, hypoglycemia, arrhythmias, nausea, and anorexia. Reversible bronchospasm has occurred w/inhalation therapy. **RARE:** Bad taste in the mouth, anemia, rash, urticaria, pruritus, dizziness w/o hypotension.

ADVERSE REACTIONS/TOXIC EFFECTS

Life-threatening/fatal hypotension, arrhythmias, hypoglycemia, or leukopenia; nephrotoxicity and renal failure; anaphylactic shock; Stevens-Johnson syndrome; toxic epidural necrolysis. Hyperglycemia and insulin-dependent diabetes mellitus (often permanent) may occur even months after therapy.

NURSING IMPLICATIONS

BASELINE ASSESSMENT:

Question history of anaphylactic reaction to pentamidine isethionate. Avoid concurrent use of nephrotoxic drugs. Establish baseline for B/P, blood glucose. Obtain specimens for diagnostic tests before giving first dose.

INTERVENTION/EVALUATION:

Monitor B/P during administration until stable for both IM and IV administration (pt should remain supine). Check glucose levels and clinical signs for hypoglycemia (sweating, nervousness, tremor, tachycardia, palpitation, lightheadedness, headache, numbness of lips, double vision, incoordination), hyperglycemia (polyuria, polyphagia, polydipsia, malaise, visual changes, abdominal pain, headache, nausea/vomiting). Evaluate IM sites for pain, redness, and induration; IV sites for phlebitis (heat, pain, red streaking over vein). Monitor renal, hepatic, and hematology test results. Assess skin for rash. Determine food tolerance. Evaluate equilibrium during ambulation. Be alert for respiratory difficulty when administering by inhalation route.

PATIENT/FAMILY TEACHING:

Remain flat in bed during administration of medication and get up slowly w/assistance when B/P stable. Notify nurse immediately of sweating, shakiness, light-headedness, palpitations. Even several months after therapy stops, drowsiness, increased urination, thirst, anorexia may develop—notify nurse/physician immediately. Mouthwash, hard candy, or gum may help w/unpleasant taste that can occur.

pentazocine

pen-tah´sew-seen
(Talwin [parenteral])

FIXED-COMBINATION(S):
W/naloxone, a narcotic antagonist (oral) (Talwin NX); w/aspirin (oral) (Talwin Compound); w/acetaminophen (oral) (Talacen)

CANADIAN AVAILABILITY:
Talwin

CLASSIFICATION

Opioid analgesic **(Schedule IV)**

PHARMACOKINETICS

	ONSET	PEAK	DURATION
PO	15-30 min	1-3 hrs	>3 hrs
SubQ	15-20 min	—	—
IM	15-20 min	1 hr	2 hrs
IV	2-3 min	15 min	1 hr

Well absorbed from GI tract; after IM, SubQ administration. Widely distributed. Protein binding: 60%. Metabolized in liver. Primarily excreted in urine. Half-life: 2-3 hrs.

ACTION

Binds w/opioid receptors within CNS, altering processes affecting pain perception, emotional response to pain. May displace opioid agonists and competitively inhibit their action (may precipitate withdrawal symptoms).

USES

Relief of moderate to severe pain. Parenteral form used preop or preanesthetic or as supplement to surgical anesthesia.

STORAGE/HANDLING

Store oral, parenteral form at room temperature.

PO/SubQ/IM/IV ADMINISTRATION

PO:

1. Scored tablets may be crushed; do not crush or break Talwin Compound caplets.
2. May give w/o regard to meals but give w/food or milk if GI distress is evident.

SubQ:

1. Give SubQ only if absolutely necessary (severe tissue damage possible at injection sites).

IM:

1. Give deep into upper outer quadrant of buttock, always rotating sites (severe sclerosing of skin, tissue and muscle damage may occur at repeated injection site).

IV:

1. Do not mix in same syringe w/soluble barbiturates (precipitation will occur).
2. May be given undiluted or diluted (each 5 mg w/1 ml sterile water for direct injection).
3. Administer each 5 mg or fraction thereof >1 min.

INDICATIONS/DOSAGE/ROUTES

NOTE: Do not mix parenteral form in same syringe w/soluble barbiturates.

Analgesia:
PO: Adults: 50 mg q3-4h. May in-

crease to 100 mg q3-4h, if needed. **Maximum:** 600 mg/day.
SubQ/IM/IV: Adults: 30 mg q3-4h. Do not exceed 30 mg IV or 60 mg SubQ/IM per dose. **Maximum:** 360 mg/day.

Usual elderly dosage:
PO: Elderly: 50 mg q4h prn.
IM: Elderly: 25 mg q4h prn.

Obstetric labor:
IM: Adults: 30 mg.
IV: Adults: 20 mg when contractions are regular. May repeat 2-3 times q2-3h.

PRECAUTIONS

CONTRAINDICATIONS: Hypersensitivity to naloxone. **CAUTIONS:** Impaired hepatic/renal function, elderly, debilitated, head injury, respiratory disease, prior to biliary tract surgery (produces spasm of sphincter of Oddi), MI w/ nausea, vomiting. **PREGNANCY/LACTATION:** Readily crosses placenta; unknown whether distributed in breast milk. Prolonged use during pregnancy may produce withdrawal symptoms (irritability, excessive crying, tremors, hyperactive reflexes, fever, vomiting, diarrhea, yawning, sneezing, seizures) in neonate. **Pregnancy Category C.**

INTERACTIONS

DRUG INTERACTIONS: Alcohol, CNS depressants may increase CNS, respiratory depression, hypotension. MAO inhibitors may produce severe, fatal reaction (reduce dose to 1/4 usual dose). Effects may be decreased w/buprenorphine. **ALTERED LAB VALUES:** May increase amylase, lipase.

SIDE EFFECTS

FREQUENT: Sedation, decreased respirations, nausea, dizziness, lightheadedness, sweaty palms, clammy skin, dry mouth, headache. **RARE:** Restlessness, crying, hallucinations, GI upset, vomiting, bitter taste, urinary urgency, skin burning/itching, blurred vision.

ADVERSE REACTIONS/TOXIC EFFECTS

Overdosage results in severe respiratory depression, skeletal muscle flaccidity, cyanosis, extreme somnolence progressing to convulsions, stupor, coma. Abrupt withdrawal after prolonged use may produce symptoms of narcotic withdrawal (abdominal cramps, rhinorrhea, lacrimation, nausea, vomiting, restlessness, anxiety, increased temperature, piloerection [goosebumps]). Tolerance to analgesic effect and physical dependence may occur w/chronic use.

NURSING IMPLICATIONS

BASELINE ASSESSMENT:

Raise bed rails. Obtain vital signs before giving medication. If respirations are 12/min or lower, withhold medication, contact physician. Assess onset, type, location, and duration of pain. Effect of medication is reduced if full pain recurs before next dose.

INTERVENTION/EVALUATION:

Encourage deep breathing and coughing exercises. Check vital signs periodically (5-10 min after IV dose). Monitor for change in respirations, B/P, change in rate/quality of pulse. Initiate deep breathing and coughing exercises, particularly in those w/impaired pulmonary function. Change pt's position q2-4h. Assess for clinical improvement and record onset of relief of pain. Contact physician if pain is not adequately relieved.

PATIENT/FAMILY TEACHING:

Change positions slowly to avoid dizziness. Head-low position may help relieve lightheadedness, nausea. Explain need for assistance if ambulating. Avoid alcohol. Request pain medication before pain fully recurs.

pentobarbital

pent-oh-bar′bih-tall

(Nembutal)

pentobarbital sodium

(Nembutal Sodium)

CANADIAN AVAILABILITY:
Nembutal, Nova-Rectal, Novopentobarb

CLASSIFICATION

Sedative-hypnotic **(Schedule II)**

PHARMACOKINETICS

	ONSET	PEAK	DURATION
PO	15-60 min	30-60 min	1-4 hrs
IM	10-25 min	—	—
IV	1 min	—	15 min
Rectal	15-60 min	—	1-4 hrs

Variably absorbed after oral, parenteral administration. Rapidly, widely distributed. Protein binding: 60-70%. Metabolized in liver. Primarily excreted in urine. Half-life: 15-50 hrs.

ACTION

CNS depressant producing all levels from mild sedation, hypnosis to deep coma.

USES

Treatment of insomnia (up to 2 wks), preop sedation, routine sedation; parenteral form to control status epilepticus, acute seizure episodes, facilitate intubation procedures, control agitated behavior in psychosis, provide hypnosis for general, spinal, regional anesthesia.

STORAGE/HANDLING

Store capsules, elixir, parenteral form at room temperature. Refrigerate suppositories. Discard parenteral solution if precipitate forms or solution becomes cloudy.

PO/IM/IV/RECTAL ADMINISTRATION

PO:

1. Give w/o regard to meals.
2. Elixir may be given w/water, milk, or fruit juice.

PARENTERAL FORM: Do not mix w/acidic solutions (produces precipitate).

IM:

1. Do not inject more than 250 mg or 5 ml in any one IM injection site.
2. Inject IM deep into gluteus maximus or lateral aspect of thigh.

IV:

1. Administer IV at rate not greater than 50 mg/min (a too rapid IV may produce severe hypotension, marked respiratory depression).
2. Monitor vital signs q3-5min during and q15min for 1-2 hrs after administration for excessive narcosis (deep unconsciousness, amnesia).

3. Inadvertent intra-arterial injection may result in arterial spasm w/severe pain, tissue necrosis. Extravasation in subcutaneous tissue may produce redness, tenderness, tissue necrosis. If either occurs, treat w/injection of 0.5% procaine solution into affected area, apply moist heat.

RECTAL:

1. Moisten suppository w/cold water before inserting well up into rectum.

INDICATIONS/DOSAGE/ROUTES

NOTE: Reduce dosage in elderly, debilitated, impaired liver function.

Hypnotic:
PO: Adults: 100-200 mg at bedtime.
IM: Adults: 150-200 mg. **Children:** 2-6 mg/kg or 125 mg/m^2. Do not exceed 100 mg.
RECTAL: Adults: 120 or 200 mg at bedtime. **Children 12-14 yrs:** 60-120 mg. **Children 5-12 yrs:** 60 mg. **Children 1-4 yrs:** 30-60 mg. **Children 2 mo-1 yr:** 30 mg.

Sedation:
PO: Adults: 20-40 mg 2-4 times daily.
PO/RECTAL: Children: 2-6 mg/kg daily in 3 divided doses.

Preanesthetic:
PO: Children 10-12 yrs: Average dose: 100 mg.
IM: Adults: 150-200 mg. **Children >10 yrs:** 5 mg/kg.
RECTAL: Children <10 yrs: 5 mg/kg.

Seizures, intubation procedures:
IV: Adults: Initially, 100 mg. Wait 1 min to determine full IV effect. Small doses may then be given up to total 200-500 mg.

PRECAUTIONS

CONTRAINDICATIONS: History of porphyria, bronchopneumonia. **CAUTIONS:** Uncontrolled pain (may produce paradoxical reaction), impaired liver function. **PREGNANCY/LACTATION:** Readily crosses placenta; distributed in breast milk. Produces respiratory depression in neonate during labor. May produce postpartum hemorrhage, hemorrhagic disease in newborn. Withdrawal symptoms may occur in neonates born to women who receive barbiturates during last trimester of pregnancy. **Pregnancy Category D.**

INTERACTIONS

DRUG INTERACTIONS: May decrease effects of glucocorticoids, digoxin, metronidazole, oral anticoagulants, quinidine, tricyclic antidepressants. Alcohol, CNS depressants may increase effect. May increase metabolism of carbamazepine. Valproic acid decreases metabolism, increases concentration, toxicity. **ALTERED LAB VALUES:** May decrease bilirubin.

SIDE EFFECTS

FREQUENT: Drowsiness, sedation, residual "hangover" effect, lethargy, irritability, nausea, anorexia, muscle aches and pains, gastric distress. **OCCASIONAL:** Paradoxical CNS hyperactivity/nervousness in children, excitement/restlessness in elderly (generally noted during first 2 wks of therapy, particularly noted in presence of uncontrolled pain).

ADVERSE REACTIONS/TOXIC EFFECTS

Abrupt withdrawal after prolonged therapy may produce effects ranging from markedly increased dreaming, nightmares and/or insomnia, tremor, sweating, vomiting, to hallucinations, delirium, seizures, status epilepticus. Skin eruptions appear as hypersensitivity reaction. Blood dyscrasias, liver disease, hypocalcemia occur rarely. Overdosage produces cold, clammy skin, hypothermia, severe CNS depression, cyanosis, rapid pulse, Cheyne-Stokes respirations. Toxicity may result in severe renal impairment.

NURSING IMPLICATIONS

BASELINE ASSESSMENT:

Assess B/P, pulse, respirations immediately before administration. *Hypnotic:* Raise bed rails, provide environment conducive to sleep (back rub, quiet environment, low lighting). *Seizures:* Review history of seizure disorder (frequency, duration, intensity, level of consciousness). Observe frequently for recurrence of seizure activity. Initiate seizure precautions.

INTERVENTION/EVALUATION:

Assess sleep pattern of pt. Assess elderly/debilitated for paradoxical reaction, particularly during early therapy. Evaluate for therapeutic response: *Insomnia:* Observe for decrease in number of nocturnal awakenings, increase in length of sleep duration time. *Seizures:* Observe for decrease in number, frequency of seizures.

PATIENT/FAMILY TEACHING:

Drowsiness usually diminishes w/continued therapy. Do not abruptly withdraw medication following long-term use. Avoid tasks that require alertness, motor skills until response to drug is established. Tolerance/dependence may occur w/prolonged use of high doses. Avoid alcohol and CNS depressants. Do not use during pregnancy, nursing.

pentostatin

pent´tah-stah-tin

(Nipent)

CLASSIFICATION

Antineoplastic

PHARMACOKINETICS

After IV administration, rapidly distributed to body tissues (poorly distributed to CSF). Protein binding: 4%. Excreted primarily in urine unchanged or as active metabolite. Half-life: 5.7 hrs (increased in decreased renal function).

ACTION

Inhibits enzyme ADA (increases intracellular levels of adenine deoxynucleotide leading to cell death). Greatest activity in T cells of lymphoid system. Inhibits ADA and RNA synthesis. Produces DNA damage.

USES

Treatment of hairy cell leukemia refractory to, or poor response to, interferon alpha therapy.

STORAGE/HANDLING

Refrigerate vial. Contains no preservatives; after reconstitution or dilution, use within 8 hrs when given at room temperature, environmental light. Discard unused portion. Follow institutional procedures for handling antineoplastic medication. Use protective clothing/gloves when handling.

IV ADMINISTRATION

NOTE: Give by IV injection or IV infusion (*never* SubQ or IM). Gloves, gowns, eye goggles recommended during preparation and administration of medication. If powder or solution come in contact w/skin, wash thoroughly. Avoid small veins, swollen/edematous extremities, and areas overlying joints, tendons.

1. Adequately hydrate pt before and immediately after (decreases risk of adverse renal effects).
2. Reconstitute each 10 mg vial w/5 ml 0.9% NaCl injection to provide a concentration of 2 mg/ml. Shake thoroughly to ensure dissolution.
3. For direct injection, give over 5 min.
4. For IV infusion, further dilute w/25-50 ml 5% dextrose or 0.9% NaCl and give over 20-30 min.

INDICATIONS/DOSAGE/ROUTES

NOTE: Dosage individualized based on clinical response, tolerance to adverse effects. When used in combination therapy, consult specific protocols for optimum dosage, sequence of drug administration.

Hairy cell leukemia:
IV: Adults, elderly: 4 mg/m^2 q2wks until complete response attained (w/o any major toxicity). Discontinue if no response in 6 mo; partial response in 12 mo.
NOTE: Withhold/discontinue in those w/severe reaction to pentostatin, nervous system toxicity, active underlying infections, increased serum creatinine, in pt w/neutrophil count $<$200/mm^3 w/baseline count $>$500/mm^3.

Dosage in renal impairment:
Only when benefits justify risks, give 2-3 mg/m^2 in pt w/Ccr 50-60 ml/min.

PRECAUTIONS

CONTRAINDICATIONS: None significant. **EXTREME CAUTION:** Preexisting myelosuppression, cardiac disease, impaired hepatic/renal function. **PREGNANCY/LACTATION:** If possible, avoid use during pregnancy (may be embryotoxic). Unknown whether drug is distributed in breast milk (advise to discontinue nursing before drug initiation). **Pregnancy Category D.**

INTERACTIONS

DRUG INTERACTIONS: May increase pulmonary toxicity w/fludarabine. May increase effects, toxicity of vidarabine. **ALTERED LAB VALUES:** May increase hemoglobin, granulocyte, platelet (particularly neutropenia) count, BUN, serum creatinine, liver function studies.

SIDE EFFECTS

FREQUENT: Nausea, vomiting, unexplained fever, fatigue, rash (occasionally severe), cough, upper respiratory infection, anorexia, diarrhea. **OCCASIONAL:** Hematuria, dysuria, headache, pharyngitis, sinusitis, myalgia, arthralgia, peripheral edema, anorexia, blurred vision, conjunctivitis, skin discoloration, sweating, easy bruising, anxiety, depression, dizziness, confusion.

ADVERSE REACTIONS/TOXIC EFFECTS

Bone marrow depression manifested as hematologic toxicity (principally leukopenia, anemia, thrombocytopenia). Doses higher

P

than recommended (20-50 mg/m^2 in divided doses >5 days) may produce severe renal, hepatic, pulmonary, or CNS toxicity, death.

NURSING IMPLICATIONS

BASELINE ASSESSMENT:

Provide emotional support to pt and family. Obtain CBC, differential count (particularly platelets, neutrophils, lymphocytes), liver function studies (esp. SGOT [AST], SGPT [ALT], LDH, GGT, alkaline phosphatase), creatinine before initiating therapy. Antiemetics may be effective in preventing, treating nausea.

INTERVENTION/EVALUATION:

Obtain CBC, differential count, liver function studies, creatinine at frequent intervals during therapy. Severe occurrence of rash, severe hematologic, blood chemistry values that have significantly changed from baseline or evidence of pulmonary or CNS toxicity may indicate need to terminate medication. Contact physician. Monitor closely for bone marrow suppression: evidence of infection (fever, sore throat), bleeding (easy bruising, unusual bleeding from any site), symptoms of anemia (excessive tiredness, weakness). Be alert for CNS toxicity (agitation, nervousness, confusion, anxiety, depression, insomnia). Avoid IM injections, rectal temperatures or other trauma that may induce bleeding.

PATIENT/FAMILY TEACHING:

Bone marrow aspiration and biopsy may be a necessary part of program at 2-3 mo intervals to assess treatment response. Do not have immunizations w/o physician's approval (drug lowers body's resistance). Avoid crowds, those w/infection. Promptly report fever, sore throat, signs of local infection, easy bruising or unusual bleeding from any site, emotional changes.

pentoxifylline

pen-tox-ih-fill´in
(Trental)

CANADIAN AVAILABILITY:
Trental

CLASSIFICATION

Hemorheologic

PHARMACOKINETICS

Completely absorbed from GI tract. Bound to erythrocyte membrane. Metabolized in erythrocytes, liver to active metabolite. Primarily excreted in urine. Half-life: 0.4-0.8 hrs; metabolite: 1-1.6 hrs.

ACTION

Reduces blood viscosity, improves erythrocyte flexibility, improves microcirculatory flow, tissue oxygen concentration.

USES

Symptomatic treatment of intermittent claudication associated w/occlusive peripheral vascular disease, diabetic angiopathies.

PO ADMINISTRATION

1. Do not crush or break film-coated tablets.
2. Give w/meals to avoid GI upset.

INDICATIONS/DOSAGE/ROUTES

Intermittent claudication:
PO: Adults, elderly: 400 mg 3

times/day. Decrease to 400 mg 2 times/day if GI or CNS side effects occur. Continue for at least 8 wks.

PRECAUTIONS

CONTRAINDICATIONS: History of intolerance to xanthine derivatives (caffeine, theophylline, theobromine). **CAUTIONS:** Coronary artery disease, cerebrovascular disease, impaired renal function. **PREGNANCY/LACTATION:** Unknown whether drug crosses placenta; distributed in breast milk. **Pregnancy Category C.**

INTERACTIONS

DRUG INTERACTIONS: May increase effect of antihypertensives. **ALTERED LAB VALUES:** None significant.

SIDE EFFECTS

OCCASIONAL: Dyspepsia (heartburn, indigestion, epigastric pain), nausea, dizziness. **RARE:** Headache, hand tremor, vomiting.

ADVERSE REACTIONS/TOXIC EFFECTS

Angina, chest pain occur rarely. May be accompanied by palpitations, tachycardia, arrhythmias. Overdosage (flushing, hypotension, nervousness, agitation, hand tremor, fever, somnolence) noted 4-5 hrs after ingestion, lasts 12 hrs.

NURSING IMPLICATIONS

INTERVENTION/EVALUATION:

Assist w/ambulation if dizziness occurs. Assess for hand tremor. Monitor for relief of symptoms of intermittent claudication (pain, aching, cramping in calf muscles, buttocks, thigh, feet). Symptoms generally occur while walking/exercising and not at rest or w/weight bearing in absence of walking/exercising. Monitor B/P, EKG.

PATIENT/FAMILY TEACHING:

Therapeutic effect generally noted in 2-4 wks. Avoid driving, tasks requiring alert response until response to drug known. Do not smoke (causes constriction and occlusion of peripheral blood vessels).

pergolide mesylate

purr´go-lied

(Permax)

CANADIAN AVAILABILITY:
Permax

CLASSIFICATION

Antiparkinson

PHARMACOKINETICS

Well absorbed from GI tract. Protein binding: 90%. Metabolized in liver (undergoes extensive first-pass effect). Primarily excreted in urine.

ACTION

Directly stimulates postsynaptic dopamine receptors, assisting in reduction in tremor, akinesia (absence of sense of movement), posture and equilibrium disorders, rigidity of parkinsonism. Also inhibits prolactin secretion.

USES

Adjunctive treatment w/levodopa/carbidopa in those w/Parkinson's disease.

PO ADMINISTRATION

1. Scored tablets may be crushed.

2. May be given w/o regard to meals.

INDICATIONS/DOSAGE/ROUTES

NOTE: Daily doses usually given in 3 divided doses.

Parkinsonism:
PO: Adults, elderly: Initially, 0.05 mg/day for 2 days. Increase by 0.1-0.15 mg/day q3days over following 12 days; then may increase by 0.25 mg/day q3days. **Maximum:** 5 mg/day. **Range:** 3-4.6 mg/day.

PRECAUTIONS

CONTRAINDICATIONS: None significant. **CAUTIONS:** Cardiac dysrhythmias. **PREGNANCY/LACTATION:** Unknown whether drug crosses placenta or is distributed in breast milk. May interfere w/lactation. **Pregnancy Category B.**

INTERACTIONS

DRUG INTERACTIONS: Haloperidol, loxapine, methyldopa, metoclopramide, phenothiazines may decrease effect. Hypotension producing medications may increase hypotensive effect. **ALTERED LAB VALUES:** May increase plasma growth hormone.

SIDE EFFECTS

FREQUENT: Dyskinesia (impairment of voluntary movement), nausea, dizziness, hallucinations, rhinitis, dystonia (muscle tone impairment), confusion, constipation, somnolence, orthostatic hypotension. **OCCASIONAL:** Insomnia, peripheral edema, body aches, diarrhea, dyspepsia, anxiety, abdominal cramping, visual changes, headache. **RARE:** Anorexia, dyspnea, tremor, asthenia (loss of strength/energy), dry mouth.

ADVERSE REACTIONS/TOXIC EFFECTS

High incidence of atrial premature contractions, sinus tachycardia. Overdosage may require supportive measures to maintain arterial B/P (monitor cardiac function, vital signs, blood gases, serum electrolytes). Activated charcoal may be more effective than emesis or lavage.

NURSING IMPLICATIONS

INTERVENTION/EVALUATION:

Be alert to neurologic effects: headache, lethargy, mental confusion, agitation. Monitor for evidence of dyskinesia (difficulty w/movement). Assess for clinical reversal of symptoms (improvement of tremor of head/hands at rest, mask-like facial expression, shuffling gait, muscular rigidity).

PATIENT/FAMILY TEACHING:

Tolerance to feeling of lightheadedness develops during therapy. To reduce hypotensive effect, rise slowly from lying to sitting position and permit legs to dangle momentarily before standing. Avoid tasks that require alertness, motor skills until response to drug is established. Dry mouth, drowsiness, dizziness may be expected responses of drug. Avoid alcoholic beverages during therapy. Coffee or tea may help reduce drowsiness.

---

perindopril (Aceon)
See supplement

---

perphenazine

per-fen´ah-zeen
(Trilafon)

FIXED-COMBINATION(S): W/amitriptyline, a tricyclic antidepressant (Etrafon, Triavil)

CANADIAN AVAILABILITY: Apo-Perphenazine, Trilafon

CLASSIFICATION

Antipsychotic

PHARMACOKINETICS

Well absorbed from GI tract. Widely distributed. Protein binding: >90%. Metabolized in liver to active metabolite. Primarily excreted in urine.

ACTION

Blocks postsynaptic dopaminergic receptors in brain. Possesses strong alpha-adrenergic blocking, anticholinergic effects.

USES

Management of psychotic disorders, control of nausea, vomiting, intractable hiccups.

STORAGE/HANDLING

Store oral, parenteral form at room temperature. Yellow discoloration of solution does not affect potency, but discard if markedly discolored or if precipitate forms.

PO/IM/IV ADMINISTRATION

PO:

1. Do not mix oral concentrate w/caffeine (coffee, cola, tea), apple juice because of physical incompatibility.
2. Mix each 5 ml oral concentrate w/60 ml water, 7-Up, carbonated orange drink, milk, V-8, pineapple, apricot, prune, orange, tomato, grapefruit juice.

NOTE: Parenteral Administration: Pt must remain recumbent for 30-60 min in head-low position w/legs raised, to minimize hypotensive effect.

IM:

1. Inject slow, deep IM into upper outer quadrant of gluteus maximus. If irritation occurs, dilute further injections w/0.9% NaCl or 2% procaine hydrochloride.
2. Massage IM injection site to reduce discomfort.

IV:

NOTE: Give by fractional IV injection or IV infusion.

1. For fractional IV, dilute each 5 mg (1 ml) w/9 ml 0.9% NaCl, producing final concentration of 0.5 mg/ml.
2. Do not give more than 1 mg per injection at slow rate at not less than 1-2 min intervals.
3. For IV infusion, dilute further and give at rate of 0.5 mg or less/min.

INDICATIONS/DOSAGE/ROUTES

NOTE: Decrease dose gradually to optimum response. Decrease to lowest effective level for maintenance. Replace parenteral therapy w/oral therapy as soon as possible.

Hospitalized psychotic:
PO: Adults, children >12 yrs: 8-16 mg 2-4 times/day. **Extended release:** 8-32 mg 2 times/day.

IM: Adults, children >12 yrs:

5 mg q6h, as needed.

Nonhospitalized:
PO: Adults, children >12 yrs: 4-8 mg 3 times/day. **Extended release:** 8-16 mg 2 times/day.

Severe nausea, vomiting, intractable hiccups:
IM: Adults: 5 mg.
IV: Adults: Up to 5 mg.

Usual elderly dosage (nonpsychotic):

PO: Elderly: Initially, 2-4 mg/day. May increase by 2-4 mg/day every 4-7 days. **Maximum:** 32 mg/day.

PRECAUTIONS

CONTRAINDICATIONS: Severe CNS depression, comatose states, severe cardiovascular disease, bone marrow depression, subcortical brain damage. **CAUTIONS:** Impaired respiratory/hepatic/renal/cardiac function, alcohol withdrawal, history of seizures, urinary retention, glaucoma, prostatic hypertrophy, hypocalcemia (increases susceptibility to dystonias). **PREGNANCY/LACTATION:** Crosses placenta; distributed in breast milk. **Pregnancy Category C.**

INTERACTIONS

DRUG INTERACTIONS: Alcohol, CNS depressants may increase CNS, respiratory depression, hypotensive effects. Tricyclic antidepressants, MAO inhibitors may increase sedative, anticholinergic effects. Antithyroid agents may increase risk of agranulocytosis. Extrapyramidal symptoms (EPS) may increase w/EPS producing medications. Hypotensives may increase hypotension. May decrease levodopa effects. Lithium may decrease absorption, produce adverse neurologic effects. **ALTERED LAB VALUES:** May produce false-positive pregnancy test, phenylketonuria (PKU). EKG changes may occur, including Q and T wave disturbances.

SIDE EFFECTS

FREQUENT: Hypotension, dizziness, fainting occur frequently after parenteral form is given and occasionally thereafter but rarely w/oral dosage. **OCCASIONAL:** Marked photosensitivity. Drowsiness during early therapy, dry mouth, blurred vision, lethargy, constipation/diarrhea, nasal congestion, peripheral edema, urinary retention. **RARE:** Ocular changes, skin pigmentation (those on high doses for prolonged periods).

ADVERSE REACTIONS/TOXIC EFFECTS

Extrapyramidal symptoms appear dose related (particularly high dosage) and are divided into 3 categories: akathisia (inability to sit still, tapping of feet, urge to move around), parkinsonian symptoms (mask-like face, tremors, shuffling gait, hypersalivation), and acute dystonias: torticollis (neck muscle spasm), opisthotonos (rigidity of back muscles), and oculogyric crisis (rolling back of eyes). Dystonic reaction may also produce profuse sweating, pallor. Tardive dyskinesia (protrusion of tongue, puffing of cheeks, chewing/puckering of the mouth) occurs rarely (may be irreversible). Abrupt withdrawal following long-term therapy may precipitate nausea, vomiting, gastritis, dizziness, tremors. Blood dyscrasias, particularly agranulocytosis, mild leukopenia may occur. May lower seizure threshold.

NURSING IMPLICATIONS

BASELINE ASSESSMENT:

Avoid skin contact w/solutions (contact dermatitis). *Antiemetic:* Assess for dehydration (poor skin turgor, dry mucous membranes, longitudinal furrows in tongue). *Antipsychotic:* Assess behavior, appearance, emotional status, response to environment, speech pattern, thought content.

INTERVENTION/EVALUATION:

Monitor B/P for hypotension. Assess for extrapyramidal symptoms. Monitor WBC, differential count for blood dyscrasias. Monitor for fine tongue movement (may be early sign of tardive dyskinesia). Supervise suicidal-risk pt closely during early therapy (as depression lessens, energy level improves increasing suicide potential. Assess for therapeutic response (interest in surroundings, improvement in self-care, increased ability to concentrate, relaxed facial expression). For antiemetic use: monitor I&O and food tolerance.

PATIENT/FAMILY TEACHING:

Full therapeutic effect may take up to 6 wks. Urine may turn pink or reddish-brown. Do not abruptly withdraw from long-term drug therapy. Report visual disturbances. Sugarless gum or sips of tepid water may relieve dry mouth. Drowsiness generally subsides during continued therapy. Avoid tasks that require alertness, motor skills until response to drug is established. Avoid alcohol and CNS depressants. Wear protective clothing, sunscreens in sunlight.

phenazopyridine hydrochloride

feen-ah-zoe-pigh´rih-deen
(Pyridium, Urodine)

FIXED-COMBINATION(S):
W/oxytetracycline, an antibiotic and sulfamethizole, a sulfonamide (Urobiotic-250); w/butabarbital, a barbiturate and hyoscyamine, an anticholinergic (Pyridium Plus); w/sulfasoxizole, a sulfonamide (Azo-Gantrisin); w/sulfamethoxazole, a sulfonamide (Azo-Gantanol)

CANADIAN AVAILABILITY:
Phenazo, Pyridium, Pyronium

CLASSIFICATION

Urinary analgesic

PHARMACOKINETICS

Well absorbed from GI tract. Partially metabolized in liver. Primarily excreted in urine.

ACTION

Exact mechanism unknown. Analgesic/local anesthetic activity on urinary tract mucosa.

USES

Symptomatic relief of pain, burning, urgency, frequency resulting from lower urinary tract mucosa irritation (may be caused by infection, trauma, surgery).

PO ADMINISTRATION

Give after meals.

INDICATIONS/DOSAGE/ROUTES

Analgesic:
PO: Adults: 200 mg 3 times/day. **Children:** 12 mg/kg/day in 3 divided doses for 3-15 days.

PRECAUTIONS

CONTRAINDICATIONS: Renal insufficiency. **CAUTIONS:** None significant. **PREGNANCY/LACTATION:** Unknown whether drug crosses placenta or is distributed in breast milk. **Pregnancy Category B.**

INTERACTIONS

DRUG INTERACTIONS: None significant. **ALTERED LAB VALUES:** May interfere w/urinalysis color reactions, e.g., urinary glucose, ketone tests; urinary protein, or determination of urinary steroids.

SIDE EFFECTS

OCCASIONAL: Headache, GI disturbance, rash, pruritus.

ADVERSE REACTIONS/TOXIC EFFECTS

Overdosage levels or those w/ impaired renal function or severe hypersensitivy may develop renal toxicity, hemolytic anemia, hepatic toxicity. Methemoglobinemia generally occurs as result of massive, acute overdosage.

NURSING IMPLICATIONS

INTERVENTION/EVALUATION:

Assess for therapeutic response: relief of pain, burning, urgency, frequency of urination.

PATIENT/FAMILY TEACHING:

A reddish-orange discoloration of urine should be expected. May stain fabric. Take after meals (reduces possibility of GI upset).

phenelzine sulfate

fen´ell-zeen
(Nardil)

CANADIAN AVAILABILITY:
Nardil

CLASSIFICATION

Antidepressant: MAO inhibitor

PHARMACOKINETICS

Well absorbed from GI tract. Metabolized in liver. Primarily excreted in urine.

ACTION

Inhibits monoamine oxidase enzyme (assists in metabolism of sympathomimetic amines) at CNS storage sites. Increased levels of epinephrine, norepinephrine, serotonin, dopamine at neuron receptor sites, producing antidepressant effect.

USES

Management of atypical, nonendogenous, neurotic depression associated w/anxiety, phobic, hypochondriacal features in those not responsive to other antidepressant therapy.

PO ADMINISTRATION

Give w/food if GI distress occurs.

INDICATIONS/DOSAGE/ROUTES

Depression:
PO: Adults $<$60 yrs: 15 mg 3 times daily. Increase rapidly to 60 mg daily until therapeutic response noted (2-6 wks). Thereafter, reduce dose gradually to maintenance level. **Elderly:** Initially, 7.5 mg. May increase by 7.5-15 mg q3-4 days. **Maintenance:** 15-60 mg/day in 3-4 divided doses.

CONTRAINDICATIONS: Pts $>$60 yrs, debilitated/hypertensive pts, cerebrovascular/cardiovascular disease, foods containing tryptophan/tyramine, within 10 days of elective surgery, pheochromocytoma, CHF, history of liver disease, abnormal liver function tests, severe renal impairment, history of severe/recurrent headache. **CAUTIONS:** Impaired renal function, history of seizures, parkinsonian syndrome, diabetic pts, hyperthyroidism. **PREGNANCY/**

LACTATION: Crosses placenta; unknown whether distributed in breast milk. **Pregnancy Category C.**

INTERACTIONS

DRUG INTERACTIONS: Alcohol, CNS depressants may increase CNS depressant effects. Tricyclic antidepressants, fluoxetine, trazodone may cause serotonin syndrome. May increase effect of oral hypoglycemics, insulin. B/P may increase w/buspirone. Caffeine containing medications may increase cardiac arrhythmias, hypertension. May precipitate hypertensive crises w/carbamazepine, cyclobenzaprine, maprotiline, other MAO inhibitors. Meperidine, other opioid analgesics may produce immediate excitation, seating, rigidity, severe hypertension or hypotension, severe respiratory distress, coma, convulsions, vascular collapse, death. May increase CNS stimulant effects of methylphenidate. Sympathomimetics may increase cardiac stimulant, vasopressor effects. Tyramine, foods w/pressor amines (e.g., aged cheese) may cause sudden, severe hypertension. **ALTERED LAB VALUES:** None significant.

SIDE EFFECTS

FREQUENT: Postural hypotension, restlessness, GI upset, insomnia, dizziness, headache, lethargy, weakness, dry mouth, peripheral edema. **OCCASIONAL:** Flushing, increased perspiration, rash, urinary frequency, increased appetite, transient impotence. **RARE:** Visual disturbances.

ADVERSE REACTIONS/TOXIC EFFECTS

Hypertensive crisis may be noted by hypertension, occipital headache radiating frontally, neck stiffness/soreness, nausea, vomiting, sweating, fever/chilliness, clammy skin, dilated pupils, palpitations. Tachycardia or bradycardia, constricting chest pain may also be present. Antidote for hypertensive crisis: 5-10 mg phentolamine IV injection.

NURSING IMPLICATIONS

BASELINE ASSESSMENT:

Periodic liver function tests should be performed in those requiring high dosage undergoing prolonged therapy. MAO inhibitor therapy should be discontinued for 7-14 days prior to elective surgery.

INTERVENTION/EVALUATION:

Assess appearance, behavior, speech pattern, level of interest, mood. Monitor for occipital headache radiating frontally and/or neck stiffness/soreness (may be first signal of impending hypertensive crisis). Monitor blood pressure diligently for hypertension. Discontinue medication immediately if palpitations or frequent headaches occur.

PATIENT/FAMILY TEACHING:

Antidepressant relief may be noted during first wk of therapy; maximum benefit noted in 2-6 wks. Report headache, neck stiffness/soreness immediately. To avoid orthostatic hypotension, change from lying to sitting position slowly and dangle legs momentarily before standing. Avoid tasks that require alertness, motor skills until response to drug is established. Avoid foods that require bacteria or molds for their preparation or preservation or those that contain tyramine, e.g., cheese, sour cream, beer, wine, pickled herring, liver, figs, raisins, bananas, avocados, soy sauce, yeast extracts, yogurt, papaya, broad beans, meat tenderizers, or excessive amounts of caffeine (coffee, tea, chocolate), or over-the-counter preparations for hay fever, colds, weight reduction. Avoid alcohol.

phenobarbital

feen-oh-bar′bih-tall

(Barbita, Sulfoton)

phenobarbital sodium

(Luminal)

FIXED-COMBINATION(S): W/phenytoin sodium, an anticonvulsant (Dilantin w/Phenobarbital Kapseals)

CLASSIFICATION

Anticonvulsant, hypnotic

PHARMACOKINETICS

	ONSET	PEAK	DURATION
PO	20-60 min	—	—
IM	10-15 min	—	4-6 hrs
IV	5 min	30 min	4-6 hrs

Well absorbed after oral, parenteral administration. Rapidly, widely distributed. Protein binding: 20-45%. Metabolized in liver. Primarily excreted in urine. Half-life: 53-118 hrs.

ACTION

CNS depressant producing all levels from mild sedation, hypnosis to deep coma. *Anticonvulsant:* Elevates seizure threshold for motor cortex to electrical/chemical stimulation.

USES

Management of generalized tonic-clonic (grand mal) seizures, partial seizures, control of acute convulsive episodes (status epilepticus, eclampsia, febrile seizures). Relieves anxiety, provides preop sedation.

STORAGE/HANDLING

Store oral, parenteral form at room temperature. Do not use oral liquid or parenteral form if solution is cloudy or contains precipitate.

PO/IM/IV ADMINISTRATION

PO:

1. Give w/o regard to meals. Tablets may be crushed. Capsules may be emptied and mixed w/food.
2. Elixir may be mixed w/water, milk, fruit juice.

IM:

PARENTERAL FORM: Do not mix w/acidic solutions (forms precipitate). May be diluted w/normal saline, 5% dextrose, lactated Ringer's, Ringer's.

1. Do not inject more than 5 ml in any one IM injection site (produces tissue irritation).
2. Inject IM deep into gluteus maximus or lateral aspect of thigh.

IV:

1. Administer at rate not greater than 60 mg/min (too rapid IV may produce severe hypotension, marked respiratory depression).
2. Monitor vital signs q3-5min during and q15min for 1-2 hrs after administration.
3. Inadvertent intra-arterial injection may result in arterial spasm

w/severe pain, tissue necrosis. Extravasation in subcutaneous tissue may produce redness, tenderness, tissue necrosis. If either occurs, treat w/injection of 0.5% procaine solution into affected area, apply moist heat.

INDICATIONS/DOSAGE/ROUTES

NOTE: When replacement by another anticonvulsant is necessary, decrease phenobarbital over 1 wk as therapy begins w/low replacement dose.

Anticonvulsant:
NOTE: Administration may be necessary for 2-3 wks before full therapeutic response is noted.
PO: Adults, elderly: 100-300 mg/day, preferably at bedtime. **Children:** 3-5 mg/kg/day.

Prevention of febrile seizures:
PO: Children: 3-4 mg/kg/day.

Status epilepticus, acute seizures:
IM/IV: Adults, elderly: 200-600 mg. **Children:** 100-400 mg. Administer until seizure stops or 20 mg/kg is reached.

Sedation:
PO: Adults, elderly: 30-120 mg daily, usually given in 2-3 divided doses. **Children:** 6 mg/kg/day in 3 divided doses.

Hypnotic:
PO/IM/IV: Adults, elderly: 100-320 mg.

Preop sedation, antianxiety:
IM: Adults, elderly: 100-200 mg. **Children:** 16-100 mg given 60-90 min before surgery.

PRECAUTIONS

CONTRAINDICATIONS: History of porphyria, bronchopneumonia. **EXTREME CAUTION:** Nephritis, renal insufficiency. **CAUTIONS:** Uncontrolled pain (may produce paradoxical reaction), impaired liver function. **PREGNANCY/LACTATION:** Readily crosses placenta; distributed in breast milk. Produces respiratory depression in neonates during labor. May cause postpartum hemorrhage, hemorrhagic disease in newborn. Withdrawal symptoms may appear in neonates born to women receiving barbiturates during last trimester of pregnancy. Lowers serum bilirubin concentration in neonates. **Pregnancy Category D.**

INTERACTIONS

DRUG INTERACTIONS: May decrease effects of glucocorticoids, digoxin, metronidazole, oral anticoagulants, quinidine, tricyclic antidepressants. Alcohol, CNS depressants may increase effect. May increase metabolism of carbamazepine. Valproic acid decreases metabolism, increases concentration, toxicity. **ALTERED LAB VALUES:** May decrease bilirubin.

SIDE EFFECTS

FREQUENT: Drowsiness, sedation, irritability, headache, restlessness, ataxia (muscular incoordination), joint aches, vertigo, anorexia, nausea, gastric distress. **OCCASIONAL:** Paradoxical CNS hyperactivity/nervousness in children, excitement/restlessness in elderly (generally noted during first 2 wks of therapy, particularly noted in presence of uncontrolled pain).

ADVERSE REACTIONS/TOXIC EFFECTS

Abrupt withdrawal after prolonged therapy may produce effects ranging from markedly in-

P

creased dreaming, nightmares and/or insomnia, tremor, sweating, vomiting, to hallucinations, delirium, seizures, status epilepticus. Skin eruptions appear as hypersensitivity reaction. Blood dyscrasias, liver disease, hypocalcemia occur rarely. Overdosage produces cold, clammy skin, hypothermia, severe CNS depression, cyanosis, rapid pulse, Cheyne-Stokes respirations. Toxicity may result in severe renal impairment.

NURSING IMPLICATIONS

BASELINE ASSESSMENT:

Assess B/P, pulse, respirations immediately before administration. Liver function tests, blood counts should be performed before therapy begins and periodically during therapy. *Hypnotic:* Raise bed rails, provide environment conducive to sleep (back rub, quiet environment, low lighting). *Seizures:* Review history of seizure disorder (length, presence of auras, level of consciousness). Observe frequently for recurrence of seizure activity. Initiate seizure precautions.

INTERVENTION/EVALUATION:

Assess elderly, debilitated, children for evidence of paradoxical reaction, particularly during early therapy. Evaluate for therapeutic response: Decrease in length, number of seizures. Monitor for therapeutic serum level (10-30 mcg/ml).

PATIENT/FAMILY TEACHING:

Drowsiness may gradually decrease/disappear w/continued use. Do not abruptly withdraw medication following long-term use (may precipitate seizures). Avoid tasks that require alertness, motor skills until response to drug is established. Tolerance/dependence may occur w/prolonged use of high doses. Strict maintenance of drug therapy is essential for seizure control. Avoid alcohol and other CNS depressants. Notify physician promptly of pregnancy.

phenolphthalein

feen-ohl-thay´leen
(Alophen, ExLax, Modane)

FIXED-COMBINATION(S):
W/mineral oil, a lubricant laxative (Agoral)

CANADIAN AVAILABILITY:
ExLax

CLASSIFICATION

Laxative: Stimulant

PHARMACOKINETICS

	ONSET	PEAK	DURATION
PO	6-12 hrs	—	—

Minimally absorbed from GI tract. Primarily eliminated in feces.

ACTION

Increases peristalsis by direct effect on colonic smooth musculature (stimulates intramural nerve plexi). Promotes fluid and ion accumulation in colon (increases laxative effect).

USES

Facilitates defecation in those w/ diminished colonic motor response, for evacuation of colon for rectal, bowel examination, elective colon surgery.

PO ADMINISTRATION

1. Give on an empty stomach (faster results).
2. Offer 6-8 glasses of water/day (aids stool softening).
3. Avoid giving within 1 hr of other oral medication (decreases drug absorption).

INDICATIONS/DOSAGE/ROUTES

Laxative:
PO: Adults, elderly: 1-2 tablets at bedtime.

PRECAUTIONS

CONTRAINDICATIONS: Abdominal pain, nausea, vomiting, appendicitis, intestinal obstruction. **CAUTIONS:** None significant. **PREGNANCY/LACTATION:** Distributed in breast milk. **Pregnancy Category C.**

INTERACTIONS

DRUG INTERACTIONS: May decrease transit time of concurrently administered oral medication, decreasing absorption. **ALTERED LAB VALUES:** May decrease calcium, potassium.

SIDE EFFECTS

FREQUENT: Pink to red discoloration of urine. **OCCASIONAL:** Some degree of abdominal discomfort, nausea, mild cramps, griping, faintness. **RARE:** Hypersensitivity reaction manifested by skin eruptions, rash, itching, burning, skin pigmentation.

ADVERSE REACTIONS/TOXIC EFFECTS

Long-term use may result in laxative dependence, chronic constipation, loss of normal bowel function. Chronic use or overdosage may result in electrolyte disturbances (hypokalemia, hypocalcemia, metabolic acidosis or alkalosis), persistent diarrhea, malabsorption, weight loss. Electrolyte disturbance may produce vomiting, muscle weakness.

NURSING IMPLICATIONS

INTERVENTION/EVALUATION:

Encourage adequate fluid intake. Assess bowel sounds for peristalsis. Monitor daily bowel activity and stool consistency (watery, loose, soft, semi-solid, solid). Assess for abdominal disturbances. Monitor serum electrolytes in those exposed to prolonged, frequent, or excessive use of medication.

PATIENT/FAMILY TEACHING:

Urine may turn pink to red (only temporary and is not harmful). Institute measures to promote defecation: Increase fluid intake, exercise, high-fiber diet. Do not take other oral medication within 1 hr of taking this medicine (decreased effectiveness). Cola, unsalted crackers, dry toast may relieve nausea.

phenoxybenzamine hydrochloride

fen-ox-ee-ben´zah-mean
(Dibenzyline)

CLASSIFICATION

Alpha-adrenergic blocking agent

PHARMACOKINETICS

	ONSET	PEAK	DURATION
PO	Several hrs	—	3-4 days

Variably absorbed from GI tract.

Metabolized in liver. Primarily excreted in urine. Half-life: 24 hrs.

ACTION

Irreversibly combines w/postganglionic alpha-adrenergic receptors, prevents or reverses effects of catecholamines in exocrine glands, smooth muscle.

USES

Control/prevent hypertension and sweating in pts w/pheochromocytoma.

PO ADMINISTRATION

Do not crush or break capsules.

INDICATIONS/DOSAGE/ROUTES

Pheochromocytoma:
PO: Adults, elderly: Initially, 10 mg 2 times/day. **Maintenance:** 20-40 mg 2-3 times/day. May increase dose every other day. **Children:** Initially, 0.2 mg/kg once daily. Maximum: 10 mg. **Maintenance:** 0.4-1.2 mg/kg/day in divided doses.

PRECAUTIONS

CONTRAINDICATIONS: Conditions when decrease in B/P is unwarranted. **CAUTIONS:** Compounds that produce further fall in B/P, marked cerebral/coronary arteriosclerosis, renal impairment/damage. **PREGNANCY/LACTATION:** Unknown whether drug crosses placenta or is distributed in breast milk. **Pregnancy Category C.**

INTERACTIONS

DRUG INTERACTIONS: May decrease effects of sympathomimetics (e.g., dopamine, phenylephrine). **ALTERED LAB VALUES:** None significant.

SIDE EFFECTS

Frequency of effects unknown: Dizziness, nasal stuffiness, miosis, postural hypotension, inhibition of ejaculation, GI distress, drowsiness.

ADVERSE REACTIONS/TOXIC EFFECTS

Severe hypotension.

NURSING IMPLICATIONS

INTERVENTION/EVALUATION:

Assist w/ambulation if dizziness, drowsiness occurs. Monitor B/P.

PATIENT/FAMILY TEACHING:

Side effects tend to diminish as therapy continues. Avoid alcoholic beverages. Avoid over-the-counter cough, cold medications. Change positions slowly to prevent postural hypotension. Avoid driving or tasks that require alert response until drug effects known.

phentolamine

fen-toll´ah-mean
(Regitine)

CANADIAN AVAILABILITY:
Rogitine

CLASSIFICATION

Alpha-adrenergic blocking agent

PHARMACOKINETICS

Excreted in urine. Half-life: 19 min.

ACTION

Antihypertensive: Antagonizes effects of epinephrine, norepinephrine producing vasodilation, decreased peripheral vascular resistance. *Heart failure:* Decreases afterload, pulmonary arterial pressure; increases cardiac output; produces positive inotropic effect.

USES

Diagnosis of pheochromocytoma. Control/prevent hypertensive episodes immediately before, during surgical excision. Prevent/treat dermal necrosis and sloughing following IV administration of norepinephrine/dopamine.

IM/IV ADMINISTRATION

NOTE: Maintain pt in supine position (preferably in quiet, darkened room) during pheochromocytoma testing. Decrease in B/P noted generally <2 min.

IV:

1. Reconstitute 5 mg vial w/1 ml sterile water to provide concentration of 5 mg/ml.
2. After reconstitution, stable for 48 hrs at room temperature or 1 wk refrigerated.
3. Inject rapidly. Monitor B/P immediately after injection, q30sec for 3 min, then q60sec for 7 min.

INDICATIONS/DOSAGE/ROUTES

Diagnosis of pheochromocytoma:
IV: Adults, elderly: 2.5-5 mg. **Children:** 1 mg.

Prevent/control hypertension in pheochromocytoma:
IV: Adults, elderly: 5 mg 1-2 hrs before surgery. May repeat. **Children:** 1 mg.

Prevent/treat necrosis/sloughing:
IV: Adults, elderly: 5-10 mg in 10 ml saline infiltrated into affected area. **Children:** 0.1-0.2 mg/kg up to maximum of 10 mg.

NOTE: 10 mg may be added to each liter of solution containing norepinephrine.

PRECAUTIONS

CONTRAINDICATIONS: Epinephrine, myocardial infarction, coronary insufficiency, angina, coronary artery disease. **CAUTIONS:** Severe coronary insufficiency, recent MI, cerebrovascular disease, chronic renal failure, Raynaud's disease, thromboangitis obliterans. **PREGNANCY/LACTATION:** Unknown whether drug crosses placenta or is distributed in breast milk. **Pregnancy Category C.**

INTERACTIONS

DRUG INTERACTIONS: May decrease effects of sympathomimetics (e.g., dopamine, phenylephrine). **ALTERED LAB VALUES:** None significant.

SIDE EFFECTS

Frequency of effects unknown: Weakness, dizziness, flushing, orthostatic hypotension, nasal stuffiness, nausea, vomiting, diarrhea.

ADVERSE REACTIONS/TOXIC EFFECTS

Tachycardia, arrhythmias, acute/prolonged hypotension may occur. Do not use epinephrine (will produce further drop in B/P.)

NURSING IMPLICATIONS

BASELINE ASSESSMENT:

Positive pheochromocytoma test indicated by decrease in B/P >35 mm Hg systolic, >25 mm Hg diastolic pressure. Negative test indicated by no B/P change, elevated B/P, or B/P elevated 35 mm Hg systolic and 25 mm Hg diastolic. Preinjection B/P generally occurs

P

within 15-30 min after administration.

INTERVENTION/EVALUATION:

Assist w/ambulation if dizziness occurs. Monitor B/P continuously during therapy/tests.

phenylbutazone

feh-nul-bu´tah-zone

(Butazolidin)

CANADIAN AVAILABILITY:
Apo-Phenylbutazone, Butazolidin, Novobutazone

CLASSIFICATION

Nonsteroidal anti-inflammatory

PHARMACOKINETICS

Rapidly absorbed from GI tract. Metabolized slowly in liver. Primarily excreted in urine. Half-life: 54-99 hrs.

ACTION

Inhibits prostaglandin synthesis. Inhibits action of cyclooxygenase, decreases formation of prostaglandin, thromboxane precursors from arachidonic acid.

USES

Relief of pain and disability associated w/acute gouty arthritis, active rheumatoid arthritis, acute osteoarthritis of hips and knees, active ankylosing spondylitis, painful shoulder.

PO ADMINISTRATION

1. May give w/food, milk, or antacids if GI distress occurs.
2. Do not crush or break capsules/film-coated tablets.

INDICATIONS/DOSAGE/ROUTES

Rheumatoid arthritis, active ankylosing spondylitis, acute attacks of osteoarthritis:
PO: Adults, elderly: Initially, 300-600 mg/day in 3-4 divided doses. **Maintenance:** 400 mg/day.

Acute gouty arthritis:
PO: Adults, elderly: Initially, 400 mg as single dose; then 100 mg q4h until relief is obtained. Do not continue drug therapy for more than 7 days.

PRECAUTIONS

CONTRAINDICATIONS: Active peptic ulcer, GI ulceration, chronic inflammation of GI tract, GI bleeding disorders, history of hypersensitivity to aspirin/NSAIDs. **CAUTIONS:** Impaired renal/hepatic function, history of GI tract disease, predisposition to fluid retention. **PREGNANCY/LACTATION:** Crosses placenta; is distributed in breast milk. Avoid use during 3rd trimester (may adversely affect fetal cardiovascular system [premature closure of ductus arteriosus]). **Pregnancy Category C.**

INTERACTIONS

DRUG INTERACTIONS: May increase effects of oral anticoagulants, heparin, thrombolytics. May decrease effect of antihypertensives, diuretics. Salicylates, aspirin may increase risk of GI side effects, bleeding. Bone marrow depressants may increase risk of hematologic reactions. May increase concentration, toxicity of lithium, phenytoin. May decrease concentration of digoxin. Penicillamine may increase risk of severe hematologic, renal adverse effects. May increase methotrexate toxicity. Probenecid may increase concentration. **ALTERED LAB VAL-**

UES: May increase glucose, sodium, liver function tests. May decrease uric acid. May prolong bleeding time.

SIDE EFFECTS

NOTE: Incidence of side effects increases after age 40. **FREQUENT:** Dyspepsia (heartburn, GI distress, abdominal distention w/flatulence, nausea, indigestion), edema. **OCCASIONAL:** Headache, dizziness, rash, pruritus.

ADVERSE REACTIONS/TOXIC EFFECTS

Peptic or intestinal ulcers have occurred in pts w/no known ulcer history. Bone marrow depression may result in aplastic anemia, agranulocytosis and is the most serious of blood dyscrasias reported. Other hematologic toxicities (leukopenia, thrombocytopenia w/purpura, petechiae, hemorrhage) may occur shortly after initiation of therapy or after prolonged use. Aplastic anemia may develop within 1-3 mo, agranulocytosis within 3 mo to 1 yr.

NURSING IMPLICATIONS

BASELINE ASSESSMENT:

Assess onset, type, location, duration of pain, inflammation. Inspect appearance of affected joints for immobility, deformities, skin condition.

INTERVENTION/EVALUATION:

Assist with ambulation if dizziness occurs. Monitor pattern of daily bowel activity and stool consistency. Monitor for evidence of dyspepsia. Check behind medial malleolus for fluid retention (usually first area noted). Evaluate for therapeutic response: Relief of pain, stiffness, swelling, increase in joint mobility, reduced joint tenderness, improved grip strength.

PATIENT/FAMILY TEACHING:

Anti-inflammatory effect noted in 3-7 days; antigout effect in 1-4 days. Avoid aspirin, alcohol during therapy (increases risk of GI bleeding). If GI upset occurs, take w/food, milk, or antacids. Avoid tasks that require alertness until response to drug is established. Do not crush or chew capsules/film-coated tablets.

P

phenylephrine hydrochloride

fen-ill-eh´frin

(Alconefrin, Neo-Synephrine, Prefrin)

FIXED-COMBINATION(S):
W/zinc sulfate, an astringent (Zincfrin); w/pyrilamine maleate, an antihistamine (Prefrin-A); w/sulfacetamide, an anti-infective (Vasosulf); w/pheniramine maleate, an antihistamine (Dristan); w/naphazoline, a vasoconstrictor, and pyrilamine, an antihistamine (4 Way Nasal Spray)

CANADIAN AVAILABILITY:
AK-Dilate, Neo-Synephrine, Prefrin

CLASSIFICATION

Sympathomimetic

PHARMACOKINETICS

	ONSET	PEAK	DURATION
Ophthalmic	Immediate	—	0.5-4 hrs
Nasal	Immediate	—	0.5-4 hrs
IV	Immediate	—	15-20 min
IM	10-15 min	—	0.5-2 hrs

Minimal absorption following intranasal, ophthalmic administration. Metabolized in liver, GI tract. Primarily excreted in urine. Half-life: 2.5 hrs.

ACTION

Acts on alpha-adrenergic receptors of vascular smooth muscle (increases systolic/diastolic blood pressure); produces constriction of blood vessels, conjunctival arterioles, nasal arterioles.

USES

Nasal: Topical application to nasal mucosa reduces nasal secretion, promoting drainage of sinus secretions. *Ophthalmic:* Topical application to conjunctiva relieves congestion, itching, minor irritation; whitens sclera of eye. *Parenteral:* Vascular failure in shock, drug-induced hypotension.

STORAGE/HANDLING

Store nasal, ophthalmic, parenteral forms at room temperature. Appears clear, colorless, slightly yellow. Do not use if discolored.

NASAL/OPHTHALMIC/IV ADMINISTRATION

NASAL:

1. Blow nose before medication is administered. W/head tilted back, apply drops in 1 nostril. Remain in same position and wait 5 min before applying drops in other nostril.
2. Sprays should be administered into each nostril w/head erect. Sniff briskly while squeezing container. Wait 3-5 min before blowing nose gently. Rinse tip of spray bottle.

OPHTHALMIC:

1. For topical ophthalmic use only.
2. Instruct pt to tilt head backward and look up.
3. Gently pull lower lid down to form pouch and instill medication.
4. Do not touch tip of applicator to lids or any surface.
5. When lower lid is released, have pt keep eye open w/o blinking for at least 30 sec.
6. Apply gentle finger pressure to lacrimal sac (bridge of the nose, inside corner of the eye) for 1-2 min.
7. Remove excess solution around eye w/tissue. Wash hands immediately to remove medication on hands.

PARENTERAL:

1. Dilute each 10 mg vial w/500 ml 5% dextrose to provide a concentration of 2 mcg/ml.

INDICATIONS/DOSAGE/ROUTES

Nasal decongestant:

PO: Adults, children >12 yrs: 2-3 drops, 1-2 sprays of 0.25-0.5% solution into each nostril. **Children 6-12 yrs:** 2-3 drops or 1-2 sprays of 0.25% solution in each nostril. **Children <6 yrs:** 2-3 drops of 0.125% solution in each nostril. Repeat q4h as needed. Do not use longer than 3 days.

Ophthalmic:

PO: Adults, children >12 yrs: 1-2 drops of 0.125% solution q3-4hrs.

Usualy elderly dosage:
NASAL: Elderly: 2-3 drops or 1-2 sprays q4h for 3 days.
OPHTHALMIC: Elderly: 1 drop (2.5%). May repeat in 1 hr.

Hypotension:
IV INFUSION: Adults, elderly: Initially, 100-180 mcg/min. **Maintenance:** 40-60 mcg/min.

PRECAUTIONS

CONTRAINDICATIONS: Idiosyncrasy to sympathomimetics manifested by insomnia, dizziness, weakness, tremor, arrhythmias, MAO inhibitor therapy. *Ophthalmic:* Angle-closure glaucoma, those w/soft-contact lenses, use of 10% solution in infants. *Nasal:* Those w/insomnia, tremor, asthenia, dizziness, arrhythmias due to previous drug doses. **CAUTIONS:** Marked hypertension, cardiac disorders, advanced arteriosclerotic disease, type I (insulin-dependent) diabetes mellitus, hyperthyroidism, children w/low body weight, elderly. **PREGNANCY/LACTATION:** Crosses placenta; is distributed in breast milk. **Pregnancy Category C.**

INTERACTIONS

DRUG INTERACTIONS: Tricyclic antidepressants, maprotiline may increase cardiovascular effects. May decrease effect of methyldopa. May have mutually inhibitory effects w/beta-blockers. May increase risk of arrhythmias w/digoxin. Ergonovine, oxytocin may increase vasoconstriction. MAO inhibitors may increase vasopressor effects. **ALTERED LAB VALUES:** None significant.

SIDE EFFECTS

FREQUENT: *Nasal:* Rebound nasal congestion due to overuse (longer than 3 days). **OCCASIONAL:** Mild CNS stimulation (restlessness, nervousness, tremors, headache, insomnia), particularly in those hypersensitive to sympathomimetics (generally, elderly patients). *Nasal:* Stinging, burning, drying of nasal mucosa. *Ophthalmic:* Transient burning/stinging, brow ache, blurred vision.

ADVERSE REACTIONS/TOXIC EFFECTS

Large doses may produce tachycardia, palpitations (particularly in those with cardiac disease), lightheadedness, nausea, vomiting. Overdosage in those >60 yrs may result in hallucinations, CNS depression, seizures. Prolonged nasal use may produce chronic swelling of nasal mucosa, rhinitis.

NURSING IMPLICATIONS

BASELINE ASSESSMENT:

If phenylephrine 10% ophthalmic is instilled into denuded or damaged corneal epithelium, corneal clouding may result.

PATIENT/FAMILY TEACHING:

Discontinue drug if adverse reactions occur. Do not use for nasal decongestion longer than 3-5 days (rebound congestion). Discontinue drug if insomnia, dizziness, weakness, tremor, or feeling of irregular heart beat occur. *Nasal:* Stinging/burning of inside nose may occur. *Ophthalmic:* Blurring of vision w/eye instillation generally subsides w/continued therapy. Discontinue medication if redness/swelling of eyelids, itching appears.

phenytoin

phen´ih-toy-in
(Dilantin)

phenytoin sodium

(Dilantin)

FIXED-COMBINATION(S):
W/phenobarbital, a barbiturate (Dilantin w/Phenobarbital)

CANADIAN AVAILABILITY:
Dilantin

CLASSIFICATION

Anticonvulsant

PHARMACOKINETICS

Slow, variably absorbed after oral administration; slow but complete absorption following IM administration. Widely distributed. Protein binding: >90%. Metabolized in liver. Primarily excreted in urine. Half-life: 22 hrs.

ACTION

Anticonvulsant: Stabilizes neuronal membranes, limits spread of seizure activity. Decreases sodium, calcium, ion influx in neurons. Decreases post-tetanic potentiation and repetitive after-discharge. *Antiarrhythmic:* Decreases abnormal ventricular automaticity (shortens refractory period, QT interval, action potential duration).

USES

Management of generalized tonic-clonic seizures (grand mal), complex partial seizures (psychomotor), cortical focal seizures, status epilepticus. Ineffective in absence seizures, myoclonic seizures, atonic epilepsy when used alone. Treatment of cardiac arrhythmias due to digitalis intoxication.

STORAGE/HANDLING

Store oral suspension, tablets, capsules, parenteral form at room temperature. Precipitate may form if parenteral form is refrigerated (will dissolve at room temperature). Slight yellow discoloration of parenteral form does not affect potency, but do not use if solution is not clear or if precipitate is present.

PO/IV ADMINISTRATION

PO:

1. Give w/food if GI distress occurs.
2. Do not chew/break capsules. Tablets may be chewed.
3. Shake oral suspension well before using.

IV:

NOTE: Give by direct IV injection. Do not add to IV infusion (precipitate may form).

1. Severe hypotension, cardiovascular collapse occurs if rate of IV injection exceeds 50 mg/min for adults. Administer 50 mg >2-3 min for elderly. In neonates, administer at rate not exceeding 1-3 mg/kg/min.
2. IV injection very painful (chemical irritation of vein due to alkalinity of solution). To minimize effect, flush vein w/sterile saline solution through same IV needle/catheter following each IV injection.
3. IV toxicity characterized by CNS depression, cardiovascular collapse.

INDICATIONS/DOSAGE/ROUTES

NOTE: Pts who are stabilized on 100 mg 3 times daily may receive

300 mg once daily w/extended release medication. When replacement by another anticonvulsant is necessary, phenytoin should be decreased over 1 wk as therapy is begun w/low dose of replacement drug.

Seizure control:
PO: Adults, elderly: Initially, 100 mg 3 times daily. May be increased in 100 mg increments q2-4wks until therapeutic response achieved. **Usual dose range:** 300-400 mg daily. **Maximum daily dose:** 600 mg daily (300 mg for extended release). **Children:** Initially, 5 mg/kg daily in 2-3 equally divided doses. **Usual maintenance dose:** 4-8 mg/kg. **Maximum daily dose:** 300 mg daily.

Status epilepticus:
IV: Adults, elderly: 150-250 mg, then 100-150 mg in 30 min, if needed. **Children:** 250 mg/m^2.

Arrhythmias:
IV: Adults, elderly: 100 mg at 5 min intervals until arrhythmias disappear or undesirable effects occur.

Management of arrhythmias:
PO: Adults, elderly: 100 mg 2-4 times daily.

PRECAUTIONS

CONTRAINDICATIONS: Seizures due to hypoglycemia, hydantoin hypersensitivity. *IV route only:* Sinus bradycardia, sinoatrial block, second- and third-degree heart block, Adam-Stokes syndrome. **EXTREME CAUTION:** *IV route only:* Respiratory depression, myocardial infarction, CHF, damaged myocardium. **CAUTIONS:** Impaired hepatic/renal function, severe myocardial insufficiency, hypotension, hyperglycemia. **PREGNANCY/LACTATION:** Crosses placenta; is distributed in small amount in breast milk. Fetal hydantoin syndrome (craniofacial abnormalities, nail/digital hypoplasia, prenatal growth deficiency) has been reported. There is increased frequency of seizures in pregnant women due to altered absorption of metabolism of phenytoin. May increase risk of hemorrhage in neonate, maternal bleeding during delivery. **Pregnancy Category D.**

INTERACTIONS

DRUG INTERACTIONS: May decrease effect of glucocorticoids. Alcohol, CNS depressants may increase CNS depression. Antacids may decrease absorption. Amiodarone, anticoagulants, cimetidine, disulfiram, isoniazid, sulfonamides may increase phenytoin concentration, effects, toxicity. Fluconazole, ketoconazole, miconazole may increase concentration. Lidocaine, propranolol may increase cardiac depressant effects. Valproic acid may increase concentration, decrease metabolism. May increase xanthine metabolism. **ALTERED LAB VALUES:** May increase alkaline phosphatase, GGT, glucose.

SIDE EFFECTS

Effects are dose related and generally occur w/larger doses. **FREQUENT:** Drowsiness, lethargy, irritability, headache, restlessness, joint aches, vertigo, anorexia, nausea, gastric distress, gingival hyperplasia (w/prolonged therapy). **OCCASIONAL:** Morbilliform rash, hypertrichosis (hair growth).

ADVERSE REACTIONS/TOXIC EFFECTS

Abrupt withdrawal may precipitate status epilepticus. Blood dyscrasias, lymphadenopathy, osteomalacia (due to interference of vitamin D metabolism) may occur. Phenytoin blood concentration of 25 mcg/ml (toxic) may produce ataxia (muscular incoordination), nystagmus (rhythmic oscillation of eyes), double vision. As level increases, extreme lethargy to comatose states occur.

NURSING IMPLICATIONS

BASELINE ASSESSMENT:

Anticonvulsant: Review history of seizure disorder (intensity, frequency, duration, level of consciousness). Initiate seizure precautions. Liver function tests, CBC, platelet count should be performed before therapy begins and periodically during therapy. Repeat CBC, platelet count 2 wks after therapy begins, and 2 wks after maintenance dose is given.

INTERVENTION/EVALUATION:

Observe frequently for recurrence of seizure activity. Assess for clinical improvement (decrease in intensity/frequency of seizures). Monitor EKG for cardiac arrhythmias. Assess B/P, EKG diligently w/IV administration. Assist w/ambulation if drowsiness, lethargy, vertigo occurs. Monitor for therapeutic serum level (10-20 mcg/ml).

PATIENT/FAMILY TEACHING:

Pain may occur w/IV injection. To prevent gingival hyperplasia (bleeding, tenderness, swelling of gums) encourage good oral hygiene care, gum massage, regular dental visits. CBC should be performed every month for 1 yr after maintenance dose is established and q3mo thereafter. Urine may appear pink, red, or red-brown. Report sore throat, fever, glandular swelling, skin reaction (hematologic toxicity). Drowsiness usually diminishes w/continued therapy. Do not abruptly withdraw medication following long-term use (may precipitate seizures). Strict maintenance of drug therapy is essential for seizure control, arrhythmias. Avoid tasks that require alertness, motor skills until response to drug is established. Avoid alcohol.

phosphates

potassium phosphate

(Neutra-phos K, K-Phosphate)

sodium phosphate

(Na-Phosphate)

potassium-sodium phosphate

(Neutraphos)

CANADIAN AVAILABILITY: Potassium phosphate, Uro-KP-Neutral

CLASSIFICATION

Electrolyte

PHARMACOKINETICS

Well absorbed from GI tract. Primarily excreted in urine.

ACTION

Modifies calcium concentration, buffer effect on acid-base equilibrium, influences renal excretion of hydrogen.

USES

Prophylactic treatment of hypophosphatemia.

PO ADMINISTRATION

1. Dissolve tablets in water.
2. Take after meals or w/food (decreases GI upset).
3. Maintain high fluid intake (prevents kidney stones).

INDICATIONS/DOSAGE/ROUTES

ELECTROLYTE REPLACEMENT:

Potassium phosphate:
IV: Adults, elderly, adolescents: 10 mmP (310 mg)/day. **Children:** 1.5-2 mmP (46.5-62 mg phosphate)/day.
PO: Adults, elderly, adolescents: 1.45 Gm (250 mg phosphate) in 75 ml water/juice 4 times/day. **Children:** 200 mg phosphate in 60 ml water/juice 4 times/day.

Sodium phosphate:
IV: Adults, elderly, adolescents: 10-15 mmP (310-465 mg phosphate)/day. **Children:** 1.5-2 mmP/kg/day.

Potassium-sodium phosphate:
PO: Adults, elderly, adolescents: 1.25 Gm (250 mg phosphate) in 75 ml water/juice 4 times/day. **Children <4 yrs:** 1 Gm (200 mg phosphate) in 60 ml water/juice 4 times/day.

PRECAUTIONS

CONTRAINDICATIONS: Addison's disease, hyperkalemia, acidification of urine in urinary stone disease, those w/infected urolithiasis or struvite stone formation, severely impaired renal function (<30% of normal), hyperphosphatemia. **CAUTIONS:** Those on sodium/potassium restricted diet, cardiac disease, dehydration, renal impairment, tissue breakdown, myotonia congenita (spasm/rigidity of muscle upon attempts at muscle movement), cardiac failure, cirrhosis/severe hepatic disease, peripheral and pulmonary edema, hypernatremia, hypertension, preeclampsia, hypoparathyroidism, osteomalacia, acute pancreatitis. **PREGNANCY/LACTATION:** Unknown whether drug crosses placenta or is distributed in breast milk. **Pregnancy Category C.**

INTERACTIONS

DRUG INTERACTIONS: Glucocorticoids w/sodium phosphate may cause edema. Antacids may decrease absorption. Calcium-containing medications may increase risk of calcium deposition in soft tissues, decrease phosphate absorption. NSAIDs, ACE inhibitors, potassium-sparing diuretics, potassium-containing medications, salt substitutes w/potassium phosphate may increase potassium concentration. Digoxin and potassium phosphate may increase risk of heart block (due to hyperkalemia). Phosphate-containing medications may increase risk of hyperphosphatemia. Sodium-containing medication w/sodium phosphate may increase risk of edema. **ALTERED LAB VALUES:** None significant.

SIDE EFFECTS

FREQUENT: Mild laxative effect first few days of therapy. **OCCASIONAL:** GI upset (diarrhea, nausea, abdominal pain, vomiting). **RARE:** Headache, dizziness, mental confusion, heaviness of legs, fatigue, muscle cramps, numbness/tingling of hands, feet, around lips, peripheral edema, irregular heartbeat, weight gain, thirst.

ADVERSE REACTIONS/TOXIC EFFECTS

High phosphate levels may produce extra skeletal calcification.

NURSING IMPLICATIONS

INTERVENTION/EVALUATION:

Monitor serum calcium, phosphorus, potassium, sodium levels routinely.

PATIENT/FAMILY TEACHING:

Report diarrhea, nausea, vomiting.

physostigmine salicylate

phy-sew-stig´meen

(Antilirium, Isopto Eserine)

physostigmine sulfate

(Eserine Sulfate)

FIXED-COMBINATION(S): Physostigmine salicylate w/pilocarpine, a miotic (Isopto P-ES)

CANADIAN AVAILABILITY: Antilirium

CLASSIFICATION

Anticholinesterase agent

PHARMACOKINETICS

	ONSET	PEAK	DURATION
IM	3-8 min	—	30 min-5 hrs
IV	<5 min	—	45-60 min
Opthalmic	2 min	1-2 hrs	12-48 hrs

Readily absorbed after IM, SubQ, ophthalmic administration. Widely distributed. Penetrates blood-brain barrier. Hydrolyzed by cholinesterases. Primarily destroyed by hydrolysis. Half-life: 1-2 hrs.

ACTION

Reversibly inhibits destruction of acetylcholine by acetylcholinesterase. Contracts iris sphincter muscle causing miosis, constricts ciliary muscle increasing accommodation. Reduces intraocular pressure by decreasing resistance to aqueous humor outflow. Increases skeletal muscle tone, produces bradycardia, increases salivation and sweat gland secretions.

USES

Antidote for reversal of toxic CNS effects due to anticholinergic drugs, tricyclic antidepressants; reduces IOP in primary glaucoma.

STORAGE/HANDLING

Store ophthalmic solutions, parenteral form at room temperature. May produce a red tint after extended contact w/metals or long exposure to heat, light, or air. May further degrade to blue/brown color. Discard if discolored.

IM/IV/OPHTHALMIC ADMINISTRATION

IM/IV:

1. For IV injection, administer at rate no more than 1 mg/min for adults, 0.5 mg/min in children. A too-rapid IV may produce bradycardia, hypersalivation, bronchospasm, seizures.

OPHTHALMIC:

1. For topical ophthalmic use only.
2. Administer at bedtime to reduce side effects.
3. Instruct pt to tilt head backward and look up.
4. Gently pull lower lid down to form pouch and instill medication.
5. Do not touch tip of applicator to lids or any surface.

6. When lower lid is released, have pt keep eye open w/o blinking for at least 30 sec.

7. Apply gentle finger pressure to lacrimal sac (bridge of the nose, inside corner of the eye) for 1-2 min.

8. Remove excess solution around eye w/a tissue. Wash hands immediately to remove medication on hands.

INDICATIONS/DOSAGE/ROUTES

Antidote:

IM/IV: Adults, elderly: Initially, 0.5-2 mg. If no response, repeat q20min until response occurs or adverse cholinergic effects occur. If initial response occurs, may give additional doses of 1-4 mg at 30-60 min intervals as life-threatening signs recur (arrhythmias, seizures, deep coma). **Children:** 0.02 mg/kg. May give additional doses at 5-10 min intervals until response occurs, adverse cholinergic effects occur, or total dose of 2 mg given.

Glaucoma:

OPHTHALMIC: Adults, elderly: *Solution:* 1-2 gtts 0.25% or 0.5% solution up to 4 times/day. *Ointment:* Apply small quantity 1-3 times/day.

PRECAUTIONS

CONTRAINDICATIONS: Asthma, gangrene, diabetes, cardiovascular disease, mechanical obstruction of intestinal/urogenital tract, vagotonic state, those receiving ganglionic blocking agents. Hypersensitivity to cholinesterase inhibitors or any component of the preparation; active uveal inflammation; angle-closure (narrow-angle) glaucoma before iridectomy; glaucoma associated w/iridocyclitis. **CAUTIONS:** Bronchial asthma, gastrointestinal disturbances, peptic ulcer, bradycardia, hypotension, recent myocardial infarction, epilepsy, parkinsonism, and other disorders that may respond adversely to vagotonic effects. Safety and efficacy in children not established. Use ophthalmic physostigmine only when shorter-acting miotics are not adequate, except in aphakics. Discontinue at least 3 wks before ophthalmic surgery. **PREGNANCY/LACTATION:** Probably crosses placenta. Unknown whether distributed in breast milk. May produce uterine irritability, induce premature labor if administered IV near term. **Pregnancy Category C.**

INTERACTIONS

DRUG INTERACTIONS: May increase effects of cholinesterases (e.g., bethanechol, carbachol). May prolong action of succinylcholine. **ALTERED LAB VALUES:** None significant.

SIDE EFFECTS

COMMON: Miosis, increased GI and skeletal muscle tone, reduced pulse rate, constriction of bronchi and ureters, salivary and sweat gland secretion. *Ophthalmic:* Stinging, burning, tearing, hypersensitivity reactions (including allergic conjunctivitis, dermatitis, or keratitis), painful ciliary/accommodative spasm, blurred vision/myopia, poor vision in dim light. **OCCASIONAL:** Slight, temporary decrease in diastolic B/P w/mild reflex tachycardia, short periods of atrial fibrillation in hyperthyroid pts. Hypertensive pts may react w/marked fall in B/P. *Ophthalmic:* Iris cysts (more frequent in children), increased visibility of floaters, headache, browache, photophobia, ocular pain. **RARE:** Allergic reaction. *Ophthalmic:* Lens

P

opacities, paradoxical increase in intraocular pressure.

ADVERSE REACTIONS/TOXIC EFFECTS

Parenteral overdosage produces a cholinergic reaction manifested as abdominal discomfort/cramping, nausea, vomiting, diarrhea, flushing, feeling of warmth/heat about face, excessive salivation and sweating, lacrimation, pallor, bradycardia/tachycardia, hypotension, urinary urgency, blurred vision, bronchospasm, pupillary contraction, involuntary muscular contraction visible under the skin (fasciculation).

Overdosage may also produce a *cholinergic crisis,* manifested by increasingly severe muscle weakness (appears first in muscles involving chewing, swallowing, followed by muscular weakness of shoulder girdle and upper extremities), respiratory muscle paralysis, followed by pelvic girdle and leg muscle paralysis. Requires a withdrawal of all anticholinergic drugs and immediate use of 0.6-1.2 mg atropine sulfate IM/IV for adults, 0.01 mg/kg in infants and children under 12 yrs. *Ophthalmic:* Conjunctivitis occurs frequently with chronic use. Retinal detachment and vitreous hemorrhage have occurred occasionally. Systemic effects (nausea, vomiting, diarrhea, abdominal cramps, respiratory difficulty, excessive salivation, bradycardia, cardiac arrhythmias) occur infrequently, require parenteral administration of atropine sulfate.

NURSING IMPLICATIONS

BASELINE ASSESSMENT:

Have tissues readily available at pt's bedside.

INTERVENTION/EVALUATION:

Parenteral therapy: Assess vital signs immediately before and every 15-30 min following administration. Monitor diligently for cholinergic reaction (sweating, irregular heartbeat, muscle weakness, abdominal pain, dyspnea, hypotension). Reduce dosage if excessive sweating, nausea occurs; discontinue if excessive salivation, vomiting, urination, defecation occurs. *Ophthalmic:* Be alert for systemic toxicity: Severe nausea, vomiting, diarrhea, frequent urination, excessive salivation, bradycardia (may trigger asthma attack in asthmatics). Assess vision acuity and provide assistance w/ambulation as needed.

PATIENT/FAMILY TEACHING:

Teach proper administration. Do not use more often than directed because of risk of overdosage. Adverse effects often subside after the first few days of therapy. Avoid night driving, activities requiring visual acuity in dim light. Avoid insecticides, pesticides; inhalation/absorption through skin may add to systemic effects of physostigmine. Report promptly any systemic effects (see above) or ocular problems.

pilocarpine

pye-loe-kar´peen

(Ocusert)

pilocarpine hydrochloride

(Pilocar, Isopto Carpine, Ocu-Carpine, Piloptic,

Adsorbocarpine, Akarpine, Pilopine, Pilostat, Salagen)

pilocarpine nitrate

(Pilagan Liquifilm)

FIXED-COMBINATION(S): W/epinephrine bitartrate, a vasoconstrictor (E-Pilo-1, 2, 3, 4 or 6); w/physostigmine salicylate, a miotic (Isopto P-ES)

CANADIAN AVAILABILITY: Isopto Carpine, Miocarpine, Ocusert, Pilopine, Spersarpine

CLASSIFICATION

Cholinergic

PHARMACOKINETICS

	ONSET	PEAK	DURATION
Decrease IOP	60 min	75 min	4-14 hrs
Miosis	10-30 min	30 min	4-8 hrs
Ocusert	—	1.5-2 hrs	7 days

Ocusert releases drug continuously over 7 day period. Spasm of accommodation occurs in 15 min; persists for 2-3 hrs.

ACTION

Directly stimulates cholinergic receptors. Contracts iris sphincter muscle causing miosis, constricts ciliary muscle increasing accommodation. Reduces intraocular pressure by decreasing resistance to aqueous humor outflow.

USES

To decrease elevated intraocular pressure (IOP) in glaucoma; to counter the effects of cycloplegics and mydriatics after surgery or ophthalmoscopic examination; to protect the lens before goniotomy or iridectomy. Treatment of xeroma.

STORAGE/HANDLING

Refrigerate Ocusert system.

OPHTHALMIC ADMINISTRATION

TOPICAL:

Ophthalmic solutions:

1. Instruct pt to lie down or tilt head backward and look up.
2. Gently pull lower lid down to form pouch and instill medication.
3. Do not touch tip of applicator to any surface.
4. When lower lid is released have pt keep eye open w/o blinking for at least 30 sec.
5. Apply gentle finger pressure to lacrimal sac (bridge of the nose, inside corner of the eye) for 1-2 min.
6. Remove excess solution around eye w/tissue. Wash hands immediately to remove medication on hands.
7. Tell pt not to close eyes tightly or blink more often than necessary.
8. Never rinse dropper.
9. Do not use solution if discolored.

Ophthalmic gel:

1. Apply as a ribbon in the lower conjunctival sac at bedtime.
2. When used in conjunction w/ pilocarpine solutions, instill solution first, wait 5 min before applying gel.

Ocular systems:

1. Place in the lower conjunctival sac at bedtime (greatest myopia during first several hours).
2. Move to upper conjunctival sac for better retention by gentle finger pressure through closed eyelid while pt rolls the eyes. Do

not move the system across the colored portion of the eye.

INDICATIONS/DOSAGE/ROUTES

Glaucoma:
OPHTHALMIC: Adults, elderly: (Solution): 1-2 drops (0.5-4% solution) up to 6 times/day. (Ocusert): Initially 20 mcg system (releases 20 mcg/hr/7 days). May increase to 40 mcg system.

Xeroma:
PO: Adults: Initially, 5 mg 3 times/day up to 10 mg 3 times/day.

PRECAUTIONS

CONTRAINDICATIONS: Hypersensitivity to any of components; any condition where miosis is undesirable (e.g., acute iritis, some forms of secondary glaucoma, acute inflammatory disease of the anterior chamber). Safety in children not established. **CAUTIONS:** Corneal abrasions, bronchial asthma, spastic GI conditions, urinary tract obstruction, peptic ulcer, severe bradycardia, hypotension, epilepsy, hyperthyroidism, recent myocardial infarction. **PREGNANCY/LACTATION:** Safety during pregnancy, lactation not known. **Pregnancy Category C.**

INTERACTIONS

DRUG INTERACTIONS: Cyclopentolate may decrease effects. **ALTERED LAB VALUES:** None significant.

SIDE EFFECTS

FREQUENT: Stinging, burning, tearing, painful ciliary/accommodative spasm, blurred vision/myopia, poor vision in dim light. **OCCASIONAL:** Iris cysts (more frequent in children), increased visibility of floaters, headache, brow ache, photophobia, ocular pain, hypersensitivity reactions (including allergic conjunctivitis, dermatitis, or keratitis). **RARE:** Lens opacities, paradoxical increase in intraocular pressure.

ADVERSE REACTIONS/TOXIC EFFECTS

Retinal detachment and vitreous hemorrhage have occurred occasionally. Systemic effects (nausea, vomiting, diarrhea, abdominal cramps, respiratory difficulty, excessive salivation, bradycardia, cardiac arrhythmias) occur infrequently, require parenteral administration of atropine sulfate.

NURSING IMPLICATIONS

BASELINE ASSESSMENT:

Question for hypersensitivity to components. Obtain baseline pulse, B/P. Assess physical appearance of eye and pt's perception of vision.

INTERVENTION/EVALUATION:

Evaluate therapeutic response. Assess for systemic reaction esp. sweating, flushing, increased salivation. Check B/P, pulse, respirations.

PATIENT/FAMILY TEACHING:

Do not drive for several hrs after administration. Avoid night driving/performing hazardous tasks in poor light. Blurred vision usually decreases w/prolonged use. W/glaucoma, probably will need medication for remainder of life. Importance of remaining under physician's care. Teach proper administration (see Ophthalmic Administration). Notify physician of difficulty breathing, change in vision, sweating, flushing.

pimozide

pim′oh-zied
(Orap)

CANADIAN AVAILABILITY:
Orap

CLASSIFICATION

Antipsychotic

PHARMACOKINETICS

Poorly absorbed from GI tract. Undergoes first-pass effect. Widely distributed. Metabolized in liver to active metabolite. Primarily excreted in urine. Half-life: 55 hrs.

ACTION

Inhibits dopamine receptors in CNS, interrupting impulse movement. Produces strong extrapyramidal, moderate anticholinergic, sedative effects.

USES

Suppression of severely compromising motor and phonic tics in those w/Tourette's disorders who have failed to respond adequately to standard treatment.

PO ADMINISTRATION

May give w/o regard to meals.

INDICATIONS/DOSAGE/ROUTES

Tourette's disorder:
PO: Adults: Initially, 1-2 mg/day in divided doses. Increase every other day. **Maintenance:** <0.2 mg/kg/day or 10 mg/day, whichever is less. **Maximum:** 0.2 mg/kg/day or 10 mg/day.

PRECAUTIONS

CONTRAINDICATIONS: Congenital QT syndrome, history of cardiac arrhythmias, administration w/other drugs that prolong QT interval, severe toxic CNS depression, comatose states. **CAUTIONS:** History of seizures, cardiovascular disease, impaired respiratory, hepatic/renal function, alcohol withdrawal, urinary retention, glaucoma, prostatic hypertrophy. **PREGNANCY/LACTATION:** Unknown whether drug crosses placenta or is distributed in breast milk. **Pregnancy Category C.**

INTERACTIONS

DRUG INTERACTIONS: Alcohol, CNS depressants may increase CNS depressant effect. Methylphenidate, pemoline may mask signs of tics. Anticholinergics may increase anticholinergic effects. Tricyclic antidepressants, phenothiazines, quinidine may increase risk of cardiac arrhythmias. Extrapyramidal symptom producing medications (EPS) may increase anticholinergic, CNS depressant, and EPS effects. **ALTERED LAB VALUES:** None significant.

SIDE EFFECTS

FREQUENT: Drowsiness, salivation, constipation, dizziness, tachycardia. **OCCASIONAL:** Nausea, sweating, dry mouth, headache, hypotension, GI upset, weight gain. **RARE:** Visual disturbances, diarrhea, rash, urinary abnormalities.

ADVERSE REACTIONS/TOXIC EFFECTS

Extrapyramidal reactions occur frequently but are usually mild and reversible (generally noted during first few days of therapy). Motor restlessness, dystonia, hyperreflexia occur much less frequently. Persistent tardive dyskinesia has occurred. Those on long-term maintenance may experience transient dyskinetic signs following abrupt withdrawal.

NURSING IMPLICATIONS

BASELINE ASSESSMENT:

Obtain baseline EKG. Potassium level should be checked and corrected if necessary.

INTERVENTION/EVALUATION:

EKG should be periodically monitored. Assess for extrapyramidal symptoms. Monitor WBC, differential count for blood dyscrasias. Monitor for fine tongue movement (may be early sign of tardive dyskinesia). Assess for therapeutic response (decreased tic activity).

PATIENT/FAMILY TEACHING:

Do not exceed prescribed dose. Do not abruptly withdraw from long-term drug therapy. Report visual disturbances. Drowsiness generally subsides during continued therapy. Avoid tasks that require alertness, motor skills until response to drug is established. Avoid alcohol and CNS depressants.

pindolol

pin´doe-lol

(Visken)

FIXED-COMBINATION(S):
W/hydrochlorothiazide, a diuretic (Viskazide)

CANADIAN AVAILABILITY:
Syn-Pindolol, Visken

CLASSIFICATION

Beta-adrenergic blocker

PHARMACOKINETICS

	ONSET	PEAK	DURATION
PO	3 hrs	—	24 hrs

Completely absorbed from GI tract. Protein binding: 40%. Metabolized in liver. Primarily excreted in urine. Half-life: 3-4 hrs (increased in decreased renal function, elderly).

ACTION

Nonselective beta-blocker. Blocks $beta_1$-adrenergic receptors, slowing sinus heart rate, decreasing cardiac output, decreasing B/P (exact mechanism unknown but may block peripheral adrenergic receptors, decrease sympathetic outflow from CNS or decrease renin release from kidney). Blocks $beta_2$-adrenergic receptors, increasing airway resistance. Decreases myocardial ischemia severity by decreasing oxygen requirements. Has moderate intrinsic sympathomimetic activity.

USES

Management of hypertension. May be used alone or in combination w/diuretic.

PO ADMINISTRATION

1. May give w/o regard to food.
2. Tablets may be crushed.

INDICATIONS/DOSAGE/ROUTES

Hypertension:
PO: Adults: Initially, 5 mg 2 times/day. Gradually increase dose by 10 mg/day at 2-4 week intervals. **Maintenance:** 10-30 mg/day in 2-3 divided doses. **Maximum:** 60 mg/day.

Usual elderly dosage:
PO: Elderly: Initially, 5 mg/day. May increase by 5 mg q3-4wks.

PRECAUTIONS

CONTRAINDICATIONS: Bronchial asthma, COPD, uncontrolled cardiac failure, sinus bradycardia, heart block greater than first degree, cardiogenic shock, CHF, unless secondary to tachyarrhythmias. **CAUTIONS:** Inadequate cardiac function, impaired renal/hepatic function, diabetes mellitus, hyperthyroidism. **PREGNANCY/LACTATION:** Readily crosses placenta; is distributed in breast milk. May produce bradycardia, apnea, hypoglycemia, hypothermia during delivery, small birthweight infants. **Pregnancy Category B.**

INTERACTIONS

DRUG INTERACTIONS: Diuretics, other hypotensives may increase hypotensive effect; sympathomimetics, xanthines may mutually inhibit effects; may mask symptoms of hypoglycemia, prolong hypoglycemic effect of insulin, oral hypoglycemics; NSAIDs may decrease anti-hypertensive effect; cimetidine may increase concentration. **ALTERED LAB VALUES:** May increase ANA titer, SGOT (AST), SGPT (ALT), alkaline phosphatase, LDH, bilirubin, BUN, creatinine, potassium, uric acid, lipoproteins, triglycerides.

SIDE EFFECTS

FREQUENT: Dizziness, fatigue, insomnia, bizarre dreams, paresthesia, visual disturbances, anxiety, peripheral edema, dyspnea, weight gain. **OCCASIONAL:** Nausea, GI distress, palpitation, coldness of extremities, syncope, tachycardia, chest pain, muscle/joint pain. **RARE:** Lethargy, hallucinations, diarrhea, vomiting, wheezing, rash, pruritus, urinary frequency, impotence.

ADVERSE REACTIONS/TOXIC EFFECTS

Abrupt withdrawal (particularly in those w/coronary artery disease) may produce angina or precipitate MI. May precipitate thyroid crisis in those w/thyrotoxicosis.

NURSING IMPLICATIONS

BASELINE ASSESSMENT:

Assess baseline renal/liver function tests. Assess B/P, apical pulse immediately before drug is administered (if pulse is 60/min or below or systolic B/P is below 90 mm Hg, withhold medication, contact physician).

INTERVENTION/EVALUATION:

Assess pulse for strength/weakness, irregular rate, bradycardia. Monitor EKG for cardiac changes. Assist w/ambulation if dizziness occurs. Assess for peripheral edema of hands, feet (usually, first area of low extremity swelling is behind medial malleolus in ambulatory, sacral area in bedridden). Monitor pattern of daily bowel activity, stool consistency. Assess skin for development of rash. Monitor any unusual changes in pt.

PATIENT/FAMILY TEACHING:

Do not abruptly discontinue medication. Compliance w/therapy regimen is essential to control hypertension. If dizziness occurs, sit or lie down immediately. Full therapeutic response may not occur for up to 2 wks. Avoid tasks that require alertness, motor skills until response to drug is established. Report excessive slow pulse rate (<60/min), peripheral numbness, dizziness. Do not use nasal decongestants, over-the-counter cold preparations (stimulants) w/o physician approval. Outpatients should monitor B/P, pulse before taking medication. Restrict salt, alcohol intake.

pipecuronium bromide

pip-eh-cure-oh´knee-um
(Arduan)

(See Classifications section under Neuromuscular blockers)

piperacillin sodium

pip-ur-ah-sill´in
(Pipracil)

CANADIAN AVAILABILITY:
Pipracil

CLASSIFICATION

Antibiotic: Penicillin

PHARMACOKINETICS

Well absorbed after IM administration. Widely distributed. Protein binding: 16-22%. Primarily excreted unchanged in urine. Removed by hemodialysis. Half-life: 0.6-1.2 hrs (increased in decreased renal function).

ACTION

Bactericidal. Binds to bacterial membranes. Inhibits cell wall synthesis.

USES

Treatment of gynecologic, skin/skin structure, respiratory, urinary tract, bone and joint, intra-abdominal infections, septicemia, gonorrhea (w/Probenecid); perioperative prophylaxis, esp. in abdominal surgery.

STORAGE/HANDLING

Solution appears clear to pale yellow; may darken (does not indicate loss of potency). IV infusion (piggyback) is stable for 24 hrs at room temperature, 7 days if refrigerated.

IM/IV ADMINISTRATION

NOTE: Space doses evenly around the clock.

IM:

1. Reconstitute each Gm w/2 ml sterile water for injection or 0.9% NaCl injection to provide concentration of 1 Gm/2.5 ml.
2. Shake well until dissolved.
3. Inject into gluteus maximus.
4. Do not exceed 2 Gm IM at any one injection site.

IV:

1. For IV injection, dilute w/5 ml sterile water for injection or 0.9% NaCl injection or other compatible diluent. Give over 3-5 min.
2. For intermittent IV infusion (piggyback), further dilute w/50-100 ml 5% dextrose, 0.9% NaCl, or other compatible IV fluid, infuse over 20-30 min.
3. Because of potential for hypersensitivity/anaphylaxis, start initial dose at few drops/min, increase slowly to ordered rate; stay w/pt first 10-15 min, then check q10min.
4. Alternating IV sites, use large veins to avoid phlebitis.

INDICATIONS/DOSAGE/ROUTES

Uncomplicated UTI:
IM/IV: Adults, elderly: 6-8 Gm/day in divided doses q6-12h.

Complicated UTI:
IV: Adults, elderly: 8-16 Gm/day in divided doses q6-8h.

Septicemia, intra-abdominal, gynecologic, skin/skin structure, nosocomial infections:
IV: Adults, elderly: 12-18 Gm/day in divided doses q4-6h.

Perioperative prophylaxis:
IV: Adults, elderly: 2 Gm 30-60 min before surgery, 2 Gm in surgery or immediately after, and 2 Gm postop q6h for up to 24 hrs postop.

Cesarean sections:
IV: Adults: 2 Gm as soon as umbilical cord clamped and 4 and 8 hrs after first dose.

Acute, uncomplicated gonococcal urethritis:
IM: Adults: 2 Gm one time w/1 Gm probenecid 30 min before injection.

Dosage in renal impairment:

Dose and/or frequency modified based on creatinine clearance and/or severity of infection.

	CREATININE CLEARANCE	
	20-40 ml/min	**<20 ml/min**
Uncomplicated UTI	No adjustment	3 Gm q12h
Complicated UTI	3 Gm q8h	3 Gm q12h
Serious infections	4 Gm q8h	4 Gm q12h

PRECAUTIONS

CONTRAINDICATIONS: Hypersensitivity to any penicillin. **CAUTIONS:** History of allergies, esp. cephalosporins, other drugs. **PREGNANCY/LACTATION:** Readily crosses placenta; appears in cord blood, amniotic fluid. Distributed in breast milk in low concentrations. May lead to allergic sensitization, diarrhea, candidiasis, skin rash in infant. **Pregnancy Category B.**

INTERACTIONS

DRUG INTERACTIONS: Probenecid may increase concentration, risk of toxicity. Hepatotoxic medications may increase hepatotoxicity. **ALTERED LAB VALUES:** May increase SGOT (AST), SGPT (ALT), alkaline phosphatase, bilirubin, LDH, sodium. May cause positive Coombs' test. May decrease potassium.

SIDE EFFECTS

FREQUENT: Rash, urticaria, pain/induration at IM injection site, phlebitis, thrombophlebitis w/IV dose. **OCCASIONAL:** Nausea, vomiting, diarrhea. **RARE:** Headache, dizziness, fatigue.

ADVERSE REACTIONS/TOXIC EFFECTS

Superinfections, potentially fatal antibiotic-associated colitis may result from bacterial imbalance. Seizures, neurologic reactions w/overdosage (more often w/renal impairment). Severe hypersensitivity reaction, including anaphylaxis, occur rarely.

NURSING IMPLICATIONS

BASELINE ASSESSMENT:

Question for history of allergies, esp. penicillins, cephalosporins, other drugs. Obtain specimen for culture and sensitivity before giving first dose (may begin therapy before results are known).

INTERVENTION/EVALUATION:

Hold medication, promptly report rash (hypersensitivity) or diarrhea (w/fever, abdominal pain, mucus and blood in stool may indicate antibiotic-associated colitis). Assess food tolerance. Evaluate IV site for phlebitis (heat, pain, red streaking over vein). Check IM injection site for pain, induration. Monitor I&O, urinalysis, renal function tests. Assess for bleeding (overt bleeding, bruising, or tissue swelling); check hematology reports. Monitor electrolytes, esp. potassium. Be alert for superinfection (increased fever, onset sore throat, diarrhea, vomiting, ulceration/other oral changes, anal/genital pruritus).

PATIENT/FAMILY TEACHING:

Continue antibiotic for full length of treatment. Space doses evenly. Discomfort may occur at IM injection site. Notify physician in event of rash, diarrhea, bleeding, bruising, other new symptom.

piperacillin sodium/tazobactam sodium

pip-ur-ah-sill'in/tay-zoe-back'tum
(Zosyn)

CANADIAN AVAILABILITY:
Zosyn

CLASSIFICATION

Antibiotic: Penicillin

PHARMACOKINETICS

Widely distributed. Protein binding: 30%. Primarily excreted unchanged in urine. Removed by hemodialysis. Half-life: 0.7-1.2 hrs (increased in decreased renal function, hepatic cirrhosis).

ACTION

Piperacillin: Bactericidal. Binds to bacterial membranes. Inhibits cell wall synthesis. *Tazobactam:* Beta-lactamase inhibitor (extends spectrum of activity, decreases MIC for bacteria, prevents bacterial overgrowth).

USES

Treatment of appendicitis (complicated by rupture or abscess), peritonitis, uncomplicated and complicated skin and skin structure infections including cellulitis, cutaneous abscesses, ischemic/diabetic foot infections, postpartum endometritis, pelvic inflammatory disease, community-acquired pneumonia (moderate severity only).

STORAGE/HANDLING

Reconstituted vials stable for 24 hrs at room temperature or 48 hrs if refrigerated. After further dilution, stable for 24 hrs at room temperature or 7 days if refrigerated.

IV ADMINISTRATION

1. Reconstitute each 1 Gm w/5 ml diluent.
2. Further dilute w/at least 50 ml 5% dextrose, 0.9% NaCl or other compatible diluent.
3. Infuse over 30 min.
4. Alternate IV sites, use large veins to prevent phlebitis.

INDICATIONS/DOSAGE/ROUTES

Usual parenteral dosage:
IV: Adults, elderly: 12 Gm/1.5 Gm/day as 3.375 Gm every 6 hrs.

Dosage in renal impairment:
Dose and/or frequency based on creatinine clearance.

CREATININE CLEARANCE	DOSAGE
20-40 ml/min	8 Gm/1 Gm/day (2.25 Gm q6h)
<20 ml/min	6 Gm/0.75 Gm/day (2.25 Gm q8h)

PRECAUTIONS

CONTRAINDICATIONS: Hypersensitivity to any penicillin. **CAUTIONS:** History of allergies, esp. cephalosporins, other drugs. **PREGNANCY/LACTATION:** Readily crosses placenta; appears in cord blood, amniotic fluid. Distributed in breast milk in low concentrations. May lead to allergic sensitization, diarrhea, candidiasis, skin rash in infant. **Pregnancy Category B.**

INTERACTIONS

DRUG INTERACTIONS: Probenecid may increase concentration, risk of toxicity. Hepatotoxic medications may increase hepatotoxicity. **ALTERED LAB VALUES:** May increase SGOT (AST), SGPT (ALT), alkaline phosphatase, bilirubin, LDH, sodium. May cause positive Coombs' test. May decrease potassium.

SIDE EFFECTS

FREQUENT: Diarrhea, headache, constipation, nausea, insomnia, rash. **OCCASIONAL:** Vomiting, dyspepsia, pruritus, fever, agitation, pain, moniliasis, dizziness, abdominal pain, edema, anxiety, dyspnea, rhinitis.

ADVERSE REACTIONS/TOXIC EFFECTS

Superinfections, potentially fatal antibiotic-associated colitis may result from bacterial imbalance. Seizures, neurologic reactions w/overdosage (more often w/renal impairment). Severe hypersensitivity reaction, including anaphylaxis, occur rarely.

NURSING IMPLICATIONS

BASELINE ASSESSMENT:

Question for history of allergies, esp. penicillins, cephalosporins, other drugs. Obtain specimen for culture and sensitivity before giving first dose (may begin therapy before results are known).

INTERVENTION/EVALUATION:

Hold medication and promptly report rash (hypersensitivity) or diarrhea (w/fever, abdominal pain, mucus and blood in stool may indicate antibiotic-associated colitis). Evaluate IV site for phlebitis (heat, pain, red streaking over vein). Monitor I&O, urinalysis, renal function tests. Monitor electrolytes, esp. potassium. Be alert for superinfection: increased fever, onset sore throat, diarrhea, vomiting, ulceration, or other oral changes, anal/genital pruritus.

PATIENT/FAMILY TEACHING:

Continue antibiotic for full length of treatment. Space doses evenly. Notify physician in event of rash, diarrhea, bleeding, bruising, other new symptom.

piroxicam

purr-ox′i-kam
(Feldene)

CANADIAN AVAILABILITY:
Apo-Piroxicam, Feldene, Novopirocam

CLASSIFICATION

Nonsteroidal anti-inflammatory

PHARMACOKINETICS

	ONSET	PEAK	DURATION
PO (analgesic)	1 hr	—	48-72 hrs
PO (antirheumatic)	7-12 days	2-3 wks	—

P

Well absorbed from GI tract. Metabolized in liver. Primarily excreted in urine. Half-life: 30-86 hrs (increased in decreased renal function).

ACTION

Inhibits prostaglandin synthesis. Inhibits action of cyclooxygenase, decreases formation of prostaglandin, thromboxane precursors from arachidonic acid.

USES

Symptomatic treatment of acute/chronic rheumatoid arthritis, osteoarthritis.

PO ADMINISTRATION

1. Do not crush or break capsule form.
2. May give w/food, milk, or antacids if GI distress occurs.

INDICATIONS/DOSAGE/ROUTES

Acute/chronic rheumatoid arthritis, osteoarthritis:
PO: Adults, elderly: Initially, 20 mg/day as single/divided doses. Some pts may require up to 30-40 mg/day.

PRECAUTIONS

CONTRAINDICATIONS: Active peptic ulcer, GI ulceration, chronic inflammation of GI tract, GI bleeding disorders, history of hypersensitivity to aspirin/NSAIDs. **CAUTIONS:** Impaired renal/hepatic function, history of GI tract disease, predisposition to fluid retention. **PREGNANCY/LACTATION:** Distributed in breast milk. Avoid use during third trimester (may adversely affect fetal cardiovascular system [premature closure of ductus arteriosus]). **Pregnancy Category C.**

INTERACTIONS

DRUG INTERACTIONS: May increase effects of oral anticoagulants, heparin, thrombolytics. May decrease effect of antihypertensives, diuretics. Salicylates, aspirin may increase risk of GI side effects, bleeding. Bone marrow depressants may increase risk of hematologic reactions. May increase concentration, toxicity of lithium. May increase methotrexate toxicity. Probenecid may increase concentration. **ALTERED LAB VALUES:** May increase serum transaminase activity. May decrease uric acid.

SIDE EFFECTS

FREQUENT: Epigastric distress, nausea. **OCCASIONAL:** Peripheral edema, anorexia, indigestion, flatulence, diarrhea, headache, malaise, rash, somnolence/dizziness.

ADVERSE REACTIONS/TOXIC EFFECTS

Peptic ulcer, GI bleeding, gastritis, severe hepatic reaction (cholestasis, jaundice) occur rarely. Nephrotoxicity (dysuria, hematuria, proteinuria, nephrotic syndrome), severe hypersensitivity reaction (fever, chills, bronchospasm), hematologic toxicity (anemia, leukopenia, eosinophilia, thrombocytopenia) may occur rarely w/long-term treatment.

NURSING IMPLICATIONS

BASELINE ASSESSMENT:

Assess onset, type, location, duration of pain/inflammation. Inspect appearance of affected joints for immobility, deformities, and skin condition.

INTERVENTION/EVALUATION:

Assist with ambulation if dizziness occurs. Monitor pattern of daily bowel activity, stool consistency. Check behind medial malleolus for fluid retention (usually first area noted). Monitor for evidence of nausea, GI distress. Assess skin for evidence of rash. Evaluate for therapeutic response (relief of pain, stiffness, swelling, increase in joint mobility, reduced joint tenderness, improved grip strength).

PATIENT/FAMILY TEACHING:

Avoid aspirin, alcohol during therapy (increases risk of GI bleeding). If GI upset occurs, take w/food, milk, or antacids. Avoid tasks that require alertness until response to drug is established. Do not crush or chew capsule form.

plasma protein fraction

(Plasmanate, Plasma-Plex, Plasmatein)

CLASSIFICATION

Plasma volume expander

ACTION

Regulates both the volume of circulating blood and tissue fluid balance. Binds and functions as a carrier of intermediate metabolites (hormones, enzymes, drugs) in the transport, exchange of tissue products.

USES

Plasma volume expansion in treatment of shock complicated by circulatory volume deficit. Management of protein deficiencies in pts with hypoproteinemia.

STORAGE/HANDLING

Store at room temperature. Liquid is typically transparent, slightly brown, and odorless. Do not use if solution has been frozen, if solution appears turbid or contains sediment, or if not used within 4 hrs of opening vial.

IV ADMINISTRATION

1. Give by IV infusion.
2. May be administered without regard to pt's blood group/Rh factor.
3. Do not administer near site of any trauma/infection.
4. Monitor blood pressure during infusion.

INDICATIONS/DOSAGE/ROUTE

Hypovolemic shock:

IV: Adults, elderly: Initially, 250-500 ml at a rate not exceeding 10 ml/min (minimizes hypotension). **Infants, children:** 20-30 ml/kg at a rate not to exceed 10 ml/min.

Hypoproteinemia:

IV: Adults, elderly: 1,000-1,500 ml/day at a rate not to exceed 5-8 ml/min (prevents hypervolemia).

PRECAUTIONS

CONTRAINDICATIONS: Severe anemia, cardiac failure, history of allergic reactions to albumin, renal insufficiency, no albumin deficiency. **CAUTIONS:** Low cardiac reserve, pulmonary disease, hepatic/renal failure. **PREGNANCY/LACTATION:** Unknown whether drug crosses placenta or is distributed in breast milk. **Pregnancy Category C.**

INTERACTIONS

DRUG INTERACTIONS: None significant. **ALTERED LAB VALUES:** None significant.

SIDE EFFECTS

OCCASIONAL: Hypotension. High dosage, repeated therapy may result in allergy or protein overload (chills, fever, flushing, low back pain, nausea, urticaria, vital sign changes).

ADVERSE REACTIONS/TOXIC EFFECTS

Fluid overload (headache, weakness, blurred vision, behavioral changes, incoordination, isolated muscle twitching) and pulmonary edema (rapid breathing, rales, wheezing, coughing, increased B/P, distended neck veins) may occur.

NURSING IMPLICATIONS

BASELINE ASSESSMENT:

Obtain B/P, pulse, respirations immediately before administration. There should be adequate hydration before albumin is administered.

INTERVENTION/EVALUATION:

Monitor B/P for hypotension. Assess frequently for evidence of fluid overload, pulmonary edema (see Adverse Reactions/Toxic Effects). Check skin for flushing, urticaria. Monitor hemoglobin, hematocrit. Monitor I & O ratio (watch for decreased output). Assess for therapeutic response (increased B/P, decreased edema).

plicamycin

ply-kah-my´sin

(Mithracin)

CLASSIFICATION

Antineoplastic, antihypercalcemic

PHARMACOKINETICS

Localized in liver, kidney, formed bone surfaces. Crosses blood-brain barrier, enters CSF. Primarily excreted in urine.

ACTION

Forms complexes w/DNA, inhibiting DNA-directed RNA synthesis. Lowers serum calcium concentration. Blocks hypercalcemic action of vitamin D and blocks action of parathyroid hormone. Decreases serum phosphate levels.

USES

Treatment of malignant testicular tumors, hypercalcemia, hypercalcuria associated w/advanced neoplasms.

STORAGE/HANDLING

NOTE: May be carcinogenic, mutagenic, or teratogenic. Handle w/extreme care during preparation/administration.

Refrigerate vials. Solutions must be freshly prepared before use; discard unused portions.

IV ADMINISTRATION

NOTE: Give by IV infusion.

1. Reconstitute 2,500 mcg (2.5 mg) vial w/4.9 ml sterile water for injection to provide concentration of 500 mcg/ml (0.5 mg/ml).
2. Dilute w/500-1,000 ml 5% dextrose or 0.9% NaCl fluid for injection. Infuse over 4-6 hrs.
3. Extravasation produces painful inflammation, induration. Sloughing may occur. Aspirate as much drug as possible. Apply warm compresses.

INDICATIONS/DOSAGE/ROUTES

NOTE: Dosage individualized based on clinical response, tolerance to adverse effects. Dose based on actual body weight. Use ideal body weight for obese or edematous pts. Do not exceed 30 mcg/kg/day or more than 10 daily doses (increases potential for hemorrhage).

Testicular tumors:
IV: Adults, elderly: 25-30 mcg/kg/day for 8-10 days. Repeat at monthly intervals.

Hypercalcemia/hyperuricemia:
IV: Adults, elderly: 15-25 mcg/kg/day for 3-4 days. Repeat at weekly or longer intervals until desired response achieved.

PRECAUTIONS

CONTRAINDICATIONS: Existing thrombocytopenia, thrombocytopathy, coagulation disorders, tendency to hemorrhage, impaired bone marrow function. **EXTREME CAUTION:** Renal/hepatic impairment. **CAUTIONS:** Electrolyte imbalance. **PREGNANCY/LACTATION:** Contraindicated during pregnancy. Breast feeding not recommended. **Pregnancy Category X.**

INTERACTIONS

DRUG INTERACTIONS: May increase effect of oral anticoagulants, heparin, thrombolytics. May increase risk of hemorrhage w/NSAIDs, aspirin, dipyridamole, sulfinpyrazone, valproic acid. Bone marrow depressants, hepatotoxic, nephrotoxic medications may increase toxicity. Calcium containing medications, vitamin D may decrease effect. Live virus vaccines may potentiate virus replication, increase vaccine side effects, decrease pt's antibody response to vaccine. **ALTERED LAB VALUES:** None significant.

SIDE EFFECTS

FREQUENT: Nausea, vomiting, anorexia, diarrhea, stomatitis. **OCCASIONAL:** Fever, drowsiness, weakness, lethargy, malaise, headache, mental depression, nervousness, dizziness, rash, acne.

ADVERSE REACTIONS/TOXIC EFFECTS

Hematologic toxicity noted by marked facial flushing, persistent nosebleeds, hemoptysis, purpura, ecchymoses, leukopenia, thrombocytopenia. Risk of bleeding tendencies increase w/higher doses and/or more than 10 doses are given. May produce electrolyte imbalance.

P

NURSING IMPLICATIONS

BASELINE ASSESSMENT:

Question for possibility of pregnancy before initiating therapy (Pregnancy Category X). Antiemetics may be effective in preventing, treating nausea. Therapy discontinued if platelet count falls below 150,000/mm^3, if WBC falls below 4,000/mm^3, or if prothrombin time is 4 sec higher than control test. Renal/hepatic studies should be performed daily in those w/impairment.

INTERVENTION/EVALUATION:

Monitor hematologic, renal, hepatic function studies; platelet count; prothrombin, bleeding times; serum calcium, phosphorus, potassium levels. Assess pattern of daily bowel activity, stool consistency. Monitor for stomatitis (burning/erythema of oral mucosa at inner margin of lips, sore throat, difficulty swallowing, oral ulceration). Monitor for thrombocytopenia (bleeding from gums, tarry stool, petechiae, small subcutaneous hemorrhages). Avoid IM injections, rectal temperatures, any trauma that may induce bleeding.

PATIENT/FAMILY TEACHING:

Maintain fastidious oral hygiene. Do not have immunizations w/o physician's approval (drug lowers body's resistance). Avoid crowds, those w/infection. Promptly report fever, sore throat, signs of local infection, easy bruising, unusual bleeding from any site. Contact physician if nausea/vomiting continues at home. Use nonhormonal contraception.

polycarbophil

pol-lee-car´bow-fill
(Fibercon, Mitrolan)

CANADIAN AVAILABILITY:
Mitrolan

CLASSIFICATION

Laxative: Bulk-forming

PHARMACOKINETICS

	ONSET	PEAK	DURATION
PO	12-72 hrs	—	—

Acts in small/large intestine.

ACTION

Laxative: Retains water in intestine, opposes dehydrating forces of the bowel (promotes well-formed stools). *Antidiarrheal:* Absorbs free fecal water (forms gel, producing formed stool).

USES

Treatment of diarrhea associated w/irritable bowel syndrome, diverticulosis, acute nonspecific diarrhea. Relieves constipation associated w/irritable or spastic bowel.

INDICATIONS/DOSAGE/ROUTES

NOTE: For severe diarrhea, give q1/2hr up to maximum daily dosage; for laxative, give w/8 oz liquid.

Laxative, antidiarrheal:
PO: Adults, elderly: 1 Gm 4 times/day, or as needed. **Maximum:** 6 Gm/24 hrs. **Children 6-12 yrs:** 500 mg 1-3 times/day, or as needed. **Maximum:** 3 Gm/24 hrs. **Children 2-6 yrs:** 500 mg 1-2 times/day, or as needed. **Maximum:** 1.5 Gm/24 hrs.

PRECAUTIONS

CONTRAINDICATIONS: Abdominal pain, nausea, vomiting, symptoms of appendicitis, partial bowel obstruction, dysphagia. **CAUTIONS:** None significant. **PREGNANCY/LACTATION:** Safe for use in pregnancy. **Pregnancy Category C.**

INTERACTIONS

DRUG INTERACTIONS: May interfere w/effects of potassium-sparing diuretics, potassium supplements. May decrease effect of oral anticoagulants, digoxin, salicylates, tetracyclines by decreasing absorption. **ALTERED LAB VALUES:** May increase glucose. May decrease potassium.

SIDE EFFECTS

RARE: Some degree of abdominal discomfort, nausea, mild cramps, griping, faintness.

ADVERSE REACTIONS/TOXIC EFFECTS

Esophageal/bowel obstruction

may occur if administered with insufficient liquid (less than 250 ml or 1 full glass).

NURSING IMPLICATIONS

INTERVENTION/EVALUATION:

Encourage adequate fluid intake. Assess bowel sounds for peristalsis. Monitor daily bowel activity, stool consistency (watery, loose, soft, semi-solid, solid) and record time of evacuation. Monitor serum electrolytes in those exposed to prolonged, frequent, or excessive use of medication.

PATIENT/FAMILY TEACHING:

Institute measures to promote defecation (increase fluid intake, exercise, high-fiber diet). Drink 6-8 glasses of water/day when used as laxative (aids stool softening).

polyethylene glycol-electrolyte solution (PEG-ES)

poly-eth'ah-leen
(Colovage, CoLyte, GoLYTELY, OCL)

CANADIAN AVAILABILITY:
CoLyte, Golytely, Peglyte

CLASSIFICATION

Bowel evacuant

ACTION

Osmotic effect. Fluid overload of bowel induces liquid stool. (Electrolytes in solution prevent water/electrolyte imbalance.) No net absorption. Onset usually in 30-60 min; completed within 4 hrs.

USES

Bowel cleansing before GI examination.

STORAGE/HANDLING

Refrigerate reconstituted solutions; use within 48 hrs.

PO ADMINISTRATION

1. May use tap water to prepare solution. Shake vigorously several minutes to ensure complete dissolution of powder.
2. Fasting should occur at least 3 hrs before ingestion of solution (solid food should always be avoided <2 hrs before administration).
3. Only clear liquids permitted after administration.
4. May give via N-G tube.
5. Rapid drinking preferred.

INDICATIONS/DOSAGE/ROUTES

Bowel evacuant:
PO: Adults: 4 liters prior to GI examination: 240 ml (8 oz) q10min until 4 liters consumed or rectal effluent clear. N-G tube: 20-30 ml/min.

PRECAUTIONS

CONTRAINDICATIONS: GI obstruction, gastric retention, bowel perforation, toxic colitis, toxic megacolon, ileus. **CAUTIONS:** Ulcerative colitis. **PREGNANCY/LACTATION:** Unknown whether drug crosses placenta or is distributed in breast milk. **Pregnancy Category C.**

INTERACTIONS

DRUG INTERACTIONS: May decrease absorption of oral medications if given within 1 hr (may be flushed from GI tract). **ALTERED LAB VALUES:** None significant.

SIDE EFFECTS

FREQUENT: Some degree of abdominal fullness, nausea, bloating. **OCCASIONAL:** Abdominal cramping, vomiting, anal irritation. **RARE:** Urticaria, rhinorrhea, dermatitis.

ADVERSE REACTIONS/TOXIC EFFECTS

None significant.

NURSING IMPLICATIONS

BASELINE ASSESSMENT:

Do not give oral medication within 1 hr of start of therapy (may not adequately be absorbed before GI cleansing).

INTERVENTION/EVALUATION:

Assess bowel sounds for peristalsis. Monitor bowel activity, stool consistency (watery, loose, soft, semi-solid, solid) and record time of evacuation. Assess for abdominal disturbances.

polymyxin B sulfate

polly-mix´in

(Aerosporin)

FIXED-COMBINATION(S): *Ophthalmic:* w/bacitracin, an antiinfective (Ocumycin, Polysporin Ophthalmic, AK-Poly-Bac); w/neomycin, an aminoglycoside (Statrol); w/neomycin and bacitracin, antiinfectives (Neosporin, AK-Spore, Ocutricin); w/neomycin and bacitracin, antiinfectives, and hydrocortisone, a corticosteroid (Coracin); w/dexamethasone, a corticosteroid, and neomycin, an aminoglycoside (AK-Trol, Dexacidin, Dex-Ide, Maxitrol); w/chloramphenicol, an antibiotic (Ophthocort). *Otic:* w/hydrocortisone, a steroid (Otobiotic, Pyocidin-Otic); w/hydrocortisone, a steroid, and neomycin, an aminoglycoside (Biotis-S, Pedi-Otic, Oti-Sone, Cortisporin Otic). *Misc:* w/neomycin, an aminoglycoside (Neosporin GU irrigant).

CANADIAN AVAILABILITY: Aerosporin

CLASSIFICATION

Antibiotic

PHARMACOKINETICS

Widely distributed in tissues; excreted unchanged in urine. Serum concentration increased, half-life prolonged in those w/renal impairment. Half-life: 4-6 hrs (increased in decreased renal function).

ACTION

Bactericidal in susceptible microorganisms due to alteration of cell membrane permeability w/ loss of essential elements.

USES

Septicemia, infections of skin, urinary tract, meninges; treatment of superficial ocular infections, minor skin abrasions, external ear canal infections, mastoidectomy cavity infections. Prevent bacteruria/ bacteremia associated w/indwelling catheters (combination w/neomycin) as irrigating solution.

STORAGE/HANDLING

After reconstitution, solution stable for 72 hrs if refrigerated. Discard if precipitate forms.

IM/IV/TOPICAL/OPHTHALMIC/ OTIC ADMINISTRATION

NOTE: Patients must be hospitalized, closely supervised by physician for parenteral administration.

IM:

1. Reconstitute each 500,000 U vial w/2 ml sterile water for injection, 0.9% NaCl injection, or 1% procaine to provide concentration of 250,000 U/ml.
2. Administer deeply into upper outer quadrant of gluteus maximus.
3. Repeat IM injections at same site not recommended (produces tissue irritation, pain).

IV:

1. For IV infusion (piggyback), further dilute w/300-500 ml 5% dextrose. Infuse over 60-90 min.
2. Alternating IV sites, use large veins to reduce risk of phlebitis.

TOPICAL:

1. Apply only to affected area(s); do not apply to large denuded areas.
2. Concomitant cortisone therapy may mask development of bacterial, fungal, viral infections.

OPHTHALMIC:

1. Place finger on lower eyelid and pull out until a pocket is formed between eye and lower lid. Hold dropper above pocket and place correct number of drops (¼-½ inch ointment) into pocket.
2. Have pt close eye gently; w/ solution, apply digital pressure to lacrimal sac for 1-2 min (minimizes draining into nose and throat, reducing risk of systemic effects).
3. W/ointment, have pt close and roll eyes in all directions (increases contact area of drug to eye).
4. Remove excess solution or ointment around eye w/tissue.

OTIC:

1. Hold container in hand for a few min to warm to near body temperature. Shake suspensions well for 10 sec.
2. Have pt lie on side or tilt the affected ear upward.
3. *Adults:* Hold the earlobe up and back. *Children:* Hold the earlobe down and back.
4. Instill prescribed number of drops, holding the dropper outside the ear canal. Do not touch the dropper to any surface.
5. Instruct pt to keep ear tilted for 2 min or insert a cotton plug.

INDICATIONS/DOSAGE/ROUTES

NOTE: Space doses evenly around the clock.

Mild to moderate infections:
IV: Adults, elderly, children >2 yrs: 15,000-25,000 U/kg/day in divided doses q12h. **Infants:** Up to 40,000 U/kg/day.
IM: Adults, elderly, children >2 yrs: 25,000-30,000 U/kg/day in divided doses q4-6h. **Infants:** Up to 40,000 U/kg/day.

Usual irrigation dosage:
CONTINUOUS BLADDER IRRIGATION: Adults, elderly: 1 ml urogenital concentrate (contains 200,000 U polymyxin B, 57 mg neomycin) added to 1,000 ml 0.9% NaCl. Give each 1,000 ml >24 hrs for up to 10 days (may increase to 2,000 ml/day when urine output >2 liters/day).

Usual ophthalmic dosage:
SOLUTION: Adults, elderly, children: 1 drop q3-4h.
OINTMENT: Adults, elderly, children: Apply thin strip to conjunctiva q3-4h.

Usual otic dosage:
OTIC: Adults, elderly: 4 drops q6-8h. **Children:** 3 drops q6-8h.

Usual topical dosage:
TOPICAL: Adults, elderly, children: Apply to affected area 2-5 times/day.

PRECAUTIONS

CONTRAINDICATIONS: Hypersensitivity to polymyxins or other components in fixed-combinations. **CAUTIONS:** Renal impairment, neuromuscular disorders. **PREGNANCY/LACTATION:** Does not cross placenta; unknown whether excreted in breast milk. **Pregnancy Category B.**

INTERACTIONS

DRUG INTERACTIONS: May produce muscle paralysis, prolonged or increased skeletal muscle relaxation w/neuromuscular blocking agents or anesthetics. Aminoglycosides, other nephrotoxic drugs may increase nephrotoxicity. **ALTERED LAB VALUES:** None significant.

SIDE EFFECTS

NOTE: It is important to know side effects of components when Polymyxin B is used in fixed-combinations.
FREQUENT: Severe pain, irritation at IM injection sites, phlebitis, thrombophlebitis w/IV administration. **OCCASIONAL:** Fever, urticaria. **RARE:** *Topical:* Hypersensitivity reaction w/inflammation, itching, burning.

ADVERSE REACTIONS/TOXIC EFFECTS

Nephrotoxicity, esp. w/concurrent/sequential use of other nephrotoxic drugs, renal impairment, concurrent/sequential use of muscle relaxants. Neurotoxicity may occur, esp w/other neurotoxic medications, following anesthesia. Superinfection, esp. w/fungi may occur.

NURSING IMPLICATIONS

BASELINE ASSESSMENT:

Question pt for history of allergies to polymyxins, other ingredients when used in fixed-combinations. Inquire about sulfite sensitivity, asthma when administering otic preparations containing potassium metabisulfite. Avoid concurrent administration of other nephrotoxic, neurotoxic drugs if possible. Obtain specimens for culture, sensitivity before giving first dose (therapy may begin before results are known).

INTERVENTION/EVALUATION:

Evaluate IV sites for phlebitis (heat, pain, red streaking over vein). Assess pain, irritation from IM injections. Check I&O, renal function tests. Monitor level of consciousness. Assess for muscle weakness, steadiness on ambulation (support as needed). Obtain vital signs, be esp. alert to respiratory depression. Watch for signs of sensitivity w/topical use (burning, itching, inflammation). W/topical preparations containing corticosteroids, consider masking effect on clinical signs.

PATIENT/FAMILY TEACHING:

Therapy must be continued for full length of treatment. Doses are spaced evenly for full effectiveness. Discomfort may occur at IM injection sites. Notify physician in event of dizziness, drowsiness, difficulty breathing, or other new symptom; w/topical, otic, or ophthalmic therapy report any increased irritation, inflammation, itching, burning.

potassium acetate
(Potassium acetate)

potassium bicarbonate/citrate
(K-Lyte)

potassium chloride
(K-Lor, K-Lyte-Cl, Klotrix, K-Dur, Kaochlor, Micro-K, Slow-K)

potassium gluconate
(Kaon)

potassium phosphate
(Potassium phosphate)

CANADIAN AVAILABILITY: Apo-K, Kaochlor, Kaon, K-Lor, Micro-K, Novolente-K, Slow-K

CLASSIFICATION

Electrolyte

PHARMACOKINETICS

Well absorbed from GI tract. Enters cells via active transport from extracellular fluid. Primarily excreted in urine.

ACTION

Primary intracellular cation. Necessary for nerve impulse conduction, contraction of cardiac, skeletal, smooth muscle; maintains normal renal function, acid-base balance. Necessary for multiple cellular metabolic processes.

USES

Treatment of potassium deficiency found in severe vomiting, diarrhea, loss of GI fluid, malnutrition, prolonged diuresis, debilitated, poor GI absorption, metabolic alkalosis, prolonged parenteral alimentation.

STORAGE/HANDLING

Store oral, parenteral forms at room temperature.

PO/IV ADMINISTRATION

PO:

1. Take w/or after meals and w/full glass of water (decreases GI upset).
2. Liquids, powder, or effervescent tablets: Mix, dissolve w/juice, water before administering.
3. Do not chew, crush tablets; swallow whole.

IV:

1. For IV infusion only, must dilute before administration/mixed well/infused slowly.
2. Generally, no more than 40 mEq/liter; no faster than 20 mEq/hr. (Higher concentrations/faster rates may sometimes be necessary.)
3. Use largest peripheral vein/small bore needle.
4. Avoid adding potassium to hanging IV.
5. Check IV site closely during infusion for evidence of phlebitis (heat, pain, red streaking of skin over vein, hardness to vein), extravasation (swelling, pain, cool skin, little or no blood return).

INDICATIONS/DOSAGE/ROUTES

Treatment/prevention hypokalemia:
NOTE: Dosage is individualized.
PO: Adults, elderly: *Prevention:* 20 mEq/day. *Treatment:* 40-100 mEq/day. **Children:** No more than 3 mEq/kg/day. **Infants:** 2-3 mEq/kg/day. Give in 2-4 divided doses.
IV: Adults, elderly, children: In-

dividualize based on EKG, serum potassium concentrations.

PRECAUTIONS

CONTRAINDICATIONS: Severe renal impairment, untreated Addison's disease, postop oliguria, shock w/hemolytic reaction and/or dehydration, hyperkalemia, those receiving potassium-sparing diuretics, digitalis toxicity, heat cramps, severe burns. **CAUTIONS:** Cardiac disease, tartrazine sensitivity (mostly noted in those w/aspirin hypersensitivity). **PREGNANCY/LACTATION:** Unknown whether drug crosses placenta or is distributed in breast milk. **Pregnancy Category C.**

INTERACTIONS

DRUG INTERACTIONS: Angiotensin-converting enzyme (ACE) inhibitors, NSAIDs, beta-adrenergic blockers, potassium sparing diuretics, heparin, potassium containing medications, salt substitutes may increase potassium concentration. Anticholinergics may increase risk of GI lesions. **ALTERED LAB VALUES:** None significant.

SIDE EFFECTS

OCCASIONAL: Nausea, vomiting, diarrhea, flatulence, abdominal discomfort w/distention, phlebitis w/IV administration (particularly when potassium concentration of more than 40 mEq/liter is infused). **RARE:** Rash.

ADVERSE REACTIONS/TOXIC EFFECTS

Hyperkalemia (observed particularly in elderly or in those w/impaired renal function) manifested as paresthesia of extremities, heaviness of legs, cold skin, grayish pallor, hypotension, mental confusion, irritability, flaccid paralysis, cardiac arrhythmias.

NURSING IMPLICATIONS

BASELINE ASSESSMENT:

Oral dose should be given w/food or after meals w/full glass of water or fruit juice (minimizes GI irritation).

INTERVENTION/EVALUATION:

Monitor serum potassium level (particularly in renal function impairment). If GI disturbance is noted, dilute preparation further or give w/meals. Be alert to decrease in urinary output (may be indication of renal insufficiency). Monitor daily bowel activity, stool consistency. Assess I&O diligently during diuresis, IV site for extravasation, phlebitis. Be alert to evidence of hyperkalemia (skin pallor/coldness, complaints of paresthesia of extremities, feeling of heaviness of legs).

PATIENT/FAMILY TEACHING:

Food rich in potassium include beef, veal, ham, chicken, turkey, fish, milk, bananas, dates, prunes, raisins, avocado, watermelon, cantaloupe, apricots, molasses, beans, yams, broccoli, brussel sprouts, lentils, potatoes, spinach. Report paresthesia of extremities, feeling of heaviness of legs.

pravastatin

pra´vah-sta-tin

(Pravachol)

CANADIAN AVAILABILITY:

Pravachol

CLASSIFICATION

Antihyperlipoproteinemic

PHARMACOKINETICS

Poorly absorbed from GI tract. Protein binding: 50%. Metabolized in liver (minimal active metabolites). Primarily excreted in feces via biliary system. Half-life: 2.7 hrs.

ACTION

Inhibits cholesterol biosynthesis by preventing the conversion of HMG-CoA reductase to mevalonate, a precursor to cholesterol. Decreases LDL cholesterol, VLDL, plasma triglycerides; increases HDL concentration.

USES

Adjunct to diet therapy to decrease elevated total, LDL cholesterol concentrations in those w/ primary hypercholesterolemia (types IIa and IIb).

PO ADMINISTRATION

1. Give w/o regard to meals.
2. Administer in evening.

INDICATIONS/DOSAGE/ROUTES

NOTE: Before initiating therapy, pt should be on standard cholesterol lowering diet for minimum of 3-6 mo. Continue diet throughout pravastatin therapy.

Hyperlipidemia:
PO: Adults: Initially, 10-20 mg/day at bedtime. **Elderly:** 10 mg/day at bedtime. **Range:** 10-40 mg/day at bedtime.

CONTRAINDICATIONS: Hypersensitivity to pravastatin or any component of the preparation, active liver disease or unexplained, persistent elevations of liver function tests. Safety and efficacy in individuals less than 18 yrs of age has not been established. **CAUTIONS:** History of liver disease, substantial alcohol consumption. Withholding/discontinuing pravastatin may be necessary when pt at risk for renal failure secondary to rhabdomyolysis. Severe metabolic, endocrine, or electrolyte disorders. **PREGNANCY/LACTATION:** Contraindicated in pregnancy (suppression of cholesterol biosynthesis may cause fetal toxicity) and lactation. Unknown whether drug is distributed in breast milk, but there is risk of serious adverse reactions in nursing infants. **Pregnancy Category X.**

INTERACTIONS

DRUG INTERACTIONS: Increased risk of rhabdomyolysis, acute renal failure w/cyclosporine, erythromycin, gemfibrozil, niacin, other immunosuppressants. **ALTERED LAB VALUES:** May increase creatinine kinase, serum transaminase concentrations.

SIDE EFFECTS

Generally well tolerated. Side effects usually mild and transient. **FREQUENT:** Nausea/vomiting, diarrhea and/or constipation, flatulence, abdominal pain, headache, localized pain, rash, pruritus. **OCCASIONAL:** Heartburn, dyspepsia, myalgia, muscle cramping, fatigue, dizziness, cardiac chest pain. **RARE:** Myopathy (myalgia and/or muscle weakness w/markedly elevated CK concentrations).

ADVERSE REACTIONS/TOXIC EFFECTS

Potential for malignancy, cataracts. Hypersensitivity syndrome has been reported rarely.

NURSING IMPLICATIONS

BASELINE ASSESSMENT:

Question for possibility of pregnancy before initiating therapy (Pregnancy Category X). Question history of hypersensitivity to pravastatin. Assess baseline lab results: Cholesterol, triglycerides, liver function tests.

INTERVENTION/EVALUATION:

Monitor cholesterol and triglyceride lab results for therapeutic response. Evaluate food tolerance. Determine pattern of bowel activity. Check for headache, dizziness (provide assistance as needed). Assess for rash, pruritus. Be alert for malaise, muscle cramping/weakness; if accompanied by fever, may require discontinuation of medication.

PATIENT/FAMILY TEACHING:

Take w/o regard to meals. Follow special diet (important part of treatment). Periodic lab tests are essential part of therapy. Do not take other medications w/o physician's knowledge. Do not stop medication w/o consulting physician. Report promptly any muscle pain/weakness, esp. if accompanied by fever or malaise. Do not drive/perform activities that require alert response if dizziness occurs. Use nonhormonal contraception.

praziquantel

pray-zih-kwon´tel
(Biltricide)

CLASSIFICATION

Anthelmintic

PHARMACOKINETICS

Rapidly absorbed from GI tract (undergoes extensive first-pass metabolism). Distributed in serum, CSF. Protein binding: 80%. Metabolized in liver. Primarily excreted in urine. Half-life: 0.8-1.5 hrs (metabolite: 4-6 hrs).

ACTION

Vermicidal. Increases cell permeability in susceptible helminths w/loss of calcium; resultant contractions and paralysis of their musculature dislodges the dead and dying worms, followed by attachment of phagocytes.

USES

Treatment of all stages of schistosomiasis (bilharziasis or fluke infections), infections due to liver flukes, clonorchiasis and opisthorchiasis.

PO ADMINISTRATION

1. Tablets must not be chewed, but can be halved or quartered.
2. Give w/meals, w/sufficient fluid to swallow w/o gagging.

INDICATIONS/DOSAGE/ROUTES

Schistosomiasis:
PO: Adults, elderly: 3 doses of 20 mg/kg as 1 day treatment. Do not give doses <4 and not >6 hrs apart.

Clonorchiasis/opisthorchiasis:
PO: Adults, elderly: 3 doses of 25 mg/kg as 1 day treatment.

PRECAUTIONS

CONTRAINDICATIONS: Ocular cysticercosis, hypersensitivity to praziquantel. **CAUTIONS:** None significant. **PREGNANCY/LACTATION:** Distributed in breast milk; nursing should be discontinued until 72 hrs after last dose (milk should be expressed, thrown away during this period). **Pregnancy Category B.**

INTERACTIONS

DRUG INTERACTIONS: None significant. **ALTERED LAB VALUES:** None significant.

SIDE EFFECTS

FREQUENT: Headache, dizziness, malaise, abdominal pain occur in 90% of pts. **OCCASIONAL:** Anorexia, vomiting, diarrhea. Severe cramping abdominal pain may occur within 1 hr of administration w/ fever, sweating, bloody stools. **RARE:** Giddiness, urticaria.

ADVERSE REACTIONS/TOXIC EFFECTS

Overdose should be treated w/ fast-acting laxative.

NURSING IMPLICATIONS

BASELINE ASSESSMENT:

Question for history of hypersensitivity to praziquantel. Obtain stool, urine specimens to confirm diagnosis.

INTERVENTION/EVALUATION:

Collect stool, urine specimens as required to monitor effectiveness of therapy. Assess food tolerance, encourage adequate nutrition. Monitor CNS reactions, provide safety measures for ambulation. Check hematology results for anemia. Assess for urticaria.

PATIENT/FAMILY TEACHING:

Complete full course of therapy. If iron supplements are ordered, continue as directed (may be up to 6 mo posttherapy). Notify physician if symptoms do not improve in a few days, or if they become worse. Follow-up office visits (several mo after therapy is complete) are essential to assure cure. Don't drive, use machinery if dizzy or drowsy.

prazosin hydrochloride

pray´zoe-sin
(Minipress)

FIXED-COMBINATION(S):
W/polythiazide, a diuretic (Minizide)

CANADIAN AVAILABILITY:
Minipress

CLASSIFICATION

Antihypertensive

PHARMACOKINETICS

	ONSET	PEAK	DURATION
PO	2 hrs	2-4 hrs	24 hrs

Well absorbed from GI tract. Widely distributed. Protein binding: 97%. Metabolized in liver. Primarily eliminated in feces and bile. Not removed by hemodialysis. Half-life: 2-3 hrs.

ACTION

Blocks alpha-adrenergic receptors. Produces vasodilation, decrease peripheral resistance.

USES

Treatment of mild to moderate hypertension. Used alone or in combination w/other antihypertensives.

PO ADMINISTRATION

1. May give w/o regard to food.
2. Administer first dose at bed-

time (minimizes risk of fainting due to "first-dose syncope").

INDICATIONS/DOSAGE/ROUTES

Hypertension (alone):
PO: Adults: Initially, 0.5-1 mg 2-3 times/day. Increase gradually up to 20-40 mg/day in divided doses. **Maintenance:** 6-15 mg/day in divided doses.

Hypertension (in combinations w/antihypertensives):
PO: Adults: 1-2 mg 3 times/day and retitrate.

Usual elderly dosage:
PO: Elderly: Initially, 1 mg 1-2 times/day.

PRECAUTIONS

CONTRAINDICATIONS: None significant. **CAUTIONS:** Chronic renal failure, impaired hepatic function. **PREGNANCY/LACTATION:** Unknown whether drug crosses placenta; distributed in small amount in breast milk. **Pregnancy Category C.**

INTERACTIONS

DRUG INTERACTIONS: Estrogen, NSAIDs, sympathomimetics may decrease effect. Hypotension-producing medications may increase anti-hypertensive effect. **ALTERED LAB VALUES:** None significant.

SIDE EFFECTS

FREQUENT: Dizziness, lightheadedness, headache, drowsiness, lassitude, weakness, palpitations, nausea. **OCCASIONAL:** Dry mouth, GI effects (diarrhea/constipation, abdominal discomfort), urinary urgency, nasal congestion.

ADVERSE REACTIONS/TOXIC EFFECTS

"First-dose syncope" (hypotension w/sudden loss of consciousness) generally occurs 30-90 min after giving initial dose of 2 mg or greater, a too-rapid increase in dose, or addition of another hypotensive agent to therapy. May be preceded by tachycardia (120-160 beats/min).

NURSING IMPLICATIONS

BASELINE ASSESSMENT:

Give first dose at bedtime. If initial dose is given during daytime, pt must remain recumbent for 3-4 hrs. Assess B/P, pulse immediately before each dose and q15-30min until stabilized (be alert to B/P fluctuations).

INTERVENTION/EVALUATION:

Monitor pulse diligently (first-dose syncope may be preceded by tachycardia). Monitor pattern of daily bowel activity and stool consistency. Assist w/ambulation if dizziness, lightheadedness occurs.

PATIENT/FAMILY TEACHING:

Dry mouth may be relieved by sugarless gum/sips of tepid water. Carbonated beverage, unsalted crackers, dry toast may relieve nausea. Nasal congestion may occur. Full therapeutic effect may not occur for 3-4 wks.

---

prednicarbate (Dermatop)
See supplement

---

prednisolone

pred-niss´oh-lone
(Prelone, Delta-Cortef)

prednisolone acetate

(Econopred, Inflamase, Pred Mild, Pred Forte, Predolone)

prednisolone sodium phosphate
(Hydeltrasol, Pediapred)

prednisolone tebutate
(Hydeltra TBA, Predalone TBA)

FIXED-COMBINATION(S): Prednisolone acetate w/sulfacetamide sodium, a sulfonamide (Blephamide Liquifilm, Isopto Cetopred); w/atropine sulfate, a mydriatic (Mydrapred); w/neomycin and polymyxin B, anti-infectives (Poly-Pred Liquifilm)

Prednisolone sodium phosphate w/sulfacetamide, a sulfonamide (Vasocidin, Optimyd)

CANADIAN AVAILABILITY: Inflamase

CLASSIFICATION

Corticosteroid

PHARMACOKINETICS

Well absorbed from GI tract, after IM administration. Widely distributed. Protein binding: 65-91%. Metabolized in liver, tissues. Primarily excreted in urine. Half-life: 3-6 hrs.

ACTION

Decreases/prevents tissue response to inflammatory process. Inhibits accumulation of inflammatory cells at inflammation sites, phagocytosis, lysosomal enzyme release, and synthesis and/or release of mediators of inflammation. Prevents/suppresses cell-mediated immune reactions.

USES

Substitution therapy in deficiency states: Acute/chronic adrenal insufficiency, congenital adrenal hyperplasia, adrenal insufficiency secondary to pituitary insufficiency. *Nonendocrine disorders:* Arthritis, rheumatic carditis; allergic, collagen, intestinal tract, liver, ocular, renal, skin diseases; bronchial asthma, cerebral edema, malignancies.

PO/IM/IV/OPHTHALMIC ADMINISTRATION

PO:

1. Give w/food or milk.
2. Single doses given before 9 AM; multiple doses at evenly spaced intervals.

IM:

1. Give deep IM in gluteus maximus.

IV:

1. May add to 5% dextrose in water or 0.9% NaCl; use within 24 hrs.
2. Prednisolone tebutate not for IV use.

OPHTHALMIC:

1. Place finger on lower eyelid and pull out until a pocket is formed between eye and lower lid. Hold dropper above pocket and place correct number of drops (¼-½ inch ointment) into pocket. Close eye gently. *Solution:* Apply digital pressure to lacrimal sac for 1-2 min (minimizes drainage into nose and throat, reducing risk of systemic effects). *Ointment:* Close eye for 1-2 min, rolling eyeball (increases contact area of drug to eye). Remove excess solution or ointment around eye w/tissue.
2. Ointment may be used at night to reduce frequency of solution administration.

3. As w/other corticoids, taper dosage slowly when discontinuing.

INDICATIONS/DOSAGE/ROUTES

NOTE: Individualize dose based on disease, pt, and response.

Usual oral dosage:
PO: Adults, elderly: 5-60 mg/day

Multiple sclerosis:
PO: Adults, elderly: 200 mg/day for 1 wk; then 80 mg every other day for 1 mo.

Prednisolone acetate:
IM: Adults, elderly: 4-60 mg/day.
INTRALESIONAL, INTRA-ARTICULAR, SOFT TISSUE: Adults, elderly: 5 mg up to 100 mg/day.

Multiple sclerosis:
IM: Adults, elderly: 200 mg/day for 7 days; then 80 mg every other day for 30 days.

Prednisolone tebutate:
INTRALESIONAL, INTRA-ARTICULAR, SOFT TISSUE: Adults, elderly: 4-30 mg.

Prednisolone sodium phosphate:
IM/IV Adults, elderly: 4-60 mg/day.
INTRALESIONAL, INTRA-ARTICULAR, SOFT TISSUE: Adults, elderly: 2-30 mg.

Multiple sclerosis:
IM: Adults, elderly: 200 mg/day for 7 days; then 80 mg every other day for 30 days.

Usual ophthalmic dosage:
OPHTHALMIC: Adults, elderly: Solution: 1-2 drops q1h during day; q2h during night; after response; decrease dose to 1 drop q4h, then 1 drop 3-4 times/day. Ointment: thin coat 3-4 times/day; after response, decrease to 2 times/day; then once daily.

PRECAUTIONS

CONTRAINDICATIONS: Hypersensitivity to any corticosteroid or tartrazine, systemic fungal infection, peptic ulcers (except life-threatening situations). Avoid live virus vaccine such as smallpox. **CAUTIONS:** Thromboembolic disorders, history of tuberculosis (may reactivate disease), hypothyroidism, cirrhosis, nonspecific ulcerative colitis, CHF, hypertension, psychosis, renal insufficiency, seizure disorders. Prolonged therapy should be discontinued slowly. **PREGNANCY/LACTATION:** Drug crosses placenta, is distributed in breast milk. May cause cleft palate (chronic use first trimester). Nursing contraindicated. **Pregnancy Category D.** *Ophthalmic:* **Pregnancy Category C:** Unknown if topical steroids could have sufficient absorption to be distributed in breast milk.

INTERACTIONS

DRUG INTERACTIONS: Amphotericin may increase hypokalemia. May decrease effect of oral hypoglycemics, insulin, diuretics, potassium supplements. May increase digoxin toxicity (due to hypokalemia). Hepatic enzyme inducers may decrease effect. Live virus vaccines may potentiate virus replication, increase vaccine side effects, decrease pt's antibody response to vaccine. **ALTERED LAB VALUES:** May decrease calcium, potassium, thyroxine. May increase cholesterol, lipids, glucose, sodium, amylase.

SIDE EFFECTS

FREQUENT: Increased appetite, exaggerated sense of well-being, abdominal distension, weight gain, insomnia, mood swings. *High dose,* *prolonged therapy:* Increased susceptibility to infection (signs/symptoms masked); slow wound healing, hypokalemia, hypocalcemia, GI distress. **OCCASIONAL:** Headache, vertigo, insomnia, mood swings, hyperglycemia, hirsutism, acne. **RARE:** Psychosis, tachycardia. *Ophthalmic:* Stinging or burning, posterior subcapsular cataracts.

ADVERSE REACTIONS/TOXIC EFFECTS

Long-term therapy: Muscle wasting (esp. arms, legs), osteoporosis, spontaneous fractures, amenorrhea, cataracts, glaucoma, peptic ulcer, CHF, growth retardation in children. Abrupt withdrawal following long-term therapy: Anorexia, nausea, fever, headache, joint pain, rebound inflammation, fatigue, weakness, lethargy, dizziness, orthostatic hypotension. Sudden discontinuance may be fatal.

NURSING IMPLICATIONS

BASELINE ASSESSMENT:

Question for hypersensitivity to any corticosteroids. Obtain baselines for height, weight, B/P, glucose, electrolytes. Check results of initial tests, e.g., TB skin test, x-rays, EKG. Never give live virus vaccine, (i.e., smallpox).

INTERVENTION/EVALUATION:

Evaluate food tolerance and bowel activity; report hyperacidity promptly. Check B/P, temperature, pulse, respiration at least 2 times/day. Be alert to infection (sore throat, fever or vague symptoms); assess mouth daily for signs of candida infection (white patches, painful tongue and mucous membranes). Monitor electrolytes. Monitor I&O, daily weight; assess for edema. Watch for hypokalemia (weakness and muscle cramps, numbness/tingling esp. lower extremities, nausea and vomiting, irritability, EKG changes) or hypocalcemia (muscle twitching, cramps, positive Trousseau's or Chvostek's signs). Assess emotional status, ability to sleep. Provide assistance w/ambulation.

PATIENT/FAMILY TEACHING:

Carry identification of drug and dose, physician's name and phone number. Do not change dose/schedule or stop taking drug, must taper off gradually under medical supervision. Notify physician of fever, sore throat, muscle aches, sudden weight gain/swelling. W/dietician give instructions for prescribed diet (may be sodium restricted, high protein and potassium). Maintain careful personal hygiene, avoid exposure to disease or trauma. Severe stress (serious infection, surgery, or trauma) may require increased dosage. Do not take any other medication w/o consulting physician. Follow-up visits, lab tests are necessary; children must be assessed for growth retardation. Inform dentist or other physicians of prednisolone therapy now or within past 12 mo. Caution against overuse of joints injected for symptomatic relief. *Ophthalmic:* Teach proper administration.

prednisone

pred´nih-sewn

(Orasone, Deltasone, Meticorten)

CANADIAN AVAILABILITY: Apo-Prednisone, Deltasone, Winpred

CLASSIFICATION

Corticosteroid

PHARMACOKINETICS

Well absorbed from GI tract. Widely distributed. Protein binding: 65-91%. Metabolized in liver (converted to prednisolone). Primarily excreted in urine. Half-life: 3.4-3.8 hrs.

ACTION

Decreases/prevents tissue response to inflammatory process. Inhibits accumulation of inflammatory cells at inflammation sites, phagocytosis, lysosomal enzyme release, and synthesis and/or release of mediators of inflammation. Prevents/suppresses cell-mediated immune reactions.

USES

Substitution therapy in deficiency states: Acute/chronic adrenal insufficiency, congenital adrenal hyperplasia, adrenal insufficiency secondary to pituitary insufficiency. *Nonendocrine disorders:* Arthritis, rheumatic carditis; allergic, collagen, intestinal tract, liver, ocular, renal, skin diseases; bronchial asthma, cerebral edema, malignancies.

PO ADMINISTRATION

1. Give w/o regard to meals (give w/food if GI upset occurs).
2. Give single doses before 9 AM, multiple doses at evenly spaced intervals.

INDICATIONS/DOSAGE/ROUTES

Usual oral dosage:
PO: Adults, elderly: 5-60 mg/day. **Children:** 0.14-2 mg/kg/day.

PRECAUTIONS

CONTRAINDICATIONS: Hypersensitivity to any corticosteroid, systemic fungal infection, peptic ulcer (except life-threatening situations), breast feeding. **CAUTIONS:** Thromboembolic disorders, history of tuberculosis (may reactivate disease), hypothyroidism, cirrhosis, nonspecific ulcerative colitis, CHF, hypertension, psychosis, renal insufficiency, seizure disorders. **PREGNANCY/LACTATION:** Crosses placenta; is distributed in breast milk. Cleft palate generally occurs w/chronic use, first trimester. **Pregnancy Category C.**

INTERACTIONS

DRUG INTERACTIONS: Amphotericin may increase hypokalemia. May decrease effect of oral hypoglycemics, insulin, diuretics, potassium supplements. May increase digoxin toxicity (due to hypokalemia). Hepatic enzyme inducers may decrease effect. Live virus vaccines may potentiate virus replication, increase vaccine side effects, decrease pt's antibody response to vaccine. **ALTERED LAB VALUES:** May decrease calcium, potassium, thyroxine. May increase cholesterol, lipids, glucose, sodium, amylase.

SIDE EFFECTS

FREQUENT: Increased appetite, exaggerated sense of well-being, abdominal distension, weight gain, insomnia, mood swings. *High dose, prolonged therapy:* Increased susceptibility to infection (signs/symptoms masked); slow wound healing, hypokalemia, hypocalcemia, GI distress. **OCCASIONAL:** Headache, vertigo. **RARE:** Increased blood coagulability, tachycardia, frequency/urgency of urination, psychosis.

ADVERSE REACTIONS/TOXIC EFFECTS

Long-term therapy: Muscle wasting (esp. arms, legs), osteoporosis, spontaneous fractures, amenorrhea, cataracts, glaucoma, peptic ulcer, CHF. Abrupt withdrawal following long-term therapy: Anorexia, nausea, fever, headache, joint pain, rebound inflammation, fatigue, weakness, lethargy, dizziness, orthostatic hypotension.

NURSING IMPLICATIONS

BASELINE ASSESSMENT:

Question for hypersensitivity to any corticosteroids. Obtain baselines for height, weight, B/P, glucose, electrolytes. Check results of initial tests, e.g., TB skin test, x-rays, EKG. Never give live virus vaccine.

INTERVENTION/EVALUATION:

Monitor I&O, daily weight; assess for edema. Check lab results for blood coagulability, clinical evidence of thromboembolism. Evaluate food tolerance, bowel activity; report hyperacidity promptly. Check B/P, temperature, pulse, respiration, at least 2 times/day. Be alert to infection: Sore throat, fever/vague symptoms. Assess mouth daily for signs of candida infection (white patches, painful tongue and mucous membranes). Monitor electrolytes. Watch for hypocalcemia (muscle twitching, cramps, positive Trousseau's or Chvostek's signs) or hypokalemia (weakness and muscle cramps, numbness/tingling, esp. lower extremities, nausea and vomiting, irritability, EKG changes). Assess emotional status, ability to sleep. Provide assistance w/ambulation.

PATIENT/FAMILY TEACHING:

Carry identification of drug and dose, physician's name and phone number. Do not change dose/schedule or stop taking drug (must taper off gradually under medical supervision). Notify physician of fever, sore throat, muscle aches, sudden weight gain/swelling. Give instructions for prescribed diet (may be sodium restricted, high protein and potassium). Maintain careful personal hygiene, avoid exposure to disease/trauma. Severe stress (serious infection, surgery, or trauma) may require increased dosage. Do not take any other medication w/o consulting physician. Follow-up visits, lab tests are necessary; children must be assessed for growth retardation. Inform dentist or other physicians of prednisone therapy now or within past 12 mo. Caution against overuse of joints injected for symptomatic relief.

primidone

pri´mih-doan
(Mysoline)

CANADIAN AVAILABILITY:

Apo-Primidone, Mysoline, Sertan

CLASSIFICATION

Anticonvulsant

PHARMACOKINETICS

Rapid, completely absorbed from GI tract. Widely distributed. Protein binding: 0-20%. Metabolized in liver to active metabolite (phenobarbital). Primarily excreted in urine. Half-life: 3-23 hrs; metabolite: 75-126 hrs.

ACTION

Elevates seizure threshold for motor cortex to electrical/chemical stimulation.

USES

Management of partial seizures w/complex symptomatology (psychomotor seizures), generalized tonic-clonic (grand mal) seizures.

PO ADMINISTRATION

1. Give w/o regard to meals.
2. Shake oral suspension well before administering (may be mixed w/food).
3. Tablets may be crushed.

INDICATIONS/DOSAGE/ROUTES

NOTE: When replacement by another anticonvulsant is necessary, decrease primidone gradually as therapy begins w/low replacement dose.

Anticonvulsant:
PO: Adults, elderly, children >8 yrs: 100-125 mg daily for 3 days at bedtime, then 100-125 mg 2 times/day for days 4-6, then 100-125 mg 3 times/day for days 7-9, then maintenance of 250 mg 3 times/day. **Children <8 yrs:** 50 mg at bedtime for 3 days, then 50 mg 2 times/day for days 4-6, then 100 mg 2 times/day for days 7-9, then maintenance of 125-250 mg 3 times/day.

PRECAUTIONS

CONTRAINDICATIONS: History of porphyria, bronchopneumonia. **EXTREME CAUTION:** Nephritis, renal insufficiency. **CAUTIONS:** Uncontrolled pain (may produce paradoxical reaction), impaired liver function. **PREGNANCY/LACTATION:** Readily crosses placenta; is distributed in breast milk in substantial quantities. Produces respiratory depression in the neonate during labor. May cause postpartum hemorrhage, hemorrhagic disease in newborn. Withdrawal symptoms may occur in neonates born to women who receive barbiturates during last trimester of pregnancy. Lowers serum bilirubin concentrations in neonates. **Pregnancy Category D.**

INTERACTIONS

DRUG INTERACTIONS: May decrease effects of glucocorticoids, digoxin, metronidazole, oral anticoagulants, quinidine, tricyclic antidepressants. Alcohol, CNS depressants may increase effect. May increase metabolism of carbamazepine. Valproic acid decreases metabolism, increases concentration, toxicity. **ALTERED LAB VALUES:** May decrease bilirubin.

SIDE EFFECTS

FREQUENT: Drowsiness, sedation, muscular incoordination. **OCCASIONAL:** Irritability, headache, restlessness, dizziness, ataxia (muscular incoordination), joint aches, vertigo, mood changes, anorexia, nausea, gastric distress.

ADVERSE REACTIONS/TOXIC EFFECTS

Abrupt withdrawal after prolonged therapy may produce effects ranging from markedly increased dreaming, nightmares and/or insomnia, tremor, sweating, vomiting, to hallucinations, delirium, seizures, status epilepticus. Skin eruptions may appear as hypersensitivity reaction. Blood dyscrasias, liver disease, hypocalcemia occur rarely. Overdosage produces cold, clammy skin, hypothermia, severe CNS depression followed by high fever, coma.

NURSING IMPLICATIONS

BASELINE ASSESSMENT:

Review history of seizure disorder (intensity, frequency, duration, level of consciousness). Observe frequently for recurrence of seizure activity. Initiate seizure precautions.

INTERVENTION/EVALUATION:

For those on long-term therapy, liver/renal function tests, blood counts should be performed periodically. Assist w/ambulation if dizziness, ataxia occur. Assess children, elderly for paradoxical reaction (particularly during early therapy). Assess for clinical improvement (decrease in intensity/frequency of seizures). Monitor for therapeutic serum level (5-12 mcg/ml).

PATIENT/FAMILY TEACHING:

Do not abruptly withdraw medication following long-term use (may precipitate seizures). Strict maintenance of drug therapy is essential for seizure control. Drowsiness usually disappears during continued therapy. If dizziness occurs, change positions slowly from recumbent to sitting position before standing. Avoid tasks that require alertness, motor skills until response to drug is established. Avoid alcohol.

probenecid

pro-ben´ah-sid
(Benemid, Probalan)

FIXED-COMBINATION(S):
W/colchicine, antigout agent (ColBenemid, Proben-C)

CANADIAN AVAILABILITY:
Benemid, Benuryl

CLASSIFICATION

Uricosuric

PHARMACOKINETICS

Rapidly, completely absorbed from GI tract. Widely distributed. Protein binding: 75-95%. Metabolized in liver to active metabolite. Primarily excreted in urine. Half-life: 3-12 hrs.

ACTION

Inhibits active reabsorption of urate at proximal renal tubule. Increases urinary excretion of uric acid.

USES

Treatment of hyperuricemia associated w/gout or gouty arthritis. Adjunctive therapy w/penicillins or cephalosporins to elevate and prolong antibiotic plasma levels.

PO ADMINISTRATION

1. May give w/or immediately after meals or milk.
2. Instruct pt to drink at least 10-12 glasses (8 oz) of water/day (prevents kidney stone development).

INDICATIONS/DOSAGE/ROUTES

Gout:
NOTE: Do not start until acute gout attack subsides; continue if acute attack occurs during therapy.
PO: Adults, elderly: Initially, 250 mg 2 times/day for 1 wk; then 500 mg 2 times/day. May increase by 500 mg q4wks. **Maximum:** 2-3 Gm/day. **Maintenance:** Dosage that maintains normal uric acid levels.

Penicillin/cephalosporin therapy:
NOTE: Do not use in presence of renal impairment.
PO: Adults, elderly: 2 Gm/day in divided doses. **Children (2-14 yrs):** Initially, 25 mg/kg. **Maintenance:** 40 mg/kg/day in 4 divided doses. **Children >50 kg:** Receive adult dosage.

PRECAUTIONS

CONTRAINDICATIONS: Blood dyscrasias, uric acid kidney stones, concurrent use w/penicillin in presence of renal impairment. **CAUTIONS:** Impaired renal function, history of peptic ulcer. **PREGNANCY/LACTATION:** Crosses placenta, appears in cord blood. Unknown whether distributed in breast milk. **Pregnancy Category C.**

INTERACTIONS

DRUG INTERACTIONS: May increase concentrations of cephalosporins, methotrexate, NSAIDs, nitrofurantoin, penicillins, zidovudine. Antineoplastics may increase risk of uric acid nephropathy. Salicylates may decrease uricosuric effect. May increase, prolong effects of heparin. **ALTERED LAB VALUES:** May inhibit renal excretion of PSP (phenolsulfonphthalein), 17-ketosteroids, BSP (sulfobromophthalein) tests.

SIDE EFFECTS

OCCASIONAL: Headache, GI distress, urinary frequency, flushing, dizziness.

ADVERSE REACTIONS/TOXIC EFFECTS

Severe hypersensitivity reactions (including anaphylaxis) occur rarely (usually within a few hrs after readministration following previous use). Discontinue immediately, contact physician. Pruritic maculopapular rash should be considered a toxic reaction. May be accompanied by malaise, fever, chills, joint pain, nausea, vomiting, leukopenia.

NURSING IMPLICATIONS

BASELINE ASSESSMENT:

Do not initiate therapy until acute gouty attack has subsided. Question pt for hypersensitivity to probenecid or if taking penicillin or cephalosporin antibiotics. Instruct pt to drink 8-10 glasses (8 oz) of fluid daily while on medication.

INTERVENTION/EVALUATION:

If exacerbation of gout recurs following therapy, use other agents for gout. Discontinue medication immediately if rash or other evidence of allergic reaction appears. Encourage high fluid intake (3,000 ml/day). Monitor I&O (output should be at least 2,000 ml/day). Assess CBC, serum uric acid levels. Assess urine for cloudiness, unusual color, odor. Assess for therapeutic response (reduced joint tenderness, swelling, redness, limitation of motion).

PATIENT/FAMILY TEACHING:

Encourage low purine food intake (reduce/omit meat, fowl, fish; use eggs, cheese, vegetables). Foods high in purine: Kidneys, liver, sweetbreads, sardines, anchovies, meat extracts. May take 1 or more wks for full therapeutic effect. Drink 8-10 glasses (8 oz) of fluid daily while on medication. Avoid tasks that require alertness, motor skills until response to drug is established. Contact physician, nurse if rash, irritation of eyes, swelling of lips/mouth occurs.

probucol

pro´byew-call
(Lorelco)

CANADIAN AVAILABILITY:
Lorelco

CLASSIFICATION

Antihyperlipoproteinemic

PHARMACOKINETICS

Variably absorbed from GI tract (food increases absorption). Primarily accumulates in adipose tissue. Primarily eliminated via biliary system. Half-life: 20 days.

ACTION

Lowers serum cholesterol (decreases LDL, HDL). Increases biliary excretion of cholesterol and fractional rate of LDL catabolism (breakdown).

USES

Adjunct to diet therapy to decrease elevated serum cholesterol in those w/primary hypercholesterolemia (elevated LDL).

PO ADMINISTRATION

Give w/meals.

INDICATIONS/DOSAGE/ROUTES

Hypercholesterolemia:
PO: Adults, elderly: 500 mg 1-2 times/day w/morning and/or evening meal.

PRECAUTIONS

CONTRAINDICATIONS: Hypersensitivity to probucol, recent or progressive myocardial damage, cardiovascular or unexplained syncope, ventricular arrhythmias, severe bradycardia, abnormally long QT interval. **CAUTIONS:** Hypokalemia or hypomagnesemia must be corrected before therapy. **PREGNANCY/LACTATION:** Unknown whether distributed in breast milk. **Pregnancy Category B.**

INTERACTIONS

DRUG INTERACTIONS: Antiarrhythmics w/QT interval prolongation (e.g., amiodarone, lidocaine, procainamide, quinidine) may be additive. May increase risk of ventricular tachycardia w/beta-adrenergic blockers, digoxin. **ALTERED LAB VALUES:** May increase SGOT (AST), SGPT (ALT), alkaline phosphatase, bilirubin, BUN, creatinine kinase, glucose, uric acid. May decrease eosinophils, Hgb, Hct.

SIDE EFFECTS

FREQUENT: Diarrhea, flatulence, nausea, vomiting, abdominal pain. **OCCASIONAL:** Dizziness, headache, numbness of face, fingers, or toes. **RARE:** Prolonged QT interval, syncope, arrhythmias, swelling of face, hands, or feet. Idiosyncratic reaction: Chest pain, palpitations, nausea and vomiting, dizziness, syncope.

ADVERSE REACTIONS/TOXIC EFFECTS

Cardiovascular toxicity.

NURSING IMPLICATIONS

BASELINE ASSESSMENT:

Question for history of hypersensitivity to probucol. Obtain specimens for baseline electrolytes, serum cholesterol, serum triglycerides. Check EKG results.

INTERVENTION/EVALUATION:

Evaluate food tolerance. Determine pattern of bowel activity. Assess for numbness or swelling of face, hands, feet. Check for headache, dizziness. Monitor EKG for changes, lab results for electrolytes, serum cholesterol, serum triglycerides.

PATIENT/FAMILY TEACHING:

Take w/meals. Do not discontinue w/o checking w/physician. Take only medications approved by physician. Follow prescribed diet; diet may affect results of therapy. Notify physician in event of new symptoms, esp. dizziness, persistent diarrhea, or swelling of face, hands or feet.

procainamide hydrochloride

pro-cane´ah-myd
(Procan-SR, Pronestyl, Rhythmin)

CANADIAN AVAILABILITY:
Pronestyl, Procan SR

CLASSIFICATION

Antiarrhythmic

PHARMACOKINETICS

Rapidly, completely absorbed from GI tract. Widely distributed. Protein binding: 15-20%. Metabolized in liver to active metabolite. Primarily excreted in urine. Removed by hemodialysis. Half-life: 2.5-4.5 hrs; metabolite: 6 hrs.

ACTION

Direct cardiac effects (decreases excitability, conduction velocity, automaticity, membrane responsiveness; prolongs refractory period).

USES

Prophylactic therapy to maintain normal sinus rhythm after conversion of atrial fibrillation and/or flutter. Treatment of premature ventricular contractions, paroxysmal atrial tachycardia, atrial fibrillation, ventricular tachycardia.

STORAGE/HANDLING

Solution appears clear, colorless to light yellow. Discard if solution darkens/appears discolored or if precipitate forms. When diluted w/ 5% dextrose, solution is stable for 24 hrs at room temperature or for 7 days if refrigerated.

PO/IM/IV ADMINISTRATION

PO:

1. Do not crush or break sustained-release tablets.

IM/IV:

NOTE: May give by IM, IV injection, or IV infusion.

1. B/P, EKG should be monitored continuously during IV administration and rate of infusion adjusted to eliminate arrhythmias.
2. For direct IV injection, dilute w/5% dextrose and, w/pt in supine position, administer at rate not exceeding 25-50 mg/min.
3. For initial loading infusion, add 1 Gm to 50 ml 5% dextrose to provide a concentration of 20 mg/ml. Infuse 1 ml/min for up to 25-30 min.
4. For IV infusion, add 1 Gm to 250-500 ml 5% dextrose to provide concentration of 2-4 mg/ml. Infuse at 1-3 ml/min.
5. Check B/P q5-10min during infusion. If fall in B/P exceeds 15 mm Hg, discontinue drug, contact physician.
6. Monitor EKG for cardiac changes, particularly widening of

QRS, prolongation of PR and QT interval. Notify physician of any significant interval changes.

INDICATIONS/DOSAGE/ROUTES

NOTE: Dose, interval of administration individualized based on underlying myocardial disease, pt's age, renal function, clinical response. Extended-release capsules used for maintenance therapy.

Usual oral dosage (to provide 50 mg/kg/day):
PO: Adults, elderly (40-50 kg): 250 mg q3h up to 500 mg q6h. **(60-70 kg):** 375 mg q3h up to 750 mg q6h. **(80-90 kg):** 500 mg q3h up to 1 Gm q6h. **(>100 kg):** 625 mg q3h up to 1.25 Gm q6h.
PO (extended release): Adults, elderly (40-50 kg): 500 mg q6h. **(60-70 kg):** 750 mg q6h. **(80-90 kg):** 1 Gm q6h. **(>100 kg):** 1.25 Gm q6h.

Usual parenteral dosage:
IM: Adults, elderly: 50 mg/kg/day in divided doses q3-6h.
IV: Adults, elderly: 100 mg q5min until arrhythmias suppressed or 500 mg administered.
IV INFUSION: Adults, elderly: Initially, loading infusion of 20 mg/ml at 1 ml/min for 25-30 min to deliver 500-600 mg procainamide. Maintenance: Infusion of 2 mg/ml at 1-3 ml/min to deliver 2-6 mg/min.

PRECAUTIONS

CONTRAINDICATIONS: Complete AV block, second- and third-degree AV block w/o pacemaker, abnormal impulses/rhythms because of escape mechanism. **CAUTIONS:** Ventricular tachycardia during coronary occlusion, renal/hepatic disease, incomplete AV nodal block, digitalis intoxication, CHF, preexisting hypotension.
PREGNANCY/LACTATION: Crosses placenta; unknown whether distributed in breast milk. **Pregnancy Category C.**

INTERACTIONS

DRUG INTERACTIONS: Pimozide, other antiarrhythmics may increase cardiac effects. May increase effects of antihypertensives (IV procainamide), neuromuscular blockers. May decrease effects of antimyasthenics on skeletal muscle. **ALTERED LAB VALUES:** May cause positive ANA, Coombs' test, EKG changes. May increase SGOT (AST), SGPT (ALT), alkaline phosphatase, bilirubin, LDH.

SIDE EFFECTS

FREQUENT: *Oral:* Abdominal pain/cramping, nausea, diarrhea, vomiting. **OCCASIONAL:** Dizziness, giddiness, weakness, hypersensitivity reaction (rash, urticaria, pruritus, flushing). **INFREQUENT:** *IV:* Transient but at times marked hypotension. **RARE:** Confusion, mental depression, psychosis.

ADVERSE REACTIONS/TOXIC EFFECTS

Paradoxical, extremely rapid ventricular rate may occur during treatment of atrial fibrillation/flutter. Systemic lupus erythematosus–like syndrome (fever, joint pain, pleuritic chest pain) w/prolonged therapy. Cardiotoxic effects occur most commonly w/IV administration, observed as conduction changes (50% widening of QRS complex, frequent ventricular premature contractions, ventricular tachycardia, complete AV block). Prolonged PR and QT intervals, flattened T waves occur less frequently (discontinue drug immediately).

NURSING IMPLICATIONS

BASELINE ASSESSMENT:

Check B/P and pulse for 1 full min (unless pt is on continuous monitor) before giving medication.

INTERVENTION/EVALUATION:

Monitor EKG for cardiac changes, particularly widening of QRS, prolongation of PR and QT interval. Assess pulse for strength/weakness, irregular rate. Monitor I&O, electrolyte serum level (potassium, chloride, sodium). Assess for complaints of GI upset, headache, dizziness, joint pain. Monitor pattern of daily bowel activity, stool consistency. Assess for dizziness. Monitor B/P for hypotension. Assess skin for evidence of hypersensitivity reaction (especially in those on high dose therapy). Monitor for therapeutic serum level (3-10 mcg/ml).

PATIENT/FAMILY TEACHING:

Take medication at evenly spaced doses around the clock. Contact physician if fever, joint pain/stiffness, signs of upper respiratory infection occur. Do not abruptly discontinue medication. Compliance w/therapy regimen is essential to control arrhythmias. Do not use nasal decongestants, over-the-counter cold preparations (stimulants) w/o physician approval. Restrict salt, alcohol intake.

procaine hydrochloride

prow´cane
(Novocain)

CANADIAN AVAILABILITY:
Novocain

(See Classifications section under Anesthetics: local)

procarbazine hydrochloride

pro-car´bah-zeen
(Matulane)

CANADIAN AVAILABILITY:
Natulan

CLASSIFICATION

Antineoplastic

PHARMACOKINETICS

Completely absorbed from GI tract. Widely distributed (crosses blood-brain barrier). Metabolized in liver to active metabolite. Primarily excreted in urine. Half-life: 10 min.

ACTION

Cell cycle-specific for S phase of cell division. Inhibits DNA, RNA, protein synthesis.

USES

Treatment of advanced Hodgkin's disease.

INDICATIONS/DOSAGE/ROUTES

NOTE: May be carcinogenic, mutagenic, or teratogenic. Handle w/extreme care during administration. Dosage individualized based on clinical response, tolerance to adverse effects. When used in combination therapy, consult specific protocols for optimum dosage, sequence of drug administration. Dosage based on actual weight.

Use ideal body weight for obese and edematous pts.

Hodgkin's disease:
PO: Adults, elderly: Initially, 2-4 mg/kg daily as single or divided dose for 1 wk, then 4-6 mg/kg day. **Children:** 50 mg/m^2 daily for 1 wk, then 100 mg/m^2 daily. Continue until maximum response, leukocyte count falls below 4,000/mm^3, or platelets fall below 100,000/mm^3.

Maintenance:
PO: Adults, elderly: 1-2 mg/kg/day. **Children:** 50 mg/m^2 daily.

Component of MOPP:
PO: Adults, elderly: 100 mg/m^2 daily on days 1-14 of 28-day cycle.

PRECAUTIONS

CONTRAINDICATIONS: Inadequate bone marrow reserve. **CAUTIONS:** Impaired renal/hepatic function. **PREGNANCY/LACTATION:** If possible, avoid use during pregnancy, especially first trimester. Breast feeding not recommended. **Pregnancy Category D.**

INTERACTIONS

DRUG INTERACTIONS: Alcohol may cause disulfiram reaction. Anticholinergics, antihistamines may increase anticholinergic effects. Tricyclic antidepressants may increase anticholinergic effects, cause hyperpyretic crisis, convulsions. May increase effects of oral hypoglycemics, insulin. Bone marrow depressants may increase bone marrow depression. May increase B/P w/buspirone, caffeine containing medications. May cause hyperpyretic crisis, seizures, death w/carbamazepine, cyclobenzaprine, maprotiline, MAO inhibitors. CNS depressants may increase CNS depression. Meperidine may produce immediate excitation, sweating, rigidity, severe hypertension or hypotension, severe respiratory distress, coma, convulsions, vascular collapse, death. Sympathomimetics may increase cardiac stimulant, vasopressor effects. **ALTERED LAB VALUES:** None significant.

SIDE EFFECTS

FREQUENT: Severe nausea, vomiting, respiratory disorders (cough, effusion), myalgia, arthralgia, drowsiness, nervousness, insomnia, nightmares, sweating, hallucinations, seizures. **OCCASIONAL:** Hoarseness, tachycardia, nystagmus, retinal hemorrhage, photophobia, photosensitivity, urinary frequency, nocturia, hypotension, diarrhea, stomatitis, paresthesia, unsteadiness, confusion, decreased reflexes, footdrop. **RARE:** Hypersensitivity reaction (dermatitis, pruritus, rash, urticaria), hyperpigmentation, alopecia.

ADVERSE REACTIONS/TOXIC EFFECTS

Major toxic effects are bone marrow depression manifested as hematologic toxicity (principally leukopenia, thrombocytopenia, anemia) and hepatotoxicity manifested by jaundice, ascites. Urinary tract infection secondary to leukopenia may occur. Therapy should be discontinued if stomatitis, diarrhea, paresthesia, neuropathies, confusion, hypersensitivity reaction occur.

NURSING IMPLICATIONS

BASELINE ASSESSMENT:

Obtain bone marrow tests, Hgb, Hct, leukocyte, differential, reticulocyte, platelet, urinalysis, serum transaminase, serum alkaline phosphatase, BUN results before

P

therapy and periodically thereafter. Therapy should be interrupted if WBC falls below 4,000/mm^3 or platelet count falls below 100,000/mm^3.

INTERVENTION/EVALUATION:

Monitor hematologic status, renal, hepatic function studies. Assess for stomatitis (burning/erythema of oral mucosa at inner margin of lips, sore throat, difficulty swallowing, oral ulceration). Monitor for hematologic toxicity (fever, sore throat, signs of local infection, easy bruising, unusual bleeding from any site), symptoms of anemia (excessive tiredness, weakness). Avoid IM injections, rectal temperatures, trauma that may induce bleeding.

PATIENT/FAMILY TEACHING:

Do not drink alcoholic beverages during or for 2 wks after therapy (Antabuse-like reaction: Severe headache, tachycardia, chest pain, stiff neck). Avoid foods with high tyramine content (i.e., yogurt, ripe cheese, smoked meat, overripe fruit). Avoid over-the-counter medications. Do not have immunizations w/o physician's approval (drug lowers body's resistance). Avoid crowds, those w/infection. Promptly report fever, sore throat, signs of local infection, easy bruising, or unusual bleeding from any site. Contact physician if nausea/vomiting continues at home. Wear protective clothing, sunscreens to protect from sun/ultraviolet light.

prochlorperazine

pro-klor-pear'ah-zeen

(Compazine suppositories)

prochlorperazine edisylate

(Compazine syrup, injection)

prochlorperazine maleate

(Compazine spansule, tablets)

CANADIAN AVAILABILITY:

Prorazin, Stemetil

CLASSIFICATION

Antiemetic, antipsychotic

PHARMACOKINETICS

	ONSET	PEAK	DURATION
Tablets, syrup (antiemetic)	30-40 min	—	3-4 hrs
Ext-Release (antiemetic)	30-40 min	—	10-12 hrs
IM (antiemetic)	10-20 min	—	3-4 hrs
Rectal (antiemetic)	60 min	—	3-4 hrs

Variably absorbed after oral administration, well absorbed after IM administration. Widely distributed. Protein binding: >90%. Metabolized in liver, GI mucosa. Primarily excreted in urine. Half-life: 23 hrs.

ACTION

Blocks postsynaptic dopaminergic receptors in brain. Acts centrally to inhibit/block dopamine receptors in chemoreceptor trigger zone and peripherally to block vagus nerve in GI tract.

USES

Control of severe nausea and vomiting, management for psychotic disorders, moderate to severe anxiety and tension in psychoneurotic pts.

STORAGE/HANDLING

Store at room temperature (including suppositories), protect from light (darkens on exposure). Slight yellow discoloration of solution does not affect potency, but discard if markedly discolored or precipitate forms.

PO/IM/IV/RECTAL ADMINISTRATION

PO:

1. Give w/o regard to meals.

PARENTERAL ADMINISTRATION: Pt must remain recumbent for 30-60 min in head-low position w/legs raised to minimize hypotensive effect.

IM:

1. Inject slow, deep IM into upper outer quadrant of gluteus maximus. If irritation occurs, further injections may be diluted w/0.9% NaCl or 2% procaine hydrochloride.
2. Massage IM injection site to reduce discomfort.

IV:

NOTE: Give by direct IV injection or IV infusion.

1. For direct IV, administer each 5 mg >1 min.
2. For IV infusion, dilute 20 mg (4 ml) prochlorperazine w/1 L 0.9% NaCl and administer 5 mg/min rate of infusion.
3. Monitor B/P diligently for hypotension during IV administration.

RECTAL:

1. Moisten suppository w/cold water before inserting well up into rectum.

INDICATIONS/DOSAGE/ROUTES

Severe nausea, vomiting:
PO: Adults, elderly: 5-10 mg 3-4 times/day. **Children 20-29 lbs, >2 yrs:** 2.5 mg q12-24h. Do not exceed 7.5 mg/day. **Children 30-39 lbs:** 2.5 mg 2-3 times/day. Do not exceed 10 mg/day. **Children 40-85 lbs:** 2.5 mg 3 times/day or 5 mg 2 times/day. Do not exceed 15 mg/day.
IM: Adults, elderly: 5-10 mg q3-4h. Do not exceed 40 mg/day. **Children >20 lbs, >2 yrs:** 0.13 mg/kg.
RECTAL: Adults, elderly: 25 mg 2 times/day. **Children <20 lbs, >2 yrs:** 0.4 mg/kg in 3-4 divided doses. **Children 20-29 lbs:** 2.5 mg 1-2 times/day. **Children 30-85 lbs:** 2.5 mg 3 times/day or 5 mg twice/day.

Severe nausea, vomiting after surgery:
IM: Adults, elderly: 5-10 mg. Repeat once in 30 min, if needed.
IV: Adults, elderly: 5-10 mg. Repeated once, if needed.

Psychotic disorders, outpatient:
PO: Adults, elderly: 5-10 mg 3-4 times/day. Increase dosage gradually every 2-3 days until therapeutic response noted.
PO/RECTAL: Children 2-12 yrs: 2.5 mg 2-3 times/day. Increase gradually to therapeutic response. **Maximum: Children 2-5 yrs:** 20 mg/day. **6-12 yrs:** 25 mg/day.

Psychotic disorders, inpatient:
PO: Adults, elderly: 10 mg 3-4 times/day.
IM: Adults, elderly: 10-20 mg q1-4h to control symptoms.

PRECAUTIONS

CONTRAINDICATIONS: Suspected Reye's syndrome, severe CNS depression, comatose states, severe cardiovascular disease, bone marrow depression, subcortical brain damage. **CAU-**

TIONS: Impaired respiratory/hepatic/renal/cardiac function, alcohol withdrawal, history of seizures, urinary retention, glaucoma, prostatic hypertrophy, hypocalcemia (increases susceptibility to dystonias). **PREGNANCY/LACTATION:** Crosses placenta; is distributed in breast milk. **Pregnancy Category C.**

INTERACTIONS

DRUG INTERACTIONS: Alcohol, CNS depressants may increase CNS, respiratory depression, hypotensive effects. Tricyclic antidepressants, MAO inhibitors may increase sedative, anticholinergic effects. Antithyroid agents may increase risk of agranulocytosis. Extrapyramidal symptoms (EPS) may increase w/EPS producing medications. Hypotensives may increase hypotension. May decrease levodopa effects. Lithium may decrease absorption, produce adverse neurologic effects. **ALTERED LAB VALUES:** None significant.

SIDE EFFECTS

FREQUENT: Hypotension, dizziness, fainting occur frequently after first injection, occasionally after subsequent injections, and rarely w/oral dosage. **OCCASIONAL:** Drowsiness during early therapy, dry mouth, blurred vision, lethargy, constipation/diarrhea, muscular aches, nasal congestion, peripheral edema, urinary retention.

ADVERSE REACTIONS/TOXIC EFFECTS

Extrapyramidal symptoms appear dose-related (particularly w/high dosage) and are divided into 3 categories: Akathisia (inability to sit still, tapping of feet, urge to move around), parkinsonian symptoms (mask-like face, tremors, shuffling gait, hypersalivation), and acute dystonias (torticollis [neck muscle spasm], opisthotonos [rigidity of back muscles], and oculogyric crisis [rolling back of eyes]). Dystonic reaction may also produce profuse sweating, pallor. Tardive dyskinesia (protrusion of tongue, puffing of cheeks, chewing/puckering of the mouth) occurs rarely (may be irreversible). Abrupt withdrawal following long-term therapy may precipitate nausea, vomiting, gastritis, dizziness, tremors. Blood dyscrasias, particularly agranulocytosis, mild leukopenia (sore mouth/gums/throat) may occur. May lower seizure threshold.

NURSING IMPLICATIONS

BASELINE ASSESSMENT:

Avoid skin contact w/solution (contact dermatitis). *Antiemetic:* Assess for dehydration (poor skin turgor, dry mucous membranes, longitudinal furrows in tongue). *Antipsychotic:* Assess behavior, appearance, emotional status, response to environment, speech pattern, thought content.

INTERVENTION/EVALUATION:

Monitor B/P for hypotension. Assess for extrapyramidal symptoms. Monitor WBC, differential count for blood dyscrasias. Monitor for fine tongue movement (may be early sign of tardive dyskinesia). Supervise suicidal-risk pt closely during early therapy (as depression lessens, energy level improves, increasing suicide potential). Assess for therapeutic response (interest in surroundings, improvement in self-care, increased ability to concentrate, relaxed facial expression).

PATIENT/FAMILY TEACHING:

Urine may turn pink or reddish-brown. Do not abruptly withdraw from long-term drug therapy. Report visual disturbances. Sugarless gum or sips of tepid water may relieve dry mouth. Drowsiness generally subsides during continued therapy. Avoid tasks that require alertness, motor skills until response to drug is established. Avoid alcohol, CNS depressants. Use sunscreen, protective clothing in sun or ultraviolet light. Use caution in hot weather (possibility of heat stroke).

progesterone

proe-jess´ter-one

(Gesterol)

CANADIAN AVAILABILITY: Progestilin

CLASSIFICATION

Progestin

PHARMACOKINETICS

Slow absorption after IM administration. Metabolized in liver. Primarily excreted in urine.

ACTION

Transforms endometrium from proliferative to secretory (in an estrogen-primed endometrium); inhibits secretion of pituitary gonadotropins, preventing follicular maturation and ovulation. Stimulates the growth of mammary alveolar tissue; relaxes uterine smooth muscle.

USES

Treatment of primary or secondary amenorrhea, abnormal uterine bleeding due to hormonal imbalance, endometriosis.

IM ADMINISTRATION

1. For IM use only.
2. Administer deep IM in large muscle.

INDICATIONS/DOSAGE/ROUTES

Amenorrhea:
IM: Adults: 5-10 mg for 6-8 days. Withdrawal bleeding expected in 48-72 hrs if ovarian activity produced proliferative endometrium.

Abnormal uterine bleeding:
IM: Adults: 5-10 mg for 6 days. (When estrogen given concomitantly, begin progesterone after 2 wks of estrogen therapy; discontinue when menstrual flow begins.)

PRECAUTIONS

CONTRAINDICATIONS: Hypersensitivity to progestins; thrombophlebitis, thromboembolic disorders, cerebral apoplexy or history of these conditions; severe liver dysfunction; breast cancer; undiagnosed vaginal bleeding; missed abortion; use as a diagnostic test for pregnancy. **CAUTIONS:** Diabetes, conditions aggravated by fluid retention (e.g., asthma, epilepsy, migraine, cardiac/renal dysfunction), history of mental depression. **PREGNANCY/LACTATION:** Not recommended during pregnancy, esp. first 4 mo (congenital heart, limb reduction defects). Distributed in breast milk. **Pregnancy Category X.**

INTERACTIONS

DRUG INTERACTIONS: May interfere w/effects of bromocriptine. **ALTERED LAB VALUES:** May increase alkaline phosphatase, LDL. May decrease HDL. May cause abnormal thyroid, metapyrone, liver, endocrine function tests, decrease glucose tolerance.

SIDE EFFECTS

FREQUENT: Breakthrough bleeding or spotting at beginning of therapy. Amenorrhea, change in menstrual flow, breast tenderness. **OCCASIONAL:** Edema, weight gain or loss, rash, pruritus, photosensitivity, skin pigmentation. **RARE:** Pain/swelling at injection site, acne, mental depression, alopecia, hirsutism.

ADVERSE REACTIONS/TOXIC EFFECTS

Thrombophlebitis, cerebrovascular disorders, retinal thrombosis, pulmonary embolism occur rarely.

NURSING IMPLICATIONS

BASELINE ASSESSMENT:

Question for possibility of pregnancy or hypersensitivity to progestins before initiating therapy. Obtain baseline weight, blood glucose level, B/P.

INTERVENTION/EVALUATION:

Check weight daily; report weekly gain of 5 lbs or more. Assess skin for rash, hives. Immediately report the development of chest pain, sudden shortness of breath, sudden decrease in vision, migraine headache, pain (esp. w/ swelling, warmth, and redness) in calves, numbness of an arm/leg (thrombotic disorders). Check B/P periodically. Note progesterone therapy on pathology specimens.

PATIENT/FAMILY TEACHING:

Importance of medical supervision. Do not take other medications w/o physician's approval. Use sunscreens, protective clothing to protect from sunlight/ultraviolet light until tolerance determined. Notify physician of abnormal vaginal bleeding or other symptoms. Teach how to perform Homans' test, signs and symptoms of blood clots (report these to physician immediately). Teach self-breast exam. Stop taking medication and contact physician at once if pregnancy suspected. Give labeling from drug package.

promethazine hydrochloride

pro-meth´ah-zeen
(Phenergan)

FIXED-COMBINATION(S):
W/codeine, a narcotic analgesic (Phenergan w/Codeine); w/dextromethorphan, an antitussive (Phenergan w/Dextromethorphan); w/meperidine, a narcotic analgesic (Mepergan); w/phenylephrine, a nasal vasoconstrictor (Phenergan VC); w/phenylephrine and codeine (Phenergan VC w/Codeine)

CANADIAN AVAILABILITY:
Histantil, Phenergan, PMS Promethazine

CLASSIFICATION

Antihistamine

PHARMACOKINETICS

	ONSET	PEAK	DURATION
PO	20 min	—	2-8 hrs
IM	20 min	—	2-8 hrs
Rectal	20 min	—	2-8 hrs
IV	3-5 min	—	2-8 hrs

Well absorbed from GI tract, after IM administration. Widely distributed. Protein binding: 65-90%. Metabolized in liver. Primarily excreted in urine.

ACTION

Antihistamine: Prevents, antagonizes most histamine effects (e.g., urticaria, pruritus). *Antiemetic:* Central anticholinergic effect: diminishes vestibular stimulation, depresses labyrinthine function, acts on chemoreceptor trigger zone. *Sedative-hypnotic:* Decreases stimulation to brain stem reticular formation.

USES

Provides symptomatic relief of allergic symptoms; sedative/antiemetic in surgery/labor; decreases postop nausea/vomiting; adjunct to analgesics in control of pain; management of motion sickness.

STORAGE/HANDLING

Store oral, parenteral forms at room temperature. Refrigerate suppositories.

PO/IM/IV/RECTAL ADMINISTRATION

PO:

1. Give w/o regard to meals. Scored tablets may be crushed.
2. Do not crush or break capsules.

IM:

NOTE: Significant tissue necrosis may occur if given SubQ. Inadvertent intra-arterial injection may produce severe arteriospasm, resulting in severe circulation impairment.

1. May be given undiluted.
2. Inject deep IM.

IV:

1. Final dilution should not exceed 25 mg/ml.
2. Administer at 25 mg/min rate thru IV infusion tube.
3. A too-rapid rate of infusion may result in transient fall in blood pressure, producing orthostatic hypotension, reflex tachycardia.
4. If pt complains of pain at IV site, stop injection immediately (possibility of intra-arterial needle placement/perivascular extravasation).

Rectal:

1. Moisten suppository w/cold water before inserting well up into rectum.

INDICATIONS/DOSAGE/ROUTES

Allergic symptoms:
PO: Adults, elderly: 25 mg at bedtime or 12.5 mg 4 times/day. **Children:** Up to 25 mg at bedtime or up to 12.5 mg 3 times/day.
RECTAL/IM/IV: Adults, elderly: 25 mg, may repeat in 2 hrs.

Motion sickness:
PO: Adults, elderly: 25 mg 30-60 min before departure; may repeat in 8-12 hrs then every morning on arising and before evening meal. **Children:** 12.5-25 mg (same regimen).

Prevention of nausea, vomiting:
PO/IM/IV/RECTAL: Adults, elderly: 12.5-25 mg q4-6h as needed. **Children:** 0.25-0.5 mg/kg q4-6h as needed.

Pre- and postop sedation; adjunct to analgesics:
IM/IV: Adults, elderly: 25-50 mg. **Children:** 12.5-25 mg.

PRECAUTIONS

CONTRAINDICATIONS: Comatose, those receiving large doses

P

of other CNS depressants, acutely ill/dehydrated children, acute asthmatic attack, vomiting of unknown etiology in children, Reye's syndrome, those receiving MAO inhibitors. **EXTREME CAUTION:** History of sleep apnea, young children, family history of sudden infant death syndrome (SIDS), those difficult to arouse from sleep. **CAUTIONS:** Narrow-angle glaucoma, peptic ulcer, prostatic hypertrophy, pyloroduodenal/bladder neck obstruction, asthma, COPD, increased intraocular pressure, cardiovascular disease, hyperthyroidism, hypertension, seizure disorders. **PREGNANCY/LACTATION:** Readily crosses placenta; unknown whether drug is excreted in breast milk. May inhibit platelet aggregation in neonates if taken within 2 wks of birth. May produce jaundice, extrapyramidal symptoms in neonates if taken during pregnancy. **Pregnancy Category C.**

INTERACTIONS

DRUG INTERACTIONS: Alcohol, CNS depressants may increase CNS depressant effects. Anticholinergics may increase anticholinergic effects. MAO inhibitors may prolong, intensify anticholinergic, CNS depressant effects. **ALTERED LAB VALUES:** May suppress wheal and flare reactions to antigen skin testing, unless discontinued 4 days before testing.

SIDE EFFECTS

HIGH INCIDENCE: Drowsiness, disorientation. Hypotension, confusion, syncope more likely noted in elderly. **FREQUENT:** Dry mouth, urinary retention, thickening of bronchial secretions. **OCCASIONAL:** Epigastric distress, flushing, visual disturbances, hearing disturbances, wheezing, paresthesia, sweating, chills. **RARE:** Dizziness, urticaria, photosensitivity, nightmares. Fixed-combination form with pseudoephedrine may produce mild CNS stimulation.

ADVERSE REACTIONS/TOXIC EFFECTS

Paradoxical reaction (particularly in children) manifested as excitation, nervousness, tremor, hyperactive reflexes, convulsions. CNS depression has occurred in infants and young children (respiratory depression, sleep apnea, SIDS). Long-term therapy may produce extrapyramidal symptoms noted as dystonia (abnormal movements), pronounced motor restlessness (most frequently occurs in children) and parkinsonian symptoms (esp. noted in elderly). Blood dyscrasias, particularly agranulocytosis, has occurred.

NURSING IMPLICATIONS

BASELINE ASSESSMENT:

Assess B/P and pulse for bradycardia/tachycardia if pt is given parenteral form. If used as an antiemetic, assess for dehydration (poor skin turgor, dry mucous membranes, longitudinal furrows in tongue).

INTERVENTION/EVALUATION:

Monitor serum electrolytes in pts w/severe vomiting. Assist w/ambulation if drowsiness, lightheadedness occur.

PATIENT/FAMILY TEACHING:

Drowsiness, dry mouth may be an expected response to drug. Sugarless gum, sips of tepid water may relieve dry mouth. Coffee/tea may help reduce drowsiness. Report visual disturbances. Avoid tasks that require alertness, motor skills until response to drug is established. Avoid alcohol and other CNS depressants. Use caution in sun-protective clothing and sunscreens.

propafenone hydrochloride

pro-pah´phen-own
(Rythmol)

CANADIAN AVAILABILITY:
Rythmol

CLASSIFICATION

Antiarrhythmic

PHARMACOKINETICS

Well absorbed from GI tract (undergoes first-pass effect). Distributed primarily to heart, liver, lung. Metabolized in liver to active metabolite. Primarily eliminated in feces. Half-life: 2-32 hrs.

ACTION

Decreases inward sodium current in Purkinje/myocardial cells. Decreases excitability, automaticity, prolongs conduction velocity, refractory period. Greatest effects on Purkinje system.

USES

Treatment of documented, life-threatening ventricular arrhythmias (e.g., sustained ventricular tachycardias).

PO ADMINISTRATION

1. Scored tablets may be crushed.
2. Give w/o regard to meals (food may increase serum concentrations).

INDICATIONS/DOSAGE/ROUTES

Usual dosage:
PO: Adults, elderly: Initially, 150 mg q8h, may increase at 3-4 day intervals to 225 mg q8h, then to 300 mg q8h. **Maximum:** 900 mg/day.

PRECAUTIONS

CONTRAINDICATIONS: Uncontrolled CHF, cardiogenic shock, sinoatrial, AV and intraventricular disorders of impulse/conductions (sick sinus syndrome [bradycardia-tachycardia], AV block) w/o presence of pacemaker, bradycardia, marked hypotension, bronchospastic disorders, manifest electrolyte imbalance. **CAUTIONS:** Impaired renal/hepatic function, recent myocardial infarction, CHF, conduction disturbances. **PREGNANCY/LACTATION:** Unknown whether drug crosses placenta or is distributed in breast milk. **Pregnancy Category C.**

INTERACTIONS

DRUG INTERACTIONS: May increase concentrations of digoxin, propranolol. May increase effects of warfarin. **ALTERED LAB VALUES:** May cause EKG changes (e.g., QRS widening, PR prolongation), positive ANA titers.

SIDE EFFECTS

FREQUENT: Dizziness, unusual taste, nausea, vomiting, constipation, blurred vision. **OCCASIONAL:** Headache, dyspepsia, weakness. **RARE:** Dry mouth, diarrhea, rash, edema, hot flashes.

ADVERSE REACTIONS/TOXIC EFFECTS

May produce/worsen existing

arrhythmias. Overdosage may produce hypotension, somnolence, bradycardia, intra-atrial and intraventricular conduction disturbances.

NURSING IMPLICATIONS

BASELINE ASSESSMENT:

Correct electrolyte imbalance before administering medication.

INTERVENTION/EVALUATION:

Assess pulse for strength/weakness, irregular rate. Monitor EKG for cardiac performance/changes, particularly widening of QRS, prolongation of PR interval. Question for visual disturbances, headache, GI upset. Monitor fluid, electrolyte serum levels. Monitor pattern of daily bowel activity, stool consistency. Assess for dizziness, unsteadiness. Monitor liver enzymes results. Monitor for therapeutic serum level (0.06-1 μ/ml).

PATIENT/FAMILY TEACHING:

Compliance w/therapy regimen is essential to control arrhythmias. Unusual taste sensation may occur. Report headache, blurred vision.

proparacaine

proe´par-ah-kane

(Ophthaine, AK-Taine, Alcaine, I-Paracaine, Kainair, Ophthetic)

FIXED-COMBINATION(S): W/fluorescein, a water-soluble dye (Fluoracaine, Parascein, Ocu-Flurcaine)

CANADIAN AVAILABILITY: Ak-Taine, Alcaine, Ophthaine, Ophthetic

(See Classifications section under Anesthetics: local)

propofol

pro-poe´foal

(Diprivan)

CANADIAN AVAILABILITY: Dipravan

CLASSIFICATION

Anesthetic: General

PHARMACOKINETICS

Rapidly, extensively distributed. Protein binding: 95-99%. Metabolized in liver. Primarily excreted in urine. Half-life: 3-12 hrs.

ACTION

Unknown. Short-acting hypnotic.

USES

Induction/maintenance of anesthesia. Continuous sedation in intubated/respiratory controlled adult pts in ICU.

STORAGE/HANDLING

Store at room temperature. Discard unused portions. Do not use if emulsion separates. Shake well before using.

IV ADMINISTRATION

NOTE: Do not give through same IV line w/blood or plasma.

1. Dilute only w/5% dextrose.
2. Do not dilute to concentration <2 mg/ml.
3. Use larger veins of forearm or antecubital fossa to minimize IV pain.
4. Transient, local pain at IV site

may be reduced w/1 ml of 1% IV lidocaine solution.

5. A too-rapid IV may produce marked severe hypotension, respiratory depression, irregular muscular movements.

6. Observe for signs of intra-arterial injection (pain, discolored skin patches, white/blue color to hand, delayed onset of drug action).

7. Inadvertent intra-arterial injection may result in arterial spasm w/severe pain, thrombosis, gangrene.

INDICATIONS/DOSAGE/ROUTES

ICU sedation:

IV: Adults, elderly: Initially, 5 mcg/kg/min for at least 5 min until onset of peak effect. May increase by increments of 5-10 mcg/kg/min over 5-10 min intervals. **Maintenance:** 5-50 mcg/kg/min (some pts may require higher dosage).

Anesthesia:

IV: Adults <55 yrs, *ASA* I & II: 2-2.5 mg/kg (about 40 mg q10sec until onset of anesthesia). **IV: Elderly, debilitated, hypovolemic or *ASA* III or IV:** 1-1.5 mg/kg q10sec until onset of anesthesia.

Maintenance:

IV: Adults <55 yrs, *ASA* I & II: 0.1-0.2 mg/kg/min. **IV: Elderly, debilitated, hypovolemic, or *ASA* III or IV:** 0.05-0.1 mg/kg/min.

PRECAUTIONS

CONTRAINDICATIONS: Increased intracranial pressure, impaired cerebral circulation. **CAUTIONS:** Debilitated, impaired respiratory, circulatory, renal, hepatic, lipid metabolism disorders. **PREGNANCY/LACTATION:** Unknown whether drug crosses placenta. Distributed in breast milk. Not recommended for obstetrics, nursing mothers. **Pregnancy Category B.**

INTERACTIONS

DRUG INTERACTIONS: Alcohol, CNS depressants may increase CNS, respiratory, depression, hypotensive effect. **ALTERED LAB VALUES:** None significant.

SIDE EFFECTS

FREQUENT: Involuntary muscular movement, apnea (common during induction; lasts >60 sec), hypotension, nausea, vomiting, burning/stinging at IV site. **OCCASIONAL:** Twitching, bucking, jerking, thrashing, headache, dizziness, bradycardia, hypertension, fever, abdominal cramping, tingling, numbness, coldness, cough, hiccups, facial flushing. **RARE:** Rash, dry mouth, agitation, confusion, myalgia, thrombophlebitis.

P

ADVERSE REACTIONS/TOXIC EFFECTS

Continuous/repeated intermittent infusion may result in extreme somnolence, respiratory/circulatory depression. A too-rapid IV may produce marked severe hypotension, respiratory depression, irregular muscular movements. Acute allergic reaction (erythema, pruritus, urticaria, rhinitis, dyspnea, hypotension, restlessness, anxiety, abdominal pain) may occur.

NURSING IMPLICATIONS

BASELINE ASSESSMENT:

Resuscitative equipment, endotracheal tube, suction, oxygen must be available. Obtain vital signs before administration.

INTERVENTION/EVALUATION:

Monitor for hypotension, bradycardia q3-5min during and after administration until recovery is achieved. Assess diligently for apnea during administration. Monitor for involuntary skeletal muscle movement.

PATIENT/FAMILY TEACHING:

Discomfort along IV route may occur.

propoxyphene hydrochloride

pro-pox´ih-feen
(Darvon)

FIXED-COMBINATION(S):
W/aspirin, caffeine (Darvon Compound-65); w/acetaminophen (Wygesic)

propoxyphene napsylate

(Darvon-N)

FIXED-COMBINATION(S):
W/acetaminophen (Darvocet-N)

CANADIAN AVAILABILITY:
Darvon-N, Novopropoxyn

CLASSIFICATION

Opioid analgesic

PHARMACOKINETICS

	ONSET	PEAK	DURATION
PO	15-60 min	—	4-6 hrs

Well absorbed from GI tract. Widely distributed. Protein binding: high. Metabolized in liver. Primarily excreted in urine. Half-life: 6-12 hrs; metabolite: 30-36 hrs.

ACTION

Binds w/opioid receptors within CNS, altering processes affecting pain perception, emotional response to pain.

USES

Relief of mild to moderate pain.

PO ADMINISTRATION

1. Give w/o regard to meals.
2. Capsules may be emptied and mixed w/food.
3. Shake oral suspension well.
4. Do not crush or break film-coated tablets.

INDICATIONS/DOSAGE/ROUTES

NOTE: Reduce initial dosage in those w/hypothyroidism, concurrent CNS depressants, Addison's disease, renal insufficiency, elderly/debilitated.

Propoxyphene hydrochloride:
PO: Adults, elderly: 65 mg q4h, as needed. **Maximum:** 390 mg/day.

Propoxyphene napsylate:
PO: Adults, elderly: 100 mg q4h, as needed. **Maximum:** 600 mg/day.

PRECAUTIONS

CONTRAINDICATIONS: None significant. **EXTREME CAUTION:** Severe CNS depression, anoxia, hypercapnia, respiratory depression, seizures, acute alcoholism, shock, untreated myxedema, respiratory dysfunction. **CAUTIONS:** Increased intracranial pressure, impaired hepatic function, acute abdominal conditions, hypothyroidism, prostatic hypertrophy, Addison's disease, urethral stricture, COPD. **PREGNANCY/LACTATION:** Crosses placenta; minimal amount distributed in breast milk. Respiratory depression may occur in neonate if mother received opiates during labor. Regular use of opiates during pregnancy may produce withdrawal symptoms in neonate (irritability, excessive crying, tremors, hyperactive reflexes, fever, vomiting, diarrhea, yawning, sneezing, seizures). **Pregnancy Category C.**

INTERACTIONS

DRUG INTERACTIONS: Alcohol, CNS depressants may increase CNS, respiratory depression, hypotension. May increase concentration, toxicity of carbamazepine. Effects may be decreased w/buprenorphine. MAO inhibitors may produce severe, fatal reaction (reduce dose to 1/4 usual dose). **ALTERED LAB VALUES:** May increase amylase, lipase, SGOT (AST), SGPT (ALT), LDH, alkaline phosphatase, bilirubin.

SIDE EFFECTS

NOTE: Effects dependent on dosage amount. Ambulatory pts and those not in moderate pain may experience dizziness, nausea, vomiting, hypotension more frequently than those in supine position or having moderate pain.
FREQUENT: Suppressed breathing depth. **OCCASIONAL:** Lightheadedness, mental clouding, dizziness, sedation, hypotension, nausea, vomiting, euphoria/dysphoria, constipation (drug delays digestion), sweating, flushing, feeling of facial and neck warmth, urinary retention.

ADVERSE REACTIONS/TOXIC EFFECTS

Overdosage results in respiratory depression, skeletal muscle flaccidity, cold, clammy skin, cyanosis, extreme somnolence progressing to convulsions, stupor, coma. Hepatotoxicity may occur w/overdosage of acetaminophen component. Tolerance to analgesic effect, physical dependence may occur w/repeated use.

NURSING IMPLICATIONS

BASELINE ASSESSMENT:

Obtain vital signs before giving medication. If respirations are 12/min or lower (20/min or lower in children), withhold medication, contact physician. Assess onset, type, location, and duration of pain. Effect of medication is reduced if full pain recurs before next dose.

INTERVENTION/EVALUATION:

Palpate bladder for urinary retention. Monitor pattern of daily bowel activity, stool consistency. Initiate deep breathing and coughing exercises, particularly in those w/impaired pulmonary function. Assess for clinical improvement, record onset of relief of pain. Contact physician if pain is not adequately relieved.

PATIENT/FAMILY TEACHING:

Change positions slowly to avoid orthostatic hypotension. Avoid tasks that require alertness, motor skills until response to drug is established. Tolerance/dependence may occur w/prolonged use of high doses.

propranolol hydrochloride

pro-pran´oh-lol
(Inderal)

FIXED-COMBINATION(S):
W/hydrochlorothiazide, a diuretic (Inderide)

CANADIAN AVAILABILITY:
Detensol, Inderal, Novopranol

CLASSIFICATION

Beta-adrenergic blocker

PHARMACOKINETICS

	ONSET	PEAK	DURATION
PO	—	60-90 min	—
PO (long acting)	—	6 hrs	—
IV	Immediate	1 min	—

Almost completely absorbed from GI tract. Widely distributed. Protein binding: 93%. Metabolized in liver. Primarily excreted in urine. Not removed by hemodialysis. Half-life: 3-5 hrs.

ACTION

Nonselective beta-blocker. Blocks $beta_1$-adrenergic receptors, slowing sinus heart rate, decreasing cardiac output, decreasing B/P (exact mechanism unknown but may block peripheral adrenergic receptors, decrease sympathetic outflow from CNS, or decrease renin release from kidney). Blocks $beta_2$-adrenergic receptors, increasing airway resistance. Exhibits antiarrhythmic activity, slowing AV conduction, increasing refractory period in AV node.

USES

Treatment of hypertension, angina, various cardiac arrhythmias, hypertrophic subaortic stenosis, migraine headache, essential tremor and as an adjunct to alpha-blocking agents in the treatment of pheochromocytoma. Used to reduce risk of cardiovascular mortality and reinfarction in pts who have previously suffered a myocardial infarction (MI).

PO/IV ADMINISTRATION

PO:

1. May crush scored tablets.
2. Give at same time each day.

IV:

1. Give undiluted for direct injection.
2. Do not exceed 1 mg/min injection rate.
3. For IV infusion, may dilute each 1 mg in 10 ml 5% dextrose in water.
4. Give 1 mg over 10-15 min.

INDICATIONS/DOSAGE/ROUTES

Hypertension:
PO: Adults, elderly: Initially, 40 mg 2 times/day or 80 mg daily as extended-release capsule. Increase at 3-7 day intervals. **Maintenance:** 120-240 mg/day as tablets or oral solution, 120-160 mg/day as extended-release capsules. **Maximum:** 640 mg/day. **Children:** Initially, 1 mg/kg/day in 2 equally divided doses. Increase at 3-5 day intervals up to 2 mg/kg/day.

Angina pectoris:
PO: Adults, elderly: Initially, 80-320 mg/day in 2-4 divided doses or 80 mg/day (sustained release). **Maximum:** 320 mg/day. **Maintenance:** 160 mg/day.

Cardiac arrhythmias:
PO: Adults, elderly: 10-30 mg 3-4 times/day.

Life-threatening arrhythmias:
IV: Adults, elderly: 0.5-3 mg. Repeat once in 2 min. Give additional doses at intervals of at least 4 hrs.

Hypertrophic subaortic stenosis:
PO: Adults, elderly: 20-40 mg in 3-4 divided doses or 80-160 mg/day as extended-release capsule.

Pheochromocytoma:
PO: Adults, elderly: 60 mg/day in divided doses w/alpha-blocker for 3 days before surgery. **Maintenance (inoperable tumor):** 30 mg/day w/alpha-blocker.

Migraine headache:
PO: Adults, elderly: 80 mg/day in divided doses or 80 mg once daily as extended-release capsule. Increase up to 160-240 mg/day in divided doses.

Myocardial infarction:
PO: Adults, elderly: 180-240 mg/day in divided doses beginning 5-21 days after MI.

Essential tremor:
PO: Adults, elderly: Initially, 40 mg 2 times/day increased up to 120-320 mg/day in 3 divided doses.

Usual pediatric dosage:
PO: Children: 2-4 mg/kg/day in 2 equally divided doses up to 16 mg/kg/day in divided doses.

PRECAUTIONS

CONTRAINDICATIONS: Bronchial asthma, COPD, uncontrolled cardiac failure, sinus bradycardia, heart block greater than first degree, cardiogenic shock, CHF, unless secondary to tachyarrhythmias, those on MAO inhibitors. **CAUTIONS:** Inadequate cardiac function, impaired renal/hepatic function, those w/Wolff-Parkinson-White syndrome, diabetes mellitus, hyperthyroidism. **PREGNANCY/LACTATION:** Crosses placenta; is distributed in breast milk. Avoid use during first trimester. May produce bradycardia, apnea, hypoglycemia, hypothermia during delivery, small birth-weight infants. **Pregnancy Category C.**

INTERACTIONS

DRUG INTERACTIONS: Diuretics, other hypotensives may increase hypotensive effect. Sympathomimetics, xanthines may mutually inhibit effects. May mask symptoms of hypoglycemia, prolong hypoglycemic effect of insulin, oral hypogycemics. NSAIDs may decrease antihypertensive effect. May increase cardiac depressant effect w/IV phenytoin. **ALTERED LAB VALUES:** May increase ANA titer, SGOT (AST), SGPT (ALT), alkaline phosphatase, LDH, bilirubin, BUN, creatinine, potassium, uric acid, lipoproteins, triglycerides.

SIDE EFFECTS

IV effects more common, severe than w/oral dose, esp. in elderly, azotemic pts. **FREQUENT:** Bradycardia. **OCCASIONAL:** Peripheral vascular insufficiency, (usually Raynaud's type), dizziness, fatigue. **RARE:** Sedation, behavioral change, hypotension, GI upset, peripheral skin necrosis, rash, rhythm and/or conduction disturbance.

ADVERSE REACTIONS/TOXIC EFFECTS

May produce profound bradycardia, hypotension. Abrupt withdrawal may result in sweating, palpitations, headache, tremulousness. May precipitate CHF, MI in those w/cardiac disease, thyroid storm in those w/thyrotoxicosis, peripheral ischemia in those w/existing peripheral vascular disease. Hypoglycemia may occur in previously controlled diabetics.

NURSING IMPLICATIONS

BASELINE ASSESSMENT:

Assess baseline renal/liver

function tests. Assess B/P, apical pulse immediately before drug is administered (if pulse is 60/min or below or systolic B/P is below 90 mm Hg, withhold medication, contact physician). *Anginal:* Record onset, type (sharp, dull, squeezing), radiation, location, intensity, and duration of anginal pain and precipitating factors (exertion, emotional stress).

INTERVENTION/EVALUATION:

Assess pulse for strength/weakness, irregular rate, bradycardia. Monitor EKG for cardiac arrhythmias. Assess fingers for color, numbness (Raynaud's). Assist w/ ambulation if dizziness occurs. Assess for evidence of CHF (dyspnea [particularly on exertion or lying down], night cough, peripheral edema, distended neck veins). Monitor I&O (increase in weight, decrease in urine output may indicate CHF). Assess for rash, fatigue, behavioral changes. Therapeutic response ranges from a few days to several weeks. Measure B/P near end of dosing interval (determines if B/P is controlled throughout day).

PATIENT/FAMILY TEACHING:

Do not abruptly discontinue medication. Compliance w/therapy regimen is essential to control hypertension, arrhythmia, anginal pain. To avoid hypotensive effect, rise slowly from lying to sitting position, wait momentarily before standing. Avoid tasks that require alertness, motor skills until response to drug is established. Report excessively slow pulse rate (<60 beats/min), peripheral numbness, dizziness. Do not use nasal decongestants, over-the-counter cold preparations (stimulants) w/o physician approval. Outpatients should monitor B/P, pulse before taking medication. Restrict salt, alcohol intake.

propylthiouracil

pro-pill-thye-oh-yoor′ah-sill
(Propylthiouracil)

CANADIAN AVAILABILITY:
Propyl-Thyracil

CLASSIFICATION

Antithyroid

PHARAMACOKINETICS

Readily absorbed from GI tract. Concentrated in thyroid. Protein binding: 80%. Metabolized in liver. Primarily excreted in urine. Minimally removed by hemodialysis. Half-life: 1-2 hrs.

ACTION

Inhibits thyroid hormone synthesis. Diverts iodine from thyroid hormone synthesis.

USES

Palliative treatment of hyperthyroidism; adjunct to ameliorate hyperthyroidism in preparation for surgical treatment or radioactive iodine therapy.

PO ADMINISTRATION

Space doses evenly.

INDICATIONS/DOSAGE/ROUTES

Hyperthyroidism:
PO: Adults, elderly: Initially: 300-400 mg/day. **Maintenance:** 100-150 mg/day; **Children (6-10 yrs):** Initially: 50-150 mg/day; **(>10 yrs):** 150-300 mg/day. **Maintenance:** Determined by pt response.

PRECAUTIONS

CONTRAINDICATIONS: Hypersensitivity to the drug. **CAUTIONS:** Pts over 40 years of age or in combination w/other agranulocytosis-inducing drugs. **PREGNANCY/LACTATION:** Do not give to nursing mothers. **Pregnancy Category D.**

INTERACTIONS

DRUG INTERACTIONS: Amiodarone, iodinated glycerol, iodine, potassium iodide may decrease response. May decrease effect of oral anticoagulants. May increase concentration of digoxin (as pt becomes euthyroid). May decrease thyroid uptake of I^{131}. **ALTERED LAB VALUES:** May increase SGOT (AST), SGPT (ALT), alkaline phosphatase, LDH, bilirubin, prothrombin time.

SIDE EFFECTS

FREQUENT: Urticaria, rash, pruritus, nausea, skin pigmentation, hair loss, headache, paresthesia. **OCCASIONAL:** Drowsiness, lymphadenopathy, vertigo. **RARE:** Drug fever, lupus-like syndrome.

ADVERSE REACTIONS/TOXIC EFFECTS

Agranulocytosis (which may occur as long as 4 mo after therapy), pancytopenia, fatal hepatitis have occurred.

NURSING IMPLICATIONS

BASELINE ASSESSMENT:

Question for hypersensitivity. Obtain baseline weight, pulse.

INTERVENTION/EVALUATION:

Monitor pulse, weight daily. Assess food tolerance. Check for skin eruptions, itching, swollen lymph glands. Be alert to hepatitis (nausea, vomiting, drowsiness, jaundice). Monitor hematology results for bone marrow suppression; check for signs of infection/bleeding.

PATIENT/FAMILY TEACHING:

Do not exceed ordered dose; follow-up w/physician is essential. Space evenly around the clock. Take resting pulse daily (teach pt/family), report as directed. Do not take other medications w/o approval of physician. Seafood, iodine products may be restricted. Report illness, unusual bleeding/bruising immediately. Inform physician of sudden/continuous weight gain, cold intolerance, or depression.

P

protamine sulfate

pro´tah-meen
(Protamine sulfate)

CANADIAN AVAILABILITY:
Protamine

CLASSIFICATION

Heparin antagonist

PHARMACOKINETICS

	ONSET	PEAK	DURATION
IV	5 min	—	2 hrs

After IV administration, protamine neutralizes heparin within 5 min (forms complex).

ACTION

Complexes w/heparin to form a stable salt resulting in reduction of anticoagulant activity of heparin.

USES

Treatment of severe heparin

overdose (causing hemorrhage). Neutralizes effects of heparin administered during extracorporeal circulation.

STORAGE/HANDLING

Keep at room temperature. Use only colorless solutions. Discard unused portions.

IV ADMINISTRATION

IV:

1. Administer *slowly,* over 1-3 min (less than 50 mg over any 10 min period).
2. Give by IV injection only.
3. May be administered undiluted or diluted w/5% dextrose/0.9% NaCl fluid for injection.

INDICATIONS/DOSAGE/ROUTES

Antidote:

IV: Adults, elderly: 1 mg protamine sulfate neutralizes 90-115 U of heparin. Heparin disappears rapidly from circulation, reducing the dosage demand for protamine as time elapses.

PRECAUTIONS

CONTRAINDICATIONS: None significant. **CAUTIONS:** History of allergy to fish, vasectomized/infertile men, those on isophane (NPH) insulin or previous protamine therapy (propensity to hypersensitivity reaction). **PREGNANCY/LACTATION:** Unknown whether drug crosses placenta or is distributed in breast milk. **Pregnancy Category C.**

INTERACTIONS

DRUG INTERACTIONS: None significant. **ALTERED LAB VALUES:** None significant.

OCCASIONAL: Hypersensitivity reaction: urticaria, angioedema (occurs in those particularly sensitive to fish, vasectomized or infertile men, those on isophane [NPH] insulin or previous protamine therapy). **RARE:** Back pain.

ADVERSE REACTIONS/TOXIC EFFECTS

A too-rapid IV injection may produce acute hypotension, bradycardia, pulmonary hypertension, dyspnea, transient flushing, feeling of warmth. Heparin rebound may occur several hrs after heparin has been neutralized by protamine (usually evident 8-9 hrs after protamine administration). Occurs most often following arterial/cardiac surgery.

NURSING IMPLICATIONS

Baseline Assessment:

Check prothrombin time, activated partial thromboplastin time (APTT) hematocrit; assess for bleeding.

Intervention/Evaluation:

Monitor pts closely after cardiac surgery for evidence of hyperheparinemia/bleeding. Monitor APTT or activated coagulation time (ACT) 5-15 min after protamine administration. Because of possibility of heparin rebound, repeat tests in 2-8 hrs. Assess hematocrit, platelet count, urine/stool culture for occult blood. Assess for decrease in B/P, increase in pulse rate, complaint of abdominal/back pain, severe headache (may be evidence of hemorrhage). Question for increase in amount of discharge during menses. Assess peripheral pulses; skin for bruises, petechiae. Check for excessive bleeding from minor cuts, scratches. Assess gums for erythema, gingival bleeding. Assess urine output for hematuria.

protriptyline hydrochloride

pro-trip'teh-leen
(Vivactil)

CANADIAN AVAILABILITY: Triptil

CLASSIFICATION

Antidepressant: Tricyclic

PHARMACOKINETICS

Well absorbed from GI tract. Widely distributed. Protein binding: 92%. Metabolized in liver (undergoes first-pass effect). Primarily excreted in urine. Half-life: 67-89 hrs.

ACTION

Increases synaptic concentration of norepinephrine and/or serotonin (inhibits reuptake by presynaptic membrane).

USES

Treatment of various forms of depression, often in conjunction w/ psychotherapy.

PO ADMINISTRATION

1. Give w/food or milk if GI distress occurs.
2. Do not break or chew tablets.

INDICATIONS/DOSAGE/ROUTES

Depression:
PO: Adults: Initially, 15-40 mg daily, given in 1-4 divided doses. Increase dosage gradually to 60 mg daily, then reduce dosage to lowest effective maintenance level. **Adolescents:** Initially, 5 mg 3 times daily.

Usual elderly dosage:
PO: Elderly: Initially, 5-10 mg/day. May increase by 5-10 mg/day q3-7days. **Maintenance:** 10-20 mg/day.

PRECAUTIONS

CONTRAINDICATIONS: Acute recovery period following MI, within 14 days of MAO inhibitor therapy. **CAUTIONS:** Prostatic hypertrophy, history of urinary retention/obstruction, glaucoma, diabetes mellitis, history of seizures, hyperthyroidism, cardiac/hepatic/renal disease, schizophrenia, increased intraocular pressure, hiatal hernia. **PREGNANCY/LACTATION:** Crosses placenta; is distributed in breast milk. **Pregnancy Category C.**

INTERACTIONS

DRUG INTERACTIONS: Alcohol, CNS depressants may increase CNS, respiratory depression, hypotensive effects. Antithyroid agents may increase risk of agranulocytosis. Phenothiazines may increase sedative, anticholinergic effects. Cimetidine may increase concentration, toxicity. May decrease effects of clonidine, guanadrel. May increase cardiac effects w/sympathomimetics. May increase risk of hypertensive crisis, hyperpyretic convulsions w/ MAO inhibitors. **ALTERED LAB VALUES:** May alter EKG readings, glucose.

SIDE EFFECTS

FREQUENT: Drowsiness, fatigue, dry mouth, blurred vision, constipation, delayed micturition, postural hypotension, excessive sweating, disturbed concentration, increased appetite, urinary retention. **OCCASIONAL:** GI disturbances (nausea, GI distress, metallic taste sensation). **RARE:** Paradoxical reaction (agitation, restlessness, nightmares, insomnia), extrapyramidal symptoms (particularly fine hand tremor).

ADVERSE REACTIONS/TOXIC EFFECTS

High dosage may produce cardiovascular effects (severe postural hypotension, dizziness, tachycardia, palpitations, arrhythmias) and seizures. May also result in altered temperature regulation (hyperpyrexia/hypothermia). Abrupt withdrawal from prolonged therapy may produce headache, malaise, nausea, vomiting, vivid dreams.

NURSING IMPLICATIONS

BASELINE ASSESSMENT:

For those on long-term therapy, liver/renal function tests, blood counts should be performed periodically.

INTERVENTION/EVALUATION:

Supervise suicidal-risk patient closely during early therapy (as depression lessens, energy level improves, increasing suicide potential). Assess appearance, behavior, speech pattern, level of interest, mood. Monitor stools; avoid constipation. Monitor B/P, pulse for hypotension, arrhythmias. Closely monitor for cardiac disturbances in elderly pts receiving more than 20 mg daily. Assess for urinary retention by bladder palpation.

PATIENT/FAMILY TEACHING:

Change positions slowly to avoid hypotensive effect. Tolerance to postural hypotension, sedative and anticholinergic effects usually develops during early therapy. Therapeutic effect may be noted within 2-5 days, maximum effect within 2-3 weeks. Photosensitivity to sun may occur; use sunscreens, wear protective clothing. Dry mouth may be relieved by sugarless gum, sips of tepid water. Report visual disturbances. Do not abruptly discontinue medication. Avoid tasks that require alertness, motor skills until response to drug is established. Avoid alcohol and other CNS depressants.

pseudoephedrine hydrochloride

sudo-eh-fed´rin

(Novafed, Sudafed)

(Afrinol Repetabs)

FIXED-COMBINATION(S):
W/acrivastine, an antihistamine (Semprex-D); w/loratidine, an antihistamine (Claritin-D)

CANADIAN AVAILABILITY:
Eltor, Pseudofrin, Sudafed

CLASSIFICATION

Sympathomimetic

PHARMACOKINETICS

	ONSET	PEAK	DURATION
Tablets, syrup	15-30 min	—	4-6 hrs
Ext-release	—	—	8-12 hrs

Well absorbed from GI tract. Partially metabolized in liver. Primarily excreted in urine. Half-life: 9-16 hrs.

ACTION

Acts directly on alpha-adrenergic receptors, and to lesser extent, on beta-adrenergic receptors, producing vasoconstriction of respiratory tract mucosa, resulting in shrinkage of nasal mucous membranes, edema, nasal congestion. Produces little, if any, rebound nasal congestion.

USES

For nasal congestion, treatment of obstructed eustachian ostia in those w/otic inflammation, infection.

PO ADMINISTRATION

Do not crush, chew extended-release tablets; swallow whole.

INDICATIONS/DOSAGE/ROUTES

Decongestant:
PO: Adults, children >12 yrs: 60 mg q4-6h. **Maximum:** 240 mg/day. **Children 6-12 yrs:** 30 mg q6h. **Maximum:** 120 mg/day. **Children 2-5 yrs:** 15 mg q6h. **Maximum:** 60 mg/day.

Usual elderly dose:
PO: Elderly: 30-60 mg q6h as needed.

Extended-release:
PO: Adults, children >12 yrs: 120 mg q12h.

PRECAUTIONS

CONTRAINDICATIONS: Severe hypertension, coronary artery disease, lactating women, MAO inhibitor therapy. **CAUTIONS:** Elderly, hyperthyroidism, diabetes, ischemic heart disease, prostatic hypertrophy. **PREGNANCY/LACTATION:** Crosses placenta; is distributed in breast milk. **Pregnancy Category C.**

INTERACTIONS

DRUG INTERACTIONS:
May decrease effects of antihypertensive, diuretics, beta-adrenergic blockers. MAO inhibitors may increase cardiac stimulant, vasopressor effects. **ALTERED LAB VALUES:** None significant.

SIDE EFFECTS

OCCASIONAL: Mild CNS stimulation (restlessness, nervousness, tremors, headache, insomnia), particularly in those hypersensitive to sympathomimetics (generally, elderly pts).

ADVERSE REACTIONS/TOXIC EFFECTS

Large doses may produce tachycardia, palpitations (particularly in those with cardiac disease), lightheadedness, nausea, vomiting. Overdosage in those >60 yrs may result in hallucinations, CNS depression, seizures.

NURSING IMPLICATIONS

PATIENT/FAMILY TEACHING:

Discontinue drug if adverse reactions occur.

psyllium

sill′ee-um
(Fiberall, Hydrocil, Konsyl, Metamucil, Perdiem)

CANADIAN AVAILABILITY:
Metamucil, Prodiem Plain, Siblin

CLASSIFICATION

Laxative: Bulk-forming

PHARMACOKINETICS

	ONSET	PEAK	DURATION
PO	12-72 hrs	—	—

Acts in small/large intestine.

ACTION

Dissolves, swells in water (provides increased bulk, moisture content in stool). Increased bulk promotes peristalsis, bowel motility.

USES

Prophylaxis in those who should not strain during defecation. Facilitates defecation in those w/diminished colonic motor response.

PO ADMINISTRATION

1. Drink 6-8 glasses of water/day (aids stool softening).
2. Do not swallow in dry form, mix w/at least 1 full glass (8 oz) liquid.

INDICATIONS/DOSAGE/ROUTES

Laxative:
PO: Adults, elderly: 1 rounded tsp, packet, or wafer in water 1-3 times/day.

PRECAUTIONS

CONTRAINDICATIONS: Abdominal pain, nausea, vomiting, symptoms of appendicitis, partial bowel obstruction, dysphagia. **CAUTIONS:** None significant. **PREGNANCY/LACTATION:** Safe for use in pregnancy. **Pregnancy Category C.**

INTERACTIONS

DRUG INTERACTIONS: May interfere w/effects of potassium-sparing diuretics, potassium supplements. May decrease effect of oral anticoagulants, digoxin, salicylates by decreasing absorption. **ALTERED LAB VALUES:** May increase glucose. May decrease potassium.

SIDE EFFECTS

RARE: Some degree of abdominal discomfort, nausea, mild cramps, griping, faintness.

ADVERSE REACTIONS/TOXIC EFFECTS

Esophageal/bowel obstruction may occur if administered with insufficient liquid (less than 250 ml or 1 full glass).

NURSING IMPLICATIONS

INTERVENTION/EVALUATION:

Encourage adequate fluid intake. Assess bowel sounds for peristalsis. Monitor daily bowel activity, stool consistency (watery, loose, soft, semi-solid, solid). Monitor serum electrolytes in those exposed to prolonged, frequent, or excessive use of medication.

PATIENT/FAMILY TEACHING:

Institute measures to promote defecation (increase fluid intake, exercise, high-fiber diet).

pyrazinamide

peer-a-zin′a-mide
(Pyrazinamide)

FIXED-COMBINATION(S):
W/isoniazid and rifampin, antituberculars (Rifater)

CANADIAN AVAILABILITY:
PMS Pyrazinamide, Tebrazid

CLASSIFICATION

Antitubercular

PHARMACOKINETICS

Rapidly, completely absorbed from GI tract. Widely distributed. Protein binding: 10-20%. Metabolized in liver to active metabolite. Primarily excreted in urine. Removed by hemodialysis. Half-life: 9.5 hrs (increased in decreased renal function).

ACTION

Exact mechanism unknown. May be bacteriostatic or bactericidal depending on its concentration at infection site and susceptibility of infecting bacteria.

USES

In conjunction w/at least one other antitubercular agent in treatment of clinical tuberculosis after failure of primary agents (isoniazid, rifampin).

INDICATIONS/DOSAGE/ROUTES

Tuberculosis:
PO: Adults: 20-35 mg/kg/day in 3-4 divided doses. **Maximum:** 3 Gm/day. **Children:** 15-30 mg/kg/day in 1 or 2 doses. **Maximum:** 1.5 Gm/day.

PRECAUTIONS

CONTRAINDICATIONS: Hypersensitivity to pyrazinamide, severe hepatic dysfunction. **CAUTIONS:** Diabetes mellitus, renal impairment, history of gout, children (safety not established). Possible cross-sensitivity w/isoniazid, ethionamide, niacin. **PREGNANCY/LACTATION:** Excreted in breast milk. **Pregnancy Category C.**

INTERACTIONS

DRUG INTERACTIONS: May decrease effects of allopurinol, colchicine, probenecid, sulfinpyrazone. **ALTERED LAB VALUES:** May increase SGOT (AST), SGPT (ALT), uric acid concentrations.

SIDE EFFECTS

FREQUENT: Arthralgia, myalgia (usually mild and self-limiting). **RARE:** Hypersensitivity (rash, urticaria, pruritus), photosensitivity.

ADVERSE REACTIONS/TOXIC EFFECTS

Hepatoxicity, thrombocytopenia, anemia occur rarely.

NURSING IMPLICATIONS

BASELINE ASSESSMENT:

Question for hypersensitivity to pyrazinamide, isoniazid, ethionamide, niacin. Assure collection of specimens for culture, sensitivity. Evaluate results of initial CBC, hepatic function tests, uric acid levels.

INTERVENTION/EVALUATION:

Monitor hepatic function results and be alert for hepatic reactions: jaundice, malaise, fever, liver tenderness, anorexia/nausea/vomiting (stop drug, notify physician promptly). Check serum uric acid levels and assess for hot, painful, swollen joints, esp. big toe, ankle, or knee (gout). Evaluate blood sugars, diabetic status carefully (pyrazinamide makes management difficult). Assess for rash, skin eruptions. Monitor CBC results for thrombocytopenia, anemia.

PATIENT/FAMILY TEACHING:

Do not skip doses; complete full length of therapy (may be months, years). Office visits, lab tests are essential part of treatment. Take w/food to reduce GI upset. Do not take any other medications w/o consulting physician. Avoid too much sun or ultraviolet light until photosensitivity is determined. Notify physician of any new symptom, immediately for yellow eyes or skin; unusual tiredness; fever; loss of appetite; hot, painful, or swollen joints.

pyridostigmine bromide

pier-id-oh-stig′meen
(Mestinon, Regonol)

CANADIAN AVAILABILITY:
Mestinon, Regonol

CLASSIFICATION

Anticholinesterase Agent

PHARMACOKINETICS

	ONSET	PEAK	DURATION
PO	30-45 min	—	3-6 hrs
IM	<15 min	—	2-4 hrs
IV	2-5 min	—	2-3 hrs

Minimally absorbed from GI tract. Protein binding: 0%. Metabolized in liver, by plasma cholinesterases. Primarily excreted in urine. Half-life: 63-112 min.

ACTION

Prevents destruction of acetylcholine by anticholinesterase. Effects include increased secretions, salivation, miosis, bradycardia, increased intestinal, skeletal muscle tone.

USES

Improvement of muscle strength in control of myasthenia gravis, reversal of effects of nondepolarizing neuromuscular blocking agents after surgery.

STORAGE/HANDLING

Store oral, parenteral forms at room temperature.

PO/IM/IV ADMINISTRATION

PO:

1. Give w/food or milk.
2. Tablets may be crushed; do not chew, crush extended-release tablets (may be broken).
3. Give larger dose at times of increased fatigue (e.g., for those w/difficulty in chewing, 30-45 min before meals).

IM/IV:

1. Give large parenteral doses concurrently w/0.6-1.2 mg atropine sulfate IV to minimize side effects.

INDICATIONS/DOSAGE/ROUTES

NOTE: Dosage, frequency of administration dependent on daily clinical pt response (remissions, exacerbations, physical and emotional stress).

Myasthenia gravis:
PO: Adults, elderly: Initially, 60 mg 3 times/day. Increase dose at intervals of 48 hrs or more until therapeutic response is achieved. When increased dosage does not produce further increase in muscle strength, reduce dose to previous dosage level. **Maintenance:** 60-1,500 mg/day. **Children:** Initially, 7 mg/kg/day in 5-6 divided doses.
EXTENDED RELEASE: Adults, elderly: 180-540 mg 1-2 times/day (must maintain at least 6 hrs between doses).
IM/IV: Adults, elderly: 2 mg q2-3h.
PO: Neonate: 5 mg q4-6h.
IM: Neonate: 0.05-0.15 mg/kg q4-6h.

Reversal nondepolarizing muscle relaxants:
IV: Adults, elderly: 10-20 mg with, or shortly after, 0.6-1.2 mg atropine sulfate or 0.2-0.6 mg glycopyrrolate.

PRECAUTIONS

CONTRAINDICATIONS:
Mechanical GI, urinary obstruc-

tion. **CAUTIONS:** Bronchial asthma, bradycardia, epilepsy, recent coronary occlusion, vagotonia, hyperthyroidism, cardiac arrhythmias, peptic ulcer. **PREGNANCY/LACTATION:** Transient muscular weakness occurs in 10-20% of neonates born to mothers treated with drug therapy for myasthenia gravis during pregnancy. Myasthenic mothers may be given 1/30 of their usual oral dose by IM or slow IV injection 1 hr before completion of second stage of labor. **Pregnancy Category C.**

INTERACTIONS

DRUG INTERACTIONS: Anticholinergics reverse/prevent effects. Cholinesterase inhibitors may increase toxicity. Antagonizes neuromuscular blocking agents. Quinidine, procainamide may antagonize action. **ALTERED LAB VALUES:** None significant.

SIDE EFFECTS

COMMON: Miosis, increased GI and skeletal muscle tone, reduced pulse rate, constriction of bronchi and ureters, salivary and sweat gland secretion. **OCCASIONAL:** Headache, slight, temporary decrease in diastolic B/P w/mild reflex tachycardia, short periods of atrial fibrillation in hyperthyroid pts. Hypertensive pts may react w/ marked fall in B/P. **RARE:** Rash.

ADVERSE REACTIONS/TOXIC EFFECTS

Overdosage produces cholinergic reaction manifested as abdominal discomfort/cramping, nausea, vomiting, diarrhea, flushing, feeling of warmth/heat about face, excessive salivation and sweating, lacrimation, pallor, bradycardia/tachycardia, hypotension, urinary urgency, blurred vision, bronchospasm, pupillary contraction, involuntary muscular contraction visible under the skin (fasciculation).

Overdosage may also produce a *cholinergic crisis,* manifested by increasingly severe muscle weakness (appears first in muscles involving chewing, swallowing, followed by muscular weakness of shoulder girdle and upper extremities), respiratory muscle paralysis followed by pelvic girdle and leg muscle paralysis. Requires withdrawal of all cholinergic drugs and immediate use of 1-4 mg atropine sulfate IV for adults, 0.01 mg/kg in infants and children under 12 yrs.

Myasthenic crisis (due to underdosage) also produces extreme muscle weakness but requires a *more* intensive drug therapy program *(differentiation between the two crises is imperative for accurate treatment).* Weakness beginning 1 hr after drug administration suggests overdosage; weakness occurring 3 hrs or more after administration suggests underdosage/resistance to anticholinesterase drugs. Extremely high doses may produce CNS stimulation followed by CNS depression. Resistance to pyridostigmine therapy may occur following prolonged treatment in myasthenic pts. Responsiveness may be restored by decreasing dose/temporarily discontinuing therapy for several days.

NURSING IMPLICATIONS

BASELINE ASSESSMENT:

Larger doses should be given at time of greatest fatigue. Assess muscle strength before testing for diagnosis of myasthenia gravis and after drug administration. Avoid large doses in those w/megacolon or reduced GI motility. Have tissues readily available at pt's bedside.

INTERVENTION/EVALUATION:

Monitor respirations closely during myasthenia gravis testing or if dosage is increased. Assess diligently for cholinergic reaction, as well as bradycardia in the myasthenic pt in crisis. Coordinate dosage time vs. periods of fatigue and increased/decreased muscle strength. Monitor for therapeutic response to medication (increased muscle strength, decreased fatigue, improved chewing, swallowing functions).

PATIENT/FAMILY TEACHING:

Report nausea, vomiting, diarrhea, sweating, increased salivary secretions, irregular heartbeat, muscle weakness, severe abdominal pain, or difficulty in breathing.

pyridoxine hydrochloride (vitamin B_6)

(Pyridoxine)

CANADIAN AVAILABILITY:
Hexa-Betalin

CLASSIFICATION

Vitamin (B_6), coenzyme

PHARMACOKINETICS

Readily absorbed primarily in jejunum. Stored in liver, muscle, brain. Metabolized in liver. Primarily excreted in urine. Removed by hemodialysis. Half-life: 15-20 days.

ACTION

Coenzyme for various metabolic functions affecting protein, carbohydrate, lipid utilization.

USES

Prevention, treatment of pyridoxine deficiency caused by inadequate diet, drug-induced (e.g., INH, penicillamine, cyclosporine) or in-born error of metabolism. Treatment of INH poisoning. Treatment of seizures in neonate unresponsive to conventional therapy. Treatment of sideroblastic anemia associated w/increased serum iron concentrations.

PO/SubQ/IM/IV ADMINISTRATION

NOTE: Give orally unless nausea, vomiting or malabsorption occurs. Avoid IV use in cardiac pts.
IV: Give undiluted or add to IV solutions and give as infusion.

INDICATIONS/DOSAGE/ROUTES

Pyridoxine deficiency:
PO: Adults, elderly: (Diet): 2.5-10 mg/day; after signs of deficiency decreased, 2.5-5 mg/day for several wks. (Drug-Induced): 10-50 mg/day (INH, penicillamine); 100-300 mg/day (cyclosporine). (Error metabolism): 100-500 mg/day.

INH toxicity (>10 Gm); with other anticonvulsants:
IV: Adults, elderly: 4 Gm, then 1 Gm IM q30min until entire dose given. Total dose: Equal to amount INH ingested.

Seizures in neonates:
IM/IV: Neonates: 10-100 mg/day; then oral therapy of 2-100 mg/day for life.

Sideroblastic anemia:
PO: Adults, elderly: 200-600 mg/

day. After adequate response, 30-50 mg/day for life.

PRECAUTIONS

CONTRAINDICATIONS: IV therapy in cardiac pts. **CAUTIONS:** Megadosage in pregnancy. **PREGNANCY/LACTATION:** Crosses placenta; is excreted in breast milk. High doses in utero may produce seizures in neonates. **Pregnancy Category A.**

INTERACTIONS

DRUG INTERACTIONS: Immunosuppressants, isoniazid, penicillamine may antagonize pyridoxine (may cause anemia/peripheral neuritis). Reverses effects of levodopa. **ALTERED LAB VALUES:** None significant.

SIDE EFFECTS

FREQUENT: Stinging at IM injection site. **RARE:** Headache, nausea, somnolence, paresthesia.

ADVERSE REACTIONS/TOXIC EFFECTS

Rare allergic reaction may produce itching, general malaise, bronchospasm. Long-term megadoses (2-6 Gm more than 2 mo) may produce sensory neuropathy (reduced deep tendon reflex, profound impairment of sense of position in distal limbs, gradual sensory ataxia). Toxic symptoms reverse w/drug discontinuance. Seizures have occurred following IV megadoses.

NURSING IMPLICATIONS

INTERVENTION/EVALUATION:

Observe for improvement of deficiency symptoms, including nervous system abnormalities (anxiety, depression, insomnia, motor difficulty, peripheral numbness and tremors), skin lesions (glossitis, seborrhea-like lesions around mouth, nose, eyes). Evaluate for nutritional adequacy.

PATIENT/FAMILY TEACHING:

Discomfort may occur w/IM injection. Foods rich in pyridoxine include legumes, soybeans, eggs, sunflower seeds, hazelnuts, organ meats, tuna, shrimp, carrots, avocado, banana, wheat germ, bran.

quazepam

quay'zah-pam

(Doral)

CLASSIFICATION

Sedative-hypnotic **(Schedule IV)**

PHARMACOKINETICS

Well absorbed from GI tract. Widely distributed. Protein binding: >95%. Metabolized in liver to active metabolite. Primarily excreted in urine. Half-life: 39 hrs.

ACTION

Enhances action of inhibitory neurotransmitter gamma-aminobutyric acid (GABA). Depressant effects occur at all levels of CNS.

USES

Short-term treatment of insomnia (up to 4 wks). Reduces sleep-induction time, number of nocturnal awakenings; increases length of sleep.

PO ADMINISTRATION

Give w/o regard to meals.

INDICATIONS/DOSAGE/ROUTES

Hypnotic:
PO: Adults: 15 mg at bedtime until pt responds; then decrease to 7.5 mg in some pts. **Elderly/debilitated/liver disease/low serum albumin:** 7.5-15 mg at bedtime, attempt to decrease dose after 2 nights.

PRECAUTIONS

CONTRAINDICATIONS: Acute narrow-angle glaucoma, acute alcohol intoxication. **CAUTIONS:** Impaired renal/hepatic function. **PREGNANCY/LACTATION:** Crosses placenta; may be distributed in breast milk. Chronic ingestion during pregnancy may produce withdrawal symptoms, CNS depression in neonates. **Pregnancy Category X.**

INTERACTIONS

DRUG INTERACTIONS: Alcohol, CNS depressants may increase CNS depressant effect. **ALTERED LAB VALUES:** None significant.

SIDE EFFECTS

FREQUENT: Drowsiness, dizziness, ataxia, sedation. Morning drowsiness may occur initially. **OCCASIONAL:** GI disturbances, nervousness, blurred vision, dry mouth, headache, confusion, skin rash, irritability, slurred speech. **RARE:** Paradoxical CNS excitement/restlessness (particularly noted in elderly/debilitated).

ADVERSE REACTIONS/TOXIC EFFECTS

Abrupt or too-rapid withdrawal may result in pronounced restlessness and irritability, insomnia, hand tremors, abdominal/muscle cramps, sweating, vomiting, seizures. Overdosage results in somnolence, confusion, diminished reflexes, coma.

NURSING IMPLICATIONS

BASELINE ASSESSMENT:

Provide environment conducive to sleep (back rub, quiet environment, low lighting). Provide protective measures, e.g., raise bed rails, place call light within easy reach.

INTERVENTION/EVALUATION:

Evaluate for therapeutic response (a decrease in number of nocturnal awakenings, increase in length of sleep duration time). Assess for paradoxical reaction, esp. during early therapy and in elderly, debilitated. Provide assistance w/ambulation, including daytime if drowsiness continues.

PATIENT/FAMILY TEACHING:

Smoking reduces drug effectiveness, increases risk of fire by falling asleep w/lighted cigarette. Do not take alcohol or other CNS depressants w/this drug. Notify physician promptly of pregnancy. Do not abruptly withdraw medication following long-term use.

quinapril hydrochloride

quin´ah-prill
(Accupril)

CLASSIFICATION

Angiotensin converting enzyme (ACE) inhibitor

PHARMACOKINETICS

	ONSET	PEAK	DURATION
PO	1 hr	2-4 hrs	—

Readily absorbed from GI tract.

Protein binding: 97%. Metabolized in liver, GI tract, extravascular tissue to active metabolite. Primarily excreted in urine. Minimal removal by hemodialysis. Half-life: 1-2 hrs; metabolite: 3 hrs (increased in decreased renal function).

ACTION

Suppresses renin-angiotensin-aldosterone system (prevents conversion of angiotensin I to angiotensin II, a potent vasoconstrictor; may also inhibit angiotensin II at local vascular and renal sites). Decreases plasma angiotensin II, increases plasma renin activity, decreases aldosterone secretion. Reduces peripheral arterial resistance.

USES

Treatment of hypertension. Used alone or in combination w/ other antihypertensives. Adjunctive therapy in management of heart failure.

PO ADMINISTRATION

1. May give w/o regard to food.
2. Tablets may be crushed.

INDICATIONS/DOSAGE/ROUTES

Hypertension (used alone):
PO: Adults: Initially, 10 mg/day. May adjust dose at least 2-wk intervals. **Maintenance:** 20-80 mg/day as single or 2 divided doses.

Hypertension (combination therapy):
NOTE: Discontinue diuretic 2-3 days before initiating quinapril therapy.
PO: Adults: Initially, 5 mg/day titrated to pt's needs.

Usual elderly dose:
PO: Elderly: Initially, 2.5-5 mg/day. May increase by 2.5-5 mg q1-2wks.

Dosage in renal impairment:
Titrate to pt need after following initial doses:

CREATININE CLEARANCE	INITIAL DOSE
>60 ml/min	10 mg
30-60 ml/min	5 mg
10-30 ml/min	2.5 mg

Heart failure:
PO: Adults, elderly: Initially, 5 mg 2 times/day. **Range:** 20-40 mg/day.

PRECAUTIONS

CONTRAINDICATIONS: MI, coronary insufficiency, angina, evidence of coronary artery disease, hypersensitivity to phentolamine, history of angioedema w/previous treatment w/ACE inhibitors. **CAUTIONS:** Renal impairment, those w/sodium depletion or on diuretic therapy, dialysis, hypovolemia, coronary/cerebrovascular insufficiency. **PREGNANCY/LACTATION:** Crosses placenta; unknown whether distributed in breast milk. May cause fetal-neonatal mortality/morbidity. **Pregnancy Category D.**

INTERACTIONS

DRUG INTERACTIONS: Alcohol, diuretics, hypotensive agents may increase effects. NSAIDs may decrease effect. Potassium sparing diuretics, potassium supplements may cause hyperkalemia. May increase lithium concentration, toxicity. **ALTERED LAB VALUES:** May increase potassium SGOT (AST), SGPT (ALT), alkaline phosphatase, bilirubin, BUN, creatinine. May decrease sodium. May cause positive ANA titer.

SIDE EFFECTS

FREQUENT: Headache. **OCCA-**

SIONAL: Dizziness, fatigue. **RARE:** Nausea, vomiting.

ADVERSE REACTIONS/TOXIC EFFECTS

Excessive hypotension (first-dose syncope) may occur in those w/CHF, severely salt/volume depleted. Angioedema (swelling of face/lips), hyperkalemia occur rarely. Agranulocytosis, neutropenia may be noted in those w/impaired renal function or collagen vascular disease (systemic lupus erythematosus, scleroderma). Nephrotic syndrome may be noted in those w/history of renal disease.

NURSING IMPLICATIONS

BASELINE ASSESSMENT:

Obtain B/P immediately before each dose in addition to regular monitoring (be alert to fluctuations). If excessive reduction in B/P occurs, place pt in supine position w/legs slightly elevated. Renal function tests should be performed before therapy begins. In those w/prior renal disease, urine test for protein by dip-stick method should be made w/first urine of day before therapy begins and periodically thereafter. In those w/renal impairment, autoimmune disease or those taking drugs that affect leukocytes/immune response, CBC and differential count should be performed before therapy begins and q2wks for 3 mo, then periodically thereafter.

INTERVENTION/EVALUATION:

Assist w/ambulation if dizziness occurs. Question for evidence of headache.

PATIENT/FAMILY TEACHING:

To reduce hypotensive effect, rise slowly from lying to sitting position and permit legs to dangle from bed momentarily before standing. Noncola carbonated beverage, unsalted crackers, dry toast may relieve nausea. Full therapeutic effect may take 1-2 wks. Report any sign of infection (sore throat, fever). Skipping doses or voluntarily discontinuing drug may produce severe rebound hypertension. Avoid driving and other tasks that require alert responses until reaction to drug known. Do not use salt substitutes w/o consulting physician.

quinidine gluconate

kwin´ih-deen

(Duraquin, Quinaglute)

polygalacturonate

(Cardioquin)

quinidine sulfate

(Cin-quin, Quinidex)

CANADIAN AVAILABILITY:

Apo-Quinidine, Cardioquin, Novoquinidin, Quinaglute, Quinidex

CLASSIFICATION

Antiarrhythmic

PHARMACOKINETICS

	ONSET	PEAK	DURATION
PO	1-3 hrs	—	6-8 hrs

Completely absorbed from GI tract. Widely distributed. Protein binding: 70-80%. Metabolized in liver. Primarily excreted in urine. Small amounts removed by hemodialysis. Half-life: 6 hrs (increased in CHF, cirrhosis, elderly).

ACTION

Direct cardiac effects (decreases excitability, conduction velocity, automaticity, membrane responsiveness; prolongs refractory period).

USES

Prophylactic therapy to maintain normal sinus rhythm after conversion of atrial fibrillation and/or flutter. Prevention of premature atrial, AV and ventricular contractions, paroxysmal atrial tachycardia, paroxysmal AV junctional rhythm, atrial fibrillation, atrial flutter, paroxysmal ventricular tachycardia not associated w/complete heart block.

STORAGE/HANDLING

For parenteral form, use only clear, colorless solution. Solution is stable for 24 hrs at room temperature when diluted w/5% dextrose.

PO/IM/IV ADMINISTRATION

PO:

1. Do not crush or chew sustained-release tablets.
2. GI upset can be reduced if given w/food.

IV:

NOTE: B/P, EKG should be monitored continuously during IV administration and rate of infusion adjusted to eliminate arrhythmias.

1. For IV infusion, dilute 800 mg w/40 ml 5% dextrose to provide concentration of 16 mg/ml.
2. Administer w/pt in supine position.
3. For IV injection, give at rate of 1 ml (16 mg)/min (too-rapid IV rate may markedly decrease arterial pressure).
4. Monitor EKG for cardiac changes, particularly prolongation of PR, QT interval, widening of QRS complex. Notify physician of any significant interval changes.

INDICATIONS/DOSAGE/ROUTES

NOTE: Extended-release capsules used only for maintenance therapy. 267 mg quinidine gluconate = 275 mg quinidine polygalacturonate or 200 mg quinidine sulfate.

Conversion of atrial fibrillation:
PO: Adults, elderly: 200 mg q2-3h for 5-8 doses. Increase dose until sinus rhythm achieved/toxicity occurs. **Maximum:** 4 Gm/day. Control ventricular rate w/digoxin before quinidine administration.

Atrial flutter:
PO: Adults, elderly: Individualize, give after digitalization.

Paroxysmal supraventricular tachycardia:
PO: Adults, elderly: 400-600 mg q2-3h.

Premature atrial/ventricular contractions:
PO: Adults, elderly: 200-300 mg 3-4 times/day.

Maintenance therapy:
PO: Adults, elderly: 200-400 mg 3-4 times/day or 300-600 mg (as extended-release tablets) q8-12h.

Usual parenteral dosage:
IM: Adults, elderly: Initially, 600 mg, then 400 mg q2h adjusting each subsequent dose according to effect achieved by previous dose.
IV: Adults, elderly: 300 mg (may give 500-750 mg) infused at initial rate of 16 mg/min (1 ml/min).

PRECAUTIONS

CONTRAINDICATIONS: Complete AV block, intraventricular conduction defects, abnormal impulses and rhythms due to escape mechanism, myasthenia gravis. **EXTREME CAUTION:** Incomplete AV block, digitalis intoxication, CHF, preexisting hypotension. **CAUTIONS:** Preexisting asthma, muscle weakness, infection w/fever, hepatic/renal insufficiency. **PREGNANCY/LACTATION:** Crosses placenta; is distributed in breast milk. **Pregnancy Category C.**

INTERACTIONS

DRUG INTERACTIONS: May increase concentration of digoxin. Pimozide, other antiarrhythmics may increase cardiac effects. Urinary alkalizers (e.g., antacids) may decrease excretion. May increase effects of oral anticoagulants, neuromuscular blockers. May decrease effects of antimyasthenics on skeletal muscle. **ALTERED LAB VALUES:** None significant.

SIDE EFFECTS

FREQUENT: Abdominal pain/cramps, nausea, diarrhea, vomiting (can be immediate, intense). **OCCASIONAL:** Mild cinchonism (ringing in ears, blurred vision, hearing loss) or severe cinchonism (headache, vertigo, sweating, lightheadedness, photophobia, confusion, delirium). **RARE:** Hypotension (particularly w/IV administration), hypersensitivity reaction (fever, anaphylaxis, thrombocytopenia).

ADVERSE REACTIONS/TOXIC EFFECTS

Cardiotoxic effects occur most commonly w/IV administration, particularly at high concentration, observed as conduction changes (50% widening of QRS complex, prolonged QT interval, flattened T waves, disappearance of P wave), ventricular tachycardia/flutter, frequent PVCs, complete AV block. Quinidine-induced syncope may occur w/usual dosage (discontinue drug). Severe hypotension may result from high doses. Atrial flutter/fibrillation pts may experience a paradoxical, extremely rapid ventricular rate (may be prevented by prior digitalization). Hepatotoxicity w/jaundice due to drug hypersensitivity.

NURSING IMPLICATIONS

BASELINE ASSESSMENT:

Check B/P and pulse for 1 full min (unless pt is on continuous monitor) before giving medication. For those on long term therapy, CBC and liver/renal function tests should be performed periodically.

INTERVENTION/EVALUATION:

Monitor EKG for cardiac changes, particularly prolongation of PR, QT interval, widening of QRS complex. Monitor I&O, CBC, serum potassium, hepatic/renal function tests. Monitor pattern of daily bowel activity, stool consistency. Assess for dizziness, syncope. Monitor B/P for hypotension (esp. in those on high-dose therapy). If cardiotoxic effect occurs (see Adverse Reactions/Toxic Effects), notify physician immediately. Monitor for therapeutic serum level (2-6 mcg/ml).

PATIENT/FAMILY TEACHING:

Report rash, fever, unusual bleeding or bruising, visual disturbances, ringing in ears. Teach pt/family to take pulse properly. Photophobia may occur—sunglasses will provide some relief.

quinine sulfate

kwye´nine

(Quin-260, Quinamm, Quiphile)

FIXED-COMBINATION(S): W/Vitamin E for nocturnal leg cramps (M-KYA, Q-vel)

CANADIAN AVAILABILITY: Novoquinine

CLASSIFICATION

Antimalarial, antimyotonic

PHARMACOKINETICS

Rapidly, completely absorbed from GI tract. Widely distributed. Protein binding: 70-90%. Metabolized in liver. Primarily excreted in urine. Minimal removal by hemodialysis. Half-life: 11 hrs.

ACTION

Antimalarial: Interferes w/function of plasmodial DNA. Depresses oxygen uptake and carbohydrate metabolism. *Antimyotonic action:* Relaxes skeletal muscle by increasing the refractory period, decreasing excitability of motor end-plates (curare-like), and affecting distribution of calcium w/muscle fiber. Produces analgesic, antipyretic, oxytocic effects.

USES

Generally replaced by more effective, less toxic antimalarials. Used alone, w/pyrimethamine and sulfonamide (or w/oral tetracycline) for treatment of chloraquine-resistant falciparum malaria. Prevention, treatment of nocturnal recumbency leg cramps.

PO ADMINISTRATION

1. Do *not* crush tablets (irritating to gastric mucosa, bitter).
2. Give w/or after meals to reduce GI distress.
3. Bedtime dose should be given w/milk or snack.

INDICATIONS/DOSAGE/ROUTES

Treatment of chloroquin-resistant malaria:

PO: Adults, elderly: 650 mg q8h for 5-7 days. **Children:** 25 mg/kg q8h for 5-7 days.

Treatment of chloroquin-sensitive malaria:

PO: Adults, elderly: 600 mg q8h for 5-7 days. **Children:** 10 mg/kg q8h for 5-7 days.

Nocturnal leg cramps:

PO: Adults, elderly: 260-300 mg at bedtime as needed.

PRECAUTIONS

CONTRAINDICATIONS: Hypersensitivity to quinine (possible cross-sensitivity to quinidine), G-6-PD deficiency, tinnitus, optic neuritis, history of thrombocytopenia during previous quinine therapy, blackwater fever. **CAUTIONS:** Cardiovascular disease (as w/quinidine), myasthenia gravis, asthma. **PREGNANCY/LACTATION:** Crosses placenta; is excreted in breast milk. Not recommended during lactation. May cause congenital malformations (i.e., deafness, limb anomalies, visceral defects, visual changes, stillbirths). **Pregnancy Category X.**

INTERACTIONS

DRUG INTERACTIONS: May increase concentration of digoxin. Mefloquine may increase seizures,

EKG abnormalities. **ALTERED LAB VALUES:** May interfere w/ 17-OH steroid determinations.

SIDE EFFECTS

FREQUENT: Nausea, headache, tinnitus, slight visual disturbances (mild cinchonism). **OCCASIONAL:** Extreme flushing of skin w/intense generalized pruritus is most typical hypersensitivity reaction; also rash, wheezing, dyspnea, angioedema. Prolonged therapy: Cardiac conduction disturbances, decreased hearing.

ADVERSE REACTIONS/TOXIC EFFECTS

Overdosage (severe cinchonism): Cardiovascular effects, severe headache, intestinal cramps w/vomiting and diarrhea, apprehension, confusion, seizures, blindness, respiratory depression. Hypoprothrombinemia, thrombocytopenic purpura, hemoglobinuria, asthma, agranulocytosis, hypoglycemia, deafness, optic atrophy occur rarely.

NURSING IMPLICATIONS

BASELINE ASSESSMENT:

Question for hypersensitivity to quinine, quinidine. Evaluate initial EKG, CBC results.

INTERVENTION/EVALUATION:

Check for hypersensitivity: Flushing, rash/urticaria, itching, dyspnea, wheezing (hold drug, inform physician at once). Assess level of hearing, visual acuity, presence of headache/tinnitus, nausea and report adverse effects promptly (possible cinchonism). Monitor CBC results for blood dyscrasias; be alert to infection (fever, sore throat) and bleeding/bruising or unusual tiredness/weakness. Assess pulse, EKG for arrhythmias. Check FBS levels and watch for hypoglycemia (cold sweating, tremors, tachycardia, hunger, anxiety).

PATIENT/FAMILY TEACHING:

For malaria, continue for full length of treatment. Take w/food; do not crush tablets. Do not take any other medication w/o consulting physician. Report *any* new symptom immediately, esp. visual/hearing difficulties, shortness of breath, rash/itching, nausea. Periodic lab tests are part of therapy. Use nonhormonal contraception.

ramipril

ram´ih-prill

(Altace)

CLASSIFICATION

Angiotensin converting enzyme (ACE) inhibitor

PHARMACOKINETICS

	ONSET	PEAK	DURATION
PO	1-2 hrs	3-6 hr	24 hrs

Well absorbed from GI tract. Protein binding: 73%. Metabolized in liver to active metabolite. Primarily excreted in urine. Half-life: 5.1 hrs.

ACTION

Suppresses renin-angiotensin-aldosterone system (prevents conversion of angiotensin I to angiotensin II, a potent vasoconstrictor; may also inhibit angiotensin II at local vascular and renal sites). Decreases plasma angiotensin II, increases plasma renin activity, decreases aldosterone secretion.

Reduces peripheral arterial resistance.

USES

Treatment of hypertension. Used alone or in combination w/ other antihypertensives.

PO ADMINISTRATION

1. May give w/o regard to food.
2. Do not chew or break capsules.

INDICATIONS/DOSAGE/ROUTES

Hypertension (used alone):
PO: Adults, elderly: Initially, 2.5 mg/day. **Maintenance:** 2.5-20 mg/day as single or in 2 divided doses.

Hypertension (combination therapy):
NOTE: Discontinue diuretic 2-3 days before initiating ramipril therapy.
PO: Adults, elderly: Initially, 1.25 mg/day titrated to pt's needs.

Dosage in renal impairment (Ccr <40 ml/min; serum creatinine >2.5 mg/dl):
Initially: 1.25 mg/day titrated up to maximum of 5 mg/day.

PRECAUTIONS

CONTRAINDICATIONS: History of angioedema w/previous treatment w/ACE inhibitors. **CAUTIONS:** Renal impairment, those w/sodium depletion or on diuretic therapy, dialysis, hypovolemia, coronary/cerebrovascular insufficiency. **PREGNANCY/LACTATION:** Crosses placenta; is distributed in breast milk. May cause fetal/neonatal mortality/morbidity. **Pregnancy Category D.**

INTERACTIONS

DRUG INTERACTIONS: Alcohol, diuretics, hypotensive agents may increase effects. NSAIDs may decrease effect. Potassium sparing diuretics, potassium supplements may cause hyperkalemia. May increase lithium concentration, toxicity. **ALTERED LAB VALUES:** May increase potassium, SGOT (AST), SGPT (ALT), alkaline phosphatase, bilirubin, BUN, creatinine. May decrease sodium. May cause positive ANA titer.

SIDE EFFECTS

FREQUENT: Cough (common), headache, dizziness, peripheral numbness. **OCCASIONAL:** Fatigue. **RARE:** GI distress, mental depression.

ADVERSE REACTIONS/TOXIC EFFECTS

Excessive hypotension (first-dose syncope) may occur in those w/CHF, severely salt/volume depleted. Angioedema (swelling of face/lips), hyperkalemia occur rarely. Agranulocytosis, neutropenia may be noted in those w/ impaired renal function or collagen vascular disease (systemic lupus erythematosus, scleroderma). Nephrotic syndrome may be noted in those w/history of renal disease.

NURSING IMPLICATIONS

BASELINE ASSESSMENT:

Obtain B/P immediately before each dose, in addition to regular monitoring (be alert to fluctuations). If excessive reduction in B/P occurs, place pt in supine position w/legs elevated. Renal function tests should be performed before therapy begins. In those w/ prior renal disease, urine test for protein by dip-stick method should be made w/first urine of day before therapy begins and periodically thereafter. In those w/renal impairment, autoimmune disease, or taking drugs that affect leukocytes/immune response, CBC and differential count should be performed before therapy begins and q2wks for 3 mo, then periodically thereafter.

INTERVENTION/EVALUATION:

Assess for cough (common effect). Assist w/ambulation if dizziness occurs. Assess lung sounds for rales, wheezing in those w/ CHF. Monitor urinalysis for proteinuria. Monitor serum potassium levels in those on concurrent diuretic therapy. Monitor pattern of daily bowel activity, stool consistency.

PATIENT/FAMILY TEACHING:

Report any sign of infection (sore throat, fever). Several wks may be needed for full therapeutic effect of B/P reduction. Skipping doses or voluntarily discontinuing drug may produce severe, rebound hypertension. To reduce hypotensive effect, rise slowly from lying to sitting position and permit legs to dangle from bed momentarily before standing.

ranitidine

rah-nih´tih-deen

(Zantac)

CANADIAN AVAILABILITY:

Apo-Ranitidine, Novoranidine, Zantac

CLASSIFICATION

Histamine H-2 receptor antagonist

PHARMACOKINETICS

Rapidly absorbed from GI tract. Widely distributed. Protein binding: 15%. Metabolized in liver. Primarily excreted in urine. Half-life: *Oral:* 2.5 hrs; *IV:* 2-2.5 hrs (increase in decreased renal function).

ACTION

Inhibits histamine action at H_2 receptors of parietal cells, inhibiting basal and nocturnal gastric acid secretion.

USES

Short-term treatment of active duodenal ulcer. Prevention of duodenal ulcer recurrence. Treatment of active benign gastric ulcer, pathologic GI hypersecretory conditions, acute gastroesophageal reflux disease (GERD) including erosive esophagitis. Maintenance of healed erosive esophagitis.

STORAGE/HANDLING

Store tablets, syrup at room temperature. IV solutions appear clear, colorless to yellow (slight darkening does not affect potency). IV infusion (piggyback) is stable for 48 hrs at room temperature (discard if discolored or precipitate forms).

PO/IM/IV ADMINISTRATION

PO:

1. Give w/o regard to meals. Best given after meals or at bedtime.
2. Do not administer within 1 hr of magnesium- or aluminum-containing antacids (decreases absorption by 33%).

IM:

1. May be given undiluted.
2. Give deep IM into large muscle mass.

IV:

1. For direct IV, dilute w/20 ml

NaCl or other compatible IV fluid. Administer over minimum of 5 min (prevents arrhythmias, hypotension).

2. For intermittent IV infusion (piggyback), dilute w/50 ml 0.9% NaCl, 5% dextrose, or other compatible IV fluid. Infuse over 15-20 min.

3. For IV infusion, dilute w/100-1,000 ml 0.9% NaCl, 5% dextrose solution. Infuse over 24 hrs.

INDICATIONS/DOSAGE/ROUTES

Active duodenal ulcer:
PO: Adults, elderly: 150 mg 2 times/day or 300 mg at bedtime. **Maintenance:** 150 mg at bedtime.

Pathologic hypersecretory conditions:
PO: Adults, elderly: 150 mg 2 times/day up to 6 Gm/day.

Benign gastric ulcer, GERD:
PO: Adults, elderly: 150 mg 2 times/day.

Erosive esophagitis:
PO: Adults, elderly: 150 mg 4 times/day.

Usual parenteral dosage:
IM/IV: Adults, elderly: 50 mg q6-8h. **Maximum:** 400 mg/day.
IV INFUSION: Adults, elderly: 150 mg/day.

Dosage in renal impairment:
Creatinine clearance <50 ml/min: *PO:* 150 mg q24h. *IM/IV:* 50 mg q18-24h.

PRECAUTIONS

CONTRAINDICATIONS: None significant. **CAUTIONS:** Impaired renal/hepatic function, elderly. **PREGNANCY/LACTATION:** Unknown whether drug crosses placenta or is distributed in breast milk. **Pregnancy Category B.**

INTERACTIONS

DRUG INTERACTIONS: Antacids may decrease absorption (do not give within 1 hr). May decrease absorption of ketoconazole (give at least 2 hrs after). **ALTERED LAB VALUES:** Interferes w/skin tests using allergen extracts. May increase liver function tests, creatinine, gamma-glutamyl transpeptidase.

SIDE EFFECTS

OCCASIONAL: Headache (may be severe). **RARE:** Malaise, vertigo, constipation, nausea, insomnia, rash; mental confusion, agitation, depression, hallucinations, particularly in elderly.

ADVERSE REACTIONS/TOXIC EFFECTS

Reversible hepatitis, blood dyscrasias occur rarely.

NURSING IMPLICATIONS

BASELINE ASSESSMENT:

Do not confuse medication w/Xanax (alprazolam).

INTERVENTION/EVALUATION:

Monitor serum SGOT (AST), SGPT (ALT) levels. Assess mental status in elderly.

PATIENT/FAMILY TEACHING:

Smoking decreases effectiveness of medication. Do not take medicine within 1 hr of magnesium- or aluminum-containing antacids. Transient burning/itching may occur w/IV administration. Report headache. Avoid alcohol, aspirin.

R

ribavirin

rye-bah-vi´rim
(Virazole)

CANADIAN AVAILABILITY: Virazole

CLASSIFICATION

Antiviral

PHARMACOKINETICS

Small amount systemically absorbed after inhalation. Rapidly absorbed from GI tract. Primarily distributed to plasma, respiratory tract secretions, RBCs. Metabolized in liver to active metabolite. Primarily excreted in urine. Half-life: 9.5 hrs.

ACTION

Appears to be virustatic through disruption of RNA and DNA synthesis, interfering w/protein synthesis, viral replication.

USES

Severe lower respiratory tract infections due to respiratory syncytial viruses in select infants, children.

STORAGE/HANDLING

Solutions appear clear and colorless, are stable for 24 hrs at room temperature. Discard solutions for nebulization after 24 hrs. Discard if discolored or cloudy.

INHALATION ADMINISTRATION

NOTE: May be given via nasal or oral inhalation.

1. Add 50-100 ml sterile water for injection or inhalation to 6 Gm vial.
2. Transfer to a flask, serving as reservoir for aerosol generator.
3. Further dilute to final volume of 300 ml, giving a solution concentration of 20 mg/ml.
4. Use only aerosol generator available from manufacturer of drug.
5. Do not give concomitantly w/ other drug solutions for nebulization.
6. Discard reservoir solution when fluid levels are low and at least q24h.
7. Controversy over safety in ventilator-dependent pts; only experienced personnel should administer.

INDICATIONS/DOSAGE/ROUTES

Severe lower respiratory tract infection caused by RSV, influenza A or B viruses:
INHALATION: Children, infants: Deliver mist containing 190 mcg/liter at rate of 12.5 liters of mist/min continuously for 12-18 hrs/day for 3-7 days.

PRECAUTIONS

CONTRAINDICATIONS:
CAUTIONS: Use care in assisted ventilation because of mechanical problems associated w/precipitate and "rainout" when fluid accumulates in tubing.

INTERACTIONS

DRUG INTERACTIONS: May have antagonistic effect w/zidovudine. **ALTERED LAB VALUES:** None significant.

SIDE EFFECTS

OCCASIONAL: Rash, conjunctivitis, reticulocytosis. **RARE:** Hypotension, digitalis toxicity.

ADVERSE REACTIONS/TOXIC EFFECTS

Cardiac arrest, apnea and ventilator dependence, bacterial pneumonia, pneumonia, pneumothorax occur rarely. If therapy exceeds 7 days, anemia may occur.

NURSING IMPLICATIONS

BASELINE ASSESSMENT:

Obtain respiratory tract secretions before giving first dose or at least during first 24 hrs of therapy. Assess respiratory status for baseline.

INTERVENTION/EVALUATION:

Monitor I&O, fluid balance carefully. Check hematology reports for anemia due to reticulocytosis when therapy exceeds 7 days. For ventilator-assisted pts watch for "rainout" in tubing and empty frequently; be alert to impaired ventilation and gas exchange due to drug precipitate. Assess skin for rash. Monitor B/P, respirations; assess lung sounds.

PATIENT/FAMILY TEACHING:

Therapy must be continued for full length of treatment. Report immediately any difficulty breathing, chest discomfort or itching/swelling/redness of eyes.

rifabutin

rye-fah-byew'tin
(Mycobutin)

CANADIAN AVAILABILITY:
Mycobutin

CLASSIFICATION

Antimycobacterial

PHARMACOKINETICS

Readily absorbed from GI tract (high-fat meals slow absorption). Widely distributed. Crosses blood-brain barrier. Extensive intracellular tissue uptake. Protein binding: 85%. Metabolized in liver to active metabolite. Excreted in urine; eliminated in feces. Half-life: 16-69 hrs.

ACTION

Antimycobacterial agent. Inhibits DNA-dependent RNA polymerase insusceptible strains of *E. coli* and *Bacillus subtilis*. Not active in mammalian cells.

USES

Prevention of disseminated *Mycobacterium avium* complex (MAC) disease in those w/advanced HIV infection.

PO ADMINISTRATION

1. May take w/o regard to food. Give w/food to decrease GI irritation.
2. May mix w/applesauce if pt is unable to swallow capsules whole.

INDICATIONS/DOSAGE/ROUTES

MAC:
PO: Adults, elderly, adolescents: 300 mg/day as single dose or in two divided doses.

R

PRECAUTIONS

CONTRAINDICATIONS: Hypersensitivity to rifabutin, other rifamycins (e.g., rifampin). Active tuberculosis. **CAUTIONS:** Safety in children not established. **PREGNANCY/LACTATION:** Unknown whether drug crosses placenta or is excreted in breast milk. **Pregnancy Category B.**

INTERACTIONS

DRUG INTERACTIONS: May decrease effects of oral contraceptives. May decrease concentration of zidovudine (does not affect inhibition of HIV by zidovudine). **ALTERED LAB VALUES:** May increase SGOT (AST), SGPT (ALT), alkaline phosphatase. May cause anemia, neutropenia, leukopenia, thrombocytopenia.

SIDE EFFECTS

Generally well tolerated. **FREQUENT:** Skin rash, nausea, vomiting. Reddish-orange discoloration of feces, urine, saliva, sputum, sweat, tears (may also discolor soft contact lenses). **RARE:** Arthralgia (joint pain); uveitis; eye pain, loss of vision (more likely in doses >1050 mg/day).

ADVERSE REACTIONS/TOXIC EFFECTS

Hepatitis, thrombocytopenia occur rarely.

NURSING IMPLICATIONS

BASELINE ASSESSMENT:

Chest x-ray, sputum or blood cultures, biopsy of suspicious node must be done to rule out active tuberculosis (given in active tuberculosis may cause resistance to both rifabutin and rifampin). Obtain baseline CBC, platelets, differential count, hepatic function tests.

INTERVENTION/EVALUATION:

Monitor CBC, platelets, differential count. Avoid IM injections, rectal temperatures, other trauma that may induce bleeding. Check temperature and notify physician of flu-like syndrome, rash, or GI intolerance. If jaundice occurs w/ nausea, vomiting, and fatigue, may indicate hepatitis.

PATIENT/FAMILY TEACHING:

Urine, feces, saliva, sputum, perspiration, tears, skin may be discolored brown-orange. Soft contact lenses may be permanently discolored. Rifabutin may decrease efficacy of oral contraceptives; nonhormonal methods should be considered. Avoid crowds, those w/infections. Notify physician immediately of signs and symptoms of MAC and tuberculosis: night sweats, fatigue, fever, weight loss, abdominal pain. Report any yellowing of skin or eyes.

rifampin

rif-am´pin

(Rifadin, Rimactane)

FIXED-COMBINATION(S):
W/isoniazid, an antitubercular (Rifamate); w/isoniazid and pyrazinamide, antituberculars (Rifater)

CANADIAN AVAILABILITY:
Rifadin, Rimactane, Rofact

CLASSIFICATION

Antitubercular

PHARMACOKINETICS

Well absorbed from GI tract (food delays absorption). Widely distributed. Protein binding: 89%. Metabolized in liver to active metabolite. Primarily eliminated via biliary system. Not removed by hemodialysis. Half-life: 3-5 hrs.

ACTION

Inhibits bacterial RNA synthesis, binds to DNA-dependent RNA polymerase. Blocks RNA transcription.

USES

In conjunction w/at least one other antitubercular agent for initial treatment and retreatment of clinical tuberculosis. Eliminate *Neisseria* meningococci from the nasopharynx of asymptomatic carriers in situations w/high risk of meningococcal meningitis (prophylaxis, not cure). Recommended by WHO as adjunctive therapy w/ dapsone for leprosy.

STORAGE/HANDLING

Store capsules at room temperature. Reconstituted vial stable for 24 hrs. Use diluted solution within 4 hrs.

PO/IV ADMINISTRATION

PO:

1. Preferably give 1 hr before or 2 hrs after meals w/8 oz water (may give w/food to decrease GI upset; will delay absorption).
2. For those unable to swallow capsules, contents may be mixed w/applesauce, jelly.
3. Administer at least 1 hr before antacids, esp, those containing aluminum.

IV:

1. For IV infusion only. Avoid IM, SubQ administration.
2. Avoid extravasation (local irritation, inflammation).
3. Reconstitute 600 mg vial w/10 ml sterile water to provide concentration of 60 mg/ml.
4. Withdraw desired dose and further dilute w/500 ml 5% dextrose; infuse over 3 hrs (may dilute w/100 ml D5W and infuse over 30 min).

INDICATIONS/DOSAGE/ROUTES

Tuberculosis:
IV/PO: Adults, elderly: 600 mg/day. **Children:** 10-20 mg/kg/day. **Maximum:** 600 mg/day.

Meningococcal carrier:
PO: Adults, elderly: 600 mg/day. **Children:** 10-20 mg/kg/day. **Maximum:** 600 mg for 4 consecutive days.

PRECAUTIONS

CONTRAINDICATIONS: Hypersensitivity to rifampin or any rifamycin, intermittent therapy. **CAUTIONS:** Hepatic dysfunction, active/treated alcoholism. Dosage not established in children under 5 yrs of age. **PREGNANCY/LACTATION:** Crosses placenta; is distributed in breast milk. **Pregnancy Category C.**

INTERACTIONS

DRUG INTERACTIONS: Alcohol, hepatotoxic medications may increase risk of hepatotoxicity. May increase clearance of aminophylline, theophylline. May decrease effects of oral anticoagulants, oral hypoglycemics, chloramphenicol, digoxin, disopyramide, mexiletine, quinidine, tocainide, fluconazole, methadone, phenytoin, verapamil. **ALTERED LAB VALUES:** May increase SGOT (AST), SGPT (ALT), alkaline phosphatase, bilirubin, BUN, uric acid.

SIDE EFFECTS

FREQUENT: Heartburn, nausea, vomiting, diarrhea. In high dosage, "flu-like" hypersensitivity syndrome: fever, chills and shivering, headache, muscle/bone pain, dyspnea. **OCCASIONAL:** Irritation, inflammation w/infiltration at IV site. Fatigue, visual disturbances, dizziness, ataxia, confusion, pruritus, urticaria/rash, sore mouth/tongue, muscle/joint/extremity pain, generalized numbness, skin blisters, conjunctivitis, menstrual disturbance. **RARE:** Hematuria.

ADVERSE REACTIONS/TOXIC EFFECTS

Hepatotoxicity (risk increased w/isoniazid combination), hepatitis, blood dyscrasias, Stevens-Johnson syndrome, antibiotic-associated colitis occur rarely.

NURSING IMPLICATIONS

Baseline Assessment:

Question for hypersensitivity to rifampin, rifamycins. Assure collection of diagnostic specimens. Evaluate initial hepatic function and CBC results.

Intervention/Evaluation:

Assess IV site at least hourly during infusion; restart at another site at the first sign of irritation/inflammation. Monitor hepatic function tests and assess for hepatitis: Jaundice, anorexia/nausea/vomiting, fatigue, weakness (hold rifampin and inform physician at once). Report hypersensitivity reactions promptly: Any type skin eruption, pruritus, flu-like syndrome w/high dosage. Monitor frequency, consistency of stools esp. w/potential for antibiotic-associated colitis. Evaluate mental status. Check for visual difficulties. Assess for dizziness, assist w/ambulation as needed. Monitor CBC results for blood dyscrasias and be alert for infection (fever, sore throat), bleeding/bruising or unusual tiredness/weakness.

Patient/Family Teaching:

Do not skip doses, take full length of treatment (may take for mo, yrs). Office visits, vision and lab tests are important part of treatment. Preferably take on empty stomach w/8 oz water 1 hr before or 2 hrs after meal (w/food if GI upset). Avoid alcohol during treatment. Do not take *any* other medications w/o consulting physician, including antacids; must take rifampin at least 1 hr before antacid. Urine, feces, sputum, sweat, tears may become red-orange; soft contact lenses may be permanently stained. Notify physician of *any* new symptom, immediately for yellow eyes/skin, fatigue, weakness, nausea/vomiting, sore throat, fever, "flu," unusual bruising/bleeding. Be certain no vision difficulty, dizziness, or other impairment exists before driving, using machinery. If taking oral contraceptives check w/physician (reliability may be affected).

rimantadine

rye-mah'tah-deen

(Flumadine)

CLASSIFICATION

Antiviral

PHARMACOKINETICS

Readily absorbed from GI tract. Protein binding: 40%. Metabolized in liver. Primarily excreted in urine. Half-life: 20-65 hrs (increased in severe liver and/or renal impairment).

ACTION

Exact mechanism unknown. Appears to exert inhibitory effects early in replication cycle. May inhibit uncoating of virus preventing replication of influenza A virus.

USES

Adults: Prophylaxis and treatment of illness due to influenza A virus. *Children:* Prophylaxis against influenza A virus.

PO ADMINISTRATION:

May take w/o regard to food.

INDICATIONS/DOSAGE/ROUTES

Prophylaxis against influenza virus A:

PO: Adults, elderly, children >10

yrs: 100 mg 2 times/day. **Pts w/ severe hepatic, renal impairment, elderly nursing home patients:** 100 mg/day. **Children <10 yrs:** 5 mg/kg once daily. **Maximum:** 150 mg.

Treatment of influenza virus A:
PO: Adults, elderly: 100 mg 2 times/day for 7 days. **Pts w/severe hepatic, renal impairment, elderly nursing home patients:** 100 mg/day for 7 days.

PRECAUTIONS

CONTRAINDICATIONS: Hypersensitivity to amantadine, rimantadine. **CAUTIONS:** Pts w/renal, liver impairment; history of seizures (increased incidence of seizures). **PREGNANCY/LACTATION:** Avoid use in nursing mothers. Potentially carcinogenic. Unknown whether drug crosses placenta or excreted in breast milk. **Pregnancy Category C.**

INTERACTIONS

DRUG INTERACTIONS: Acetaminophen, aspirin may decrease concentrations. Cimetidine may increase concentrations. **ALTERED LAB VALUES:** None significant.

SIDE EFFECTS

OCCASIONAL: Insomnia, dizziness, headache, nervousness, fatigue, asthenia. Nausea, vomiting, anorexia, dry mouth, abdominal pain. **RARE:** Diarrhea, dyspepsia, agitation, impaired concentration, ringing in ears, dyspnea.

ADVERSE REACTIONS/TOXIC EFFECTS

None significant.

NURSING IMPLICATIONS

INTERVENTION/EVALUATION:

Assess for nervousness and evaluate sleep pattern for insomnia. Provide assistance if dizziness occurs. Check food tolerance. When administering for illness, monitor temperature.

PATIENT/FAMILY TEACHING:

Avoid contact w/those who are at high risk for influenza A (rimantadine-resistant virus may be shed during therapy). Do not drive or perform tasks that require alert response if dizziness or decreased concentration occurs. Do not take aspirin, acetaminophen, or compounds containing these drugs.

---

rimexolone (Vexol)
See supplement

---

risperidone

ris-pear'ih-doan
(Risperdal)

CLASSIFICATION

Antipsychotic

PHARMACOKINETICS

Well absorbed from GI tract (unaffected by food). Extensively metabolized in liver to active metabolite. Protein binding: 90% (metabolite: 77%). Primarily excreted in urine. Half-life: 3-20 hrs; metabolite: 21-30 hrs (increased in elderly).

ACTION

Exact mechanism unknown. Action may be due to dopamine and serotonin receptor antagonism.

USES

Management of manifestations of psychotic disorders.

PO ADMINISTRATION

May take w/o regard to food.

INDICATIONS/DOSAGE/ROUTES

Antipsychotic:

PO: Adults: Initially, 1 mg 2 times/day for 1 day; then, 2 mg 2 times/day for 1 day; then, 3 mg 2 times/day for 1 day. Further adjustments of 1 mg 2 times/day made at at least 1 wk intervals. Maximum effect in range of 4-6 mg/day. **Elderly, debilitated, pts w/severe liver, renal impairment, risk of hypotension:** Initially, 0.5 mg 2 times/day for 1 day; then, 1 mg 2 times/day for 1 day; then, 1.5 mg 2 times/day for 1 day. Further adjustments made at at least 1 wk intervals.

PRECAUTIONS

CONTRAINDICATIONS: Hypersensitivity to risperidone. **CAUTIONS:** Cardiac pts (e.g., history of MI, ischemia, CHF, conduction abnormality); pts w/cerebrovascular disease, dehydration, hypovolemia, use of antihypertensives. History of seizures. Safety in children unknown. May mask signs of drug overdose, intestinal obstruction. **PREGNANCY/LACTATION:** Unknown whether drug crosses placenta or is excreted in breast milk. Recommend against breast feeding. **Pregnancy Category C.**

INTERACTIONS

DRUG INTERACTIONS: May decrease effects of levodopa, dopamine agonists. Carbamazepine may decrease concentration. Clozapine may increase concentration. **ALTERED LAB VALUES:** May increase creatine phosphokinase, uric acid, triglycerides, SGOT (AST), SGPT (ALT), prolactin. May decrease potassium, sodium, protein, glucose. May cause ECG changes.

SIDE EFFECTS

FREQUENT: Extrapyramidal symptoms (EPS), insomnia, agitation, anxiety, stuffy nose. **OCCASIONAL:** Somnolence, constipation, nausea, dyspepsia, vomiting. **RARE:** Abdominal pain.

ADVERSE REACTIONS/TOXIC EFFECTS

Neuroleptic malignant syndrome (NMS): hyperpyrexia, muscle rigidity, change in mental-status, irregular pulse, B/P, tachycardia, diaphoresis, cardiac dysrhythmias, elevated creatine phosphokinase, rhabdomyolysis, acute renal failure. Tardive dyskinesia: irreversible, involuntary, dyskinetic movements. Extension of action: drowsiness, sedation, tachycardia, hypotension, EPS.

NURSING IMPLICATIONS

BASELINE ASSESSMENT:

Renal and liver function tests should be done before therapy. Assess behavior, appearance, emotional status, response to environment, speech pattern, thought content.

INTERVENTION/EVALUATION:

Monitor for fine tongue movement (may be first sign of tardive dyskinesia, which may be irreversible: protrusion of tongue, puffing of cheeks, chewing/puckering of the mouth). Supervise suicidal risk pt closely during early therapy (as depression lessens, energy level improves, increasing suicide potential). Smallest prescription possible reduces risk of overdose. Assess for therapeutic response (greater interest in surroundings, improved self-care, increased ability to concentrate, relaxed facial expression). Monitor for potential NMS: fever, muscle rigidity, irregular B/P or pulse, altered mental status. Possible antiemetic effect may mask signs and symptoms of other conditions.

PATIENT/FAMILY TEACHING:

Change positions slowly to prevent hypotensive effect. Wear protective clothing, use sunscreens to protect from sunlight, ultraviolet light. Do not drive or perform tasks requiring alert response until assured that drug does not cause impairment. Consult physician before taking any other medications. Inform physician if become or plan to become pregnant; do not breast-feed.

ritodrine

rih´toe-dreen
(Yutopar)

CANADIAN AVAILABILITY:
Yutopar

CLASSIFICATION

Uterine relaxant

PHARMACOKINETICS

Well absorbed from GI tract. Undergoes first-pass metabolism. Protein binding: low. Metabolized in liver. Primarily excreted in urine. Removed by hemodialysis. Half-life: *Oral:* 12 hrs; *IV:* 15-17 hrs.

ACTION

Beta$_2$-adrenergic stimulant that inhibits uterine contractions by relaxing uterine muscle.

USES

To prolong gestation by inhibiting uterine contractions in preterm labor.

STORAGE/HANDLING

Stable for 48 hrs at room temperature after dilutions of 150 mg in 500 ml 0.9% NaCl or 5% dextrose in water. Do not use if discolored or precipitate forms.

PO/IV ADMINISTRATION

IV:

1. Hospitalization advised.
2. Place pt in left lateral position to prevent hypotension.
3. Dilute 15 ml of concentrate for injection (150 mg) in 500 ml of 5% dextrose injection (provides solution of 0.3 mg/ml). Because of potential for pulmonary edema, NaCl-containing solutions are used only when dextrose medically undesirable (e.g., diabetes mellitus).
4. Use infusion device to carefully control rate of flow.

PO:

1. Usually begin oral ritodrine about 30 min before termination of IV infusion.

INDICATIONS/DOSAGE/ROUTES

Usual parenteral dosage:
IV INFUSION: Adults: Initially, 0.1 mg/min (20 ml/hr); gradually increase by 0.05 mg/min (10 ml/hr) q10min until desired result reached. Range: 0.15-0.35 mg/min (30-70 ml/hr). Continue for 12 hrs after uterine contractions cease.

Usual oral dosage:
PO: Adults: Initially, 10 mg (about 30 min before termination of IV) then 10 mg q2h for 24 hrs; then 10-20 mg q4-6h. **Maximum:** 120 mg/day. Continue as long as it is desirable to prolong pregnancy.

PRECAUTIONS

CONTRAINDICATIONS: Before 20th week of pregnancy. Preexisting medical conditions for mother that would be adversely affected by the effects of ritodrine: Cardiac arrhythmias, uncontrolled hypertension, bronchial asthma treated w/betamimetics or steroids, hypovolemia. When continuation of pregnancy is hazardous to mother or fetus: Eclampsia, severe preeclampsia, antepartum hemorrhage, intrauterine fetal death, pulmonary hypertension, pheochromocytoma, hyperthyroidism, cardiac disease, chorioamnionitis, uncontrolled diabetes mellitus. W/ injection, sulfite sensitivity (often w/aspirin sensitivity). **CAUTIONS:** Migraine headache, diabetes mellitus, concomitant use of potassium-depleting diuretics. **PREGNANCY/LACTATION:** Drug crosses placenta; unknown whether distributed in breast milk. **Pregnancy Category B.**

INTERACTIONS

DRUG INTERACTIONS: Beta-adrenergic blockers antagonize effects. Glucocorticoids enhance fetal lung maturity; may increase risk of pulmonary edema in mother. **ALTERED LAB VALUES:** May increase SGOT (AST), SGPT (ALT), FFA, blood glucose, serum insulin. May decrease potassium.

SIDE EFFECTS

Effects are associated more w/ IV administration and are dose related. **FREQUENT:** (80-100%): Increased maternal and fetal heart rates widening maternal pulse pressure; palpitations (33%); nausea, vomiting, headache, erythema (10-15%). **OCCASIONAL:** Tremors, jitteriness. **INFREQUENT:** Chest pain/tightness, constipation, diarrhea, bloating, sweating, chills, weakness. *Neonate:* Hypo/hyperglycemia, ileus, hypocalcemia, hypotension. **RARE:** Impaired liver function.

ADVERSE REACTIONS/TOXIC EFFECTS

Ketoacidosis occurs infrequently. Pulmonary edema (may be fatal, esp. w/preexisting cardiopulmonary disease or concomitant use of corticosteroids), anaphylactic shock, hepatitis occur rarely.

NURSING IMPLICATIONS

BASELINE ASSESSMENT:

Question for hypersensitivity to ritodrine, sulfite, or aspirin. Assess baselines for temperature, pulse, respiration, B/P, glucose and potassium levels, EKG, fetal heart rate. Check lungs, determine hydration status. Determine frequency, duration, and strength of contractions.

INTERVENTION/EVALUATION:

IV administration: Take temperature at start and conclusion of IV infusion. B/P, pulse, respirations, and fetal heart rate are monitored every 15 min until stable, then hourly until infusion complete. Check uterine contractions frequently throughout the infusion. Assess lungs for rales; pay particular attention to evidence of impending pulmonary edema (persistent tachycardia, fluid retention [I&O], increased respiratory rate/shortness of breath). Monitor potassium and glucose levels. Evaluate for palpitations, chest pain/tightness, nausea/vomiting, headache, jitteriness.

Patient/Family Teaching:

Keep pt, family informed of therapeutic response during infusion. Explain importance of left lateral position during IV infusion. For discharge on oral ritodrine, teach pt to take own pulse, report increase of rate (over 100/min or as advised by physician) or irregularity. Also notify physician if contractions resume or palpitations, shortness of breath, other symptoms occur. Do not take any other medications w/o physician approval.

rocuronium bromide

(Zemuron)

(See Classifications section under Neuromuscular blockers)

salicylate salts

sal-ih'sah-late

choline salicylate

(Arthropan)

magnesium salicylate

(Magan, Mobidin)

sodium salicylate

(Trilisate combination)

CANADIAN AVAILABILITY: Back-Ese

CLASSIFICATION

Nonsteroidal anti-inflammatory

PHARMACOKINETICS

Rapidly, completely absorbed from GI tract. Protein binding: high. Hydrolyzed in GI tract, liver, blood; further metabolized in liver. Primarily excreted in urine. Removed by hemodialysis. Half-life: dose dependent (*low-dose:* 2-3 hrs; *high dose:* 20 hrs).

ACTION

Produces analgesic and anti-inflammatory effect by inhibiting prostaglandin synthesis, reducing inflammatory response and intensity of pain stimulus reaching sensory nerve endings. Antipyresis produced by drug's effect on hypothalamus, producing vasodilation, decreasing elevated body temperature.

USES

Relieves mild to moderate musculoskeletal, arthritic pain of low to moderate intensity; reduces fever.

PO ADMINISTRATION

1. May give w/food, milk, or antacids if GI distress occurs.
2. Choline salicylate may be mixed w/water, fruit juice, carbonated beverage to mask taste (do not mix w/antacid).

INDICATIONS/DOSAGE/ROUTES

Analgesic, Antipyretic:

Choline salicylate:
PO: Adults, elderly, children >11 yrs: 2.5-5 ml q4h as needed. **Children, 2-11 yrs:** 11.5 ml/m^2/day in 4-6 divided doses.

Magnesium salicylate:
PO: Adults, elderly, children >11 yrs: 300-600 mg q4h as needed. **Children, 2-11 yrs:** 150-450 mg q4h as needed.

S

Sodium salicylate:
PO: Adults, elderly, children >11 yrs: 325-650 mg q4h as needed. **Children, 2-11 yrs:** 25-50 mg/kg/day in 4-6 divided doses.

RHEUMATOID ARTHRITIS, OSTEOARTHRITIS, INFLAMMATORY CONDITIONS:

Choline salicylate:
PO: Adults, elderly: 5-10 ml up to 20-40 ml/day in divided doses. **Children:** 0.6-0.8 ml/kg/day in divided doses.

Magnesium salicylate:
PO: Adults, elderly: 545-1200 mg 3-4 times/day.

Sodium salicylate:
PO: Adults, elderly: 3.6-5.4 Gm/day in divided doses. **Children:** 80-100 mg/kg/day up to 130 mg/kg/day in divided doses.

PRECAUTIONS

CONTRAINDICATIONS: Chickenpox or flu in children/teenagers, GI bleeding/ulceration, bleeding disorders, history of hypersensitivity to aspirin/NSAIDs, impaired hepatic function. **CAUTIONS:** Vitamin K deficiency, chronic renal insufficiency, those w/"aspirin triad" (rhinitis, nasal polyps, asthma). **PREGNANCY/LACTATION:** Readily crosses placenta, is distributed in breast milk. Avoid use during last trimester (may adversely affect fetal cardiovascular system: Premature closure of ductus arteriosus). **Pregnancy Category C.**

INTERACTIONS

DRUG INTERACTIONS: Alcohol, NSAIDs may increase risk of GI effects (e.g., ulceration). Urinary alkalinizer, antacids increase excretion. Anticoagulants, heparin, thrombolytics increase risk of bleeding. Large dose may increase effect of insulin, oral hypoglycemics. Valproic acid, platelet aggregation inhibitors may increase risk of bleeding. May increase toxicity of methotrexate, zidovudine. Ototoxic medications, vancomycin may increase ototoxicity. May decrease effect of probenecid, sulfinpyrazone. **ALTERED LAB VALUES:** May alter SGOT (AST), SGPT (ALT), alkaline phosphatase, uric acid; prolong prothrombin time, bleeding time. May decrease cholesterol, potassium, T_3, T_4.

SIDE EFFECTS

OCCASIONAL: Dyspepsia (cramping, heartburn, abdominal distention, mild nausea).

ADVERSE REACTIONS/TOXIC EFFECTS

High doses may produce GI bleeding and/or gastric mucosal lesions. Low-grade toxicity characterized by ringing in ears, generalized pruritus (may be severe), decreased hearing ability, headache, dizziness, flushing, tachycardia, hyperventilation, sweating, thirst. Febrile, dehydrated children can reach toxic levels quickly. Marked intoxication may be manifested by hyperthermia, restlessness, abnormal breathing pattern, convulsions, respiratory failure, coma.

NURSING IMPLICATIONS

BASELINE ASSESSMENT:

Do not give to children/teenagers who have flu/chickenpox (increases risk of Reye's syndrome). Assess onset, type, location, and duration of pain, fever, or inflammation. Inspect appearance of affected joints for immobility, deformities and skin condition.

INTERVENTION/EVALUATION:

In long-term therapy, monitor plasma salicylic acid concentration. Monitor urinary pH (sudden acidification [pH from 6.5 to 5.5] may result in toxicity). Assess skin for evidence of bruising. If given as an antipyretic, assess temperature directly before and 1 hr after giving medication. Evaluate for therapeutic response: Relief of pain, stiffness, swelling, increase in joint mobility, reduced joint tenderness, improved grip strength.

PATIENT/FAMILY TEACHING:

Take w/food if GI distress is noted. Minimize or avoid other NSAIDs, alcohol during therapy (increases possibility of GI irritation).

salmeterol

sal-met'er-all
(Serevent)

CANADIAN AVAILABILITY:
Serevent

CLASSIFICATION

Bronchodilator

PHARMACOKINETICS

	ONSET	PEAK	DURATION
Inhalation	10-20 min	3 hrs	12 hrs

Primarily acts in lung; low systemic absorption. Protein binding: 94-98%. Metabolized by hydroxylation. Primarily eliminated in feces. Half-life: 5.5 hrs.

ACTION

Stimulates beta$_2$-adrenergic receptors in lung (relaxes bronchial smooth muscle by increasing cAMP). Inhibits release of mast cell mediators (e.g., histamine). Inhibits both early and late phase allergen-induced bronchoconstriction.

USES

Long-term twice daily maintenance treatment of asthma; prevention of bronchospasm; prevention of exercise-induced bronchospasm.

INHALATION ADMINISTRATION

1. Shake container well, then remove cap from mouthpiece.
2. Position mouthpiece to bottom, tilt head back.
3. Breath out through mouth to functional volume.
4. Place mouthpiece in mouth or hold 1-2 inches away from open mouth.
5. Activate inhaler while breathing in slowly and deeply.
6. Hold breath 5-10 sec (or as long as possible).
7. Remove inhaler from mouth and breath out slowly.
8. Wait 1-10 min before second inhalation.

INDICATIONS/DOSAGE/ROUTES

Maintenance of bronchodilation, prevention of asthma symptoms:
INHALATION: Adults, elderly: 2 puffs (42 mcg) 2 times/day, morning and evening about 12 hrs apart.

Prevention of exercise-induced bronchospasm:
INHALATION: Adults, elderly: 2 puffs at least 30-60 min before exercise.

PRECAUTIONS

CONTRAINDICATIONS: History

of hypersensitivity to salmeterol. **CAUTIONS:** Not for acute symptoms. May cause paradoxical bronchospasm. pts w/cardiovascular disorders (e.g., coronary insufficiency, arrhythmias, hypertension), seizure disorder, thyrotoxicosis. Safety in children <12 yrs not known. **PREGNANCY/LACTATION:** Unknown whether excreted in breast milk. **Pregnancy Category C.**

INTERACTIONS

DRUG INTERACTIONS: Tricyclic antidepressants may increase cardiovascular effects. MAO inhibitors may increase risk of hypertensive crisis. May decrease effects of beta-adrenergic blockers. Digoxin, sympathomimetics may increase risk of arrhythmias. **ALTERED LAB VALUES:** May decrease serum potassium levels.

SIDE EFFECTS

FREQUENT: Headache. **OCCASIONAL:** Tremor, cough, dizziness, giddiness.

ADVERSE REACTIONS/TOXIC EFFECTS

Tachycardia, arrhythmias, tremor, headache, muscle cramps. May prolong QT interval (may lead to ventricular arrhythmias). May cause hypokalemia, hyperglycemia.

NURSING IMPLICATIONS

INTERVENTION/EVALUATION:

Monitor rate, depth, rhythm, tape of respiration; quality and rate of pulse, B/P. Assess lungs for wheezing, rales, rhonchi. Periodically evaluate potassium levels.

PATIENT/FAMILY TEACHING:

Not for relief of acute episodes. Keep canister at room temperature (cold decreases effects). Teach pt correct use of aerosol. Do not stop medication or exceed recommended dosage. Notify physician promptly of chest pain, dizziness, or failure to respond to medication. Wait at least one full minute before second inhalation. Administer dose 30 to 60 min before exercise when used to prevent exercise induced bronchospasm. Avoid excessive use of caffeine derivatives: coffee, tea, colas, chocolate.

salsalate

sal´sah-late

(Disalcid, Mono-Gesic)

CLASSIFICATION

Nonsteroidal anti-inflammatory

PHARMACOKINETICS

Rapidly, completely absorbed from GI tract. Protein binding: 90%. Hydrolyzed in GI tract, liver, blood; further metabolized in liver. Primarily excreted in urine. Removed by hemodialysis. Half-life: dose dependent (*low-dose:* 7-8 hrs; *high dose:* 15-30 hrs).

ACTION

Produces analgesic, anti-inflammatory effect by inhibiting prostaglandin synthesis, reducing inflammatory response and intensity of pain stimulus reaching sensory nerve endings.

USES

Symptomatic treatment of acute and/or chronic rheumatoid arthritis and osteoarthritis, related inflammatory conditions.

PO ADMINISTRATION

Give w/food/large amount of water.

INDICATIONS/DOSAGE/ROUTES

Rheumatoid arthritis, osteoarthritis:
PO: Adults, elderly: Initially: 3 Gm/day in 2-3 divided doses. **Maintenance:** 2-4 Gm/day.

PRECAUTIONS

CONTRAINDICATIONS: History of hypersensitivity to salicylates; chickenpox/flu in children/teenagers. **CAUTIONS:** None significant. **PREGNANCY/LACTATION:** Avoid use during last trimester (may adversely affect fetal cardiovascular system: Premature closure of ductus arteriosus). **Pregnancy Category C.**

INTERACTIONS

DRUG INTERACTIONS: Alcohol, NSAIDs may increase risk of GI effects (e.g., ulceration). Urinary alkalinizers, antacids increase excretion. Anticoagulants, heparin, thrombolytics increase risk of bleeding. Large dose may increase effect of insulin, oral hypoglycemics. Valproic acid, platelet aggregation inhibitors may increase risk of bleeding. May increase toxicity of methotrexate, zidovudine. Ototoxic medications, vancomycin may increase ototoxicity. May decrease effect of probenecid, sulfinpyrazone. **ALTERED LAB VALUES:** May alter SGOT (AST), SGPT (ALT), alkaline phosphatase, uric acid; prolong prothrombin time, bleeding time. May decrease cholesterol, potassium, T_3, T_4.

SIDE EFFECTS

OCCASIONAL: Nausea, dyspepsia (heartburn, indigestion, epigastric pain).

ADVERSE REACTIONS/TOXIC EFFECTS

Tinnitus may be first sign that blood salicylic acid concentration is reaching/exceeding upper therapeutic range. May also produce vertigo, headache, confusion, drowsiness, sweating, hyperventilation, vomiting, diarrhea. Severe overdosage may result in electrolyte imbalance, hyperthermia, dehydration, blood pH imbalance. Low incidence of GI bleeding, peptic ulcer.

NURSING IMPLICATIONS

BASELINE ASSESSMENT:

Do not give to children/teenagers who have flu/chickenpox (increases risk of Reye's syndrome). Assess type, location, duration of pain, inflammation. Inspect appearance of affected joints for immobility, deformities, and skin condition.

INTERVENTION/EVALUATION:

Monitor pattern of daily bowel activity, stool consistency. Assess skin for evidence of bruising. Check behind medial malleolus for evidence of fluid retention. Assess for evidence of nausea, dyspepsia. Evaluate for therapeutic response: Relief of pain, stiffness, swelling, increase in joint mobility, reduced joint tenderness, improved grip strength.

PATIENT/FAMILY TEACHING:

Do not crush/chew capsules or film-coated tablets. Report ringing/roaring in ears. Avoid antacids (decreases drug effectiveness).

sargramostim

sar-gra-moh′stim
(Leukine, Prokine)

CLASSIFICATION

Colony stimulating factor

PHARMACOKINETICS

Half-life: *IV:* 2 hrs, *SubQ:* 3 hrs.

ACTION

Stimulates proliferation/differentiation of hematopoietic progenitor cells in the granulocyte-macrophage pathways. May also activate mature granulocytes/macrophages. Chemotactic, antifungal, and antiparasite activities increase. Increases cytotoxicity of monocytes to certain neoplastic cell lines; activates polymorphonuclear neutrophils to inhibit tumor cell growth.

USES

Accelerates myeloid recovery in pt w/non-Hodgkin's lymphoma, acute lymphoblastic leukemia, and Hodgkin's disease undergoing autologous bone marrow transplantation. In pts w/allogenic or autologous bone marrow transplantation where engraftment is delayed or has failed.

STORAGE/HANDLING

Refrigerate powder, reconstituted solution, diluted solution for injection. Do not shake. Do not use past expiration date. Reconstituted solutions are clear, colorless. Use within 6 hrs; discard unused portions. Use 1 dose/vial; do not reenter vial.

IV ADMINISTRATION

1. To 250 mg/500 mg vial, add 1 ml sterile water for injection (preservative-free).

2. Direct sterile water to side of vial, gently swirl contents to avoid foaming; do not shake/vigorously agitate.

3. After reconstitution, further dilute w/0.9% NaCl. If final concentration <10 mcg/ml, add 1 mg albumin/ml 0.9% NaCl to provide a final albumin concentration of 0.1%. **Note:** Albumin is added before addition of sargramostim (prevents drug adsorption to components of drug delivery system).

4. Administer within 6 hrs of preparation/dilution.

5. Monitor for supraventricular arrhythmias during administration (particularly in those w/history of cardiac arrhythmias).

6. Assess closely for dyspnea during and immediately following infusion (particularly in those w/history of lung disease). If dyspnea occurs during infusion, cut infusion rate by half. If dyspnea continues, stop infusion immediately.

7. If neutrophil count exceeds 20,000 cells/mm^3 or platelet count exceeds 500,000/mm^3, stop infusion or reduce dose by half, based on clinical condition of pt.

INDICATIONS/DOSAGE/ROUTES

NOTE: Administer by IV infusion.

Usual parenteral dosage:
IV INFUSION: Adults, elderly: 250 mcg/m^2/day for 21 days (as a 2 hr infusion). Begin 2-4 hrs after autologous bone marrow infusion and not less than 24 hrs after last dose of chemotherapy or not less than 12 hrs after last radiation treatment. Discontinue if blast cells appear or underlying disease progresses.

Bone marrow transplantation failure/engraftment delay:
IV INFUSION: Adults, elderly: 250 mcg/m^2/day for 14 days. Infuse over 2 hrs. May repeat after 7 days off therapy if engraftment not occurred w/500 mcg/m^2/day for 14 days.

PRECAUTIONS

CONTRAINDICATIONS: Excessive leukemic myeloid blasts in bone marrow/peripheral blood (greater/equal to 10%), known hypersensitivity to GM-CSF, yeast-derived products, any component of drug, 24 hrs before/after chemotherapy, 12 hrs before/after radiation therapy. **CAUTIONS:** Preexisting cardiac disease, hypoxia, preexisting fluid retention, pulmonary infiltrates, CHF, impaired renal/hepatic function. **PREGNANCY/LACTATION:** Unknown whether drug crosses placenta or is distributed in breast milk. **Pregnancy Category C.**

INTERACTIONS

DRUG INTERACTIONS: Lithium, steroids may increase effect. **ALTERED LAB VALUES:** May decrease albumin. May increase bilirubin, creatinine, liver enzymes.

SIDE EFFECTS

Generally well tolerated. **OCCASIONAL:** Diarrhea, fatigue, weakness, redness, irritation at local injection site, peripheral edema, rash.

ADVERSE REACTIONS/TOXIC EFFECTS

Pleural/pericardial effusion occurs rarely following infusion.

NURSING IMPLICATIONS

BASELINE ASSESSMENT:

Assess renal, hepatic function tests before initial therapy and biweekly. Note that excessive blood counts return to normal or baseline 3-7 days after discontinuation of therapy. Obtain baseline weight.

INTERVENTION/EVALUATION:

Monitor urinalysis reports, alkaline phosphatase, serum creatinine, bilirubin, SGOT (AST), SGPT (ALT) levels, CBC w/differential diligently. Monitor body weight. Assess for peripheral edema, particularly behind medial malleolus (usually first area showing peripheral edema), skin turgor, mucous membranes for hydration status. Note skin temperature, moisture. Assess muscle strength. Monitor daily bowel activity, stool consistency (watery, loose, soft, semisolid, solid). Assess injection site for redness, irritation.

scopolamine

sco-pawl´ah-meen
(Scopolamine, Transderm Scop)

scopolamine bromide

(Isopto Hyoscine)

CANADIAN AVAILABILITY:
Busecopan, Transderm-V

CLASSIFICATION

Anticholinergic

PHARMACOKINETICS

Rapidly absorbed after IM administration. Protein binding: low. Metabolized in liver. Primarily excreted in urine. Half-life: 8 hrs. *Mydriasis:* Peak 20-30 min; recovery 3-7 days. *Cycloplegia:* Peak 30-60 min; recovery 3-7 days. After IM administration, inhibition of salivation occurs within 30 min, peaks in 1-2 hrs, persists for up to 4-6 hrs.

ACTION

Inhibits action of acetylcholine on structures innervated by postganglionic sites: smooth, cardiac muscle, SA, AV nodes, exocrine glands. Larger doses may decrease motility, secretory activity of GI system, tone of ureter, urinary bladder. Blocks responses of sphincter muscle and accommodation muscle in ciliary body producing mydriasis, cycloplegia. *Antiemetic:* reduces excitability of labyrinthine receptors, depressing conduction in vestibular cerebellar pathway.

USES

Prevention of nausea/vomiting induced by motion. Used preoperatively to inhibit salivation, excessive secretion of respiratory tract. Prevents cholinergic effect during surgery (cardiac arrhythmias, hypotension, bradycardia). Used preoperatively in obstetrics w/analgesics or sedatives to produce tranquilization, amnesia.

OPHTHALMIC/TRANSDERMAL/SubQ/IM/IV ADMINISTRATION

OPHTHALMIC:

1. Do not use ophthalmic solutions for injection.
2. Place finger on lower eyelid and pull out until pocket is formed between eye and lower lid.
3. Hold dropper above pocket and place prescribed number of drops into pocket. Close eye gently.
4. Apply digital pressure to lacrimal sac for 1-2 min (minimizes drainage into nose and throat, reducing risk of systemic effects).
5. Remove excess solution around eye w/tissue.

TRANSDERMAL:

1. Apply patch at least 4 hrs before anticipated motion.
2. Apply firmly to clean dry area behind ear. Avoid touching exposed adhesive layer of patch. Thoroughly wash hands w/soap and water after application.
3. Only one system to be worn at any one time.
4. Rotate sites of application.

IM:

1. May be given SubQ or IM.

IV:

1. Dilute w/sterile water before administration.
2. Give by direct IV injection.

INDICATIONS/DOSAGE/ROUTES

Usual parenteral dosage:
IM/IV/SubQ: Adults, elderly: 0.3-0.65 mg. **Children:** 0.006 mg/kg. **Maximum:** 0.3 mg.

Usual topical dosage:
TRANSDERMAL: Adults, elderly: One system (0.5 mg) q72hrs.

Refraction:
OPHTHALMIC: Adults, elderly: 1-2 drops 1 hr before refraction.

Inflammation:
OPHTHALMIC: Adults, elderly: 1-2 drops up to 4 times/day.

PRECAUTIONS

CONTRAINDICATIONS: Children (transdermal system), narrow-angle glaucoma, severe ulcerative colitis, toxic megacolon, paralytic ileus, obstructive disease of GI tract, paralytic ileus, intestinal atony, myasthenia gravis in those not treated w/neostigmine, tachycardia secondary to cardiac insufficiency/thyrotoxicosis, cardiospasm, unstable cardiovascular status in acute hemorrhage, bladder neck obstruction, pyloric obstruction. **EXTREME CAUTION:** Autonomic neuropathy, known/suspected GI infections, diarrhea, mild to moderate ulcerative colitis, metabolic, hepatic, renal dysfunction; elderly (scopolamine-induced mental confusion). **CAUTIONS:** Glaucoma w/transdermal system; hyperthyroidism, hypertension, tachyarrhythmias, CHF, coronary artery disease, gastric ulcer, esophageal reflux/hiatal hernia associated w/reflux esophagitis, infants, children (particularly susceptible to systemic administration), those w/COPD. **PREGNANCY/LACTATION:** Crosses placenta; unknown whether distributed in breast milk. If given before onset of labor, may produce CNS depression in neonate, contribute to neonatal hemorrhage (decreased vitamin K-dependent clotting factors in neonate). **Pregnancy Category C.**

INTERACTIONS

DRUG INTERACTIONS: Antacids, antidiarrheals may decrease absorption. Anticholinergics may increase effects. May decrease absorption of ketoconazole. May increase severity of GI lesions with KCl (wax matrix). CNS depressants may increase sedative effect. Antiglaucoma medications (e.g., carbachol, pilocarpine) action may be antagonized. **ALTERED LAB VALUES:** None significant.

SIDE EFFECTS

FREQUENT: Dry mouth (sometimes severe), decreased sweating, constipation, pupillary dilation, temporary paralysis of accommodation. **OCCASIONAL:** Blurred vision, bloated feeling, urinary hesitancy, drowsiness (w/high dosage), headache, intolerance to light, loss of taste, nervousness, flushing, insomnia, impotence, mental confusion/excitement (particularly in elderly, children). Parenteral form may produce temporary lightheadedness, local irritation. **RARE:** Dizziness, faintness.

ADVERSE REACTIONS/TOXIC EFFECTS

May produce excessive susceptibility to scopolamine: Complete disorientation to active delirium. Marked somnolence may be noted. Overdosage may produce temporary paralysis of ciliary muscle, pupillary dilation, tachycardia, palpitation; hot/dry/flushed skin; absence of bowel sounds, hyperthermia, increased respiratory rate, EKG abnormalities, nausea, vomiting, rash over face/upper trunk; CNS stimulation, psychosis (agitation, restlessness, rambling speech, visual hallucination, paranoid behavior, delusions) followed by depression.

NURSING IMPLICATIONS

BASELINE ASSESSMENT:

Before giving medication, instruct pt to void (reduces risk of urinary retention).

INTERVENTION EVALUATION:

Monitor stool consistency, frequency. Palpate bladder for urinary retention. Monitor changes in B/P, temperature. Assess skin turgor, mucous membranes to evaluate hydration status (encourage adequate fluid intake), bowel sounds for peristalsis. Be alert for fever (increased risk of hyperthermia).

Patient/Family Teaching:

Use care not to become overheated during exercise or hot weather (may result in heat stroke). Avoid hot baths, saunas. Avoid tasks that require alertness, motor skills until response to drug is established. Sugarless gum, sips of tepid water may relieve dry mouth. Do not take antacids/medicine for diarrhea within 1 hr of taking this medication (decreases effectiveness). Wash hands well w/soap, water after transdermal system use (contamination of fingers, eyes may result in blurred vision). Protect eyes from light by wearing sunglasses. Avoid alcohol and CNS depressants.

secobarbital sodium

seek-oh-bar′bih-tall
(Seconal)

FIXED-COMBINATION(S):
W/amobarbital, a barbiturate (Tuinal)

CANADIAN AVAILABILITY:
Novosecobarb, Seconal

CLASSIFICATION

Sedative-hypnotic **(Schedule II)**

PHARMACOKINETICS

	ONSET	PEAK	DURATION
PO	15 min	—	1-4 hrs
IM	7-10 min	—	—
IV	1-3 min	—	15 min
Rectal	15-30 min	—	1-4 hrs

Variably absorbed after oral, parenteral administration. Rapidly, widely distributed. Protein binding: 46-70%. Metabolized in liver. Primarily excreted in urine. Half-life: 15-40 hrs.

ACTION

CNS depressant, producing all levels from mild sedation, hypnosis to deep coma.

USES

Short-term treatment of insomnia (up to 2 wks), preop sedation, routine sedation. Parenteral form used to control status epilepticus/acute seizure episodes, to facilitate intubation procedures, control of agitated behavior in psychosis, provide hypnosis for general, spinal, regional anesthesia. Used rectally to produce anesthesia in children.

STORAGE/HANDLING

Store oral form at room temperature. Refrigerate parenteral form, suppositories. Discard parenteral solution if precipitate forms or solution becomes cloudy.

PO/IM/IV/RECTAL ADMINISTRATION

PO:

1. Best absorbed if given on empty stomach, but may be given w/food.
2. Capsules may be emptied and mixed w/food.

PARENTERAL FORM:

1. Do not mix w/acidic solutions (produces precipitate).

IM:

1. May be diluted w/sterile water for injection, 0.9% NaCl, Ringer's injection. Do NOT use lactated Ringer's injection.
2. Do not inject more than 5 ml in any one IM injection site (produces tissue irritation).

3. Inject IM deep into gluteus maximus or lateral aspect of thigh.

IV:

1. Administer IV at rate not greater than 50 mg/15 seconds (1 ml of 5% concentration).
2. A too-rapid IV may produce marked respiratory depression, severe hypotension, apnea, laryngospasm, bronchospasm.
3. Monitor vital signs q3-5min during and q15min for 1-2 hrs after administration.
4. Inadvertent intra-arterial injection may result in arterial spasm w/severe pain, tissue necrosis. Extravasation in SubQ tissue may produce redness, tenderness, tissue necrosis. If either occurs, treat w/ injection of 0.5% procaine solution into affected area, apply moist heat.

RECTAL:

1. Moisten suppository w/cold water before inserting well up into rectum.

INDICATIONS/DOSAGE ROUTES

NOTE: Reduce dosage in elderly, debilitated, impaired liver function.

Hypnotic:
PO/IM: Adults, elderly: 100-200 mg.
IM: Children: 3-5 mg/kg. **Maximum:** 100 mg.

Preop sedation:
PO: Adults, elderly: 100-300 mg given 1-2 hrs before surgery. **Children:** 50-100 mg.
IM: Children: 4-5 mg/kg.
RECTAL: Children over 3 yrs: 60-120 mg. **Children 6 mo-3 yrs:** 60 mg. **Children <6 mo:** 30-60 mg.

Status epilepticus:
IM/IV: Adults, elderly: 250-350 mg. If no response in 5 min, additional dose may be administered. Do not exceed total IV dosage of 500 mg.

Acute seizures:
IM/IV: Adults, elderly: 5.5 mg/kg. May repeat q3-4h as needed.

PRECAUTIONS

CONTRAINDICATIONS: History of porphyria, bronchopneumonia. **CAUTIONS:** Uncontrolled pain (may produce paradoxical reaction), impaired liver function. **PREGNANCY/LACTATION:** Readily crosses placenta; is distributed in breast milk. Produces respiratory depression in neonates during labor. May cause postpartum hemorrhage, hemorrhagic disease in newborn. Withdrawal symptoms may occur in neonates born to women who receive barbiturates during last trimester of pregnancy. **Pregnancy Category D.**

INTERACTIONS

DRUG INTERACTIONS: May decrease effects of glucocorticoids, digoxin, metronidazole, oral anticoagulants, quinidine, tricyclic antidepressants. Alcohol, CNS depressants may increase effect. May increase metabolism of carbamazepine. Valproic acid may decrease metabolism, increase concentration, toxicity. **ALTERED LAB VALUES:** May decrease bilirubin.

SIDE EFFECTS

FREQUENT: Drowsiness, sedation, residual "hangover" effect, lethargy, irritability, nausea, anorexia, muscle aches and pains, gastric distress. **OCCASIONAL:** Paradoxical CNS hyperactivity/ nervousness in children, excitement/restlessness in elderly (generally noted during first 2 wks of therapy, particularly noted in presence of uncontrolled pain).

ADVERSE REACTIONS/TOXIC EFFECTS

Abrupt withdrawal after prolonged therapy may produce effects ranging from markedly increased dreaming, nightmares and/or insomnia, tremor, sweating, vomiting, to hallucinations, delirium, seizures, status epilepticus. Skin eruptions appear as hypersensitivity reaction. Blood dyscrasias, liver disease, hypocalcemia occur rarely. Overdosage produces cold, clammy skin, hypothermia, severe CNS depression, cyanosis, rapid pulse, Cheyne-Stokes respirations. Toxicity may result in severe renal impairment.

NURSING IMPLICATIONS

BASELINE ASSESSMENT:

Assess B/P, pulse, respirations immediately before administration. *Hypnotic:* Raise bed rails, provide environment conducive to sleep (back rub, quiet environment, low lighting). *Seizures:* Review history of seizure disorder (length, intensity, frequency, duration, level of consciousness). Observe frequently for recurrence of seizure activity. Initiate seizure precautions.

INTERVENTION/EVALUATION:

Assess sleep pattern of pt. Assess elderly/debilitated for paradoxical reaction, particularly during early therapy. Evaluate for therapeutic response. *Insomnia:* A decrease in number of nocturnal awakenings, increase in length of sleep duration time. *Seizures:* A decrease in number, frequency of seizures.

PATIENT/FAMILY TEACHING:

Drowsiness usually diminishes w/continued therapy. Do not abruptly withdraw medication following long-term therapy (may precipitate seizures). Avoid tasks that require alertness, motor skills until response to drug is established. Tolerance/dependence may occur w/prolonged use of high doses. Strict maintenance of drug therapy is essential for seizure control. Avoid alcohol.

selegiline hydrochloride

sell-eh´geh-leen

(Eldepryl)

CANADIAN AVAILABILITY:

Deprenyl, Eldepryl

CLASSIFICATION

Antiparkinson

PHARMACOKINETICS

Rapidly absorbed from GI tract. Crosses blood-brain barrier. Metabolized in liver to active metabolites. Primarily excreted in urine. Half-life: 16-69 hrs.

ACTION

Irreversibly inhibits monoamine oxidase type B activity. Increases dopaminergic action, assisting in reduction in tremor, akinesia (absence of sense of movement), posture and equilibrium disorders, rigidity of parkinsonism.

USES

Adjunctive to levodopa/carbidopa in treatment of Parkinson's disease.

PO ADMINISTRATION

May be given w/meals.

INDICATIONS/DOSAGE/ROUTES

NOTE: Therapy should begin w/ lowest dosage, then be increased in gradual increments over 3-4 weeks.

Parkinsonism:
PO: Adults: 10 mg/day in divided doses (5 mg at breakfast and lunch). **Elderly:** Initially, 5 mg in morning. May increase up to 10 mg/day.

PRECAUTIONS

CONTRAINDICATIONS: None significant. **CAUTIONS:** Cardiac dysrhythmias. **PREGNANCY/LACTATION:** Unknown whether drug crosses placenta or is distributed in breast milk. **Pregnancy Category C.**

INTERACTIONS

DRUG INTERACTIONS: Fluoxetine may cause mania, serotonin syndrome (mental changes, restlessness, diaphoresis, diarrhea, fever). Meperidine may cause a potentially fatal reaction (e.g., excitation, sweating, rigidity, hypertension or hypotension, coma and death). Tyramine rich foods may produce hypertensive reactions. **ALTERED LAB VALUES:** None significant.

SIDE EFFECTS

FREQUENT: Nausea, dizziness, lightheadedness, faintness, abdominal discomfort. **OCCASIONAL:** Confusion, hallucinations, dry mouth, vivid dreams, dyskinesia (impairment of voluntary movement). **RARE:** Headache, generalized aches.

ADVERSE REACTIONS/TOXIC EFFECTS

Overdosage may vary from CNS depression (sedation, apnea, cardiovascular collapse, death) to severe paradoxical reaction (hallucinations, tremor, seizures). Impaired motor coordination (loss of balance, blepharospasm [eye blinking], facial grimace, feeling of heavy leg/stiff neck, involuntary movements), hallucinations, confusion, depression, nightmares, delusions, overstimulation, sleep disturbance, anger occurs in some pts.

NURSING IMPLICATIONS

INTERVENTION/EVALUATION:

Be alert to neurologic effects (headache, lethargy, mental confusion, agitation). Monitor for evidence of dyskinesia (difficulty w/movement). Assess for clinical reversal of symptoms (improvement of tremor of head/hands at rest, mask-like facial expression, shuffling gait, muscular rigidity.

PATIENT/FAMILY TEACHING:

Tolerance to feeling of lightheadedness develops during therapy. To reduce hypotensive effect, rise slowly from lying to sitting position and permit legs to dangle momentarily before standing. Avoid tasks that require alertness, motor skills until response to drug is established. Dry mouth, drowsiness, dizziness may be an expected response of drug. Avoid alcoholic beverages during therapy. Coffee/tea may help reduce drowsiness. Inform other physicians, dentist of Eldepryl therapy.

senna

sen′ah

(Senokot, Senolax)

FIXED-COMBINATION(S): W/docusate, a stool softener (Gentlax-S, Senokap DSS, Senokot-S)

CANADIAN AVAILABILITY: Senokot

CLASSIFICATION

Laxative: Stimulant

PHARMACOKINETICS

	ONSET	PEAK	DURATION
PO	6-12 hrs	—	—
Rectal	0.5-2 hrs	—	—

Minimal absorption after oral administration. Hydrolyzed to active form by enzymes of colonic flora. Absorbed drug metabolized in liver; eliminated in feces via biliary system.

ACTION

Increases peristalsis by direct effect on intestinal smooth musculature (stimulates intramural nerve plexi). Promotes fluid and ion accumulation in colon to increase laxative effect.

USES

Facilitates defecation in those w/ diminished colonic motor response, for evacuation of colon for rectal, bowel examination, elective colon surgery.

PO/RECTAL ADMINISTRATION

PO:

1. Give on an empty stomach (faster results).
2. Offer at least 6-8 glasses of water/day (aids stool softening).
3. Avoid giving within 1 hr of other oral medication (decreases drug absorption).

RECTAL:

1. If suppository is too soft, chill for 30 min in refrigerator or run cold water over foil wrapper.
2. Moisten suppository w/cold water before inserting well up into rectum.

INDICATIONS/DOSAGE/ROUTES

Laxative:

PO: Adults, elderly: 2 tablets (or 1 tsp granules) at bedtime. **Maximum:** 4 tablets (2 tsp) 2 times/day. **Children:** 1 tablet (1/2 tsp granules) at bedtime.

PO: Adults, elderly: (Syrup): 10-15 ml at bedtime. **Children 5-15 yrs:** 5-10 ml at bedtime. **Children 1-5 yrs:** 2.5-5 ml at bedtime. **Children 1 mo-1 yr:** 1.25-2.5 ml at bedtime.

RECTAL: Adults, elderly: 1 suppository at bedtime, may repeat in 2 hrs. **Children:** 1/2 suppository at bedtime.

PRECAUTIONS

CONTRAINDICATIONS: Abdominal pain, nausea, vomiting, appendicitis, intestinal obstruction. **CAUTIONS:** None significant. **PREGNANCY/LACTATION:** Unknown whether distributed in breast milk. **Pregnancy Category C.**

INTERACTIONS

DRUG INTERACTIONS: May decrease transit time of concurrently administered oral medication, decreasing absorption. **ALTERED LAB VALUES:** None significant.

SIDE EFFECTS

FREQUENT: Pink-red, red-violet,

red-brown, or yellow-brown discoloration of urine. **OCCASIONAL:** Some degree of abdominal discomfort, nausea, mild cramps, griping, faintness.

ADVERSE REACTIONS/TOXIC EFFECTS

Long-term use may result in laxative dependence, chronic constipation, loss of normal bowel function. Chronic use/overdosage may result in electrolyte disturbances (hypokalemia, hypocalcemia, metabolic acidosis/alkalosis), persistent diarrhea, malabsorption, weight loss. Electrolyte disturbance may produce vomiting, muscle weakness.

NURSING IMPLICATIONS

INTERVENTION/EVALUATION:

Encourage adequate fluid intake. Assess bowel sounds for peristalsis. Monitor stool frequency, consistency (watery, loose, soft, semi-solid, solid). Assess for abdominal disturbances. Monitor serum electrolytes in those exposed to prolonged, frequent, or excessive use of medication.

PATIENT/FAMILY TEACHING:

Urine may turn pink-red, red-violet, red-brown, or yellow-brown (is only temporary and is not harmful). Institute measures to promote defecation (increase fluid intake, exercise, high-fiber diet). Laxative effect generally occurs in 6-12 hrs, but may take 24 hrs. Suppository produces evacuation in 30 min to 2 hrs. Do not take other oral medication within 1 hr of taking this medicine (decreased effectiveness).

sertraline hydrochloride

sir´trah-leen
(Zoloft)

CLASSIFICATION

Antidepressant

PHARMACOKINETICS

Incompletely, slowly absorbed from GI tract (food increases absorption). Widely distributed. Protein binding: 87%. Undergoes extensive first-pass metabolism in liver to active compound. Excreted in urine, eliminated in feces. Half-life: 26 hrs.

ACTION

Blocks reuptake of neurotransmitter, serotonin at CNS neuronal presynaptic membranes, increasing availability at postsynaptic receptor sites.

S

USES

Treatment of major depressive disorders.

PO ADMINISTRATION

Give w/food or milk if GI distress occurs.

INDICATIONS/DOSAGE/ROUTES

Antidepressant:
PO: Adults: Initially, 50 mg/day w/morning or evening meal. May increase at intervals no sooner than 1 wk. **Elderly:** Initially, 25 mg/day. May increase by 25 mg q2-3days. **Maximum:** 200 mg/day.

PRECAUTIONS

CONTRAINDICATIONS: During or within 14 days of MAO inhibitor antidepressant therapy. **CAUTIONS:** Severe hepatic/renal impairment. **PREGNANCY/LACTATION:** Unknown whether drug crosses placenta or is distributed in breast milk. **Pregnancy Category B.**

INTERACTIONS

DRUG INTERACTIONS: May increase concentration, toxicity of highly protein bound medications (e.g., digoxin, warfarin). MAO inhibitors may cause serotonin syndrome (mental changes, restlessness, diaphoresis, shivering, diarrhea, fever), confusion, agitation, hyperpyretic convulsions. **ALTERED LAB VALUES:** May increase SGOT (AST), SGPT (ALT), total cholesterol, triglycerides. May decrease uric acid.

SIDE EFFECTS

FREQUENT: Nausea, headache, diarrhea, insomnia, dry mouth, sexual dysfunction (male), dizziness, tremor, fatigue. **OCCASIONAL:** Increased sweating, constipation, dyspepsia, agitation, flatulence, anorexia, nervousness, rhinitis, abnormal vision. **RARE:** Palpitations, paresthesia, rash, vomiting, frequent urination, twitching.

ADVERSE REACTIONS/TOXIC EFFECTS

None significant.

NURSING IMPLICATIONS

BASELINE ASSESSMENT:

For those on long-term therapy, liver/renal function tests, blood counts should be performed periodically.

INTERVENTION/EVALUATION:

Supervise suicidal-risk pt closely during early therapy (as depression lessens, energy level improves, increasing suicide potential. Assess appearance, behavior, speech pattern, level of interest, mood. Monitor pattern of daily bowel activity, stool consistency. Assist w/ambulation if dizziness occurs.

PATIENT/FAMILY TEACHING:

Dry mouth may be relieved by sugarless gum or sips of tepid water. Report headache, fatigue, tremor, sexual dysfunction. Avoid tasks that require alertness, motor skills until response to drug is established. Take w/food if nausea occurs. Inform physician if become pregnant. Avoid alcohol. Do not take over-the-counter medications w/o consulting physician.

silver sulfadiazine

sul-fah-dye´ah-zeen

(Silvadene, Flint SSD)

CANADIAN AVAILABILITY:
Flamazine

CLASSIFICATION

Burn preparation

PHARMACOKINETICS

Variably absorbed. Significant systemic absorption may occur if applied to extensive burns. Absorbed medication excreted unchanged in urine. Half-life: 10 hrs (increased in decreased renal function).

ACTION

Acts upon cell wall and cell membrane to produce bactericidal effect. Silver is released slowly in concentrations selectively toxic to bacteria.

USES

Prevention, treatment of infection in second and third degree burns, protection against conversion from partial to full thickness wounds (infection causes extended tissue destruction).

TOPICAL ADMINISTRATION

1. Apply to cleansed, debrided burns using sterile glove.
2. Keep burn areas covered w/ silver sulfadiazine cream at all times; reapply to areas where removed by pt activity.
3. Dressings may be ordered on individual basis.

INDICATIONS/DOSAGE/ROUTES

Usual topical dosage:
TOPICAL: Adults, elderly: Apply 1-2 times/day.

PRECAUTIONS

CONTRAINDICATIONS: Hypersensitivity to silver sulfadiazine, components of preparation. **CAUTIONS:** Impaired renal/hepatic function, G-6-PD deficiency, premature neonates, infants <2 mos. Cross-sensitivity w/other sulfonamides unknown. **PREGNANCY/LACTATION:** Not recommended during pregnancy unless burn area is greater than 20% of body surface. Unknown whether distributed in breast milk. Risk of kernicterus in neonates. **Pregnancy Category C.**

INTERACTIONS

DRUG INTERACTIONS: Collagenase, papain, sutilains may be inactivated. **ALTERED LAB VALUES:** None significant.

SIDE EFFECTS

OCCASIONAL: Pain, burning, itching, localized rash. Side effects characteristic of all sulfonamides may occur when systemically absorbed, e.g., extensive burn areas (over 20% of body surface): Anorexia, nausea, vomiting, headache, diarrhea, dizziness, photosensitivity, joint pain.

ADVERSE REACTIONS/TOXIC EFFECTS

Less often but serious are hemolytic anemia, hypoglycemia, diuresis, peripheral neuropathy, Stevens-Johnson syndrome, agranulocytosis, disseminated lupus erythematosus, anaphylaxis, hepatitis, toxic nephrosis. Fungal superinfections may occur. Interstitial nephritis occurs rarely.

NURSING IMPLICATIONS

BASELINE ASSESSMENT:

Question for hypersensitivity to silver sulfadiazine/components, other sulfonamides. Determine initial CBC, renal/hepatic function test results.

INTERVENTION/EVALUATION:

Evaluate fluid balance, renal function: Check I&O, renal function tests and report changes promptly. Monitor vital signs. Check serum sulfonamide concentrations carefully. Assess burns, surrounding areas for pain, burning, itching, rash (antihistamines may provide relief, silver sulfadiazine therapy continued unless reactions severe). Check CBC results.

PATIENT/FAMILY TEACHING:

Therapy must be continued until

healing is satisfactory or the site is ready for grafting.

simethicone

sye-meth´ih-cone

(Mylicon, Phazyme, Silain)

FIXED-COMBINATION(S): W/aluminum and magnesium hydroxide, antacids (Digel, Gelusil, Maalox Plus, Mylanta); w/magaldrate, an antacid (Riopan)

CANADIAN AVAILABILITY: Ovol, Phazyme

CLASSIFICATION

Antiflatulent

KINETICS

Does not appear to be absorbed from GI tract. Excreted unchanged in feces.

ACTION

Disperses, prevents formation of gas pockets in GI tract. Changes surface tension of gas bubbles (allowing easier elimination of gas).

USES

Treatment of flatulence, gastric bloating, postop gas pain or when gas retention may be problem (i.e., peptic ulcer, spastic colon, air swallowing).

PO ADMINISTRATION

1. Give after meals and at bedtime as needed. Chewable tablets are to be chewed thoroughly before swallowing. Enteric coated tablets are swallowed whole; do not crush.
2. Shake suspension well before using.

INDICATIONS/DOSAGE/ROUTES

Antiflatulent:

PO: Adults, elderly: (capsules): 125 mg 4 times/day; (tablets): 50-125 mg 4 times/day; (suspension): 40 mg (0.6 ml) 4 times/day; (chewable tablets): 40-80 mg 4 times/day.

PRECAUTIONS

CONTRAINDICATIONS: None significant. **CAUTIONS:** None significant. **PREGNANCY/LACTATION:** Unknown whether drug crosses placenta or is distributed in breast milk. **Pregnancy Category C.**

INTERACTIONS

DRUG INTERACTIONS: None significant. **ALTERED LAB VALUES:** None significant.

SIDE EFFECTS

None significant.

ADVERSE REACTIONS/TOXIC EFFECTS

None significant.

NURSING IMPLICATIONS

INTERVENTION/EVALUATION:

Evaluate for therapeutic response: Relief of flatulence, abdominal bloating.

simvastatin

sim´vah-sta-tin

(Zocor)

CANADIAN AVAILABILITY: Zocor

CLASSIFICATION

Antihyperlipoproteinemic

PHARMACOKINETICS

Well absorbed from GI tract. Undergoes extensive first-pass metabolism. Hydrolyzed to active metabolite. Protein binding: 95%. Primarily eliminated in feces.

ACTION

Inhibits HMG-CoA preventing conversion of HMG-CoA to mevalonate (early step in cholesterol synthesis). Decreases LDL, cholesterol, VLDL, plasma triglycerides, slight increase in HDL concentration.

USES

Adjunct to diet therapy to decrease elevated total and LDL cholesterol concentrations in those w/ primary hypercholesterolemia (types IIa and IIb).

PO ADMINISTRATION

1. Give w/o regard to meals.
2. Administer in evening.

INDICATIONS/DOSAGE/ROUTES

NOTE: Before initiating therapy, pt should be on standard cholesterol lowering diet for minimum of 3-6 mo. Continue diet throughout simvastatin therapy.

Hyperlipidemia:
PO: Adults: Initially, 5-10 mg/day in evening. Dosage adjustment at 4 wk intervals. **Elderly:** Initially, 5 mg/day. May increase by 5-10 mg/day q4wks. **Range:** 5-40 mg/day. **Maximum:** 40 mg/day.

PRECAUTIONS

CONTRAINDICATIONS: Hypersensitivity to simvastatin/any component of the preparation, active liver disease or unexplained, persistent elevations of liver function tests. Safety and efficacy in individuals less than 18 yrs of age has not been established. **CAUTIONS:** History of liver disease, substantial alcohol consumption. Withholding/discontinuing simvastatin may be necessary when pt at risk for renal failure secondary to rhabdomyolysis. Severe metabolic, endocrine, or electrolyte disorders. **PREGNANCY/LACTATION:** Contraindicated in pregnancy (suppression of cholesterol biosynthesis may cause fetal toxicity) and lactation. Unknown whether drug is distributed in breast milk, but there is risk of serious adverse reactions in nursing infants. **Pregnancy Category X.**

INTERACTIONS

DRUG INTERACTIONS: Increased risk of rhabdomyolysis, acute renal failure w/cyclosporine, erythromycin, gemfibrozil, niacin, other immunosuppressants. **ALTERED LAB VALUES:** May increase creatinine kinase, serum transaminase concentrations.

SIDE EFFECTS

Generally well tolerated. Side effects usually mild and transient. **OCCASIONAL:** Abdominal pain, headache, constipation, upper respiratory infection. **RARE:** Diarrhea, flatulence, asthenia (loss of strength and energy), nausea/vomiting.

ADVERSE REACTIONS/TOXIC EFFECTS

Potential for lens opacities. Hypersensitivity reaction, hepatitis occurs rarely.

NURSING IMPLICATIONS

BASELINE ASSESSMENT:

Question for possibility of pregnancy before initiating therapy (Pregnancy Category X). Question history of hypersensitivity to simvastatin. Assess baseline lab results: Cholesterol, triglycerides, liver function tests.

INTERVENTION/EVALUATION:

Monitor cholesterol and triglyceride lab results for therapeutic response. Evaluate food tolerance. Determine pattern of bowel activity. Check for headache, dizziness (provide assistance as needed). Assess for rash, pruritus. Be alert for malaise, muscle cramping/weakness; if accompanied by fever, may require discontinuation of medication.

PATIENT/FAMILY TEACHING:

Take w/o regard to meals. Follow special diet (important part of treatment). Periodic lab tests are essential part of therapy. Do not take other medications w/o physician knowledge. Do not stop medication w/o consulting physician. Report promptly any muscle pain/weakness, esp. if accompanied by fever/malaise. Do not drive or perform activities that require alert response if dizziness occurs.

sodium bicarbonate

(Sodium bicarbonate)

CANADIAN AVAILABILITY:
Sodium bicarbonate

CLASSIFICATION

Antacid, alkalinizing agent

PHARMACOKINETICS

After administration, sodium bicarbonate dissociates to sodium and bicarbonate ions. Forms/excretes CO_2 (w/increased hydrogen ions combines to form carbonic acid then dissociates to carbon dioxide, which is excreted by lungs). Plasma concentrations regulated by kidney (ability to excrete/make bicarbonate).

ACTION

Systemic alkalizer: Increases plasma bicarbonate, buffers excess hydrogen ion concentration, increases pH, reverses acidosis. *Urinary alkalizer:* Increases excretion of free bicarbonate in urine, increases urinary pH. *Antacid:* Neutralizes existing quantities of stomach acid, increases pH of stomach contents.

USES

Corrects metabolic acidosis occurring in severe renal disease and for advanced cardiac life support during cardiopulmonary resuscitations. Used in treatment of drug intoxicants and as adjunct in treatment of hyperkalemia. Used to increase urinary pH to aid solubility and prevent nephrotoxicity.

PO/IV ADMINISTRATION

PO:

1. Individualize dose (based on neutralizing capacity of antacids).
2. Chewable tablets: Thoroughly chew tablets before swallowing (follow w/glass of water or milk).

IV:

1. The 4%, 4.2%, 7.5%, and 8.4% solutions can be used for direct IV administration.
2. For IV injection, give up to 1 mEq/kg over 1-3 min for cardiac arrest.
3. The 5% solution is administered by IV piggyback.

4. For IV infusion, do not exceed rate of infusion of 50 mEq/hr. For children <2 yrs, premature infants, neonates, administer by slow infusion, up to 8 mEq/daily.

INDICATIONS/DOSAGE/ROUTES

NOTE: May give by direct IV, IV infusion, or orally. Dose individualized (based on severity of acidosis, laboratory values, pt age, weight, clinical conditions). Do not fully correct bicarbonate deficit during first 24 hrs (may cause metabolic alkalosis).

Cardiac arrest:
IV: Adults, elderly: Initially, 1 mEq/kg (as 7.5-8.4% solution). May repeat w/0.5 mEq/kg q10min during continued arrest. Postresuscitation phase based on arterial blood pH, $Paco_2$ base deficit. **Children, infants:** Initially, 1 mEq/kg.

Metabolic acidosis (less severe):
IV INFUSION: Adults, elderly, older children: 2-5 mEq/kg over 4-8 hrs. May repeat based on laboratory values.

Acidosis (associated w/chronic renal failure):
NOTE: Give when plasma bicarbonate <15 mEq/L.
PO: Adults, elderly: Initially, 20-36 mEq/day in divided doses.

Renal tubular acidosis (prevent renal failure, osteomalacia):
PO: Adults, elderly: 4-6 Gm/day in divided doses or 0.5-10 mEq/kg/day in divided doses (higher doses for proximal renal tubular acidosis).

Alkalinization of urine:
PO: Adults, elderly: Initially, 4 Gm, then 1-2 Gm q4h. **Maximum:** 16 Gm/day. **Children:** 84-840 mg/kg/day in divided doses.

Antacid:
PO: Adults, elderly: 300 mg to 2 Gm 1-4 times/day.

PRECAUTIONS

CONTRAINDICATIONS: Metabolic/respiratory alkalosis, hypocalcemia, excessive chloride loss due to vomiting/diarrhea/GI suction. **CAUTIONS:** CHF, edematous states, renal insufficiency, those on corticosteroid therapy. **PREGNANCY/LACTATION:** May produce hypernatremia, increase tendon reflexes in neonate/fetus whose mother is a chronic, high dose user. May be distributed in breast milk. **Pregnancy Category C.**

INTERACTIONS

DRUG INTERACTIONS: May decrease excretion of quinidine, ketoconazole, tetracyclines. Calcium-containing products, milk, milk products may result in milk-alkali syndrome. May increase excretion of salicylates, lithium. May decrease effect of methenamine. **ALTERED LAB VALUES:** May increase serum, urinary pH.

SIDE EFFECTS

FREQUENT: Abdominal distention, flatulence, belching. Extravasation may occur at IV site, resulting in necrosis, ulceration.

ADVERSE REACTIONS/TOXIC EFFECTS

Excessive/chronic use may produce metabolic alkalosis (irritability, twitching, numbness/tingling of extremities, cyanosis, slow/shallow respiration, headache, thirst, nausea). Fluid overload results in headache, weakness, blurred vision, behavioral changes, incoordination, muscle twitching, rise in B/P, decrease in pulse rate, rapid respirations, wheezing, coughing, distended neck veins.

NURSING IMPLICATIONS

BASELINE ASSESSMENT:

Do not give other oral medication within 1-2 hrs of antacid administration.

INTERVENTION/EVALUATION:

Monitor blood and urine pH, CO_2 level, serum electrolytes, plasma bicarbonate, and P_{CO_2} levels. Watch for signs of metabolic alkalosis, fluid overload. Assess for clinical improvement of metabolic acidosis (relief from hyperventilation, weakness, disorientation). Assess pattern of daily bowel activity, stool consistency. Monitor serum phosphate, calcium, uric acid levels. Assess for relief of gastric distress.

PATIENT/FAMILY TEACHING:

Chewable tablets: Chew tablets thoroughly before swallowing (may be followed by water or milk). Tablets may discolor stool. Maintain adequate fluid intake.

sodium chloride

(Salinex, Ocean Mist)

CANADIAN AVAILABILITY:
Sodium chloride

CLASSIFICATION

Electrolyte

PHARMACOKINETICS

Well absorbed from GI tract. Widely distributed. Primarily excreted in urine.

ACTION

Sodium is a major cation of extracellular fluid. Primarily in control of water distribution, fluid/electrolyte balance, osmotic pressure of body fluids. Association with chloride and bicarbonate in maintaining acid-base balance.

USES

Parenteral: Source of hydration; prevent/treats sodium and chloride deficiencies (hypertonic for severe deficiencies). Prevents muscle cramps/heat prostration occurring w/excessive perspiration. Hypotonic: Hydrating solution, used to assess renal function status and manage hyperosmolar diabetes. Diluent for reconstitution. *Nasal:* Restores moisture, relieves dry and inflamed nasal membranes. *Ophthalmic:* Therapy in reduction of corneal edema, diagnostic aid in ophthalmoscopic exam.

STORAGE/HANDLING

Store nasal, ophthalmic, parenteral forms at room temperature.

PO/NASAL/OPHTHALMIC/IM/IV ADMINISTRATION

PO:

1. Do not crush or break enteric-coated or extended-release tablets.

NASAL:

1. Instruct pt to begin inhaling slowly just before releasing medication into nose.
2. Inhale slowly, then release air gently through mouth.
3. Continue technique for 20-30 sec.

OPHTHALMIC:

1. Position pt w/head tilted back, looking up.

2. Gently pull lower lid down to form pouch and instill drops (or apply thin strip of ointment).
3. Do not touch tip of applicator to lids or any surface.
4. When lower lid is released, have pt keep eye open w/o blinking for at least 30 sec for solution; for ointment have pt close eye and roll eyeball around to distribute medication.
5. Apply gentle finger pressure to lacrimal sac (bridge of the nose, inside corner of the eye) for 1-2 min after administration of solution.
6. Remove excess solution around eye w/tissue.

IV:

1. Hypertonic solutions (3 or 5%) administered via large vein; avoid infiltration; do not exceed 100 ml/hr.
2. Vials containing 2.5-4 mEq/ml (concentrated NaCl) must be diluted before administration.

INDICATIONS/DOSAGE/ROUTES

Usual parenteral dosage:
NOTE: Dosage based on age, weight, clinical condition, fluid, electrolyte, acid-base status.
IV INFUSION: Adults, elderly: (0.9 or 0.45%): 1-2 liters/day. (3 or 5%): 100 ml over 1 hr; assess serum electrolyte concentration before additional fluid given.

Usual oral dosage:
PO: Adults, elderly: 1-2 Gm 3 times/day.

Usual nasal dosage:
INTRANASAL: Adults, elderly: Take as needed.

Usual ophthalmic dosage:
OPHTHALMIC: Adults, elderly: (Solution): 1-2 drops q3-4h. (Ointment): Once/day or as directed.

PRECAUTIONS

CONTRAINDICATIONS: Hypernatremia, fluid retention. **CAUTIONS:** CHF, circulatory insufficiency, kidney dysfunction, hypoproteinemia. Do not use NaCl preserved w/benzyl alcohol in neonates. **PREGNANCY/LACTATION: Pregnancy Category C.**

INTERACTIONS

DRUG INTERACTIONS: Hypertonic saline and oxytocics may cause uterine hypertonus, possible uterine ruptures or lacerations. **ALTERED LAB VALUES:** None significant.

SIDE EFFECTS

OCCASIONAL: Fever, irritation/phlebitis/extravasation at injection site.

ADVERSE REACTIONS/TOXIC EFFECTS

Too rapid administration may produce peripheral edema, CHF, pulmonary edema. Excessive dosage produces hypokalemia, hypervolemia, hypernatremia.

NURSING IMPLICATIONS

BASELINE ASSESSMENT:

Assess fluid balance (I&O, edema).

INTERVENTION/EVALUATION:

Monitor fluid balance (e.g., I&O, daily weight, edema, lung sounds), IV site for extravasation. Monitor serum electrolytes, acid-base balance, B/P. Hypernatremia associated w/edema, weight gain, elevated B/P; hyponatremia associated w/muscle cramps, nausea, vomiting, dry mucous membranes.

PATIENT/FAMILY TEACHING:

Temporary burning, irritation

may occur upon instillation of eye medication. Discontinue eye medication if severe pain, headache, rapid change in vision (side and straight ahead), sudden appearance of floating spots, acute redness of eyes, pain on exposure to light, or double vision occurs and contact physician.

sodium polystyrene sulfonate

(SPS, Kayexalate)

CANADIAN AVAILABILITY: Kayexalate

CLASSIFICATION

Cation exchange resin

ACTION

Resin passes through intestine or is retained in colon, releases sodium ions in exchange for primarily potassium ions. Occurs from 2-12 hrs after oral administration, longer after rectal administration.

USES

Treatment of hyperkalemia.

STORAGE/HANDLING

After preparation, suspension stable for 24 hrs.

PO/RECTAL ADMINISTRATION

PO:

1. Give w/20-100 ml sorbitol (facilitates passage of resin through intestinal tract, prevents constipation, aids in potassium removal, increases palatability).
2. Do not mix w/foods, liquids containing potassium.

RECTAL:

1. Initial cleansing enema, then insert large rubber tube into rectum well into sigmoid colon, tape in place.
2. Introduce suspension (w/100 ml sorbitol) via gravity.
3. Flush w/50-100 ml fluid and clamp.
4. Retain for several hrs if possible.
5. Irrigate colon w/nonsodium-containing solution to remove resin.

INDICATIONS/DOSAGE/ROUTES

Hyperkalemia:
PO: Adults, elderly: 60 ml (15 Gm) 1-4 times/day.
RECTAL: Adults, elderly: 30-50 Gm as needed q6h.

Usual pediatric dosage:
PO/RECTAL: Children: Based on 1 Gm resin binding approximately 1 mEq potassium.

PRECAUTIONS

CONTRAINDICATIONS: None significant. **CAUTIONS:** Those who cannot tolerate increase in sodium (CHF, severe hypertension, marked edema). **PREGNANCY/LACTATION:** Unknown whether drug crosses placenta or is distributed in breast milk. **Pregnancy Category C.**

INTERACTIONS

DRUG INTERACTIONS: Cation-donating antacids, laxatives (e.g., magnesium hydroxide) may decrease effect, cause systemic alkalosis (pts w/renal impairment). **ALTERED LAB VALUES:** May decrease magnesium, calcium.

SIDE EFFECTS

High doses may produce anorexia, nausea, vomiting, constipation, w/diarrhea occurring less often.

ADVERSE REACTIONS/TOXIC EFFECTS

Serious potassium deficiency may occur. Early signs of hypokalemia: Irritable confusion, delayed thought processes, often associated w/lengthened QT interval and widening, flattening, or conversion of T wave and prominent U waves. Arrhythmias, severe muscle weakness may be noted.

NURSING IMPLICATIONS

BASELINE ASSESSMENT:

Does not rapidly correct severe hyperkalemia (may take hours to days). Consider other measures in medical emergency (IV calcium, IV sodium bicarbonate, glucose, insulin, dialysis).

INTERVENTION/EVALUATION:

Frequent potassium levels within each 24 hrs should be maintained, monitored. Assess pt's clinical condition, EKG (valuable in determining when treatment should be discontinued). Besides checking serum potassium, monitor magnesium, calcium levels. Monitor daily bowel activity, stool consistency (fecal impaction may occur in those on high doses, particularly in elderly).

somatrem

soe´ma-trem

(Protropin)

CANADIAN AVAILABILITY:
Protropin

CLASSIFICATION

Growth stimulator

PHARMACOKINETICS

Well absorbed following SubQ, IM administration. Metabolized in liver. Eliminated in feces via biliary system, excreted in urine. Half-life: *IV:* 20 minutes, *IM/SubQ:* 3-5 hrs.

ACTION

Stimulates linear growth. Increases number, size of muscle cells, increases red cell mass. Affects carbohydrate metabolism (antagonizes action of insulin), fats (increases mobilization of fats), and proteins (increases cellular protein synthesis).

USES

Long-term treatment of children who have growth failure due to endogenous growth hormone deficiency.

STORAGE/HANDLING

Refrigerate vials. After reconstitution, use within 7 days. Avoid freezing.

IM ADMINISTRATION

1. Reconstitute each 5 mg vial w/1-5 ml of bacteriostatic water for injection (benzyl alcohol preserved only). For newborns (because of toxicity w/benzyl alcohol) reconstitute w/water for injection.
2. To prepare solution, inject diluent into vial aiming the stream of liquid against the glass wall. Swirl gently until dissolved. DO NOT SHAKE.
3. Use one dose per vial; discard unused portion.
4. Do not administer if solution is cloudy/contains particulate matter.
5. To prevent contamination,

use disposable needle/syringe for each entry into vial.

INDICATIONS/DOSAGE/ROUTES

Usual parenteral dosage:
IM/SubQ: Up to 0.1 mg/kg (0.26 IU/kg) 3 times/wk.

PRECAUTIONS

CONTRAINDICATIONS: Pts w/ closed epiphyses, known sensitivity to benzyl alcohol, active neoplasia (intracranial tumors must be inactive and antitumor therapy complete before somatrem therapy; discontinue if tumor growth recurs). **CAUTIONS:** Diabetes mellitus, hypothyroidism, pts whose growth hormone deficiency is secondary to an intracranial lesion.

INTERACTIONS

DRUG INTERACTIONS: Glucocorticoids (chronic use) may decrease effects. **ALTERED LAB VALUES:** May increase fatty acid, phosphate concentration. May decrease glucose tolerance, thyroid function tests.

SIDE EFFECTS

FREQUENT: 30% of pts develop persistent antibodies to growth hormone (generally does not cause failure to respond to somatrem). **OCCASIONAL:** Insulin resistance w/hyperglycemia. **RARE:** Pain, swelling at injection site.

ADVERSE REACTIONS/TOXIC EFFECTS

Hypothyroidism (must be treated or will interfere w/response to somatrem).

NURSING IMPLICATIONS

BASELINE ASSESSMENT:

Question sensitivity to benzyl alcohol. Baseline blood glucose, thyroid function, and bone age determinations should be established.

INTERVENTION/EVALUATION:

Monitor blood glucose levels and check for hyperglycemia (polyuria, polydipsia, polyphagia). Assess for developing hypothyroidism: Forgetfulness, dry skin and hair, feeling cold, apathy, lethargy, weight gain, bradycardia.

PATIENT/FAMILY TEACHING:

Somatrem therapy may continue for years, as long as pt is responsive, until mature adult height is reached or epiphyses close. Importance of regular visits to the physician, tests during therapy. Record height, weight as directed by physician. Signs and symptoms of hypothyroidism, hyperglycemia; report promptly.

somatropin

soe-mah-troe´pin
(Humatrope, Nutropin)

CANADIAN AVAILABILITY:
Humatrope

CLASSIFICATION

Growth stimulator

PHARMACOKINETICS

Well absorbed following SubQ, IM administration. Metabolized in liver. Eliminated in feces via biliary system, excreted in urine. Half-life: *IV:* 20 min, *IM/SubQ:* 3-5 hrs.

ACTION

Stimulates linear growth. Increases number, size of muscle cells, increases red cell mass. Affects carbohydrate metabolism (antagonizes action of insulin), fats (increases mobilization of fats), and proteins (increases cellular protein synthesis).

USES

Long-term treatment of children who have growth failure due to endogenous growth hormone deficiency or associated w/chronic renal insufficiency (Nutropin only).

STORAGE/HANDLING

Refrigerate vials. After reconstitution, stable for 14 days refrigerated. Avoid freezing.

SubQ/IM ADMINISTRATION

1a. *Humatrope:* Reconstitute each 5 mg vial w/1.5-5 ml diluent or sterile water for injection. (If sterile water used, use 1 dose/vial, refrigerate solution if not used immediately, use within 24 hrs, discard unused portion.)

1b. *Nutropin:* Reconstitute 5 mg vial w/1-5 mg (10 mg w/1-10 ml) bacteriostatic water for injection.

2. DO NOT SHAKE.

3. Do not inject if solution is cloudy or contains particulate matter.

INDICATIONS/DOSAGE/ROUTES

Growth hormone deficiency:
IM/SubQ: *(Humatrope):* Up to 0.06 mg/kg 3 times/wk.
SubQ: *(Nutropin):* 0.3 mg/kg/wk.

Chronic renal insufficiency:
SubQ: *(Nutropin):* 0.35 mg/kg/wk.

PRECAUTIONS

CONTRAINDICATIONS: Pts w/ closed epiphyses, active neoplasia (intracranial tumors must be inactive and antitumor therapy complete before somatropin therapy; discontinue if tumor growth recurs). Do not use supplied diluent when sensitivity to m-cresol or glycerin is known. **CAUTIONS:** Diabetes mellitus, hypothyroidism, pts whose growth hormone deficiency is secondary to an intracranial lesion.

INTERACTIONS

DRUG INTERACTIONS: Glucocorticoids (chronic use) may decrease effects. **ALTERED LAB VALUES:** May increase fatty acid, phosphate concentration. May decrease glucose tolerance, thyroid function tests.

SIDE EFFECTS

FREQUENT: Development of persistent antibodies to growth hormone (generally does not cause failure to respond to somatropin); hypercalciuria during first 2-3 mo of therapy. **OCCASIONAL:** Insulin resistance w/hyperglycemia. **RARE:** Pain, swelling at injection site.

ADVERSE REACTIONS/TOXIC EFFECTS

Hypothyroidism (must be treated or will interfere w/response to somatrem).

NURSING IMPLICATIONS

BASELINE ASSESSMENT:

Question sensitivity to m-cresol, glycerin. Baseline blood glucose, thyroid function, and bone age determinations should be established.

INTERVENTION/EVALUATION:

Monitor blood glucose levels and check for hyperglycemia (polyuria, polydipsia, polyphagia). Assess for developing hypothyroidism: Forgetfulness, dry skin and hair, feeling cold, apathy, lethargy, weight gain, bradycardia. During early therapy, be alert to renal calculi associated w/hypercalciuria (flank pain and colic, chills, fever, urinary frequency, hematuria).

PATIENT/FAMILY TEACHING:

Somatropin therapy may continue for years, as long as pt is responsive, until mature adult height is reached or epiphyses close. Importance of regular visits to the physician, tests during therapy. Record height, weight as directed by physician. Signs and symptoms of hypothyroidism, hyperglycemia, renal calculi; report promptly.

sotalol

sew'tah-lol
(Betapace)

CANADIAN AVAILABILITY:
Sotocor

CLASSIFICATION

Beta-adrenergic blocking agent

PHARMACOKINETICS

Well absorbed from GI tract. Widely distributed. Protein binding: 0%. Primarily excreted unchanged in urine. Half-life: 12 hrs (increased in elderly, pts w/decreased renal function).

ACTION

Antiarrhythmic: Decreases heart rate, AV nodal conduction; increases AV nodal refractoriness. Prolongs action potential and effective refractory period, QT interval.

USES

Treatment of documented, life-threatening ventricular arrhythmias.

PO ADMINISTRATION

May give w/o regard to food.

INDICATIONS/DOSAGE/ROUTES

Antiarrhythmic:
PO: Adults, elderly: Initially, 80 mg 2 times/day. May increase gradually at 2-3 day intervals. **Range:** 240-320 mg/day.
NOTE: Some patients may require 480-640 mg/day. Dosing more than 2 times/day usually not necessary due to long half-life.

Dosage in renal impairment:

CREATININE CLEARANCE	DOSAGE INTERVAL
30-60 ml/min	24 hrs
10-30 ml/min	36-48 hr
<10 ml/min	Individualized

PRECAUTIONS

CONTRAINDICATIONS: Bronchial asthma, uncontrolled cardiac failure, sinus bradycardia, second- and third-degree heart block, cardiogenic shock, long QT syndrome (unless functioning pacemaker present). **CAUTIONS:** Pts w/history of ventricular tachycardia, ventricular fibrillation, cardiomegaly, CHF, diabetes mellitus, excessive prolongation of QT interval, hypokalemia, and hypomagnesium. Severe, prolonged diarrhea. Pts w/sick sinus syndrome; pts at risk of developing thyrotoxicosis. Avoid abrupt withdrawal. **PREGNANCY/LACTATION:** Crosses placenta; excreted in breast milk. **Pregnancy Category B.**

INTERACTIONS

DRUG INTERACTIONS: Antiarrhythmics, phenothiazine, tricyclic antidepressants, terfenadine, astemizole may increase prolonged QT interval. May increase proarrhythmia w/digoxin. Calcium channel blockers may increase effect on AV conduction, B/P. May mask signs of hypoglycemia, prolong effect of insulin, oral hypoglycemics. May inhibit effects of sympathomimetics. May potentiate rebound hypertension seen after discontinuing clonidine. **ALTERED LAB VALUES:** May increase glucose, alkaline phosphatase, LDH, SGOT (AST), SGPT (ALT), lipoproteins, triglycerides.

SIDE EFFECTS

FREQUENT: Bradycardia, palpitations. **OCCASIONAL:** Breathing difficulty, irregular heartbeat, CHF (swelling ankles, feet, lower legs), cold hands, feet. Anxiety, nervousness, constipation, diarrhea, dizziness, drowsiness, nausea, vomiting, itching, nightmares, stomach discomfort, unusual tiredness or weakness. **RARE:** Skin rash, chest pain, mental depression.

ADVERSE REACTIONS/TOXIC EFFECTS

Bradycardia, CHF, hypotension, bronchospasms, hypoglycemia, prolonged QT interval, torsade de pointes, ventricular tachycardia, premature ventricular complexes.

NURSING IMPLICATIONS

BASELINE ASSESSMENT:

Pt must be on continuous cardiac monitoring upon initiation of therapy. Establish baseline B/P and pulse. Do not administer w/o consulting physician if pulse is below 60 beats/min.

INTERVENTION/EVALUATION:

Monitor B/P for hypotension, pulse for bradycardia. Assess for CHF: dyspnea, peripheral edema, jugular vein distention, increase weight, rales in lungs, decreased urine output.

PATIENT/FAMILY TEACHING:

May have lightheadedness; do not drive or perform tasks that require alert response if this occurs. Carry identification bracelet/card. Teach pt/family to correctly take B/P, pulse before dosing; contact physician if below parameters, usually systolic B/P of 90 mm Hg, pulse of 60 beats/ min. Change positions slowly to prevent orthostatic hypotension. Do not take over-the-counter cold medications, nasal decongestants. Restrict sodium and alcohol as ordered. Do not stop taking drug suddenly. Report chest pain, fatigue, shortness of breath.

S

spectinomycin hydrochloride

speck-tin-oh-my′sin
(Trobicin)

CANADIAN AVAILABILITY:
Trobicin

CLASSIFICATION

Antibiotic

PHARMACOKINETICS

Rapidly, completely absorbed after IM administration. Primarily concentrated in urine. Excreted in urine. Removed by hemodialysis. Half-life: 1-3 hrs (increased in decreased renal function).

ACTION

Inhibits protein synthesis by interaction w/30S subunit of bacterial cells.

USES

Treatment of acute gonococcal urethritis, proctitis in males, acute gonococcal cervicitis and proctitis in females.

STORAGE/HANDLING

Following reconstitution, stable for 24 hrs at room temperature. Use within 24 hrs.

IM ADMINISTRATION

1. For IM injection, reconstitute each 2 Gm vial w/3.2 ml bacteriostatic water for injection containing 0.9% benzyl alcohol (6.2 ml to 4 Gm vial) to provide concentration of 400 mg/ml.
2. Shake vigorously.
3. Inject deep IM into upper outer quadrant of gluteal muscle (use 20 gauge needle).
4. Do not inject more than 5 ml in one site.
5. Observe pt for 1 hr after injection for potential anaphylaxis.

INDICATIONS/DOSAGE/ROUTES

Usual adult dosage:
IM: Adults: 2 Gm once. In areas where antibiotic resistance is known to be prevalent, 4 Gm (10 ml) divided between 2 injection sites is preferred.

PRECAUTIONS

CONTRAINDICATIONS: None significant. **CAUTIONS:** History of allergies. **PREGNANCY/LACTATION:** Unknown whether drug crosses placenta or is distributed in breast milk. **Pregnancy Category B.**

INTERACTIONS

DRUG INTERACTIONS: None significant. **ALTERED LAB VALUES:** None significant.

SIDE EFFECTS

FREQUENT: Pain at injection site. **OCCASIONAL:** Dizziness, insomnia. **RARE:** Decreased urine output.

ADVERSE REACTIONS/TOXIC EFFECTS

Hypersensitivity reaction characterized as chills, fever, nausea, vomiting, urticaria.

NURSING IMPLICATIONS

BASELINE ASSESSMENT:

Question pt for history of allergies, particularly to spectinomycin. Obtain culture and sensitivity test before giving first dose (therapy may begin before results are known). Serologic test for syphilis should be completed before therapy.

INTERVENTION/EVALUATION:

Observe pt for 1 hr after injection because of potential for anaphylaxis.

PATIENT/FAMILY TEACHING:

May have discomfort at injection site.

---

spirapril (Renormax)
See supplement

---

spironolactone

spear-own-oh-lak´tone
(Aldactone)

FIXED-COMBINATION(S):
W/hydrochlorothiazide, a thiazide diuretic (Aldactazide, Spironazide)

CANADIAN AVAILABILITY: Aldactone, Novospiroton

CLASSIFICATION

Diuretic: Potassium-sparing

PHARMACOKINETICS

	ONSET	PEAK	DURATION
PO	24-48 hrs	48-72 hrs	48-72 hrs

Well absorbed from GI tract (increased w/food). Protein binding: >90%. Metabolized in liver to active metabolite. Primarily excreted in urine. Half-life: 9-24 hrs.

ACTION

Competitively inhibits action of aldosterone. Interferes w/sodium reabsorption in distal tubule, increasing sodium and water excretion and increasing potassium retention.

USES

Treatment of excessive aldosterone production, essential hypertension, decreasing edema due to CHF, cirrhosis of liver/nephrotic syndrome. Adjunct to potassium-losing diuretics or to potentiate action of other diuretics. Diagnosis of hyperaldosteronism.

STORAGE/HANDLING

Oral suspension containing crushed tablets in cherry syrup is stable for up to 30 days if refrigerated.

PO ADMINISTRATION

1. Cherry suspension available for pediatric administration.
2. Drug absorption enhanced if taken w/food.
3. Scored tablets may be crushed.
4. Do not crush or break film-coated tablets.

INDICATIONS/DOSAGE/ROUTES

NOTE: Use loading dose to prevent delay in therapeutic effect (may take up to 3 days).

Edema:
PO: Adults: 25-200 mg daily. Give in single or equally divided doses. **Children:** 3.3 mg/kg daily.

Hypokalemia:
PO: Adults: 25-100 mg daily.

Hypertension:
PO: Adults: 50-100 mg daily.

Usual elderly dosage:
PO: Elderly: Initially, 25-50 mg/day. May increase by 25-50 mg/day every 5 days.

Diagnosis of primary aldosteronism:
PO: Adults: 400 mg daily for 3-4 wks. Increase in potassium and reduction in hypertension point to primary aldosteronism. This dosage may be tried for 4 days w/increase in potassium levels during use as the diagnostic indicator. **Children:** 125-375 mg/m^2 over 24 hrs.

Preoperative or maintenance therapy for hyperaldosteronism:
PO: Adults: 100-400 mg daily for preoperative therapy; 400 mg initial dose followed by lowest therapeutic dose at 100-300 mg/day for maintenance if surgery cannot be done.

PRECAUTIONS

CONTRAINDICATIONS: Acute renal insufficiency/impairment, anuria, BUN/creatinine over twice normal values levels, hyperkalemia. **CAUTIONS:** Hepatic/renal impairment. **PREGNANCY/LACTATION:** Active metabolite excreted in breast milk—nursing not advised. **Pregnancy Category C.**

INTERACTIONS

DRUG INTERACTIONS: May decrease effect of anticoagulants, heparin. NSAIDs may decrease anti-hypertensive effect. ACE inhibitors (e.g., captopril), potassium containing medications, potassium supplements may increase potassium. May decrease lithium clearance, increase toxicity. May increase digoxin half-life. **ALTERED LAB VALUES:** May increase BUN, calcium excretion, creatinine, glucose, magnesium, potassium, uric acid. May decrease sodium.

SIDE EFFECTS

FREQUENT: Hyperkalemia for those on potassium supplements or those w/renal insufficiency; dehydration, hyponatremia, lethargy. **OCCASIONAL:** Nausea, vomiting, anorexia, cramping, diarrhea, headache, ataxia, drowsiness, confusion, fever. *Male:* Gynecomastia, impotence, decreased libido. *Females:* Menstrual irregularities/amenorrhea, postmenopausal bleeding, breast tenderness. **RARE:** Rash, urticaria, hirsutism. Those w/primary aldosteronism may experience rapid weight loss, severe fatigue during high-dose therapy.

ADVERSE REACTIONS/TOXIC EFFECTS

Severe hyperkalemia may produce arrhythmias, bradycardia, tented T waves, widening QRS, ST depression. These can proceed to cardiac standstill or ventricular fibrillation. Cirrhosis pts at risk for hepatic decompensation if dehydration/hyponatremia occurs.

NURSING IMPLICATIONS

BASELINE ASSESSMENT:

Weigh pt; initiate strict I&O. Evaluate hydration status by assessing mucous membranes, skin turgor. Baseline electrolytes, renal/hepatic functions, urinalysis should be obtained. EKG may be ordered. Assess for edema, note location and extent. Check baseline vital signs, note pulse rate/regularity.

INTERVENTION/EVALUATION:

Monitor electrolyte values, esp. for increased potassium. Monitor B/P levels. Monitor for hyponatremia: Mental confusion, thirst, cold/clammy skin, drowsiness, dry mouth. Monitor for hyperkalemia: Colic, diarrhea, muscle twitching followed by weakness/paralysis, arrhythmias. Obtain daily weight. Note changes in edema, skin turgor.

PATIENT/FAMILY TEACHING:

Expect increase in volume, frequency of urination. Therapeutic effect takes several days to begin and can last for several days when drug is discontinued. This may not apply if pt is on a potassium-losing drug concomitantly (diet and use of supplements should be established by physician). Notify physician for irregular/slow pulse, electrolyte imbalance (signs noted above). Avoid foods high in potassium such as whole grains (cereals), legumes, meat, bananas, apricots, orange juice, potatoes (white, sweet), raisins.

---

stavudine (Zerit)
See supplement

---

streptokinase

strep-toe-kine´ace
(Kabikinase, Streptase)

CANADIAN AVAILABILITY:
Streptase

CLASSIFICATION

Thrombolytic

PHARMACOKINETICS

Rapidly cleared from plasma by antibodies, reticuloendothelial system. Route of elimination unknown. Duration of action continues for several hrs after discontinuing medication. Half-life: 23 min.

ACTION

Activates fibrinolytic system by converting plasminogen to plasmin (enzyme that degrades fibrin clots). Acts indirectly by forming complex w/plasminogen, which converts plasminogen to plasmin. Action occurs within thrombus, on its surface, and in circulating blood.

USES

Management of acute myocardial infarction (lyses thrombi obstructing coronary arteries, decreases infarct size, improves ventricular function after MI, decreases CHF, mortality associated w/AMI). Lysis of diagnosed pulmonary emboli, acute, extensive thrombi of deep veins, and acute arterial thrombi/emboli. Clears total/partially occluded arteriovenous cannulae.

STORAGE/HANDLING

Store vials at room temperature. Reconstitute vials immediately before use. Solution for direct IV administration may be used within 8 hrs of reconstitution. Discard unused portion.

IV/INTRACORONARY ADMINISTRATION

NOTE: Must be administered within 12-14 hrs of clot formation (little effect on older, organized clots).

IV:

1. Give by direct IV/IV infusion (via infusion pump). Infuse into selected thrombosed coronary artery, intra-arterially, or by cannula.
2. Reconstitute vial w/5 ml 5% dextrose or 0.9% NaCl solution. (Add diluent slowly to side of vial, roll and tilt to avoid foaming. Do not shake vial.)
3. Slight flocculation may occur, does not affect safe use of the drug.
4. Further dilute w/50-500 ml 5% dextrose or 0.9% NaCl.
6. If minor bleeding occurs at puncture sites, apply pressure for 30 min, then apply pressure dressing.
7. Monitor B/P during infusion (hypotension may be severe, occurs in 1-10%). Decrease of infusion rate may be necessary.
8. If uncontrolled hemorrhage occurs, discontinue infusion immediately (slowing rate of infusion may produce worsening hemorrhage). Do not use dextran to control hemorrhage.

INTRACORONARY:

1. Monitor for arrhythmias during and immediately after infusion (atrial/ventricular).

INDICATIONS/DOSAGE/ROUTES

NOTE: Do not use from 5 days to 6 mo of previous streptokinase treatment of streptococcal infection (pharyngitis, rheumatic fever, acute glomerulonephritis secondary to streptococcal infection).

Acute evolving transmural myocardial infarction (give as soon as possible after symptoms occur):

IV INFUSION: Adults, elderly:

(1.5 million U diluted to 45 ml): 1,500,000 IU infused over 60 min.
INTRACORONARY INFUSION: Adults, elderly: 250,000 U diluted to 125 ml): Initially, 20,000 IU (10 ml) bolus; then, 2,000 IU/min for 60 min. Total dose: 140,000 IU.

Pulmonary embolism, deep vein thrombosis, arterial thrombosis/embolism (give within 7 days after onset):
IV INFUSION: Adults, elderly: (1.5 million U diluted to 90 ml): Initially, 250,000 IU infused over 30 min; then, 100,000 IU/hr for 24-72 hrs for arterial thrombosis/embolism, 24-72 hrs for pulmonary embolism, 72 hrs for deep vein thrombosis.
INTRACORONARY INFUSION: Adults, elderly: (1.5 million U diluted to 45 ml): Initially: 250,000 IU infused over 30 min; then, 100,000 IU/hr for maintenance.

Arteriovenous cannulae occlusion:

Instill 100,000-250,000 IU into each occluded cannula limb; clamp for 2 hrs. Aspirate contents of infused cannula limb; flush w/ saline, reconnect cannula.

PRECAUTIONS

CONTRAINDICATIONS: Active internal bleeding, recent (within 2 mo) cerebrovascular accident, intracranial/intraspinal surgery, intracranial neoplasm, severe uncontrolled hypertension. **CAUTIONS:** Recent (10 days) major surgery/GI bleeding, obstetrical delivery, organ biopsy, trauma (cardiopulmonary resuscitation); uncontrolled arterial hypertension, left heart thrombus, endocarditis, severe hepatic/renal disease, pregnancy, elderly, cerebrovascular disease, diabetic retinopathy, thrombophlebitis, occluded AV cannula at infected site. **PREGNANCY/LACTATION:** Use only when benefit outweighs potential risk to fetus. Unknown whether drug crosses placenta or is distributed in breast milk. **Pregnancy Category C.**

INTERACTIONS

DRUG INTERACTIONS: Anticoagulants, heparin may increase risk of hemorrhage. Platelet aggregation inhibitors (e.g., aspirin) may increase risk of bleeding. **ALTERED LAB VALUES:** Decreases plasminogen and fibrinogen level during infusion, decreasing clotting time (confirms presence of lysis).

SIDE EFFECTS

OCCASIONAL: Minor breathing difficulty, eye swelling (periorbital swelling), mild allergic reaction (urticaria, itching, flushing), aches/pains.

ADVERSE REACTIONS/TOXIC EFFECTS

Severe internal hemorrhage may occur. Lysis of coronary thrombi may produce atrial/ventricular arrhythmias.

NURSING IMPLICATIONS

BASELINE ASSESSMENT:

Assess Hct, platelet count, thrombin (TT), activated thromboplastin (APTT), prothrombin (PT) time, fibrinogen level, before therapy is instituted. If heparin is component of treatment, discontinue before streptokinase is instituted (TT/APTT should be less than twice normal value before institution of therapy).

INTERVENTION/EVALUATION:

Monitor EKG continuously. Assess clinical response, vital signs (pulse, temperature, respiratory rate, B/P) q4h or per protocol. Handle pt carefully and infrequently as possible to prevent bleeding. Do not obtain B/P in lower extremities (possible deep vein thrombi). Monitor TT, PT, APTT, fibrinogen level q4h after initiation of therapy. Check stool for occult blood. Assess for decrease in B/P, increase in pulse rate, complaint of abdominal/back pain, severe headache (may be evidence of hemorrhage). Question for increase in amount of discharge during menses. Assess area of thromboembolus for color, temperature. Assess peripheral pulses, skin for bruises and petechiae. Check for excessive bleeding from minor cuts, scratches. Assess urine output for hematuria.

streptomycin sulfate

strep-tow-my'sin
(Streptomycin)

CLASSIFICATION

Antibiotic: Aminoglycoside

PHARMACOKINETICS

Rapidly, completely absorbed following IM administration. Widely distributed, does not cross blood-brain barrier. Protein binding: 0-10%. Primarily excreted unchanged in urine. Removed by hemodialysis. Half-life: 2-4 hrs (increased in decreased renal function).

ACTION

Bactericidal because of receptor binding action, interfering w/ protein synthesis in susceptible microorganisms.

USES

In conjunction w/at least one other antitubercular agent in the treatment of tuberculosis.

STORAGE/HANDLING

Store vials at room temperature. After reconstitution, stable for 2-28 days at room temperature, 14 days refrigerated. Solutions are colorless to yellow; may darken upon exposure to light (does not affect potency).

IM ADMINISTRATION

1. Reconstitute each vial w/sterile water for injection or 0.9% NaCl for injection to provide concentration of 200 to 500 mg/ml.
2. To minimize discomfort, give deep IM slowly. Less painful if injected into gluteus maximus rather than lateral aspect of thigh.

INDICATIONS/DOSAGE/ROUTES

Tuberculosis:
IM: Adults: 1 Gm/day. May reduce to 1 Gm 2-3 times/wk. **Range:** 1 Gm 2 times/wk up to 2 Gm/day. **Elderly:** 500-750 mg/day. **Children:** 20 mg/kg once daily. **Maximum:** 1 Gm/day.

S

PRECAUTIONS

CONTRAINDICATIONS: Hypersensitivity to streptomycin, other aminoglycosides. Pts w/myasthenia gravis, parkinsonism, eighth cranial nerve damage. **CAUTIONS:** Elderly, neonates because of renal insufficiency, immaturity; young infants (may cause CNS depression). **PREGNANCY/LACTATION:** Crosses placenta, may be nephrotoxic in human fetus. May cause total, irreversible, bilateral congenital deafness in children when mothers received streptomycin during pregnancy. Excreted in breast milk. **Pregnancy Category D.**

INTERACTIONS

DRUG INTERACTIONS: Other aminoglycosides, nephrotoxic, ototoxic producing medications may increase toxicity. May increase effects of neuromuscular blocking agents. **ALTERED LAB VALUES:** May increase SGOT (AST), SGPT (ALT), alkaline phosphatase, LDH, bilirubin, BUN, creatinine. May decrease serum calcium, magnesium, potassium, sodium concentrations.

SIDE EFFECTS

FREQUENT: Nephrotoxicity (e.g., change in frequency of urine, increased thirst, decreased appetite, nausea, vomiting). Neurotoxicity (e.g., muscle numbness, tingling, twitching, seizures). Ototoxicity, vestibular (e.g., dizziness, clumsiness, unsteadiness). Peripheral neuritis (burning of face or mouth). Ototoxicity, auditory (e.g., loss of hearing, ringing in ears, full feeling in ears). **OCCASIONAL:** Hypersensitivity (e.g., itching, rash, swelling). Any loss of vision. **RARE:** Neuromuscular blockade (breathing difficulty, weakness, drowsiness).

ADVERSE REACTIONS/TOXIC EFFECTS

Nephrotoxicity (evidenced by increased BUN and serum creatinine, decreased creatinine clearance) may be reversible if drug stopped at first sign of symptoms; irreversible otoxicity (tinnitus, dizziness, ringing/roaring in ears, reduced hearing) and neurotoxicity (headache, dizziness, lethargy, tremors, visual disturbances) occur occasionally. Risk is greater w/ higher dosages, prolonged therapy.

NURSING IMPLICATIONS

BASELINE ASSESSMENT:

Dehydration must be treated before aminoglycoside therapy. Establish pt's baseline hearing acuity before beginning therapy. Question for history of allergies, esp. to aminoglycosides. Obtain specimens for culture, sensitivity before giving the first dose (therapy may begin before results are known). Maintain adequate hydration.

INTERVENTION/EVALUATION:

Monitor I&O (maintain hydration), urinalysis (casts, RBCs, WBCs, decrease in specific gravity). Monitor results of peak/trough blood tests. Be alert to ototoxic and neurotoxic symptoms. Check IM injection site for pain, induration. Assess for skin rash. Assess for superinfection, particularly genital/anal pruritus, changes of oral mucosa, diarrhea. When treating pts w/neuromuscular disorders, assess respiratory response carefully.

PATIENT/FAMILY TEACHING:

Continue antibiotic for full length of treatment, at least 1 year w/tuberculosis therapy (assure adequate support system for daily injections). Discomfort may occur w/ IM injection. Notify physician in event of hearing, visual, balance, urinary problems even after therapy is completed. Do not take other medication w/o consulting physician. Lab tests are an essential part of therapy.

streptozocin

strep-to-zoe´sin
(Zanosar)

CANADIAN AVAILABILITY:
Zanosar

CLASSIFICATION

Antineoplastic

PHARMACOKINETICS

Rapidly distributed primarily in liver, kidneys, intestine, pancreas. Metabolized in liver. Primarily excreted in urine. Half-life: 35 min; metabolite: 40 min.

ACTION

Cell cycle-phase nonspecific. Cross-links strands of DNA, inhibiting DNA synthesis.

USES

Treatment of metastatic islet cell carcinoma of pancreas.

STORAGE/HANDLING

NOTE: May be carcinogenic, mutagenic, or teratogenic. Handle w/ extreme care during preparation/ administration.

Refrigerate unopened vials. Solutions are clear to pale gold. Discard if color changes to dark brown (indicates decomposition). Discard solution within 12 hrs after reconstitution.

IV ADMINISTRATION

NOTE: May give by IV injection or infusion. Wear gloves when preparing solution (topical contact may be carcinogenic hazard). If powder or solution come in contact w/skin, wash immediately, thoroughly w/soap, water.

1. Reconstitute 1 Gm vial w/9.5 ml 5% dextrose or 0.9% NaCl injection to provide concentration of 100 mg/ml.
2. For IV injection, administer over 10-15 min.
3. For IV infusion, further dilute w/10-200 ml 5% dextrose or 0.9% NaCl solution and infuse over 15 min-6 hrs.
4. Extravasation may produce severe tissue necrosis. Apply warm compresses to reduce severity of irritation at IV site.

INDICATIONS/DOSAGE/ROUTES

NOTE: Dosage individualized based on clinical response, tolerance to adverse effects. When used in combination therapy, consult specific protocols for optimum dosage, sequence of drug administration. Dosage based on body surface area (BSA).

Daily:
IV: Adults, elderly: 500 mg/m^2 of BSA for 5 consecutive days q6wks.

Weekly:
IV: Adults, elderly: Initially, 1 Gm/m^2 BSA weekly for 2 wks. May increase up to 1.5 Gm/m^2 BSA.

PRECAUTIONS

CONTRAINDICATIONS: None significant. **EXTREME CAUTION:** Impaired renal function. **CAUTION:** Impaired hepatic function. **PREGNANCY/LACTATION:** If possible, avoid use during pregnancy, esp. first trimester. Unknown whether distributed in breast milk. Breast feeding not recommended. **Pregnancy Category C.**

INTERACTIONS

DRUG INTERACTIONS: Nephrotoxic medications may increase nephrotoxicity. May decrease effects of phenytoin. Live virus vaccines may potentiate virus replication, increase vaccine side effects, decrease pt's antibody response to vaccine. **ALTERED LAB VALUES:** May increase SGOT (AST), SGPT (ALT), alkaline phosphatase, bilirubin, LDH, BUN, creatinine, urinary protein. May decrease albumin, phosphate concentrations.

SIDE EFFECTS

FREQUENT: Severe nausea, vomiting (usually begins 1-4 hrs after administration; may persist over 24 hrs). **OCCASIONAL:** A burning sensation originating at IV site and moving up arm (occurs particularly w/rapid IV injection), diarrhea, confusion, lethargy, depression, particularly in those receiving continuous IV infusion over 5 days.

ADVERSE REACTIONS/TOXIC EFFECTS

High incidence of nephrotoxicity manifested by azotemia, anuria, proteinuria, hyperchloremia, hypophosphatemia. Proximal renal tubular acidosis evidenced by glycosuria, acetonuria, aminoaciduria. Mild to moderate bone marrow depression manifested as hematologic toxicity (leukopenia, thrombocytopenia, anemia). Severe myelosuppression, hepatotoxicity occur rarely.

NURSING IMPLICATIONS

BASELINE ASSESSMENT:

Phenothiazine antiemetics only minimally effective in preventing/reducing nausea, vomiting; droperidol, metoclopramide appear to be more effective. Obtain renal function tests, electrolytes, CBC before and weekly during therapy. Obtain hepatic function tests before therapy.

INTERVENTION/EVALUATION:

Monitor urinalysis, creatinine clearance, BUN, serum creatinine, electrolyte, CBC. (Earliest sign of renal toxicity is mild proteinuria, glycosuria.) Inform physician if urine is positive for proteinuria or if vomiting exceeds 600-800 ml/8 hrs. Monitor for hematologic toxicity (fever, sore throat, signs of local infection, easy bruising, unusual bleeding from any site), symptoms of anemia (excessive tiredness, weakness).

PATIENT/FAMILY TEACHING:

Do not have immunizations w/o physician's approval (drug lowers body's resistance). Avoid contact w/those who have recently received live virus vaccine. Promptly report fever, sore throat, signs of local infection, easy bruising/unusual bleeding from any site. Increase fluid intake (decreases risk of nephrotoxicity). A burning sensation may be noted w/IV administration. Contact physician if nausea/vomiting continues at home.

succinylcholine chloride

suc-sin-eel-co´leen
(Anectine, Quelicin)

CANADIAN AVAILABILITY:
Anectine, Quelicin

(See Classifications section under Neuromuscular blockers)

sucralfate

sue-kral´fate
(Carafate)

CANADIAN AVAILABILITY:
Sulcrate

CLASSIFICATION

Antiulcer

PHARMACOKINETICS

Minimally absorbed from GI tract. Eliminated in feces w/small amount excreted in urine.

ACTION

Forms adhesive gel that adheres to ulcer site. Gel protects damaged mucosa from further destruction by absorbing gastric acid, pepsin, bile salts and reacting w/exudation of proteins.

USES

Short-term treatment (up to 8 wks) of duodenal ulcer. Maintenance therapy of duodenal ulcer after healing of acute ulcers.

PO ADMINISTRATION

1. Administer 1 hr before meals and at bedtime.
2. Tablets may be crushed/dissolved in water.
3. Avoid antacids ½ hr before or 2 hrs after giving sucralfate.

INDICATIONS/DOSAGE/ROUTES

NOTE: 1 Gm = 10 ml suspension.

Duodenal ulcers, active:
PO: Adults, elderly: 1 Gm 4 times/day (before meals and at bedtime) for up to 8 wks.

Duodenal ulcers, maintenance:
PO: Adults, elderly: 1 Gm 2 times/day.

PRECAUTIONS

CONTRAINDICATIONS: None significant. **CAUTIONS:** None significant. **PREGNANCY/LACTATION:** Unknown whether drug crosses placenta or is distributed in breast milk. **Pregnancy Category B.**

INTERACTIONS

DRUG INTERACTIONS: Antacids may interfere w/binding (do not give within 1/2 hr). May decrease absorption of digoxin, phenytoin, quinolones (e.g., ciprofloxacin), theophylline (do not give within 2-3 hrs of sucralfate). **ALTERED LAB VALUES:** None significant.

SIDE EFFECTS

RARE: Constipation, dry mouth.

ADVERSE REACTIONS/TOXIC EFFECTS

None significant.

NURSING IMPLICATIONS

INTERVENTION EVALUATION:

Monitor stool consistency and frequency.

PATIENT/FAMILY TEACHING:

Take medication on an empty stomach. Antacids may be given as an adjunct but should not be taken for 30 min before or after sucralfate (formation of sucralfate gel is activated by stomach acid). Dry mouth may be relieved by sour hard candy or sips of tepid water.

sufentanil citrate

sue-fen´tah-nil
(Sufenta)

CANADIAN AVAILABILITY:
Sufenta

(See Classifications section under Opioid analgesics)

sulconazole nitrate

sul-con´ah-zole
(Exelderm)

CLASSIFICATION

Antifungal

PHARMACOKINETICS

Minimal systemic absorption.

ACTION

Alters cell membrane permeability w/leakage of essential elements. Broad spectrum antifungal agent w/antifungal and antiyeast activity.

USES

Treatment of Tinea pedis (athlete's foot), T. cruris (jock itch), T. corporis (ringworm), T. versicolor.

INDICATIONS/DOSAGE/ROUTES

Tinea corporis, T. cruris, T. versicolor:
TOPICAL: Adults, elderly: 1-2 times/day for 3 wks.

Tinea pedis:
TOPICAL: Adults, elderly: 2 times/day for 4 wks.

PRECAUTIONS

CONTRAINDICATIONS: Hypersensitivity to sulconazole/any component of the preparation. **CAUTIONS:** Safety and efficacy in children not established. **PREGNANCY/LACTATION:** Unknown whether excreted in breast milk. **Pregnancy Category C.**

INTERACTIONS

DRUG INTERACTIONS: None significant. **ALTERED LAB VALUES:** None significant.

SIDE EFFECTS

OCCASIONAL: Stinging, burning, itching, redness at fungal site.

ADVERSE REACTIONS/TOXIC EFFECTS

None significant.

NURSING IMPLICATIONS

BASELINE ASSESSMENT:

Question for hypersensitivity to sulconazole/components of preparation. Confirm that culture and/or smears were done for accurate diagnosis; therapy may begin before results known.

INTERVENTION/EVALUATION:

Assess for therapeutic response or burning, itching, stinging.

PATIENT/FAMILY TEACHING:

Gently rub small amount of preparation into affected and surrounding areas. For external use; avoid getting in eyes. Do not interrupt/stop treatment (may take several weeks). Do not apply any other preparations/occlusive covering w/o consulting physician. Keep areas clean, dry; wear light clothing for ventilation. Separate personal items in contact w/affected areas. Thorough hand washing. Notify physician of increased burning, itching, or other symptom.

sulfacetamide sodium

sul-fah-see´tah-mide
(AK-Sulf, Bleph-10, Isopto Cetamide, Ophthacet, Sodium Sulamyd, Sulfair)

FIXED-COMBINATION(S): W/phenylephrine hydrochloride, a sympathomimetic (Vasosulf); w/ prednisolone, a steroid (Blephamide, Cetapred, Metimyd, Optimyd, Sulphrin, Vasocidin)

CANADIAN AVAILABILITY: AK-Sulf, Balsulph, Bleph-10, Sodium Sulamyd, Sulfex

CLASSIFICATION

Sulfonamide

PHARMACOKINETICS

Minimal absorption after ophthalmic administration.

ACTION

Interferes w/the biosynthesis of folic acid by inhibiting utilization of *p*-aminobenzoic acid in susceptible bacteria (only bacteria that synthesize own folic acid are affected). Bacteriostatic.

USES

Treatment of corneal ulcers, conjunctivitis and other superficial infections of the eye, prophylaxis after injuries to the eye/removal of foreign bodies, adjunctive therapy for trachoma and inclusion conjunctivitis. *Topical lotion:* Seborrheic dermatitis, seborrheic sicca (dandruff), secondary bacterial skin infections.

STORAGE/HANDLING

Protect from light. May develop a yellow-brown or reddish-brown color. Do not use if color change occurs/precipitate forms.

OPHTHALMIC ADMINISTRATION

1. Place finger on lower eyelid and pull out until a pocket is formed between eye and lower lid.
2. Hold dropper above pocket and place correct number of drops (¼-½ inch ointment) into pocket. Close eye gently.
3. For solution: Apply digital pressure to lacrimal sac for 1-2 min (minimizes drainage into nose and throat, reducing risk of systemic effects). For ointment: Close eye for 1-2 min, rolling eyeball (increases contact area of drug to eye).
4. Remove excess solution/ointment around eye w/tissue.

INDICATIONS/DOSAGE/ROUTES

Usual ophthalmic dosage:
OPHTHALMIC: Adults, elderly: Ointment: Apply small amount in lower conjunctival sac 1-4 times/day and at bedtime. Solution: 1-3 drops to lower conjunctival sac q2-3hr.

Usual topical dosage:
TOPICAL: Adults, elderly: Apply 1-4 times/day.

PRECAUTIONS

CONTRAINDICATIONS: Hypersensitivity to sulfonamides or any component of preparation (some products contain sulfite). **CAUTIONS:** Extremely dry eye. Application of lotion to large infected, denuded, or debrided areas. **PREGNANCY/LACTATION:** Unknown whether excreted in breast milk. **Pregnancy Category C.**

INTERACTIONS

DRUG INTERACTIONS: Silver-containing preparations are incompatible. **ALTERED LAB VALUES:** None significant.

SIDE EFFECTS

FREQUENT: Transient burning, stinging w/ophthalmic application. **OCCASIONAL:** Headache, local irritation. **RARE:** Hypersensitivity: Erythema, rash, itching, swelling.

Retarded corneal healing, photosensitivity.

ADVERSE REACTIONS/TOXIC EFFECTS

Superinfection, drug-induced lupus erythematosus, Stevens-Johnson syndrome occur rarely; nephrotoxicity w/high dermatologic concentrations.

NURSING IMPLICATIONS

BASELINE ASSESSMENT:

Question for hypersensitivity to sulfonamides, any ingredients of preparation (e.g., sulfite).

INTERVENTION/EVALUATION:

Withhold medication and notify physician at once of hypersensitivity reaction (redness, itching, urticaria, rash). Assess for fever, joint pain, or sores in mouth—discontinue drug and inform physician immediately.

PATIENT/FAMILY TEACHING:

Continue therapy as directed. May have transient burning, stinging upon ophthalmic application; may cause sensitivity to light—wear sunglasses, avoid bright light. Notify physician of *any* new symptom, esp. swelling, itching, rash, joint pain, fever. For topical skin/scalp treatment, cleanse (shampoo) area before application to ensure direct contact w/affected areas.

sulfamethoxazole

sul-fah-meth-ox´ah-zole
(Gantanol)

FIXED-COMBINATION(S): W/trimethoprim, an antibacterial (Bactrim, Septra, Sulfamethoprim, Cotrimoxizole); w/phenazopyridine, a urinary tract analgesic (Azo Gantanol, Azo-Sulfamethoxazole)

CANADIAN AVAILABILITY: Apo-Methoxazole, Gantanol

CLASSIFICATION

Sulfonamide

PHARMACOKINETICS

Rapid, well absorbed from GI tract. Widely distributed. Protein binding: 60-70%. Metabolized in liver. Primarily excreted in urine. Removed by hemodialysis. Half-life: 6-12 hrs (increased in decreased renal function).

ACTION

Interferes w/biosynthesis of folic acid by inhibiting utilization of *p*-aminobenzoic acid in susceptible bacteria (only bacteria that synthesize own folic acid are affected). Bacteriostatic.

USES

Treatment of urinary tract infections, nocardiosis, meningococcal meningitis prophylaxis (group A strains only), inclusion conjunctivitis, trachoma, chancroid, adjunctive therapy for malaria, toxoplasmosis, and acute otitis media.

PO ADMINISTRATION

1. Space doses evenly around clock.
2. Administer 1 hr before or 2 hrs after meals.
3. Give w/8 oz water; encourage several glasses of water between meals.

INDICATIONS/DOSAGE/ROUTES

Mild to moderate infections:
PO: Adults, elderly: Initially, 2

Gm, then 1 Gm 2 times/day (morning and evening).

Severe infections:
PO: Adults, elderly: Initially, 2 Gm, then 1 Gm 3 times/day.

Usual dosage for children:
PO: Children: Initially, 50-60 mg/kg, then 25-30 mg/kg 2 times/day (morning and evening).

PRECAUTIONS

CONTRAINDICATIONS: Hypersensitivity to sulfonamides or chemically related drugs (e.g., sulfonylureas, thiazides, acetazolamide, probenecid, some goitrogens), severe renal/hepatic dysfunction, porphyria, infants <2 mo (except for congenital toxoplasmosis), group A beta-hemolytic strep infections, chronic renal disease in children <6 yrs. **CAUTIONS:** Severe allergies, bronchial asthma, impaired renal/hepatic function, G-6-PD deficiency. **PREGNANCY/LACTATION:** Crosses placenta; is distributed in breast milk. Competes w/bilirubin for protein binding sites. May cause kernicterus. Contraindicated at term, in lactation. **Pregnancy Category C.**

INTERACTIONS

DRUG INTERACTIONS: May increase effects of oral anticoagulants, anticonvulsants, oral hypoglycemics, methotrexate. Hemolytics may increase toxicity. Hepatotoxic medications may increase hepatotoxicity. **ALTERED LAB VALUES:** May increase SGOT (AST), SGPT (ALT), bilirubin, BUN, creatinine.

SIDE EFFECTS

FREQUENT: Anorexia, nausea, vomiting, fever (7-10 days after initial dose), pruritus, rash. **OCCASIONAL:** Crystalluria/hematuria/oliguria (related to urinary concentration), diarrhea, dizziness, drowsiness, photosensitivity, headache, joint pain, urticaria, bronchospasm, insomnia, tinnitus. **RARE:** Hypoglycemia, diuresis, goiter production.

ADVERSE REACTIONS/TOXIC EFFECTS

Hematologic toxicity (thrombocytopenia, leukopenia, agranulocytosis, hemolytic anemia, aplastic anemia), Stevens-Johnson syndrome, anaphylaxis, peripheral neuropathy, disseminated lupus erythematosus, nephrotoxicity, hepatotoxicity, superinfection occur rarely.

NURSING IMPLICATIONS

BASELINE ASSESSMENT:

Question for hypersensitivity to any of the sulfonamides, chemically related drugs. Check initial urinanalysis (UA)/renal, CBC, hepatic function tests. Assure that specimens for culture and sensitivity have been obtained (therapy may begin before results are known).

INTERVENTION/EVALUATION:

Assess for rash (discontinue drug/notify physician at first sign). Be alert to hypersensitivity: Fever, joint pain, rash/urticaria, bronchospasm. Check I&O, UA/renal function tests; assure adequate hydration (minimum output 1,500 ml/24 hr) to prevent nephrotoxicity. Monitor CBCs closely; assess for/report immediately hematologic effects: Bleeding, bruising, fever, sore throat, pallor, weakness, purpura, jaundice. Evaluate for dizziness, provide ambulatory assistance. Assess food tolerance. Monitor temperature, report new/increased fever immediately. Check pattern of bowel activity, stool consistency. Monitor culture/sensitivity tests for therapeutic response.

PATIENT/FAMILY TEACHING:

Space doses evenly around clock; continue full length of treatment. Take w/8 oz water 1 hr before or 2 hrs after meals; if upset stomach occurs take w/meals. Drink several glasses of water between meals. Do not take any other medications (including vitamins) w/o consulting physician. Follow-up, lab tests are essential. In event of dental/other surgery inform dentist/surgeon of sulfa therapy. Notify physician of *any* new symptom, immediately for fever, sore throat, difficulty breathing, rash, any bleeding, ringing in ears. Avoid exposure to sun/ultraviolet light until photosensitivity determined (may last for months after last dose).

sulfasalazine

sul-fah-sal'ah-zeen
(Azulfidine, Azulfidine EN-tabs)

CANADIAN AVAILABILITY:
PMS Sulfasalazine, Salazopyrin, SAS-500

CLASSIFICATION

Sulfonamide, anti-inflammatory

PHARMACOKINETICS

Poorly absorbed from GI tract. Cleaved in colon by intestinal bacterial forming sulfapyridine and mesalamine (5-ASA). Absorbed in colon. Widely distributed. Protein binding: sulfapyridine: 50%, 5-ASA: 43%. Metabolized in liver. Primarily excreted in urine. Half-life: sulfapyridine: 6-14 hrs; 5-ASA: 0.6-1.4 hrs.

ACTION

Mesalamine: Blocks prostaglandin synthesis in colon. Produces local inhibitory effect on arachidonic acid metabolite production (increase in pts w/chronic inflammatory bowel disease).

USES

Treatment of ulcerative colitis.

PO ADMINISTRATION

1. Space doses evenly (intervals not to exceed 8 hrs).
2. Administer after meals if possible (prolong intestinal passage).
3. Swallow enteric-coated tablets whole, do not chew.
4. Give w/8 oz water; encourage several glasses of water between meals.

INDICATIONS/DOSAGE/ROUTES

Ulcerative colitis:
PO: Adults, elderly: Initially, 1-4 Gm/day in divided doses. **Maintenace:** 2 Gm/day in 4 divided doses. **Children >2 yrs:** Initially, 40-60 mg/kg/day in 4-6 divided doses. **Maintenance:** 20-30 mg/kg in 4 divided doses. **Maximum:** 2 Gm/day.

PRECAUTIONS

CONTRAINDICATIONS: Hypersensitivity to salicylates, sulfonamides, or chemically related drugs (e.g., sulfonylureas, thiazides, acetazolamide, probenecid, some goitrogens); severe hepatic/renal dysfunction, porphyria, intestinal/urinary tract obstruction, children <2 yrs. **CAUTIONS:** Severe allergies, bronchial asthma, impaired hepatic/renal function, G-6-PD deficiency. **PREGNANCY/LACTATION:** Crosses placenta; minimal distribution in breast milk. Risk of kernicterus is low. **Pregnancy Category C.**

INTERACTIONS

DRUG INTERACTIONS: May increase effects of oral anticoagulants, anticonvulsants, oral hypoglycemics, methotrexate. Hemolytics may increase toxicity. Hepatotoxic medications may increase hepatotoxicity. **ALTERED LAB VALUES:** None significant.

SIDE EFFECTS

FREQUENT: Anorexia, nausea, vomiting, headache, oligospermia (generally reversed by withdrawal of drug). **OCCASIONAL:** Hypersensitivity reaction: rash, urticaria, pruritus, fever, anemia. **RARE:** Tinnitus, hypoglycemia, diuresis, goiter production, photosensitivity.

ADVERSE REACTIONS/TOXIC EFFECTS

Increased urinary concentration produces crystalluria, hematuria, oliguria. Anaphylaxis, Stevens-Johnson syndrome, hematologic toxicity (leukopenia, agranulocytosis), hepatotoxicity, nephrotoxicity occur rarely.

NURSING IMPLICATIONS

BASELINE ASSESSMENT:

Question for hypersensitivity to salicylates, sulfonamides, or chemically related drugs (e.g., thiazides, sulfonylureas, acetazolamide, probenecid, goitrogens). Check initial urinalysis (UA)/renal, CBC, hepatic function tests. Assure that specimens for culture/sensitivity have been obtained (therapy may begin before results are known).

INTERVENTION/EVALUATION:

Check I&O, UA/renal function tests; assure adequate hydration (minimum output 1,500 ml/24 hr) to prevent nephrotoxicity. Evaluate food tolerance (distribute doses more evenly or consult physician regarding enteric-coated tablets, reduction of dose). Assess skin for rash (discontinue drug/notify physician at first sign). Check pattern of bowel activity, stool consistency (dosage may need to be increased if diarrhea continues/recurs). Monitor CBCs closely; assess for/report immediately hematologic effects: Bleeding, bruising, fever, sore throat, pallor, weakness, purpura, jaundice.

PATIENT/FAMILY TEACHING:

May cause orange-yellow discoloration of urine, skin. Space doses evenly around the clock. Take after food w/8 oz water; drink several glasses of water between meals. Continue for full length of treatment; may be necessary to take drug even after symptoms relieved. Do not take any other medications (including vitamins) w/o consulting physician. Follow-up, lab tests are essential. In event of dental/other surgery inform dentist/surgeon of sulfasalazine therapy. Notify physician of any new symptom, immediately for fever, sore throat, shortness of breath, rash, any bleeding, ringing in ears. Avoid exposure to sun/ultraviolet light until photosensitivity determined (may last for months after last dose).

sulindac

suel-in´dak
(Clinoril)

CANADIAN AVAILABILITY: Apo-Sulin, Clinoril, Novo Sundac

CLASSIFICATION

Nonsteroidal anti-inflammatory

PHARMACOKINETICS

	ONSET	PEAK	DURATION
PO (anti-rheumatic):	7 days	2-3 wks	—

Well absorbed from GI tract. Protein binding: >90%. Metabolized in liver to active metabolite. Primarily excreted in urine. Half-life: 7.8 hrs; metabolite: 16.4 hrs.

ACTION

Inhibits prostaglandin synthesis. Inhibits action of cyclooxygenase, decreases formation of prostaglandin, thromboxane precursors from arachidonic acid.

USES

Treatment of pain of rheumatoid arthritis, osteoarthritis, ankylosing spondylitis, acute painful shoulder, bursitis/tendonitis, acute gouty arthritis.

PO ADMINISTRATION

May give w/food, milk, or antacids if GI distress occurs.

INDICATIONS/DOSAGE/ROUTES

Rheumatoid arthritis, osteoarthritis, ankylosing spondylitis:
PO: Adults, elderly: Initially, 150 mg 2 times/day, up to 400 mg/day.

Acute painful shoulder, gouty arthritis, bursitis, tendonitis:
PO: Adults, elderly: 200 mg 2 times/day.

PRECAUTIONS

CONTRAINDICATIONS: Active peptic ulcer, GI ulceration, chronic inflammation of GI tract, GI bleeding disorders, history of hypersensitivity to aspirin/nonsteroidal anti-inflammatory agent. **CAUTIONS:** Impaired renal/hepatic function, history of GI tract disease, predisposition to fluid retention. **PREGNANCY/LACTATION:** Unknown whether drug is excreted in breast milk. Avoid use during third trimester (may adversely affect fetal cardiovascular system: Premature closure of ductus arteriosus). **Pregnancy Category C.**

INTERACTIONS

DRUG INTERACTIONS: May increase effects of oral anticoagulants, heparin, thrombolytics. May decrease effect of antihypertensives, diuretics. Salicylates, aspirin may increase risk of GI side effects, bleeding. Bone marrow depressants may increase risk of hematologic reactions. May increase concentration, toxicity of lithium. May increase methotrexate toxicity. Probenecid may increase concentration. Antacids may decrease concentration. **ALTERED LAB VALUES:** May increase alkaline phosphatase, liver function tests.

SIDE EFFECTS

NOTE: Age increases possibility of side effects.
FREQUENT: Diarrhea/constipation, indigestion, nausea, maculopapular rash, dermatitis, dizziness, headache. **OCCASIONAL:** Anorexia, GI cramps, flatulence.

ADVERSE REACTIONS/TOXIC EFFECTS

GI bleeding, peptic ulcer occur infrequently. Nephrotoxicity (glomerular nephritis, interstitial nephritis, and nephrotic syndrome) may occur in those w/preexisting impaired renal function. Acute hypersensitivity reaction (fever, chills, joint pain) occurs rarely.

NURSING IMPLICATIONS

BASELINE ASSESSMENT:

Assess onset, type, location, and duration of pain, fever, or inflammation. Inspect appearance of affected joints for immobility, deformities, and skin condition.

INTERVENTION/EVALUATION:

Assist w/ambulation if dizziness occurs. Monitor pattern of daily bowel activity, stool consistency. Assess for evidence of rash. Evaluate for therapeutic response: Relief of pain, stiffness, swelling, increase in joint mobility, reduced joint tenderness, improved grip strength.

PATIENT/FAMILY TEACHING:

Therapeutic antiarthritic effect noted 1-3 wks after therapy begins. Avoid aspirin, alcohol during therapy (increases risk of GI bleeding). If GI upset occurs, take w/food, milk.

sumatriptan succinate injection

sew-mah-trip'tan

(Imitrex)

CLASSIFICATION

Serotonin selective agonist (5-HT_1)

PHARMACOKINETICS

	ONSET	PEAK	DURATION
SubQ	<10 min	<2 hrs	—

Rapidly absorbed after SubQ administration. Widely distributed, protein binding (10-21%). Undergoes first-pass hepatic metabolism; excreted in urine. Half-life: 2 hrs.

ACTION

Binds selectively to vascular 5-HT_1 receptors producing a vasoconstrictive effect on cranial blood vessels. Vasoconstriction is associated w/relief of migraine. Efficiency of relief unaffected by aura, duration of attack, concurrent use of other antimigraine medications (e.g., beta blockers).

USES

Acute treatment of migraine headache w/ or w/o aura.

STORAGE/HANDLING

Store at room temperature.

INDICATIONS/DOSAGE/ROUTES

Vascular headache:

SubQ: Adults, elderly: 6 mg. **Maximum:** No more than two 6 mg injections within a 24-hr period separated by at least 1 hr between injections.

PRECAUTIONS

CONTRAINDICATIONS: IV use, those w/ischemic heart disease (angina pectoris, history of myocardial infarction), silent ischemia, Prinzmetal's angina, uncontrolled hypertension, concurrent ergotamine-containing preparations, hemiplegic or basilar migraine. **CAUTIONS:** Hepatic, renal impairment. Pt profile suggesting cardiovascular risks. **PREGNANCY/LACTATION:** Unknown whether distributed in breast milk. **Pregnancy Category C.**

INTERACTIONS

DRUG INTERACTIONS: Ergotamine-containing drugs may produce vasospastic reaction. Monoamine oxidase inhibitors may increase concentration, half-life. **ALTERED LAB VALUES:** None significant.

SIDE EFFECTS

FREQUENT: Discomfort, redness at site of injection (usually lasts <1 hr). **OCCASIONAL:** Tingling, feeling of heat, facial flushing, feeling of heaviness or pressure, numbness, mouth/jaw/neck/nasal discomfort. **RARE:** Drowsiness, cold sensation, anxiety.

ADVERSE REACTIONS/TOXIC EFFECTS

Excessive dosage may produce tremor, redness of extremities, reduced respirations, cyanosis, convulsions, paralysis. Serious arrhythmias occur rarely, but particularly in those w/hypertension, obesity, smokers, diabetics and those w/strong family history of coronary artery disease.

NURSING IMPLICATIONS

BASELINE ASSESSMENT:

Question pt regarding history of peripheral vascular disease, renal/hepatic impairment, or possibility of pregnancy. Question pt regarding onset, location, and duration of migraine and possible precipitating symptoms.

INTERVENTION/EVALUATION:

Evaluate for relief of migraine headache and resulting photophobia, phonophobia (sound sensitivity), nausea and vomiting.

PATIENT/FAMILY TEACHING:

Teach pt proper loading of autoinjector, injection technique, and discarding of syringe. Do not use more than 2 injections during any 24-hr period and allow at least 1 hr between injections. If experience wheezing, heart throbbing, skin rash, swelling of eyelids, face, or lips, pain/tightness in chest or throat, contact physician immediately.

suprofen

sue-pro´fen

(Profenal)

CLASSIFICATION

Nonsteroidal anti-inflammatory

PHARMACOKINETICS

Penetrates cornea after ophthalmic administration. May be systemically absorbed.

ACTION

Inhibits prostaglandin synthesis. Prevents, reduces miosis by relaxing iris sphincter.

USES

Inhibition of intraoperative miosis.

OPHTHALMIC ADMINISTRATION

1. Place finger on lower eyelid and pull out until pocket is formed between eye and lower lid. Hold dropper above pocket and place prescribed number of drops into pocket. Close eye gently. Apply digital pressure to lacrimal sac for 1-2 min (minimized drainage into nose and throat, reducing risk of systemic effects). Remove excess solution w/tissue.

INDICATIONS/DOSAGE/ROUTES

Ophthalmic:

PO: Adults, elderly: Apply 2 drops into conjunctival sac 3, 2, and 1 hr before surgery or 2 drops q4h while awake, day before surgery.

PRECAUTIONS

CONTRAINDICATIONS: Epithelial herpes simplex keratitis (dendritic keratitis). **CAUTIONS:** Surgical pts w/known bleeding tendencies. **PREGNANCY/LACTATION:** Distributed in low concentration in breast milk. **Pregnancy Category C.**

INTERACTIONS

DRUG INTERACTIONS: May decrease effect of acetylcholine, carbachol. May decrease antiglaucoma effect of epinephrine, other antiglaucoma medications. **ALTERED LAB VALUES:** None significant.

SIDE EFFECTS

FREQUENT: Burning, stinging on instillation, keratitis, elevated intraocular pressure.

ADVERSE REACTIONS/TOXIC EFFECTS

None significant.

NURSING IMPLICATIONS

PATIENT/FAMILY TEACHING:

Report eye irritation.

tacrine

tay'crin
(Cognex)

CLASSIFICATION

Cholinergic agent

PHARMACOKINETICS

Rapidly absorbed from GI tract. Protein binding: 55%. Undergoes first-pass metabolism in liver. Half-life: 2-4 hrs.

ACTION

Enhances cholinergic function by inhibiting acetylcholinesterase. May also selectively block potassium channels in CNS, change phosphorylation, block both pre- and postsynaptic muscarinic and nicotinic receptors.

USES

Symptomatic treatment of pts w/ Alzheimer's disease.

PO ADMINISTRATION

May take w/o regard to food.

INDICATIONS/DOSAGE/ROUTES

Alzheimer's disease:
PO: Adults, elderly: Initially, 10 mg 4 times/day for 6 wks; then 20 mg 4 times/day for 6 wks; then 30 mg 4 times/day for 12 wks; then to maximum of 40 mg 4 times/day if needed.
NOTE: If medication is stopped for >14 days, must retitrate as noted above.

PRECAUTIONS

CONTRAINDICATIONS: Known hypersensitivity to cholinergics; current treatment w/other cholinesterase inhibitors; severe, active liver disease; active, untreated gastric/duodenal ulcers; mechanical obstruction of intestine/urinary tract; pregnancy, nursing, or childbearing potential. **CAUTIONS:** Known liver dysfunction, asthma, COPD, seizure disorders, bradycardia, hyperthyroidism, cardiac arrhythmias, history of gastric/intestinal ulcers, alcohol abuse. **PREGNANCY/LACTATION:** May cause fetal harm; unknown whether secreted in breast milk. **Pregnancy Category X.**

INTERACTIONS

DRUG INTERACTIONS: May increase theophylline concentration; cimetidine may increase tacrine concentrations; may interfere w/ anticholinergics; may increase adverse effects of NSAIDs. **ALTERED LAB VALUES:** Increase SGOT (AST), SGPT (ALT); alters hematocrit, hemoglobin, electrolytes.

SIDE EFFECTS

FREQUENT: Nausea, vomiting, diarrhea, dizziness, headache. **OCCASIONAL:** Dyspepsia, constipation, myalgia, rhinitis, depression, anorexia, fatigue, chest pain. **RARE:** Agitation, rash, confusion, ataxia, insomnia, urinary frequency/incontinence.

ADVERSE REACTIONS/TOXIC EFFECTS

Overdose can cause cholinergic crises (increased salivation, lacrimation, urination, defecation, bradycardia, hypotension, increased muscle weakness). Treatment aimed at general supportive measures, use of anticholinergics (e.g., atropine).

NURSING IMPLICATIONS

Baseline Assessment:

Assess cognitive, behavioral, and functional deficits of pt. Assess liver function.

Intervention/Evaluation:

Monitor cognitive, behavioral, and functional status of pt. Monitor SGOT (AST), SGPT (ALT). ECG evaluation, periodic rhythm strips in pts w/underlying arrhythmias. Monitor for symptoms of ulcer, GI bleeding.

Patient/Family Teaching:

Take at regular intervals, between meals (may take w/meals if GI upset occurs). Do not reduce or stop medication; do not increase dosage w/o physician direction. Report increasing or new symptoms. Do not smoke (reduces plasma concentration of tacrine). Periodic lab tests are essential. Inform family of local chapter of Alzheimer's Disease Association (provides a guide to services for these pts).

---

tacrolimus (Prograf)
See supplement

---

tamoxifen citrate

tam-ox´ih-fen
(Nolvadex)

CANADIAN AVAILABILITY:
Apo-Tamox, Nolvaldex-D, Novo-Tamoxifen, Tamofen, Tamone

CLASSIFICATION

PHARMACOTHERAPEUTIC: Nonsteroidal, antiestrogen

CLINICAL: Antineoplastic

PHARMACOKINETICS

Well absorbed from GI tract. Metabolized in liver. Primarily eliminated in feces via biliary system. Half-life: 7 days.

ACTION

Competes w/estradiol for binding to estrogen receptors in tissues containing high concentration of receptors (e.g., breasts, uterus, vagina). Receptor complexes translocated to nucleus, reducing DNA synthesis, estrogen responses.

USES

Treatment of metastatic breast carcinoma in women/men. Effective in delaying recurrence following total mastectomy and axillary dissection or segmental mastectomy, axillary dissection and breast irradiation in women w/axillary node–negative breast carcinoma.

INDICATIONS/DOSAGE/ROUTES

Usual dosage:
PO: Adults, elderly: 10-20 mg 2 times/day in morning and evening.

PRECAUTIONS

CONTRAINDICATIONS: None significant. **CAUTIONS:** Leukopenia, thrombocytopenia, increased risk of uterine cancer. **PREGNANCY/LACTATION:** If possible, avoid use during pregnancy, esp. first trimester. May cause fetal harm. Breast feeding not recommended. **Pregnancy Category D.**

INTERACTIONS

DRUG INTERACTIONS: Estrogens may decrease effect. **ALTERED LAB VALUES:** May increase calcium, cholesterol, triglycerides.

SIDE EFFECTS

FREQUENT: Hot flashes, nausea, vomiting, vaginal bleeding/discharge, pruritus vulvae, skin rash. **OCCASIONAL:** Transient increase in bone pain, size of soft tissue tumor (sometimes w/erythema and surrounding soft tissue site), peripheral edema, distaste for food, mental depression, leg cramps, dizziness, weakness, lightheadedness, headache. In those w/bone metastases, hypercalcemia may be noted during initial therapy.

ADVERSE REACTIONS/TOXIC EFFECTS

Retinopathy, corneal opacity, decreased visual acuity noted in those receiving extremely high doses (240-320 mg/day) for >17 mo.

NURSING IMPLICATIONS

BASELINE ASSESSMENT:

An estrogen receptor assay should be done before therapy is begun. CBC, platelet count, serum calcium levels should be checked before and periodically during therapy.

INTERVENTION/EVALUATION:

Be alert to increased bone pain and assure adequate pain relief. Monitor I&O, weight; check for edema, esp. of dependent areas. Assess for hypercalcemia (increased urine volume, excessive thirst, nausea, vomiting, constipation, hypotonicity of muscles, deep-bone or flank pain, renal stones).

PATIENT/FAMILY TEACHING:

Report vaginal bleeding/discharge/itching, leg cramps, weight gain, shortness of breath, weakness. May initially experience increase in bone, tumor pain (appears to indicate good tumor response). Contact physician if nausea/vomiting continues at home. Nonhormone contraceptives are recommended during treatment. Have regular gynecologic exams. Report menstrual irregularities, pelvic pain, pressure.

---

teicoplanin (Targocid)
See supplement

---

temazepam

tem-az´eh-pam
(Restoril)

CANADIAN AVAILABILITY:
Restoril

CLASSIFICATION

Sedative-hypnotics

PHARMACOKINETICS

Well absorbed from GI tract. Widely distributed. Crosses blood-brain barrier. Protein binding: 96%. Metabolized in liver. Primarily excreted in urine. Half-life: 8-15 hrs.

ACTION

Enhances action of inhibitory neurotransmitter gamma-aminobutyric acid (GABA). Depressant effects occur at all levels of CNS.

USES

Short-term treatment of insomnia (up to 5 wks). Reduces sleep-induction time, number of nocturnal awakenings; increases length of sleep.

PO ADMINISTRATION

1. Give w/o regard to meals.
2. Capsules may be emptied and mixed w/food.

INDICATIONS/DOSAGE/ROUTES

Hypnotic:
PO: Adults >18 yrs: 15-30 mg at bedtime. **Elderly/debilitated:** 15 mg at bedtime.

PRECAUTIONS

CONTRAINDICATIONS: Acute narrow-angle glaucoma, acute alcohol intoxication. **CAUTIONS:** Impaired renal/hepatic function. **PREGNANCY/LACTATION:** Crosses placenta; may be distributed in breast milk. Chronic ingestion during pregnancy may produce withdrawal symptoms, CNS depression in neonates. **Pregnancy Category X.**

INTERACTIONS

DRUG INTERACTIONS: Alcohol, CNS depressants may increase CNS depressant effect. **ALTERED LAB VALUES:** None significant.

SIDE EFFECTS

FREQUENT: Drowsiness, sedation, rebound insomnia (may occur for 1-2 nights after drug is discontinued), dizziness, confusion, euphoria. **OCCASIONAL:** Weakness, anorexia, diarrhea. **RARE:** Paradoxical CNS excitement, restlessness (particularly noted in elderly/debilitated).

ADVERSE REACTION/TOXIC EFFECTS

Abrupt or too-rapid withdrawal may result in pronounced restlessness, irritability, insomnia, hand tremors, abdominal/muscle cramps, sweating, vomiting, seizures. Overdosage results in somnolence, confusion, diminished reflexes, coma.

NURSING IMPLICATIONS

BASELINE ASSESSMENT:

Assess B/P, pulse, respirations immediately before administration. Raise bed rails. Provide environment conducive to sleep (back rub, quiet environment, low lighting).

INTERVENTION/EVALUATION:

Assess sleep pattern of pt. Assess elderly/debilitated for paradoxical reaction, particularly during early therapy. Evaluate for therapeutic response: Decrease in number of nocturnal awakenings, increase in length of sleep.

PATIENT/FAMILY TEACHING:

Do not exceed prescribed dosage. Smoking reduces drug effectiveness. Do not abruptly withdraw medication following long-term use. Rebound insomnia may occur when drug is discontinued after short-term therapy. Avoid alcohol and other CNS depressants. Inform physician if you are or are planning to become pregnant.

teniposide

ten-ih'poe-side
(Vumon)

CANADIAN AVAILABILITY:
Vumon

CLASSIFICATION

Antineoplastic

PHARMACOKINETICS

Does not efficiently cross blood-brain barrier. Protein binding: >99%. Metabolized extensively in liver. Primarily excreted in urine. Half-life: 5 hrs.

ACTION

Inhibits topoisomerase II causing single and double strand DNA breaks halting cell division. Phase specific acting in late S and early G_2 phases of cell cycle.

USES

In combination w/other antineoplastic agents, induction therapy in pts w/refractory childhood acute lymphoblastic leukemia.

STORAGE/HANDLING

Refrigerate unopened ampules. Protect from light. Reconstituted solutions stable for 24 hrs at room temperature. Discard if precipitation occurs. Use 1 mg/ml solutions within 4 hrs of preparation (reduces potential for precipitation). Do not refrigerate reconstituted solutions.

IV ADMINISTATION

NOTE: Administer by slow IV infusion. Wear gloves when preparing solution. If powder or solution come in contact w/skin, wash immediately and thoroughly w/soap, water.

1. Dilute teniposide w/5% dextrose, 0.9 NaCl injection to provide final concentration of 0.1, 0.2, 0.4 or 1 mg/ml.
2. Avoid contact of undiluted teniposide w/plastic (may cause softening/cracking and possible drug leakage).
3. Prepare/administer in non-DEHP containing LVP containers such as glass or polyolefin plastic bags/containers. Avoid use of PVC containers.
4. Give over at least 30-60 min (decreases hypotension). Do not give by rapid IV injection.
5. Avoid contact w/other drugs/fluids.
6. Monitor for anaphylactic reaction during infusion (chills, fever, dyspnea, sweating, lacrimation, sneezing, throat/back/chest pain).

T

INDICATIONS/DOSAGE/ROUTES

Dosage individualized based on clinical response, tolerance to adverse effects. When used in combination therapy, consult specific protocols for optimum dosage, sequence of drug administration.

PRECAUTIONS

CONTRAINDICATIONS: Hypersensitivity to etoposide, teniposide, or Cremophor EL (polyoxyethylated castor oil); platelet count <50,000/mm^3; absolute neutrophil count <500/mm^3. **CAUTIONS:** Pts w/brain tumors/neuroblastoma (increase risk of anaphylaxis). Retreating pts w/hypersensitivity reaction to teniposide. Pts w/Down's syndrome, decrease liver function. **PREGNANCY/LACTATION:** If possible, avoid use during pregnancy, esp. during first trimester. May cause fetal harm. Breast feeding not recommended. Unknown whether excreted in breast milk. **Pregnancy Category D.**

INTERACTIONS

DRUG INTERACTIONS: May increase intracellular accumulation of methotrexate. May increase severity of peripheral neuropathy w/vincristine. Bone marrow depressants may increase bone marrow depression. Live virus vaccines may potentiate virus replication, increase vaccine side effects, decrease pt's antibody response to vaccine. **ALTERED LAB VALUES:** None significant.

SIDE EFFECTS

FREQUENT: Mucositis, nausea, vomiting, diarrhea, anemia. **OCCASIONAL:** Alopecia, rash. **RARE:** Liver dysfunction, fever, renal dysfunction, peripheral neurotoxicity.

ADVERSE REACTIONS/TOXIC EFFECTS

Bone marrow depression manifested as hematologic toxicity (principally leukopenia, neutropenia, thrombocytopenia) w/increased risk of infection or bleeding. Hypersensitivity reaction, including anaphylaxis (chills, fever, tachycardia, bronchospasm, dyspnea, facial flushing).

NURSING IMPLICATIONS

BASELINE ASSESSMENT:

Assess hematology (platelet count, Hgb, WBC, differential), renal and hepatic function tests before and frequently during therapy.

INTERVENTION/EVALUATION:

Have antihistamines, corticosteroids, epinephrine, IV fluids, and other supportive measures readily available for first dose (possible life threatening anaphylaxis as evidenced by chills, fever, tachycardia, bronchospasm, dyspnea, hyper/hypotension, facial flushing). Monitor for myelosuppression: infection (fever, sore throat, signs of local infection); unusual bleeding or bruising; anemia (excessive tiredness, weakness). Pretreat w/antiemetics for nausea, vomiting but be alert to hypotension and CNS depression that may occur w/these drug combinations (because of benzyl alcohol in teniposide, esp. w/high doses).

PATIENT/FAMILY TEACHING:

Avoid crowds, those w/infection. Do not have immunizations w/o physician's approval. Promptly report fever, signs of infection, easy bruising or unusual bleeding from any site, difficulty breathing. Avoid pregnancy. Alopecia is reversible, but new hair growth may have different color or texture.

terazosin hydrochloride

tear-ah-zoe´sin

(Hytrin)

CANADIAN AVAILABILITY:

Hytrin

CLASSIFICATION

Antihypertensive

PHARMACOKINETICS

	ONSET	PEAK	DURATION
PO	15 min	1-2 hrs	12-24 hrs

Rapid, complete absorption from GI tract. Protein binding: 90-94%. Metabolized in liver to active metabolite. Primarily eliminated in feces via biliary system; excreted in urine. Half-life: 12 hrs.

ACTION

Blocks alpha-adrenergic receptors. *HTN:* Produces vasodilation, decrease peripheral resistance. *BPH:* Relaxes smooth muscle in bladder neck and prostate.

USES

Treatment of mild to moderate hypertension. Used alone or in combination w/other antihypertensives. Treatment of benign prostatic hypertrophy.

PO ADMINISTRATION

1. May give w/o regard to food.
2. Tablets may be crushed.
3. Administer first dose at bedtime (minimizes risk of fainting due to "first-dose syncope").

INDICATIONS/DOSAGE/ROUTES

NOTE: If medication is discontinued for several days, retitrate initially using 1 mg dose at bedtime.

Hypertension:
PO: Adults, elderly: Initially, 1 mg at bedtime. Slowly increase dose to desired levels. **Range:** 1-5 mg/day as single or 2 divided doses. **Maximum:** 20 mg.

Benign prostatic hypertrophy:
PO: Adults, elderly: Initially, 1 mg at bedtime. May increase up to 10 mg/day. **Maximum:** 20 mg/day.

PRECAUTIONS

CONTRAINDICATIONS: None significant. **CAUTIONS:** Chronic renal failure, impaired hepatic function. **PREGNANCY/LACTATION:** Unknown whether drug crosses placenta or is distributed in breast milk. **Pregnancy Category C.**

INTERACTIONS

DRUG INTERACTIONS: Estrogen, NSAIDs, sympathomimetics may decrease effect. Hypotension-producing medications may increase anti-hypertensive effect. **ALTERED LAB VALUES:** May decrease albumin, total protein, Hgb, Hct, WBC.

SIDE EFFECTS

FREQUENT: Dizziness, headache, asthenia (weakness, tiredness, lassitude, fatigue). **OCCASIONAL:** Nasal congestion, peripheral edema, nausea, palpitations, extremity pain, dyspnea, sinusitis. **RARE:** Paresthesia, back pain, nervousness, blurred vision.

ADVERSE REACTIONS/TOXIC EFFECTS

"First-dose syncope" (hypotension w/sudden loss of consciousness) generally occurs 30-90 min after giving initial dose of ≥2 mg, a too-rapid increase in dose, or addition of another hypotensive agent to therapy. May be preceded by tachycardia (120-160 beats/min).

NURSING IMPLICATIONS

BASELINE ASSESSMENT:

Give first dose at bedtime. If initial dose is given during daytime, pt must remain recumbent for 3-4 hrs. Assess B/P, pulse immediately before each dose, and q15-30min until stabilized (be alert to B/P fluctuations).

INTERVENTION/EVALUATION:

Monitor pulse diligently ("first-dose syncope" may be preceded by tachycardia). Assist w/ambulation if dizziness occurs. Assess for peripheral edema of hands, feet (usually, first area of low extremity swelling is behind medial malleolus in ambulatory, sacral area in bedridden).

PATIENT/FAMILY TEACHING:

Noncola carbonated beverage, unsalted crackers, dry toast may relieve nausea. Nasal congestion may occur. Full therapeutic effect may not occur for 3-4 wks.

terbinafine hydrochloride

tur-bin'ah-feen
(Lamisil)

CLASSIFICATION

Antifungal

PHARMACOKINETICS

Minimal systemic absorption following topical administration.

ACTION

Fungicidal. Interferes w/sterol biosynthesis through inhibition of the enzyme squalene epoxidase, resulting in decreased ergosterol, accumulation of squalene in cells, fungal cell death.

USES

Treatment of *Tinea cruris* (jock itch), *T. pedis* (athlete's foot), *T corporis* (ringworm).

INDICATIONS/DOSAGE/ROUTES

NOTE: Therapy for minimum 1 wk not to exceed 4 wks.

Tinea pedis:
TOPICAL: Adults, elderly, adolescents: Apply 2 times/day until signs/symptoms significantly improved.

Tinea cruris, T. corporis:
TOPICAL: Adults, elderly, adolescents: Apply 1-2 times/day until signs/symptoms significantly improved.

PRECAUTIONS

CONTRAINDICATIONS: Hypersensitivity to terbinafine or any component in formulation. Safety in children <12 yrs not established. **CAUTIONS:** Confirm diagnosis by direct microscopic exam or culture. For external use only. Not for oral, ophthalmic, intravaginal use. **PREGNANCY/LACTATION:** Unknown whether excreted in breast milk. Avoid application to the breast. **Pregnancy Category B.**

INTERACTIONS

DRUG INTERACTIONS: None significant. **ALTERED LAB VALUES:** None significant.

SIDE EFFECTS

OCCASIONAL: Irritation, burning, itching, dryness.

ADVERSE REACTIONS/TOXIC EFFECTS

None significant.

NURSING IMPLICATIONS

BASELINE ASSESSMENT:

Assure that diagnostic tests have been completed, e.g., culture or direct microscopic examination of scrapings from infected tissue.

INTERVENTION/EVALUATION:

Check for therapeutic response. Notify physician if local reaction occurs (irritation, redness, swelling, itching, oozing, blistering, burning).

PATIENT/FAMILY TEACHING:

Complete full course of treatment. Use only as directed for the time indicated. Keep areas clean and dry; wear light clothing to promote ventilation. Separate personal items. For external use only. Avoid contact w/eyes, nose, mouth, or other mucous membranes. Rub well into affected, surrounding area. Do not cover w/occlusive dressing or use other preparations w/o consulting physician. Notify physician of local reaction (see above).

terbutaline sulfate

tur-byew'ta-leen

(Brethaire, Brethine, Bricanyl)

CANADIAN AVAILABILITY:
Bricanyl

CLASSIFICATION

Sympathomimetic

PHARMACOKINETICS

	ONSET	PEAK	DURATION
PO	30 min	1-3 hrs	4-8 hrs
SubQ	15 min	30-60 min	1.5-4 hrs
Inhalation	5-30 min	1-2 hrs	3-4 hrs

Moderately absorbed from GI tract; well absorbed after SubQ administration. Metabolized in liver. Primarily excreted in urine. Half-life: 11-16 hrs.

ACTION

Stimulates $beta_2$-adrenergic receptors in lungs (relaxes bronchial smooth muscle, relieves bronchospasm, reduces airway resistance). Relaxes uterine muscle, inhibiting uterine contractions.

USES

Symptomatic relief of reversible bronchospasm due to bronchial asthma, bronchitis, emphysema. Delays premature labor.

STORAGE/HANDLING

Store oral, parenteral form at room temperature. Do not use if solution appears discolored.

PO/INHALATION/SubQ ADMINISTRATION

PO:

1. May give w/o regard to food (take w/food if GI upset occurs).
2. Tablets may be crushed.

INHALATION:

1. Shake container well, exhale completely. Holding mouthpiece 1 inch away from lips, inhale and hold breath as long as possible before exhaling.
2. Wait 1-10 min before inhaling second dose (allows for deeper bronchial penetration).
3. Rinse mouth w/water immediately after inhalation (prevents mouth/throat dryness).

SubQ:

1. Inject SubQ into lateral deltoid region.

INDICATIONS/DOSAGE/ROUTES

Bronchospasm:

PO: Adults, elderly, children >15

T

yrs: Initially, 2.5 mg 3-4 times/day. **Maintenance:** 2.5-5 mg 3 times/day q6h while awake. **Maximum:** 15 mg/day. **Children 12-15 yrs:** 2.5 mg 3 times/day. **Maximum:** 7.5 mg/day.

INHALATION: Adults, elderly, children >12 yrs: 2 inhalations q4-6h. Allow at least 1 min between inhalations.

SubQ: Adults: Initially, 0.25 mg. Repeat in 15-30 min if substantial improvement does not occur. **Maximum:** No more than 0.5 mg/4 hrs.

Premature labor:

PO: Adults: 2.5 mg q4-6h until term.

IV INFUSION: Adults: Initially, 10 mcg/min, increase by 5 mcg/min q10min up to maximum of 80 mcg/min or until contractions cease. (After contractions cease for 1/2 - 1 hr, decrease by 5 mcg/min to lowest effective dose).

SubQ: Adults: 0.25 mg q1h until contractions cease.

PRECAUTIONS

CONTRAINDICATIONS: History of hypersensitivity to sympathomimetics. **CAUTIONS:** Impaired cardiac function, diabetes, mellitus, hypertension, hyperthyroidism, history of seizures. **PREGNANCY/LACTATION:** Transient hypokalemia, pulmonary edema, hypoglycemia may occur if given during labor. Hypoglycemia may be found in neonate. Distributed in breast milk. **Pregnancy Category B.**

INTERACTIONS

DRUG INTERACTIONS: Tricyclic antidepressants may increase cardiovascular effects. MAO inhibitors may increase risk of hypertensive crises. May decrease effects of beta-blockers. Digoxin, sympathomimetics may increase risk of arrhythmias. **ALTERED LAB VALUES:** May decrease serum potassium levels.

SIDE EFFECTS

FREQUENT: Shakiness, restlessness, increased heart rate, and mild, transient nausea if taken on an empty stomach. Drying or irritation of oropharynx noted w/inhalation therapy.

ADVERSE REACTIONS/TOXIC EFFECTS

Too-frequent or excessive use may lead to loss of bronchodilating effectiveness and/or severe, paradoxical bronchoconstriction. Excessive sympathomimetic stimulation may cause palpitations, extrasystoles, tachycardia, chest pain, slight increase in B/P followed by a substantial decrease, chills, sweating, and blanching of skin.

NURSING IMPLICATIONS

BASELINE ASSESSMENT:

Offer emotional support (high incidence of anxiety due to difficulty in breathing and sympathomimetic response to drug).

INTERVENTION/EVALUATION:

Monitor rate, depth, rhythm, type of respiration; quality and rate of pulse. Assess lung sounds for rhonchi, wheezing, rales. Monitor arterial blood gases. Observe lips, fingernails for blue or dusky color in light-skinned patients; gray in dark-skinned pts. Observe for clavicular retractions, hand tremor. Evaluate for clinical improvement (quieter, slower respirations, relaxed facial expression, cessation of clavicular retractions).

PATIENT/FAMILY TEACHING:

Increase fluid intake (decreases lung secretion viscosity). Do not take more than 2 inhalations at any one time (excessive use may produce paradoxical bronchoconstriction, or a decreased bronchodilating effect). Rinsing mouth w/water immediately after inhalation may prevent mouth/throat dryness. Avoid excessive use of caffeine derivatives (chocolate, coffee, tea, cola, cocoa).

terconazole

ter-con´ah-zole
(Terazol)

CANADIAN AVAILABILITY
Terazol

CLASSIFICATION

Antifungal

PHARMACOKINETICS

Systemic absorption minimal following intravaginal administration.

ACTION

Alters cell membrane permeability w/leakage of essential elements (e.g., amino acids, potassium) and impaired uptake of precursor molecules (e.g., purine and pyrimidine precursors to DNA). Inhibits cytochrome, leading to accumulation of sterols and decreased concentrations of ergosterol. Usually fungicidal against *Candida albicans.*

USES

Treatment of vulvovaginal candidiasis (moniliasis).

INTRAVAGINAL ADMINISTRATION

1. Use disposable gloves; always wash hands thoroughly after application.
2. Follow manufacturer's directions for use of applicator.
3. Insert suppository, applicator high in vagina.
4. Administration at bedtime is preferred.

INDICATIONS/DOSAGE/ROUTES

Vulvovaginal candidiasis:
INTRAVAGINAL: Adults, elderly: 1 applicatorful at bedtime for 7 days.

PRECAUTIONS

CONTRAINDICATIONS: Hypersensitivity to terconazole or any component of the cream or suppository. **CAUTIONS:** Safety and efficacy in children not established. **PREGNANCY/LACTATION:** Unknown whether excreted in breast milk. **Pregnancy Category C.**

INTERACTIONS

DRUG INTERACTIONS: None significant. **ALTERED LAB VALUES:** None significant.

SIDE EFFECTS

FREQUENT: Headache (26% of pts). **OCCASIONAL:** Body pain; vulvovaginal pain, burning, itching, irritation. **RARE:** Flu-like syndrome: Fever, chills, headache, and/or hypotension, occasionally w/vertigo and nausea.

ADVERSE REACTIONS/TOXIC EFFECTS

None significant.

NURSING IMPLICATIONS

BASELINE ASSESSMENT:

Question for hypersensitivity to

terconazole or components of preparation. Confirm that a potassium hydroxide (KOH) culture and/or smear were done for accurate diagnosis; therapy may begin before results known. For suppository, inquire about use of vaginal contraceptives (such as diaphragm) since base of suppository interacts w/rubber latex.

INTERVENTION/EVALUATION:

Monitor temperature at least daily. Assess for therapeutic response or burning, itching, pain, or irritation.

PATIENT/FAMILY TEACHING:

Do not interrupt or stop regimen, even during menses. Teach pt proper insertion. Not affected by oral contraception. Notify physician of increased itching, irritation, burning. Consult physician about sexual intercourse, douching, or the use of other vaginal products. Do not use vaginal contraceptive diaphragms, condoms within 72 hours after treatment. Avoid contact w/eyes. Wash hands thoroughly after application.

terfenadine

turr-phen´ah-deen

(Seldane)

FIXED-COMBINATION(S):
W/pseudoephedrine, a sympathomimetic (Seldane-D)

CANADIAN AVAILABILITY:
Seldane

CLASSIFICATION

Antihistamine

PHARMACOKINETICS

	ONSET	PEAK	DURATION
PO	1-2 hrs	3-6 hrs	>12 hrs

Well absorbed from GI tract. Undergoes first-pass metabolism. Primarily distributed in liver, lungs, GI tract. Protein binding: 97%. Metabolized in liver to active metabolite. Primarily eliminated in feces. Half-life: 20.3 hrs.

ACTION

Prevents, antagonizes most histamine effects (e.g., urticaria, pruritus).

USES

Relief of seasonal allergic rhinitis (hay fever). Provides symptomatic relief of rhinorrhea, sneezing, oronasopharyngeal irritation, itching, lacrimation, red/irritated/itching eyes.

PO ADMINISTRATION

1. May give w/food (decreases GI distress).
2. Do not crush, chew extended-release tablets.

INDICATIONS/DOSAGE/ROUTES

Allergic rhinitis:
PO: Adults, children >12 yrs: 60 mg 2 times/day. **Children 7-12 yrs:** 30 mg 2 times/day. **Children 3-6 yrs:** 15 mg 2 times/day.

Usual elderly dosage:
PO: Elderly: 60 mg 1-2 times/day.

PRECAUTIONS

CONTRAINDICATIONS: Acute asthmatic attack, those receiving MAO inhibitors. **CAUTIONS:** Narrow-angle glaucoma, peptic ulcer, prostatic hypertrophy, pyloroduodenal or bladder neck obstruction, asthma, COPD, increased intraocular pressure, cardiovascular disease, hyperthyroidism, hypertension, seizure disorders. **PREGNANCY/LACTATION:** Unknown whether drug crosses placenta or is detected in breast milk. Increased risk of seizures in neonates, premature infants if used during third trimester of pregnancy. May prohibit lactation. **Pregnancy Category C.**

INTERACTIONS

DRUG INTERACTIONS: Alcohol, CNS depressants may increase CNS depressant effects. Anticholinergics may increase anticholinergic effects. MAO inhibitors may increase anticholinergic, CNS depressant effects. Erythromycin, ketoconazole may increase risk of cardiotoxic effects. **ALTERED LAB VALUES:** May suppress wheal and flare reactions to antigen skin testing. Discontinue at least 4 days before testing.

SIDE EFFECTS

OCCASIONAL: Headache, nausea, vomiting, constipation/diarrhea, increased appetite, insomnia, paresthesia, tremor, reduced concentration, nightmares, mental depression, confusion. **RARE:** Irritability, incoordination, vertigo, dizziness, muscular weakness, hypersensitivity reaction (rash, urticaria, bronchospasm) skin dryness, photosensitivity reaction, sweating.

ADVERSE REACTIONS/TOXIC EFFECTS

Children may experience dominant paradoxical reaction (restlessness, insomnia, euphoria, nervousness, tremors). Hypersensitivity reaction (eczema, pruritus, rash, photosensitivity) may occur.

NURSING IMPLICATIONS

BASELINE ASSESSMENT:

If pt is undergoing allergic reaction, obtain history of recently ingested foods, drugs, environmental exposure, recent emotional stress. Monitor rate, depth, rhythm, type of respiration; quality and rate of pulse. Assess lung sounds for rhonchi, wheezing, rales.

INTERVENTION/EVALUATION:

Monitor B/P, esp. in elderly (increased risk of hypotension). Monitor children closely for paradoxical reaction.

PATIENT/FAMILY TEACHING:

Tolerance to antihistaminic effect generally does not occur; tolerance to sedative effect may occur. Avoid tasks that require alertness, motor skills until response to drug is established. Dry mouth, drowsiness, dizziness may be an expected response of drug. Avoid alcoholic beverages during antihistamine therapy. Sugarless gum, sips of tepid water may relieve dry mouth. Coffee/tea may help reduce drowsiness.

T

testolactone

tes-tah-lack´tone
(Teslac)

CLASSIFICATION

Antineoplastic

PHARMACOKINETICS

Pharmacokinetics unknown. Well absorbed from GI tract. Metabolized in liver; excreted in urine.

ACTION

Inhibits steroid aromatase activity (reduces estrone synthesis). Estrone is major source of estrogen in postmenopausal women.

USES

Adjunctive therapy in treatment of advanced disseminated breast carcinoma in postmenopausal women when hormonal therapy is indicated, and in premenopausal women where ovarian function has been terminated.

INDICATIONS/DOSAGE/ROUTES

Breast carcinoma:
PO: Adults, elderly: 250 mg 4 times/day.

PRECAUTIONS

CONTRAINDICATIONS: Breast cancer in men. **CAUTIONS:** Renal, liver, cardiac disease. **PREGNANCY/LACTATION:** If possible, avoid use during pregnancy, esp. first trimester. Breast feeding not recommended. **Pregnancy Category C.**

INTERACTIONS

DRUG INTERACTIONS: May increase effects of oral anticoagulants. **ALTERED LAB VALUES:** May increase calcium, creatinine, 17-ketosteroids. May decrease estradiol.

SIDE EFFECTS

RARE: Maculopapular erythema, increase in B/P, alopecia, nail growth disturbances, paresthesia, aches, edema of extremities, glossitis, anorexia, hot flashes, nausea, vomiting, diarrhea.

ADVERSE REACTIONS/TOXIC EFFECTS

None significant.

NURSING IMPLICATIONS

INTERVENTION/EVALUATION:

Monitor plasma calcium levels (hypercalcemia is evidence of active remission of bone metastasis). Assess for signs of hypercalcemia (decreased muscle tone, bone/flank pain, thirst, excessive urination). Assess skin for maculopapular erythema.

PATIENT/FAMILY TEACHING:

Therapeutic effects usually noted in 6-12 wks. Therapy should continue for at least 3 mo. If alopecia occurs, it is reversible, but new hair growth may have different color or texture. Contact physician if nausea/vomiting continues at home.

---

testosterone

tess-toss´ter-one
(Andronaq, Histerone)

testosterone cypionate

(Depotest, Depo-Testosterone)

testosterone enanthate

(Delatest)

testosterone propionate

(Testex)

testosterone transdermal

(Testoderm)

FIXED-COMBINATION(S): Testosterone cypionate w/estradiol cypionate, an estrogen (depAndrogyn, Duratestrin, De-Comberol); testosterone enanthate w/ estradiol cypionate (Deladumone)

CANADIAN AVAILABILITY: Delatestryl, Deladumone, Malogen

CLASSIFICATION

Androgen

PHARMACOKINETICS

Well absorbed after IM administration. Protein binding: 99%. Metabolized in liver (undergoes first-pass metabolism). Primarily excreted in urine. Half-life: 10-20 min.

ACTION

Stimulates spermatogenesis, development of male secondary sex characteristics, sexual maturation at puberty. Stimulates production of RBCs.

USES

Treatment of delayed puberty; testicular failure due to cryptorchidism, bilateral orchism, orchitis, vanishing testis syndrome or orchidectomy; hypogonadotropic hypogonadism due to pituitary/hypothalamic injury (tumors, trauma, or radiation), idiopathic gonadotropin or luteinizing hormone releasing hormone deficiency. Palliative therapy in women 1-5 years postmenopausal w/advancing, inoperable metastatic breast cancer or premenopausal women who have benefited from oophorectomy and have a hormone-responsive tumor. Prevention of postpartum breast pain and engorgement. In combination w/estrogens for management of moderate to severe vasomotor symptoms associated w/ menopause when estrogens alone are not effective.

IM/SubQ PELLET ADMINISTRATION

IM:

1. Give deep in gluteal muscle.
2. Do *not* give IV.
3. Warming and shaking redissolves crystals that may form in long-acting preparations.
4. Wet needle of syringe may cause solution to become cloudy; this does not affect potency.

SubQ PELLETS:

1. Physician injects using Kearns Pellet Injector or implants after surgical incision.
2. Used only after parenteral dosage established.

INDICATIONS/DOSAGE/ROUTES

TESTOSTERONE, TESTOSTERONE PROPIONATE:

Androgen replacement therapy:
IM: Adults: 25-50 mg 2-3 times/wk.

Palliation of mammary cancer:
IM: Adults, elderly: 50-100 mg 3 times/wk.

Postpartum breast engorgement (propionate):
IM: Adults: 25-50 mg/day for 3-4 days (begin at time of delivery).

TESTOSTERONE CYPIONATE, TESTOSTERONE ENANTHATE:

Male hypogonadism (replacement therapy):
IM: Adults: 50-400 mg q2-4wks.

Males (delayed puberty):
IM: Adults: 50-200 mg q2-4wks.

Females (palliation of inoperable breast cancer):
IM: Adults, elderly: 200-400 mg q2-4wks.

TESTOSTERONE TRANSDERMAL

Males (replacement therapy): **TOPICAL: Adults:** 6 mg/day system.

PRECAUTIONS

CONTRAINDICATIONS: Hypersensitivity to drug or components of preparation, serious cardiac, renal, or hepatic dysfunction. Do not use for men w/carcinomas of the breast or prostate. **EXTREME CAUTION:** In children because of bone maturation effects. **CAUTIONS:** Epilepsy, migraine, or other conditions aggravated by fluid retention; metastatic breast cancer or immobility increases risk of hypercalcemia. **PREGNANCY/LACTATION:** Contraindicated during lactation. **Pregnancy Category X.**

INTERACTIONS

DRUG INTERACTIONS: May increase effect of oral anticoagulants. Hepatotoxic medications may increase hepatotoxicity. **ALTERED LAB VALUES:** May increase SGOT (AST), alkaline phosphatase, bilirubin, calcium, potassium, sodium, Hgb, Hct, LDL. May decrease HDL.

SIDE EFFECTS

FREQUENT: Gynecomastia, acne, amenorrhea or other menstrual irregularities. Females: hirsutism, deepening of voice, clitoral enlargement (may not be reversible when drug discontinued). **OCCASIONAL:** Edema, nausea, insomnia, oligospermia, priapism, male pattern of baldness, bladder irritability, hypercalcemia in immobilized pts or those w/breast cancer, hypercholesterolemia, inflammation and pain at IM injection site. Implanted pellets may slough out. **RARE:** Polycythemia w/high dosage, hypersensitivity.

ADVERSE REACTIONS/TOXIC EFFECTS

Peliosis hepatitis (liver, spleen replaced w/blood-filled cysts), hepatic neoplasms and hepatocellular carcinoma have been associated w/prolonged high dosage, anaphylactoid reactions.

NURSING IMPLICATIONS

BASELINE ASSESSMENT:

Question for hypersensitivity to testosterone. Establish baseline weight, B/P, Hgb, and Hct. Check liver function test results, electrolytes, and cholesterol if ordered. Wrist x-rays may be ordered to determine bone maturation in children.

INTERVENTION/EVALUATION:

Weigh daily and report weekly gain of more than 5 lbs.; evaluate for edema. Monitor I&O. Check B/P at least 2 times/day. Assess electrolytes, cholesterol, Hgb and Hct (periodically for high dosage), liver function test results. W/ breast cancer or immobility, check for hypercalcemia (lethargy, muscle weakness, confusion, irritability). Assure adequate intake of protein, calories. Assess for virilization. Monitor sleep patterns. Check injection site for redness, swelling, or pain.

PATIENT/FAMILY TEACHING:

Regular visits to physician and monitoring tests are necessary. Do not take any other medications w/o consulting physician. Teach diet high in protein, calories. Food may be tolerated better in small, frequent feedings. Weigh daily, report 5 lb/gain/week. Notify physician if nausea, vomiting, acne, or ankle swelling occurs. Female pts: Promptly report menstrual irregularities, hoarseness, deepening of voice. Males: Report frequent erections, difficulty urinating, gynecomastia.

tetracaine

tet´-rah-kane
(Pontocaine)

tetracaine hydrochloride

(Pontocaine Hydrochloride)

CANADIAN AVAILABILITY:
Pontocaine, Tetracaine Minims

(See Classifications section under Anesthetics: local)

tetracycline hydrochloride

tet-rah-sigh´clean
(Achromycin, Actisite, Panmycin, Robitet, Sumycin, Topicycline)

chlortetracycline hydrochloride

(Aureomycin)

CANADIAN AVAILABILITY:
Achromycin, Aureomycin, Tetracyn, Novotetra

CLASSIFICATION

Antibiotic: Tetracycline

PHARMACOKINETICS

Readily absorbed from GI tract. Widely distributed. Protein binding: 65%. Excreted in urine; eliminated in feces via biliary system. Slowly removed by hemodialysis. Half-life: 6-11 hrs (increased in decreased renal function).

ACTION

Bacteriostatic due to binding to ribosomes, inhibiting protein synthesis.

USES

Treatment of uncomplicated gonorrhea, syphilis (when allergic to penicillin), adjunctive therapy for acne, urinary tract infection, Rocky Mountain spotted fever, typhus, Q fever, cholera, psittacosis, brucellosis, yaws, bejel, pinta, anthrax, actinomycosis, Whipple's disease, rat bite fever. *Topical:* Inflammatory acne vulgaris, superficial infections. *Ophthalmic:* Prophylaxis of ophthalmia neonatorum, superficial eye infections (blepharitis, conjunctivitis, keratitis), adjunctive therapy for trachoma, inclusion conjunctivitis.

STORAGE/HANDLING

Store capsules, oral suspension at room temperature. IM solution stable for 6-24 hrs at room temperature, 24 hrs if refrigerated. Once reconstituted, use IV solution immediately. Discard if precipitate forms.

PO/IM/IV/TOPICAL/OPHTHALMIC ADMINISTRATION

NOTE: Replace parenteral therapy w/oral as soon as possible.

PO:

1. Give capsules, tablets w/full glass of water 1 hr before or 2 hrs after meals, milk.

IM:

1. Reconstitute each 100 or 250 mg vial w/2 ml sterile water or 0.9% NaCl for injection to provide

concentration of 50 or 125 mg/ml respectively.

2. To minimize discomfort, give deep IM slowly. Less painful to inject into gluteus maximus rather than lateral aspect of thigh.

IV:

1. Reconstitute each 250 mg vial w/5 ml sterile water for injection (10 ml for a 500 mg vial) to provide concentration of 50 mg/ml.
2. Further dilute w/100-1,000 ml 5% dextrose, 0.9% NaCl, or other compatible IV fluid.

TOPICAL:

1. Cleanse area gently before application.
2. Apply only to affected area.

OPHTHALMIC:

1. Place finger on lower eyelid and pull out until a pocket is formed between eye and lower lid.
2. Hold dropper above pocket and place correct number of drops (¼-½ inch ointment) into pocket. Have pt close eye gently.
3. *Suspension:* Apply digital pressure to lacrimal sac for 1-2 min (minimizes drainage into nose and throat, reducing risk of systemic effects). *Ointment:* Instruct pt to close eye for 1-2 min, rolling eyeball (increases contact area of drug to eye).
4. Remove excess suspension or ointment around eye w/tissue.

INDICATIONS/DOSAGE/ROUTES

NOTE: Space doses evenly around the clock.

Usual dosage:

PO: Adults, elderly: 1-3 Gm/day in 2-4 divided doses. **Children >8 yrs:** 25-50 mg/kg/day in 2-4 divided doses.

IM: Adults, elderly: 250 mg one time or 300 mg in 2-3 divided doses. **Children >8 yrs:** 15-25 mg/kg/day in 2-3 divided doses. **Maximum:** 250 mg.

IV: Adults, elderly: 250-500 mg q12h up to 500 mg q6h. **Children >8 yrs:** 12 mg/kg/day in 2 divided doses up to 20 mg/kg/day.

Usual ophthalmic dosage:

OPHTHALMIC OINTMENT: Adults, elderly: 1 cm to conjunctiva q2-4h.

OPHTHALMIC SUSPENSION: Adults, elderly: 1 drop to conjunctiva q6-12h.

Usual topical dosage:

TOPICAL: Adults, elderly: Apply 2 times/day in morning, evening.

PRECAUTIONS

CONTRAINDICATIONS: Hypersensitivity to tetracyclines, sulfite, children ≤age 8 yrs. **CAUTIONS:** Sun/ultraviolet light exposure (severe photosensitivity reaction). **PREGNANCY/LACTATION:** Readily crosses placenta, is distributed in breast milk. Avoid use in women during last half of pregnancy. May produce permanent teeth discoloration, enamel hypoplasia, inhibit fetal skeletal growth in children <8 yrs. **Pregnancy Category D.**

INTERACTIONS

DRUG INTERACTIONS: Cholestyramine, colestipol may decrease absorption. May decrease effect of oral contraceptives. Carbamazepine, phenytoin may decrease concentrations. **ALTERED LAB VALUES:** May increase BUN, SGOT (AST), SGPT (ALT), alkaline phosphatase, amylase, bilirubin concentrations.

SIDE EFFECTS

FREQUENT: Pain, induration w/

IM injection; thrombophlebitis w/ IV administration; nausea, vomiting, diarrhea, dysphagia. **OCCASIONAL:** Rash, urticaria, anal/genital pruritus, vaginal candidiasis. *Ophthalmic:* Preparations may cause stinging, burning, tearing, or feeling of foreign body in eye. **RARE:** *Topical:* Dermatitis.

ADVERSE REACTIONS/TOXIC EFFECTS

Superinfection (esp. fungal), anaphylaxis, increased intracranial pressure, bulging fontanelles occur rarely in infants.

NURSING IMPLICATIONS

BASELINE ASSESSMENT:

Question for history of allergies, esp. tetracyclines, sulfite. Obtain specimens for culture and sensitivity before giving first dose (therapy may begin before results are known).

INTERVENTION/EVALUATION:

Assess IM injection site for pain, induration. Check IV site for phlebitis (heat, pain, red streaking over vein). Assess skin for rash. Determine pattern of bowel activity and stool consistency. Monitor food intake, tolerance. Be alert for superinfection: Diarrhea, ulceration, or changes of oral mucosa, anal/genital pruritus. Monitor B/P and level of consciousness because of potential for increased intracranial pressure.

PATIENT/FAMILY TEACHING:

Continue antibiotic for full length of treatment. Space doses evenly. Take oral doses on empty stomach (1 hr before or 2 hrs after food/beverages). Drink full glass of water w/capsules and avoid bedtime doses. Discomfort may occur w/IM injection. Notify physician in event of diarrhea, rash, other new symptom. Protect skin from sun exposure. Consult physician before taking any other medication. *Topical:* Skin may turn yellow w/Topicycline application (washing removes solution); fabrics may be stained by heavy application. Do not apply to deep/open wounds. *Ophthalmic:* Consult physician before applying eye makeup. Temporarily blurred vision frequently occurs w/application of ointment. Do not share medication/items in contact w/eye.

tetrahydrozyline hydrochloride

tet-rah-high-droz´ah-leen
(Visine, Tyzine)

FIXED-COMBINATION(S):
W/benzalkonium chloride, a wetting agent, and edetate disodium, a chelating agent (Murine Plus, Visine A.C.)

T

CLASSIFICATION

Sympathomimetic

PHARMACOKINETICS

	ONSET	PEAK	DURATION
Ophthalmic	Several min	—	4-8 hrs
Intranasal	Several min	—	4-8 hrs

May be systemically absorbed. Metabolic, elimination fates unknown.

ACTION

Stimulates alpha-adrenergic receptors in conjunctiva, nasal mucosa producing vasoconstriction. *Intranasal:* Constriction of dilated arterioles and reduction in nasal blood flow, congestion. *Ophthalmic:* Constriction of small arterioles and relief of conjunctival congestion w/minimal mydriasis.

USES

Ophthalmic: Relief of congestion, itching, minor irritation and to control hyperemia in pts w/superficial corneal vascularity. Combination solutions relieve discomfort due to minor eye irritations and symptoms related to dry eyes. *Intranasal:* Relief of nasal congestion of rhinitis, the common cold, sinusitis, hay fever, or other allergies; reduce swelling and improve visualization for surgery or diagnostic procedures; open obstructed eustachian ostia in pts w/ear inflammation.

OPHTHALMIC/INTRANASAL ADMINISTRATION

OPHTHALMIC:

1. Instruct pt to tilt head backward and look up.
2. Gently pull lower lid down to form pouch and instill medication.
3. Do not touch tip of applicator to lids or any surface.
4. After releasing lower lid, have pt close eyes w/o squeezing.
5. Apply gentle finger pressure to lacrimal sac (bridge of the nose, inside corner of the eye) for 1-2 min.
6. Remove excess solution around eye w/tissue. Wash hands immediately to remove medication on hands.

INTRANASAL:

NOTE: Nasal sprays are preferable to drops because of decreased risk of swallowing and systemic absorption (except in young children in whom sprays are difficult to use). Use only clear, colorless solutions.

1. Drops should be administered w/pt in lateral, head-low position or reclining w/head tilted back as far as possible.
2. Pt should maintain same position for 5 min, then drops applied to other nostril.
3. Sprays should be administered w/pt's head erect; 3-5 min later the nose should be thoroughly blown.
4. Droppers and spray containers should be used by only one person; tips of dispensers or droppers should be rinsed well w/hot water after use.

INDICATIONS/DOSAGE/ROUTES

Usual nasal dosage:

INTRANASAL: Adults, elderly, children >6 yrs: 2-4 drops (0.1% solution) to each nostril q4-6h (no sooner than q3h). **Children, 2-6 yrs:** 2-3 drops (0.05% solution) to each nostril q4-6h (no sooner than q3h).

Usual ophthalmic dosage:

OPHTHALMIC: Adults, elderly, children: 1-2 drops (0.05%) 2-4 times/day.

PRECAUTIONS

CONTRAINDICATIONS: Known hypersensitivity to tetrahydrozyline or components of preparation; children <2 yrs of age (the 0.1% nasal solution is contraindicated in children <6 yrs of age; pts w/angle-closure glaucoma or other serious eye diseases. **CAUTIONS:** Some caution should be taken when using w/cardiac disease, hyperthyroidism, hypertension, diabetes mellitus, cerebral arteriosclerosis, bronchial asthma, monoamine oxidase inhibitors. **PREGNANCY/LACTATION:** Safety in pregnancy and lactation has not been established. **Pregnancy Category C.**

INTERACTIONS

DRUG INTERACTIONS: Maprotiline, tricyclic antidepressants may increase pressor effects. MAO inhibitors may cause severe hypertensive reaction. **ALTERED LAB VALUES:** None significant.

SIDE EFFECTS

OCCASIONAL: *Intranasal:* Transient burning, stinging, sneezing, dryness of mucosa. *Ophthalmic:* Irritation, blurred vision, mydriasis. Systemic sympathomimetic effects may occur w/either route: Headache, hypertension, weakness, sweating, palpitations, tremors. Prolonged use may result in rebound congestion.

ADVERSE REACTIONS/TOXIC EFFECTS

Overdosage may result in CNS depression w/drowsiness, decreased body temperature, bradycardia, hypotension, coma, apnea.

NURSING IMPLICATIONS

PATIENT/FAMILY TEACHING:

Discard if solution becomes cloudy or discolored. Overuse of vasoconstrictors may produce rebound congestion, hyperemia. Avoid excessive dosage, prolonged or too frequent use. *Ophthalmic:* Do not use w/glaucoma unless under advice and direction of physician. Remove contact lenses before administration. Do not use w/wetting agents for contact lenses. Discontinue and consult physician immediately if ocular pain or visual changes occur, if condition worsens or continues for more than 72 hrs. *Intranasal:* Discontinue and consult physician if rebound congestion occurs.

thiamine hydrochloride (vitamin B_1)

thigh'ah-min
(Betalin)

CANADIAN AVAILABILITY:
Betaxin, Bewon

CLASSIFICATION

Vitamin: B-complex

PHARMACOKINETICS

Readily absorbed from GI tract primarily in duodenum, after IM administration. Widely distributed. Metabolized in liver. Primarily excreted in urine.

ACTION

Combines w/adenosine triphosphate (ATP) in liver, kidney, leukocytes to form thiamine diphosphate, which is necessary for carbohydrate metabolism.

USES

Prevention/treatment of thiamine deficiency (e.g., beriberi, alcoholic w/altered sensorium).

STORAGE/HANDLING

Store oral, parenteral form at room temperature.

PO/IM/IV ADMINISTRATION

NOTE: IM/IV administration used only in acutely ill or those unresponsive to oral route (GI malabsorption syndrome). IM route preferred to IV use. Give by direct IV, or add to most IV solution and give as infusion.

INDICATIONS/DOSAGE/ROUTES

Dietary supplement:
PO: Adults, elderly: 1-2 mg/day. **Children:** 0.5-1 mg/day. **Infants:** 0.3-0.5 mg/day.

Thiamine deficiency:
PO: Adults, elderly: 5-30 mg/day, in single or 3 divided doses, for 1 mo. **Children:** 10-50 mg/day in 3 divided doses.

Critically ill/malabsorption syndrome:
IM/IV: Adults, elderly: 5-100 mg, 3 times/day. **Children:** 10-25 mg/day.

Metabolic disorders:
PO: Adults, elderly, children: 10-20 mg/day; up to 4 Gm in divided doses/day.

PRECAUTIONS

CONTRAINDICATIONS: None significant. **CAUTIONS:** None significant. **PREGNANCY/LACTATION:** Crosses placenta; unknown whether excreted in breast milk. **Pregnancy Category A.**

INTERACTIONS

DRUG INTERACTIONS: None significant. **ALTERED LAB VALUES:** None significant.

SIDE EFFECTS

FREQUENT: Pain, induration, tenderness at IM injection site.

ADVERSE REACTIONS/TOXIC EFFECTS

Rare, severe hypersensitivity reaction w/IV administration may result in feeling of warmth, pruritus, urticaria, weakness, sweating, nausea, restlessness, tightness of throat, angioedema (swelling of face/lips), cyanosis, pulmonary edema, GI tract bleeding, cardiovascular collapse.

NURSING IMPLICATIONS

INTERVENTION/EVALUATION:

Monitor lab values for erythrocyte activity, EKG readings. Assess for clinical improvement (improved sense of well being, weight gain). Observe for reversal of deficiency symptoms (*neurologic:* Peripheral neuropathy, hyporeflexia, nystagmus, ophthalmoplegia, ataxia, muscle weakness; *cardiac:* Venous hypertension, bounding arterial pulse, tachycardia, edema; *mental:* Confused state).

PATIENT/FAMILY TEACHING:

Discomfort may occur w/IM injection. Foods rich in thiamine include pork, organ meats, whole grain and enriched cereals, legumes, nuts, seeds, yeast, wheat germ, rice bran.

thiethylperazine maleate

thigh-eth-yl-pear′ah-zeen
(Torecan)

CANADIAN AVAILABILITY:
Torecan

CLASSIFICATION

Antiemetic

PHARMACOKINETICS

	ONSET	PEAK	DURATION
PO	30-60 min	—	4 hrs
IM	30 min	—	4 hrs
Rectal	30-60 min	—	4 hrs

Well absorbed after oral, rectal, IM administration. Widely distributed, primarily in CNS. Metabolized in liver. Excreted in urine.

ACTION

Exact mechanism unknown. May have direct effect on vomiting center/chemoreceptor trigger zone in CNS.

USES

Control of nausea and vomiting.

STORAGE/HANDLING

Store oral, rectal, parenteral form at room temperature.

PO/IM/RECTAL ADMINISTRATION

PO:

1. Give w/o regard to meals.

IM:

1. Give deep IM into large muscle mass, preferably upper outer gluteus maximus.

RECTAL:

1. If suppository is too soft, chill for 30 min in refrigerator or run cold water over foil wrapper.
2. Moisten suppository w/cold water before inserting well into rectum.

INDICATIONS/DOSAGE/ROUTES

NOTE: Do not use IV route (produces severe hypotension).

Nausea, vomiting:
PO, RECTAL, IM: Adults, elderly: 10 mg, 1-3 times/day.

PRECAUTIONS

CONTRAINDICATIONS: Severe CNS depression, comatose states, hypersensitivity to phenothiazines, pregnancy. **CAUTIONS:** Elderly, debilitated, dehydration, electrolyte imbalance, high fever. **PREGNANCY/LACTATION:** Unknown whether drug crosses placenta or is distributed in breast milk. Contraindicated during pregnancy. **Pregnancy Category unknown.**

INTERACTIONS

DRUG INTERACTIONS: Alcohol, CNS depressants may increase CNS, respiratory depression, increase hypotension. May block alpha-adrenergic effects of epinephrine (causing hypotension, tachycardia). Extrapyramidal symptom (EPS) producing medications may increase risk of EPS. May inhibit effects of levodopa. May increase cardiac effects w/quinidine. **ALTERED LAB VALUES:** None significant.

SIDE EFFECTS

OCCASIONAL: Dizziness, headache, fever, restlessness, dry mouth/nose. *IM injection:* Postural hypotension, drowsiness. **RARE:** Blurred vision, tinnitus (ringing/roaring in ears), peripheral edema of hands/arms/face.

ADVERSE REACTIONS/TOXIC EFFECTS

Extrapyramidal symptoms manifested as torticollis (neck muscle spasm), oculogyric crisis (rolling back of eyes), akathisia (motor restlessness, anxiety) occur rarely.

NURSING IMPLICATIONS

BASELINE ASSESSMENT:

Assess for dehydration if excessive vomiting occurs (poor skin turgor, dry mucous membranes, longitudinal furrows in tongue).

INTERVENTION EVALUATION:

Monitor B/P esp. before dosing. Assist w/ambulation if dizziness or hypotension occurs. Assess for improvement of dehydration status. Monitor I&O. Monitor for evidence of fever. Assess any vomitus. Be alert for extrapyramidal symptoms.

PATIENT/FAMILY TEACHING:

Report visual disturbances, headache. Dry mouth is expected response to medication. Relief from nausea/vomiting generally occurs within 30 min of drug administration. Avoid alcohol and other CNS depressants. Change positions slowly to prevent postural hypotension. Avoid tasks requiring alert response until assured drug does not cause impairment

thioguanine

thigh-oh-guan´een
(Thioguanine)

CANADIAN AVAILABILITY:
Lanvis

CLASSIFICATION

Antineoplastic

PHARMACOKINETICS

Incompletely, variably absorbed from GI tract. Metabolized in liver. Primarily excreted in urine. Half-life: 25-240 min.

ACTION

Cell cycle-specific for S phase of cell division. Action may include inhibition of DNA, RNA synthesis.

USES

Treatment of acute myelogenous leukemia, chronic myelogenous leukemia.

INDICATIONS/DOSAGE/ROUTES

NOTE: May be carcinogenic, mutagenic, or teratogenic. Handle w/ extreme care during administration.

Dosage individualized based on clinical response, tolerance to adverse effects. When used in combination therapy, consult specific protocols for optimum dosage, sequence of drug administration.

Initial treatment:
PO: Adults, elderly, children: 2 mg/kg/day as single dose. Increase to 3 mg/kg/day after 4 wks if no leukocyte, platelet depression appears and no clinical improvement obvious.

Maintenance:
PO: Adults, elderly, children: 2-3 mg/kg/day.

PRECAUTIONS

CONTRAINDICATIONS: Disease resistance to prior therapy w/ drug. **EXTREME CAUTION:** Preexisting liver disease, pts receiving other hepatotoxic drugs. **PREGNANCY/LACTATION:** If possible, avoid use during pregnancy, esp. first trimester. May cause fetal harm. Unknown whether distributed in breast milk. Breast feeding not recommended. **Pregnancy Category D.**

INTERACTIONS

DRUG INTERACTIONS: May decrease effect of antigout medications. Bone marrow depressants may increase bone marrow depression. Live virus vaccines may potentiate virus replication, increase vaccine side effects, decrease pt's antibody response to vaccine. **ALTERED LAB VALUES:** May increase uric acid.

SIDE EFFECTS

FREQUENT: Hyperuricemia. **OCCASIONAL:** Nausea, vomiting, anorexia, stomatitis, diarrhea (particularly with excessive dosage), rash, dermatitis, unsteady gait, loss of vibration sensitivity, jaundice.

ADVERSE REACTIONS/TOXIC EFFECTS

Major effects are bone marrow depression manifested as leukopenia, thrombocytopenia, anemia, pancytopenia, hepatotoxicity manifested as jaundice, hepatomegaly, veno-occlusive liver disease.

NURSING IMPLICATIONS

BASELINE ASSESSMENT:

Obtain liver function tests weekly during initial therapy, monthly intervals thereafter. Obtain hematology tests at least weekly during therapy. Discontinue therapy if abnormally large/rapid decrease (over few days) of WBC, platelet, Hgb level occur or at first sign of clinical jaundice.

INTERVENTION/EVALUATION:

Monitor serum transaminase, alkaline phosphatase, bilirubin, blood uric acid, Hgb, Hct, WBC, differential, platelet count. Assess skin, sclera for evidence of jaundice. Encourage fluid intake. Monitor for stomatitis (burning/erythema of oral mucosa at inner margin of lips, sore throat, difficulty swallowing, oral ulceration). Monitor for hematologic toxicity; infection (fever, sore throat, signs of local infection), easy bruising, unusual bleeding from any site), symptoms of anemia (excessive tiredness, weakness). Assess pattern of daily bowel activity and stool consistency.

PATIENT/FAMILY TEACHING:

Drink plenty of fluid. Maintain fastidious oral hygiene. Do not have immunizations w/o physician's approval (drug lowers body's resistance). Avoid crowds, those w/infection. Use nonhormonal contraceptive during therapy; notify physician at once if pregnancy is suspected. Promptly report fever, sore throat, signs of local infection, easy bruising, unusual bleeding from any site, yellowing of skin or eyes, flank pain. Contact physician if nausea/vomiting continues at home.

thiopental sodium

thigh-oh-pen´tall
(Pentothal)

CANADIAN AVAILABILITY:
Pentothal

(See Classifications section under Anesthetics: general)

thioridazine

thigh-or-rid´ah-zeen
(Mellaril-S)

thioridazine hydrochloride

(Mellaril)

CANADIAN AVAILABILITY:
Apo-Thioridazine, Mellaril, Novoridazine

CLASSIFICATION

Antipsychotic

PHARMACOKINETICS

Variably absorbed from GI tract. Widely distributed. Protein binding: >90%. Metabolized in liver to some active metabolites. Excreted in urine, eliminated in feces.

ACTION

Blocks postsynaptic dopaminergic receptors in brain. Possesses strong anticholinergic, sedative effects.

USES

Management of psychotic disorders, severe behavioral disturbances in children, including those w/excessive motor activity, conduct disorders. Used in short-term treatment of moderate to marked depression w/variable degrees of anxiety.

PO ADMINISTRATION

1. Dilute oral concentrate solution in water or fruit juice just before administration.
2. Do not crush, chew, or break tablets.

INDICATIONS/DOSAGE/ROUTES

Psychotic disorders:
PO: Adults: 50-100 mg 3 times/day in hospitalized pts. May gradually increase to 800 mg/day maximum. Dosage from 200-800 mg/day should be divided in 2-3 divided doses. Reduce dose gradually when therapeutic response is achieved.

Depression w/anxiety:
PO: Adults: 25 mg 3 times/day. **Total dose range/day:** 10 mg 2 times/day to 50 mg 3-4 times/day.

Usual elderly dosage (nonpsychotic):
PO: Elderly: Initially, 10-25 mg 1-2 times/day. May increase by 10-25 mg q4-7days. **Maximum:** 400 mg/day.

Moderate behavioral disturbances:
PO: Children 2-12 yrs: Initially, 10 mg 3 times/day in hospitalized children.

PRECAUTIONS

CONTRAINDICATIONS: Severe CNS depression, comatose states, severe cardiovascular disease, bone marrow depression, subcortical brain damage. **CAUTIONS:** Impaired respiratory/hepatic/renal/cardiac function, alcohol withdrawal, history of seizures, urinary retention, glaucoma, prostatic hypertrophy, hypocalcemia (increases susceptibility to dystonias). **PREGNANCY/LACTATION:** Crosses placenta; distributed in breast milk. **Pregnancy Category C.**

INTERACTIONS

DRUG INTERACTIONS: Alcohol, CNS depressants may increase CNS, respiratory depression, hypotensive effects. Tricyclic antidepressants, MAO inhibitors may increase sedative, anticholinergic effects. Antithyroid agents may increase risk of agranulocytosis. Extrapyramidal symptoms (EPS) may increase w/EPS producing medications. Hypotensives may increase hypotension. May decrease levodopa effects. Lithium may decrease absorption, produce adverse neurologic effects. **ALTERED LAB VALUES:** May cause EKG changes.

SIDE EFFECTS

Generally well-tolerated w/only mild and transient effects. **OCCASIONAL:** Drowsiness during early therapy, dry mouth, blurred vision, lethargy, constipation or diarrhea, nasal congestion, peripheral edema, urinary retention. **RARE:** Ocular changes, skin pigmentation (those on high doses for prolonged periods).

ADVERSE REACTIONS/TOXIC EFFECTS

Extrapyramidal symptoms appear dose-related (particularly high dosage) and are divided into 3 categories: Akathisia (inability to sit still, tapping of feet, urge to move around), parkinsonian symptoms (mask-like face, tremors, shuffling gait, hypersalivation), and acute dystonias: Torticollis (neck muscle spasm), opisthotonos (rigidity of back muscles), and oculogyric crisis (rolling back of eyes). Dystonic reaction may also produce profuse sweating, pallor. Tardive dyskinesia (protrusion of tongue, puffing of cheeks, chewing/puckering of the mouth) occurs rarely (may be irreversible). Abrupt withdrawal following long-term therapy may precipitate nausea, vomiting, gastritis, dizziness, tremors. Blood dyscrasias, particularly agranulocytosis, mild leukopenia (sore mouth/gums/throat) may occur. May lower seizure threshold.

NURSING IMPLICATIONS

BASELINE ASSESSMENT:

Avoid skin contact w/solution (contact dermatitis). Assess behavior, appearance, emotional status, response to environment, speech pattern, thought content.

INTERVENTION EVALUATION:

Monitor B/P for hypotension. Assess for extrapyramidal symptoms. Monitor WBC, differential count for blood dyscrasias. Monitor for fine tongue movement (may be early sign of tardive dyskinesia). Supervise suicidal-risk pt closely during early therapy (as depression lessens, energy level improves, but suicide potential increases). Assess for therapeutic response (interest in surroundings, improvement in self-care, increased ability to concentrate, relaxed facial expression).

PATIENT/FAMILY TEACHING:

Full therapeutic effect may take up to 6 wks. Urine may darken. Do not abruptly withdraw from long-term drug therapy. Report visual disturbances. Sugarless gum or sips of tepid water may relieve dry mouth. Drowsiness generally subsides during continued therapy. Avoid tasks that require alertness, motor skills until response to drug is established.

thiotepa

thigh-oh-teh´pah
(Thiotepa)

T

CANADIAN AVAILABILITY:

Thiotepa

CLASSIFICATION

Antineoplastic

PHARMACOKINETICS

Variable systemic absorption occurs following local administration. Primarily excreted in urine as metabolites.

ACTION

Cell cycle-phase nonspecific. Binds w/many intracellular structures. Cross-links strands of DNA, RNA. Inhibits protein synthesis.

USES

Treatment of superficial papillary carcinoma of urinary bladder, adenocarcinoma of breast and ovary, Hodgkin's disease, lymphosarcoma. Intracavitary injection to control pleural, pericardial, or peritoneal effusions due to metastatic tumors.

STORAGE/HANDLING

NOTE: May be carcinogenic, mutagenic, or teratogenic. Handle w/ extreme care during preparation/ administration.

Refrigerate unopened vials. Reconstituted solutions appear clear to slightly opaque; stable for 5 days if refrigerated. Discard if solution grossly opaque or precipitate forms.

PARENTERAL ADMINISTRATION

NOTE: Give by IV, intrapleural, intraperitoneal, intrapericardial, or intratumor injection, intravesical instillation.

1. Reconstitute 15 mg vial w/1.5 ml sterile water for injection to provide concentration of 10 mg/ml.
2. For IV injection, administer over 1 min.
3. Further dilute w/5% dextrose, 0.9% NaCl injection for intracavitary use, IV infusion, perfusion therapy.

INDICATIONS/DOSAGE/ROUTES

NOTE: Dosage individualized based on clinical response, tolerance to adverse effects. When used in combination therapy, consult specific protocols for optimum dosage, sequence of drug administration.

Initial treatment:

IV: Adults, elderly: 0.3-0.4 mg/kg q1-4wks. Maintenance dose adjusted weekly on basis of blood counts.

INTRACAVITARY: Adults, elderly: 0.6-0.8 mg/kg q1-4wks.

INTRATUMOR: Adults, elderly: Initially, 0.6-0.8 mg/kg given directly into tumor. **Maintenance:** 0.7-0.8 mg/kg q1-4wks.

INTRAVESICAL: Adults, elderly: 30-60 mg in 30-60 ml sterile water instilled by catheter into bladder of pt who has been dehydrated for 8-12 hrs. Retain in bladder for 2 hrs. Reposition pt q15min for maximum area contact. Repeat once weekly for 4 wks.

PRECAUTIONS

CONTRAINDICATIONS: Existing hepatic, renal, bone marrow damage unless drug administered in low doses, concurrent use w/ alkylating agents or radiation therapy until pt recovers from myelosuppression. **CAUTIONS:** None significant. **PREGNANCY/LACTATION:** If possible, avoid use during pregnancy, esp. first trimester. Breast feeding not recommended. **Pregnancy Category C.**

INTERACTIONS

DRUG INTERACTIONS: May decrease effect of antigout medications. Bone marrow depressants may increase bone marrow depression. Live virus vaccines may potentiate virus replication, increase vaccine side effects, decrease pt's antibody response to vaccine. **ALTERED LAB VALUES:** May increase uric acid.

SIDE EFFECTS

OCCASIONAL: Pain at injection site, headache, dizziness, tightness of throat, amenorrhea, decreased spermatogenesis, hives, skin rash, nausea, vomiting, anorexia. **RARE:**

Alopecia, cystitis, hematuria following intravesical dosing.

ADVERSE REACTIONS/TOXIC EFFECTS

Hematologic toxicity manifested as leukopenia, anemia, thrombocytopenia, pancytopenia due to bone marrow depression. Although WBC falls to lowest point at 10-14 days after initial therapy, bone marrow effects not evident for 30 days. Stomatitis, ulceration of intestinal mucosa may be noted.

NURSING IMPLICATIONS

BASELINE ASSESSMENT:

Interrupt therapy if WBC falls below 3,000/mm^3, platelet count below 150,000/mm^3, WBC or platelet counts declines rapidly. Obtain hematologic status at least weekly during therapy and for 3 wks after therapy discontinued.

INTERVENTION/EVALUATION:

Monitor uric acid serum levels, hematology tests. Assess for stomatitis (burning/erythema of oral mucosa at inner margin of lips, sore throat, difficulty swallowing, oral ulceration). Monitor for hematologic toxicity: infection (fever, sore throat, signs of local infection), easy bruising, unusual bleeding from any site), symptoms of anemia (excessive tiredness, weakness). Assess skin for rash, hives.

PATIENT/FAMILY TEACHING:

Discomfort may occur w/IV administration. Maintain fastidious oral hygiene. Do not have immunizations w/o physician's approval (drug lowers body's resistance). Avoid crowds, those w/infection. Promptly report fever, sore throat, signs of local infection, easy bruising, unusual bleeding from any site. Contact physician if nausea/vomiting continues at home.

thiothixene

thigh-oh-thick´seen

(Navane caps)

thiothixene hydrochloride

(Navane solution, injection)

CANADIAN AVAILABILITY:

Navane

CLASSIFICATION

Antipsychotic

PHARMACOKINETICS

	ONSET	PEAK	DURATION
IM	—	1-6 hrs	—

Well absorbed from GI tract, after IM administration. Widely distributed. Protein binding: 90-99%. Metabolized in liver. Primarily excreted in urine. Half-life: 34 hrs.

ACTION

Blocks postsynaptic dopamine receptors. Has alpha-adrenergic blocking effects; depresses release of hypothalamic, hypophyseal hormones.

USES

Symptomatic management of psychotic disorders.

STORAGE/HANDLING

Reconstituted solutions stable for 48 hrs at room temperature.

PO/IM ADMINISTRATION

PO:

1. Give w/o regard to meals.
2. Avoid skin contact w/oral solution (contact dermatitis).

IM:

1. Following parenteral form, pt must remain recumbent for 30-60 min in head-low position w/legs raised, to minimize hypotensive effect.
2. For IM injection, reconstitute 10 mg thiothixene hydrochloride w/2.2 ml sterile water for injection, yielding final solution of 5 mg/ml.
3. Inject slow, deep IM into upper outer quadrant of gluteus maximus or midlateral thigh.

INDICATIONS/DOSAGE/ROUTES

NOTE: Reduce dosage gradually to optimum response, then decrease to lowest effective level for maintenance. Replace parenteral therapy w/oral therapy as soon as possible.

Mild to moderate symptoms:
PO: Adults: 2 mg 3 times/day. May be increased gradually to 15 mg/day.

Severe symptoms:
PO: Adults: 5 mg 2 times/day. Increase gradually to 60 mg if needed. **Usual dose range:** 20-30 mg/day.
IM: Adults: 4 mg 2-4 times/day. May increase to maximum 30 mg/day. **Usual dose range:** 16-20 mg/day.

Usual elderly dosage (nonpsychotic):
PO: Elderly: Initially, 1-2 mg 1-2 times/day. May increase by 1-2 mg q4-7days. **Maximum:** 30 mg/day.

PRECAUTIONS

CONTRAINDICATIONS: Comatose states, circulatory collapse, CNS depression, blood dyscrasias. **EXTREME CAUTION:** History of seizures. **CAUTIONS:** Severe cardiovascular disorders, alcoholic withdrawal, pt exposure to extreme heat, glaucoma, prostatic hypertrophy. **PREGNANCY/LACTATION:** Crosses placenta; distributed in breast milk. **Pregnancy Category C.**

INTERACTIONS

DRUG INTERACTIONS: Alcohol, CNS depressants may increase CNS, respiratory depression, increase hypotension. Extrapyramidal symptom (EPS) producing medications may increase risk of EPS. May inhibit effects of levodopa. may increase cardiac effects w/quinidine. **ALTERED LAB VALUES:** May decrease uric acid.

SIDE EFFECTS

Hypotension, dizziness, and fainting occur frequently after first injection, occasionally after subsequent injections, and rarely w/oral dosage. **FREQUENT:** Transient drowsiness, dry mouth, constipation, blurred vision, nasal congestion. **OCCASIONAL:** Diarrhea, peripheral edema, urinary retention, nausea. **RARE:** Ocular changes, skin pigmentation (those of high doses for prolonged periods).

ADVERSE REACTIONS/TOXIC EFFECTS

Frequently noted extrapyramidal symptom is akathisia (motor restlessness, anxiety). Occurring less frequently is akinesia (rigidity, tremor, salivation, mask-like facial expression, reduced voluntary movements). Infrequently noted are dystonias: Torticollis (neck muscle spasm), opisthotonos (rigidity of back muscles), and oculogyric crisis (rolling back of eyes). Tardive dyskinesia (protrusion of tongue, puffing of cheeks, chewing/puckering of mouth) occurs rarely but may be irreversible. Risk is greater in female geriatric pts. Grand mal seizures may occur in epileptic pts (risk higher w/IM administration).

NURSING IMPLICATIONS

BASELINE ASSESSMENT:

Assess behavior, appearance, emotional status, response to environment, speech pattern, thought content.

INTERVENTION/EVALUATION:

Supervise suicidal-risk pt closely during early therapy (as depression lessens, energy level improves, increasing suicide potential. Monitor B/P for hypotension. Assess for peripheral edema behind medial malleolus (sacral area in bedridden pts). Assess stools; prevent constipation. Monitor for EPS, tardive dyskinesia (see Adverse Reactions) and potentially fatal, rare neuroleptic malignant syndrome: fever, irregular pulse or B/P, muscle rigidity, altered mental status. Assess for therapeutic response (interest in surroundings, improvement in self-care, increased ability to concentrate, relaxed facial expression).

PATIENT/FAMILY TEACHING:

Full therapeutic effect may take up to 6 wks. Report visual disturbances. Sugarless gum or sips of tepid water may relieve dry mouth. Drowsiness generally subsides during continued therapy. Avoid tasks that require alertness, motor skills until response to drug is established. Avoid alcohol and other CNS depressants.

thyroid

thye´royd
(S-P-T, Thyrar, Armour Thyroid)

CANADIAN AVAILABILITY:
Thyroid

CLASSIFICATION

Thyroid

PHARMACOKINETICS

Well absorbed from GI tract. Widely distributed. Protein binding: 99%. Metabolized in liver. Undergoes enterohepatic circulation. Primarily excreted in urine. Half-life: T_3: 1-2 days; T_4: 6-7 days.

ACTION

Involved in normal metabolism, growth, and development (esp. CNS). Possesses catabolic and anabolic effects. Increases basal metabolic rate, enhances gluconeogenesis, stimulates protein synthesis.

USES

Replacement in decreased or absent thyroid function (partial or complete absence of gland, primary atrophy, functional deficiency, effects of surgery, radiation or antithyroid agents, pituitary or hypothalamic hypothyroidism); management of simple (nontoxic) goiter and chronic lymphocytic thyroiditis; treatment of thyrotoxicosis (w/antithyroid drugs) to prevent goitrogenesis and hypothyroidism. Management of thyroid cancer.

PO ADMINISTRATION

1. Give at the same time each day to maintain hormone levels.
2. Administer before breakfast to prevent insomnia.

INDICATIONS/DOSAGE/ROUTES

Hypothyroidism:
PO: Adults, elderly: Initially, 30 mg/day; increase w/15 mg q2-3wks. **Maintenance:** 60-120 mg/day.

Thyroid cancer:
PO: Adults, elderly: Larger doses required than that used for replacement therapy.

Congenital hypothyroidism:
PO: Children (>12 yrs): >90 mg/day; **(6-12 yrs):** 60-90 mg/day; **(1-5 yrs):** 45-60 mg/day; **(6-12 mos):** 30-45 mg/day; **(0-6 mos):** 15-30 mg/day.

PRECAUTIONS

CONTRAINDICATIONS: Thyrotoxicosis and myocardial infarction uncomplicated by hypothyroidism; hypersensitivity to any component; treatment of obesity. **CAUTIONS:** Elderly, angina pectoris, hypertension or other cardiovascular disease. Signs and symptoms of diabetes mellitus, diabetes insipidus, adrenal insufficiency, hypopituitarism may become intensified. Begin therapy w/small doses, gradually increase. Treat w/adrenocortical steroids before thyroid therapy in coexisting hypothyroidism and hypoadrenalism. **PREGNANCY/LACTATION:** Drug does not cross placenta; minimal excretion in breast milk. **Pregnancy Category A.**

INTERACTIONS

DRUG INTERACTIONS: May alter effects of oral anticoagulants. Cholestyramine, colestipol may decrease absorption. Sympathomimetics may increase effects, coronary insufficiency. **ALTERED LAB VALUES:** None significant.

SIDE EFFECTS

OCCASIONAL: Most reactions are due to excessive dosage w/signs, symptoms of hyperthyroidism: weight loss, palpitations, increased appetite, tremors, nervousness, tachycardia, increased B/P, headache, insomnia, menstrual irregularities. Children may have reversible hair loss upon initiation. **RARE:** Skin reactions, GI intolerance.

ADVERSE REACTIONS/TOXIC EFFECTS

Cardiac arrhythmias, possibly death due to cardiac failure.

NURSING IMPLICATIONS

BASELINE ASSESSMENT:

Question for hypersensitivities. Obtain baseline weight, vital signs. Check results of thyroid function tests.

INTERVENTION/EVALUATION:

Monitor pulse for rate, rhythm (report pulse of 100 or marked increase). Assess for tremors, nervousness. Check appetite and sleep pattern.

PATIENT/FAMILY TEACHING:

Do not discontinue; replacement for hypothyroidism is lifelong. Follow-up office visits and thyroid function tests are essential. Take medication at the same time each day, preferably in the morning. Teach pt/family to take pulse correctly, report marked increase, pulse of 100 or above, change of rhythm. Do not change brands (not equivalent). Take other medications only on advice of physician. Notify physician promptly of chest pain, weight loss nervousness or tremors, insomnia. Children may have reversible hair loss/increased aggressiveness during the first few months of therapy.

ticarcillin disodium

tie-car-sill´in
(Ticar)

CANADIAN AVAILABILITY:
Ticar

CLASSIFICATION

Antibiotic: Penicillin

PHARMACOKINETICS

Well absorbed after IM administration. Widely distributed. Protein binding: 50-60%. Minimal metabolism in liver. Primarily excreted unchanged in urine. Moderately removed by hemodialysis. Half-life: 1-1.2 hrs (increased in decreased renal function).

ACTION

Bactericidal. Binds to bacterial cell wall inhibiting bacterial cell wall synthesis causing cell lysis, death.

USES

Treatment of gynecologic, skin/skin structure, respiratory, urinary tract (UTI), bone and joint, intra-abdominal infections, septicemia; perioperative prophylaxis, particularly abdominal surgery.

STORAGE/HANDLING

IM solution is stable for 24 hrs at room temperature, 72 hrs if refrigerated; IV infusion (piggyback) is stable for 48-72 hrs at room temperature, 14 days if refrigerated. Discard if precipitate forms or solution darkens (indicates loss of potency).

IM/IV ADMINISTRATION

NOTE: Space doses evenly around the clock.

IM:

1. Reconstitute each Gm w/2 ml sterile water for injection or 0.9% NaCl injection to provide concentration of 1 Gm/2.5 ml.
2. Use solution for IM injection promptly.
3. Inject as slowly as possible into large muscle mass.
4. Do not inject more than 2 Gm at any one injection site.

IV:

1. For IV injection, reconstitute each Gm w/4 ml sterile water for injection. Further dilute to make concentration of 50 mg/ml. Give as slowly as possible to avoid vein irritation.
2. For intermittent IV infusion (piggyback), further dilute w/50-100 ml 5% dextrose, 0.9% NaCl or other compatible IV fluid. Infuse over 30-120 min.
3. Because of potential for hypersensitivity/anaphylaxis, start initial dose at few drops/min, increase slowly to ordered rate; stay w/pt first 10-15 min, then check q10min.
4. Alternating IV sites, use large veins to avoid phlebitis.

INDICATIONS/DOSAGE/ROUTES

Uncomplicated UTI:
IM/IV: Adults, elderly, children

>40 kg: 1 Gm q6h. **Children <40 kg:** 50-100 mg/kg/day in divided dose q6-8h.

Complicated UTI:
IV: Adults, elderly, children: 3 Gm q6h.

Respiratory tract, septicemia, intra-abdominal, skin/skin structure infections, infections of female pelvis and genital tract:
IV: Adults, elderly, children: 3 Gm q3, 4, or 6h.

Usual dosage (neonates):
IM/IV: Neonates (0-7 days): 75 mg/kg q8-12h. **Neonates (7-28 days):** 75-100 mg/kg q8h.

Dosage in renal/hepatic impairment:
Dose and/or frequency may be modified based on creatinine clearance and/or severity of infection. After an initial dose of 3 Gm:

CREATININE CLEARANCE	DOSAGE
30-60 ml/min	2 Gm IV q4h
10-30 ml/min	2 Gm IV q8h
<10 ml/min	2 Gm IV q12h (or 1 Gm IM q6h)
<10 ml/min w/ liver impairment	2 Gm IV q24h (or 1 Gm IM q12h)

PRECAUTIONS

CONTRAINDICATIONS: Hypersensitivity to any penicillin. **CAUTIONS:** History of allergies, esp. cephalosporins. **PREGNANCY/LACTATION:** Readily crosses placenta, appears in cord blood, amniotic fluid. Distributed in breast milk in low concentrations. May lead to allergic sensitization, diarrhea, candidiasis, skin rash in infant. **Pregnancy Category B.**

INTERACTIONS

DRUG INTERACTIONS: Anticoagulants, heparin, thrombolytics, NSAIDs may increase risk of hemorrhage w/high doses of ticarcillin. Probenecid may increase concentration, risk of toxicity. **ALTERED LAB VALUES:** May cause positive Coombs' test. May increase SGOT (AST), SGPT (ALT), alkaline phosphatase, bilirubin, creatinine, LDH, bleeding time. May decrease potassium, sodium, uric acid.

SIDE EFFECTS

FREQUENT: Rash, urticaria, pain, and induration at IM injection site, phlebitis, thrombophlebitis w/IV dose. **OCCASIONAL:** Nausea, vomiting, diarrhea. **RARE:** Bleeding w/high IV dosage; hypokalemia, fatigue, hallucinations.

ADVERSE REACTIONS/TOXIC EFFECTS

Superinfections, potentially fatal antibiotic-associated colitis may result from bacterial imbalance. Seizures, neurologic reactions may occur w/overdosage (more often w/renal impairment). Severe hypersensitivity reactions, including anaphylaxis, occur rarely.

NURSING IMPLICATIONS

BASELINE ASSESSMENT:

Question for history of allergies, esp. penicillins, cephalosporins. Obtain specimen for culture and sensitivity before giving first dose (therapy may begin before results are known).

INTERVENTION/EVALUATION:

Hold medication and promptly report rash (hypersensitivity) or diarrhea (w/fever, abdominal pain, mucus and blood in stool may indicate antibiotic-associated colitis). Assess food tolerance. Evaluate IV site for phlebitis (heat, pain, red streaking over vein). Check IM injection site for pain, induration. Monitor I&O, urinalysis, renal function tests. Assess for bleeding: Overt bleeding, bruising, or tissue swelling; check hematology reports. Monitor electrolytes, particularly potassium. Be alert for superinfection: Increased fever, onset of sore throat, diarrhea, vomiting, ulceration, or other changes in oral mucosa, anal/genital pruritus.

PATIENT/FAMILY TEACHING:

Continue antibiotic for full length of treatment. Space doses evenly. Discomfort may occur at IM injection site. Notify physician in event of rash, diarrhea, bleeding, bruising, other new symptom.

ticarcillin disodium/ clavulanate potassium

ty-car-sill'in/klah-view'lah-nate

(Timentin)

CANADIAN AVAILABILITY: Timentin

CLASSIFICATION

Antibiotic: Penicillin

PHARMACOKINETICS

Widely distributed. Protein binding: 50-60%. Minimal metabolism in liver. Primarily excreted unchanged in urine. Moderately removed by hemodialysis. Half-life: 1-1.2 hrs (increased in decreased renal function.

ACTION

Bactericidal. Binds to bacterial cell wall inhibiting bacterial cell wall synthesis causing cell lysis, death. *Clavulanate:* Inhibits bacterial beta-lactamase protecting ticarcillin from enzymatic degradation.

USES

Treatment of septicemia, skin/skin structure, bone and joint, lower respiratory, urinary tract infections, endometritis.

STORAGE/HANDLING

Solution appears colorless to pale yellow (if solution darkens, indicates loss of potency). IV infusion (piggyback) stable for 24 hrs at room temperature, 3 days if refrigerated. Discard if precipitate forms.

IV ADMINISTRATION

NOTE: Space doses evenly around the clock.

1. For IV infusion (piggyback), reconstitute each 3.1 Gm vial w/13 ml sterile water for injection or 0.9% NaCl injection to provide concentration of 200 mg ticarcillin and 6.7 mg clavulanic acid per ml.
2. Shake vial to assist reconstitution.
3. Further dilute w/50-100 ml 5% dextrose, 0.9% NaCl or other IV fluid. Infuse over 30 min.
4. Because of potential for hypersensitivity/anaphylaxis, start initial dose at few drops/min, increase slowly to ordered rate; stay w/pt first 10-15 min, then check q10min.
5. Alternating IV sites, use large veins to reduce risk of phlebitis.

INDICATIONS/DOSAGE/ROUTES

Systemic and urinary tract infections:
IV: Adults >60 kg: 3.1 Gm q4-6h. **Adults <60 kg, children >12 yrs:** 200-300 mg/kg/day in divided doses q4-6h.

Gynecologic infections:
IV: Adults >60 kg: 200 mg/kg/day in divided doses q6h up to 300 mg/kg/day in divided doses q4h.

Dosage in renal/hepatic impairment:

Hepatic impairment alone usually requires no change. Renal impairment alone, administer 3.1 Gm initially, then modify dose and/or frequency based on creatinine clearance and/or severity of infection.

CREATININE CLEARANCE	DOSAGE
30-60 ml/min	2 Gm IV q4h
10-30 ml/min	2 Gm q8h
<10 ml/min	2 Gm q12h
<10 ml/min w/liver impairment	2 Gm q24h

PRECAUTIONS

CONTRAINDICATIONS: Hypersensitivity to any penicillin. **CAUTIONS:** History of allergies, esp. cephalosporins. **PREGNANCY/LACTATION:** Readily crosses placenta, appears in cord blood, amniotic fluid. Distributed in breast milk in low concentrations. May lead to allergic sensitization, diarrhea, candidiasis, skin rash in infant. **Pregnancy Category B.**

INTERACTIONS

DRUG INTERACTIONS: Anticoagulants, heparin, thrombolytics, NSAIDs may increase risk of hemorrhage w/high doses of ticarcillin. Probenecid may increase concentration, risk of toxicity. **ALTERED LAB VALUES:** May cause positive Coombs' test. May increase SGOT (AST), SGPT (ALT), alkaline phosphatase, bilirubin, creatinine, LDH, bleeding time. May decrease potassium, sodium, uric acid.

SIDE EFFECTS

FREQUENT: Phlebitis, thrombophlebitis w/IV dose, rash, urticaria, pruritus, taste/smell disturbances. **OCCASIONAL:** Nausea, diarrhea, vomiting, flatulence. **RARE:** Headache, bleeding, hyperkalemia, or hypokalemia.

ADVERSE REACTIONS/TOXIC EFFECTS

Seizures, neurologic reactions w/overdosage (more often w/renal impairment). Superinfections, potentially fatal antibiotic-associated colitis may result from bacterial imbalance. Severe hypersensitivity reactions, including anaphylaxis, occur rarely.

NURSING IMPLICATIONS

BASELINE ASSESSMENT:

Question for history of allergies, esp. penicillins, cephalosporins. Obtain specimen for culture and sensitivity before giving first dose (therapy may begin before results are known).

INTERVENTION/EVALUATION:

Hold medication and promptly report rash (hypersensitivity) or diarrhea (w/fever, abdominal pain, mucus and blood in stool may indicate antibiotic-associated colitis). Assess food tolerance. Provide mouth care, sugarless gum or hard candy to offset taste, smell effects. Evaluate IV site for phlebitis (heat, pain, red streaking over vein). Monitor I&O, urinalysis, renal function tests. Assess for bleeding: Overt bleeding, bruising or tissue swelling, and check hematology reports. Monitor electrolytes, particularly potassium. Be alert for superinfection: Increased fever, onset of sore throat, diarrhea, vomiting, ulceration or other oral changes, anal/genital pruritus.

PATIENT/FAMILY TEACHING:

Continue antibiotic for full length of treatment. Space doses evenly. Notify physician in event of rash, diarrhea, bleeding, bruising, or other new symptom.

ticlopidine hydrochloride

tie-clow´pih-deen

(Ticlid)

CANADIAN AVAILABILITY:
Ticlid

CLASSIFICATION

Platelet aggregation inhibitor

PHARMACOKINETICS

Rapid, well absorbed from GI tract (absorption increases after meals). Protein binding: 98%. Metabolized in liver to active metabolite. Primarily excreted in urine. Half-life: single dose: 7.9-12.6 hrs; repeated doses: 4-5 days.

ACTION

Inhibits platelet aggregation. Inhibits release of platelet granule constituents, platelet-platelet interactions, and adhesion to endothelium and atheromatous plaque.

USES

To reduce risk of stroke in those who have experienced stroke-like warnings or those w/history of thrombotic stroke.

PO ADMINISTRATION

Give w/food or just after meals (bioavailability increased, GI discomfort decreased).

INDICATIONS/DOSAGE/ROUTES

Prevention of stroke:
PO: Adults, elderly: 250 mg 2 times/day.

PRECAUTIONS

CONTRAINDICATIONS: Hematopoietic disorders (neutropenia, thrombocytopenia), presence of hemostatic disorder, active pathologic bleeding (bleeding peptic ulcer, intracranial bleeding), severe liver impairment. **CAUTIONS:** Those at risk of increased bleeding from trauma, surgery, pathologic conditions. **PREGNANCY/LACTATION:** Unknown whether drug crosses placenta or is distributed in breast milk. **Pregnancy Catetory B.**

INTERACTIONS

DRUG INTERACTIONS: May increase risk of bleeding w/oral anticoagulants, heparin, thrombolytics, aspirin. **ALTERED LAB VALUES:** May increase alkaline phosphatase, bilirubin, liver function tests, cholesterol, triglycerides. May prolong bleeding time. May decrease neutrophil, platelet count.

SIDE EFFECTS

FREQUENT: Diarrhea, nausea, dyspepsia, rash, GI discomfort. **OCCASIONAL:** Neutropenia, purpura, vomiting. **RARE:** Flatulence, pruritus, dizziness.

ADVERSE REACTIONS/TOXIC EFFECTS

Overdosage produces peripheral vasodilation resulting in hypotension.

NURSING IMPLICATIONS

BASELINE ASSESSMENT:

Drug should be discontinued 10-14 days before surgery if antiplatelet effect is not desired.

INTERVENTION/EVALUATION:

Assist w/ambulation if dizziness occurs. Monitor heart sounds by auscultation. Assess B/P for hypotension. Assess skin for flushing, rash.

PATIENT/FAMILY TEACHING:

If nausea occurs, cola, unsalted crackers, or dry toast may relieve effect. Therapeutic response may not be achieved before 2-3 mos of continuous therapy.

timolol maleate

tim´oh-lol

(Blocadren, Timoptic, Timoptic XE)

FIXED-COMBINATION(S): W/hydrochlorothiazide, a diuretic (Timolide)

CANADIAN AVAILABILITY: Apo-Timol, Blocadren, Timoptic

CLASSIFICATION

Beta-adrenergic blocker

PHARMACOKINETICS

	ONSET	PEAK	DURATION
Eye drops	30 min	1-2 hrs	12-24 hrs

Well absorbed from GI tract. Minimal absorption following ophthalmic administration. Protein binding: <10%. Metabolized in liver. Primarily excreted in urine. Not removed by hemodialysis. Half-life: 4 hrs. *Ophthalmic:* Systemic absorption may occur.

ACTION

Nonselective beta-adrenergic blocking agent. Blocks $beta_1$-adrenergic receptors, slowing sinus heart rate, decreasing cardiac output, decreasing B/P (exact mechanism unknown but may block peripheral adrenergic receptors, decrease sympathetic outflow from CNS or decrease renin release from kidney). Blocks $beta_2$-adrenergic receptors, increasing airway resistance. Decreases myocardial ischemia severity by decreasing oxygen requirements. Reduces intraocular pressure (IOP).

USES

Management of mild to moderate hypertension. Used alone or in combination w/diuretics, especially thiazide-type. Reduces cardiovascular mortality in those w/definite/suspected acute MI. Prophylaxis of migraine headache. *Ophthalmic:* Reduces IOP in management of open-angle glaucoma, aphakic glaucoma, ocular hypertension, secondary glaucoma.

STORAGE/HANDLING

Store oral form, ophthalmic solution at room temperature.

PO/OPHTHALMIC ADMINISTRATION

PO:

1. May be given w/o regard to meals.
2. Tablets may be crushed.

OPHTHALMIC:

1. Place finger on lower eyelid and pull out until pocket is formed between eye and lower lid.
2. Hold dropper above pocket and place prescribed number of drops into pocket. Instruct pt to close eyes gently so medication will not be squeezed out of sac.
3. Apply gentle finger pressure to the lacrimal sac at inner canthus for 1 min following installation (lessens risk of systemic absorption).

INDICATIONS/DOSAGE/ROUTES

Hypertension:
PO: Adults, elderly: Initially, 10 mg 2 times/day, alone or in combination w/other therapy. Gradually increase at intervals of not less than 1 wk. **Maintenance:** 20-60 mg/day in 2 divided doses.

Myocardial infarction:
PO: Adults, elderly: 10 mg 2 times/day, beginning within 1-4 weeks after infarction.

Migraine prophylaxis:
PO: Adults, elderly: Initially, 10 mg 2 times/day. **Range:** 10-30 mg/day.

Glaucoma:
EYE DROPS: Adults, elderly: 1 drop of 0.25% solution in affected eye(s) 2 times/day. May be increased to 1 drop of 0.5% solution in affected eye(s) 2 times/day. When IOP is controlled, dosage may be reduced to 1 drop 1 time/day. If pt is transferred to timolol from another antiglaucoma agent, administer concurrently for 1 day. Discontinue other agent on following day. *Timoptic XE:* 1 drop/day.

PRECAUTIONS

Precautions apply to oral and ophthalmic administration (because of systemic absorption of ophthalmic). **CONTRAINDICATIONS:** Bronchial asthma, COPD, uncontrolled cardiac failure, sinus bradycardia, heart block greater than first degree, cardiogenic shock, CHF, unless secondary to tachyarrhythmias, those on MAO inhibitors. **CAUTIONS:** Inadequate cardiac function, impaired renal/hepatic function, hyperthyroidism. **PREGNANCY/LACTATION:** Distributed in breast milk; not for use in nursing women because of potential for serious adverse effect on nursing infant. Avoid use during first trimester. May produce bradycardia, apnea, hypoglycemia, hypothermia during delivery, small birth weight infants. **Pregnancy Category C.**

INTERACTIONS

DRUG INTERACTIONS: Diuretics, other hypotensives may increase hypotensive effect. Sympathomimetics, xanthines may mutually inhibit effects. May mask symptoms of hypoglycemia, prolong hypoglycemic effect of insulin, oral hypoglycemics. NSAIDs may decrease antihypertensive effect. **ALTERED LAB VALUES:** May increase ANA titer, SGOT (AST), SGPT (ALT), alkaline phosphatase, LDH, bilirubin, BUN, creatinine, potassium, uric acid, lipoproteins, triglycerides.

SIDE EFFECTS

Generally well tolerated. **FREQUENT:** *Oral:* Bradycardia. *Oph-*

thalmic: Eye irritation, visual disturbances. **OCCASIONAL:** Hypotension manifested as dizziness, nausea, diaphoresis, headache, fatigue; peripheral vascular insufficiency, nervousness, insomnia. **RARE:** GI discomfort, nausea, constipation, paresthesia, arthralgia.

ADVERSE REACTIONS/TOXIC EFFECTS

Oral form may produce profound bradycardia, hypotension, bronchospasm. Abrupt withdrawal may result in sweating, palpitations, headache, tremulousness. May precipitate CHF, myocardial infarction in those w/cardiac disease, thyroid storm in those w/thyrotoxicosis, peripheral ischemia in those w/existing peripheral vascular disease. Hypoglycemia may occur in previously controlled diabetics. Ophthalmic overdosage may produce bradycardia, hypotension, bronchospasm, acute cardiac failure.

NURSING IMPLICATIONS

BASELINE ASSESSMENT:

Assess B/P, apical pulse immediately before drug is administered (if pulse is 60/min or below, or systolic B/P is below 90 mm Hg, withhold medication, contact physician).

INTERVENTION/EVALUATION:

Monitor B/P for hypotension, respiration for shortness of breath. Assess pulse for strength/weakness, irregular rate, bradycardia. Monitor EKG for cardiac arrhythmias, particularly PVCs. Monitor stool frequency and consistency. Assist w/ambulation if dizziness occurs. Assess for evidence of CHF: Dyspnea (particularly on exertion or lying down), night cough, peripheral edema, distended neck veins. Monitor I&O (increase in weight, decrease in urine output may indicate CHF). Assess for nausea, diaphoresis, headache, fatigue. *Ophthalmic:* Monitor B/P and pulse regularly.

PATIENT/FAMILY TEACHING:

Do not abruptly discontinue medication. Compliance w/therapy regimen is essential to control glaucoma, hypertension, angina, arrhythmias. To avoid hypotensive effect, rise slowly from lying to sitting position, wait momentarily before standing. Avoid tasks that require alertness, motor skills until response to drug is established. Report shortness of breath, excessive fatigue, prolonged dizziness/headache. Do not use nasal decongestants, over-the-counter cold preparations (stimulants) w/o physician approval. Monitor B/P, pulse before taking medication. Restrict salt, alcohol intake. *Ophthalmic:* Teach pt how to correctly instill drops, how to take pulse. Importance of maintaining regimen, of keeping office visits to check IOP. Transient stinging, discomfort may occur upon instillation. Report difficulty breathing immediately.

tioconazole

tie-oh-con´ah-zole
(Vagistat)

CANADIAN AVAILABILITY:
Gyno-Trosyd

CLASSIFICATION

Antifungal

PHARMACOKINETICS

Systemic absorption minimal.

ACTION

Fungistatic. Inhibits biosynthesis of ergosterol, other sterols, damaging fungal cell membrane. Alters cell membrane permeability w/leakage of essential elements and impaired uptake of precursor molecules.

USES

Treatment of vulvovaginal candidiasis (moniliasis).

INTRAVAGINAL ADMINISTRATION

1. Use disposable gloves, always wash hands thoroughly after application.
2. Follow manufacturer's directions for use of applicator.
3. Insert applicator high in vagina.
4. Administer preferably at bedtime.

INDICATIONS/DOSAGE/ROUTES

Vulvovaginal candidiasis:
INTRAVAGINAL: Adults, elderly: 1 applicatorful just before bedtime as a single dose.

PRECAUTIONS

CONTRAINDICATIONS: Hypersensitivity to tioconazole, other imidazole antifungal agents, or any component of the cream/suppository. **CAUTIONS:** Safety and efficacy in children and diabetic pts not established. **PREGNANCY/LACTATION:** Unknown whether excreted in breast milk. **Pregnancy Category C.**

INTERACTIONS

DRUG INTERACTIONS: None significant. **ALTERED LAB VALUES:** None significant.

SIDE EFFECTS

FREQUENT: Headache (26% of pts). **OCCASIONAL:** Body pain, vulvovaginal pain, burning, itching, irritation. **RARE:** Flu-like syndrome: fever, chills, headache, and/or hypotension, occasionally w/vertigo and nausea.

ADVERSE REACTIONS/TOXIC EFFECTS

None significant.

NURSING IMPLICATIONS

BASELINE ASSESSMENT:

Question for hypersensitivity to tioconazole, other imidazole antifungal agents, or components of preparation. Confirm that potassium hydroxide culture and/or smears were done for accurate diagnosis, therapy may begin before results known. Inquire about use of rubber/latex contraceptives since there is interaction between such products and the medication.

INTERVENTION/EVALUATION:

Assess for therapeutic response or burning, itching, pain, or irritation.

PATIENT/FAMILY TEACHING:

Do not interrupt/stop regimen, even during menses. Teach pt proper insertion. Not affected by oral contraception. Notify physician of increased itching, irritation, burning. Consult physician about sexual intercourse, douching, or the use of other vaginal products. Do not use vaginal contraceptive diaphragms, condoms within 72 hrs after treatment. Avoid contact w/eyes. Wash hands thoroughly after application.

---

tirilazad (Freedox)
See supplement

tobramycin sulfate

tow-bra-my′sin
(Nebcin, Tobrex)

FIXED-COMBINATION(S):
W/dexamethasone, a steroid (TobraDex)

CANADIAN AVAILABILITY:
Nebcin, Tobrex

CLASSIFICATION

Antibiotic: Aminoglycoside

PHARMACOKINETICS

Rapid, complete absorption after IM administration. Widely distributed (does not cross blood-brain barrier, low concentrations in CSF). Protein binding: 10%. Excreted unchanged in urine. Removed by hemodialysis. Half-life: 2-4 hrs (increased in decreased renal function, neonates; decreased in cystic fibrosis, burn or febrile pts).

ACTION

Irreversibly binds to protein on 30S subunit of bacterial ribosome, interfering in protein synthesis of susceptible microorganisms.

USES

Skin/skin structure, bone, joint, respiratory tract infections; post-op, burn, intra-abdominal infections, complicated urinary tract infections, septicemia, meningitis. *Ophthalmic:* Superficial eye infections: Blepharitis, conjunctivitis, keratitis, corneal ulcers.

STORAGE/HANDLING

Store vials, ophthalmic ointment, solution at room temperature. Solutions may be discolored by light/air (does not affect potency). Intermittent IV infusion (piggyback) stable for 24 hrs at room temperature. Discard if precipitate forms.

IM/IV/OPHTHALMIC ADMINISTRATION

NOTE: Coordinate peak and trough lab draws w/administration times.

IM:

1. To minimize discomfort, give deep IM slowly. Less painful if injected into gluteus maximus rather than lateral aspect of thigh.

IV:

1. Dilute w/50-200 ml 5% dextrose, 0.9% NaCl, or other compatible fluid. Amount of diluent for infants, children depends upon individual need.
2. Infuse over 20-60 min.
3. Alternating IV sites, use large veins to reduce risk of phlebitis.

OPHTHALMIC:

1. Place finger on lower eyelid and pull out until a pocket is formed between eye and lower lid.
2. Hold dropper above pocket and place correct number of drops (¼-½ inch ointment) into pocket. Have pt close eye gently.
3. *Solution:* Apply digital pressure to lacrimal sac for 1-2 min (minimizes drainage into nose and throat, reducing risk of systemic effects.) *Ointment:* Close eye for 1-2 min, rolling eyeball (increases contact area of drug to eye).
4. Remove excess solution or ointment around eye w/tissue.

INDICATIONS/DOSAGE/ROUTES

NOTE: Space parenteral doses evenly around the clock. Dosage based on ideal body weight. Peak, trough level is determined periodically to maintain desired serum concentrations (minimizes risk of toxicity). *Recommended peak level:* 4-10 mcg/ml; *trough level:* 1-2 mcg/ml.

Moderate to severe infections:
IM/IV: Adults, elderly: 3 mg/kg/day in divided doses q8h.

Life-threatening infections:
IM/IV: Adults, elderly: Up to 5 mg/kg/day in divided doses q6-8h.

Usual dosage for children, infants:
IM/IV: Children, infants: 6-7.5 mg/kg/day in 3-4 divided doses.

Dosage in renal impairment:
Dose and/or frequency is modified based on degree of renal impairment, serum concentration of drug. After loading dose of 1-2 mg/kg, maintenance dose/frequency based on serum creatinine/creatinine clearance.

Usual ophthalmic dosage:
OPHTHALMIC OINTMENT: Adults, elderly: Thin strip to conjunctiva q8-12h (q3-4h for severe infections). **OPHTHALMIC SOLUTION: Adults, elderly:** 1-2 drops q4h (2 drops every hr for severe infections).

PRECAUTIONS

CONTRAINDICATIONS: Hypersensitivity to tobramycin, other aminoglycosides (cross-sensitivity). **CAUTIONS:** Elderly, neonates because of renal insufficiency/immaturity; neuromuscular disorders (potential for respiratory depression), prior hearing loss, vertigo, renal impairment. Cumulative effects may occur w/concurrent ophthalmic and systemic administration. **PREGNANCY/LACTATION:** Readily crosses placenta; is distributed in breast milk. May cause fetal nephrotoxicity. **Pregnancy Category D.** Ophthalmic form should not be used in nursing mothers and only when specifically indicated in pregnancy. **Pregnancy Category B.**

INTERACTIONS

DRUG INTERACTIONS: Other aminoglycosides, nephrotoxic, ototoxic producing medications may increase toxicity. May increase effects of neuromuscular blocking agents. **ALTERED LAB VALUES:** May increase BUN, SGPT (ALT), SGOT (AST), bilirubin, creatinine, LDH concentrations; may decrease serum calcium, magnesium, potassium, sodium concentrations.

SIDE EFFECTS

OCCASIONAL: Pain, induration at IM injection site; phlebitis, thrombophlebitis w/IV administration; hypersensitivity reactions (rash, fever, urticaria, pruritus). *Ophthalmic:* Tearing, itching, redness, swelling of eyelid. **RARE:** Hypotension, nausea, vomiting.

ADVERSE REACTIONS/TOXIC EFFECTS

Nephrotoxicity (evidenced by increased BUN and serum creatinine, decreased creatinine clearance) may be reversible if drug stopped at first sign of symptoms; irreversible ototoxicity (tinnitus, dizziness, ringing/roaring in ears, reduced hearing) and neurotoxicity (headache, dizziness, lethargy, tremors, visual disturbances) occur occasionally. Risk is greater w/higher dosages, prolonged therapy, or if solution is applied directly to mucosa. Superinfections, particularly w/fungi, may result from bacterial imbalance via any route of administration; anaphylaxis.

NURSING IMPLICATIONS

Baseline Assessment:

Dehydration must be treated before parenteral therapy is begun. Question for history of allergies, esp. to aminoglycosides and sulfite (and parabens for topical/ophthalmic routes). Establish baseline for hearing acuity. Obtain specimens for culture, sensitivity before giving first dose (therapy may begin before results are known).

Intervention/Evaluation:

Monitor I&O (maintain hydration), urinalysis (casts, RBCs, WBCs, decrease in specific gravity). Monitor results of peak/trough blood tests. Be alert to ototoxic and neurotoxic symptoms (see Adverse Reactions/Toxic Effects). Check IM injection site for pain, induration. Evaluate IV site for phlebitis (heat, pain, red streaking over vein). Assess for rash (*ophthalmic*—assess for redness, swelling, itching, tearing). Be alert for superinfection particularly genital/anal pruritus, changes of oral mucosa, diarrhea. When treating pts w/neuromuscular disorders, assess respiratory response carefully.

Patient/Family Teaching:

Continue antibiotic for full length of treatment. Space doses evenly. Discomfort may occur w/IM injection. Notify physician in event of any hearing, visual, balance, urinary problems even after therapy is completed. Do not take other medication w/o consulting physician. Lab tests are an essential part of therapy. *Ophthalmic:* Blurred vision/tearing may occur briefly after application. Contact physician if tearing, redness, or irritation continue.

tocainide hydrochloride

toe-kayn′eyed

(Tonocard)

CANADIAN AVAILABILITY:
Tonocard

CLASSIFICATION

Antiarrhythmic

PHARMACOKINETICS

Completely absorbed from GI tract. Widely distributed. Protein binding: 10%. Metabolized in liver. Primarily excreted in urine. Removed by hemodialysis. Half-life: 15 hrs (increased in decreased renal function).

ACTION

Blocks sodium channels in cardiac tissues, particularly Purkinje fibers. Reduces action potential, decreases automaticity, shortens action potential duration, decreases effective refractory period.

USES

Suppression, prevention of ventricular arrhythmias including frequent unifocal/multifocal coupled premature ventricular contractions and paroxysmal ventricular tachycardia.

PO ADMINISTRATION

1. Do not crush or break film-coated tablets.

2. May give w/food (decreases GI upset).

3. Monitor EKG for cardiac changes, particularly, shortening of QT interval. Notify physician of any significant interval changes.

INDICATIONS/DOSAGE/ROUTES

NOTE: When giving tocainide in those receiving IV lidocaine, give single 600 mg dose 6 hrs before cessation of lidocaine and repeat in 6 hrs. Then give standard tocainide maintenance doses.

Ventricular arrhythmias:
PO: Adults, elderly: Initially, 400 mg q8h. **Maintenance:** 1.2-1.8 Gm/day in divided doses q8h. **Maximum:** 2,400 mg/day

PRECAUTIONS

CONTRAINDICATIONS: Hypersensitivity to local anesthetics, second- or third-degree AV block. **CAUTIONS:** CHF, elderly, severe respiratory depression, bradycardia, incomplete heart block. **PREGNANCY/LACTATION:** Unknown whether drug crosses placenta or is distributed in breast milk. **Pregnancy Category C.**

INTERACTIONS

DRUG INTERACTIONS: Other antiarrhythmics may increase risk of adverse cardiac effects. Beta-adrenergic blockers may increase pulmonary wedge pressure, decrease cardiac index. **ALTERED LAB VALUES:** None significant.

SIDE EFFECTS

Generally well tolerated. **FREQUENT:** Minor, transient lightheadedness, dizziness, nausea, paresthesia, rash, tremor. **OCCASIONAL:** Clammy skin, night sweats, joint pain. **RARE:** Restlessness, nervousness, disorientation, mood changes, ataxia (muscular incoordination), visual disturbances.

ADVERSE REACTIONS/TOXIC EFFECTS

High dosage may produce bradycardia/tachycardia, hypotension, palpitations, increased ventricular arrhythmias, PVCs, chest pain, exacerbation of CHF.

NURSING IMPLICATIONS

BASELINE ASSESSMENT:

Assess pulse for strength/weakness, irregular rate. Monitor EKG for cardiac changes, particularly shortening of QT interval. Notify physician of any significant interval changes. Monitor fluid and electrolyte serum levels. Assess hand movement for sign of tremor (usually first clinical sign that maximum dose is being reached). Assess sleeping pt for night sweats. Question for tingling/numbness in hands/feet. Assess skin for rash, clamminess. Observe for CNS disturbances (restlessness, disorientation, mood changes, incoordination). Assist w/ambulation if lightheadedness, dizziness occur. Assess for evidence of CHF: Dyspnea (particularly on exertion or lying down), night cough, peripheral edema, distended neck veins. Monitor I&O (increase in weight, decrease in urine output may indicate CHF). Monitor for therapeutic serum level (3-10 mcg/ml).

PATIENT/FAMILY TEACHING:

Avoid tasks that require alertness, motor skills until response to drug is established. Side effects generally disappear w/continued therapy. Unsalted crackers, dry toast may relieve nausea.

tolazamide

tole-az′ah-mide
(Tolinase, Tolamide)

CLASSIFICATION

Hypoglycemic: Oral

PHARMACOKINETICS

	ONSET	PEAK	DURATION
PO	4-6 hrs	—	10 hrs

Rapidly absorbed from GI tract. Protein binding: 90%. Metabolized in liver to active metabolite. Primarily excreted in urine. Half-life: 7 hrs.

ACTION

Promotes release of insulin from beta cells of pancreas, decreases hepatic glycogenolysis and gluconeogenesis, increases insulin sensitivity at peripheral sites.

USES

As adjunct to diet/exercise in management of stable, mild to moderately severe noninsulin dependent diabetes mellitus (type II, NIDDM). May be used to supplement insulin in pts w/type I diabetes mellitus.

PO ADMINISTRATION

May give w/food. Responses are better if given 15-30 min before meals.

INDICATIONS/DOSAGE/ROUTES

Diabetes mellitus:
PO: Adults, elderly: Initially, 100 mg/day up to 1,000 mg/day in 1-2 doses. **Maintenance:** 250 mg/day. Pts on 500 mg or less usually take 1 dose/day.

PRECAUTIONS

CONTRAINDICATIONS: Sole therapy for: Type I diabetes mellitus, diabetic complications (ketosis, acidosis, diabetic coma), stress situations (severe infection, trauma, surgery); hypersensitivity to drug; severe renal, endocrine, or hepatic impairment; uremia. **CAUTIONS:** Elderly, malnourished/debilitated, those w/renal or hepatic dysfunction, cardiac disease, pituitary/adrenal insufficiency, history of hepatic porphyria. Cardiovascular risks may be increased. **PREGNANCY/LACTATION:** Insulin is drug of choice during pregnancy; tolazamide given within 2 wks of delivery may cause neonatal hypoglycemia. Drug crosses placenta; is excreted in breast milk. **Pregnancy Category C.**

INTERACTIONS

DRUG INTERACTIONS: May have disulfiram reaction w/alcohol. May increase effect of oral anticoagulants. Chloramphenicol, MAOIs, salicylates, sulfonamides may increase effect. Beta-adrenergic blockers may increase hypoglycemic effect, mask signs of hypoglycemia. May increase effect of insulin. **ALTERED LAB VALUES:** May increase alkaline phosphatase, SGOT (AST), LDH, creatinine, BUN. May decrease uric acid.

SIDE EFFECTS

FREQUENT: Nausea, heartburn, epigastric fullness. **OCCASIONAL:** Vomiting, diarrhea, constipation, skin reactions characterized as pruritus, photosensitivity, urticaria. **RARE:** Headache, dizziness, malaise, weakness, vertigo.

ADVERSE REACTIONS/TOXIC EFFECTS

Hypoglycemia may occur due to

overdosage, insufficient food intake esp. w/increased glucose demands. Cholestatic hepatic jaundice, blood dyscrasias, disulfiram-like reaction occur rarely.

NURSING IMPLICATIONS

BASELINE ASSESSMENT:

Question for hypersensitivity to tolazamide. Check blood glucose level. Discuss lifestyle to determine extent of learning, emotional needs.

INTERVENTION/EVALUATION:

Monitor blood glucose and food intake. Assess for hypoglycemia (cool wet skin, tremors, dizziness, anxiety, headache, tachycardia, numbness in mouth, hunger, diplopia) or hyperglycemia (polyuria, polyphagia, polydipsia; nausea and vomiting; dim vision; fatigue; deep rapid breathing). Monitor stools for diarrhea, constipation. Check for adverse skin reactions, jaundice. Monitor hematology reports. Assess for bleeding/bruising. Be alert to conditions altering glucose requirements (fever, increased activity/stress, surgical procedure).

PATIENT/FAMILY TEACHING:

Prescribed diet is principal part of treatment; do not skip/delay meals. Diabetes mellitus requires life-long control. Check blood glucose/urine as ordered. Signs and symptoms, treatment of hypo/hyperglycemia. Carry candy, sugar packets, or other sugar supplements for immediate response to hypoglycemia. Wear, carry medical alert identification. Check w/ physician when glucose demands change, e.g., fever, infection, trauma, stress, heavy physical activity. Avoid alcoholic beverages. Do not take other medication w/o consulting physician. Weight control, exercise, hygiene (including foot care) and nonsmoking are essential part of therapy. Protect skin, limit sun exposure. Avoid exposure to infections. Select clothing, positions that do not restrict blood flow. Notify physician promptly of skin eruptions, itching, bleeding, yellow skin, dark urine. Inform dentist, physician, or surgeon of this medication before any treatment. (Assure follow-up instruction if pt/family does not thoroughly understand diabetes management or glucose testing techniques.)

tolazoline hydrochloride

toll-ah´zoh-lean

(Priscoline)

CLASSIFICATION

Antihypertensive

PHARMACOKINETICS

Rapidly, completely absorbed. Concentrated primarily in liver, kidney. Excreted unchanged in urine. Half-life: 3-10 hrs.

ACTION

Directly relaxes vascular smooth muscle (causes vasodilation, decreases peripheral resistance). Has moderate alpha-adrenergic blocking activity.

USES

Treatment of persistent pulmonary vasoconstriction and hypertension of newborn (persistent fetal circulation). Improves oxygenation.

PARENTERAL ADMINISTRATION

Monitor B/P diligently for systemic hypotension. If hypotension occurs, place in supine position w/feet elevated, give IV fluids. Do not administer epinephrine. Tolazoline may cause "epinephrine reversal" (further B/P decrease followed by rebound hypertension).

INDICATIONS/DOSAGE/ROUTES

Persistent fetal circulation:
IV: Newborn: Initially, 1-2 mg/kg via scalp vein over 10 min; then, IV infusion of 1-2 mg/kg/hr.

PRECAUTIONS

CONTRAINDICATIONS: None significant. **CAUTIONS:** Known/suspected mitral stenosis. **PREGNANCY/LACTATION:** Unknown whether drug crosses placenta or is distributed in breast milk. **Pregnancy Category C.**

INTERACTIONS

DRUG INTERACTIONS: Antagonizes vasoconstriction caused by dopamine. Decreases effects of metaraminol, ephedrine, phenylephrine. **ALTERED LAB VALUES:** None significant.

SIDE EFFECTS

Frequency of effects unknown: Flushing, vomiting, diarrhea, rash.

ADVERSE REACTIONS/TOXIC EFFECTS

Overdosage may produce increased pilomotor activity (goose bumps), skin flushing. Profound hypotension, arrhythmias, tachycardia, rebound hypertension, GI hemorrhage, pulmonary hemorrhage, hepatitis, thrombocytopenia, leukopenia, edema, oliguria, hematuria may occur.

NURSING IMPLICATIONS

BASELINE ASSESSMENT:

Obtain B/P immediately before each dose, in addition to regular monitoring (be alert to fluctuations). If excessive reduction in B/P occurs, place pt in supine position w/feet elevated, give IV fluids.

INTERVENTION/EVALUATION:

Monitor vital signs, oxygenation, acid-base balance, fluid and electrolytes.

tolbutamide

tole-byoo´tah-mide
(Orinase, Oramide)

CANADIAN AVAILABILITY:
Apo-Tolbutamide, Mobenol, Novobutamide, Orinase

CLASSIFICATION

Hypoglycemic: Oral

PHARMACOKINETICS

	ONSET	PEAK	DURATION
PO	—	5-8 hrs	24 hrs

Rapidly absorbed from GI tract. Protein binding: 90%. Metabolized in liver. Primarily excreted in urine. Half-life: 4.5-6.5 hrs.

ACTION

Promotes release of insulin from beta cells of pancreas, decreases hepatic glycogenolysis and gluconeogenesis, increases insulin sensitivity at peripheral sites.

USES

As adjunct to diet/exercise in management of stable, mild to moderately severe noninsulin dependent diabetes mellitus (type II, NIDDM). May be used to supplement insulin in pts w/type I diabetes mellitus.

PO ADMINISTRATION

May give w/food. Responses are better if given 15-30 min before meals.

INDICATIONS/DOSAGE/ROUTES

Diabetes mellitus:
PO: Adults: Initially, 500 mg/day up to 3,000 mg/day in 2-3 divided doses. **Maintenance:** 1,500 mg/day.

Usual elderly dosage:
PO: Elderly: 250 mg 1-3 times/day. **Range:** 500-2000 mg/day. **Maximum:** 3000 mg/day.

PRECAUTIONS

CONTRAINDICATIONS: Sole therapy for: Type I diabetes mellitus, diabetic complications (ketosis, acidosis, diabetic coma), stress situations (severe infection, trauma, surgery), hypersensitivity to drug, severe renal/hepatic impairment. **CAUTIONS:** Elderly, malnourished/debilitated, those w/renal or hepatic dysfunction, cardiac disease, adrenal/pituitary insufficiency, history of hepatic porphyria. Cardiovascular risks may be increased. **PREGNANCY/LACTATION:** Insulin is drug of choice during pregnancy, tolbutamide given within 2 wks of delivery may cause neonatal hypoglycemia. Drug crosses placenta. Excreted in breast milk. **Pregnancy Category C.**

INTERACTIONS

DRUG INTERACTIONS: May have disulfiram reaction w/alcohol. May increase effect of oral anticoagulants. Chloramphenicol, MAO inhibitors, salicylates, sulfonamides may increase effect. Beta-adrenergic blockers may increase hypoglycemic effect, mask signs of hypoglycemia. May increase effect of insulin. **ALTERED LAB VALUES:** May increase alkaline phosphatase, SGOT (AST), LDH, creatinine, BUN. May decrease uric acid.

SIDE EFFECTS

FREQUENT: Nausea, heartburn, epigastric fullness, taste alteration. **OCCASIONAL:** Anorexia, vomiting, diarrhea, skin reactions characterized as pruritus, photosensitivity, urticaria, headache.

ADVERSE REACTIONS/TOXIC EFFECTS

Hypoglycemia may occur due to overdosage, insufficient food intake esp. w/increased glucose demands. Cholestatic hepatic jaundice, blood dyscrasias, disulfiram-like reaction occur rarely.

NURSING IMPLICATIONS

BASELINE ASSESSMENT:

Question for hypersensitivity to tolbutamide. Check blood glucose level. Discuss lifestyle to determine extent of learning, emotional needs.

INTERVENTION/EVALUATION:

Monitor blood glucose and food intake. Assess for hypoglycemia (cool wet skin, tremors, dizziness, anxiety, headache, tachycardia, numbness in mouth, hunger, diplopia) or hyperglycemia (polyuria, polyphagia, polydipsia; nausea and vomiting; dim vision; fatigue; deep rapid breathing). Check I&O, assess for water retention. Be alert to conditions altering glucose requirements (fever, increased activity/stress, surgical procedure). Monitor stools for diarrhea, constipation. Check for adverse skin reactions, jaundice. Monitor hematology reports. Assess for bleeding/bruising.

PATIENT/FAMILY TEACHING:

Prescribed diet is a principal part of treatment; do not skip/delay meals. Diabetes mellitus requires life-long control. Check blood glucose/urine as ordered. Signs and symptoms, treatment of hypo/hyperglycemia. Carry candy, sugar packets, or other sugar supplements for immediate response to hypoglycemia. Wear, carry medical alert identification. Check w/physician when glucose demands change, e.g., fever, infection, trauma, stress, heavy physical activity. Avoid alcoholic beverages. Do not take other medication w/o consulting physician. Weight control, exercise, hygiene (including foot care) and nonsmoking are essential part of therapy. Protect skin, limit sun exposure. Avoid exposure to infections. Select clothing, positions that do not restrict blood flow. Notify physician promptly of shortness of breath, swelling, skin eruptions, bleeding, yellow skin, dark urine. Inform dentist, physician, or surgeon of this medication before any treatment. (Assure follow-up instruction if pt/family does not thoroughly understand diabetes management or glucose testing techniques.)

tolmetin sodium

toll´meh-tin

(Tolectin)

CANADIAN AVAILABILITY:
Tolectin

CLASSIFICATION

Nonsteroidal anti-inflammatory

PHARMACOKINETICS

	ONSET	PEAK	DURATION
PO (anti-rheumatic):	7 days	1-2 wks	—

Rapidly, completely absorbed from GI tract. Protein binding: >90%. Metabolized in liver. Excreted in urine. Half-life: 5 hrs.

ACTION

Inhibits prostaglandin synthesis. Inhibits action of cyclooxygenase, decreases formation of prostaglandin, thromboxane precursors from arachidonic acid.

USES

Relief of pain, disability associated w/rheumatoid arthritis, juvenile rheumatoid arthritis, osteoarthritis.

PO ADMINISTRATION

May give w/food, milk, or antacids if GI distress occurs.

INDICATIONS/DOSAGE/ROUTES

Rheumatoid arthritis, osteoarthritis:

PO: Adults, elderly: Initially, 400 mg 3 times/day (including 1 dose upon arising, 1 dose at bedtime).

Adjust dose at 1-2 wk intervals. **Maintenance:** 600-1,800 mg/day in 3-4 divided doses.

Juvenile rheumatoid arthritis:
PO: Children >2 yrs: Initially, 20 mg/kg/day in 3-4 divided doses. **Maintenance:** 15-30 mg/kg/day in 3-4 divided doses.

PRECAUTIONS

CONTRAINDICATIONS: History of hypersensitivity to aspirin or other NSAIDs, those severely incapacitated, bedridden, wheelchair-bound. **CAUTIONS:** Impaired renal function, impaired cardiac function, coagulation disorders, history of upper GI disease. **PREGNANCY/LACTATION:** Distributed in breast milk. Avoid use during third trimester (may adversely affect fetal cardiovascular system [premature closure of ductus arteriosus]). **Pregnancy Category C.**

INTERACTIONS

DRUG INTERACTIONS: May increase effects of oral anticoagulants, heparin, thrombolytics. May decrease effect of antihypertensives, diuretics. Salicylates, aspirin may increase risk of GI side effects, bleeding. Bone marrow depressants may increase risk of hematologic reactions. May increase concentration, toxicity of lithium. May increase methotrexate toxicity. Probenecid may increase concentration. Antacids may decrease concentration. **ALTERED LAB VALUES:** May increase BUN, potassium, liver function tests. May decrease Hgb, Hct. May prolong bleeding time.

SIDE EFFECTS

FREQUENT: Nausea, indigestion, GI distress, diarrhea, flatulence, vomiting, headache, loss of strength (asthenia), increased B/P, mild peripheral edema, dizziness, weight gain/loss.

ADVERSE REACTIONS/TOXIC EFFECTS

Peptic ulcer, GI bleeding, gastritis, severe hepatic reaction (cholestasis, jaundice) occur rarely. Nephrotoxicity (dysuria, hematuria, proteinuria, nephrotic syndrome) and severe hypersensitivity reaction (fever, chills, bronchospasm) occur rarely.

NURSING IMPLICATIONS

BASELINE ASSESSMENT:

Assess onset, type, location, and duration of pain/inflammation. Inspect appearance of affected joints for immobility, deformities, and skin condition.

INTERVENTION/EVALUATION:

Monitor pattern of daily bowel activity, stool consistency. Assist w/ambulation if dizziness occurs. Monitor for evidence of GI distress. Evaluate for therapeutic response (relief of pain, stiffness, swelling; increase in joint mobility, reduced joint tenderness, improved grip strength).

PATIENT/FAMILY TEACHING:

Therapeutic effect noted in 1-3 wks. Avoid tasks that require alertness, motor skills until response to drug is established. If GI upset occurs, take w/food, milk. Avoid aspirin, alcohol during therapy (increases risk of GI bleeding). Report headache, GI distress.

tolnaftate

tole-naf´tate
(Tinactin, Aftate)

CANADIAN AVAILABILITY:
Pitrex, Tinactin

CLASSIFICATION

Antifungal

ACTION

Distorts hyphae and stunts mycelial growth in susceptible fungi. Fungistatic/fungicidal; exact mechanism unknown.

USES

Treatment of *Tinea pedis, T. cruris, T. corporis, T. manuum, T. versicolor.* Also, superficial fungal infections of skin, mild fungus infections of scalp *(T. capitis).*

INDICATIONS/DOSAGE/ROUTES

Usual topical dosage:
TOPICAL: Adults, elderly: 2 times/day, morning and evening, to affected area for 2-6 wks.

PRECAUTIONS

CONTRAINDICATIONS: Hypersensitivity to tolnaftate, components of preparation. **PREGNANCY/LACTATION: Pregnancy Category C.**

INTERACTIONS

DRUG INTERACTIONS: None significant. **ALTERED LAB VALUES:** None significant.

SIDE EFFECTS

OCCASIONAL: Stinging when spray solution applied. **Rare:** Increased local irritation.

ADVERSE REACTIONS/TOXIC EFFECTS

None significant.

NURSING IMPLICATIONS

BASELINE ASSESSMENT:

Question for history of hypersensitivity to tolnaftate or ingredients of preparation.

INTERVENTION/EVALUATION:

Assess for therapeutic response or increased local irritation.

PATIENT/FAMILY TEACHING:

Rub cream well into affected areas. Deliberate concentration, inhaling of aerosol contents can be harmful or fatal. Do not use occlusive covering or use other preparations w/o consulting physician. Avoid contact w/eyes. Continue full course of therapy (may take several wks). Keep areas clean, dry; wear light clothing to promote ventilation. Separate personal items, linens. Notify physician of increased irritation.

torsemide

tore'seh-mide
(Demadex)

CLASSIFICATION

Diuretic: Loop

PHARMACOKINETICS

	ONSET	PEAK	DURATION
PO	1 hr	1-2 hrs	6-8 hrs
IV	20 min	1 hr	6-8 hrs

Rapidly, well absorbed from GI tract. Protein binding: 97-99%. Metabolized in liver. Primarily excreted in urine. Half-life: 3.3 hrs.

ACTION

Inhibits electrolyte reabsorption in thick ascending limb of loop of Henle. Inhibits the sodium/potassium/chloride carrier system (increases excretion of sodium, chloride, water; reduces effect on potassium excretion).

USES

Treatment of hypertension either alone or in combination w/ other antihypertensives. Edema associated w/CHF, renal disease, hepatic cirrhosis.

STORAGE/HANDLING

Store oral, parenteral form at room temperature.

PO/IV ADMINISTRATION

PO:

1. May take w/o regard to food. Give w/food to avoid GI upset, preferably w/breakfast (prevents nocturia).

IV:

1. Give slowly over 2 min.
2. Give high doses slowly (minimizes ototoxicity).

INDICATIONS/DOSAGE/ROUTES

Hypertension:
PO: Adults, elderly: Initially, 5 mg/day. May increase to 10 mg/day if no response in 4-6 wks. If no response, additional antihypertensive added.

Congestive heart failure:
IV/PO: Adults, elderly: Initially, 10-20 mg/day. May increase by approximately doubling dose until desired diuretic dose attained. (Dose >200 mg not adequately studied.)

Chronic renal failure:
IV/PO: Adults, elderly: Initially, 20 mg/day. May increase by approximately doubling dose until desired diuretic dose attained. (Dose >200 mg not adequately studied.)

Hepatic cirrhosis:
IV/PO: Adults, elderly: Initially, 5 mg/day (w/aldosterone antagonist or potassium sparing diuretic). May increase by approximately doubling dose until desired diuretic dose attained. (Dose >40 mg not adequately studied.)

PRECAUTIONS

CONTRAINDICATIONS: Anuria, hepatic coma, severe electrolyte depletion. **EXTREME CAUTION:** Hypersensitivity to sulfonamides. **CAUTIONS:** Elderly, cardiac pts, pts w/history of ventricular arrhythmias, pts w/hepatic cirrhosis, ascites. Renal impairment, systemic lupus erythematosus. Safety in children not known. **PREGNANCY/LACTATION:** Unknown whether drug is excreted in breast milk. **Pregnancy Category B.**

INTERACTIONS

DRUG INTERACTIONS: May increase antihypertensive effect of other antihypertensives. NSAIDs, probenecid may decrease effect. May increase risk of digoxin induced arrhythmias (due to hypokalemia). **ALTERED LAB VALUES:** May increase uric acid, BUN, creatinine. May decrease calcium, chloride, magnesium, potassium, sodium.

SIDE EFFECTS

FREQUENT: Headache, dizziness, rhinitis. **OCCASIONAL:** Asthenia, insomnia, nervousness, diarrhea, constipation, nausea, dyspepsia, edema, EKG changes, sore throat, cough, arthralgia, myalgia. **RARE:** Syncope, hypotension, arrhythmias.

ADVERSE REACTIONS/TOXIC EFFECTS

Acute, profound water loss, volume and electrolyte depletion, dehydration, decreased blood vol-

T

ume, circulatory collapse. Ototoxicity may occur: high IV doses must be given slowly to minimize ototoxicity.

NURSING IMPLICATIONS

BASELINE ASSESSMENT:

Assess B/P for hypotension. Check electrolyte levels, esp. potassium. Obtain baseline weight, check for edema, rales in lungs.

INTERVENTION/EVALUATION:

Monitor B/P, electrolytes (esp. potassium), I&O, weight. Notify physician of any hearing abnormality. Note extent of diuresis. Assess lungs for rales. Check for signs of edema, particularly of dependent areas. Although less potassium is lost w/torsemide than furosemide, assess for signs of hypokalemia (change of muscle strength, tremor, muscle cramps, change in mental status, cardiac arrhythmias).

PATIENT/FAMILY TEACHING:

Take medication in morning to prevent nocturia. Expect increased frequency and volume of urination. Report irregular heartbeats, signs of hypokalemia (see above). Change positions slowly to prevent orthostatic hypotension. Do not take other medications (including over-the-counter drugs) w/o consulting physician. Eat foods high in potassium such as whole grains (cereals), legumes, meat, bananas, apricots, orange juice, potatoes (white, sweet), raisins.

tramadol (Ultram)
See supplement

tranylcypromine sulfate

tran-ill-cy′proe-meen
(Parnate)

CANADIAN AVAILABILITY:
Parnate

CLASSIFICATION

Antidepressant: MAO inhibitor

PHARMACOKINETICS

Well absorbed from GI tract. Metabolized in liver. Primarily excreted in urine. Half-life: 1.5-3 hrs.

ACTION

Inhibits MAO enzyme (assists in metabolism of sympathomimetic amines) at CNS storage sites. Levels of epinephrine, norepinephrine, serotonin, dopamine increased at neuron receptor sites, producing antidepressant effect.

USES

Symptomatic treatment of severe depression in hospitalized or closely supervised pts who have not responded to other antidepressant therapy, including electroconvulsive therapy.

PO ADMINISTRATION

Give w/food if GI distress occurs.

INDICATIONS/DOSAGE/ROUTES

PO: Adults, elderly: 20 mg daily (10 mg in morning, 10 mg in afternoon) for 2 wks. If no response, increase to 30 mg/day (20 mg in morning, 10 mg in afternoon) for 1 wk. Thereafter, reduce dosage gradually to maintenance level of 10-20 mg/day.

PRECAUTIONS

CONTRAINDICATIONS: Pts >60 yrs, debilitated/hypertensive pts, cerebrovascular / cardiovascular disease, foods containing tryptophan/tyramine, within 10 days of elective surgery, pheochromocytoma, congestive heart failure, history of liver disease, abnormal liver function tests, severe renal impairment, history of severe/recurrent headache. **CAUTIONS:** Impaired renal function, history of seizures, parkinsonian syndrome, diabetic pts, hyperthyroidism. **PREGNANCY/LACTATION:** Crosses placenta; unknown whether distributed in breast milk. **Pregnancy Category C.**

INTERACTIONS

DRUG INTERACTIONS: Alcohol, CNS depressants may increase CNS depressant effects. Tricyclic antidepressants, fluoxetine, trazodone may cause serotonin syndrome. May increase effect of oral hypoglycemics, insulin. B/P may increase w/buspirone. Caffeine containing medications may increase cardiac arrhythmias, hypertension. May precipitate hypertensive crises w/carbamazepine, cyclobenzaprine, maprotiline, other MAO inhibitors. Meperidine, other opioid analgesics may produce immediate excitation, sweating, rigidity, severe hypertension or hypotension, severe respiratory distress, coma, convulsions, vascular collapse, death. May increase CNS stimulant, vasopressor effects. Tyramine, foods w/pressor amines (e.g., aged cheese) may cause sudden, severe hypertension. **ALTERED LAB VALUES:** None significant.

SIDE EFFECTS

FREQUENT: Postural hypotension, restlessness, GI upset, insomnia, dizziness, lethargy, weakness, dry mouth, peripheral edema. **OCCASIONAL:** Flushing, increased perspiration, rash, urinary frequency, increased appetite, transient impotence. **RARE:** Visual disturbances.

ADVERSE REACTIONS/TOXIC EFFECTS

Hypertensive crisis may be noted by hypertension, occipital headache radiating frontally, neck stiffness/soreness, nausea, vomiting, sweating, fever/chilliness, clammy skin, dilated pupils, palpitations. Tachycardia/bradycardia, constricting chest pain may also be present. Antidote for hypertensive crisis: 5-10 mg phentolamine IV injection.

NURSING IMPLICATIONS

BASELINE ASSESSMENT:

Periodic liver function tests should be performed in those requiring high dosage and/or undergoing prolonged therapy. MAO inhibitor therapy should be discontinued for 7-14 days before elective surgery.

INTERVENTION/EVALUATION:

Assess appearance, behavior, speech pattern, level of interest, mood. Monitor for occipital headache radiating frontally, and/or neck stiffness or soreness (may be first signal of impending hypertensive crisis). Monitor blood pressure diligently for hypertension. Assess skin temperature for fever. Discontinue medication immediately if palpitations or frequent headaches occur.

PATIENT/FAMILY TEACHING:

Antidepressant relief may be

noted during first week of therapy; maximum benefit noted within 3 wks. Report headache, neck stiffness/soreness immediately. To avoid orthostatic hypotension, change from lying to sitting position slowly and dangle legs momentarily before standing. Avoid tasks that require alertness, motor skills until response to drug is established. Avoid foods that require bacteria/molds for their preparation/preservation or those that contain tyramine, e.g., cheese, sour cream, beer, wine, pickled herring, liver, figs, raisins, bananas, avocados, soy sauce, yeast extracts, yogurt, papaya, broad beans, meat tenderizers, or excessive amounts of caffeine (coffee, tea, chocolate), or over-the-counter preparations for hay fever, colds, weight reduction.

trazodone hydrochloride

tray´zeh-doan

(Desyrel)

CANADIAN AVAILABILITY: Desyrel

CLASSIFICATION

Antidepressant

PHARMACOKINETICS

Well absorbed from GI tract. Protein binding: 89-95%. Metabolized in liver. Primarily excreted in urine. Half-life: 5-9 hrs.

ACTION

Selectively inhibits serotonin reuptake in brain. Alters serotonin receptor binding.

USES

Treatment of major depression often w/psychotherapy.

PO ADMINISTRATION

1. Give shortly after snack, meal (reduces risk of dizziness, lightheadedness).
2. Tablets may be crushed.

INDICATIONS/DOSAGE/ROUTES

Antidepressant:

PO: Adults: Initially, 150 mg daily in equally divided doses. Increase by 50 mg/day at 3-4 day intervals until therapeutic response is achieved. Do not exceed 400 mg/day for outpatients, 600 mg/day for hospitalized pts.

Usual elderly dosage:

PO: Elderly: Initially, 25-50 mg at bedtime. May increase by 25-50 mg q3-7days. **Range:** 75-150 mg/day.

PRECAUTIONS

CONTRAINDICATIONS: Recovery phase of MI, surgical pts, electroconvulsive therapy. **CAUTIONS:** Cardiovascular disease, MAO inhibitor therapy. **PREGNANCY/LACTATION:** Crosses placenta; minimally distributed in breast milk. **Pregnancy Category C.**

INTERACTIONS

DRUG INTERACTIONS: Alcohol, CNS depression producing medications may increase CNS depression. May increase effects of antihypertensives. May increase concentration of digoxin, phenytoin. **ALTERED LAB VALUES:** May decrease neutrophil, leukocyte counts.

SIDE EFFECTS

COMMON: Drowsiness, dry

mouth, lightheadedness/dizziness, headache, blurred vision, nausea/vomiting. **OCCASIONAL:** Nervousness, fatigue, constipation, generalized aches and pains, mild hypotension.

ADVERSE REACTIONS/TOXIC EFFECTS

Priapism (painful, prolonged penile erection), decreased/increased libido, retrograde ejaculation, impotence have been noted rarely. Appears to be less cardiotoxic than other antidepressants, although arrhythmias may occur in pts w/preexisting cardiac disease.

NURSING IMPLICATIONS

Baseline Assessment:

For those on long-term therapy, liver/renal function tests, blood counts should be performed periodically.

Intervention/Evaluation:

Supervise suicidal-risk pt closely during early therapy (as depression lessens, energy level improves, increasing suicide potential). Assess appearance, behavior, speech pattern, level of interest, mood. Monitor WBC and neutrophil count (drug should be stopped if levels fall below normal). Assist w/ambulation if dizziness or lightheadedness occurs.

Patient/Family Teaching:

Immediately discontinue medication and consult physician if priapism occurs. Change positions slowly to avoid hypotensive effect. Tolerance to sedative and anticholinergic effects usually develops during early therapy. Photosensitivity to sun may occur. Dry mouth may be relieved by sugarless gum, sips of tepid water. Report visual disturbances. Do not abruptly discontinue medication. Avoid tasks that require alertness, motor skills until response to drug is established. Avoid alcohol.

tretinoin

tret´ih-noyn
(Retin-A)

FIXED-COMBINATION(S):
W/octyl methoxycinnamate and oxybenzone, moistures, and SPF-12, a sunscreen (Retin-A Regimen Kit)

CANADIAN AVAILABILITY:
Retin-A, Stieva-A, Vitamin A Acid

CLASSIFICATION

Antiacne agent

PHARMACOKINETICS

Minimally absorbed following topical application.

ACTION

Acts as an irritant to decrease cohesiveness of follicular epithelial cells w/subsequent reduction of microcomedone formation; increases turnover of follicular epithelial cells, causing extrusion of comedones. Bacterial skin counts are not altered.

USES

Topical application in the treatment of acne vulgaris, esp. grades I-III in which comedones, papules, pustules predominate.

TOPICAL ADMINISTRATION

1. Thoroughly cleanse area before applying tretinoin.
2. Lightly cover entire affected

area. Liquid may be applied w/fingertip, gauze, or cotton, taking care to avoid running onto unaffected skin.

3. Wash hands immediately.

INDICATIONS/DOSAGE/ROUTES

Acne:

TOPICAL: Adults: Apply once daily at bedtime.

PRECAUTIONS

CONTRAINDICATIONS: Hypersensitivity to any component of the preparation. **EXTREME CAUTION:** Eczema. **CAUTIONS:** Those w/considerable sun exposure in their occupation or hypersensitivity to sun. **PREGNANCY/LACTATION:** Use during pregnancy only if clearly needed. Unknown whether excreted in breast milk; exercise caution in nursing mother. **Pregnancy Category B.**

INTERACTIONS

DRUG INTERACTIONS: Topical keratolytic agents (e.g., sulfur, benzoyl peroxide, salicylic acid) may increase skin irritation. **ALTERED LAB VALUES:** None significant.

SIDE EFFECTS

Local inflammatory reactions are to be expected and are reversible w/discontinuation of tretinoin. **FREQUENT:** Transient feeling of warmth or stinging, redness, and scaling. **OCCASIONAL:** Temporary hyperpigmentation, severe erythema, crusting, blistering, edema. **RARE:** Contact allergy.

ADVERSE REACTIONS/TOXIC EFFECTS

Possible tumorigenic potential when combined w/ultraviolet radiation.

NURSING IMPLICATIONS

PATIENT/FAMILY TEACHING:

If medications containing keratolytic agents (resorcinol, sulfur, benzoyl peroxide, or salicylic acid) have been used it is advisable to "rest" the skin until effects subside. Use of keratolytic agents concomitantly is discouraged due to possible interactions. Keep tretinoin away from eyes, mouth, angles of nose and mucous membranes. Minimize sunlight, sunlamp exposure; use sunscreens and protective clothing. Affected areas should also be protected from wind, cold. Do not use medicated, drying, or abrasive soaps; wash face no more than 2-3 times/day with bland soap. Avoid use of preparations containing alcohol, menthol, spice, or lime such as shaving lotions, astringents, perfume. Application may cause temporary warmth or stinging feeling. Mild redness, peeling are expected; decrease frequency or discontinue medication if excessive reaction occurs. Nonmedicated cosmetics may be used; however, cosmetics must be removed before tretinoin application.

triamcinolone

trye-am-sin´oh-lone

(Aristocort, Kenacort)

triamcinolone diacetate

(Amcort, Aristocort Intralesional, Trilone)

triamcinolone acetonide

(Aristocort, Azmacort, Kenalog)

triamcinolone hexacetonide

(Aristospan)

FIXED-COMBINATION(S): Triamcinolone acetonide w/Nystatin, an anti-fungal (Myco-Aricin, Myco II, Myco-Biotic, Mycogen II, Nystolone)

CANADIAN AVAILABILITY: Aristocort, Azmacort, Kenalog, Triaderm

CLASSIFICATION

Corticosteroid

PHARMACOKINETICS

Rapidly absorbed after inhalation. Completely absorbed from GI tract; well absorbed after IM administration. Widely distributed. Protein binding: 65-90%. Metabolized in liver. Primarily excreted in urine. Half-life: 2-5 hrs.

ACTION

Decreases/prevents tissue response to inflammatory process. Inhibits accumulation, inflammatory cells at inflammation sites, phagocytosis, lysosomal enzyme release and synthesis and/or release of mediators of inflammation. Prevents/suppresses cell-mediated immune reactions.

USES

Substitution therapy in deficiency states: Acute/chronic adrenal insufficiency, congenital adrenal hyperplasia, adrenal insufficiency secondary to pituitary insufficiency. Nonendocrine disorders: Arthritis, rheumatic carditis, allergic, collagen, intestinal tract, liver, ocular, renal, and skin diseases, bronchial asthma, cerebral edema, malignancies.

PO/IM/ORAL/INHALATION/ TOPICAL ADMINISTRATION

PO:

1. Give w/food or milk.
2. Single doses given before 9 AM; multiple doses at evenly spaced intervals.

IM:

1. Do *not* give IV.
2. Give deep IM in gluteus maximus.

ORAL INHALATION:

1. Shake and inhale immediately before use.
2. Pt should exhale completely; place mouthpiece 2 fingers–width away from mouth.
3. Tilt head back; while activating inhaler, take slow, deep breath for 3-5 sec.
4. Pt should hold breath as long as possible (5-10 sec) then exhale slowly.
5. Wait 1 min between inhalations when multiple inhalations ordered.
6. Following treatment, pt should thoroughly rinse mouth w/ water or mouthwash.

TOPICAL:

1. Gently cleanse area before application.
2. Use occlusive dressings only as ordered.
3. Apply sparingly and rub into area thoroughly.

INDICATIONS/DOSAGE/ROUTES

NOTE: Individualize dose based on disease, pt, and response.

Usual oral dosage:
PO: Adults, elderly: 4-60 mg/day.

Triamcinolone diacetate:
IM: Adults, elderly: 40 mg/wk.
INTRA-ARTICULAR, INTRASYNOVIAL: Adults, elderly: 5-40 mg.

Triamcinolone acetonide:
IM: Initially, 2.5-60 mg/day.
INTRA-ARTICULAR: Adults, elderly: Initially, 2.5-40 mg up to 100 mg.

Triamcinolone hexacetonide:
INTRA-ARTICULAR: Adults, elderly: 2-20 mg.

Control of bronchial asthma:
INHALATION: Adults, elderly: 2 inhalations 3-4 times/day. **Children 6-12 yrs:** 1-2 inhalations 3-4 times/day. **Maximum:** 12 inhalations/day.

Usual topical dosage:
TOPICAL: Adults, elderly: Sparingly 2-4 times/day. May give 1-2 times/day or intermittent therapy.

PRECAUTIONS

CONTRAINDICATIONS: Hypersensitivity to any corticosteroid or tartrazine, systemic fungal infection, peptic ulcers (except life-threatening situations). IM injection, oral inhalation not for children <6 yrs of age. Avoid immunizations, smallpox vaccination. *Topical:* marked circulation impairment. **CAUTIONS:** History of tuberculosis (may reactivate disease), hypothyroidism, cirrhosis, nonspecific ulcerative colitis, CHF, hypertension, psychosis, renal insufficiency. Prolonged therapy should be discontinued slowly. **PREGNANCY/LACTATION:** Drug crosses placenta, distributed in breast milk. May cause cleft palate (chronic use during first trimester). Nursing contraindicated. **Pregnancy Category C.**

INTERACTIONS

DRUG INTERACTIONS: Amphotericin may increase hypokalemia. May decrease effect of oral hypoglycemics, insulin, diuretics, potassium supplements. May increase digoxin toxicity (due to hypokalemia). Hepatic enzyme inducers may decrease effect. Live virus vaccines may potentiate virus replication, increase vaccine side effects, decrease pt's antibody response to vaccine. **ALTERED LAB VALUES:** May decrease calcium, potassium, thyroxine. May increase cholesterol, lipids, glucose, sodium, amylase.

SIDE EFFECTS

FREQUENT: Increased appetite, exaggerated sense of well-being, abdominal distension, weight gain, insomnia, mood swings. *High dose, prolonged therapy:* Increased susceptibility to infection (signs/symptoms masked); slow wound healing; hypokalemia, hypocalcemia; GI distress. **OCCASIONAL:** Headache, vertigo. **RARE:** Increased blood coagulability, tachycardia, frequency or urgency of urination, psychosis. *Topical:* allergic contact dermatitis.

ADVERSE REACTIONS/TOXIC EFFECTS

Long-term therapy: muscle wasting (esp. arms, legs), osteoporosis, spontaneous fractures, amenorrhea, cataracts, glaucoma, peptic ulcer, CHF. *Abrupt withdrawal following long-term therapy:* Anorexia, nausea, fever, headache, joint pain, rebound inflammation, fatigue, weakness, lethargy, dizziness, orthostatic hypotension. Anaphylaxis w/parenteral administration. Sudden discontinuance may be fatal. Blindness has occurred rarely after intralesional injection around face, head.

NURSING IMPLICATIONS

BASELINE ASSESSMENT:

Question for hypersensitivity to any of the corticosteroids or tartrazine (Kenacort). Obtain baselines for height, weight, B/P, glucose, electrolytes. Check results of initial tests, e.g., TB skin test, x-rays, EKG.

INTERVENTION/EVALUATION:

Monitor I&O, daily weight; assess for edema. Evaluate food tolerance and bowel activity; promptly report hyperacidity. Check B/P, temperature, pulse, respiration at least 2 times/day. Be alert to infection: Sore throat, fever, or vague symptoms. Monitor electrolytes. Watch for hypocalcemia (muscle twitching, cramps, positive Trousseau's or Chvostek's signs) or hypokalemia (weakness and muscle cramps, numbness/tingling, esp. in lower extremities, nausea and vomiting, irritability, EKG changes). Assess emotional status, ability to sleep. Check lab results for blood coagulability and clinical evidence of thromboembolism. Provide assistance w/ambulation.

PATIENT/FAMILY TEACHING:

Take w/food or milk. Carry identification of drug and dose, physician name and phone number. Do not change dose/schedule or stop taking drug, must taper off gradually under medical supervision. Notify physician of fever, sore throat, muscle aches, sudden weight gain/swelling. W/dietician give instructions for prescribed diet (usually sodium restricted w/ high vitamin D, protein and potassium). Maintain careful personal hygiene, avoid exposure to disease or trauma. Severe stress (serious infection, surgery, or trauma) may require increased dosage. Do not take any other medication w/o consulting physician. Follow-up visits, lab tests are necessary; children must be assessed for growth retardation. Inform dentist or other physicians of triamcinolone therapy now or within past 12 mo. Caution against overuse of joints injected for symptomatic relief. Teach proper oral inhalation technique. *Topical:* Apply after shower/bath for best absorption. Do not cover unless physician orders; do not use tight diapers, plastic pants or coverings. Avoid contact w/eyes. Do not expose treated area to sunlight.

triamterene

try-am´tur-een

(Dyrenium)

FIXED-COMBINATION(S):

W/hydrochlorothiazide, a thiazide diuretic (Dyazide, Maxzide)

CANADIAN AVAILABILITY:

Dyrenium

CLASSIFICATION

Diuretic: Potassium-sparing

PHARMACOKINETICS

	ONSET	PEAK	DURATION
PO	2-4 hrs	6-8 hrs	12-16 hrs

Incompletely absorbed from GI

tract. Widely distributed. Protein binding: 67%. Metabolized in liver. Primarily eliminated in feces via biliary route. Half-life: 1.5-2 hrs (increased in decreased renal function).

ACTION

Directly interferes w/sodium reabsorption in distal tubule, increasing sodium and water excretion and decreasing potassium excretion. Initial decrease in B/P due to decreased plasma and extracellular fluid volume.

USES

Treatment of edema associated w/CHF, hepatic cirrhosis, nephrotic syndrome, steroid-induced edema, idiopathic edema, edema due to secondary hyperaldosteronism. May be used alone or w/other diuretics.

PO ADMINISTRATION

1. May give w/food if GI disturbances occur.
2. Do not crush or break capsules.
3. Scored tablets may be crushed.

INDICATIONS/DOSAGE/ROUTES

NOTE: Fixed-combination medication should not be used for initial therapy but rather for maintenance therapy.

Dyrenium:
PO: Adults: Initially, 100 mg twice daily after meals. **Maintenance:** 100 mg/day or every other day. **Maximum:** 300 mg/day. When used concurrently w/other diuretics, decrease dosage of each drug initially; adjust to pt's needs.

Usual elderly dosage:
PO: Elderly: Initially, 50 mg/day. **Maximum:** 100 mg/day in 1-2 doses.

Dyazide, Maxzide:
PO: Adults: 1-2 capsules/tablets per day.

PRECAUTIONS

CONTRAINDICATIONS: Severe or progressive renal disease, severe hepatic disease, preexisting or drug-induced hyperkalemia. **CAUTIONS:** Impaired hepatic or kidney function, history of renal calculi, diabetes mellitus. **PREGNANCY/LACTATION:** Crosses placenta; is distributed in breast milk. Nursing is not advised. **Pregnancy Category B.**

INTERACTIONS

DRUG INTERACTIONS: May decrease effect of anticoagulants, heparin. NSAIDs may decrease antihypertensive effect. ACE inhibitors (e.g., catopril), potassium containing medications, potassium supplements may increase potassium. May decrease lithium clearance, increase toxicity. **ALTERED LAB VALUES:** May increase BUN, calcium excretion, creatinine, glucose, magnesium, potassium, uric acid. May decrease sodium.

SIDE EFFECTS

EXPECTED RESPONSE: Frequent urination, polyuria. **OCCASIONAL:** Tiredness, nausea, diarrhea, abdominal distress, leg aches, headache. **RARE:** Anorexia, weakness, rash, dizziness.

ADVERSE REACTIONS/TOXIC EFFECTS

Severe hyperkalemia may produce irritability, anxiety, heaviness of legs, paresthesia, hypotension, bradycardia, tented T waves, widening QRS, ST depression.

NURSING IMPLICATIONS

BASELINE ASSESSMENT:

Assess baseline electrolytes, particularly check for low potassium. Assess renal/hepatic functions. Assess edema (note location, extent), skin turgor, mucous membranes for hydration status. Assess muscle strength, mental status. Note skin temperature, moisture. Obtain baseline weight. Initiate strict I&O. Note pulse rate/regularity.

INTERVENTION/EVALUATION:

Monitor B/P, vital signs, electrolytes (particularly potassium), I&O, weight. Note extent of diuresis. Watch for changes from initial assessment (hyperkalemia may result in muscle strength changes, tremor, muscle cramps), change in mental status (orientation, alertness, confusion), cardiac arrhythmias. Monitor potassium level, particularly during initial therapy. Weigh daily. Assess lung sounds for rhonchi, wheezing.

PATIENT/FAMILY TEACHING:

Expect increase in volume and frequency of urination. Therapeutic effect takes several days to begin and can last for several days when drug is discontinued. High potassium diet/potassium supplements can be dangerous, esp. if pt has renal/hepatic problems.

triazolam

try-a-zoe´lam
(Halcion)

CANADIAN AVAILABILITY:
Apo-Triazo, Halcion, Novotriolam

CLASSIFICATION

Sedative-hypnotic **(Schedule IV)**

PHARMACOKINETICS

Well absorbed from GI tract. Widely distributed (crosses blood-brain barrier). Protein binding: 89%. Metabolized in liver (undergoes first-pass liver extraction). Primarily excreted in urine. Half-life: 1.5-5.5 hrs.

ACTION

Enhances action of inhibitory neurotransmitter gamma-aminobutyric acid (GABA). Depressant effects occur at all levels of CNS.

USES

Short-term treatment of insomnia (up to 6 wks). Reduces sleep-induction time, number of nocturnal awakenings; increases length of sleep.

PO ADMINISTRATION

1. Give w/o regard to meals.
2. Tablets may be crushed.

T

INDICATIONS/DOSAGE/ROUTES

Hypnotic:
PO: Adults >18 yrs: 0.125-0.5 mg at bedtime. **Elderly:** 0.0625-0.125 mg at bedtime.

PRECAUTIONS

CONTRAINDICATIONS: Acute narrow-angle glaucoma, acute alcohol intoxication. **CAUTIONS:** Impaired renal/hepatic function. **PREGNANCY/LACTATION:** May cross placenta; may be distributed in breast milk. Chronic ingestion during pregnancy may produce withdrawal symptoms. CNS depression in neonates. **Pregnancy Category X.**

INTERACTIONS

DRUG INTERACTIONS: Alcohol, CNS depressants may increase CNS depressant effect. **ALTERED LAB VALUES:** None significant.

SIDE EFFECTS

FREQUENT: Drowsiness, sedation, headache, dizziness, nervousness, lightheadedness, incoordination, nausea. **OCCASIONAL:** Euphoria, tachycardia, abdominal cramps, visual disturbances. **RARE:** Paradoxical CNS excitement, restlessness, particularly noted in elderly, debilitated.

ADVERSE REACTIONS/TOXIC EFFECTS

Abrupt or too-rapid withdrawal may result in pronounced restlessness, irritability, insomnia, hand tremors, abdominal/muscle cramps, sweating, vomiting, seizures. Overdosage results in somnolence, confusion, diminished reflexes, coma.

NURSING IMPLICATIONS

BASELINE ASSESSMENT:

Assess B/P, pulse, respirations immediately before administration. Raise bedrails. Provide environment conducive to sleep (backrub, quiet environment, low lighting).

INTERVENTION/EVALUATION:

Assess sleep pattern of pt. Assess elderly/debilitated for paradoxical reaction, particularly during early therapy. Evaluate for therapeutic response to insomnia: A decrease in number of nocturnal awakenings, increase in length of sleep.

PATIENT/FAMILY TEACHING:

Smoking reduces drug effectiveness. Do not abruptly withdraw medication following long-term use. Rebound insomnia may occur when drug is discontinued after short-term therapy. Avoid alcohol.

trifluoperazine hydrochloride

try-floo-oh-pear′ah-zeen
(Stelazine)

CANADIAN AVAILABILITY:
Apo-Trifluoperazine, Stelazine

CLASSIFICATION

Antipsychotic

PHARMACOKINETICS

Variably absorbed after oral administration, well absorbed after IM administration. Widely distributed. Protein binding: >90%. Metabolized in liver to some active metabolites. Primarily excreted in urine.

ACTION

Blocks postsynaptic dopaminergic receptors in brain. Has strong extrapyramidal, antiemetic action; weak anticholinergic, sedative effects.

USES

Management of psychotic disorders, nonpsychotic anxiety.

STORAGE/HANDLING

Store oral solutions, parenteral form at room temperature. Slight yellow discoloration of solutions does not affect potency, but discard if markedly discolored or if precipitate forms.

PO/IM ADMINISTRATION

PO:

1. Add oral concentrate to 60 ml tomato or fruit juice, milk, carbonated beverages, coffee, tea, water. May also add to semi-solid food.

IM:

1. **Parenteral administration:** Pt must remain recumbent for 30-60 min in head-low position w/legs raised, to minimize hypotensive effect.
2. Inject slow, deep IM into upper outer quadrant of gluteus maximus. If irritation occurs, further injections may be diluted w/0.9% NaCl or 2% procaine hydrochloride.

INDICATIONS/DOSAGE/ROUTES

NOTE: Decrease dosage gradually to optimum response, then decrease to lowest effective level for maintenance. Replace parenteral therapy w/oral therapy as soon as possible.

Psychotic disorders (hospitalized):
PO: Adults: 2-5 mg twice daily. Gradually increase to average daily dose of 15-20 mg (up to 40 mg may be required in severe cases). **Children 6-12 yrs:** 1 mg 1-2 times/day. Gradually increase to maximum daily dose of 15 mg.
IM: Adults: 1-2 mg q4-6h. Do not exceed 6 mg/24 hrs. **Children 6-12 yrs:** 1 mg 1-2 times/day.

Psychotic disorders (outpatient):
PO: Adults: 1-2 mg 2 times/day.

Nonpsychotic anxiety:
PO/IM: Adults: 1-2 mg 2 times/day.

Usual elderly dosage (nonpsychotic):
PO: Elderly: Initially, 1-5 mg 2 times/day. **Range:** 15-20 mg/day. **Maximum:** 40 mg/day.
IM: Elderly: Initially, 1 mg q4-6h as needed. **Maximum:** 6 mg/day.

PRECAUTIONS

CONTRAINDICATIONS: Severe CNS depression, comatose states, severe cardiovascular disease, bone marrow depression, subcortical brain damage. **CAUTIONS:** Impaired respiratory/hepatic/renal/cardiac function, alcohol withdrawal, history of seizures, urinary retention, glaucoma, prostatic hypertrophy, hypocalcemia (increases susceptibility to dystonias). **PREGNANCY/LACTATION:** Crosses placenta; distributed in breast milk. **Pregnancy Category C.**

INTERACTIONS

DRUG INTERACTIONS: Alcohol, CNS depressants may increase CNS, respiratory depression, hypotensive effects. Tricyclic antidepressants, MAO inhibitors may increase sedative, anticholinergic effects. Antithyroid agents may increase risk of agranulocytosis. Extrapyramidal symptoms (EPS) may increase w/EPS producing medications. Hypotensives may increase hypotension. May decrease levodopa effects. Lithium may decrease absorption, produce adverse neurologic effects. **ALTERED LAB VALUES:** May cause EKG changes.

SIDE EFFECTS

FREQUENT: Hypotension, dizziness, and fainting occur frequently after first injection, occasionally after subsequent injections, and rarely w/oral dosage. **OCCASIONAL:** Drowsiness during early therapy, dry mouth, blurred vision, lethargy, constipation or diarrhea, nasal congestion, peripheral edema, urinary retention. **RARE:** Ocular changes, skin pigmentation (those on high doses for prolonged periods).

ADVERSE REACTIONS/TOXIC EFFECTS

Extrapyramidal symptoms appear dose-related (particularly high dosage), and is divided into 3 categories: Akathisia (inability to sit still, tapping of feet, urge to move around), parkinsonian symptoms (mask-like face, tremors, shuffling gait, hypersalivation), and acute dystonias: Torticollis (neck muscle spasm), opisthotonos (rigidity of back muscles), and oculogyric crisis (rolling back of eyes). Dystonic reaction may also produce profuse sweating, pallor. Tardive dyskinesia (protrusion of tongue, puffing of cheeks, chewing/puckering of the mouth) occurs rarely (may be irreversible). Abrupt withdrawal following long-term therapy may precipitate nausea, vomiting, gastritis, dizziness, tremors. Blood dyscrasias, particularly agranulocytosis, mild leukopenia (sore mouth/gums/throat) may occur. May lower seizure threshold.

NURSING IMPLICATIONS

BASELINE ASSESSMENT:

Avoid skin contact w/solution (contact dermatitis). Assess behavior, appearance, emotional status, response to environment, speech pattern, thought content.

INTERVENTION/EVALUATION:

Monitor B/P for hypotension. Assess for extrapyramidal symptoms. Monitor WBC, differential count for blood dyscrasias. Monitor for fine tongue movement (may be early sign of tardive dyskinesia). Supervise suicidal-risk pt closely during early therapy (as depression lessons, energy level improves, increasing suicide potential). Assess for therapeutic response (interest in surroundings, improvement in self-care, increased ability to concentrate, relaxed facial expression).

PATIENT/FAMILY TEACHING:

Maximum therapeutic response occurs in 2-3 wks. Urine may darken. Do not abruptly withdraw from long-term drug therapy. Report visual disturbances. Sugarless gum or sips of tepid water may relieve dry mouth. Drowsiness generally subsides during continued therapy. Avoid tasks that require alertness, motor skills until response to drug is established. Avoid alcohol.

trifluridine

trye-flure´ih-deen

(Viroptic)

CANADIAN AVAILABILITY:

Viroptic

CLASSIFICATION

Antiviral

PHARMACOKINETICS

Intraocular penetration occurs after instillation. Half-life: 12-18 min.

ACTION

Incorporated into DNA causing increased rate of mutation and errors in protein formation w/inhibition of viral replication.

USES

Recurrent epithelial keratitis and primary keratoconjunctivitis caused by herpes simplex types 1 and 2. Treatment of epithelial keratitis not responding to idoxuridine or resistant to vidarabine.

STORAGE/HANDLING

1. Refrigerate ophthalmic solution.

OPHTHALMIC ADMINISTRATION

1. Place finger on lower eyelid and pull out until pocket is formed between eye and lower lid.
2. Hold dropper above pocket and place correct number of drops into pocket. Have pt close eye gently.
3. Apply digital pressure to lacrimal sac for 1-2 min (minimizes drainage into nose and throat, reducing risk of systemic effects).

INDICATIONS/DOSAGE/ROUTES

Usual ophthalmic dosage:

OPHTHALMIC: Adults, elderly: 1 drop onto cornea q2h while awake. **Maximum:** 9 drops/day. Continue until corneal ulcer has completely re-epithelialized; then, 1 drop q4h while awake (minimum: 5 drops/day) for an additional 7 days.

PRECAUTIONS

CONTRAINDICATIONS: Hypersensitivity to trifluridine or any component of the preparation. **PREGNANCY/LACTATION:** Not recommended during pregnancy or lactation because of mutagenic effects in vitro. **Pregnancy Category C.**

INTERACTIONS

DRUG INTERACTIONS: None significant. **ALTERED LAB VALUES:** None significant.

SIDE EFFECTS

FREQUENT: Transient stinging or burning w/instillation. **OCCASIONAL:** Edema of eyelid. **RARE:** Hypersensitivity reaction: Itching, redness, swelling, increased irritation; superficial punctate keratopathy, increased intraocular pressure, keratitis sicca.

ADVERSE REACTIONS/TOXIC EFFECTS

Ocular toxicity if used longer than 21 days.

NURSING IMPLICATIONS

BASELINE ASSESSMENT:

Question for hypersensitivity to trifluridine or components of preparation.

INTERVENTION/EVALUATION:

Evaluate for therapeutic response or burning/stinging, edema of eyelid, hypersensitivity reaction.

PATIENT/FAMILY TEACHING:

Use only as directed by physician (assure proper administration); do not stop or increase frequency of doses. Contact physician if no improvement after 7 days or complete healing after 14. Do not continue longer than 21 days. Refrigerate; avoid freezing. Mild, transient burning, stinging may occur when instilled. Promptly report itching, swelling, redness, or any increased irritation. Medication and personal items in contact w/ eye should not be shared. Do not use any other products, including makeup, around the eye w/o advice of physician.

trihexyphenidyl hydrochloride

try-hex-eh-fen′ih-dill
(Artane)

CANADIAN AVAILABILITY:
Apo-Trihex, Artane, Novohexidyl

CLASSIFICATION

Anticholinergic, antiparkinsonism

PHARMACOKINETICS

	ONSET	PEAK	DURATION
PO	1 hr	2-3 hrs	6-12 hrs

Well absorbed from GI tract. Primarily excreted in urine. Half-life: 5.6-10.2 hrs.

ACTION

Blocks central cholinergic receptors (aids in balancing cholinergic and dopaminergic activity). Decreases salivation, relaxes smooth muscle.

USES

Adjunctive treatment for all forms of Parkinson's disease, including postencephalitic, arteriosclerotic, idiopathic types. Controls symptoms of drug-induced extrapyramidal symptoms.

PO ADMINISTRATION

1. May take w/o regard to food; give w/food if GI distress occurs.
2. Scored tablets may be crushed; do not crush or break sustained-release capsules.

INDICATIONS/DOSAGE/ROUTES

Parkinsonism:
NOTE: Do not use sustained-release capsules for initial therapy. Once stabilized, may switch, on mg-for-mg basis, giving a single daily dose after breakfast or 2 divided doses 12 hrs apart.
PO: Adults, elderly: Initially, 1 mg on first day. May increase by 2 mg/day at 3-5 day intervals up to 6-10 mg/day (12-15 mg/day in pts w/ postencephalitic parkinsonism).

Drug-induced extrapyramidal symptoms:
PO: Adults, elderly: Initially, 1 mg/day. **Range:** 5-15 mg/day.

PRECAUTIONS

CONTRAINDICATIONS: Angle-closure glaucoma, GI obstruction, paralytic ileus, intestinal atony, severe ulcerative colitis, prostatic hypertrophy, myasthenia gravis, megacolon. **CAUTIONS:** Treated open-angle glaucoma, autonomic neuropathy, pulmonary disease, esophageal reflux, hiatal hernia, heart disease, hyperthyroidism, hypertension. **PREGNANCY/LACTATION:** Unknown whether drug crosses placenta; is distributed in breast milk. **Pregnancy Category C.**

INTERACTIONS

DRUG INTERACTIONS: Alcohol, CNS depressants may increase sedative effect. Amantadine, anticholinergics, MAO inhibitors may increase anticholinergic effects. Antacids, antidiarrheals may decrease absorption, effects. **ALTERED LAB VALUES:** None significant.

SIDE EFFECTS

NOTE: Elderly (>60 yrs) tend to develop mental confusion, disorientation, agitation, psychotic-like symptoms.
FREQUENT: Drowsiness, dizziness, muscular weakness, dry mouth/nose/throat/lips, urinary

retention, thickening of bronchial secretions. Sedation, dizziness, hypotension more likely noted in elderly. **OCCASIONAL:** Epigastric distress, flushing, visual disturbances, hearing disturbances, paresthesia, sweating, chills.

ADVERSE REACTIONS/TOXIC EFFECTS

Children may experience dominant paradoxical reaction (restlessness, insomnia, euphoria, nervousness, tremors). Overdosage in children may result in hallucinations, convulsions, death. Hypersensitivity reaction (eczema, pruritus, rash, cardiac disturbances, photosensitivity) may occur. Overdosage may vary from CNS depression (sedation, apnea, cardiovascular collapse, death) to severe paradoxical reaction (hallucinations, tremor, seizures).

NURSING IMPLICATIONS

Baseline Assessment:

If pt is undergoing allergic reaction, obtain history of recently ingested foods, drugs, environmental exposure, recent emotional stress. Monitor rate, depth, rhythm, type of respiration; quality and rate of pulse. Assess lung sounds for rhonchi, wheezing, rales.

Intervention/Evaluation:

Be alert to neurologic effects: Headache, lethargy, mental confusion, agitation. Monitor children closely for paradoxical reaction. Assess for clinical reversal of symptoms (improvement of tremor of head/hands at rest, masklike facial expression, shuffling gait, muscular rigidity).

Patient/Family Teaching:

Avoid tasks that require alertness, motor skills until response to drug is established. Dry mouth, drowsiness, dizziness may be an expected response of drug. Avoid alcoholic beverages during therapy. Sugarless gum, sips of tepid water may relieve dry mouth. Coffee/tea may help reduce drowsiness.

trimeprazine tartrate

trim-eh´prah-zeen
(Temaril)

CANADIAN AVAILABILITY:
Panectyl

CLASSIFICATION

Antihistamine

PHARMACOKINETICS

	ONSET	PEAK	DURATION
PO	15-60 min	1-2 hrs	3-6 hrs

Well absorbed from GI tract. Widely distributed (primarily concentrated in lungs). Protein binding: 65-90%. Metabolized in liver. Primarily excreted in urine. Half-life: 10-14 hrs.

ACTION

Antihistamine: Prevents, antagonizes most histamine effects (e.g., urticaria, pruritus).

USES

Relief of pruritus associated w/ urticaria, various skin conditions.

PO ADMINISTRATION

1. Give w/o regard to meals.
2. Do not crush or chew ex-

tended-release or film-coated tablets.

INDICATIONS/DOSAGE/ROUTES

Allergic condition:
PO: Adults: 2.5 mg 4 times/day. **Elderly:** 2.5 mg 2 times/day. **Children >3 yrs:** 2.5 mg at bedtime or 2.5 mg 3 times/day, if needed. **Children 6 mo-3 yrs:** 1.25 mg at bedtime or 1.25 mg 3 times/day, if needed.

Extended release:
PO: Adults: 5 mg q12h. **Children >6 yrs:** 5 mg once/day.

PRECAUTIONS

CONTRAINDICATIONS: Acute asthmatic attack, pts receiving MAO inhibitors. **EXTREME CAUTION:** History of sleep apnea, young children, family history of sudden infant death syndrome (SIDS), those w/difficulty waking. **CAUTIONS:** Narrow-angle glaucoma, peptic ulcer, prostatic hypertrophy, pyloroduodenal or bladder neck obstruction, asthma, COPD, increased intraocular pressure, cardiovascular disease, hyperthyroidism, hypertension, seizure disorders. **PREGNANCY/LACTATION:** Readily crosses placenta; unknown whether drug is excreted in breast milk. May inhibit platelet aggregation in neonates if taken within 2 wks of delivery. May produce jaundice, extrapyramidal symptoms in neonates if taken during pregnancy. **Pregnancy Category C.**

INTERACTIONS

DRUG INTERACTIONS: Alcohol, CNS depressants may increase CNS depressant effects. Anticholinergics may increase anticholinergic effects. MAO inhibitors may prolong, intensify anticholinergic, CNS depressant effects. **ALTERED LAB VALUES:** May suppress wheal and flare reactions to antigen skin testing, unless antihistamines are discontinued 4 days before testing.

SIDE EFFECTS

HIGH INCIDENCE: Drowsiness, disorientation. Hypotension, confusion, syncope more likely noted in elderly. **FREQUENT:** Dry mouth/nose/throat/lips, urinary retention, thickening of bronchial secretions. **OCCASIONAL:** Epigastric distress, flushing, visual disturbances, hearing disturbances, wheezing, paresthesia, sweating, chills. **RARE:** Dizziness, urticaria, photosensitivity, nightmares.

ADVERSE REACTIONS/TOXIC EFFECTS

CNS depression (respiratory depression, sleep apnea, SIDS) has occurred in infants, young children. Long-term therapy may produce extrapyramidal symptoms noted as dystonia (abnormal movements), pronounced motor restlessness (most frequently noted in children) and parkinsonian symptoms (esp. noted in elderly). Paradoxical reaction (particularly in children) manifested as excitation, nervousness, tremor, hyperactive reflexes, convulsions. Blood dyscrasias (particularly agranulocytosis) has occurred.

NURSING IMPLICATIONS

BASELINE ASSESSMENT:

If pt is undergoing allergic reaction, obtain history of recently ingested foods, drugs, environmental exposure, recent emotional stress. Monitor rate, depth, rhythm, type of respiration; quality and rate of pulse. Assess lung sounds for rhonchi, wheezing, rales.

INTERVENTION/EVALUATION:

Monitor B/P, esp. in elderly (increased risk of hypotension). Monitor children closely for paradoxical reaction.

PATIENT/FAMILY TEACHING:

Tolerance to antihistaminic effect generally does not occur; tolerance to sedative effect may occur. Avoid tasks that require alertness, motor skills until response to drug is established. Dry mouth, drowsiness, dizziness may be an expected response of drug. Avoid alcoholic beverages during antihistamine therapy. Sugarless gum, sips of tepid water may relieve dry mouth. Coffee or tea may help reduce drowsiness.

trimethaphan camsylate

try-meth'ah-fan
(Arfonad)

CANADIAN AVAILABILITY:
Arfonad

CLASSIFICATION

Antihypertensive

PHARMACOKINETICS

May be metabolized by pseudocholinesterase. Primarily excreted unchanged in urine. B/P reduction occurs immediately; returns to pretreatment level 10 min after trimethaphan discontinued.

ACTION

Competes w/acetylcholine for postsynaptic receptors. May cause direct peripheral vasodilation, release of histamine.

USES

Rapid reduction of B/P in hypertensive emergencies. Produces controlled hypotension in surgical procedures of head and neck to reduce bleeding.

STORAGE/HANDLING

Refrigerate. After dilution, solution is stable for 24 hrs at room temperature. Discard unused portion.

IV ADMINISTRATION

1. Administer by IV infusion via infusion pump.
2. Dilute 500 mg ampoule w/500 ml 5% dextrose to provide concentration of 1 mg/ml.
3. Use immediately after preparation.
4. Administer after pt is anesthesized; discontinue before wound closure (allows B/P to return to normal). Systolic B/P should not go below 60 mm Hg.

INDICATIONS/DOSAGE/ROUTES

Controlled hypotension during anesthesia:
IV: Adults, elderly: Initially, 3-4 mg/min to maintain B/P. **Range:** 0.3-6 mg/min.

Hypertensive emergencies:
IV: Adults, elderly: Initially, 0.5-1 mg/min, adjusted to pt's response. **Maintenance:** 1-15 mg/min.

PRECAUTIONS

CONTRAINDICATIONS: Anemia, glaucoma, hypovolemia, shock (incipient or frank), asphyxia, respiratory insufficiency, any condition that may subject pt to undue risk. **EXTREME CAUTION:** Arteriosclerosis, cardiac

T

disease, hepatic or renal disease, degenerative disease of CNS, Addison's disease, diabetes mellitus, corticosteroid-dependent pts. **CAUTIONS:** History of allergies, elderly, debilitated, children. **PREGNANCY/LACTATION:** Crosses placenta. May decrease fetal GI motility, resulting in meconium ileus or paralytic ileus. **Pregnancy Category C.**

INTERACTIONS

DRUG INTERACTIONS: May interfere w/effects of ambenonium, neostigmine, pyridostigmine. May prolong effects of neuromuscular blockers. **ALTERED LAB VALUES:** May decrease potassium.

SIDE EFFECTS

None significant.

ADVERSE REACTIONS/TOXIC EFFECTS

None significant.

NURSING IMPLICATIONS

INTERVENTION/EVALUATION:

Monitor B/P diligently; do not allow systolic B/P to go below 60 mm Hg.

trimethobenzamide hydrochloride

try-meth-oh-benz′ah-mide
(Tigan)

CLASSIFICATION

Antiemetic

PHARMACOKINETICS

	ONSET	PEAK	DURATION
PO	10-40 min	—	3-4 hrs
IM	15-30 min	—	2-3 hrs

Partially absorbed from GI tract. Distributed primarily to liver. Metabolic fate unknown. Excreted in urine.

ACTION

Inhibits emetic impulses at the chemoreceptor trigger zone in CNS (medulla oblongata).

USES

Control of nausea and vomiting.

STORAGE/HANDLING

Store oral, rectal, parenteral form at room temperature.

PO/IM/RECTAL ADMINISTRATION

PO:

1. Give w/o regard to meals.
2. Do not crush or break capsule form.

IM:

Give deep IM into large muscle mass, preferably upper outer gluteus maximus.

RECTAL:

1. If suppository is too soft, chill for 30 min in refrigerator or run cold water over foil wrapper.
2. Moisten suppository w/cold water before inserting well up into rectum.

INDICATIONS/DOSAGE/ROUTES

NOTE: Do not use IV route (produces severe hypotension).

Nausea, vomiting:
PO: Adults, elderly: 250 mg 3-4

times/day. **Children 30-100 lbs:** 100-200 mg 3-4 times/day.
IM: Adults, elderly: 200 mg 3-4 times/day.
RECTAL: Adults, elderly: 200 mg 3-4 times/day. **Children 30-100 lbs:** 100-200 mg 3-4 times/day. **Children <30 lbs:** 100 mg 3-4 times/day. Do not use in premature or newborn infants.

PRECAUTIONS

CONTRAINDICATIONS: Hypersensitivity to benzocaine or similar local anesthetics; parenteral form in children, suppositories in premature infants or neonates. **CAUTIONS:** Elderly, debilitated, dehydration, electrolyte imbalance, high fever. **PREGNANCY/LACTATION:** Unknown whether drug crosses placenta or is distributed in breast milk. **Pregnancy Category C.**

INTERACTIONS

DRUG INTERACTIONS: CNS depression producing medications may increase CNS depression. **ALTERED LAB VALUES:** None significant.

SIDE EFFECTS

NOTE: Elderly (>60 yrs) tend to develop mental confusion, disorientation, agitation, psychotic-like symptoms.
FREQUENT: Drowsiness, dizziness, muscular weakness, dry mouth/nose/throat/lips, urinary retention, thickening of bronchial secretions. Sedation, dizziness, hypotension more likely noted in elderly. **OCCASIONAL:** Epigastric distress, flushing, visual disturbances, hearing disturbances, paresthesia, sweating, chills. *IM injection*: Pain, burning, redness, swelling at injection site, hypotension.

ADVERSE REACTIONS/TOXIC EFFECTS

Hypersensitivity reaction manifested as extrapyramidal symptoms (muscle rigidity, allergic skin reactions) occur rarely. Children may experience dominant paradoxical reaction (restlessness, insomnia, euphoria, nervousness, tremors). Overdosage may vary from CNS depression (sedation, apnea, cardiovascular collapse, death) to severe paradoxical reaction (hallucinations, tremor, seizures).

NURSING IMPLICATIONS

BASELINE ASSESSMENT:

Assess for dehydration if excessive vomiting occurs (poor skin turgor, dry mucous membranes, longitudinal furrows in tongue).

INTERVENTION/EVALUATION:

Check B/P, esp. in elderly (increased risk of hypotension). Assess children closely for paradoxical reaction. Monitor serum electrolytes in those with severe vomiting. Assess skin turgor, mucous membranes to evaluate hydration status. Assess for extrapyramidal symptoms (hypersensitivity). Measure I&O and assess any vomitus.

PATIENT/FAMILY TEACHING:

Report visual disturbances, headache. Dry mouth is expected response to medication. Relief from nausea/vomiting generally occurs within 30 min of drug administration.

trimethoprim

try-meth′oh-prim
(Proloprim, Trimpex)

FIXED-COMBINATION(S): W/sulfamethoxazole, a sulfonamide (Bactrim, Septra)

CANADIAN AVAILABILITY: Proloprim

CLASSIFICATION

Anti-infective

PHARMACOKINETICS

Rapidly, completely absorbed from GI tract. Widely distributed including CSF. Protein binding: 45%. Metabolized in liver. Primarily excreted in urine. Moderately removed by hemodialysis. Half-life: 8-10 hrs (increased in decreased renal function, newborns; decreased in children).

ACTION

Blocks conversion of dihydrofolic acid to tetrahydrofolic acid. Depletion of folic acid interferes w/bacterial nucleic acid, protein production.

USES

Treatment of initial acute uncomplicated urinary tract infections (UTIs).

PO ADMINISTRATION

1. Space doses evenly to maintain constant level in urine.
2. Give w/o regard to meals (if stomach upset occurs, give w/food).

INDICATIONS/DOSAGE/ROUTES

Acute, uncomplicated UTIs:
PO: Adults, elderly: 100 mg q12h or 200 mg once daily for 10 days.

Dosage in renal impairment:
The dose and/or frequency is modified in response to degree of renal impairment, severity of infection, and serum concentration of drug.

CREATININE CLEARANCE	DOSAGE
>30 ml/min	No change
15-30 ml/min	50 mg q12h

PRECAUTIONS

CONTRAINDICATIONS: Hypersensitivity to trimethoprim, infants <2 mo, megaloblastic anemia due to folic acid deficiency. **CAUTIONS:** Impaired renal or hepatic function, children who have X chromosome w/mental retardation, pts who have possible folic acid deficiency. **PREGNANCY/LACTATION:** Readily crosses placenta; is distributed in breast milk. **Pregnancy Category C.**

INTERACTIONS

DRUG INTERACTIONS: Folate antagonists (e.g., methotrexate) may increase risk of myeloblastic anemia. **ALTERED LAB VALUES:** May increase BUN, SGOT (AST), SGPT (ALT), serum bilirubin, creatinine concentration.

SIDE EFFECTS

FREQUENT: Rash, pruritus, unpleasant taste, nausea, vomiting, epigastric discomfort. **OCCASIONAL:** Photosensitivity.

ADVERSE REACTIONS/TOXIC EFFECTS

Stevens-Johnson syndrome, erythema multiforme, exfoliative dermatitis, anaphylaxis, occur rarely. Hematologic toxicity (thrombocytopenia, neutropenia, leukopenia, megaloblastic anemia) more likely to occur in elderly, debilitated, alcoholics, those w/impaired renal function or receiving prolonged high dosage.

NURSING IMPLICATIONS

BASELINE ASSESSMENT:

Question for history of hypersensitivity to trimethoprim. Obtain specimens for diagnostic tests before giving first dose (therapy may begin before results are known). Identify hematology baseline reports.

INTERVENTION/EVALUATION:

Assess skin for rash. Evaluate food tolerance. Monitor hematology reports, renal, hepatic test results if ordered. Check for developing signs of hematologic toxicity: Pallor, fever, sore throat, malaise, bleeding, or bruising.

PATIENT/FAMILY TEACHING:

Space doses evenly. Complete full length of therapy (may be 10-14 days). May take on empty stomach or w/food if stomach upset occurs. Avoid sun/ultraviolet light; use sunscreen, wear protective clothing. Immediately report to physician pallor, tiredness, sore throat, bleeding, bruising or discoloration of skin, fever.

---

trimetrexate (Neutrexin)
See supplement

---

tropicamide

troe-pick´a-mide
(Mydriacyl, Tropicacyl)

CANADIAN AVAILABILITY:
Mydriacyl, Tropicacyl, Tropicamide Minims

CLASSIFICATION

Mydriatic, cycloplegic

PHARMACOKINETICS

	ONSET	PEAK	DURATION
Mydriasis	—	20-40 min	6-7 hrs
Cycloplegia	—	20-35 min	1-6 hrs

ACTION

Blocks cholinergic stimulation of the sphincter muscle of the iris (dilation of the pupil) and accommodative ciliary muscle of the lens (paralysis of accommodation).

USES

For mydriasis and cycloplegia before ophthalmoscopic examinations. Treatment of some cases of acute iritis, iridocyclitis, and keratitis.

OPHTHALMIC ADMINISTRATION

1. Place finger on lower eyelid and pull out until pocket is formed between eye and lower lid.
2. Hold dropper above pocket and instill prescribed number of drops. Take care to avoid contamination of solution container.
3. Instruct pt to close eyes. Apply gentle finger pressure to the lacrimal sac at inner canthus for 1-2 min following instillation (lessens risk of systemic absorption).

INDICATIONS/DOSAGE/ROUTES

Mydriasis:
OPHTHALMIC: Adults, elderly: 1-2 drops (0.5% solution) 15-20 min before examination. May repeat q30min as necessary.

Cycloplegia:
OPHTHALMIC: Adults, elderly: Initially, 1-2 drops (1% solution), repeat in 5 min. If examination not performed in 20-30 min, administer 1 drop of 1% solution.

PRECAUTIONS

CONTRAINDICATIONS: Hypersensitivity to tropicamide or any ingredient of the preparation. Known or suspected angle-closure glaucoma. **EXTREME CAUTION:** Safety for use in children not established. Infants and children are esp. prone to potentially dangerous CNS and cardiopulmonary side effects. **CAUTIONS:** Elderly, because of potential for undiagnosed glaucoma. **PREGNANCY/LACTATION:** Safety for use during pregnancy has not been established; use only if potential benefit outweighs potential hazards to the fetus. Excreted in breast milk; not recommended during nursing because of potential serious adverse reactions in nursing infant. **Pregnancy Category C.**

INTERACTIONS

DRUG INTERACTIONS: None significant. **ALTERED LAB VALUES:** None significant.

SIDE EFFECTS

FREQUENT: Transient stinging, blurred vision, photophobia, dry mouth, headache, tachycardia, increased intraocular pressure. **OCCASIONAL:** Prolonged use may cause irritation (e.g., hyperemia, follicular conjunctivitis, allergic lid reactions, eczematoid dermatitis). **RARE:** Allergic reactions.

ADVERSE REACTIONS/TOXIC EFFECTS

Psychotic reactions, behavioral disturbances have been reported in children and in those hypersensitive to anticholinergic drugs. Tropicamide may cause dangerous CNS disturbances and cardiorespiratory collapse in children. Other systemic reactions are symptoms of atropine toxicity: Flushing/dryness of skin (rash may be present in children), photophobia, blurred vision, rapid irregular pulse, fever, distended abdomen in infants, headache, mental aberration followed by retrograde amnesia, urinary retention, decreased GI motility, hypotension, cardiac dysrhythmias, progressive respiratory depression. Overdosage is treated w/parenteral physostigmine.

NURSING IMPLICATIONS

BASELINE ASSESSMENT:

Have epinephrine 1:1,000 immediately available before initial administration.

INTERVENTION/EVALUATION:

Assess pt for systemic reaction.

PATIENT/FAMILY TEACHING:

May experience transient stinging upon instillation. Blurred vision, increased sensitivity to light may occur for several hrs after administration; do not drive or perform tasks requiring visual acuity during this period. Discontinue use and report eye pain immediately.

tubocurarine chloride

two-bow-cure-are´een

CANADIAN AVAILABILITY: Tubarine

(See Classifications section under Neuromuscular blockers)

urokinase

your-oh-kine´ace
(Abbokinase)

CLASSIFICATION

Thrombolytic

PHARMACOKINETICS

Rapidly cleared from circulation by liver. Small amounts eliminated in urine and via bile. Half-life: 20 min.

ACTION

Acts directly on the fibrinolytic system to convert plasminogen to plasmin (an enzyme that degrades fibrin clots, fibrinogen, and other plasma proteins).

USES

Lysis of acute pulmonary emboli, pulmonary emboli accompanied by unstable hemodynamics, acute thrombi obstructing coronary arteries associated with evolving transmural myocardial infarction. Restores patency to IV catheters obstructed by clotted blood or fibrin.

STORAGE/HANDLING

Refrigerate vials. Reconstitute immediately before use. After reconstitution, solution is stable for 24 hours at room temperature or if refrigerated. Solutions are clear, colorless to light straw. Do not use if solution is highly colored; discard unused portions.

IV ADMINISTRATION

NOTE: Must be administered within 12-14 hrs of clot formation (little effect on older, organized clots).

IV:

1. Give by IV infusion via pump; via coronary catheter into thrombosed coronary artery; or via syringe into occluded IV catheter.
2. For IV infusion, reconstitute each 250,000 IU vial with 5 ml sterile water for injection to provide a concentration of 50,000 IU/ml. Further dilute up to 200 ml with 5% dextrose or 0.9% NaCl.
3. For intracoronary administration, reconstitute three 250,000 IU vials with 5 ml sterile water for injection for each vial. Further dilute with 500 ml 5% dextrose or 0.9% NaCl to provide a concentration of 1,500 IU/ml.
4. Gently roll and tilt vial (minimizes formation of filaments). Do not shake vial.
5. Solutions may be filtered through an 0.45 micron or smaller filter.
6. If minor bleeding occurs at puncture sites, apply pressure for 30 min, then apply pressure dressing.
7. If uncontrolled hemorrhage occurs, discontinue infusion immediately (slowing rate of infusion may produce worsening hemorrhage). Do not use dextran to control hemorrhage.
8. Avoid undue pressure when drug is injected into catheter (can rupture catheter or expel clot into circulation).

INDICATIONS/DOSAGE/ROUTES

Pulmonary embolism:
IV: Adults, elderly: Initially, 4,400 IU/kg at rate of 90 ml/hr over 10 min; then, 4,400 IU/kg at rate of 15 ml/hr for 12 hrs. Flush tubing. Follow with anticoagulant therapy.

Coronary artery thrombi:
INTRACORONARY: Adults, elderly: 6,000 IU/min for up to 2 hrs. **NOTE:** Before therapy, give 2,500-10,000 U heparin by IV injection; continue heparin after artery is opened.

Occluded IV catheter:
Disconnect IV tubing from catheter; attach a 1 ml TB syringe with 5,000 U urokinase to catheter; inject urokinase slowly (equal to vol-

ume of catheter). Wait 5 min. Connect empty 5 ml syringe; aspirate residual clot. When patency is restored; aspirate 4-5 ml blood. Irrigate with 0.9% NaCl; reconnect IV tubing to catheter.

PRECAUTIONS

CONTRAINDICATIONS: Active internal bleeding, recent (within 2 mo) cerebrovascular accident, intracranial/intraspinal surgery, intracranial neoplasm. **CAUTIONS:** Recent (within 10 days) major surgery/GI bleeding, OB delivery, organ biopsy, recent trauma (cardiopulmonary resuscitation, uncontrolled arterial hypertension, left ventricular thrombus), endocarditis, severe hepatic/renal disease, pregnancy, elderly, cerebrovascular disease, diabetic retinopathy, thrombophlebitis, occluded AV cannula at infected site. **PREGNANCY/LACTATION:** Use only when benefit outweighs potential risk to fetus. Unknown whether drug crosses placenta or is distributed in breast milk. **Pregnancy Category B.**

INTERACTIONS

DRUG INTERACTIONS: Anticoagulants, heparin may increase risk of hemorrhage. NSAIDs, platelet aggregate inhibitors may increase risk of bleeding. Antifibrinolytics (e.g., aminocaproic acid) may antagonize effects. **ALTERED LAB VALUES:** Decreases plasminogen and fibrinogen level during infusion, decreasing clotting time (confirms presence of lysis).

SIDE EFFECTS

FREQUENT: Superficial or surface bleeding at puncture sites (venous cutdowns, arterial punctures, surgical sites, IM sites, retroperitoneal/intracerebral sites); internal bleeding (GI/GU tract, vaginal). **RARE:** Mild allergic reaction (rash, wheezing).

ADVERSE REACTIONS/TOXIC EFFECTS

Severe internal hemorrhage may occur. Lysis of coronary thrombi may produce atrial/ventricular arrhythmias.

NURSING IMPLICATIONS

BASELINE ASSESSMENT:

Avoid arterial invasive technique before and during treatment. If arterial puncture is necessary, use upper extremity vessels. Assess Hct, platelet count, thrombin (TT), activated thromboplastin (APTT), prothrombin time (PT), fibrinogen level before therapy is instituted.

INTERVENTION/EVALUATION:

Handle pt as carefully and infrequently as possible to prevent bleeding. Never give urokinase via IM injection route. Monitor clinical response, vital signs (pulse, temperature, respiratory rate, B/P) q4h. Do not obtain B/P in lower extremities (possible deep vein thrombi). Monitor TT, PT, APTT, fibrinogen level q4h or per protocol after initiation of therapy, stool culture for occult blood. Assess for decrease in B/P, increase in pulse rate, complaint of abdominal/back pain, severe headache (may be evidence of hemorrhage). Question for increase in amount of discharge during menses. Assess peripheral pulses; assess skin for bruises, petechiae. Check for excessive bleeding from minor cuts, scratches. Assess urine for hematuria.

ursodiol (ursodeoxycholic acid)

er-sew´dee-ol
(Actigall)

CLASSIFICATION

Gallstone solubilizing agent

PHARMACOKINETICS

Readily absorbed from small bowel. Undergoes first-pass hepatic extraction. Distributed primarily in liver, bile, intestinal lumen. Protein binding: high. Metabolized in liver. Excreted into bile and eliminated in feces.

ACTION

Suppresses liver synthesis, secretion of cholesterol. Inhibits intestinal absorption of cholesterol. Solubilizes and causes dispersion of cholesterol as liquid crystals.

USES

Dissolution of radiolucent, noncalcified gallstones when cholecystectomy is an unacceptable method of treatment.

INDICATIONS/DOSAGE/ROUTES

Usual dosage:
PO: Adults, elderly: 8-10 mg/kg/day in 2-3 divided doses. Treatment may require months of therapy. Obtain ultrasound image of gallbladder at 6-mo intervals for first year. If dissolved, continue therapy and repeat ultrasound within 1-3 mo.

PRECAUTIONS

CONTRAINDICATIONS: Calcified cholesterol stones, radiopaque stones, radiolucent bile pigment stones, allergy to bile acids, chronic liver disease. **CAUTIONS:** None significant. **PREGNANCY/LACTATION:** Unknown whether drug crosses placenta or is distributed in breast milk. **Pregnancy Category B.**

INTERACTIONS

DRUG INTERACTIONS: Aluminum-containing antacids, cholestyramine, colestipol may decrease absorption, effects. Estrogens, oral contraceptives, clofibrate may decrease effect. **ALTERED LAB VALUES:** May alter liver function tests.

SIDE EFFECTS

None significant.

ADVERSE REACTIONS/TOXIC EFFECTS

None significant.

NURSING IMPLICATIONS

Baseline Assessment:

SGOT (AST) and SGPT (ALT) liver function tests should be obtained before therapy begins, after 1 and 3 mo of therapy, and q6mo thereafter. Those w/significant liver test abnormalities should be monitored more frequently.

Intervention/Evaluation:

Monitor liver function tests in those w/impaired liver function (metabolic acidosis may occur during infusion).

Patient/Family Teaching:

Treatment requires months of therapy.

valacyclovir (Valtrex)
See supplement

valproic acid

val-pro´ick
(Depakene)

V

valproate sodium

(Depakene syrup)

divalproex sodium

(Depakote)

CANADIAN AVAILABILITY: Divalproex sodium (Epival), valproic acid (Depakene)

CLASSIFICATION

Anticonvulsant

PHARMACOKINETICS

Well absorbed from GI tract. Protein binding: 90-95%. Metabolized in liver. Primarily excreted in urine. Half-life: 6-16 hrs (may be increased in decreased liver function, elderly, children <18 months).

ACTION

Directly increases concentration of inhibitory neurotransmitter gamma-aminobutyric acid (GABA). May also act on postsynaptic receptor sites.

USES

Prophylaxis of absence seizures (petit mal), myoclonic, tonic-clonic seizure control. Used principally as adjunct w/other anticonvulsant agents.

PO ADMINISTRATION

1. Give w/food if GI distress occurs.
2. Do not crush, chew, or break enteric-coated tablets.
3. Do not mix solution w/carbonated drinks (may produce local mouth irritation, unpleasant taste).

INDICATIONS/DOSAGE/ROUTES

Anticonvulsant:

PO: Adults, elderly, children: Initially, 15 mg/kg daily (if dosage exceeds 250 mg daily, give in two or more equally divided doses). Increase at 1-wk intervals by 5-10 mg/kg daily until seizures are controlled or unacceptable effects occur. **Maximum daily dose:** 60 mg/kg.

PRECAUTIONS

CONTRAINDICATIONS: Hepatic disease. **CAUTIONS:** History of hepatic disease, bleeding abnormalities. **PREGNANCY/LACTATION:** Crosses placenta; is distributed in breast milk. **Pregnancy Category D.**

INTERACTIONS

DRUG INTERACTIONS: Alcohol, CNS depressants may increase CNS depressant effects. May increase risk of bleeding w/anticoagulants, heparin, thrombolytics, platelet aggregation inhibitors. May increase concentration of primidone. Carbamazepine may decrease concentration. Hepatotoxic medications may increase risk of hepatotoxicity. May alter phenytoin protein binding increasing toxicity. Phenytoin may decrease effect. **ALTERED LAB VALUES:** May increase SGOT (AST), SGPT (ALT), LDH, bilirubin.

SIDE EFFECTS

FREQUENT: Transient nausea, vomiting, indigestion (high incidence in children). **OCCASIONAL:** Abdominal cramps, diarrhea, or constipation. Sedation and drowsiness may be seen in those on adjunctive therapy.

ADVERSE REACTIONS/TOXIC EFFECTS

Hepatotoxicity may occur, particularly in the first 6 mo of therapy. May not be preceded by abnormal liver function tests, but may be noted as loss of seizure control, malaise, weakness, lethargy, anorexia, and vomiting. Blood dyscrasias may occur.

NURSING IMPLICATIONS

BASELINE ASSESSMENT:

Review history of seizure disorder (intensity, frequency, duration, level of consciousness). Initiate safety measures, quiet, dark environment. CBC, platelet count should be performed before and 2 wks after therapy begins, then 2 wks after maintenance dose is given.

INTERVENTION/EVALUATION:

Observe frequently for recurrence of seizure activity. Monitor liver function, CBC, platelet count. Assess skin for bruising, petechiae. Monitor for clinical improvement (decrease in intensity or frequency of seizures).

PATIENT/FAMILY TEACHING:

Do not abruptly withdraw medication following long-term use (may precipitate seizures). Strict maintenance of drug therapy is essential for seizure control. Drowsiness usually disappears during continued therapy. Avoid tasks that require alertness, motor skills until response to drug is established. Avoid alcohol.

vancomycin hydrochloride

van-koe-my´sin

(Vancocin, Vancoled)

CANADIAN AVAILABILITY:
Vancocin

CLASSIFICATION

Antibiotic

PHARMACOKINETICS

Oral: Poorly absorbed from GI tract. Primarily eliminated in feces. *Parenteral:* Widely distributed. Protein binding: 55%. Primarily excreted unchanged in urine. Not removed by hemodialysis. Half-life: 4-11 hrs (increased in decreased renal function).

ACTION

Bactericidal. Inhibits bacterial cell wall synthesis by binding to cell wall. May alter cell wall permeability, inhibit RNA synthesis.

USES

Treatment of respiratory tract, bone, skin/soft tissue infections, endocarditis, peritonitis, septicemia. Given prophylactically to those at risk for bacterial endocarditis (if penicillin contraindicated) when undergoing dental, respiratory, GI, GU, biliary surgery/invasive procedures. Treatment of choice for methcillin-resistant *Staphylococcus aureus* infections, staphylococcal enterocolitis, antibiotic-associated colitis.

STORAGE/HANDLING

Store capsules at room temperature. Oral solutions stable for 2 wks if refrigerated. IV infusion (piggyback) stable for 24 hrs at room temperature, 96 hrs if refrigerated. Discard if precipitate forms.

PO/IV ADMINISTRATION

NOTE: Space doses evenly around the clock.

PO:

1. Generally not given for sys-

temic infections because of poor absorption from GI tract; however, some pts w/colitis may have effective absorption.

2. Powder for oral solution may be reconstituted, given by mouth or nasogastric tube.

3. Do not use powder for oral solution for IV administration.

IV:

NOTE: Give by intermittent IV infusion (piggyback), continuous IV infusion. Do not give IV push (may result in exaggerated hypotension).

1. For intermittent IV infusion (piggyback), reconstitute each 500 mg vial w/10 ml sterile water for injection (20 ml for 1 Gm vial) to provide concentration of 50 mg/ml.

2. Further dilute each 500 mg w/ at least 100 ml 5% dextrose, 0.9% NaCl, or other compatible IV fluid. Infuse over at least 1 hr.

3. For IV infusion, add 1-2 Gm reconstituted vancomycin to sufficient amount 5% dextrose or 0.9% NaCl to infuse over 24 hrs.

4. Monitor B/P closely during IV infusion.

5. ADD-Vantage vials should not be used in neonates, infants, children requiring less than 500 mg dose.

6. Alternating IV sites, use large veins every 2-3 days to reduce risk of phlebitis.

INDICATIONS/DOSAGE/ROUTES

Usual parenteral dosage:
IV: Adults, elderly: 500 mg q6h or 1 Gm q12h. **Children >1 mo:** 40 mg/kg/day in divided doses. **Maximum:** 2 Gm/day. **Neonates:** 15 mg/kg initially, then 10 mg/kg q8-12hr.

Dosage in renal impairment:
After a loading dose, subsequent dose and/or frequency is modified based on degree of renal impairment, severity of infection, serum concentration of drug.

***Staphylococcal enterocolitis, antibiotic-associated pseudomembranous colitis caused by* Closteridium difficile:**
PO: Adults, elderly: 0.5-2 Gm/day in 3-4 divided doses for 7-10 days. **Children:** 40 mg/kg/day in 3-4 divided doses for 7-10 days. **Maximum:** 2 Gm/day.

PRECAUTIONS

CONTRAINDICATIONS: None significant. **CAUTIONS:** Renal dysfunction, preexisting hearing impairment, concurrent therapy w/ other ototoxic/nephrotoxic medications. **PREGNANCY/LACTATION:** Drug crosses placenta; unknown whether distributed in breast milk. **Pregnancy Category C.**

INTERACTIONS

DRUG INTERACTIONS: *Oral:* Cholestyramine, colestipol may decrease effect. *Parenteral:* Aminoglycosides, amphotericin, aspirin, bumetanide, carmustine, cisplatin, cyclosporine, ethacrynic acid, furosemide, streptozocin may increase ototoxicity and/or nephrotoxicity. **ALTERED LAB VALUES:** May increase BUN.

SIDE EFFECTS

FREQUENT: Phlebitis, thrombophlebitis, pain at IV site. Necrosis may occur w/extravasation. **RARE:** Dizziness, vertigo, tinnitus, chills, fever, rash.

ADVERSE REACTIONS/TOXIC EFFECTS

Nephrotoxicity (uremia), ototoxicity (deafness due to damage to auditory branch of eighth cranial nerve), anaphylaxis occurs rarely.

NURSING IMPLICATIONS

BASELINE ASSESSMENT:

Question pt for history of allergy to vancomycin. Avoid other ototoxic and nephrotoxic medications if possible. Obtain culture and sensitivity test before giving first dose (therapy may begin before results are known).

INTERVENTION/EVALUATION:

Evaluate IV site for phlebitis (heat, pain, red streaking over vein). Monitor renal function tests, I&O. Assess skin for rash. Check hearing acuity, balance. Monitor B/P carefully during infusion.

PATIENT/FAMILY TEACHING:

Continue therapy for full length of treatment. Doses should be evenly spaced. Notify physician in event of tinnitus, rash, other new symptom. Lab tests are important part of total therapy.

vasopressin

vay-soe-press´in
(Pitressin)

vasopressin tannate

(Pitresin Tannate in Oil)

CANADIAN AVAILABILITY:
Pitressin, Pressyn

CLASSIFICATION

Vasopressor, antidiuretic

PHARMACOKINETICS

	ONSET	PEAK	DURATION
IM/SubQ	—	—	2-8 hrs
IV	—	—	0.5-1 hr
In oil	—	—	48-96 hrs

Absorption of tannate erratic after IM/SubQ. Distributed throughout extracellular fluid. Metabolized in liver, kidney. Primarily excreted in urine. Half-life: 10-20 min.

ACTION

Increases reabsorption of water by the renal tubules resulting in increased urine osmolality and decreased urinary flow rate. Urea is also reabsorbed by the collecting ducts. Directly stimulates contraction of smooth muscle. Causes vasoconstriction w/reduced blood flow, esp. in portal and splanchnic vessels, also coronary, peripheral, cerebral, and pulmonary vessels. In large doses may cause mild uterine contractions.

USES

Prevent/control polydipsia, polyuria, dehydration in pts w/ neurogenic diabetes insipidus. To stimulate peristalsis in the prevention or treatment of postop abdominal distention, intestinal paresis. Unlabeled: Adjunct in treatment of acute, massive hemorrhage.

V

SubQ/IM/IV ADMINISTRATION

SubQ/IM:

1. Vasopressin tannate may be given IM; *never* administer IV.
2. Vasopressin tannate ampoule should be warmed to body temperature and shaken vigorously to disperse evenly in oil base.
3. Give 1-2 glasses of water at time of administration to reduce side effects.

IV INFUSION:

1. Dilute w/5% dextrose in water or 0.9% NaCl to concentration of 0.1-1 U/ml.

INDICATIONS/DOSAGE/ROUTES

Diabetes insipidus (vasopressin):
NOTE: May administer intranasally on cotton pledgets, by nasal spray; individualize dosage:
IM/SubQ: Adults, elderly: 5-10 U, 2-4 times/day. Range: 5-60 U/day. **Children:** 2.5-10 U, 2-4 times/day.

Chronic diabetes insipidus (vasopressin tannate in oil):
IM: Adults, elderly: 1.5-5 U every 2-3 days. **Children:** 1.25-2.5 U every 2-3 days, preferably at bedtime.

Abdominal distention:
IM: Adults, elderly: Initially, 5U. Subsequent doses of 10 U q3-4h.

GI hemorrhage:
IV INFUSION: Adults, elderly: Initially, 0.2-0.4 U/min progressively increased to 0.9 U/min.

PRECAUTIONS

CONTRAINDICATIONS: Anaphylaxis or hypersensitivity to vasopressin or components (e.g., peanut oil), chronic nephritis w/nitrogen retention. **CAUTIONS:** Migraine, epilepsy, heart failure, asthma, or any condition in which rapid addition of extracellular water may be a risk. Extreme caution in pts w/vascular disease, esp. coronary artery disease. **PREGNANCY/LACTATION:** Caution in giving to nursing woman. **Pregnancy Category C.**

INTERACTIONS

DRUG INTERACTIONS: Carbamazepine, chlorpropamide, clofibrate may increase effects. Demeclocycline, lithium, norepinephrine may decrease effect. **ALTERED LAB VALUES:** None significant.

SIDE EFFECTS

FREQUENT: Pain at injection site w/vasopressin tannate. **OCCASIONAL:** Stomach cramps, nausea, vomiting, diarrhea, dizziness, diaphoresis, paleness, circumoral pallor, trembling, "pounding" in head, eructation, and flatulence. **RARE:** Chest pain, confusion. Allergic reactions: Rash or hives, pruritus, wheezing or difficulty breathing, swelling of mouth, face, feet, hands. Sterile abscess w/vasopressin tannate.

ADVERSE REACTIONS/TOXIC EFFECTS

Anaphylaxis, myocardial infarction and water intoxication have occurred. Elderly and very young at higher risk for water intoxication.

NURSING IMPLICATIONS

BASELINE ASSESSMENT:

Question for hypersensitivity to vasopressin, components. Establish baselines for weight, B/P, pulse, electrolytes, urine specific gravity.

INTERVENTION/EVALUATION:

Monitor I&O closely, restrict intake as necessary to prevent water intoxication. Weigh daily if indicated. Check B/P and pulse 2 times/day. Monitor electrolytes, urine specific gravity. Evaluate injection site for erythema, pain, abscess. Report side effects to physician for dose reduction. Be alert for early signs of water intoxication (drowsiness, listlessness, headache). Hold medication and report immediately any chest pain/allergic symptoms.

PATIENT/FAMILY TEACHING:

Promptly report headache, chest pain, shortness of breath, or other symptom. Stress importance of I&O.

vecuronium bromide

veh-cure-oh´knee-um
(Norcuron)

CANADIAN AVAILABILITY:
Norcuron

(See Classifications section under Neuromuscular blockers)

venlafaxine

ven-lah-fah′zeen
(Effexor)

CLASSIFICATION

Antidepressant

PHARMACOKINETICS

Well absorbed from GI tract. Protein binding: 25-29%. Metabolized in liver to active metabolite. Primarily excreted in urine. Half-life: 3-7 hrs; metabolite: 9-13 hrs (increased in pts w/liver and/or renal disease).

ACTION

Potentiates CNS neurotransmitter activity. Inhibits reuptake of serotonin, norepinephrine (weakly inhibits dopamine reuptake).

USES

Treatment of depression w/psychotherapy.

PO ADMINISTRATION

1. May give w/o regard to food. Give w/food or milk if GI distress occurs.
2. Scored tablet may be crushed.

INDICATIONS/DOSAGE/ROUTES

NOTE: Decrease dose by 50% in pts w/moderate liver impairment; 25% in mild-moderate renal impairment (50% in pts on dialysis, withholding dose until completion of dialysis). When discontinuing the medication, taper slowly over 2 wks.

Depression:
PO: Adults, elderly: Initially, 75 mg/day in 2-3 divided doses w/food. May increase by 75 mg/day no sooner than 4 day intervals. **Maximum:** 375 mg/day in 3 divided doses.

PRECAUTIONS

CONTRAINDICATIONS: Hypersensitivity to venlafaxine. Children <18 yrs of age (safety unknown). Pts currently receiving MAO inhibitors (see Drug Interactions). **CAUTIONS:** Renal, hepatic impairment. History of mania, seizures, those w/metabolic or hemodynamic disease, hypertension, history of drug abuse. **PREGNANCY/LACTATION:** Unknown whether excreted in breast milk. **Pregnancy Category C.**

INTERACTIONS

DRUG INTERACTIONS: MAO inhibitors (MAOIs) may cause hyperthermia, rigidity, myoclonus, autonomic instability (including rapid fluctuations of vital signs), mental status changes, coma, extreme agitation. May cause neuroleptic malignant syndrome (wait 14 days after discontinuing MAOIs to start or wait 7 days after discontinuing venlafaxine before starting MAOIs). **ALTERED LAB VALUES:** May increase serum cholesterol, uric acid, alkaline phosphatase, SGOT (AST), SGPT (ALT), bilirubin, BUN. May decrease sodium, phosphate. May alter glucose, potassium.

SIDE EFFECTS

FREQUENT: Nausea, somnolence, headache, dry mouth. **OCCASIONAL:** Dizziness, insomnia, constipation, sweating, nervousness, asthenia (loss of strength, energy), ejaculatory disturbance, anorexia. **RARE:** Anxiety, blurred vision, diarrhea, vomiting, tremor, abnormal dreams, impotence.

ADVERSE REACTIONS/TOXIC EFFECTS

Sustained increase in diastolic B/P (10-15 mm Hg) occurs occasionally.

NURSING IMPLICATIONS

BASELINE ASSESSMENT:

Obtain initial weight and B/P.

INTERVENTION/EVALUATION:

Check B/P regularly for hypertension. Monitor weight and encourage small, frequent meals of favorite foods to prevent weight loss, esp. in underweight pts. Assess sleep pattern for insomnia. Check during waking hours for somnolence or dizziness and anxiety; provide assistance as necessary. Prescriptions should be for smallest amount possible to reduce risk of suicide. Supervise suicidal-risk pt closely during early therapy (as depression lessens, energy level improves, increasing suicide potential). Assess appearance, behavior, speech pattern, level of interest, mood for therapeutic response.

PATIENT/FAMILY TEACHING:

Take w/food. Do not increase, decrease, or suddenly stop medication. Venlafaxine may decrease appetite and cause weight loss. Do not drive or perform tasks that require alert response until certain drug does not cause impairment. Inform physician if breast-feeding, pregnant or planning to become pregnant. Avoid alcohol. Do not take any other medication including over-the-counter preparations w/o consulting physician. Report rash, hives, or other allergic responses promptly.

verapamil hydrochloride

ver-ap´ah-mill

(Calan, Isoptin, Verelan)

CANADIAN AVAILABILITY:
Apo-Verap, Isoptin, Novoveramil

CLASSIFICATION

Calcium channel blocker

PHARMACOKINETICS

	ONSET	PEAK	DURATION
PO	30 min	1-2 hrs	6-8 hrs
Ext. rel.	30 min	—	—
IV	1-2 min	3-5 min	10-60 min

Well absorbed from GI tract. Undergoes first-pass metabolism in liver. Protein binding: 90%. Metabolized in liver to active metabolite.

Primarily excreted in urine. Not removed by hemodialysis. Half-life: *oral:* 2.8-7.4 hrs; *IV:* 2-5 hrs.

ACTION

Inhibits calcium ion entry across cell membranes of cardiac and vascular smooth muscle (may dilate coronary arteries, peripheral arteries, arterioles). May decrease heart rate, myocardial contractility, slow SA and AV conduction. Decreases total peripheral vascular resistance by vasodilation.

USES

Parenteral: Management of supraventricular tachyarrhythmias, temporary control of rapid ventricular rate in atrial flutter/fibrillation. *Oral:* Management of spastic (Prinzmetal's variant) angina, unstable (crescendo, preinfarction) angina, chronic stable angina (effort-associated angina), hypertension, prevention of recurrent PSVT, and (w/digoxin) control of ventricular resting rate in those w/ atrial flutter and/or fibrillation.

PO/IV ADMINISTRATION

PO:

1. Give sustained-release tablets w/food. Verelan may be taken w/o regard to food.
2. Do not crush or break sustained-released tablets. Do not break capsules.

IV:

1. Administer direct IV >2 min for adults, children (administer >3 min for elderly).
2. Continuous EKG monitoring during IV injection is required for children, recommended for adults.
3. Monitor EKG for rapid ventricular rates, extreme bradycardia, heart block, asystole, prolongation of PR interval. Notify physician of any significant changes.
4. Monitor B/P q5-10min.
5. Pt should remain recumbent for at least 1 hr following IV administration.

INDICATIONS/DOSAGE/ROUTES

Supraventricular tachyarrhythmias:
IV: Adults, elderly: Initially, 5-10 mg, repeat in 30 min w/10 mg dose. **Children 1-15 yrs:** 2-5 mg, repeat in 30 min up to 10 mg. **Children <1 yr:** 0.75-2 mg, repeat after 30 min. Maximum single dose: 10 mg.

Arrhythmias:
PO: Adults, elderly: 240-480 mg/day in 3-4 divided doses.

Angina:
PO: Adults, elderly: Initially, 80-120 mg 3 times/day (40 mg in elderly, pts w/liver dysfunction). Titrate to optimal dose. **Maintenance:** 240-480 mg/day in 3-4 divided doses.

Hypertension:
PO: Adults, elderly: Initially, 40-80 mg 3 times/day. **Maintenance:** Up to 480 mg/day.
EXTENDED-RELEASE TABLETS: 120-240 mg/day up to 480 mg/day in 2 divided doses.

PRECAUTIONS

CONTRAINDICATIONS: Sick sinus syndrome/second- or third-degree AV block (except in presence of pacemaker), cardiogenic shock, severe hypotension (<90 mm Hg, systolic), severe CHF (unless secondary to supraventricular tachycardia). **CAUTIONS:** Impaired renal, hepatic function. **PREGNANCY/LACTATION:** Crosses placenta; is distributed in breast milk. Breast feeding not recommended. **Pregnancy Category C.**

INTERACTIONS

DRUG INTERACTIONS: Beta-blockers may have additive effect. May increase digoxin concentration. Procainamide, quinidine may increase risk of QT interval prolongation. Carbamazepine, quinidine, theophylline may increase concentration, toxicity. Disopyramide may increase negative inotropic effect. **ALTERED LAB VALUES:** PR interval may be increased.

SIDE EFFECTS

Oral: **COMMON:** Constipation. **FREQUENT:** Dizziness, hypotension, peripheral edema, bradycardia, headache, fatigue. **OCCASIONAL:** Nausea. *IV:* **OCCASIONAL:** Hypotension, bradycardia, dizziness, headache. **RARE:** Severe tachycardia.

ADVERSE REACTIONS/TOXIC EFFECTS

Rapid ventricular rate in atrial flutter/fibrillation, marked hypotension, extreme bradycardia, CHF, asystole, and second- and third-degree AV block occur rarely.

NURSING IMPLICATIONS

BASELINE ASSESSMENT:

Concurrent therapy of sublingual nitroglycerin may be used for relief of anginal pain. Record onset, type (sharp, dull, squeezing), radiation, location, intensity, and duration of anginal pain and precipitating factors (exertion, emotional stress). Check B/P for hypotension, pulse for bradycardia, immediately before giving medication.

INTERVENTION/EVALUATION:

Assess pulse for strength/weakness, irregular rate. Monitor EKG for cardiac changes, particularly, prolongation of PR interval. Notify physician of any significant interval changes. Assist w/ambulation if dizziness occurs. Assess for peripheral edema behind medial malleolus (sacral area in bedridden pts). For those taking oral form, check stool consistency, frequency. Monitor for therapeutic serum level (0.1-0.3 mcg/ml).

PATIENT/FAMILY TEACHING:

Do not abruptly discontinue medication. Compliance w/therapy regimen is essential to control anginal pain. To avoid hypotensive effect, rise slowly from lying to sitting position, wait momentarily before standing. Avoid tasks that require alertness, motor skills until response to drug is established. Contact physician/nurse if irregular heart beat, shortness of breath, pronounced dizziness, nausea, or constipation occurs.

vidarabine

vy-dare´ah-been
(Ara-A, Vira-A)

CANADIAN AVAILABILITY:
Vira-A

CLASSIFICATION

Antiviral

PHARMACOKINETICS

Rapidly deaminated to arabinosyl hypoxanthine, and active metabolite. Widely distributed. Crosses blood-brain barrier. Primarily excreted in urine. Half-life: 1.5 hrs; metabolite: 3.3 hrs (increased in decreased renal function). *Ophthalmic:* Trace amounts in aqueous humor only if there is an epithelial defect in cornea.

ACTION

Appears to interfere w/DNA synthesis by inhibiting DNA polymerase of susceptible viruses.

USES

Herpes simplex encephalitis, localized (skin, eyes, mouth) or disseminated herpes simplex virus (HSV) infection in neonates; herpes zoster (shingles), varicella zoster (chickenpox) in immunocompromised pts. *Ophthalmic:* Keratitis, keratoconjunctivitis caused by HSV-1, HSV-2.

STORAGE/HANDLING

Store at room temperature. IV solution stable for 2 wks at room temperature. Use solutions within 48 hrs. Do not refrigerate.

IV/OPHTHALMIC ADMINISTRATION

IV:

1. Administered only by IV infusion.
2. Shake initial suspension well.
3. Dilute each 1 mg w/2.22 ml 0.9% NaCl or other compatible IV fluid. Infuse >12-24 hrs.
4. For neonates, initially dilute 200 mg/ml vial w/9 ml sterile water for injection or 0.9% NaCl injection for concentration of 20 mg/ml.
5. Further dilute each 1 mg w/2.22 ml 0.9% NaCl or other compatible IV fluid. Infuse >12-24 hrs.
6. Use inline membrane filter w/pore size 0.45 mcg or smaller.
7. Take extreme care to administer slowly.

OPHTHALMIC:

1. Place finger on lower eyelid and pull out until a pocket is formed between eye and lower lid.
2. Place ¼-½ inch ointment into pocket.
3. Have pt close eye for 1-2 min, rolling eyeball (increases contact area of drug to eye).
4. Remove excess ointment around eye w/tissue.

INDICATIONS/DOSAGE/ROUTES

Herpes simplex encephalitis:
IV: Adults, elderly, children, neonates: 15 mg/kg/day for 10 days.

Herpes zoster, varicella-zoster (chickenpox) infections:
IV: Adults, elderly, children: 10 mg/kg/day for 5 days.

HSV infections in neonates:
IV: Neonates: 15 mg/kg/day for 10-14 days.

Dosage in renal impairment:
Dose is modified based on degree of renal impairment. Recommended dose is 75% with usual interval if glomerular filtration rate is <10 ml/min.

Usual ophthalmic dosage:
OPHTHALMIC: Adults, elderly: 0.5 inch into lower conjunctival sac 5 times/day at 3-hr intervals. After reepithelialization, treat additional 7 days at dosage of 2 times/day.

PRECAUTIONS

CONTRAINDICATIONS: Hypersensitivity to vidarabine, components of preparation. **CAUTIONS:** Renal/hepatic dysfunction, pts at risk for fluid overload or cerebral edema (vidarabine must be administered in large amounts of fluid). **PREGNANCY/LACTATION:** Unknown whether distributed in breast milk. **Pregnancy Category C.**

INTERACTIONS

DRUG INTERACTIONS: Allopurinol may interfere w/vidarabine metabolism. **ALTERED LAB VALUES:** May decrease reticulocyte count, Hgb, Hct, WBC, and platelet counts.

SIDE EFFECTS

FREQUENT: Anorexia, nausea, vomiting, hematemesis, diarrhea. *Ophthalmic:* Burning, itching, irritation. **OCCASIONAL:** Hemoglobin, hematocrit may be depressed; weakness, dizziness, tremors, confusion, headache, hallucinations, psychosis are usually dose related and subside w/drug discontinuance. *Ophthalmic:* Foreign body sensation, tearing, sensitivity, pain, photophobia.

ADVERSE REACTIONS/TOXIC EFFECTS

Fluid overload may pose serious threat. Doses in excess of 20 mg/kg/day may produce bone marrow depression w/leukopenia, thrombocytopenia.

NURSING IMPLICATIONS

BASELINE ASSESSMENT:

Question history of allergy to vidarabine, components of preparation. Obtain specimens for diagnostic tests before giving first dose (therapy may begin before results are known). Establish hematology baselines. Evaluate tolerance for large volumes of fluid.

INTERVENTION/EVALUATION:

Assess food tolerance. Determine frequency and consistency of stools. Evaluate mental status, equilibrium. Monitor I&O. Assess lungs, tissue for signs of fluid overload. Check hematology reports; assess for bleeding. Assure slow administration of IV fluids. *Ophthalmic:* Assess for irritation, itching, burning.

PATIENT/FAMILY TEACHING:

Medication must infuse slowly; report any increase in rate. Notify nurse immediately of any shortness of breath. Therapy will continue about 2 wks. Do not take other medications w/o physician approval. Report bleeding or onset of new symptoms. *Ophthalmic:* Assure proper administration. Notify physician if there is no improvement in 7 days or if burning, irritation, pain develop. Do not stop or increase doses. Ointment should be continued for 5-7 days after infection is gone to prevent recurrence of infection. A temporary haze may occur after application to eye; sunglasses will decrease sensitivity to light. Use other eye products, including makeup, only w/advice of physician. Refrigerate, avoid freezing; if using another eye ointment, wait at least 10 min between dosing.

---

vigabatrin (Sabril)
See supplement

---

vinblastine sulfate

vin-blass′teen
(Alkaban-AQ, Velban, Velsar)

CANADIAN AVAILABILITY:
Velbe

CLASSIFICATION

Antineoplastic

PHARMACOKINETICS

Does not cross blood-brain barrier. Protein binding: 75%. Metabolized in liver to active metabolite. Primarily eliminated in feces via biliary system. Half-life: 24.8 hrs.

ACTION

Blocks mitosis by arresting cells in metaphase of cell division. Interferes w/amino acid metabolism, synthesis of nucleic acids, protein. Cell cycle–specific for M phase of cell division. Has some immunosuppressive activity.

USES

Treatment of disseminated Hodgkin's disease, non-Hodgkin's lymphoma, advanced stage of mycosis fungoides, advanced carcinoma of testis, Kaposi's sarcoma, Letterer-Siwe disease, breast carcinoma, choriocarcinoma.

STORAGE/HANDLING

NOTE: May be carcinogenic, mutagenic, or teratogenic. Handle w/ extreme care during preparation/ administration.

Refrigerate unopened vials. Solutions are clear, colorless. Following reconstitution w/bacteriostatic 0.9% NaCl, solution stable for 30 days if refrigerated. Discard if precipitate forms, discoloration occurs.

IV ADMINISTRATION

NOTE: Give by IV injection. Leakage from IV site into surrounding tissue may produce extreme irritation. Avoid eye contact w/solution (severe eye irritation, possible corneal ulceration may result). If eye contact occurs, immediately irrigate eye w/water.

1. Reconstitute 10 mg vial w/10 ml 0.9% NaCl injection preserved w/phenol or benzyl alcohol to provide concentration of 1 mg/ml.
2. Inject into tubing of running IV infusion or directly into vein over 1 min.
3. Do not inject into extremity w/ impaired or potentially impaired circulation caused by compression or invading neoplasm, phlebitis, varicosity.
4. Rinse syringe, needle w/venous blood before withdrawing needle (minimized possibility of extravasation).
5. Extravasation may result in cellulitis, phlebitis. Large amount of extravasation may result in tissue sloughing. If extravasation occurs, give local injection of hyaluronidase and apply warm compresses.

INDICATIONS/DOSAGE/ROUTES

NOTE: Dosage individualized based on clinical response, tolerance to adverse effects. When used in combination therapy, consult specific protocols for optimum dosage, sequence of drug administration. Reduce dose if serum bilirubin >3 mg/dl. Repeat dosage at intervals of no less than 7 days and if the WBC count is at least 4,000/ mm^3.

V

Induction remission:

IV: Adults, elderly: Initially, 3.7 mg/m^2 as single dose. Increase dose at weekly intervals of about 1.8 mg/ml until desired response is attained, WBC count falls below 3,000/mm^3, or maximum weekly dose of 1.8 mg/m^2 is reached. **Children:** Initially, 2.5 mg/m^2 as single dose. Increase dose at weekly intervals of about 1.25 mg/m^2 until desired response is attained, WBC count falls below 3,000/mm^3, or maximum weekly dose of 7.5-12.5 mg/m^2 is reached.

Maintenance dose:
IV: Adults, elderly, children: Use one increment less than dose required to produce leukocyte count of 3,000/mm^3. Each subsequent dose given when leukocyte count returns to 4,000/mm^3 and at least 7 days has elapsed since previous dose.

PRECAUTIONS

CONTRAINDICATIONS: Severe leukopenia, bacterial infection, significant granulocytopenia unless a result of disease being treated. **EXTREME CAUTION:** Debilitated, elderly (high susceptibility to leukopenia). **PREGNANCY/LACTATION:** If possible, avoid use during pregnancy, esp. first trimester. Breast feeding not recommended. **Pregnancy Category D.**

INTERACTIONS

DRUG INTERACTIONS: May decrease effect of antigout medications. Bone marrow depressants may increase bone marrow depression. Live virus vaccines may potentiate virus replication, increase vaccine side effects, decrease pt's antibody response to vaccine. **ALTERED LAB VALUES:** May increase uric acid.

SIDE EFFECTS

FREQUENT: Nausea, vomiting, alopecia. **OCCASIONAL:** Constipation/diarrhea, rectal bleeding, paresthesia, headache, malaise, weakness, dizziness, pain at tumor site, jaw/face pain, mental depression, dry mouth. GI distress, headache, paresthesia occurs 4-6 hrs after administration, persists for 2-10 hrs. **RARE:** Dermatitis, stomatitis, phototoxicity, hyperuricemia.

ADVERSE REACTIONS/TOXIC EFFECTS

Hematologic toxicity manifested most commonly as leukopenia, less frequently as anemia. WBC falls to lowest point 4-10 days after initial therapy w/recovery within another 7-14 days (high doses may require 21-day recovery period). Thrombocytopenia usually slight, transient, w/rapid recovery within few days. Hepatic insufficiency may increase risk of toxicity. Acute shortness of breath, bronchospasm may occur, particularly when administered concurrently with mitomycin.

NURSING IMPLICATIONS

BASELINE ASSESSMENT:

Nausea, vomiting easily controlled by antiemetics. Discontinue therapy if WBC, thrombocyte counts fall abruptly (unless drug is clearly destroying tumor cells in bone marrow). Obtain CBC weekly or before each dosing.

INTERVENTION/EVALUATION:

If WBC falls below 2,000/mm^3, assess for signs of infection diligently. Assess for stomatitis (burning/erythema of oral mucosa at inner margin of lips, sore throat, difficulty swallowing, oral ulceration). Monitor for hematologic toxicity: infection (fever, sore throat, signs of local infection); easy bruising, unusual bleeding from any site; symptoms of anemia (excessive tiredness, weakness). Assess frequency and consistency of stools; avoid constipation.

PATIENT/FAMILY TEACHING:

Immediately report any pain or burning at injection site during administration. Pain at tumor site may occur during or shortly after injection. Do not have immunizations w/o physician approval (drug lowers body's resistance). Avoid crowds, those w/infection. Promptly report fever, sore throat, signs of local infection, easy bruising, unusual bleeding from any site. Alopecia is reversible, but new hair growth may have different color or texture. Contact physician if nausea/vomiting continues at home. Avoid constipation by increasing fluids, bulk in diet, exercise as tolerated.

vincristine sulfate

vin-cris´teen
(Oncovin, Vincasar PFS)

CANADIAN AVAILABILITY:
Oncovin

CLASSIFICATION

Antineoplastic

PHARMACOKINETICS

Does not cross blood-brain barrier. Protein binding: 75%. Metabolized in liver. Primarily eliminated in feces via biliary system. Half-life: 10-37 hrs.

ACTION

Blocks mitosis by arresting cells in metaphase stage, inhibiting cellular division. Interferes w/amino acid metabolism, nucleic acid synthesis. Cell cycle–specific for M phase of cell division. Has some immunosuppressive effect.

USES

Treatment of acute leukemia, disseminated Hodgkin's disease, advanced non-Hodgkin's lymphomas, neuroblastoma, rhabdomyosarcoma, Wilm's tumor.

STORAGE/HANDLING

NOTE: May be carcinogenic, mutagenic, or teratogenic. Handle w/ extreme care during preparation/ administration.

Refrigerate unopened vials. Solutions appear clear, colorless. Discard if precipitate forms or discoloration occurs.

IV ADMINISTRATION

NOTE: Give by IV injection. Use extreme caution in calculating, administering vincristine. Overdose may result in serious or fatal outcome.

1. Inject dose into tubing of running IV infusion or directly into vein >1 min.
2. Do not inject into extremity w/ impaired or potentially impaired circulation caused by compression or invading neoplasm, phlebitis, varicosity.
3. Extravasation produces stinging, burning, edema at injection site. Terminate immediately, locally inject hyaluronidase and apply heat (disperses drug, minimizes discomfort, cellulitis).

INDICATIONS/DOSAGE/ROUTES

NOTE: Dosage individualized based on clinical response, tolerance to adverse effects. When used in combination therapy, consult specific protocols for optimum dosage, sequence of drug administration.

Usual dosage (administer at weekly intervals):
IV: Adults, elderly: 0.4-1.4 mg/m^2. **Maximum:** 2 mg. **Children:** 1.5-2 mg/m^2. **Children <10 kg or body surface area <1 m^2:** 0.05 mg/kg.

Hepatic function impairment:

Reduce dose by 50% in those w/ direct serum bilirubin concentration <3 mg/dl.

PRECAUTIONS

CONTRAINDICATIONS: Those receiving radiation therapy through ports that include liver. **EXTREME CAUTION:** Hepatic impairment. **PREGNANCY/LACTATION:** If possible, avoid use during pregnancy, esp. first trimester. May cause fetal harm. Breast feeding not recommended. **Pregnancy Category D.**

INTERACTIONS

DRUG INTERACTIONS: May decrease effect of antigout medications. Live virus vaccines may potentiate virus replication, increase vaccine side effects, decrease pt's antibody response to vaccine. Asparaginase, neurotoxic medications may increase neurotoxicity. Doxorubicin may increase myelosuppression. **ALTERED LAB VALUES:** May increase uric acid.

SIDE EFFECTS

Peripheral neuropathy occurs in nearly every pt (first clinical sign: Depression of Achilles tendon reflex). **FREQUENT:** Peripheral paresthesia, alopecia, constipation or obstipation (upper colon impaction w/empty rectum), abdominal cramps, headache, jaw pain, hoarseness, double vision, ptosis (drooping of eyelid), urinary tract disturbances. **OCCASIONAL:** Nausea, vomiting, diarrhea, abdominal distention, stomatitis, fever. **RARE:** Mild leukopenia, mild anemia, thrombocytopenia.

ADVERSE REACTIONS/TOXIC EFFECTS

Acute shortness of breath, bronchospasm may occur (esp. when used in combination w/mitomycin). Prolonged or high-dose therapy may produce foot/wrist drop, difficulty walking, slapping gait, ataxia, muscle wasting. Acute uric acid nephropathy may be noted.

NURSING IMPLICATIONS

BASELINE ASSESSMENT:

Monitor serum uric acid levels, renal, hepatic function studies, hematologic status. Assess Achilles tendon reflex. Assess stools for consistency, frequency. Monitor for ptosis, blurred vision. Question pt regarding urinary changes.

PATIENT/FAMILY TEACHING:

Immediately report any pain or burning at injection site during administration. Alopecia is reversible, but new hair growth may have different color/texture. Contact physician if nausea/vomiting continues at home. Teach signs of peripheral neuropathy.

---

vinorelbine (Navelbine)
See supplement

---

vitamin A

(Aquasol A)

CANADIAN AVAILABILITY:
Aquasol A

CLASSIFICATION

Vitamin

PHARMACOKINETICS

Absorption dependent on bile salts, pancreatic lipase, dietary fat. Transported in blood to liver, stored in parenchymal liver cells, then transported in plasma as retinol, as needed. Metabolized in liver. Excreted in bile and to a lesser amount in urine.

ACTION

May be a cofactor in biochemical reactions. Essential for normal function of retina. Necessary for visual adaptation to darkness, bone growth, testicular and ovarian function, embryonic development.

USES

Treatment of vitamin A deficiency (biliary tract or pancreatic disease, sprue, colitis, hepatic cirrhosis, celiac disease, regional enteritis, extreme dietary inadequacy, partial gastrectomy, cystic fibrosis).

STORAGE/HANDLING

Store oral, parenteral form at room temperature.

PO/IM ADMINISTRATION

NOTE: IM administration used only in acutely ill or those unresponsive to oral route (GI malabsorption syndrome).

PO:

1. Do not crush or break capsule form.
2. May take w/o regard to food.

INDICATIONS/DOSAGE/ROUTES

Severe deficiency:
PO: Adults, elderly: 10,000-25,000 IU/day for 1-2 wks.

Severe deficiency w/ xerophthalmia (thickening of cornea):
PO: Adults, elderly, children >8 yrs: 500,000 IU/day for 3 days, then 50,000 IU/day for 2 wks; then 10,000-20,000 IU/day for 2 mo. **Children <8 yrs:** 5,000 IU/kg for 5 days or until recovery occurs.

Dietary supplement:
PO: Adults, elderly: 4,000-5,000 IU/day. **Children 7-10 yrs:** 3,300-3,500 IU/day. **Children 4-6 yrs:** 2,500 IU/day. **Children 6 mo-3 yrs:** 1,500-2,000 IU/day. **Neonates to 6 mo:** 1,500 IU/day.

PRECAUTIONS

CONTRAINDICATIONS: Hypervitaminosis A, oral use in malabsorption syndrome. **CAUTIONS:** Renal impairment. **PREGNANCY/LACTATION:** Crosses placenta; is distributed in breast milk. **Pregnancy Category X.**

INTERACTIONS

DRUG INTERACTIONS: Cholestyramine, colestipol, mineral oil may decrease absorption. Isotretinoin may increase toxicity. **ALTERED LAB VALUES:** May increase BUN, calcium, cholesterol, triglycerides. May decrease erythrocyte, leukocyte counts.

SIDE EFFECTS

None significant.

ADVERSE REACTIONS/TOXIC EFFECTS

Chronic overdosage produces malaise, nausea, vomiting, drying/cracking of skin/lips, inflammation of tongue/gums, irritability, loss of hair, night sweats. Bulging fontanelles in infants noted.

NURSING IMPLICATIONS

INTERVENTION/EVALUATION:

Closely supervise for overdosage symptoms during prolonged daily administration over 25,000 IU. Monitor for therapeutic serum vitamin A levels (80-300 IU/ml).

PATIENT/FAMILY TEACHING:

Foods rich in vitamin A include

cod, halibut, tuna, shark (naturally occurring vitamin A found only in animal sources). Avoid taking mineral oil, cholestyramine (Cholybar, Questran) while taking vitamin A.

vitamin D

calcifediol

(Calderol)

calcitriol

(Calcijex, Rocaltrol)

cholecalciferol

(Delta-D)

dihydrotachysterol

(DHT, Hytakerol)

ergocalciferol

(Calciferol, Deltalin, Drisdol)

CANADIAN AVAILABILITY:
Calciferol, Calcijex, Drisdol, Hytakerol, Rocaltrol

CLASSIFICATION

Vitamin

PHARMACOKINETICS

Readily absorbed from small intestine. Concentrated primarily in liver, fat depots. Activated in liver, kidney. Eliminated via biliary system; excreted in urine. Half-life: *calcifediol:* 10-22 days; *calcitriol:* 3-6 hrs; *ergocalciferol:* 19-48 hrs.

ACTION

Essential for absorption and utilization of calcium and phosphate, normal calcification of bone, regulation of serum calcium concentration (w/parathyroid, calcitonin).

USES

Prevention/treatment of rickets or osteomalacia; management of hypocalcemia associated w/hypoparathyroidism.

PO ADMINISTRATION

1. May take w/o regard to food.
2. Swallow whole; do not crush/chew.

INDICATIONS/DOSAGE/ROUTES

CALCIFEDIOL:

Metabolic bone disease, hypocalcemia (dialysis pts):
PO: Adults, elderly: Initially, 300-350 mcg/wk given daily or every other day. May increase at 4-wk intervals. **Maintenance:** 50-100 mcg/day or 100 and 200 mcg on alternate days.

CALCITRIOL:

Hypocalcemia (dialysis pts):
PO: Adults, elderly: Initially, 0.25 mcg/day. May increase by 0.25 mcg/day q4-8wks. **Range:** 0.25-1 mcg/day.

Hypoparathyroidism:
PO: Adults, elderly, children: Initially, 0.25 mcg/day. May increase at 2-4 wk intervals. **Maintenance: Adults, children >6 yrs:** 0.5-2 mcg/day. **Children 1-5 yrs:** 0.25-0.75 mcg/day.

CHOLECALCIFEROL:

Dietary supplement, deficiency:
PO: Adults, elderly: 400-1,000 IU/day.

DIHYDROTACHYSTEROL:

Postop tetany, idiopathic tetany, hypoparathyroidism:
PO: Adults, elderly: Initially, 0.8-2.4 mg/day for several days. **Maintenance:** 0.2-1 mg/day.

Ergocalciferol:

Familial hypophosphatemia:
PO: Adults, elderly: 10,000-80,000 IU/day plus 1-2 Gm/day elemental phosphorus.

Hypoparathyroidism:
PO: Adults, elderly: 50,000-200,000 IU/day plus 500 mg elemental calcium 6 times/day.

Refractory rickets:
PO: Adults, elderly: 12,000-500,000 IU/day.

PRECAUTIONS

CONTRAINDICATIONS: Hypercalcemia, vitamin D toxicity, malabsorption syndrome, hypervitaminosis D, decreased renal function, abnormal sensitivity to vitamin D effects (those w/idiopathic hypercalcemia). **CAUTIONS:** Those w/kidney stones, coronary disease, renal function impairment, arteriosclerosis, hypoparathyroidism, those w/tartrazine sensitivity. **PREGNANCY/LACTATION:** Unknown whether drug crosses placenta; is distributed in breast milk. **Pregnancy Category C.**

INTERACTIONS

DRUG INTERACTIONS: Aluminum containing antacid (long-term use) may increase aluminum concentration, aluminum bone toxicity. Magnesium containing antacids may increase magnesium concentration. Calcium containing preparations, thiazide diuretics may increase risk of hypercalcemia. **ALTERED LAB VALUES:** May increase calcium, cholesterol, phosphate, magnesium. May decrease alkaline phosphatase.

SIDE EFFECTS

None significant.

ADVERSE REACTIONS/TOXIC EFFECTS

Early signs of overdosage manifested as weakness, headache, somnolence, nausea, vomiting, dry mouth, constipation, muscle and bone pain, metallic taste sensation. Later signs of overdosage evidenced by polyuria, polydipsia, anorexia, weight loss, nocturia, photophobia, rhinorrhea, pruritus, disorientation, hallucinations, hyperthermia, hypertension, cardiac arrhythmias.

NURSING IMPLICATIONS

Baseline Assessment:

Therapy should begin at lowest possible dose.

Intervention/Evaluation:

Monitor serum calcium and urinary calcium levels, serum phosphate, magnesium, creatinine, alkaline phosphatase and BUN determinations (therapeutic serum calcium level: 9-10 mg/dl). Estimate daily dietary calcium intake. Encourage adequate fluid intake.

Patient/Family Teaching:

Foods rich in vitamin D include vegetable oils, vegetable shortening, margarine, leafy vegetables, milk, eggs, meats. Do not take mineral oil while on vitamin D therapy. If on chronic renal dialysis, do not take magnesium-containing antacids during vitamin D therapy. Drink plenty of liquids.

vitamin E

(Aquasol E)

CANADIAN AVAILABILITY: Aquasol E

CLASSIFICATION

Vitamin

PHARMACOKINETICS

Variably absorbed from GI tract (requires bile salts, dietary fat, normal pancreatic function). Primarily concentrated in adipose tissue. Metabolized in liver. Primarily eliminated via biliary system.

ACTION

Essential nutritional element. An antioxidant, protects cells from oxidation. Protects red blood cells against hemolysis. May act as cofactor in enzyme systems.

USES

Treatment of vitamin E deficiency.

PO ADMINISTRATION

1. Do not crush or break tablets/capsules.
2. May take w/o regard to food.

INDICATIONS/DOSAGE/ROUTES

Vitamin E deficiency:
PO: Adults, elderly: 60-75 IU/day. **Children:** 1 IU/kg/day.

PRECAUTIONS

CONTRAINDICATIONS: None significant. **CAUTIONS:** None significant. **PREGNANCY/LACTATION:** Unknown whether drug crosses placenta or is distributed in breast milk. **Pregnancy Category C.**

INTERACTIONS

DRUG INTERACTIONS: May impair hematologic response in pts w/iron deficiency anemia. Iron (large doses) may increase vitamin E requirements. Cholestyramine, colestipol, mineral oil may decrease absorption. **ALTERED LAB VALUES:** None significant.

SIDE EFFECTS

None significant.

ADVERSE REACTIONS/TOXIC EFFECTS

Chronic overdosage produces fatigue, weakness, nausea, headache, blurred vision, flatulence, diarrhea.

NURSING IMPLICATIONS

PATIENT/FAMILY TEACHING:

Foods rich in vitamin E include vegetable oils, vegetable shortening, margarine, leafy vegetables, milk, eggs, meats.

vitamin K

phytonadione (vitamin K_1)

fy-toe-na-dye´own
(AquaMEPHYTON, Konakion, Mephyton)

menadiol sodium diphosphate (vitamin K_4)

(Synkayvite)

CANADIAN AVAILABILITY: Konakion

CLASSIFICATION

CLINICAL: Nutritional supplement, antidote (drug-induced hypoprothrombinemia), antihemorrhagic

PHARMACOKINETICS

Readily absorbed from GI tract (duodenum), after IM, SubQ administration. Metabolized in liver. Excreted in urine, eliminated via biliary system. *Parenteral:* Controls hemorrhage within 3-6 hrs, normal prothrombin time in 12-14 hrs. *Oral:* Effect in 6-10 hrs. Menadiol response may take 8-24 hrs.

ACTION

Necessary for hepatic formation of coagulation factors II, VII, IX, and X, which are essential for normal clotting of blood.

USES

Prevention, treatment of hemorrhagic states in neonates; antidote for hemorrhage induced by oral anticoagulants, hypoprothombinemic states due to vitamin K deficiency. Will not counteract anticoagulation effect of heparin.

PO/SubQ/IM/IV ADMINISTRATION

PO:

1. Scored tablets may be crushed.

SubQ/IM:

1. Inject into anterolateral aspect of thigh/deltoid region.

IV:

NOTE: Restrict to emergency use only.

1. May dilute w/preservative-free NaCl or 5% dextrose immediately before use. Do not use other diluents. Discard unused portions.
2. Administer slow IV at rate of 1 mg/min.
3. Monitor continuously for hypersensitivity, anaphylactic reaction during and immediately following IV administration.

INDICATIONS/DOSAGE/ROUTES

MENADIOL:

Hypoprothrombinemia:
PO: Adults, elderly: 5-10 mg/day.

Usual parenteral dosage:
IM/SubQ/IV: Adults, elderly: 5-15 mg 1-2 times/day. **Children:** 5-10 mg 1-2 times/day.

PHYTONADIONE:

Anticoagulant-induced hypoprothrombinemia:
PO/IM/SubQ/IV: Adults, elderly: 2.5-10 mg up to 25 mg. Subsequent dosage based on pt condition, prothrombin time.

Hemorrhagic disease of newborn:
IM: Infants: 0.5-1 mg in first hr of birth.

PRECAUTIONS

CONTRAINDICATIONS: Last few wks of pregnancy or neonates (vitamin K_4). **CAUTIONS:** Those w/asthma (vitamin K_4), impaired hepatic function. **PREGNANCY/LACTATION:** Vitamin K_4 (menadiol sodium diphosphate) may produce severe hemorrhagic disease in neonates. **Pregnancy Category X.** Vitamin K_1 (phytonadione): Crosses placenta; distributed in breast milk. **Pregnancy Category C.**

INTERACTIONS

DRUG INTERACTIONS: Broad-spectrum antibiotics, high-dose salicylates may increase vitamin K requirements. May decrease effect of oral anticoagulants. Cholestyramine, colestipol, mineral oil, sucralfate may decrease absorption. **ALTERED LAB VALUES:** None significant.

SIDE EFFECTS

NOTE: Oral or SubQ administration less likely to produce side effects than IM or IV route.

OCCASIONAL: *Vitamin K_1 (phytonadione):* Pain, soreness, swelling at IM injection site; repeated injections: Pruritic erythema. *Vitamin K_4 (menadiol sodium diphosphate):* GI upset, rash, urticaria.

ADVERSE REACTIONS/TOXIC EFFECTS

May produce hyperbilirubinemia in newborn (esp. premature infants). Rarely, severe reaction occurs immediately following IV administration (cramp-like pain, chest pain, dyspnea, facial flushing, dizziness, rapid/weak pulse, rash, profuse sweating, hypotension. May progress to shock, cardiac arrest).

NURSING IMPLICATIONS

INTERVENTION/EVALUATION:

Monitor prothrombin time routinely in those taking anticoagulants. Assess skin for bruises, petechiae. Assess gums for gingival bleeding, erythema. Monitor urine output for hematuria. Assess hematocrit, platelet count, urine/stool culture for occult blood. Assess for decrease in B/P, increase in pulse rate, complaint of abdominal or back pain, severe headache (may be evidence of hemorrhage). Question for increase in amount of discharge during menses. Assess peripheral pulses, skin for bruises, petechiae. Check for excessive bleeding from minor cuts, scratches. Assess urine output for hematuria.

PATIENT/FAMILY TEACHING:

Discomfort may occur w/parenteral administration. Adults: Use electric razor, soft toothbrush to prevent bleeding. Report any sign of red or dark urine, black or red stool, coffee-ground vomitus, red-speckled mucus from cough. Do not use any over-the-counter medication w/o physician approval (may interfere w/platelet aggregation). Foods rich in vitamin K_1 (phytonadione) include leafy green vegetables, meat, cow's milk, vegetable oil, egg yolks, tomatoes.

warfarin sodium

war´fair-in

(Coumadin, Panwarfin, Sofarin)

CANADIAN AVAILABILITY: Coumadin, Warfilone

CLASSIFICATION

PHARMACOTHERAPEUTIC: Coumarin derivative

CLINICAL: Anticoagulant

PHARMACOKINETICS

	ONSET	PEAK	DURATION
PO	—	1.5-3 days	2-5 days

Well absorbed from GI tract. Protein binding: 99%. Metabolized in liver. Primarily excreted in urine. Half-life: 1.5-2.5 days.

ACTION

Indirect-acting anticoagulant. Blocks hepatic formation of coagulation factors II, VII, IX, X by inhibiting vitamin K action.

USES

Prophylaxis, treatment of venous

thrombosis, pulmonary embolism. Treatment of thromboembolism associated w/chronic atrial fibrillation. Adjunct in treatment of coronary occlusion. Prophylaxis/treatment of thromboembolic complications associated w/cardiac valve replacement.

PO ADMINISTRATION

1. Scored tablets may be crushed.
2. May give w/o regard to food. If GI upset occurs, give w/food.

INDICATIONS/DOSAGE/ROUTES

NOTE: Dosage highly individualized, based on prothrombin time (PT) level.
PO: Adults: Initially, 10-15 mg, then adjust dose. **Maintenance:** 2-10 mg/day based on prothrombin determinations.

Usual elderly dosage:
PO: Elderly: 2-5 mg/day (maintenance).

PRECAUTIONS

CONTRAINDICATIONS: Bleeding abnormalities, hemophilia, thrombocytopenia, brain/spinal cord surgery, spinal anesthesia, eye surgery, bleeding from GI, respiratory, or GU tract, threatened abortion, aneurysm, ascorbic acid deficiency, acute nephritis, cerebrovascular hemorrhage, eclampsia, preeclampsia, blood dyscrasias, hypertension, severe hepatic disease, pericardial effusion, bacterial endocarditis, visceral carcinoma, following spinal puncture, IUD insertion, or any potential for bleeding abnormalities. **CAUTIONS:** Factors increasing risk of hemorrhage, active tuberculosis, severe diabetes, GI tract ulcer disease, during menstruation, postpartum period. **PREGNANCY/LACTATION:** Contraindicated in pregnancy (fetal/neonatal hemorrhage, intrauterine death). Crosses placenta; is distributed in breast milk. **Pregnancy Category X.**

INTERACTIONS

DRUG INTERACTIONS: *Increased effect with:* Allopurinol, amiodarone, anabolic steroids, androgens, aspirin, cefamandole, cefoperazone, chloral hydrate, chloramphenicol, cimetidine, clofibrate, danazol, dextrothyroxine, diflunisal, disulfiram, erythromycin, fenoprofen, gemfibrozil, indomethacin, methimazole, metronidazole, oral hypoglycemics, phenytoin, plicamycin, PTU, quinidine, salicylates, sulfinpyrazone, sulfonamides, sulindac. *Decreased effect with:* Barbiturates, carbamazepine, cholestyramine, colestipol, estramustine, estrogens, griseofulvin, primidone, rifampin, vitamin K. **ALTERED LAB VALUES:** None significant.

SIDE EFFECTS

OCCASIONAL: GI distress (nausea, anorexia, abdominal cramps, diarrhea). **RARE:** Hypersensitivity reaction (dermatitis, urticaria, esp. in those sensitive to aspirin).

ADVERSE REACTIONS/TOXIC EFFECTS

Bleeding complications ranging from local ecchymoses to major hemorrhage occur more frequently in high dose therapy, intermittent IV infusion, and in women >60 yrs. Drug should be discontinued immediately and vitamin K (phytonadione) administered. Mild hemorrhage: 2.5-10 mg PO/IM/IV. Severe hemorrhage: 10-15 mg IV and repeated q4h, as necessary. Hepatotoxicity, blood dyscrasias, necrosis, vasculitis, local thrombosis occur rarely.

NURSING IMPLICATIONS

BASELINE ASSESSMENT:

Cross-check dose w/co-worker. Determine PT before administration and daily after therapy initiation. When stabilized, follow w/PT determination q4-6wks.

INTERVENTION/EVALUATION:

Monitor PT reports diligently. Assess Hct, platelet count, urine/stool culture for occult blood, SGOT (AST), SGPT (ALT), regardless of route of administration. Be alert to complaints of abdominal back pain, severe headache (may be signs of hemorrhage). Decrease in B/P, increase in pulse rate may also be sign of hemorrhage. Question for increase in amount of discharge during menses. Assess area of thromboembolus for color, temperature. Assess peripheral pulses, skin for bruises, petechiae. Check for excessive bleeding from minor cuts, scratches. Assess gums for erythema, gingival bleeding. Assess urine output for hematuria.

PATIENT/FAMILY TEACHING:

Take medication exactly as prescribed. Do not take or discontinue any other medication except on advice of physician. Avoid alcohol, salicylates, or drastic dietary changes. Do not change from one brand to another. Consult w/physician before surgery or dental work. Urine may become red-orange. Notify physician if bleeding, bruising, red or brown urine, black stools occur. Use electric razor, soft toothbrush to prevent bleeding. Report any sign of red or dark urine, black or red stool, coffee-ground vomitus, red-speckled mucus from cough. Do not use any over-the-counter medication w/o physician approval (may interfere w/platelet aggregation).

zalcitabine

zal-site'ah-bean

(Hivid)

CLASSIFICATION

Antiviral

PHARMACOKINETICS

Readily absorbed from GI tract (food decreases absorption). Protein binding: <4%. Undergoes phosphorylation intracellularly to the active metabolite. Primarily excreted in urine. Unknown whether removed by hemodialysis. Half-life: 1-3 hrs; metabolite: 2.6-10 hrs (increased in decreased renal function).

ACTION

Intracellularly converted to active metabolite. Inhibits viral replication via inhibition of viral DNA synthesis.

USES

Management of adult pts w/advanced HIV infection (CD4 cell count of $\leq 300/mm^3$) demonstrating significant clinical/immunologic deterioration. Given as monotherapy or in combination w/zidovudine.

PO ADMINISTRATION

1. Best taken on empty stomach (food decreases absorption).
2. May take w/food to decrease GI distress.
3. Space doses evenly around the clock.

INDICATIONS/DOSAGE/ROUTES

HIV infection:

PO: Adults: 0.75 mg q8h (may be given w/zidovudine).

Dosage in renal impairment:

Based on creatinine clearance.

CREATININE CLEARANCE	DOSE
10-40 ml/min	0.75 mg q12h
<10 ml/min	0.75 mg q24h

PRECAUTIONS

CONTRAINDICATIONS: Hypersensitivity to zalcitabine or components of preparation. Pts w/moderate/severe peripheral neuropathy. Children <13 yrs (safety not known). **EXTREME CAUTION:** Those w/low (<50/mm^3) CD4 cell counts (risk of peripheral neuropathy is greater). **CAUTIONS:** Pts w/history of pancreatitis or increased amylase, history of ethanol abuse. History of CHF, baseline cardiomyopathy, decreased renal function, liver disease. **PREGNANCY/LACTATION:** Unknown whether it crosses the placenta or is distributed in breast milk. Avoid breast-feeding in HIV-positive women. **Pregnancy Category C.**

INTERACTIONS

DRUG INTERACTIONS: Medications associated w/peripheral neuropathy may increase risk (e.g., cisplatin, disulfiram, phenytoin, vincristine). Medications causing pancreatitis may increase risk (e.g., IV pentamidine). **ALTERED LAB VALUES:** May increase SGOT (AST), SGPT (ALT), alkaline phosphatase concentrations. May cause leukopenia, neutropenia, eosinophilia, thrombocytopenia.

SIDE EFFECTS

FREQUENT: Mouth ulcers, various rashes, headache, fatigue. **OCCASIONAL:** Nausea, pruritus, myalgia, difficulty swallowing (dysphagia). **RARE:** Anorexia, abdominal pain, pharyngitis, vomiting, diarrhea.

ADVERSE REACTIONS/TOXIC EFFECTS

Peripheral neuropathy occurs commonly (17-31%), characterized by numbness, tingling, burning, and pain of lower extremities. May be followed by sharp shooting pain and progress to severe continuous burning pain that may be irreversible if the drug is not discontinued in time. Pancreatitis occurs rarely.

NURSING IMPLICATIONS

BASELINE ASSESSMENT:

Monitor CBC, triglycerides and serum amylase levels before and during therapy.

INTERVENTION/EVALUATION:

Stop medication and notify physician immediately if signs and symptoms of peripheral neuropathy develop: numbness, tingling, burning, or shooting pains of extremities, loss of vibratory sense or ankle reflex. Although it is rare, be alert to impending potentially fatal pancreatitis: increasing serum amylase, rising triglycerides, nausea, vomiting, abdominal pain (withhold medication and notify physician). Assess for therapeutic response: weight gain, increased energy, decreased fatigue.

PATIENT/FAMILY TEACHING:

Not a cure for HIV; may continue to contract illnesses associated w/advanced HIV infection. Does not preclude the need to continue practices to prevent transmission of HIV. Report promptly any signs and symptoms of peripheral neuropathy or pancreatitis (see above). Women of childbearing age should use contraception.

zidovudine

zye-dough´view-deen
(AZT, Retrovir)

CANADIAN AVAILABILITY:
Apo-Zidovudine, Novo-AZT, Retrovir

CLASSIFICATION

Antiviral

PHARMACOKINETICS

Rapidly, completely absorbed from GI tract. Undergoes first-pass metabolism in liver. Widely distributed. Crosses blood-brain barrier, CSF. Protein binding: 30-38%. Primarily excreted in urine. Minimal removal by hemodialysis. Half-life: 0.8-1.2 hrs (increased in decreased renal function).

ACTION

Virustatic. Activated intracellularly. Inhibits viral DNA replication (competes w/natural substrate for incorporation into viral RNA-dependent DNA polymerase).

USES

IV: Management of select adult pts w/symptomatic HIV infection (AIDS, advanced HIV disease) who have a cytologically confirmed history of *Pneumocystis carinii* pneumonia or an absolute CD4 (T4 helper/inducer) lymphocyte count below 200/mm^3 (peripheral blood) before therapy. *PO:* Management of pts w/HIV infection having evidence of impaired immunity (CD4 cell count of ≤500/mm^3 before therapy. HIV-infected children (>3 mo) who have HIV-related symptoms or asymptomatic w/abnormal lab values showing significant HIV-related immunosuppression. Prevent maternal-fetal HIV transmission.

STORAGE/HANDLING

Capsules kept in cool, dry place. Protect from light. After dilution, IV solution stable for 24 hrs at room temperature; 48 hrs if refrigerated. Recommend use within 8 hrs if stored at room temperature; 24 hrs if refrigerated. Do not use if particulate matter present or discoloration occurs.

PO/IV ADMINISTRATION

PO:

1. Food, milk do not affect GI absorption.
2. Space doses evenly around the clock.

IV:

1. Must dilute before administration.
2. Calculated dose added to D5W to provide a concentration no greater than 4 mg/ml.
3. Infuse over 1 hr.

INDICATIONS/DOSAGE/ROUTES

Symptomatic HIV infections:
PO: Adults, elderly: Initially, 200 mg q4h around the clock. May decrease dose to 100 mg q4h after 1 mo.

Asymptomatic HIV infection:
PO: Adults, elderly: 100 mg q4h while awake (500 mg/day).

Usual dose for children:
PO: Children >3 mo: Initially, 180 mg/mm^3 q6h up to 200 mg q6h.

Usual parenteral dosage:
IV: Adults, elderly: 1-2 mg/kg q4h around the clock.

Dosage adjustment:
Significant anemia w/o granulocytopenia may necessitate dose interruption until some evidence of bone marrow recovery observed.

PRECAUTIONS

CONTRAINDICATIONS: Life-threatening allergies to zidovudine or components of preparation. **CAUTIONS:** Bone marrow compromise, renal and hepatic dysfunction, decreased hepatic blood flow. Safety in children not established. **PREGNANCY/LACTATION:** Unknown whether crosses placenta or is distributed in breast milk. Unknown whether fetal harm or effects on fertility can occur. **Pregnancy Category C.**

INTERACTIONS

DRUG INTERACTIONS: Bone marrow depressants, ganciclovir may increase myelosuppression. Clarithromycin may decrease concentrations. Probenecid may increase concentrations, risk of toxicity. **ALTERED LAB VALUES:** May increase mean corpuscular volume.

SIDE EFFECTS

COMMON: Headache, nausea, malaise. **FREQUENT:** Anorexia, dizziness. **OCCASIONAL:** Myopathy, diarrhea, abdominal pain, asthenia (loss of strength and energy), diarrhea, rash. **RARE:** Insomnia, constipation, paresthesia, dyspnea.

ADVERSE REACTIONS/TOXIC EFFECTS

Anemia (occurring most commonly after 4-6 wks of therapy) and granulocytopenia, particularly significant in those w/pretherapy low baselines, occur rarely.

NURSING IMPLICATIONS

BASELINE ASSESSMENT:

Question history of allergy to zidovudine or components of preparation. Avoid drugs that are nephrotoxic, cytotoxic, or myelosuppressive—may increase risk of toxicity. Obtain specimens for viral diagnostic tests before starting therapy (therapy may begin before results are obtained). Check hematology reports for accurate baseline.

INTERVENTION/EVALUATION:

Monitor hematology reports for anemia and granulocytopenia; check for bleeding. Assess for headache, dizziness. Determine pattern of bowel activity. Evaluate skin for acne or rash. Be alert to development of opportunistic infections, e.g., fever, chills, cough, myalgia. Assess food tolerance. Monitor I&O, renal and liver function tests. Check for insomnia.

PATIENT/FAMILY TEACHING:

Continue therapy for full length of treatment. Doses should be evenly spaced around the clock. Zidovudine does not cure AIDS or HIV disease, acts to reduce symptomatology and slow/arrest progress of disease. Avoid sexual activity; do not share needles (zidovudine does not prevent spread of infection). Do not take any medications w/o physician approval; even acetaminophen/aspirin may have serious consequence. Bleeding from gums, nose, or rectum may occur and should be reported to physician immediately. Blood counts are essential because of bleeding potential. Dental work should be done before therapy or after blood counts return to normal (often weeks after therapy has stopped). Report any new symptoms to physician.

zolpidem tartrate

zewl'pih-dem
(Ambiem)

CLASSIFICATION

Sedative-hypnotic

PHARMACOKINETICS:

Rapidly absorbed from GI tract. Metabolized in liver; excreted in urine. Half-life: 1.4-4.5 hrs (increased in decreased liver function).

ACTION

Interacts with GABA receptor, inducing sleep w/fewer nightly awakenings, improvement of sleep quality.

USES

Short-term treatment of insomnia.

PO ADMINISTRATION

1. Do not break/crush capsule form.
2. For faster sleep onset, do not give w/or immediately after a meal.

INDICATIONS/DOSAGE/ROUTES

Hypnotic:
PO: Adults: 10 mg at bedtime. **Elderly, debilitated:** 5 mg at bedtime.

PRECAUTIONS

CONTRAINDICATIONS: None significant. **CAUTIONS:** Impaired hepatic function. **PREGNANCY/LACTATION:** Unknown whether drug crosses placenta or is distributed in breast milk. **Pregnancy Category B.**

INTERACTIONS

DRUG INTERACTIONS: Potentiated effects when used w/other CNS depressants. **ALTERED LAB VALUES:** None significant.

SIDE EFFECTS

Generally well tolerated w/only mild and transient effects. **OCCASIONAL:** Residual hangover, headache, dizziness, drowsiness, lightheadedness.

ADVERSE REACTIONS/TOXIC EFFECTS

Overdosage may produce somnolence, confusion, slurred speech, severe incoordination, respiratory depression, coma. Abrupt withdrawal of drug after long-term use may produce weakness, facial flushing, sweating, vomiting, tremor. Tolerance/dependence may occur w/prolonged use of high doses.

NURSING IMPLICATIONS

BASELINE ASSESSMENT:

Assess B/P, pulse, respirations. Raise bed rails, lower bed, need call-light. Provide environment conducive to sleep (back rub, quiet environment, low lighting).

INTERVENTION/EVALUATION:

Assess sleep pattern of pt. Evaluate for therapeutic response to insomnia: a decrease in number of nocturnal awakenings, increase in length of sleep.

PATIENT/FAMILY TEACHING:

Do not abruptly withdraw medication following long-term use. Avoid alcohol, tasks that require alertness, motor skills until response to drug is established. Tolerance/dependence may occur w/prolonged use of high doses.

Drug Classifications Contents

DRUG CLASSIFICATIONS

anesthetics: general

ACTION

General anesthetics produce loss of consciousness and loss of response to all sensations including pain, touch, taste, temperature. General anesthetics can be classified as inhalation anesthetics and IV anesthetics. Inhalation anesthetics are further classified as gases and volatile liquids. IV anesthetics can be used alone or to supplement inhalation anesthetics. They decrease dosage of inhalation anesthetics and produce effects not achieved by inhalation anesthetics.

Ideally, an inhalation general anesthetic would produce unconsciousness, analgesia, muscle relaxation, and amnesia w/o side effects. Because no agent possesses all of these properties, medications are combined to achieve what inhalation anesthetics can't do alone and to reduce side effects. These medications include short-acting barbiturates (induce anesthesia), neuromuscular blocking agents (causes muscle relaxation), opioid analgesics, and nitrous oxide (provides analgesia).

Adjuncts to anesthesia are combined to enhance beneficial effects of inhalation anesthetics, reduce side effects and include:

Benzodiazepines: Reduce anxiety, enhance amnesia.
Barbiturates: Decrease anxiety, induce sedation.
Opioids: Relieve pain both preop and postop.
Anticholinergics: Decrease risk of bradycardia.
Antiemetics: Reduce nausea, vomiting.
Neuromuscular blocking agents: Cause skeletal muscle relaxation.

SIDE EFFECTS

Inhalation anesthetics: Respiratory cardiac depression (most pts require mechanical ventilation support). May increase sensitivity of heart to catecholamine stimulation (may cause dysrhythmias). Malignant hyperthermia (muscle rigidity, profound temperature increase). Aspiration of gastric fluid (may cause bronchospasm, pneumonia—prevented by use of endotracheal tube).

INTERACTIONS

Opioid analgesics may decrease the dose of inhalation anesthetic. CNS depressants may cause additive CNS depression. CNS stimulants may increase the dose of inhalation anesthetic.

NURSING IMPLICATIONS

Preop:

BASELINE ASSESSMENT: Obtain thorough history of drug use (drugs affecting cardiovascular, respiratory system may affect response to anesthetics, accurate drug history may decrease risk of possible drug interactions), history of any disease of cardiovascular, respiratory system. Obtain baseline B/P, heart rate, respiratory rate. Assure preop medications are administered 30-60 min before surgery.

Postop:

BASELINE ASSESSMENT: Obtain information about all medications pt received during surgery (anesthetics/adjunctive medication), which assists in anticipated time of emergence from anesthesia. **EVALUATION/INTERVENTION:** Position pt on side or w/head to side (decreases risk of aspiration). Monitor vital signs (B/P, pulse rate, respiratory rate) until recovery complete. Observe for cardiovascular, respiratory distress. Employ side rails or straps to prevent accidental falls. Assist in ambulation. Monitor bowel function, urine output. Assess need for opioid analgesics in management of postop pain. Assistance w/ambulation, another driver necessary upon discharge.

ANESTHETICS: GENERAL

Generic Name	Brand Name(s)	Class	Type
desflurane	Suprane	Inhalation anesthetic	Volatile liquid
enflurane	Ethrane	Inhalation anesthetic	Volatile liquid
etomidate	Amidate	IV anesthetic	Hypnotic
halothane	Fluothane	Inhalation anesthetic	Volatile liquid
isoflurane	Forane	Inhalation anesthetic	Volatile liquid
ketamine	Ketalar	IV anesthetic	Miscellaneous
methohexital	Brevital	IV anesthetic	Barbiturate
methoxyflurane	Penthrane	Inhalation anesthetic	Volatile liquid
midazolam	Versed	IV anesthetic	Benzodiazepine
nitrous oxide	—	Inhalation anesthetic	Gas
propofol	Diprivan	IV anesthetic	Sedative-hypnotic
thiamylal	Surital	IV anesthetic	Barbiturate
thiopental	Pentothal	IV anesthetic	Barbiturate

anesthetics: local

ACTION

Blocks initiation and conduction of nerve impulses (decreases membrane permeability to sodium) that inhibits depolarization and action potential w/conduction blockade (occurs only in neurons located near site of administration). May also cause CNS depression and/or stimulation. May depress cardiac conduction, excitability and cause peripheral vasodilation. Does not cause generalized depression.

Local anesthetics can be classified based on their structure: esters or amides. Amide-type have a lower incidence of allergic reaction and are metabolized by liver enzymes; esters are metabolized by enzymes in plasma.

USES

Local anesthetics may be given topically (surface anesthesia) and by injection (local infiltration, peripheral nerve-block [axillary], IV regional [Bier block], epidural, and spinal anesthesia).

Topical:

Applied to skin to relieve pain, itching, soreness to mucous membranes of nose, mouth, pharynx, larynx, trachea, bronchi, vagina, urethra.

Injection:

Local infiltration: Inject directly into tissue to be incised or stimulated mechanically.

Peripheral nerve block (axillary): Inject into/near nerves supplying surgical field, but at a site distant from surgical field.

LOCAL ANESTHETICS

Generic Name	Brand Name(s)	Type	Uses	Onset	Peak	Duration
benzocaine	Many	Ester	Top: skin, mucous membrane	—	1 min	30-60 min
bupivacaine	Marcaine Sensorcaine	Amide	Infiltration Epidural Nerve block Spinal	5 min	—	2-4 hrs
butamben	Butesin	Ester	Top: skin	—	—	—
chloroprocaine	Nesacaine	Ester	Nerve block Epidural	6-12 min	—	15-30 min
cocaine		Ester	Top: mucous membrane	—	2-5 min	30-120 min
dibucaine	Nupercainal	Amide	Top: skin	—	<15 min	3-4 hrs
lidocaine	Xylocaine	Amide	Top: skin, mucous membrane	—	2-5 min	30-60 min
			Infiltration Nerve block IV Regional Epidural Spinal	0.5-1 min	—	30-60 min
mepivacaine	Carbocaine Polocaine	Amide	Nerve block Infiltration Epidural	3-5 min	—	45-90 min
procaine	Novocain	Ester	Infiltration Nerve block	2-5 min	—	15-30 min
tetracaine	Pontocaine	Ester	Top: skin	—	3-8 min	30-60 min
			Spinal	≤15 min	—	2-3 hrs

Top, topical.

IV regional (Bier block): Used to anesthesize limbs, injecting into distal vein of area or leg. Before administration, blood is removed from vein (apply Esmarch bandage) and tourniquet applied to limb, preventing anesthetic from entering general circulation. After administration, anesthetic diffuses from vasculature, becoming evenly distributed to all areas of occluded limb. After loosening of tourniquet, about 15-30% anesthetic is released into systemic circulation.

Epidural: Inject into epidural space (within spinal column outside dura mater). Diffusion across dura into subarachnoid space producing anesthesia of nerve roots and spinal cord.

Spinal: Inject into subarachnoid space (lumbar region below the termination of the cord).

PRECAUTIONS

CONTRAINDICATIONS: Hypersensitivity to local anesthetics. Pts w/ complete heart block, severe hemorrhage, severe hypotension, shock. Local infection at site of lumbar puncture, septicemia. **CAUTIONS:** Pts w/cardiovascular function impairment, drug sensitivity. Inflammation and/or infection in region of injection. CNS disease, coagulation defects caused by anticoagulant therapy or hematologic disorders. With preparations containing a vasoconstrictor, pts w/cardiac disease, arrhythmias, hyperthyroidism, hypertension, or peripheral vascular disease.

INTERACTIONS

CNS depression producing medications may cause additive depressant effect. Use vasoconstrictors (e.g., epinephrine) cautiously (if at all) when anesthetizing areas w/end arteries (e.g., toes, fingers).

SIDE EFFECTS

Allergic reactions ranging from dermatitis to anaphylaxis are more likely w/ester-type. No cross sensitivity between esters and amides. Cardiac depression (bradycardia, AV heart block, decreased contractility, and possibly cardiac arrest), peripheral vasodilation (may cause hypotension) can occur. CNS toxicity (stimulation followed by depression). Stimulation may cause convulsions. Depression may result in drowsiness, unconsciousness, even respiratory depression.

NURSING IMPLICATIONS

BASELINE ASSESSMENT: Resuscitative medication and equipment should be readily available. Inform pts they may experience temporary loss of sensation. **INTERVENTION/EVALUATION:** Monitor cardiovascular status, respirations, and state of consciousness closely during and after drug is administered. If ECG shows arrhythmias, prolongation of PR interval, QRS complex, inform physician immediately. Assess pulse for irregular rate, strength/weakness, bradycardia. Assess B/P for evidence of hypotension. **PATIENT/FAMILY TEACHING:** If medication used for dental procedure, avoid chewing solid foods or testing anesthetized site by biting or probing. Caution against activities that might cause unintentional harm.

angiotensin converting enzyme (ACE) inhibitors

ACTION

Suppresses renin-angiotensin-aldosterone system (prevents conversion of angiotensin I to angiotensin II, a potent vasoconstrictor).

Hypertension: Inhibits activity of angiotensin I converting enzyme. Decreases conversion of angiotensin I to angiotensin II, a potent vasoconstrictor. Results in increase in plasma renin activity and decreased aldosterone secretion. Reduces peripheral vascular resistance.

CHF: Decreases peripheral vascular resistance (afterload), pulmonary capillary wedge pressure (preload), pulmonary vascular resistance. Increases cardiac output, exercise tolerance.

USES

Treatment of hypertension alone or in combination w/other antihypertensives. Adjunctive therapy for CHF (in combination w/cardiac glycosides, diuretics).

PRECAUTIONS

CONTRAINDICATIONS: History of angioedema w/previous treatment w/ACE inhibitors. **CAUTIONS:** Renal impairment, those w/sodium depletion or on diuretic therapy, dialysis, hypovolemia, coronary or cerebrovascular insufficiency. Safety in pregnancy, lactation not established.

INTERACTIONS

May increase lithium concentrations, toxicity. Hyperkalemia may occur w/potassium-sparing diuretics, potassium supplements or potassium-containing salt substitutes. Alcohol, diuretics, hypotensive agents may increase antihypertensive effect. NSAIDs, aspirin may decrease hypotensive effect.

SIDE EFFECTS

Rash and/or urticaria, change or decrease in sense of taste, orthostatic hypotension during initial therapy. Urinary frequency. Cough, proteinuria (mostly occurs in those w/history of renal disease), dry mouth, GI distress, headache, dizziness.

TOXIC EFFECTS/ADVERSE REACTIONS

Excessive hypotension ("first-dose syncope") may occur in those w/ CHF, severely salt/volume depleted. Angioedema (swelling of face/ lips), hyperkalemia occur rarely. Agranulocytosis, neutropenia may be noted in those w/impaired renal function or collagen vascular disease (systemic lupus erythematosus, scleroderma). Nephrotic syndrome may be noted in those w/history of renal disease.

NURSING IMPLICATIONS

GENERAL: Use cardiac monitor for IV administration and preferably for initiation of oral therapy. **BASELINE ASSESSMENT:** Initial B/P, apical pulse. **INTERVENTION/EVALUATION:** Monitor B/P and apical pulse before giving drug and p.r.n.; notify physician before administration if B/P or pulse are not within agreed parameters. If excessive hypotension, place pt in supine position w/legs elevated. Assess extremities for edema; weigh daily; check lungs for rales. Monitor I&O. Check lab results, esp. electrolytes and drug levels. Monitor frequency, consistency of stools; prevent constipation. **PATIENT/FAMILY TEACHING:** Teach how to take B/P, pulse correctly. Change position slowly to prevent orthostatic hypotension. Do not take over-the-counter cold preparations, nasal decongestants w/o consulting physician. Restrict sodium and alcohol as ordered. Do not skip dose or stop taking medication; rebound hypertension may occur.

ACE INHIBITORS

Generic Name	Brand Name(s)	Use	Decrease B/P Onset (hrs)	Decrease B/P Duration (hrs)	Rte Adm	Dosage Range (mg/day)
benazepril	Lotensin	Hypertension	1	24	PO	20-80
captopril	Capoten	Hypertension	0.25	(dose	PO	50-450
		CHF		related)		12.5-450
cilazapril	Inhibace	Hypertension	1-2	24	PO	2.5-5
		CHF			PO	10
enalapril	Vasotec	Hypertension	1	24	PO	10-40
					IV	5-20
		CHF			PO	5-20
fosinopril	Monopril	Hypertension	1	24	PO	20-80
lisinopril	Prinivil	Hypertension	1	24	PO	20-40
	Zestril	CHF			PO	5-20
perindopril	Aceon	Hypertension	1	24	PO	2-16
quinapril	Accupril	Hypertension CHF	1	24	PO	20-80
ramipril	Altace	Hypertension	1	24	PO	2.5-20
spirapril	Renormax	Hypertension	1	24	PO	6-24

HTN, hypertension.

antacids

ACTION

Antacids act primarily in stomach to neutralize gastric acid (increase pH). The ability to increase pH is dependent upon dose, dosage form used, presence or absence of food in stomach, and acid neutralizing capacity (ANC). ANC is the number of mEq of hydrochloric acid that can be neutralized by a particular weight or volume of antacid. There are 4 major groups of antacids: (1) aluminum compounds, (2) magnesium compounds, (3) sodium compounds, and (4) calcium compounds.

USES

Symptomatic relief of heartburn, acid indigestion; treatment of peptic ulcer disease, prevention of aspiration pneumonia before anesthesia, prophylaxis vs. stress ulceration; symptomatic relief of gastroesophageal reflux disease (GERD), gastritis, hiatal hernia. In addition, aluminum carbonate used for hyperphosphatemia; calcium carbonate for calcium deficiency states; and magnesium oxide for magnesium deficiency states.

PRECAUTIONS

CONTRAINDICATIONS: Sensitivity to any components, first trimester of pregnancy, renal dysfunction, young children. **CAUTIONS:** Specific selection of antacid should consider preexisting bowel status, components (e.g., sodium) in relation to other medical conditions. Administer with care in elderly.

INTERACTIONS

Antacids may interact with medication by increasing gastric pH (affects absorption); absorbing or binding to medications, or increasing urinary pH (affects rate of elimination). Interactions may be prevented by avoiding concurrent use and taking antacids 2 hrs before or after ingestion of other medications.

SIDE EFFECTS

Diarrhea or constipation, depending on specific drug administered.

TOXIC EFFECTS/ADVERSE REACTIONS

Aluminum compounds in large amounts may cause severe constipation, hypophosphatemia, and osteomalacia. Magnesium compounds may cause hypermagnesemia and profound diarrhea. Calcium antacids may cause acid rebound, alkalosis, and renal calculi. W/sodium compounds, there is risk of systemic alkalosis, sodium overload with retention, and rebound hypersecretion.

NURSING IMPLICATIONS

GENERAL: Avoid sodium-based compounds for pts on low sodium diets; calcium or magnesium compounds for pts with renal impairment. Do not give other oral medication within 1-2 hrs of antacid administration. **INTERVENTION/EVALUATION:** Monitor stools for diarrhea or constipation. Assess for relief of gastric distress. **PATIENT/FAMILY TEACHING:** For best results, take 1-3 hrs after meals. Chewable tablets should be chewed thoroughly before swallowing (may be followed by water or

ANTACIDS

Brand Name	Active Ingredient Al(OH)$_2$ (mg)	Mg(OH)$_2$ (mg)	CaCO$_3$ (mg)	Other	Sodium Content (mEq/5 mL)	ANC
Amphojel	320	—	—	—	<2.3	10
Alternagel	600	—	—	Simethicone	<2.5	16
Dialume	500	—	—	—	<1.2	10
Gelusil	200	200	—	Simethicone	0.7	12
Maalox	225	200	—	—	1.4	13.3
Maalox TC	600	300	—	Sorbitol	0.8	27.2
Mag-Ox 400	—	400	—	—	—	—
MOM	—	390	—	—	0.12	14
Mylanta	200	200	—	Simethicone	0.68	12.7
Mylanta II	400	400	—	Simethicone	1.14	25.4
Riopan Plus	—	—	—	Magaldrate Simethicone	<0.1	15
Tums	—	—	500	—	<2.0	10

ANC, acid neutralizing capacity.

milk). Maintain adequate fluid intake. Eat small, frequent meals free of coffee and other caffeine products. Avoid alcohol.

antianxiety

ACTION

Benzodiazepines are the largest and most frequently prescribed group of antianxiety agents. Exact mechanism unknown; may increase the inhibiting effect of gamma-aminobutyric acid (GABA) (inhibiting nerve impulse transmission) as well as other inhibitory transmitters by binding to specific benzodiazepine receptors in various areas of the CNS.

USES

Treatment of anxiety. Additionally, some benzodiazepines are used as hypnotics, anticonvulsants to prevent delirium tremors during alcohol withdrawal and as adjunctive therapy for relaxation of skeletal muscle spasms. Midazolam, a short-acting injectable form, is used for preop sedation, relieving anxiety for short diagnostic, endoscopic procedures.

PRECAUTIONS

CONTRAINDICATIONS: Hypersensitivity, renal or hepatic dysfunction, CNS depression, history of drug abuse, pregnancy, glaucoma, lactation, young children, within 14 days of MAO inhibitors, myasthenia gravis.

ANTIANXIETY

GENERIC NAME	BRAND NAME(S)	USES	DOSAGE RANGE (MG/DAY)
alprazolam	Xanax	Anxiety Panic disorder	PO: 0.75-4
chlordiazepoxide	Librium Libritabs	Anxiety Alcohol withdrawal Preop	PO: 15-100
clonazepam	Klonopin	Anticonvulsant	PO: 1.5-20
clorazepate	Tranxene	Anxiety Alcohol withdrawal Anticonvulsant	PO: 15-60
diazepam	Valium	Anxiety Alcohol withdrawal Anticonvulsant Muscle relaxant	PO: 4-40
lorazepam	Ativan	Anxiety Preanesthetic	PO: 2-4
oxazepam	Serax	Anxiety	PO: 30-120

CAUTION: Elderly or debilitated; pts w/COPD. Drugs should be withdrawn slowly.

INTERACTIONS

CNS depressants (e.g., alcohol, barbiturates, narcotics) may increase CNS effects of benzodiazepines (e.g., sedation).

SIDE EFFECTS

Drowsiness is the most common side effect; usually disappears w/ continued use. Dizziness, hypotension occur frequently.

TOXIC EFFECTS/ADVERSE REACTIONS

Incidence of toxicity is very low when antianxiety drugs are taken alone. Confusion, hypersensitivity reactions, headache, stupor, paradoxical excitement, nausea and vomiting, blood dyscrasias, jaundice (hepatic dysfunction) are rare effects. These vary according to individual drug. IV administration may cause respiratory depression, apnea.

NURSING IMPLICATIONS

GENERAL: Provide restful environment and measures for comfort. Comply w/federal narcotic laws regarding Schedule IV drugs. Consider potential for abuse/dependence. For IV administration, have respiratory equipment available; keep pt recumbent. Most antianxiety drugs should not be mixed w/other drugs in a syringe. **INTERVENTION/EVALUATION:** Monitor B/P. Assess for therapeutic response (according to reason for use, e.g., seizure activity, anxiety, alcohol withdrawal) or paradoxical reaction. Take safety precautions for drowsiness, dizziness. **PATIENT/FAMILY TEACHING:** Avoid smoking; may interfere w/drug action. Do not drive or perform tasks requiring mental acuity until response to medication is controlled. Consult physician before taking other medications. Do not take alcohol. Medication must not be stopped abruptly. Inform other physicians, dentist of drug therapy.

antiarrhythmics

ACTION

Antiarrhythmics are classified according to electrophysiological effects they produce and/or their presumed mechanism of action.

Class IA: Inhibit inward sodium current, depress phase 0 depolarization, slows conduction velocity in myocardial Purkinje fibers.

Class IB: Inhibit inward sodium current, slight change phase 0 depolarization/slows conduction velocity in Purkinje system. Effects markedly intensified when membrane depolarized or frequency of excitation is increased. Hastens repolarization.

Class IC: Marked depression phase 0, slowing impulse conduction, suppressing inward sodium current and spontaneous ventricular premature complexes.

Class II: Depress phase IV depolarization; block excessive sympathetic activity.

Class III: Prolong action potential duration and refractoriness in Purkinje and ventricular muscle fibers.

Class IV: Depress Ca^{+2} dependent action potentials, slow conduction in AV node.

Digoxin: Decreases maximal diastolic potential and action potential duration.

Adenosine: Slows conduction time through AV node, may interrupt reentry pathways through AV node.

USES

Prevention and treatment of cardiac arrhythmias, such as premature ventricular contractions, ventricular tachycardia, premature atrial contractions, paroxysmal atrial tachycardia, atrial fibrillation and flutter.

PRECAUTIONS

CONTRAINDICATIONS: Hypersensitivity, pregnancy, lactation, children, severe bradycardia, second- or third-degree AV block, severe CHF, aortic stenosis, hypotension, cardiogenic shock, hepatic or renal dysfunction. **CAUTIONS:** Elderly generally require lowered dosage. Administer w/caution to pts w/diabetes mellitus, acute myocardial infarctions, and liver dysfunction. Have emergency cart readily available when administering agents through IV.

ANTIARRHYTHMICS

Generic Name	Brand Name(s)	Class	Antiarrhythmic Onset	Antiarrhythmic Duration	Dosage Range
acebutolol*	Sectral	II	—	24-30 hrs	600-1,200 mg/day
adenosine	Adenocard		34 sec	1-2 min	IV: 6 mg, MR w/ 12 mg at 1-2 min intervals
amiodarone	Cordarone	III	1-3 wks	—	Initial: 800-1,600 mg/day for 1-3 wks Maintenance: 600-800 mg/day
bretylium	Bretylol	III	—	6-8 hrs	IV: 1-2 mg/min
digoxin*	Lanoxin		0.5-2 hrs	>24 hrs	0.125-0.375 mg/day
disopyramide	Norpace Norpace-SR	IA	0.5 hr	6-7 hrs	400-800 mg/day
esmolol*	Brevibloc	II	<5 min	Short	IV: 50-200 mcg/kg/min
flecainide	Tambocor	IC	—	—	200-400 mg/day
lidocaine	Xylocaine	IB	—	0.25 hr	IV: 50-100 mg bolus, 1-4 mg/min infusion
mexiletine	Mexitil	IB	0.5-2 hrs	8-12 hrs	600-1,200 mg/day
moricizine	Ethmozine	IA	2 hrs	10-24 hrs	600-900 mg/day
phenytoin*	Dilantin	1B	0.5-1 hr	>24 hrs	IV: 100-1,000 mg PO:100 mg q6-12h
procainamide	Pronestyl	IA	0.5 hr	>3 hrs	PO: 250-500 mg q3h
	Procan SR		—	6 hrs	SR: 250-750 mg q6h
propafenone	Rhythmol	IC	—	—	450-900 mg/day
propranolol*	Inderal	II	0.5 hr	3-5 hrs	10-30 mg 3-4×/day
quinidine	Cardioquin	IA	0.5 hr	6-8 hrs	PO: 200-600 mg q2-4h
	Quinaglute Quinidex		—	8-12 hrs	SR: 300-600 mg q8h
sotalol*	Betapace	III	—	—	160-640 mg/day
tocainide	Tonocard	IB	1-2 hrs	8-12 hrs	1,200-1,800 mg/day
verapamil*	Calan Isoptin	IV	0.5 hr	6 hrs	IV:5-10 mg

*These agents are also discussed w/other classifications.

CLASSIFICATION

INTERACTIONS

Interactions are specific to each agent, which should be noted before administration. Please refer to individual monographs.

SIDE EFFECTS

Hypotension, bradycardia, drowsiness, lightheadedness. Other side effects are specific to individual drug.

TOXIC EFFECTS/ADVERSE REACTIONS

Visual disturbances, tinnitus or difficulty hearing, vomiting, constipation or diarrhea, headache, confusion, diaphoresis, anginal attack, rapid rhythm, cardiac arrest. Other signs specific to each drug.

NURSING IMPLICATIONS

GENERAL: Use cardiac monitor for IV administration and preferably for initiation of oral therapy. **BASELINE ASSESSMENT:** Initial B/P, apical pulse. **INTERVENTION/EVALUATION:** Monitor B/P and apical pulse before giving drug and p.r.n.; notify physician before administration if B/P or pulse are not within agreed parameters. Assess extremities for edema; weigh daily; check lungs for rales. Monitor I&O. Check lab results, esp. electrolytes and drug levels. Monitor frequency, consistency of stools; prevent constipation. **PATIENT/FAMILY TEACHING:** Teach how to take pulse correctly. Change position slowly to prevent orthostatic hypotension. Do not take other medications, including over-the-counter w/o consulting physician. Restrict sodium and alcohol as ordered.

antibiotics

ACTION

Antibiotics (antimicrobial agents) are natural or synthetic compounds that have the ability to kill or suppress the growth of microorganisms. Narrow-spectrum agents are effective against few microorganisms, whereas broad-spectrum agents are effective against a wide variety. Antimicrobial agents may also be classified based on their mechanism of action.

1. Agents that inhibit cell wall synthesis or activate enzymes that disrupt cell wall causing weakening in the cell wall, cell lysis, and death. Includes penicillins, cephalosporins, vancomycin, and imidazole antifungal agents.
2. Agents that act directly on cell wall, affecting permeability of cell membranes, causing leakage of intracellular substances. Includes antifungal agents, amphotericin and nystatin; polymixin, and colistin.
3. Agents that bind to ribosomal subunits altering protein synthesis eventually causing cell death. Includes aminoglycosides.

4. Agents that affect bacterial ribosome function altering protein synthesis causing slow microbial growth. Does not cause cell death. Includes chloramphenicol, clindamycin, erythromycin, tetracyclines.

5. Agents that inhibit nucleic acid metabolism by binding to nucleic acid or interacting with enzymes necessary for nucleic acid synthesis. Inhibits DNA or RNA synthesis. Includes rifampin, metronidazole, quinolones (e.g., ciprofloxacin).

6. Agents that inhibit specific metabolic steps necessary for microorganisms, causing a decrease in essential cell components or synthesis of nonfunctional analogs of normal metabolites. Includes trimethoprim and sulfonamides.

7. Agents that inhibit viral DNA synthesis by binding to viral enzymes necessary for DNA synthesis, preventing viral replication. Includes acyclovir, vidarabine.

SELECTION OF ANTIMICROBIAL AGENTS

Goal of therapy is to produce a favorable therapeutic result by achieving antimicrobial action at the site of infection sufficient to inhibit the growth of the microorganism. The agent selected should be the most active against the most likely infecting organism, least likely to cause toxicity or allergic reaction. Factors to consider in selection of an antimicrobial agent include:

1. Sensitivity pattern of the infecting microorganism.
2. Location and severity of infection (may determine the route of administration).
3. Pt's ability to eliminate the drug (status of renal and liver function).
4. Pt's defense mechanisms (includes both cellular and humoral immunity).
5. Pt's age, pregnancy, genetic factors, allergy, disorder of CNS, preexisting medical problems.

USES

Treat wide range of gram-positive or gram-negative bacterial infections; suppress intestinal flora before surgery; control acne; prophylactically to prevent rheumatic fever; prophylactically in high-risk situations (e.g., some surgical procedures or medical states to prevent bacterial infection).

PRECAUTIONS

CONTRAINDICATIONS: Hypersensitivity to prescribed antibiotics, others in its family, or components of the drug. Some antibiotics are contraindicated in infants and children (e.g., tetracyclines, quinolones). **EXTREME CAUTION:** Pregnancy and lactation (avoid unless benefits clearly outweigh risks). **CAUTIONS:** Renal or hepatic dysfunction. Elderly and very young may be more sensitive to effects of these drugs and may require adjusted dosage. Extra care w/gastrointestinal diseases and bleeding disorders.

INTERACTIONS

Concurrent use w/other antibiotics or drugs that add to or potentiate toxic effects is to be avoided. Alcohol should not be taken w/antibiotics; several may interact w/alcohol to produce a disulfiram reaction. Antacids should be administered 2 hrs before or after oral antibiotics to prevent interference w/absorption. Refer to specific classification pages or individual monographs.

SIDE EFFECTS

Side effects most commonly associated w/antibiotics are anorexia, nausea, vomiting, and diarrhea. Some, such as tetracyclines, produce photosensitivity. Refer to individual monographs.

TOXIC EFFECTS/ADVERSE REACTIONS

Skin rash, seen most often w/penicillins and cephalosporins, is a sign of hypersensitivity. Sensitivity reactions may range from mild rash to anaphylaxis. Superinfections may result from alteration of bacterial environment. Ototoxicity and nephrotoxicity are potential adverse reactions of a number of antibiotics, esp. the aminoglycosides. Tetracyclines combine w/calcium in forming teeth to produce discoloration. Severe diarrhea, antibiotic-associated colitis have occurred from several of the antimicrobials (clindamycin has a particular risk for this reaction).

NURSING IMPLICATIONS

GENERAL: Administer drugs on schedule to maintain blood levels. Initiate IV solutions slowly w/close observation for sensitivity response. **BASELINE ASSESSMENT:** Question for history of previous drug reaction. Culture/sensitivity must be done before first dose (may give before results are obtained). Assess WBC results, temperature, pulse, respiration. **INTERVENTION/EVALUATION:** Monitor lab results, particularly WBC and culture/sensitivity reports. Assess for adverse reactions. **PATIENT/FAMILY TEACHING:** Space doses evenly. Continue therapy for full duration. Avoid alcohol, antacids, or other medication w/o consulting physician. Notify physician of diarrhea, rash, or other new symptom.

antibiotic: aminoglycosides

ACTION

Bactericidal. Transported across bacterial cell membrane, irreversibly binds to specific receptor proteins of bacterial ribosomes. Interferes w/protein synthesis, preventing cell reproduction and eventually causing cell death.

USES

Treatment of serious infections when other less toxic agents are not effective, are contraindicated, or require adjunctive therapy (e.g., w/ penicillins or cephalosporins). Used primarily in the treatment of infections caused by gram-negative microorganisms, such as those caused by *Proteus, Klebsiella, Pseudomonas, Escherichia coli, Serratia* and *Enterobacter.* Inactive against most gram-positive microorganisms. Not well absorbed systemically from GI tract (must be administered parenterally for systemic infections). Oral agents are given to suppress intestinal bacteria.

PRECAUTIONS

CONTRAINDICATIONS: Hypersensitivity to any of the aminoglycosides; pregnancy and lactation. Not to be given orally to pts w/bowel obstruction. **CAUTIONS:** Elderly, infants, and children. Those w/dehy-

AMINOGLYCOSIDES

Generic Name	Brand Name(s)	Rte Adm	Blood Levels: Peak (mcg/ml)	Blood Levels: Trough (mcg/ml)	Dosage Range*
amikacin	Amikin	IM, IV	15-30	5-10	Adults: 15 mg/kg/day Children: 15 mg/kg/day
gentamicin	Garamycin Jenamicin	IM, IV, Topical Opthalmic	4-10	1-2	Adults: 3-5 mg/kg/day Children: 6-7.5 mg/kg/day
kanamycin	Kantrex Klebcil	PO, Irrigation	—	—	PO: 8-12 Gm/day
neomycin	Mycifradin Neobiotic	PO, Topical Ophthalmic			PO: 1 Gm × 3 dose preop
netilmicin	Netromycin	IM, IV	6-12	0.5-2	Adults: 3-6.5 mg/kg/day Children: 5.5-8 mg/kg/day
streptomycin	Streptomycin	IM	—	—	Adults: 15 mg/kg/day; maximum: 1 Gm Children: 20-40 mg/kg/day; maximum: 1 Gm
tobramycin	Nebcin	IM, IV, Ophthalmic	4-10	1-2	Adults: 3-5 mg/kg/day Children: 6-7.5 mg/kg/day

*Dosage, interval based on serum drug concentration.

dration or renal dysfunction must be monitored very closely. Use for pts w/Parkinson's disease or myasthenia gravis may result in further muscle weakness.

INTERACTIONS

Other aminoglycosides, nephrotoxic, ototoxic producing medications may increase toxicity. May increase effects of neuromuscular blocking agents.

SIDE EFFECTS

Nausea or diarrhea w/oral administration. Headache, increased salivation, anorexia. Photosensitivity when administered topically.

TOXIC EFFECTS/ADVERSE REACTIONS

Serious toxicity, primarily ototoxicity and nephrotoxicity, is a major factor in limiting the usefulness of the aminoglycosides. Ototoxicity is suggested by dizziness, vertigo, tinnitus, hearing loss. Nephrotoxicity may be signaled by proteinuria, increased BUN, oliguria. Neuromuscular blockade can occur w/high doses, resulting in weakness, shortness of breath, and even respiratory paralysis. Hypersensitivity reactions may occur. Note also that systemic effects may result from wound irrigation or topical application.

NURSING IMPLICATIONS

GENERAL: Administer on schedule to maintain blood levels. Initiate IV solutions slowly at first w/close observation for sensitivity response. **BASELINE ASSESSMENT:** Inquire about previous reactions to aminoglycosides. Culture/sensitivity must be done before first dose (may give before results are known). Assess WBC results, temperature, pulse, respiration. **INTERVENTION/EVALUATION:** Maintain good hydration and I&O. Monitor plasma concentration levels (peak and trough values) to determine continued dosage. Check WBC and culture/sensitivity results. Assess temperature, pulse, respiration, esp. rate, depth and ease of respirations. Be alert for adverse reactions: Ototoxicity, nephrotoxicity, neuromuscular blockade, allergic reaction. **PATIENT/FAMILY TEACHING:** Space doses evenly. Continue therapy for full duration. Avoid taking even over-the-counter medications w/o physician direction. Notify physician in event of any hearing, visual, balance, urinary problems even after therapy is completed.

antibiotic: cephalosporins

ACTION

Cephalosporins inhibit cell wall synthesis or activate enzymes that disrupt cell wall causing a weakening in the cell wall, cell lysis, and cell death. May be bacteriostatic or bactericidal. Most effective against rapidly dividing cells.

USES

Broad-spectrum antibiotics, which, like penicillins, may be used in a number of diseases including: Respiratory diseases, skin and soft tissue infection, bone/joint infections, genitourinary infections, prophylactically in some surgical procedures.

First generation cephalosporins have good activity against gram-positive organisms and moderate activity against gram-negative organisms including *Escherichia coli, Klebsiella pneumoniae, Proteus mirabilis.*

Second generation cephalosporins have increased activity against gram-negative organisms.

Third generation cephalosporins are less active against gram-positive organisms but more active against the Enterobacteriaceae w/some activity against *Pseudomonas aeruginosa.*

Fourth generation cephalosporins have good activity against gram-positive organisms (e.g., *Staphylococcus aureus)* and gram-negative organisms (e.g., *Pseudomonas aeruginosa).*

PRECAUTIONS

CONTRAINDICATIONS: Hypersensitivity to cephalosporins or penicillins. **CAUTION:** Careful monitoring is essential in bleeding disorders, gastrointestinal disease, renal and hepatic dysfunction. See individual monographs for pregnancy, lactation precautions.

INTERACTIONS

Interaction between alcohol and some of the cephalosporins (e.g., cefamandole, cefoperazone, cefotetan) may cause buildup of acetaldehyde in the blood w/disulfiram-like reaction: Headache, palpitations, chest pain, hypotension, nausea, vomiting, and abdominal pain. Alcohol in any form is to be avoided up to 72 hours after drug administration. Bacteriostatic drugs may decrease effects of cephalosporins. Probenecid increases blood levels; aminoglycosides and several diuretics may increase risk of renal toxicity. Cefamandole, cefoperazone, cefotetan may increase hypoprothrombinemic effect of oral anticoagulants.

SIDE EFFECTS

Mild nausea, vomiting, or diarrhea, esp. w/oral administration.

TOXIC EFFECTS/ADVERSE REACTIONS

Hypersensitivity reactions, particularly skin rash, may progress to anaphylaxis; superinfections, including antibiotic-associated colitis. Hypoprothrombinemia and thrombocytopenia may occur w/potential for hemorrhage. Nephrotoxicity may occur, esp. w/high dosages.

NURSING IMPLICATIONS

GENERAL: Administer on schedule to maintain blood levels. Initiate IV

CEPHALOSPORINS

Generic Name	Brand Name(s)	Generation	Rte Admin	Dosage Range
cefaclor	Ceclor	Second	PO	Adults: 250-500 mg q8h Children: 20-40 mg/kg/day
cefadroxil	Duricef Ultracef	First	PO	Adults: 1-2 Gm/day Children: 30 mg/kg/day
cefamandole	Mandol	Second	IM, IV	Adults: 1.5-12 Gm/day Children: 50-150 mg/kg/day
cefazolin	Ancef Kefzol Zolicef	First	IM, IV	Adults: 0.75-6 Gm/day Children: 25-100 mg/kg/day
cefepime	Maxipime	Fourth	IM, IV	Adults: 1-6 Gm/day
cefixime	Suprax	Third	PO	Adults: 400 mg/day Children: 8 mg/kg/day
cefmetazole	Zefazone	Second	IM, IV	Adults: 4-8 Gm/day
cefonicid	Monocid	Second	IM, IV	Adults: 1-2 Gm/day
cefoperazone	Cefobid	Third	IM, IV	Adults: 2-12 Gm/day
cefotaxime	Claforan	Third	IM, IV	Adults: 2-12 Gm/day Children: 100-200 mg/kg/day
cefotetan	Cefotan	Second	IM, IV	Adults: 1-6 Gm/day
cefoxitin	Mefoxin	Second	IM, IV	Adults: 3-12 Gm/day Children: 80-160 mg/kg/day
cefpodoxime	Vantin	Second	PO	Adults: 200-800 mg/day Children: 10 mg/kg/day
cefprozil	Cefzil	Second	PO	Adults: 0.5-1 Gm/day Children: 30 mg/kg/day
ceftazidime	Fortaz Tazicef Tazidime	Third	IM, IV	Adults: 0.5-6 Gm/day Children: 90-150 mg/kg/day
ceftizoxime	Cefizox	Third	IM, IV	Adults: 1-12 Gm/day Children: 150-200 mg/kg/day
ceftriaxone	Rocephin	Third	IM, IV	Adults: 1-4 Gm/day Children: 50-100 mg/kg/day

CEPHALOSPORINS *Continued*

Generic Name	Brand Name(s)	Generation	Rte Admin	Dosage Range
cefuroxime	Ceftin Kefurox Zinacef	Second	PO, IM, IV	Adults(PO): 0.25-1 Gm/day Adults(IM, IV): 2.25-9 Gm/day Children(PO): 250-500 mg/day Children(IM, IV): 50-100 mg/kg/day
cephalexin	Keftab Keflet Keflex	First	PO	Adults: 1-4 Gm/day Children: 25-100 mg/kg/day
cephalothin	Keflin Seffin	First	IM, IV	Adults: 2-12 Gm/day Children: 80-160 mg/kg/day
loracarbef	Lorabid	Second	PO	Adults: 200-800 mg/day Children: 15-30 mg/kg/day

solutions slowly at first w/close observation for sensitivity response. **BASELINE ASSESSMENT:** Inquire about previous reactions to cephalosporins, penicillins. W/history of penicillin allergy, have emergency equipment, medications available. Culture/sensitivity must be done before first dose (may give before results are known). Assess WBC results, temperature, pulse, respiration. **INTERVENTION/ASSESSMENT:** Monitor WBC results, temperature, pulse, respiration. Assess for adverse reactions, esp. allergic reaction, superinfections including antibiotic-associated colitis. **PATIENT/FAMILY TEACHING:** Space doses evenly. Continue therapy for full duration. Avoid alcohol, antacids, or other medications w/o consulting physician. Notify physician promptly of rash or diarrhea.

antibiotic: penicillins

ACTION

Penicillins inhibit cell wall synthesis or activate enzymes, which disrupt cell wall causing a weakening in the cell wall, cell lysis, and cell death. May be bacteriostatic or bactericidal. Most effective against rapidly dividing cells.

PENICILLINS

Generic Name	Brand Names(s)	Type	Rte Admin	Dosage Range
amoxicillin	Amoxil Polymox Trimox Wymox	Broad spectrum	PO	Adult: 0.75-1.5 Gm/day Children: 20-40 mg/kg/day
amoxicillin/clavulanate	Augmentin	Broad spectrum	PO	Adult: 0.75-1.5 Gm/day Children: 20-40 mg/kg/day
ampicillin	Omnipen Polycillin Principen	Broad spectrum	PO, IM, IV	Adult: 1-12 Gm/day Children: 50-200 mg/kg/day
ampicillin/sulbactam	Unasyn	Broad spectrum	IM, IV	Adult: 6-12 Gm/day
bacampicillin	Spectrobid	Broad spectrum	PO	Adult: 800-1600 mg/day Children: 25-50 mg/kg/day
carbenicillin	Geocillin	Extended spectrum	PO	Adult: 382-764 mg 4 × /day
cloxacillin	Cloxapen Tegopen	Penicillinase resistant	PO	Adult: 1-2 Gm/day Children: 50-100 mg/kg/day
dicloxacillin	Dynapen Pathocil	Pencillinase resistant	PO	Adult: 1-2 Gm/day Children: 12.5-25 mg/kg/day
methicillin	Staphcillin	Penicillinase resistant	IM, IV	Adult: 4-12 Gm/day Children: 100-300 mg/kg/day
mezlocillin	Mezlin	Extended spectrum	IM, IV	Adult: 6-18 Gm/day Children: 150-300 mg/kg/day
nafcillin	Nafcil Unipen	Penicillinase resistant	PO, IM, IV	Adult (PO): 1-6 Gm/day Adult (IM, IV): 2-6 Gm/day Children (PO): 25-50 mg/kg/day Children (IM, IV): 50 mg/kg/day
oxacillin	Bactocill Prostaphlin	Penicillinase resistant	PO, IM, IV	Adult (PO): 2-6 Gm/day Adult (IM, IV): 2-6 Gm/day Children (PO): 50-100 mg/kg/day Children (IM, IV): 50-100 mg/kg/day
penicillin G benzathine	Bicillin Permapen	Natural	IM	Adult: 1.2 million U/day Children: 0.3-1.2 million U/day

PENICILLINS *Continued*

Generic Name	Brand Names(s)	Type	Rte Admin	Dosage Range
penicillin G postassium	Pentids Pfizerpen	Natural	PO, IM, IV	Adult (PO): 0.5-2 Gm/day Adult (IM, IV): 2-24 million U/day Children (PO): 25,000-90,000 U/kg/day Children (IM, IV): 100,000-250,000 U/kg/day
penicillin G procaine	Crysticillin A.S. Wycillin	Natural	IM	Adult: 0.6-1.2 million U/day Children: 0.6-1.2 million U/day
penicillin V potassium	Pen-Vee K V-Cillin K Veetids	Natural	PO	Adult: 0.5-2 Gm/day Children: 25-50 mg/kg/day
piperacillin	Pipracil	Extended spectrum	IM, IV	Adult: 6-18 Gm/day Children: 200-300 mg/kg/day
piperacillin tazobactam	Zosyn	Extended spectrum	IV	Adults: 3.375 Gm q6h
ticarcillin	Ticar	Extended spectrum	IM, IV	Adult: 12-24 Gm/day Children: 50-300 mg/kg/day
ticarcillin clavulanate	Timentin	Extended spectrum	IM, IV	Adult: 3.1 Gm q4-6h

USES

Penicillins may be used to treat a large number of infections including pneumonia and other respiratory diseases, urinary tract infections, septicemia, meningitis, intra-abdominal infections, gonorrhea and syphilis, bone/joint infection.

Natural penicillins are very active against gram-positive cocci but ineffective against most strains of *Staphylococcus aureus* (inactivated by enzyme penicillinase).

Penicillinase-resistant penicillins are effective against penicillinase-producing *Staphylococcus aureus* but less effective against gram-positive cocci than the natural penicillins.

Broad-spectrum penicillins are effective against gram-positive cocci and some gram-negative bacteria (e.g., *Hemophilus influenzae, Escherichia coli, Proteus mirabilis).*

Extended-spectrum penicillins are effective against *Pseudomonas aeruginosa, Enterobacter, Proteus* species, *Klebsiella,* and some other gram-negative microorganisms.

PRECAUTIONS

CONTRAINDICATIONS: Hypersensitivity to penicillin, cephalosporins, or components. **CAUTIONS:** Extreme caution w/history of allergies, asthma; gastrointestinal disease; renal dysfunction; bleeding disorders; and (for some penicillins) hepatic dysfunction.

INTERACTIONS

Bacteriostatic antibiotics (e.g., tetracyclines) may decrease bactericidal effects of penicillins. Concurrent use w/allopurinol and ampicillin increases risk of skin rash. Pts should be advised that estrogen contraceptives may have decreased effectiveness when given w/penicillin. Anticoagulants may increase potential for bleeding w/high dose penicillin therapy. Probenecid increases effects by interfering w/excretion.

SIDE EFFECTS

Mild nausea, vomiting, or diarrhea; sore tongue or mouth.

TOXIC EFFECTS/ADVERSE REACTIONS

Hypersensitivity/allergic reactions ranging from skin rashes, urticaria, itching to full anaphylaxis. Superinfections, including antibiotic-associated colitis. Neurotoxicity, hematologic effects may occur in select drugs.

NURSING IMPLICATIONS

GENERAL: Administer drugs on proper schedule to maintain blood levels. Initiate IV solutions slowly at first w/close observation for sensitivity response. **BASELINE ASSESSMENT:** Question for history of hypersensitivity to penicillin or cephalosporins. W/history of cephalosporin reaction, have emergency equipment, medications available. Culture/sensitivity must be done before first dose (may give before results are obtained). Assess WBC results, temperature, pulse, respiration. **INTERVENTION/EVALUATION:** Monitor temperature, lab results, particularly WBC and culture/sensitivity reports. Assess for adverse reactions, esp. allergic reactions, superinfection. **PATIENT/FAMILY TEACHING:** Space doses evenly. Continue therapy for full duration, usually 7-10 days. Avoid alcohol, antacids, or other medications w/o consulting physician. Promptly notify physician of rash or diarrhea.

anticholinergics

ACTION

These agents are known as anticholinergics, antimuscarinics, or parasympatholytics. Competitively block muscarinic receptors. Inhibit action of acetylcholine. Prevent stimulation of receptors by muscarinic agonists. Areas affected include:

Eye: Cause mydriasis (pupil dilation), cycloplegia (paralysis of ciliary muscle).

Heart: Increase heart rate.

Gastrointestinal: Decrease salivary secretion, gastric secretion; decrease tone and motility of gastrointestinal tract.

Respiratory: Decrease secretion of nose, mouth, pharynx, bronchi; cause relaxation of bronchi.

Urinary tract: Decrease tone, contraction of ureter and urinary bladder.

USES

Management of peptic ulcer, ophthalmic administration (produce mydriasis/cycloplegia), asthma (induce bronchodilation), antagonize reflex vagal-mediated bradycardia, Parkinson's disease, administered before general anesthetic to decrease excessive salivation/secretion of respiratory tract, spastic disorders of biliary tract, antidote/antagonize effects of anticholinesterase agents; antidote for mushroom poisoning.

PRECAUTIONS

CONTRAINDICATIONS: Hypersensitivity, glaucoma, hepatic or renal dysfunction, tachycardia, ulcerative colitis, intestinal obstruction, paralytic ileus, bladder neck obstruction, myasthenia gravis, asthma. **CAUTIONS:** Pts w/cardiac disease, elderly, infants, and young children (who are particularly susceptible to toxic effects) should be monitored closely. Drugs cross placenta and are excreted in breast milk. May inhibit lactation.

INTERACTIONS

Antacids, antidiarrheals, may decrease absorption. Anticholinergics may increase effects. May decrease absorption of ketoconazole. May increase severity of gastrointestinal lesions w/potassium chloride (wax matrix).

SIDE EFFECTS

Antisalivary (dry mouth), blurred vision, urinary hesitation/retention, constipation, flushing, lightheadedness, mild tachycardia.

TOXIC EFFECTS/ADVERSE REACTIONS

CNS excitation, nausea and vomiting, hypertension, increased intraocular pressure, rash, elevated temperature, thick respiratory secretions and respiratory difficulties, impotence.

NURSING IMPLICATIONS

GENERAL: For long term therapy, change medication gradually. **BASELINE ASSESSMENT:** Check B/P, pulse, respirations. **INTERVENTION/EVALUATION:** Assess bowel activity, abdominal distention, bowel sounds. Monitor I&O, check for urination, palpate for distended bladder.

ANTICHOLINERGICS

Generic Name	Brand Name(s)	Rte Adm	Dosage Range
atropine	Atropine	IM, IV, SubQ	Adults: 0.3-1.2 mg Children: 0.01 mg/kg
dicyclomine	Bentyl	PO, IM	Adults: PO: 80-160 mg/day Adults: IM: 80 mg/day
glycopyrrolate	Robinul	PO, IM, IV	Adults: PO: 2-6 mg/day; IM, IV: 0.1-0.2 mg
scopolamine	Scopolamine	IM, IV, SubQ	Adults: 0.3-0.65 mg Children: 0.006 mg/kg
		Topical	Adults: 0.5 mg/72 hrs

Check B/P, pulse, respirations, EKG. Assess for adverse reactions, esp. in geriatric pts and those w/chronic lung conditions. **PATIENT/FAMILY TEACHING:** Mouthwash, cold drinks, hard candy or gum (if permitted) may be used for dry mouth. Take safety precautions w/drowsiness, blurred vision, or lightheadedness; do not drive or perform activities requiring mental acuity. Increased fluid intake to decrease viscosity of secretions, aid in bowel elimination. *Ophthalmic:* Protect eyes from light; wear sunglasses.

anticoagulants / antiplatelets / thrombolytics

ACTION

Anticoagulants: Inhibit blood coagulation by preventing the formation of new clots and extension of existing ones. *Do not dissolve formed clots.* Anticoagulants are subdivided into the two common classes: *Heparin:* Directly interferes w/blood coagulation by blocking the conversion of prothrombin to thrombin and fibrinogen to fibrin. *Coumarin:* Acts indirectly to prevent synthesis in the liver of vitamin K–dependent clotting factors.

Antiplatelets: Interfere w/platelet aggregation. Effects are irreversible for life of platelet.

Thrombolytics: Act directly or indirectly on fibrinolytic system to dissolve clots (converting plasminogen to plasmin, an enzyme that digests fibrin clot).

USES

Anticoagulants: Primarily decrease risk of venous thromboembolism.
Antiplatelets: Primarily decrease risk of arterial thromboembolism.
Thrombolytics: Lyse existing clots.

ANTICOAGULANTS/ANTIPLATELETS/THROMBOLYTICS

Generic Name	Brand Names(s)	Class	Dosage Range
alteplase	Activase	Thrombolytic	Adults: IV infusion: 100 mg over 3 hrs (2 hrs for pulmonary embolism)
anistreplase	Eminase	Thrombolytic	Adults: IV push: 30 U over 2-5 min
aspirin	—	Antiplatelet	Adults: 300-325 mg/day
dalteparin	Fragmin	Anticoagulant	Adults: SubQ: 200 IU/kg once daily or 100 IU/kg q12h
dipyridamole	Persantine	Antiplatelet	Adults: 75-100 mg 4 times/day
enoxaparin	Lovenox	Anticoagulant	Adults: 30 mg q12h
heparin	—	Anticoagulant	Adults: IV bolus: 5,000 U then IV infusion of 20,000-40,000 U/day Children: IV bolus: 50 U/kg then IV infusion of 20,000 U/m^2/24 hrs
streptokinase	Kabikinase Streptase	Thrombolytic	Adults: (AMI) 1.5 million U over 60 min
ticlopidine	Ticlid	Antiplatelet	Adults: 250 mg 2 times/day
urokinase	Abbokinase	Thrombolytic	Adults: IV: 4,400 IU/kg over 10 min, then 4,400 IU/kg/min for 12-24 hrs
warfarin	Coumadin	Anticoagulant	Adults: Initially, 5-10 mg/day, then 2-10 mg/day

Treatment and prevention of venous thromboembolism, acute myocardial infarction, acute cerebral embolism; reduces risk of acute myocardial infarction, total mortality in pts w/unstable angina; occlusion of saphenous grafts following open heart surgery; embolism in select pts w/atrial fibrillation, prosthetic heart valves, valvular heart disease, cardiomyopathy. Heparin also used for acute/chronic consumption coagulopathies (disseminated intravascular coagulation).

PRECAUTIONS

CONTRAINDICATIONS: Hypersensitivity, active bleeding, blood dyscrasias and bleeding tendencies, pregnancy. **CAUTIONS:** Renal, hepatic dysfunction; alcoholism; history of allergy.

INTERACTIONS

Anticoagulants interact with many drugs and foods. Pts should be cautioned against smoking, alcohol consumption, and use of over-the-counter drugs. Aspirin, many nonsteroidal anti-inflammatory drugs, antihistamines, diuretics, antibiotics, estrogen contraceptives are among the drugs that affect anticoagulant action. Any medication taken with an anticoagulant should be checked for interaction. Prothrombin time (PT) may be shortened by high-fat diet or sudden increase in foods rich in vitamin K. Antidote for heparin: Protamine sulfate; for coumarins: Vitamin K.

SIDE EFFECTS

Not common. Local reactions w/parenteral administration. Nausea, vomiting, anorexia, and diarrhea w/oral administration.

TOXIC EFFECTS/ADVERSE REACTIONS

Minor bleeding to major hemorrhage. Thrombocytopenia and alopecia are transient and reversible. Jaundice, hepatitis, increased serum transaminase levels w/coumarin therapy. Hypersensitivity reactions are rare: Fever, chills, urticaria.

NURSING IMPLICATIONS

GENERAL: Do not discontinue abruptly. Monitor coagulation test results before administration: For heparin therapy, the activated partial thromboplastin time (APTT); for coumarin therapy, the PT. Consult physician for targeted coagulation range for individual pt (generally, dosage is adjusted to keep results about 1.5-2 times control value for APTT, 1.5 times control value for PT). **INTERVENTION/EVALUATION:** Assess for bleeding: Vital signs, bruises, overt bleeding, and blood in sputum, urine, and feces. Check for headache, abdominal or back pain. **PATIENT/FAMILY TEACHING:** Importance of taking drug as directed and periodic lab tests to determine response to medication. Explain how to check for bleeding signs. Carry identification indicating anticoagulant therapy. Avoid large quantities of vitamin K–rich food, such as green leafy vegetables, liver, fish, bananas, cauliflower, tomatoes (decrease effects of oral anticoagulants). Consult physician before taking other medications (including aspirin). Avoid alcohol. Avoid activities w/high risk of injury. Inform physician, dentist of anticoagulant therapy before surgical/dental procedures.

anticonvulsants

ACTION

Seizures consist of abnormal and excessive discharges from the brain. Anticonvulsants can prevent or reduce excessive discharge of neurons w/seizure foci or decrease the spread of excitation from seizure foci to normal neurons. Exact mechanism unknown. Anticonvulsants include the hydantoins, barbiturates, succinimides, oxazolidinediones, benzodiazepines, and several miscellaneous agents.

USES

Anticonvulsants are generally effective in the treatment of *absence*

ANTICONVULSANTS

Generic Name	Brand Names(s)	Class	Uses	Dosage Range
carbamazepine	Tegretol	Miscellaneous	Complex partial, tonic-clonic, mixed seizures, trigeminal neuralgia	Adults: 800-1200 mg/day Children: 400-800 mg/day
clonazepam	Klonopin	Benzodiazepine	Petit mal, akinetic, myoclonic, absence	Adults: 1.5-20 mg/day Children: 0.01-0.2 mg/kg/day
clorazepate	Tranxene	Benzodiazepine	Partial seizures	Adults: 7.5-90 mg/day Children: 7.5-60 mg/day
diazepam	Valium	Benzodiazepine	Adjunctive therapy status epilepticus	Adults: PO: 4-40 mg/day IM/IV: 5-30 mg Children: PO: 3-10 mg/day IM/IV: 1-10 mg
ethosuximide	Zarontin	Succinimide	Absence seizures	Children: 20 mg/kg/day
felbamate	Felbatol	Miscellaneous	Partial seizures Lennox-Gustaut syndrome	Adults: 1200-3600 mg/day Children ≥14 yrs: 1200-3600 mg/day
gabapentum	Neurontin	Miscellaneous	Partial seizures	Adults: 900-1800 mg/day Children >12 yrs: 900-1800 mg/day
lamotrigine	Lamictal	Miscellaneous	Partial seizures	Adults: 100-500 mg/day

Continued.

(petit mal) seizures (brief, abrupt loss of consciousness, some clonic motor activity ranging from eyelid blinking to jerking of entire body), *tonic-clonic (grand mal) seizures* (major convulsions, usually beginning w/spasm of all body musculature, then clonic jerking, followed by depression of all central function), and *complex partial seizures* (confused behavior, impaired consciousness, bizarre generalized EEG activity). Other types of seizures generally respond poorly to anticonvulsant therapy.

ANTICONVULSANTS *Continued*

Generic Name	Brand Names(s)	Class	Uses	Dosage Range
phenobarbital	Luminal	Barbiturate	Tonic-clonic, partial, status epilepticus	Adults: PO: 100-300 mg/day IM/IV: 200-600 mg Children: PO: 3-5 mg/kg/day IM/IV: 100-400 mg
phenytoin	Dilantin	Hydantoin	Tonic-clonic, complex partial, autonomic seizures, status epilepticus	Adults: PO: 300-600 mg/day IV: 150-250 mg Status epilepticus: 15-18 mg/kg Children: PO: 4-8 mg/kg/day Status epilepticus: 10-15 mg/kg
primidone	Mysoline	Miscellaneous	Complex partial, partial, akinetic, tonic-clonic	Adults: 0.75-2 Gm/day Children: 10-25 mg/kg/day
valproic acid	Depakene Depakote	Miscellaneous	Absence, multiple seizure types	Adults, children: 15-60 mg/kg/day
vigabatrin	Sabril	Miscellaneous	Complex partial seizures	Adults: 1-4 Gm/day Children: 50-150 mg/kg/day

PRECAUTIONS

CONTRAINDICATIONS: Hypersensitivity, hepatic, renal, or thyroid dysfunction, alcoholism, blood dyscrasias; diabetes mellitus, cardiac disease/impairment, lactation. **CAUTIONS:** Pregnancy—risk benefit must be weighed in relation to congenital abnormalities. Elderly, children, and debilitated.

INTERACTIONS

Drug interactions are extensive; any other medication administered should be carefully checked for interaction w/anticonvulsants. Teach pts never to take medication w/o consulting physician. Effects are increased by CNS depressants; decreased w/tricyclic antidepressants, phenothiazine antipsychotics, antacids. Refer to individual monographs.

SIDE EFFECTS

Drowsiness, sedation, mild dizziness, gingival hyperplasia, anorexia, nausea, vomiting, hyperglycemia, and glycosuria.

TOXIC EFFECTS/ADVERSE REACTIONS

Visual disturbances, unusual excitement, confusion, skin disorders. Stevens-Johnson syndrome (headache, arthralgia, skin lesions w/other symptoms), liver damage, hirsutism, blood dyscrasias, enlarged lymph glands in neck and under arms.

NURSING IMPLICATIONS

GENERAL: Status epilepticus is a life-threatening emergency that requires immediate IV medication (diazepam is the drug of choice). *Never mix parenteral solutions w/other drugs or IV fluids—should be administered via slow IV push.* When discontinued, gradual reduction is recommended. Provide protection against injury. **INTERVENTION/EVALUATION:** Monitor B/P, pulse, respirations, serum drug levels. Assess neurologic status. Identify characteristics of seizures if they occur. **PATIENT/FAMILY TEACHING:** Therapy is usually several years to life. Take w/food or fluids to minimize GI irritation. Important to take as directed. Do not take other medications w/o consulting physician. Avoid alcohol. Do not drive or engage in activities requiring mental acuity until physician approves (seizures and response to drug are controlled). Carry identification card/bracelet indicating anticonvulsant therapy.

antidepressants

ACTION

Antidepressants are classified as tricyclic, monoamine oxidase (MAO) inhibitors, or miscellaneous. Depression may be due to reduced functioning of monoamine neurotransmitters in the CNS (decreased amount and/or decreased effects at receptor sites).

Antidepressants block metabolism, increase amount/effects of monoamine neurotransmitters (e.g., norepinephrine, serotonin [5-HT]) and act at receptor sites (change responsiveness/sensitivities of both pre- and postsynaptic receptor sites).

Miscellaneous, Tricyclics: Block reuptake of neurotransmitter at presynaptic nerve endings. Potency/selectivity varies w/these agents.

MAO inhibitors: Inhibit enzyme MAO, thus interfering w/degradation of monoamine neurotransmitters.

USES

Used primarily for the treatment of depression. Imipramine is also used for childhood enuresis, clomipramine is used only for obsessive-com-

ANTIDEPRESSANTS

Generic Name	Brand Names(s)	Type	Amine Uptake Blockage	Dosage Range (mg/day)
amitriptyline	Elavil Endep	Tricyclic	Norepinephrine Serotonin	PO: 40-300
amoxapine	Asendin	Tricyclic	Norepinephrine Serotonin	PO: 100-600
bupropion	Wellbutrin	Miscellaneous	—	PO: 200-450
clomipramine	Anafranil	Tricyclic	Norepinephrine Serotonin	PO: 25-250
desipramine	Norpramin Pertofrane	Tricyclic	Norepinephrine Serotonin	PO: 25-100
doxepin	Adapin Sinequan	Tricyclic	Norepinephrine Serotonin	PO: 75-300
fluoxetine	Prozac	Miscellaneous	Serotonin	PO: 20-80
fluvoxamine	Luvox	Miscellaneous	Serotonin	PO: 100-300
imipramine	Janimine Tofranil	Tricyclic	Norepinephrine Serotonin	PO: 30-300
maprotiline	Ludiomil	Miscellaneous	Norepinephrine	PO: 25-225
nefazodone	Serzone	Miscellaneous	Serotonin Serotonin receptor	PO: 200
nortriptyline	Aventyl Pamelor	Tricyclic	Norepinephrine Serotonin	PO: 25-100
paroxetine	Paxil	Miscellaneous	Serotonin	PO: 20-50 mg/day
phenelzine	Nardil	MAO inhibitor	—	PO: 15-90
protriptyline	Vivactil	Tricyclic	Norepinephrine Serotonin	PO: 15-60
sertraline	Zoloft	Miscellaneous	Serotonin	PO: 50-200
tranylcypromine	Parnate	MAO inhibitor	—	PO: 30-60
trazodone	Desyrel	Miscellaneous	Serotonin	PO: 50-600
venlafaxine	Effexor	Miscellaneous	Norepinephrine Serotonin	PO: 75-375 mg/day

pulsive disorder (OCD). MAO inhibitors are rarely used as initial therapy except for pts unresponsive to other therapy or when other therapy is contraindicated.

PRECAUTIONS

CONTRAINDICATIONS: Pregnancy, lactation, children <16 yrs of age (exception: Imipramine to treat enuresis in children >6 yrs of age), hypersensitivity, liver dysfunction, renal dysfunction, glaucoma, elderly, CHF. **CAUTIONS:** Never use MAO inhibitors and tricyclic antidepressants together—can result in death. Effects of antidepressants can last 2-3 wks after discontinuation.

INTERACTIONS

Tricyclic antidepressants: Alcohol, CNS depressants may increase CNS, respiratory depression, hypotensive effects. Antithyroid agents may increase risk of agranulocytosis. Phenothiazines may increase sedative, anticholinergic effects. Cimetidine may increase concentration, toxicity. May decrease effects of clonidine, guanadrel. May increase cardiac effects w/sympathomimetics. May increase risk of hypertensive crisis, hyperpyretic, convulsion w/MAO inhibitors.

MAO inhibitors: Alcohol, CNS depressants may increase CNS depressant effects. Tricyclic antidepressants, fluoxetine, trazodone may cause serotonin syndrome. May increase effect of oral hypoglycemics, insulin, B/P may increase w/buspirone, Caffeine containing medications may increase cardiac arrhythmias, hypertension. May precipitate hypertensive crises w/carbamazepine, cyclobenzaprine, maprotiline, other MAO inhibitors. Meperidine, other opioid analgesics may produce immediate excitation, sweating, rigidity, severe hypertension or hypotension, severe respiratory distress, coma, convulsions, vascular collapse, death. May increase CNS stimulant, vasopressor effects. Tyramine, foods w/pressor amines (e.g., aged cheese) may cause sudden, severe hypertension.

SIDE EFFECTS

Tricyclic antidepressants: Dizziness, drowsiness, dry mouth, headache, weight gain, photosensitivity. *MAO inhibitors:* Dizziness, and orthostatic hypotension, blurred vision, constipation, difficulty w/urination, mild headache, weight gain, insomnia.

TOXIC EFFECTS/ADVERSE REACTIONS

Tricyclic antidepressants: Severe drowsiness, confusion, hallucinations, seizures, tachycardia or bradycardia, difficulty breathing. *MAO inhibitors:* Severe drowsiness or dizziness, hypertension or hypotension, tachycardia, difficulty sleeping, hallucinations, respiratory depression.

NURSING IMPLICATIONS

GENERAL: Closely supervise pts (potential for suicide increases when emerging from depression). Elderly should be observed carefully for increased response; small doses are usually indicated. **BASELINE ASSESSMENT:** Determine initial B/P. Assess pt and environment for support needed. **INTERVENTION/EVALUATION:** Monitor B/P. Assess mental status. Check bowel activity; avoid constipation. **PATIENT/FAMILY TEACHING:** Change positions slowly to avoid orthostatic hypotension. Take medication as ordered; do not stop taking or increase dosage. Avoid driving or performing tasks that require mental acuity until response to drug controlled. Extremely important to refrain from alcohol and other medications during therapy and for 2-3 wks thereafter. Omit foods rich in tyramine, such as products containing yeast, beer/wine, aged cheese (list of foods to avoid should be given); ingestion of such foods and antidepressant may cause hypertensive crisis. Inform other physicians or dentist of antidepressant therapy. Use protection from sunlight w/ specific drugs. To the extent possible, drugs that cause drowsiness should be taken at bedtime, those causing insomnia should be taken in the morning.

antidiarrheals

ACTION

Systemic agents: Act at smooth muscle receptors (enteric) disrupting peristaltic movements, decreasing GI motility, increasing transit time of intestinal contents.

Local agents: Adsorb toxic substances and fluids to large surface areas of particles in the preparation. Some of these agents coat and protect irritated intestinal walls. May have local anti-inflammatory action.

USES

Acute diarrhea, chronic diarrhea of inflammatory bowel disease, reduction of fluid from ileostomies.

PRECAUTIONS

CONTRAINDICATIONS: Children <2 years of age, hypersensitivity to any component. Safety not established in pregnancy, lactation. **CAUTIONS:** Young children, elderly. Not for antibiotic-associated colitis or ulcerative colitis.

INTERACTIONS

Vary according to components of individual agents. CNS depressants, anticholinergics, antihistamines increase effects of antidiarrheals.

SIDE EFFECTS

Constipation, drowsiness w/systemic agents (nausea and dry mouth w/diphenoxylate hydrochloride w/atropine sulfate).

TOXIC EFFECTS/ADVERSE REACTIONS

Adverse reactions are infrequent w/proper dosage. Abdominal distention and cramps, dizziness, nausea and vomiting, drug dependence w/long-term use (atropine side effects w/diphenoxylate w/atropine).

NURSING IMPLICATIONS

GENERAL: Discontinue medication when diarrhea controlled or if abdominal distention occurs. Maintain hydration (offer 2,000-3,000 ml of fluid/day to adults). **INTERVENTION/EVALUATION:** Monitor stool frequency and consistency (watery, loose, soft, semi-solid, solid). Check I&O and assess hydration, esp. in very young and old. **PATIENT/FAMILY TEACHING:** Avoid tasks that require alertness, motor skills until response to drug is established. Do not ingest alcohol or barbiturates,

ANTIDIARRHEALS

Generic Name	Brand Names(s)	Type	Dosage Forms	Dosage Range
bismuth subsalicylate	Pepto-Bismol	Local	Suspension Tablets	Adults: 2 tablets or 30 ml Children: (9-12 yrs): 1 tablet or 15 ml Children: (6-9 yrs): ⅔ tablet or 10 ml Children: (3-6 yrs): ⅓ tablet or 5 ml
diphenoxylate (w/atropine)	Lomotil	Systemic	Liquid Tablets	Adults: 5 mg 4 × /day Children (liquid only): 0.3-0.4 mg/kg/day in 4 divided doses
kaolin (w/pectin)	Kaopectate	Local	Suspension	Adults: 60-120 ml after each BM Children (6-12 yrs): 30-60 ml Children (3-6 yrs): 15-30 ml
loperamide	Imodium	Systemic	Capsules Liquid	Adults: Initially 4 mg, max: 16 mg/day Children (8-12 yrs): 2 mg 3 × /day Children (5-8 yrs): 2 mg 2 × /day Children (2-5 yrs): 1 mg 3 × /day (liquid)

esp. w/drugs containing atropine. Contact physician for diarrhea that persists more than 2 days, high fever, blood in stool, or abdominal distension.

antihistamines

ACTION

Antihistamines (H_1 antagonists) inhibit vasoconstrictor effects and vasodilator effects on endothelial cells of histamine. Blocks increased capillary permeability, formation of edema/wheal caused by histamine. Many antihistamines can bind to receptors in CNS causing primarily depression (decreased alertness, slowed reaction times, somnolence) but also stimulation (restless, nervousness, inability to sleep). Some may counter motion sickness.

ANTIHISTAMINES

Generic Name	Brand Names(s)	Dosage Range
astemizole	Hismanal	Adults, children >12 yrs: 10 mg/day
brompheniramine	Dimetane	Adults: 4 mg q4-6h Children 6-12 yrs: 2 mg q4-6h
cetirizine	Reactine	Adults: 5-20 mg/day
chlorpheniramine	Chlor-Trimeton	Adults, children >12 yrs: 4 mg q4-6h Children 6-12 yrs: 2 mg q4-6h
clemastine	Tavist	Adults, children >12 yrs: 1.34 mg 2×/day up to 2.68 mg 3×/day
cyproheptadine	Periactin	Adults: 4-20 mg/day Children 7-14 yrs: 4 mg 2-3×/day Children 2-7 yrs: 2 mg 2-3×/day
dexchlorpheniramine	Polaramine	Adults: 2 mg q4-6h Children 6-11 yrs: 1 mg q4-6h
diphenhydramine	Benadryl	Adults: 25-50 mg q6-8h Children >10 kg: 12.5-25 mg 3-4×/day
loratidine	Claritin	Adults: 10 mg/day Children >12 yrs: 10 mg/day
promethazine	Phenergan	Adults: 25 mg at hs or 12.5 mg 3-4×/day Children: 25 mg at hs or 6.25-12.5 mg 3-4×/day
terfenadine	Seldane	Adults: 60 mg q12h
trimeprazine	Temaril	Adults: 2.5 mg 4×/day Children >3 yrs: 2.5 mg at hs or 3×/day if needed Children 6 mo-3 yrs: 1.25 mg at hs or 3×/day if needed

hs, bedtime.

USES

Symptomatic relief of upper respiratory allergic disorders. Allergic reactions associated w/other drugs respond to antihistamines as do blood transfusion reactions. Used as a second choice drug in the treatment of angioneurotic edema. Effective in treatment of acute urticaria and other dermatologic conditions. May also be used for preop sedation. Parkinson's disease and motion sickness.

PRECAUTIONS

CONTRAINDICATIONS: Hypersensitivity-cross sensitivity, infants, asthma, narrow-angle glaucoma, prostatic hypertrophy, bladder neck obstruction, CNS depression, hypertension, third trimester of pregnancy, lactation. **CAUTIONS:** Young children, elderly experience exaggerated results: Children, paradoxical excitement; elderly, heavy sedation. Care should be exercised w/cardiovascular disease, hyperthyroidism, and convulsive disorders. Safety during first and second trimester of pregnancy not established.

INTERACTIONS

Alcohol, CNS depressants may increase CNS depressant effects. Anticholinergics may increase anticholinergic effects. MAO inhibitors may increase anticholinergic, CNS depressant effects. Erythromycin, ketoconazole may increase risk of cardiotoxic effect w/astemizole, terfenadine.

SIDE EFFECTS

Sedation, headache, dizziness, nervousness, restlessness, irritability, loss of appetite, palpitations, urinary retention, constipation.

TOXIC EFFECTS/ADVERSE REACTIONS

Convulsions, hallucinations, tight chest w/shortness of breath, incoordination, flushing of face, hyperthermia, CNS may demonstrate overstimulation or depression. Children are particularly susceptible to overdosage.

NURSING IMPLICATIONS

GENERAL: Take safety precautions when given concurrently w/narcotic analgesics (use side rails; assist w/ambulation). **BASELINE ASSESSMENT:** Determine initial B/P, temperature, pulse, respiration. **INTERVENTION/EVALUATION:** Monitor B/P, temperature, pulse, respiration. Assess therapeutic response to medication; be alert to adverse reactions. Check lung sounds. Maintain I&O; assess for urinary retention. Monitor bowel activity; avoid constipation. **PATIENT/FAMILY TEACHING:** Take oral doses w/meals. Drink 8 or more glasses of fluid/day to decrease viscosity of secretions and help prevent constipation. Do not drive or engage in activities that may be affected by sedative effects. For motion sickness, take ½ to 1 hour before traveling. Avoid alcohol and other medications unless physician approves. Explain adverse reactions, need to report immediately.

antihyperlipoproteinemics

ACTION

Hyperlipoproteinemias are conditions in which the concentration of cholesterol or triglycerides carrying lipoprotein exceeds normal limits. These elevations can accelerate development of atherosclerosis and may lead to thrombosis or myocardial infarction. Cholesterol and triglycerides are transported in lipoproteins including chylomicrons, very low-density lipoprotein (VLDL), which transport triglycerides, low-density lipoproteins (LDL) and high-density lipoproteins (HDL), which transport cholesterol. Agents used in the treatment of hyperlipoproteinemia include:

HMG CoA reductase inhibitors: Block synthesis of cholesterol in liver. Produce a dose-related decrease in the concentration of LDL cholesterol; decreases triglyceride concentration; increases HDL cholesterol.

Fibric acids: Reduce plasma triglycerides by decreasing concentration of VLDL. Primary effect is to increase lipoprotein lipase (promotes VLDL catabolism). May decrease hepatic synthesis/secretion of VLDL.

Bile-acid sequestrants: Decrease concentration of cholesterol by lowering LDL levels. Bind bile acids in intestine causing increased fecal excretion, which causes increased production of bile acids from cholesterol.

USES

HMG CoA reductase inhibitors: Adjunctive therapy for reducing elevated total and LDL cholesterol in pts w/primary hypercholesterolemia (types IIa and IIb). *Fibric acids:* Treatment of hypertriglyceridemia in pts w/type IV and V hyperlipidemia. *Bile-acid sequestrants:* Adjunctive therapy for reducing elevated serum cholesterol in pts w/primary hypercholesterolemia (types IIa and IIb).

PRECAUTIONS

CONTRAINDICATIONS: Pregnancy, lactation, hypersensitivity to drug or components, liver disease, biliary cirrhosis or obstruction, severe renal dysfunction. **CAUTIONS:** History of liver disease, substantial alcohol consumption. Safety and efficacy in children not established.

INTERACTIONS

HMG CoA reductase inhibitor: Increased risk of rhabdomyolysis, acute renal failure w/cyclosporine, erythromycin, gemfibrozil, niacin, other immunosuppressants.

Fibric acid: May increase effects of oral anticoagulants, hypoglycemics.

Bile acid sequestrants: May increase effects of anticoagulants by decreasing vitamin K. May decrease warfarin absorption. May bind, decrease absorption of digoxin, thiazides, penicillins, propranolol, tetracyclines, folic acid, thyroid hormones, other medications. Binds, decreases effect of oral vancomycin.

SIDE EFFECTS

GI effects usually lessen or disappear w/continued therapy: Constipation, hemorrhoid irritation, diarrhea, abdominal distention, belching, nausea, vomiting. Headache, urticaria, rash. *HMG CoA reductase inhibitors:* Myalgia. Blurred vision w/lovastatin and gemfibrozil.

TOXIC EFFECTS/ADVERSE REACTIONS

Severe constipation w/fecal impaction, GI bleeding, cholelithiasis,

ANTIHYPERLIPOPROTEINEMICS

Generic Name	Brand Names(s)	Type	Dosage Range
cholestyramine	Colybar Questran	Bile acid sequestrant	4-24 Gm/day
colestipol	Colestid	Bile acid sequestrant	5-30 Gm/day
clofibrate	Atromid-S	Fibric acid	2 Gm/day
fenofibrate	Lipidil	Fibric acid	100-300 mg/day
fluvastatin	Lescol	HMG CoA reductase inhibitor	20-40 mg/day
gemfibrozil	Lopid	Fibric acid	1,200 mg/day
lovastatin	Mevacor	HMG CoA reductase inhibitor	20-80 mg/day
pravastatin	Pravachol	HMG CoA reductase inhibitor	10-40 mg/day
probucol	Lorelco	—	0.5-1 Gm/day
simvastatin	Zocor	HMG CoA reductase inhibitor	5-40 mg/day

acute appendicitis. Angina and cardiac arrhythmias have occurred w/ some drugs; MIs w/dextrothyroxine.

NURSING IMPLICATIONS

GENERAL: Dietary corrections should be attempted before initiating drug therapy. **BASELINE ASSESSMENT:** Determine serum cholesterol and triglyceride levels. **INTERVENTION/EVALUATION:** Monitor GI effects, esp. constipation or diarrhea. Check serum cholesterol and triglyceride levels periodically. **PATIENT/FAMILY TEACHING:** Complete full course; do not omit or change doses. Importance of diet in therapy: Reduce fats, sugars, and cholesterol. Eat high-fiber foods (whole grain cereals, fruits, vegetables) to reduce potential for constipation. Drink several glasses of water between meals. Promptly report bleeding, constipation, or muscle pain/tenderness (esp. w/fever or malaise).

antihypertensives

ACTION

There are many groups of medications used in the treatment of hypertension. In addition to the alpha-adrenergic central agonists and peripheral antagonists and vasodilators discussed below, please refer to the classifications of diuretics, beta-blockers, calcium antagonists and ACE inhibitors or individual monographs of drugs.

Alpha agonists (central action): Stimulate $alpha_2$-adrenergic receptors in cardiovascular centers of CNS, reducing sympathetic outflow and producing antihypertensive effect.

Alpha antagonists (peripheral action): Block $alpha_1$-adrenergic receptors in arterioles, veins inhibiting vasoconstriction, decreasing peripheral vascular resistance, causing a fall in B/P.

ANTIHYPERTENSIVES

Generic Name	Brand Name(s)	Antihypertensive Effect Onset (hrs)	Peak (hrs)	Duration (hrs)	Dosage Range
Central Action					
clonidine	Catapres Catapres-TTS	0.5-1	2-4	12-24	PO: 0.2-0.8 mg/day Topical: 0.1-0.6 mg/wk
guanabenz	Wytensin	1	2-4	6-12	PO: 8-32 mg/day
guanfacine	Tenex	—	1-4	24	PO: 1-3 mg/day
methyl-dopa	Aldomet	2	4-6	12-24	PO: 0.5-3 Gm/day
Peripheral Action					
doxazosin	Cardura	—	—	—	PO: 2-16 mg/day
guanadrel	Hylorel	0.5-2	4-6	9-14	PO: 20-75 mg/day
prazosin	Minipress	2	1-3	6-12	PO: 6-20 mg/day
terazosin	Hytrin	0.25	1-2	12-24	PO: 1-20 mg/day
Vasodilators					
hydralazine	Apresoline	0.75	0.5-2	6-8	PO: 40-300 mg/day
minoxidil	Loniten	0.5	2-3	24-72	PO: 10-40 mg/day

Vasodilators: Directly relax arteriolar smooth muscle, decreasing vascular resistance. Exact mechanism unknown.

USES

Treatment of mild to severe hypertension, depending on agent selected.

PRECAUTIONS

CONTRAINDICATIONS: Hypersensitivity; severe hepatic dysfunction; pheochromocytoma; advanced renal disease; rheumatic heart disease; systemic lupus erythematosus. **CAUTIONS:** Renal impairment, children, pregnancy, lactation, elderly, angina or ischemic heart disease, after myocardial infarction.

INTERACTIONS

Diuretics, other antihypertensive agents, alcohol increase hypotensive effects. Sympathomimetics may decrease hypotensive effect. Please refer to individual monographs for additional information.

SIDE EFFECTS

Specific reactions vary according to the agent given. Weakness, postural hypotension, headache, fatigue, drowsiness, nausea are common.

TOXIC EFFECTS/ADVERSE REACTIONS

Bradycardia and tachycardia; palpitations; hypersensitivity reactions; nausea, vomiting, diarrhea or constipation, arthralgia, reduced hemoglobin, leukopenia, edema. Other reactions per specific agent.

NURSING IMPLICATIONS

GENERAL: For IV administration, monitor pt carefully, place on cardiac monitor and prevent extravasation. **BASELINE ASSESSMENT:** Determine initial B/P and apical pulse. **INTERVENTION/EVALUATION:** Monitor apical pulse and B/P; check w/physician for B/P or pulse below parameters set for that pt. Check for edema of hands, feet. **PATIENT/FAMILY TEACHING:** Teach pt and/or family how to take B/P and pulse. Make position changes slowly (decrease orthostatic hypotension). Follow diet and control weight. Restrict sodium as indicated. Avoid alcohol. Cease smoking. Do not take other medications w/o consulting physician. Do not stop taking medication. Need for lifelong control.

antineoplastics

ACTION

Most antineoplastics inhibit cell replication by interfering w/supply of nutrients or genetic components of the cell (DNA or RNA). Some antineoplastics, referred to as cell cycle–specific (CCS), are particularly effective during a specific phase of cell reproduction (e.g., antimetabolites and plant alkaloids). Other antineoplastics, referred to as cell cycle–nonspecific, act independently of a specific phase of cell division (e.g., alkylating agents and antibiotics). Some hormones are also classified as antineoplastics. Although not cytotoxic, they act to depress cancer growth by altering the hormone environment. In addition there are a number of miscellaneous agents acting through different mechanisms.

Alkylating agents: Highly reactive compounds forming a bond or cross-link w/DNA, and then damaging cells, likely causing cell death.

Antimetabolites: Capable of inhibiting enzymes necessary for synthesis of essential cellular components or being incorporated into DNA, disrupting DNA function.

Antibiotics: Interacts w/DNA, inhibits DNA synthesis, DNA-dependent RNA synthesis, delays or inhibits mitosis.

Hormones: Noncytotoxic, inhibit proliferation by interfering at cellular membrane. May suppress lymphocytes in leukemias/lymphomas, altering hormonal balance in malignancies related to these hormones (e.g., tumors of breast).

Mitotic Inhibitors: Act specifically during M (mitosis) phase of cell cycle, preventing cell division.

ANTINEOPLASTICS

Generic Name	Brand Name(s)	Type	Cell-Cycle Specific	Uses
aldesleukin	Proleukin	Miscellaneous	No	Metastatic renal cell carcinoma
altretamine	Hexalen	Miscellaneous	No	Ovarian cancer
asparaginase	Elspar	Miscellaneous	No	Acute lymphocytic leukemia
BCG	TheraCys TICE BCG	Miscellaneous	No	Carcinoma in situ of urinary bladder
bleomycin	Blenoxane	Antibiotic	Yes	Squamous cell carcinoma, lymphomas, testicular carcinoma
busulfan	Myleran	Alkylating	No	Chronic myelogenous leukemia
carboplatin	Paraplatin	Alkylating	No	Ovarian carcinoma
carmustine	BCNU	Alkylating	No	Brain tumors, multiple myeloma, Hodgkin's, non-Hodgkin's lymphomas
chlorambucil	Leukeran	Alkylating	No	Chronic lymphocytic leukemia, malignant lymphomas
cisplatin	Platinol	Alkylating	No	Metastatic testicular, ovarian tumors, advanced bladder cancer
cladribine	Leustatin	Miscellaneous	No	Hairy cell leukemia
cyclophosphamide	Cytoxan	Alkylating	No	Adenocarcinoma ovary, breast cancer, malignant lymphomas, retinoblastoma, multiple myeloma, leukemias, mycosis fungoides, neuroblastoma
cytarabine	Cytosar	Antimetabolite	Yes	Acute, chronic myelocytic leukemia, acute lymphocytic leukemia
dacarbazine	DTIC	Miscellaneous	No	Metastatic malignant melanoma, Hodgkin's disease
dactinomycin	Cosmegen	Antibiotic	No	Wilms' tumor, rhabdomyosarcoma, choriocarcinoma, testicular carcinoma, Ewing's sarcoma
daunorubicin	Cerubidine	Antibiotic	No	Acute lymphocytic, nonlymphocytic leukemia
diethylstilbestrol	Diethylstilbestrol	Hormone	No	Breast cancer, prostatic carcinoma

ANTINEOPLASTICS *Continued*

Generic Name	Brand Name(s)	Type	Cell-Cycle Specific	Uses
doxorubicin	Adriamycin Rubex	Antibiotic	No	Acute lymphoblastic leukemia, acute myeloblastic leukemia, Wilms' tumor, neuroblastoma, soft tissue and bone sarcomas, breast, ovarian carcinoma, transitional cell bladder carcinoma, thyroid carcinoma, Hodgkin's, non-Hodgkin's lymphomas, bronchogenic carcinoma, gastric carcinoma
estramustine	Emcyt	Hormone	No	Carcinoma of prostate
etoposide	VePesid	Mitotic inhibitor	Yes	Refractory testicular tumor, small cell lung cancer
floxuridine	FUDR	Antimetabolite	No	GI adenocarcinoma metastatic to liver
fludarabine	Fludara	Antimetabolite	No	Chronic lymphocytic leukemia
fluorouracil	Adrucil Efudex	Antimetabolite	No	Cancer of colon, rectum, breast, stomach, and pancreas
flutamide	Eulexin	Hormone	No	Meastatic prostatic carcinoma
goserelin	Zoladex	Hormone	No	Carcinoma of prostate
hydroxyurea	Hydrea	Miscellaneous	No	Melanoma, chronic myelocytic leukemia, carcinoma of ovary
idarubicin	Idamycin	Antibiotic	No	Acute myeloid leukemia
ifosfamide	Ifex	Alkylating	No	Germ cell testicular cancer
interferon alfa-2a	Roferon-A	Miscellaneous	No	Hairy cell leukemia, AIDS-related Kaposi's sarcoma
interferon alfa-2b	Intron A	Miscellaneous	No	Hairy cell leukemia, condylomata acuminata, AIDS-related Kaposi's sarcoma
interferon alfa-n3	Alferon N	Miscellaneous	No	Condylomata acuminata
leuprolide	Lupron	Hormone	No	Advanced prostatic cancer, endometriosis

Continued.

CLASSIFICATION

Generic Name	Brand Name(s)	Type	Cell-Cycle Specific	Uses
levamisole	Ergamisol	Miscellaneous	No	Duke's stage C colon cancer
lomustine	CeeNu	Alkylating	No	Brain tumors, Hodgkin's disease
mechlor-ethamine	Mustargen	Alkylating	No	Polycythemia vera, mycosis fungoides, Hodgkin's disease, lymphosarcoma, chronic myelocytic/lymphocytic leukemia bronchogenic cancer
medroxy-progester-one	Depo-Provera	Hormone	No	Endometrial, renal carcinoma
megestrol	Megace	Hormone	No	Breast, endometrial carcinoma
melphalan	Alkeran	Alkylating	No	Multiple myeloma, ovarian carcinoma
mercapto-purine	Purinethol	Antimetabolite	Yes	Acute lymphatic myelogenous leukemia
methotrexate	Folex	Antimetabolite	Yes	Gestational choriocarcinoma, choriocarcinoma destruens, hydatiform mole, acute lymphocytic leukemia
mitomycin	Mutamycin	Antibiotic	No	Disseminated adenocarcinoma of stomach, pancreas
mitotane	Lysodren	Miscellaneous	No	Adrenal cortical carcinoma
mitoxantrone	Novantrone	Antibiotic	No	Acute, nonlymphocytic leukemia
paclitaxol	Taxol	Miscellaneous	No	Metastatic carcinoma of ovary
pegaspar-gase	Oncaspar	Miscellaneous	Yes	Acute lymphoblastic leukemia
pentostatin	Nipent	Antibiotic	No	Hairy cell leukemia
plicamycin	Mithracin	Antibiotic	No	Malignant testicular tumors
procarbazine	Maltulane	Miscellaneous	No	Hodgkin's disease
streptozocin	Zanosar	Alkylating	No	Metastatic islet cell cancer of pancreas
tamoxifen	Nolvadex	Hormone	No	Metastatic breast cancer
teniposide	Vumen	Mitotic inhibitor	Yes	Refractory acute lymphoblastic leukemia (ALL)
testolactone	Teslac	Hormone	No	Breast carcinoma
thioguanine	Thioguanine	Antimetabolite	Yes	Acute nonlymphocytic leukemia

Generic Name	Brand Name(s)	Type	Cell-Cycle Specific	Uses
thiotepa	Thiotepa	Alkylating	No	Adenocarcinoma of breast, ovary; papillary cancer of urinary bladder
vinblastine	Velban	Mitotic inhibitor	Yes	Hodgkin's disease, lymphocytic lymphoma, histiocytic lymphoma, mycosis fungoides, advanced testicular carcinoma, Kaposi's sarcoma, breast cancer
vincristine	Oncovin	Mitotic inhibitor	Yes	Acute leukemia, Hodgkin's disease, non-Hodgkin's malignant lymphoma, rhabdomyosarcoma, neuroblastoma, Wilms' tumor
vinorelbine	Navelbine	Mitotic inhibitor	Yes	Metastatic breast cancer, non-small cell lung cancer, ovarian cancer, Hodgkin's disease

USES

Treatment of a wide variety of cancers; may be palliative or curative. Treatment of choice in hematologic cancers. Frequently used as adjunctive therapy, e.g., w/surgery or irradiation; most effective when tumor mass has been removed or reduced by radiation. Often used in combinations to increase therapeutic results, decrease toxic effects. Certain agents may be used in nonmalignant conditions; polycythemia vera, psoriasis, rheumatoid arthritis, or immunosuppression in organ transplantation (used only in select cases that are severe and unresponsive to other forms of therapy). Refer to individual monographs.

PRECAUTIONS

CONTRAINDICATIONS: Known hypersensitivity, hepatic or renal insufficiency, severe leukopenia, thrombocytopenia, anemia, pregnancy, lactation, (other per individual drug). **CAUTION:** Elderly or very young, infection, radiation therapy, use of other antineoplastics.

INTERACTIONS

Highly complex agents; therefore, check the interactions of each carefully. Anticoagulants and other bone marrow depressants (including other antineoplastics) may increase the risk of myelosuppression effects. Refer to specific monographs.

SIDE EFFECTS

Stomatitis, nausea and vomiting, diarrhea, alopecia w/several drugs, myelosuppression (see Toxic Effects/Adverse Reactions), hyperuricemia effects on reproduction or local tissue injury.

TOXIC EFFECTS/ADVERSE REACTIONS

Narrow margin of safety between therapeutic and toxic response. Generally proportional to dosage and length of therapy. Myelosuppression (reduction in leukocytes, lymphocytes, thrombocytes, and erythrocytes) may precipitate life-threatening hemorrhage, infection, or anemia. Extravasation at IV site. Toxicity often a major factor in continuing therapy.

NURSING IMPLICATIONS

GENERAL: Take special precautions in handling agents to protect self and others (these drugs are highly toxic and may be inhaled or absorbed through skin; also cause local tissue damage upon contact): (1) Wear gloves, perhaps gown/mask/eye protectors (NIH guidelines). (2) Avoid contaminating articles w/agents. (3) Dispose of all contaminated materials in specifically identified containers. Administer precisely according to schedule. Use strict asepsis and protect pt from infection. When platelet count drops, avoid even the slightest trauma (such as injection or rectal temperature). **BASELINE ASSESSMENT:** Baseline lab values for RBC/WBC, platelets, vital signs are essential. **INTERVENTION/EVALUATION:** Monitor laboratory results, esp. RBC, WBC, and platelet counts; promptly report significant changes. Assess for bleeding, signs of infection, anemia. Infuse IV solutions, medications carefully to prevent extravasation. Extravasation is an EMERGENCY (standing orders and antidote kits must be available before administration). Monitor I&O. Assess response to medication; provide interventions, e.g., mouth care to relieve stomatitis; small, frequent meals of preferred foods/antiemetics for nausea and vomiting. **PATIENT/FAMILY TEACHING:** Individualized nature of therapy and need for lab tests. Explain that alopecia is reversible, but new hair may have different color, texture. Assist in supporting body image. Despite possible infertility from drug, need for appropriate contraception due to risk of fetal abnormalities; inform physician immediately if pregnancy is suspected. Avoid crowds, persons w/known infections; report signs of infection at once (fever, malaise, flu-like symptoms, etc.). Avoid contact w/anyone who recently received live virus vaccine; do not receive vaccinations. Promptly notify physician of bleeding, bruising, unexplained swelling.

antipsychotics

ACTION

Effects of these agents occur at all levels of the CNS. Antipsychotic mechanism unknown, but may antagonize dopamine action as a neurotransmitter in basal ganglia and limbic system. Antipsychotics may block postsynaptic dopamine receptors, inhibit dopamine release, increase dopamine turnover. These medications can be divided into the phenothiazines and nonphenothiazines (miscellaneous). In addition to their use in symptomatic treatment of psychiatric illness, some have antiemetic, antinausea, antihistamine, anticholinergic, and/or sedative effects.

USES

Antipsychotics are primarily used in managing psychotic illness (esp. those w/increased psychomotor activity). They are also used to treat manic phase of bipolar disorder, behavioral problems in children, nausea and vomiting, intractable hiccups, anxiety and agitation, as adjunct in treatment of tetanus, and to potentiate effects of narcotics.

PRECAUTIONS

CONTRAINDICATIONS: Alcoholism or other CNS depression, hepatic dysfunction, bone marrow depression, hypotension, glaucoma, cardiovascular disease, peptic ulcer, young children, hypersensitivity to any of the phenothiazines, pregnancy, lactation. **CAUTIONS:** Administer cautiously to elderly and debilitated pts; this group is more sensitive to effects and requires lower dosage. Drug should be withdrawn slowly; should be discontinued at least 48 hrs before surgery.

INTERACTIONS

Alcohol, CNS depressants may increase CNS, respiratory depression, hypotensive effects. Tricyclic antidepressants, MAO inhibitors may increase sedative, anticholinergic effects. Antithyroid agents may increase risk of agranulocytosis. Extrapyramidal symptoms (EPS) may increase w/ EPS producing medications. Hypotensives may increase hypotension. May decrease levodopa effects. Lithium may decrease absorption, produce adverse neurologic effects.

SIDE EFFECTS

Orthostatic hypotension, drowsiness, blurred vision, constipation, nasal congestion, photosensitivity.

TOXIC EFFECTS/ADVERSE REACTIONS

Hyperpyrexia, depression, insomnia, convulsions, hypertension, adynamic ileus, laryngospasm, bronchospasm, urticaria, menstrual irregularities, impotence, urinary retention, blood dyscrasias, systemic lupus-like reaction, extrapyramidal reactions.

NURSING IMPLICATIONS

GENERAL: Do not mix parenteral solution w/other drugs in the same syringe; give deep IM injections. Have pt remain recumbent for at least 30 min, following parenteral dose, arise slowly and w/assistance. Avoid skin contact w/solutions (contact dermatitis). **BASELINE ASSESSMENT:** Determine initial B/P, pulse, respirations. Assess pt and environment for necessary supports. **INTERVENTION/EVALUATION:** Monitor B/P. As-

ANTIPSYCHOTICS

Generic Name	Brand Name(s)	Side Effects: Sedation	Side Effects: Hypotension	Side Effects: Anticholinergic	Side Effects: EPS	Dosage (mg/day)
chlorpromazine	Thorazine	High	High	Moderate	Moderate	30-800
clozapine	Clozaril	High	High	High	Low	25-900
fluphenazine	Prolixin	Low	Low	Low	High	0.5-50
haloperidol	Haldol	Low	Low	Low	High	1-100
loxapine	Loxitane	Moderate	Moderate	Low	High	20-100
mesoridazine	Serentil	High	Moderate	High	Low	30-400
molindone	Moban	Low	Low	Low	High	50-225
perphenazine	Trilafon	Low	Low	Low	High	12-64
pimozide	Orap	Moderate	Low	Moderate	High	1-10
risperidone	Risperdal	Low	Low	Low	Moderate	4-6
thioridazine	Mellaril	High	High	High	Low	150-800
thiothixene	Navane	Low	Low	Low	High	6-60
trifluoperazine	Stelazine	Low	Low	Low	High	4-40

ESP, extrapyramidal symptoms

sess mental status, response to surroundings. Be alert to suicide potential as energy increases. Assure that oral medication is swallowed. Check bowel activity; avoid constipation. Promptly notify physician of extrapyramidal reactions (usually dose related; more frequent in female geriatric pts). **PATIENT/FAMILY TEACHING:** Take medication as ordered; do not stop taking or increase dosage. Do not drive or perform activities requiring motor skill until response has been controlled. Side effects usually subside after approximately 2 wks of therapy or can be eliminated/minimized by dosage adjustment. Avoid temperature extremes. Avoid alcohol, other medications. Inform other physicians, dentist of drug therapy. Change positions slowly to prevent orthostatic hypotension.

beta–adrenergic blockers

ACTION

Beta-adrenergic blockers competitively block beta$_1$-adrenergic receptors, located primarily in myocardium, and beta$_2$-adrenergic receptors, located primarily in bronchial and vascular smooth muscle. By occupying beta-receptor sites, these agents prevent naturally occurring or administered epinephrine/norepinephrine from exerting their effects. The results are basically opposite to that of sympathetic stimulation.

Effect of beta$_1$-blockade includes slowing heart rate, decreasing cardiac output and contractility; effect of beta$_2$-blockade includes bronchoconstriction, increased airway resistance in those w/asthma or COPD. Beta-blockers can affect cardiac rhythm/automaticity (decrease sinus rate, SA, AV conduction; increase refractory period in AV node). Decreases systolic and diastolic B/P; exact mechanism unknown but may block peripheral receptors, decrease sympathetic outflow from CNS, or decrease renin release from kidney. All beta-blockers mask tachycardia that occurs w/hypoglycemia. When applied to the eye, reduces intraocular pressure and aqueous production.

USES

Management of hypertension, angina pectoris, arrhythmias, hypertrophic subaortic stenosis, migraine headaches, myocardial infarction (prevention), glaucoma.

PRECAUTIONS

CONTRAINDICATIONS: Severe renal or hepatic disease, history of allergy, hyperthyroidism, asthma, emphysema, CHF, cerebrovascular accident, hypotension, sinus bradycardia, pregnancy. Safety in lactation not established. **CAUTIONS:** Diabetes mellitus, elderly, peptic ulcer.

INTERACTIONS

Diuretics, other hypotensives may increase hypotensive effect. Sympathomimetics, xanthines may mutually inhibit effects. May mask symptoms of hypoglycemia, prolong hypoglycemic effect of insulin, oral hypoglycemics. NSAIDs may decrease antihypertensive effect. Cimetidine may increase concentration.

SIDE EFFECTS

Postural hypotension, lightheadedness, fatigue, weakness, reflex tachycardia.

TOXIC EFFECTS/ADVERSE REACTIONS

Severe hypotension, nausea and vomiting, bradycardia, heart block, circulatory failure.

NURSING IMPLICATIONS

GENERAL: Use cardiac monitor for IV administration and preferably for initiation of oral therapy. **BASELINE ASSESSMENT:** Initial B/P, apical pulse. **INTERVENTION/EVALUATION:** Monitor B/P and apical pulse before giving drug; notify physician before administration if B/P or pulse are not within agreed parameters. Assess for CHF (dyspnea, peripheral edema, jugular venous distention, increased weight, rales in lungs, decreased urine output). Assess extremities for peripheral circulation (warmth, color, quality of pulses). **PATIENT/FAMILY TEACHING:** Teach how to take B/P, pulse correctly. Change position slowly to prevent orthostatic hypotension. Do not take over-the-counter cold medications,

BETA-BLOCKERS

Generic Name	Brand Name(s)	Selectivity	Uses	Dosage Range
acebutolol	Sectral	$Beta_1$	HTN Arrhythmias	HTN: 200-1200 mg/day Arrhythmias: 600-1200 mg/day
atenolol	Tenormin	$Beta_1$	HTN Angina MI	HTN: 50-100 mg/day Angina: 50-200 mg/day MI: 50-100 mg/day
betaxolol	Kerlone Betoptic	$Beta_1$	HTN Ocular HTN, glaucoma	HTN: 10-20 mg/day Ophth: 1 drop 2×/day
bisoprolol	Zebeta	$Beta_1$	HTN	HTN: 2.5-20 mg/day
carteolol	Cartrol	$Beta_1$, $beta_2$	HTN	HTN: 2.5-10 mg/day
celiprolol	Selecor	$Beta_1$	HTN Angina	HTN: 200-500 mg/day Angina: 300-600 mg/day
esmolol	Brevibloc	$Beta_1$	Arrhythmias	Arrhythmias: 50-200 mcg/kg/min
labetalol	Normodyne Trandate	$Beta_1$, $beta_2$ $Alpha_1$	Hypertension	HTN: 200-400 mg/day
levobunolol	Betagan	$Beta_1$, $beta_2$	Ocular HTN, glaucoma	Ophth: 1 drop 1-2×/day
metipranolol	Opti-Pranolol	$Beta_1$, $beta_2$	Ocular HTN, glaucoma	Ophth: 1 drop 2×/day
metoprolol	Lopressor	$Beta_1$	HTN Angina MI	HTN: 100-450 mg/day Angina: 100-400 mg/day MI: 50 mg q6h
nadolol	Corgard	$Beta_1$, $beta_2$	HTN Angina	HTN: 40-320 mg/day Angina: 40-240 mg/day
penbutolol	Levotol	$Beta_1$, $beta_2$	HTN	HTN: 10-40 mg/day
pindolol	Visken	$Beta_1$, $beta_2$	HTN	HTN: 10-60 mg/day
propranolol	Inderal	$Beta_1$, $beta_2$	HTN, angina, arrhythmias, MI, migraine, tremors	HTN: 120-640 mg/day Angina: 80-320 mg/day

Generic Name	Brand Name(s)	Selectivity	Uses	Dosage Range
				Arrhythmias: 10-30 mg 3-4×/day MI: 180-240 mg/day
sotalol	Betapace	$Beta_1$, $beta_2$	Arrhythmias	Arrhythmias: 160-640 mg/day
timolol	Blocadren Timoptic	$Beta_1$, $beta_2$	HTN, MI, migraine, glaucoma	HTN: 10-60 mg/day MI: 10 mg 2×/day Ophth: 1 drop 1-2×/day

HTN, hypertension; MI, myocardial infarction.

nasal decongestants. Restrict sodium and alcohol as ordered. Do not stop taking drug suddenly. Report chest pain, fatigue, shortness of breath.

bronchodilators

ACTION

Asthma (reversible airway obstruction) is the most common breathing disorder.

Methylxanthines: Directly relax smooth muscle of bronchial airway, pulmonary blood vessels (relieve bronchospasm, increase vital capacity). Increase cyclic 3,5-adenosine monophosphate.

$Beta_2$-adrenergic agonists: Stimulate beta-receptors in lung, relax bronchial smooth muscle, increase vital capacity, decrease airway resistance.

Anticholinergics: Inhibit cholinergic receptors on bronchial smooth muscle (block acetylcholine action).

USES

Relief of bronchospasm occurring during anesthesia, in bronchial asthma, bronchitis, or emphysema.

PRECAUTIONS

CONTRAINDICATIONS: Hypersensitivity to that agent or intolerance to others in the classification, components of preparation. Severe renal or hepatic dysfunction. **CAUTIONS:** Pregnancy, lactation, elderly, hepatic disease, CHF, or other cardiac conditions that would be adversely affected by cardiac stimulation.

INTERACTIONS

Methylxanthines: Glucocorticoids may produce hypernatremia. Phe-

BRONCHODILATORS

GENERIC NAME	BRAND NAME(S)	ROUTE OF ADMINISTRATION	TYPE
albuterol	Proventil Ventolin	Inhalation Oral	$Beta_2$ agonist
aminophylline	—	Oral Intravenous	Methylxanthine
bitolterol	Tornalate	Inhalation	$Beta_2$ agonist
epinephrine	Adrenalin	SubQ Intravenous	$Beta_2$ agonist
ipratropium	Atrovent	Inhalation	Anticholinergic
isoetharine	Bronkosol	Inhalation	$Beta_2$ agonist
isoproterenol	Isuprel	Inhalation	$Beta_2$ agonist
metaproterenol	Alupent	Inhalation	$Beta_2$ agonist
salmeterol	Serevent	Inhalation	$Beta_2$ agonist
terbutaline	Brethine Bricanyl	Inhalation Oral SubQ	$Beta_2$ agonist
theophylline	Aerolate Slo-Bid Slo-Phyllin Theo-24 Theo-Dur Theolair Uniphyl	Oral	Methylxanthine

nytoin, primidone, rifampin may increase metabolism. Beta-blockers may decrease effects. Cimetidine, ciprofloxacin, erythromycin, norfloxacin may increase concentration, toxicity. Smoking may decrease concentration.

$Beta_2$-adrenergic agonists: General anesthetics may increase risk of arrhythmias. Tricyclic antidepressants, maprotiline may increase cardiovascular effects. May have mutually inhibitory effects w/beta-adrenergic blockers. May increase risk of arrhythmias w/digoxin.

Anticholinergics: None significant.

SIDE EFFECTS

Nausea, increased pulse rate, nervousness, weakness, trembling, insomnia.

TOXIC EFFECTS/ADVERSE REACTIONS

Tachycardia, irregular heartbeat, headache, nausea and vomiting, severe weakness, increased B/P.

NURSING IMPLICATIONS

GENERAL: Administer oral agents on regular schedule. Assist pt in identifying what triggered an acute bronchospasm attack. **INTERVENTION/EVALUATION:** Monitor arterial blood gases, serum levels for aminophylline, theophylline. Assess lung sounds, B/P, pulse, respirations.

Encourage fluid intake to decrease viscosity of secretions. **PATIENT/FAMILY TEACHING:** Demonstrate correct use of inhalers. Drink 8 or more glasses of fluid/day. Avoid caffeine-containing products, e.g., coffee, tea, colas, chocolate (cause further CNS stimulation). Do not smoke. Use other medications only after consulting physician. Teach effective deep breathing and coughing. Notify physician if symptoms are not relieved or worsen. Report adverse reactions.

calcium channel blockers

ACTION

Calcium channel blockers inhibit the flow of extracellular Ca^{+2} ions across cell membrane of cardiac cells, vascular tissue. Calcium channel blockers relax arterial smooth muscle, depress the rate of sinus node pacemaker, slow AV conduction, decrease heart rate, produce negative inotropic effect (rarely seen clinically due to reflex response). All calcium channel blockers decrease coronary vascular resistance, increase coronary blood flow, reduce myocardial oxygen demand. Degree of action varies w/individual agent.

USES

Treatment of essential hypertension, treatment and prophylaxis of angina pectoris (including vasospastic, chronic stable, unstable), prevent/control supraventricular tachyarrhythmias, prevent neurologic damage due to subarachnoid hemorrhage.

PRECAUTIONS

CONTRAINDICATIONS: Renal or hepatic dysfunction, heart block, hypotension, extreme bradycardia, aortic stenosis, sick sinus syndrome, severe left ventricular dysfunction, pregnancy, lactation. **CAUTIONS:** Administer cautiously to elderly because half-life may be increased. Liver enzymes should be periodically monitored.

INTERACTIONS

Beta-adrenergic blockers may have additive effect. May increase digoxin concentration. Procainamide, quinidine may increase risk of QT interval prolongation. Carbamazepine, quinidine, theophylline may increase concentration, toxicity.

SIDE EFFECTS

Headache, nausea, dizziness or lightheadedness, hypotension, constipation.

CALCIUM CHANNEL BLOCKERS

Generic Name	Brand Name(s)	Onset Action	Uses	Rte Admin	Dosage Range
amlodipine	Norvasc	—	Angina Hypertension	PO	2.5-10 mg/day
bepridil	Vascor	1hr	Angina	PO	200-400 mg/day
diltiazem	Cardizem Cardizem CD	30-60 min	Angina Hypertension Arrhythmias	PO, IV	PO: 120-360 mg/day IV: 20-25 mg IV bolus; 5-15 mg/hr IV infusion
felodipine	Plendil	2-5 hrs	Hypertension	PO	5-10 mg/day
isradipine	DynaCirc	2 hrs	Hypertension	PO	5-20 mg/day
nicardipine	Cardene	20 min	Angina Hypertension	PO	60-120 mg/day
nifedipine	Adalat Procardia	20 min	Angina Hypertension	SL, PO	PO: 30-120 mg/day XL: 30-60 mg/day
nimodipine	Nimotop	—	Subarachnoid hemorrhage	PO	60 mg q4h × 21 days
verapamil	Calan Isoptin Verelan	30 min	Angina Hypertension Arrhythmias	PO, IV	PO: 120-480 mg/day IV: 5-10 mg, max: 10 mg/dose

XL, sustained release.

TOXIC EFFECTS/ADVERSE REACTIONS

Peripheral edema, palpitations, bradycardia, dyspnea, wheezing w/ possible pulmonary edema, severe hypotension, second- or third-degree heart block (rare). Administered IV for tachyarrhythmias, verapamil, nicardipine, diltiazem have the greatest potential for severe reactions.

NURSING IMPLICATIONS

GENERAL: Parenteral administration requires close cardiac monitoring w/emergency equipment close by. Discontinuation should be gradual. Be alert to potential for hypotension, esp. when pt is taking other antihypertensive drugs or beta-adrenergic blockers. **BASELINE ASSESSMENT:** Assess initial B/P and apical pulse. **INTERVENTION/EVALUATION:** Monitor B/P and apical pulse before administration; notify physician before giving dose if not within agreed parameters. Check frequency, consistency of stools; avoid constipation. Assess lungs for rales, extremities for peripheral edema. Check I&O. **PATIENT/FAMILY TEACHING:** Teach how to take B/P and pulse correctly. Change position slowly to avoid orthostatic hypotension. Restrict sodium as ordered. Avoid alcohol, other medications w/o consulting physician. Do not overexert when anginal pain relieved. Do not stop taking medication. Report irregular heartbeat, dizziness, shortness of breath. Angina can occur if medication is abruptly stopped.

cardiac glycosides

ACTION

Direct action on myocardium causes increased force of contraction, resulting in increased stroke volume and cardiac output. Depression of SA node, decreased conduction time through AV node, and decreased electrical impulses due to vagal stimulation slow heart rate. Improved myocardial contractility is probably due to improved transport of calcium, sodium, and potassium ions across cell membranes.

USES

CHF, atrial fibrillation, atrial flutter, paroxysmal atrial tachycardia and treatment of cardiogenic shock w/pulmonary edema.

PRECAUTIONS

CONTRAINDICATIONS: History of hypersensitivity, digitalis toxicity, ventricular fibrillation, ventricular tachycardia (unless due to CHF), severe myocarditis. **CAUTIONS:** Renal insufficiency, hypokalemia, incomplete AV block, infants and children, elderly and debilitated pts. Safety in pregnancy, lactation not established.

INTERACTIONS

Glucocorticoids, amphotericin, potassium depleting diuretics may increase toxicity (due to hypokalemia). Amiodarone may increase concentration, toxicity; additive effect on SA, AV nodes. Antiarrhythmics, parenteral calcium, sympathomimetics may increase risk of arrhythmias. Antidiarrheals, cholestyramine, colestipol may decrease absorption. Diltiazem, verapamil, quinidine may increase concentrations. Parenteral magnesium may cause conduction changes, heart block.

SIDE EFFECTS

The margin of safety between a therapeutic and toxic dose is very narrow.

TOXIC EFFECTS/ADVERSE REACTIONS

Anorexia, nausea and vomiting, abdominal pain, and diarrhea occur commonly. Arrhythmias, such as premature ventricular contractions (PVCs) and bradycardia, also may signal overdosage. CNS effects are most common in elderly pts; headache, drowsiness, confusion, and visual disturbances such as halos around objects, altered color perception, blurring and flickering dots. In children arrhythmias are the most reliable sign; other effects are rarely seen.

NURSING IMPLICATIONS

GENERAL: Parenteral administration requires close cardiac monitoring.

BASELINE ASSESSMENT: Establish initial B/P and apical pulse. **INTERVENTION/EVALUATION:** Assess apical pulse before giving each dose; withhold and notify physician if pulse below 60 or above 100 for adults. Measure I&O; weigh daily. Check for dependent edema; auscultate lungs for rales. Monitor potassium. **PATIENT/FAMILY TEACHING:** Take as prescribed; do not miss dose or take extra dose. Teach pt/family to take pulse and report pulse outside parameters determined by physician. Restrict sodium and alcohol as ordered. Cease smoking. Avoid over-the-counter cold preparations, nasal decongestants, coffee, tea, colas, chocolates (stimulants).

cholinergic agonists/anticholinesterase

ACTION

CHOLINERGIC AGONISTS: These agents may be referred to as muscarinics or parasympathetics and consist of two basic drug groups: Choline esters and cholinomimetic alkaloids. Primary action is to mimic action of acetylcholine at postganglionic parasympathetic nerves. Primary properties include: *Cardiovascular system:* Vasodilation, decreased cardiac rate, decreased conduction in SA, AV nodes, decreased force of myocardial contraction. *Gastrointestinal:* Increased tone, motility of GI smooth muscle, increased secretory activity of GI tract. *Urinary tract:* Increase contraction of detrusor muscle of urinary bladder, resulting in micturitio *Eye:* Miosis, contraction of ciliary muscle.

ANTICHOLINESTERASE (anti-ChE) also known as cholinesterase inhibitors: Inactivates cholinesterase, which prevents acetylcholine breakdown causing acetylcholine to accumulate at cholinergic receptor sites. These agents can be considered indirect-acting cholinergic agonists. Primary properties include action of cholinergic agonists noted above. *Skeletal neuromuscular junction:* Effects are dose-dependent. At therapeutic doses, increases force of skeletal muscle contraction; at toxic doses, reduce muscle strength.

USES

Paralytic ileus and atony of urinary bladder. Treatment of primary, and some secondary, glaucoma. Myasthenia gravis (weakness, marked fatigue of skeletal muscle). Terminates, reverses effects of neuromuscular blocking agents.

CONTRAINDICATIONS: Intestinal or urinary tract obstructions, known hypersensitivity, pregnancy, lactation, acute peptic ulcer, hyperthyroidism, peritonitis, bronchial asthma. **CAUTIONS:** Have atropine readily available in case of cholinergic crisis.

CHOLINERGIC AGONISTS

Generic Name	Brand Name(s)	Type	Use	Dosage Range
acetylcholine	Miochol	Cholinergic	Miotic	Ophth: 0.5-2 ml
bethanechol	Urecholine	Cholinergic	Nonobstructive urinary retention	PO: 10-50 mg 3-4 × /day SubQ: 2.5-5 mg 3-4 × /day
carbachol	Carbachol	Cholinergic	Miotic Glaucoma	Ophth: 0.5 ml Ophth: 1-2 drops up to 4 × /day
demecarium	Humorsol	Anti-ChE	Glaucoma	Ophth: 1-2 drops 2 × /day to 2 drops/wk
echothiophate	Phospholine	Anti-ChE	Glaucoma	Ophth: 1 drop qOd to 2 × /day
edrophonium	Tensilon	Anti-ChE	Dx, myasthenia gravis Reverse tubocurarine	IV: 10 mg in 30-45 sec; Max: 40 mg
isoflurophate	Floropryl	Anti-ChE	Glaucoma	Ophth ointment: q8-72h
neostigmine	Prostigmin	Anti-ChE	Dx/tx, myasthenia gravis Antidote Neuromuscular blocker	PO: 15-375 mg/day SubQ, IM: 0.5 mg; 0.01-0.04 mg/kg IV: 0.5-2 mg
physostigmine	Eserine	Anti-ChE	Glaucoma Antidote	Ophth: 1-2 drops up to 4 × /day IM, IV: 0.5-2 mg
pilocarpine	Isopto Carpine Ocusert	Cholinergic	Glaucoma	Ophth: 1-2 drops up to 6 × /day Every 7 days
pyridostigmine	Mestinon	Anti-ChE	Tx, myasthenia gravis Reverse tubocurarine	PO: 60-1500 mg/day IM: 0.5-1.5 mg/kg IV: 0.1-0.25 mg/kg

INTERACTIONS

Given with other cholinergics—increased effects w/greater potential for toxicity. Ganglionic blocking agents, used concurrently with cholinergics, may produce significant fall in B/P. Anticholinergics antagonize effects of cholinergics.

SIDE EFFECTS

Increased urinary frequency, salivation, belching, nausea, dizziness. Side effects infrequent, more likely w/subcutaneous injection or high doses.

TOXIC EFFECTS/ADVERSE REACTIONS

Overdose (cholinergic crisis): Abdominal cramps, diarrhea, excessive salivation, diaphoresis, muscle weakness, respiratory difficulty. Requires immediate treatment.

NURSING IMPLICATIONS

GENERAL: Have atropine readily available in case of cholinergic crisis. **BASELINE ASSESSMENT:** Check pulse, respirations. **INTERVENTION/ EVALUATION:** Monitor pulse, respiration; be alert for signs/symptoms of cholinergic crisis. Assess for therapeutic results: (1) In abdominal distention or paralytic ileus, listen for bowel sounds, check passing of flatus or stool, measure abdomen for decreased distention. (2) For urinary retention, palpate bladder and check for urination. Implement measures that support urination, e.g., running water, pouring warm water over perineum, privacy. If urination does not occur, determine whether catheterization is needed. Determine cause of urinary retention, e.g., trauma from surgical manipulation or narcotics given for pain. (3) For myasthenia gravis, observe for improved muscle tone and subsequently greater activity, less fatigue. **PATIENT/FAMILY TEACHING:** Explain purpose of medication. Increased salivation is to be expected. Call for assistance to bathroom after subcutaneous injection.

corticosteroids

ACTION

Synthesized by adrenal cortex, the corticosteroids can be divided into glucocorticoids (hepatic glycogen deposition) and mineralocorticoids (sodium retention). Corticosteroids have numerous effects including: *Carbohydrate, protein metabolism:* increase glucose formation, decrease peripheral utilization, enhance glycogen storage, increase gluconeogenesis (transformation of protein to glucose). *Lipid metabolism:* redistributes body fat, lipolysis of triglyceride of adipose tissue. *Electrolyte/water balance:* enhance sodium reabsorption, potassium excretion, increase extracellular volume. *Formed elements:* increase hemoglobin, red blood cell count, decrease number of lymphocytes, eosinophils, monocytes, basophils, increase polymorphonuclear leukocytes. *Anti-inflammatory:* inhibit anti-inflammatory process (edema, capillary dilatation, migration of leukocytes into inflamed area, phagocytic activity). *Immunosuppression:* inhibits early steps in immunity.

CORTICOSTEROIDS

Generic Name	Brand Name(s)	Rte Admin
alclometasone	Acolvate	Topical
amcinonide	Cyclocort	Topical
beclomethasone	Beclovent, Vanceril Beconase, Vancenase	Inhalation, intranasal
betamethasone	Celestone, Diprosone Uticort, Valisone	Topical, oral, IV, intralesional, intra-articular
budesonide	Rhinocort	Intranasal
clobetasol	Temovate	Topical
cortisone	Cortone	Topical, oral
desonide	Tridesilone	Topical
desoximetasone	Topicort	Topical
dexamethasone	Decadron	Topical, oral, IM, IV, ophthalmic, intanasal, inhalation
fludrocortisone	Florinef	Oral
flunisolide	Aerobid, Nasalide	Inhalation, intranasal
fluocinolone	Synalar, Synemol	Topical
fluorometholone	FML	Ophthalmic
flurandrenolide	Cordran	Topical
fluticasone	Cutivate, Flonase	Topical, intranasal
halcinonide	Halog	Topical
halobetasol	Ultravate	Topical
hydrocortisone	Cort-Dome, Cortef, Hydrocortone, Solu-Cortef	Topical, oral, IM, IV, SubQ, rectal
methylprednisolone	Medrol, Solu-Medrol	Topical, oral, IM, IV
mometasone	Elocon	Topical
prednicarbate	Dermatop	Topical
prednisolone	Delta-Cortef, Hydeltra, Hydeltrasol	Oral, IM, IV, intralesional, intra-articular
prednisone	Deltasone, Meticorten, Orasone	Oral
rimexolone	Vexol	Ophthalmic
triamcinolone	Azmacort, Kenalog, Nasacort	Oral, inhalation, intranasal

nytoin, primidone, rifampin may increase metabolism. Beta-blockers may decrease effects. Cimetidine, ciprofloxacin, erythromycin, norfloxacin

USES

Replacement therapy in adrenal insufficiency, including Addison's disease. Symptomatic treatment of multiorgan disease/conditions. Rheumatoid and osteoarthritis, severe psoriasis, ulcerative colitis, lupus erythematosus, anaphylactic shock, status asthmaticus, organ transplant.

PRECAUTIONS

CONTRAINDICATIONS: Hypersensitivity; peptic ulcer, tuberculosis, or any suspected infection; blood clotting disorders; severe renal or hepatic impairment; CHF or hypertension, lactation. **CAUTIONS:** Cautious administration in children, geriatric, and postmenopausal pts. Safe use during pregnancy has not been established.

INTERACTIONS

Amphotericin may increase hypokalemia. May decrease effect of oral hypoglycemics, insulin, diuretics, potassium supplements. May increase digoxin toxicity (due to hypokalemia). Hepatic enzyme inducers may decrease effect. Live virus vaccines may potentiate virus replication, increase vaccine side effects, decrease pt's antibody response to vaccine.

SIDE EFFECTS

Rarely cause side effects w/short term high dose or replacement therapy. Sodium/water retention, increased appetite.

TOXIC EFFECTS/ADVERSE REACTIONS

Long-term therapy causes numerous adverse reactions; peptic ulcer and steroid diabetes are the most serious. Osteoporosis, petechiae, hirsutism, acne, menstrual irregularities. Cushing-like symptoms (moon face, excess fat deposits of trunk, neck, and shoulders w/buffalo hump, wasting of arms and legs). Edema, hypertension. May have depression, personality change, and insomnia; cataracts or glaucoma, delayed healing, suppressed immune response.

NURSING IMPLICATIONS

GENERAL: Take precautions to avoid infection; recognize that these agents mask signs and symptoms of developing illness. Administer oral drugs w/food or milk in early morning in a single dose. Withdraw medication slowly. **BASELINE ASSESSMENT:** Determine initial B/P, temperature, pulse, respiration, weight, blood glucose, electrolytes, EKG and TB skin test results. **INTERVENTION/EVALUATION:** Monitor B/P, temperature, pulse, respiration, daily weight, I&O, blood glucose, and electrolytes (esp. potassium and calcium). Be alert for signs and symptoms of hypokalemia, hypocalcemia. Check dependent areas for edema. Assess for mood, personality change. **PATIENT/FAMILY TEACHING:** Follow-up visits and lab tests are essential. Carry identification of drug and dose, physician name and phone number. Do not change dose/schedule or stop taking drug; must taper off gradually under medical supervision. Report severe symptoms (visual disturbances or severe gastric distress) to physician immediately. Promptly report sudden weight gain or swelling, sore throat, fever, or other signs of infection. Wounds may heal slowly. Avoid crowds, persons w/known infections. Do not receive vaccinations. Do not take aspirin or any other medication w/o consulting physician. Give instructions for diet (usually sodium restricted w/high vitamin D, protein, and potassium). Inform dentist or other physicians of glucocorticoid therapy now or within past 12 mo. Do not overuse joint that was injected for symptomatic relief. For topical application, apply after shower for best absorption; do not cover; avoid sunlight on treated area.

corticosteroids: topical

ACTION

Diffuses across cell membranes, forms complexes w/cytoplasm. Complexes stimulate protein synthesis of inhibitory enzymes responsible for anti-inflammatory effects (e.g., inhibits edema, erythema, pruritus, capillary dilation, phagocytic activity).

Topical corticosteroids can be classified based on potency:

Low: Modest antiinflammatory effect, safest for chronic application, facial and intertriginous application, w/occlusion, for infants/young children.

Medium: For moderate inflammatory conditions (e.g., chronic eczematous dermatoses). May use for facial and intertriginous application for only limited time.

High: For more severe inflammatory conditions (e.g., lichen simplex chronicus, psoriasis). May use for facial and intertriginous application for short time only. Used in areas of thickened skin due to chronic conditions.

Very high: Alternative to systemic therapy for local effect (e.g., chronic lesions caused by psoriasis). Increased risk of skin atrophy. Used for short periods on small areas. Avoid occlusive dressings.

USES

Provides relief of inflammation/pruritus associated w/corticosteroid responsive disorders: e.g., contact dermatitis, eczema, insect bite reactions, first and second degree localized burns/sunburn.

PRECAUTIONS

CONTRAINDICATIONS: Hypersensitivity to corticosteroids. Do not use on preexisting skin atrophy, infection at treatment site w/o antibiotics, herpes simplex. Treatment of rosacea, perioral dermatitis or acne. Prolonged use (may cause glaucoma, cataracts). **CAUTIONS:** Use smallest therapeutic dose for children (chronic use may interfere w/growth and development). Local irritation: discontinue. Skin infection: treat w/appropriate antifungal or antibacterial agent.

INTERACTIONS

None significant.

SIDE EFFECTS

Contact dermatitis (burning/itching of skin). Painful, red, itchy, pus-containing blisters; thinning of skin w/easy bruising. Dryness, irritation, skin redness or scaling of skin lesions, skin rash.

CORTICOSTEROIDS: TOPICAL

Generic Name	Brand Name(s)	Potency	Dosage Forms
alclometasone	Aclovate	Low	Cream, ointment
amcinonide	Cyclocort	High	Cream, ointment, lotion
betamethasone benzoate	Uticort	Medium	Cream, lotion, gel
betamethasone dipropionate	Diprosone Maxivate	High	Ointment, cream, lotion, aerosol
betamethasone dipropionate (augmented)	Diprolene	Very high	Ointment, cream, gel, lotion
betamethasone valerate	Valisone	High	Ointment, cream, lotion
clobetasol	Temovate	Very high	Ointment, cream
desonide	Tridesilon	Low	Ointment, cream, lotion
desoximetasone	Topicort	High	Ointment, cream, gel
dexamethasone	Decadron	Medium	Cream
fluocinolone	Synalar	High	Ointment, cream, solution
fluocinonide	Lidex	High	Cream, ointment, solution, gel
flurandrenolide	Cordran	Medium	Ointment, cream, lotion
fluticasone	Cutivate	Medium	Ointment, cream
halcinonide	Halog	High	Ointment, cream, solution
halobetasol	Ultravate	Very high	Ointment, cream
hydrocortisone	Cort-Dome Hytone	Medium	Ointment, cream, lotion, gel
mometasone	Elocon	Medium	Ointment, cream, lotion
prednicarbate	Dermatop	—	Cream
triamcinolone	Aristocort Kenalog	Medium	Ointment, cream, lotion

TOXIC EFFECTS/ADVERSE REACTIONS

None significant.

NURSING IMPLICATIONS

BASELINE ASSESSMENT: Question for hypersensitivity to corticosteroid. Establish baseline assessment of skin disorder. **INTERVENTION/EVALUATION:** Assess involved area for therapeutic response or irritation. **PATIENT/FAMILY TEACHNG:** Apply after shower or bath for best absorption; rub thin film gently into affected area. Do not cover; do not use tight diapers, plastic pants, or coverings. Do not apply to weepy, denuded areas. Do not expose treated areas to sunlight (severe sunburn may occur). Use only for prescribed area and no longer than ordered. Report adverse local reactions. Avoid contact w/eyes.

diuretics

ACTION

Diuretics act to increase the excretion of water/sodium and other electrolytes via the kidneys. Exact mechanism of antihypertensive effect unknown; may be due to reduced plasma volume or decreased peripheral vascular resistance. Subclassifications of diuretics are based on their mechanism and site of action.

Thiazides: Acts at the cortical diluting segment of nephron, blocks reabsorption of Na, Cl and water; promotes excretion of Na, Cl, K, and water.

Loop: Act primarily at the thick ascending limb of Henle's loop to inhibit Na, Cl, and water absorption.

Potassium-sparing: Spironolactone blocks aldosterone action on distal nephron (causes K retention, Na excretion). Triamterene, amiloride act on distal nephron decreasing Na reuptake, reducing K secretion.

Osmotic: Elevate osmolarity of glomerular filtrate preventing reabsorption of water, increased excretion of Na, Cl.

USES

Thiazides: Management of edema resulting from a number of causes (e.g., CHF, hepatic cirrhosis); hypertension either alone or in combination w/other antihypertensives.

Potassium-sparing: Adjunctive treatment w/thiazides, loop diuretics in treatment of CHF and hypertension.

Osmotics: Reduction of intraocular pressure for ophthalmic surgery, edema, elevated intracranial pressure, and facilitating excretion of toxic substances.

Loop: Management of edema associated w/CHF, cirrhosis of liver, and renal disease. Furosemide used in treatment of hypertension alone or in combination w/other antihypertensives.

PRECAUTIONS

CONTRAINDICATIONS: Severe hepatic or renal dysfunction. Hypersensitivity to the drug (sensitivity to sulfonamides when giving thiazides). Potassium-sparing diuretics should not be given in hyperkalemia; osmotics are contraindicated in intracranial bleeding. Dehydration, pregnancy, infants and children, lactation. **CAUTIONS:** Administer cautiously to elderly, pts w/diabetes mellitus, gout or hyperuricemia, history of lupus erythematosus (may cause exacerbation).

INTERACTIONS

Thiazides: Cholestyramine, colestipol may decrease absorption, effects. May increase digoxin toxicity (due to hypokalemia). May increase lithium toxicity.

Loop: Amphotericin, ototoxic, nephrotoxic agents may increase toxicity. May decrease effect of anticoagulants, heparin. Hypokalemia caus-

DIURETICS

Generic Name	Brand Name(s)	Diuretic Effect: Type	Onset	Peak	Duration	Dosage Range
amiloride	Midamor	K-sparing	2 hrs	6-10 hrs	24 hrs	HTN: 5-20 mg/day Edema: 5-20 mg/day
bumetanide	Bumex	Loop	0.5-1 hr	1-2 hrs	4-6 hrs	Edema: 0.5-10 mg/day
chlorothiazide	Diuril	Thiazide	1-2 hrs	4 hrs	6-12 hrs	HTN: 0.5-2 Gm/day Edema: 0.5-2 Gm 1-2× /day
chlorthalidone	Hygroton	Thiazide	2 hrs	2-6 hrs	24-72 hrs	HTN: 25-100 mg/day Edema: 50-200 mg/day
ethacrynic acid	Edecrin	Loop	0.5 hrs	2 hrs	6-8 hrs	Edema: 50-200 mg/day
furosemide	Lasix	Loop	1 hr	1-2 hrs	6-8 hrs	HTN: 40 mg 2× /day Edema: up to 600 mg/day
glycerin	Glycerin	Osmotic	10-30 min	1-1.5 hrs	4-5 hrs	Edema: 1-1.5 Gm/kg
hydrochlorothiazide	Esidrix Hydro-Diunil Oretic	Thiazide	2 hrs	4-6 hrs	6-12 hrs	HTN: 25-100 mg/day Edema: 25-200 mg/day
indapamide	Lozol	Thiazide	1-2 hrs	2 hrs	Up to 36 hrs	HTN: 2.5-5 mg/day Edema: 2.5-5 mg/day
mannitol	Mannitol	Osmotic	0.5-1 hr	1 hr	6-8 hrs	Edema: 50-200 Gm/day
metolazone	Diulo Zaroxolyn	Thiazide	1 hr	2 hrs	12-24 hrs	HTN: 2.5-5 mg/day Edema: 5-20 mg/day
spironolactone	Aldactone	K-sparing	24-48 hrs	48-72 hrs	48-72 hrs	HTN: 50-100 mg/day Edema: 25-200 mg/day
torsemide	Demadex	Loop	10-60 min	1-2 hrs	6-8 hrs	HTN: 5-10 mg/day Edema: 10-200 mg/day
triamterene	Dyrenium	K-sparing	2-4 hrs	6-8 hrs	12-16 hrs	HTN: up to 300 mg/day Edema: up to 300 mg/day

HTN, hypertension.

ing agents may increase hypokalemia. May increase risk of lithium toxicity.

Potassium-sparing: May decrease anticoagulants, heparin effects. NSAIDs may decrease antihypertensive effect. ACE inhibitors (e.g., captopril), potassium containing medications, potassium supplements may increase potassium. May increase digoxin, lithium toxicity.

SIDE EFFECTS

Orthostatic hypotension, dizziness, anorexia or nausea, headache, lethargy.

TOXIC EFFECTS/ADVERSE REACTIONS

Unusual weakness, heaviness of legs, weak pulse indicate electrolyte (potassium) imbalance. Dehydration; hyperkalemia w/potassium-sparing diuretics; tinnitus and hearing loss w/loop diuretics; hypotension. Hypersensitivity reactions rarely. Impotence, GI bleeding.

NURSING IMPLICATIONS

GENERAL: If possible, administer dose in morning to avoid disturbing sleep w/urination. Provide assistance to bathroom, if needed; be sure pts confined to bed have call light handy. **INTERVENTION/EVALUATION:** Monitor I&O, weight. Check B/P and apical pulse, potassium levels. Assess for edema of dependent areas. Auscultate lungs for rales. **PATIENT/FAMILY TEACHING:** Medication will cause increased urination. Consult physician regarding alcohol and other medications. Eat foods high in potassium such as whole grains (cereals), legumes, meat, bananas, apricots, orange juice, potatoes (white, sweet), raisins (except w/potassium-sparing diuretics).

H_2 antagonists

ACTION

Inhibit gastric acid secretion by interfering w/histamine at the histamine H_2 receptors in parietal cells. Also inhibits acid secretion caused by gastrin. Inhibition occurs w/basal (fasting), nocturnal, food stimulated, or fundic distention secretion. H_2 antagonists decrease both the volume and H^+ concentration of gastric juices.

USES

Short-term treatment of duodenal ulcer, active benign gastric ulcer; maintenance therapy of duodenal ulcer; pathologic hypersecretory conditions (e.g., Zollinger-Ellison syndrome); gastroesophageal reflux disease; and prevention of upper GI bleeding in critically ill pts.

H_2 ANTAGONISTS

Generic Name	Brand Name(s)	Rte Admin	Use: Dosage
cimetidine	Tagamet	PO, IM, IV, IV infusion	Tx duodenal ulcer: 800 mg/hs, 400 mg 2×/day, 300 mg 4×/day Maintenance duodenal ulcer: 400 mg/hs Tx gastric ulcer: 800 mg/hs; 300 mg 4×/day GERD: 1600 mg/day Hypersecretory conditions: 1200-2400 mg/day Prevents upper GI bleeding: 50 mg/hr as IV infusion
famotidine	Pepcid	PO, IV	Tx duodenal ulcer: 40 mg/day Maintenance duodenal ulcer: 20 mg/day Tx gastric ulcer: 40 mg/day GERD: 40-80 mg/day Hypersecretory conditions: 80-640 mg/day
nizatidine	Axid	PO	Tx duodenal ulcer: 300 mg/day Maintenance duodenal ulcer: 150 mg/day
ranitidine	Zantac	PO, IM, IV IV infusion	Tx duodenal ulcer: 300 mg/day Maintenance duodenal ulcer: 150 mg/day Tx gastric ulcer: 300 mg/day GERD: 300 mg/day Hypersecretory conditions: 0.3-6 Gm/day

GERD, gastroesophageal reflux disease; Tx, treatment; hs, bedtime.

PRECAUTIONS

CONTRAINDICATIONS: Cross-sensitivity. Pregnancy and lactation; children. **CAUTIONS:** Elderly pts and those w/reduced renal or hepatic function.

INTERACTIONS

NOTE: Interactions more likely to occur w/cimetidine.

Antacids may decrease absorption (avoid use within 1/2-1 hr). May decrease ketoconazole absorption (given at least 2 hrs after). May decrease metabolism, increase concentration of oral anticoagulants, tricyclic antidepressants, oral hypoglycemics, metoprolol, metronidazole, phenytoin, propranolol, theophylline, calcium channel blockers, cyclosporine, lidocaine.

SIDE EFFECTS

Dizziness, headache, muscle cramps, rash, diarrhea or constipation. Confusion, esp. in elderly, debilitated, those w/renal or hepatic dysfunction.

TOXIC EFFECTS/ADVERSE REACTIONS

Unusual weakness or tiredness (may suggest blood dyscrasias), bradycardia or tachycardia, unusual bleeding; decreased sexual ability—esp. w/Zollinger-Ellison syndrome.

NURSING IMPLICATIONS

GENERAL: Administer oral agents w/meals and at bedtime for maximal effects. Antacids should not be taken within 1 hr of histamine receptor antagonists. Infuse IV solution slowly. **BASELINE ASSESSMENT:** Determine baselines for B/P, pulse. **INTERVENTION/EVALUATION:** Assess for abdominal pain, discomfort. Monitor B/P, pulse (esp. w/IV route). Check stools and emesis for blood. Assess for confusion, esp. in elderly, debilitated, and those w/renal or hepatic dysfunction. **PATIENT/FAMILY TEACHING:** Avoid alcohol, aspirin, spicy foods, and other foods known to cause distress. Need to cease smoking. Importance of completing therapy. Notify physician of abdominal or epigastric pain, blood in stool or emesis, dark tarry stools.

hematinic preparations

ACTION

Iron supplements are provided to assure adequate supplies for the formation of hemoglobin, which is needed for erythropoiesis and O_2 transport.

USES

To prevent or treat iron deficiency resulting from improper diet, pregnancy, impairment of absorption, or prolonged blood loss.

PRECAUTIONS

CONTRAINDICATIONS: Peptic ulcers, anemias caused by other factors, multiple blood transfusions, ulcerative colitis, cirrhosis, hypersensitivity to agent, hepatitis. **CAUTIONS:** Pts w/allergy, rheumatoid arthritis.

INTERACTIONS

Antacids, cimetidine, tetracycline may decrease iron absorption; iron may decrease absorption of methyldopa, quinolones, tetracycline.

SIDE EFFECTS

Nausea, vomiting, diarrhea or constipation, heartburn, hypersensitivity reactions: Rash, urticaria, pruritus.

TOXIC EFFECTS/ADVERSE REACTIONS

Severe gastrointestinal effects, anaphylactic reactions, fever, chills, arthralgia, hypotension, local abscess at IM injection site.

IRON PREPARATIONS

Generic Name	Brand Name(s)	Iron (%)	Dose Providing 100 mg Iron
ferrous fumarate	Feostat	33	300
ferrous gluconate	Fergon	11.6	860
ferrous sulfate	Mol-Iron Fer-In-Sol liquid Feosol liquid	20	500
ferrous sulfate exsiccated	Fer-In-Sol caps Feosol tabs/caps Slow FE	30	330

NURSING IMPLICATIONS

GENERAL: Give oral iron on empty stomach, w/food to reduce gastrointestinal symptoms. Provide straw w/oral liquid form to avoid tooth discoloration. Inject IM iron into gluteus maximus w/Z-track method to reduce tissue damage. **INTERVENTION/EVALUATION:** Laboratory results (hemoglobin, blood counts). Assess skin color, esp. at nail beds, ear lobes, sublingual areas. Check for fatigue, increased respirations (low hemoglobin may cause hypoxia). **PATIENT/FAMILY TEACHING:** Stools will be discolored (dark green or black). Importance of balanced diet; identify foods high in iron: Egg yolks, dried fruits, meats (esp. organ meats), whole grains, and dark-green leafy vegetables.

hypoglycemics

ACTION

Insulin: A hormone synthesized and secreted by beta cells of Langerhans' islet in the pancreas. Controls storage and utilization of glucose, amino acids, and fatty acids by activated transport systems/enzymes. Inhibits breakdown of glycogen, fat, protein. Insulin lowers blood glucose by inhibiting glycogenolysis and gluconeogenesis in liver; stimulates glucose uptake by muscle, adipose tissue. Activity of insulin is initiated by binding to cell surface receptors.

Oral hypoglycemics: Stimulates release of insulin from beta cells; increases sensitivity of insulin to peripheral tissue. Endogenous insulin must be present for oral hypoglycemics to be effective.

USES

Insulin: Treatment of insulin-dependent diabetes (type I) and noninsulin-dependent diabetes (type II). Also used in acute situations such as ketoacidosis, severe infections, major surgery in otherwise noninsulin-

HYPOGLYCEMICS: INSULIN

	Brand Name(s)	Hypoglycemic Effect Onset (hrs)	Peak (hrs)	Duration (hrs)
Rapid Acting				
regular insulin	Humulin R Novolin R Velosulin	0.5-1	—	6-8
semilente insulin	Semilente	1-1.5	5-10	12-16
Intermediate Acting				
lente insulin	Humulin L Novolin L	1-2.5	7-15	24
NPH insulin	Humulin N Insulintard Novolin N	1-1.5	4-12	24
Long Acting				
protamine zinc insulin (PZI)	PZI	4-8	14-24	36
ultralente insulin	Humulin U Ultralente	4-8	10-30	>36

dependent diabetics. Administered to pts receiving parenteral nutrition. Drug of choice during pregnancy.

Oral hypoglycemics: Controls hyperglycemia in type II diabetes not controlled by weight and diet alone. Chlorpropamide also used in adjunctive treatment of neurogenic diabetes insipidus.

PRECAUTIONS

CONTRAINDICATIONS: *Oral hypoglycemics:* Hypersensitivity to sulfonamides, pregnancy, severe stress or infection, before surgical procedures, in type I insulin-dependent diabetes; hepatic or renal dysfunction; hypoglycemia; lactation. *Insulin:* Hypersensitivity to animal proteins (human insulin available). Hypoglycemia. **CAUTION:** Elderly or debilitated pts. Renal or hepatic impairment; alcoholics; cardiac impairment.

INTERACTION

Insulin: Glucocorticoids, thiazide diuretics may increase blood glucose. Alcohol may increase insulin effect. Beta-adrenergic blockers may increase risk of hypo/hyperglycemia, mask signs of hypoglycemia, prolong period of hypoglycemia.

Oral hypoglycemics: May increase effects of oral anticoagulants. Chloramphenicol, MAO inhibitors, salicylates, sulfonamides may increase effects. Beta-blockers may increase hypoglycemic effect, may mask signs of hypoglycemia.

SIDE EFFECTS

Mild hypoglycemia; fatigue, headache, weakness, hunger, nervousness, drowsiness.

HYPOGLYCEMICS: ORAL HYPOGLYCEMICS

Generic Name	Brand Name(s)	Hypoglycemic Effect: Onset (hrs)	Hypoglycemic Effect: Duration (hrs)	Dosage: Initial (mg)	Dosage: Range (Average) (mg)
acetohexamide	Dymelor	1	12-24	250	250-1500 (1000)
chlorpropamide	Diabinese	1	24-72	100	100-750 (250)
glipizide	Glucotrol	1-1.5	16-24	2.5-5	2.5-40 (10)
glyburide	Diabeta Micronase	2-4	18-24	1.25-5	1.25-20 (7.5)
	Glynase (micronized)	1	24	0.75-3	0.75-12 (4.5)
metformin	Glucophage	—	—	500	500-300 (1500)
tolazamide	Tolinase	4-6	12-24	100	100-1000 (250)
tolbutamide	Orinase	1	6-12	500	500-3000 (1500)

TOXIC EFFECTS/ADVERSE REACTIONS

Severe hypoglycemia (due to hyperinsulinism) may occur in overdose of insulin, decrease or delay of food intake, excessive exercise or those w/brittle diabetes. Oral hypoglycemics: Urticaria or rash; mild anemia, thrombocytopenia, hepatic impairment. Diabetic ketoacidosis may result from stress, illness, omission of insulin dose or long-term poor insulin control.

NURSING IMPLICATIONS

GENERAL: Administer per schedule; rotate insulin injection sites. Recognize peak action times (see grid) as hypoglycemic reactions may occur at these times. Provide meals on time. **INTERVENTION/EVALUATION:** Monitor blood glucose levels, food consumption. Check for hypoglycemia: Cool, wet skin; tremors; dizziness; headache; anxiety; tachycardia; numbness in mouth; hunger; diplopia; restlessness, diaphoresis in sleeping pt. Check for hyperglycemia: Polyuria, polyphagia, polydipsia, nausea and vomiting, dim vision, fatigue, deep rapid breathing. **PATIENT/FAMILY TEACHING:** Diabetes mellitis requires lifelong control. Prescribed diet is essential part of treatment; do not skip or delay meals. Weight control, exercise, hygiene (including foot care) and nonsmoking are integral part of therapy. Significance of illness, stress, and exercise on regime. Teach how to handle, administer insulin. Oral hypoglycemics should be taken 15-30 min before meal. Carry candy, sugar packets, or other sugar supplements for immediate response to hypoglycemia. Wear, carry medical alert identification. Avoid alcohol; do not take other medication w/o consulting physician. Protect skin; limit sun exposure. Select clothing, positions that do not restrict blood flow. Avoid injuries, exposure to infections. Inform dentist, physician of this medication before any treatment.

immunizations

DIPHTHERIA TOXOID

INDICATIONS

Active immunity against diphtheria in children and adults.

DOSAGE:

IM: Children >6 wks and <7 yrs: Two injections of 0.5 ml at intervals of 4-8 wks, followed by third dose of 0.5 ml 6-12 months later. If initiated during first year of life, booster shot given at 4-6 yrs of age. **NOTE:** Use Diphtheria and Tetanus Toxoids Adsorbed—Pediatric.
IM: Adults, children >7 yrs: Two injections of 0.5 ml at intervals of 4-8 wks followed by third dose of 0.5 ml 6-12 months later. Booster dose of 0.5 ml should be given at 10 yr intervals to maintain immunity. **NOTE:** Use Tetanus and Diphtheria Adsorbed Adult.
IM: Children >8 wks-<7 yrs (if using DPT [Diphtheria-Pertussis-Tetanus]): Three 0.5 ml doses at 4-8 wk intervals, followed by a fourth dose of 0.5 ml 6-12 months after third dose.

CONTRAINDICATIONS

Acute respiratory infection or other active infection *except* for emergency booster doses.

ADVERSE EFFECTS

Mild to moderate tenderness, redness, and induration at injection site.

HAEMOPHILUS INFLUENZAE type b CONJUGATE VACCINE

INDICATIONS

Routine immunization of children against invasive disease caused by *H. influenzae* type b (bacterial meningitis, epiglottis, sepsis, septic arthritis, osteomyelitis, pericarditis, pneumonia).

DOSAGE

NOTE: Dosage dependent on vaccine formulation/manufacturer. Do not give in children >5 yrs unless high risk is present (children at day care centers, anatomic or functional asplenia, HIV infected or immunosuppressed children). May give with DPT, MMR, oral polio vaccine, or inactivated poliovirus vaccine.
IM: Pedvax HIB (Merck): 0.5 ml at 2, 4, and 12 months. **HibTITER (LEDERLE):** 0.5 ml at 2, 4, 6, and 15 months. **ProHIBit (Connaught):** 0.5 ml at 15 months.

ADVERSE EFFECTS

Erythema, induration, fever, diarrhea, vomiting.

HEPATITIS B VACCINE

INDICATIONS

Immunization against infection caused by all known subtypes hepatitis B virus for persons of all ages esp. those at increased risk of infection (e.g., health care workers who may be exposed via blood or pts' specimens; household and sexual contacts of hepatitis B carriers, dialysis, renal failure pts, hematology/oncology units, infants born of HBsAg-positive mothers whether HBsAg positive or negative, military personnel, persons at increased risk due to sexual practices).

DOSAGE

Children of HBsAg-negative mothers:
IM: *Recombivax HB:* 2.5 mcg at birth, 1 month, and 6 months. *Engerix-B:* 10 mcg at birth, 1 month, and 6 months (or at 2, 4, and 6 months).

Children of HBsAg-positive mothers:
NOTE: Hepatitis B immune globulin (HBIG) given within 12 hrs of birth.
IM: *Recombivax HB:* 5 mcg at birth, 1 month, and 6 months. *Engerix-B:* 10 mcg at birth, 1 month, and 6 months (or 4 doses: at birth, 1 month, 2 months, and 12 months).

Adolescents, adults:
Recombivax HB:
IM: 11-19 yrs: 0.5 ml (5 mcg) initially, 1 and 6 months after initial dose. **20 yrs or greater:** 1 ml (10 mcg) initially, then 1 and 6 months after initial dose.

Engerix-B:
IM: >11 yrs: 1 ml (20 mcg) initially, then 1 and 6 months after initial dose.

ADVERSE EFFECTS

Soreness at injection site.

HEPATITIS B IMMUNE GLOBULIN (HBIG)

INDICATIONS

Postexposure prophylaxis for hepatitis B infection. Provides passive immunization following exposure to hepatitis B virus and for infants born to mothers who are hepatitis B surface antigen positive (HBsAg-positive).

DOSAGE

Infants of HBsAg-positive mothers:
IM: 0.5 ml within 12 hours of birth.

Postexposure prophylaxis:
IM: Adults: 0.06 ml/kg (usually 3-5 ml) within 24 hrs if possible after exposure. Begin hepatitis B vaccine as soon as possible but within 7 days of exposure.

ADVERSE REACTIONS

Local pain, tenderness, urticaria.

INFLUENZAE VIRUS VACCINE

INDICATIONS

Annual vaccination for adults w/chronic cardiovascular/pulmonary diseases, metabolic disease, nursing home residents, health care workers dealing w/high-risk pts, healthy adults >65 yrs, children w/chronic metabolic or cardiopulmonary disease.

DOSAGE

IM: Adults, elderly, children >9 yrs: 0.5 ml as single dose. **Children 3-9 yrs:** 0.5 ml one or two times (1 month apart). **Children 6-35 months:** 0.25 ml one or two times (1 month apart). **NOTE:** Give two doses to children <9 yrs when receiving vaccine for first time.

CONTRAINDICATIONS

History of allergy to eggs. Defer immunization in presence of acute respiratory disease or other active infection or febrile illness.

ADVERSE EFFECTS

Local tenderness, low-grade fever.

MEASLES VACCINE, LIVE

INDICATIONS

Active immunization against measles (rubeola) in persons 15 months or older. A second dose is recommended.

DOSAGE

SubQ: Adults, children ≥15 months: 0.5 ml into outer aspect of upper arm. Usually given as MMR (Measles, Mumps, Rubella) for most vaccinations. **NOTE:** Centers for Disease Control (CDC) recommends routine second trivalent dose (MMR) at entry into kindergarten or first grade. American Academy of Pediatrics (AAP) recommends second trivalent dose (MMR) at entry into middle or junior high school.

Monovalent measles vaccine may be given as early as 6 months but two doses of trivalent vaccine still to be given w/first at age 15 months.

CONTRAINDICATIONS

Immunosuppressed pts, pregnant women, history of egg allergy, hypersensitivity to neomycin (contained in product). Any febrile respiratory infection or other active febrile infection. Active untreated TB. Pts w/ blood dyscrasias, leukemia, lymphomas, malignant neoplasms affecting bone marrow or lymphatic system.

ADVERSE EFFECTS

Febrile reaction (rarely above 39.4° C), transient rash.

MUMPS VIRUS VACCINE, LIVE

INDICATIONS

Active immunity against mumps in persons ≥12 months of age.

DOSAGE

SubQ: Adults, children ≥15 months: 0.5 ml into outer aspect of upper arm. Usually given as MMR for most vaccinations. **NOTE:** CDC recommends routine second trivalent dose (MMR) at entry into kindergarten or first grade. AAP recommends second trivalent dose (MMR) at entry into middle or junior high school.

Those born after 1/1/57 should receive two trivalent doses (MMR).

CONTRAINDICATIONS

Immunosuppressed pts, pregnant women, history of egg allergy, hypersensitivity to neomycin (contained in product). Any febrile respiratory infection or other active febrile infection. Active untreated TB. Pts w/ blood dyscrasias, leukemia, lymphomas, malignant neoplasms affecting bone marrow or lymphatic system.

ADVERSE EFFECTS

Rarely: rash, pruritus, purpura.

PERTUSSIS

INDICATION

Prevention of pertussis (whooping cough).

DOSAGE

Primary immunization:
IM: Children >8 wks to <7 yrs: 0.5 ml given at 2, 4, 6, and 18 months with a booster at age 4-6 years. Not recommended after age of 7 (risk of pertussis diminishes). Generally given w/diphtheria and tetanus toxoids (DPT vaccine).

CONTRAINDICATIONS

Acute infection or febrile illness. Occurrence of any neurologic symptoms following administration of DPT for further use. History of seizures, any evolving or changing disorder affecting the CNS.

ADVERSE EFFECTS

Local reactions, fever, prolonged crying, convulsions (1 in 1750) and acute neurologic illness w/33% rate of sequalae (1 in 110,000).

PNEUMOCOCCAL VACCINE, POLYVALENT

INDICATIONS

Immunization against pneumococcal pneumonia/bacteremia caused by types of pneumococci in vaccine. Indicated in pts at increased risk of pneumococcal disease: immunocompromised (e.g., Hodgkin's disease, renal failure, HIV infection), pts w/splenic dysfunction or anatomic asplenia, chronic cardiovascular or pulmonary disease, alcoholism, elderly (esp. institutionalized).

DOSAGE

IM/SubQ: Adults, children ≥2 yrs: 0.5 ml as single dose.

CONTRAINDICATION

Hypersensitivity, previous immunization w/any polyvalent pneumococcal vaccine.

CAUTION

Adults w/documented/suspected pneumococcal infection would wait 2-3 months after episode before immunization.

ADVERSE EFFECTS

Erythema, induration, soreness at injection site.

POLIO VACCINE, LIVE, ORAL

INDICATIONS

Prevention of poliomyelitis caused by poliovirus 1, 2, 3. Immunization recommended for all children and young adults up to 18 years.

RECOMMENDATIONS FOR IMMUNIZATION OF INFANTS/CHILDREN

	Birth	1 Mo	2 Mo	4 Mo	6 Mo	12 Mo	15 Mo	18 Mo	4-6 Yrs
Diphtheria[1,2]			x	x	x			x	x
Tetanus[1,2]			x	x	x			x	x
Pertussis[1,2]			x	x	x			x	x
Measles[3]							x		x
Mumps[3]							x		x
Rubella[3]							x		x
Haemophilus[4]									
HibTITER			x	x	x		x		
ProHIBit							x		
PedvaxHIB			x	x		x			
Hepatitis B									
HBsAg-negative[5] mothers	x	x			x				
HBsAg-positive mothers	x	x			x				
Poliovirus			x	x				x	x

[1] Usually given as diphtheria and tetanus toxoid combined w/pertussis vaccine.

[2] Booster given at 10 yr intervals to maintain immunity.

[3] Usually given as combined measles, mumps, rubella (MMR) vaccine.

[4] Dosage schedule dependent on vaccine formulation and manufacturer used.

[5] See monograph for alternate schedule.

DOSAGE

PO: Three doses of 0.5 ml initially at 6-8 wks of age, 6-8 wks after first dose and third dose 8-12 months after second dose. Older children may receive third dose 6-12 months after the second dose. Fourth dose given upon entering elementary school (not required if third dose given on or after fourth birthday).

CONTRAINDICATIONS

Pts w/immunosuppression or household members (e.g., leukemia, lymphoma, lowered resistance to infection from steroid therapy). Defer in presence of any acute illness, vomiting, diarrhea, and in pts w/advanced debilitated disease (inactivated poliovirus vaccine recommended).

ADVERSE EFFECTS

No immediate effect seen.

Rh_o(D) IMMUNE GLOBULIN (RDIG)

INDICATIONS

Suppresses immune response of nonsensitized Rh_o(D) negative pts who receive Rh_o(D) positive blood due to fetomaternal hemorrhage, abdominal trauma, amniocentesis, abortion, or full-term delivery. RDIG prevents future chance of erythroblastosis fetalis in subsequent pregnancies with a Rh_o(D) positive fetus.

DOSAGE

Term delivery:
IM: 300 mcg within 72 hours.

After amniocentesis, miscarriage, abortion, ectopic pregnancy >13 wks:
IM: 300 mcg one time.

Before delivery:
IM: 300 mcg at 28 wks, 300 mcg within 72 hrs of delivery.

Transfusion accident:
IM: Dependent on volume of packed red cells or whole blood transfused.

Termination of pregnancy (<13 wks):
IM: 50 mcg within 72 hours.
NOTE: Do not give to individuals that are positive Rh_o(D) and D^u antigens or those w/anti-Rh_o(D) antibodies.

ADVERSE EFFECTS

Fever, injection site tenderness.

RUBELLA VIRUS VACCINE, LIVE (GERMAN MEASLES)

INDICATIONS

Active immunization against rubella (German measles). Intended to reduce occurrence of congenital rubella syndrome among offspring or women contracting rubella during pregnancy. Indicated for children >1 year; >12 yrs w/o evidence of wild virus infection, women of childbearing potential for whom serologic testing unavailable (up to 45 yrs of age), those at substantial risk for exposure.

DOSAGE

SubQ: Adults, children ≥15 months: 0.5 ml into outer aspect of upper arm. Usually given as MMR for most vaccinations. **NOTE:** CDC recommends routine second trivalent dose (MMR) at entry into kindergarten or first grade. AAP recommends second trivalent dose (MMR) at entry into middle or junior high school.

CONTRAINDICATIONS

Immunosuppressed pts, pregnant women, history of egg allergy, hypersensitivity to neomycin (contained in product). Any febrile respiratory infection or other active febrile infection. Active untreated TB. Pts w/

blood dyscrasias, leukemia, lymphomas, malignant neoplasms affecting bone marrow or lymphatic system.

ADVERSE EFFECTS

Increase w/age of pt. Lymphadenopathy, rash, urticaria, fever, malaise, sore throat, headache, myalgia, paresthesia of extremities.

TETANUS TOXOID ADSORBED (TTA)

INDICATION

Active immunity against tetanus (esp. military personnel, farm/utility workers, those working w/horses, firemen, occupations that render liable to even minor lacerations/abrasions).

DOSAGE

IM: Adults, children >6 wks: Two injections of 0.5 ml 4-8 wks apart and third dose of 0.5 ml approximately 6-12 months after second injection. Booster doses of 0.5 ml recommended every 10 yrs. In event of injury for which tetanus is indicated, a booster dose of 0.5 ml should be given.
IM: Children >8 wks to <7 yrs (if using DPT): Three 0.5 ml doses at 4-8 wk intervals, followed by a fourth dose of 0.5 ml 6-12 months after third dose.

CONTRAINDICATIONS

Acute respiratory infection or other active infection except for emergency booster doses.

ADVERSE EFFECTS

Local reactions at injection site (warmth, redness, induration).

laxatives

ACTION

Laxatives ease or stimulate defecation. Mechanisms by which this is accomplished include: 1. Attracting, retaining fluid in colonic contents due to hydrophilic or osmotic properties; 2. Acting directly or indirectly on mucosa to decrease absorption of water and NaCl; or 3. Increasing intestinal motility, decreasing absorption of water and NaCl by virtue of decreased transit time.

Bulk-forming: Act primarily in small/large intestine. Retains water in stool, may bind water, ions in colonic lumen (soften feces, increase bulk); may increase colonic bacteria growth (increases fecal mass). Produces soft stool in 1-3 days.

LAXATIVES

Generic Name	Brand Name(s)	Type	Dosage Range
bisacodyl	Dulcolax	Stimulant	Adults (PO): 10-15 mg; (Rectal): 10 mg Children >6 yrs (PO): 5-10 mg Children <2 yrs (Rectal): 5 mg
cascara	Cascara	Stimulant	Adults: 1 tablet or 5 ml
castor oil	Castor Oil	Stimulant	Adults: 15-60 ml Children (6-12 yrs): 5-15 ml
docusate CA	Surfak	Surfactant	Adults: 240 mg/day Children >6 yrs: 50-150 mg/day
docusate K	Dialose	Surfactant	Adults: 100-300 mg/day Children > 6 yrs: 100 mg at hs
docusate Na	Colace	Surfactant	Adults: 50-500 mg/day Children 6-12 yrs: 40-120 mg; 3-6 yrs: 20-60 mg; <3 yrs: 10-40 mg
lactulose	Cephulac	Osmotic	Adults: 30-45 ml 3-4 × /day Children: 40-90 ml/day in divided doses Infants: 2.5-10 ml/day in divided doses
magnesium citrate	Citro-Nesia	Saline	Adults: 240 ml as needed Children: 120 ml as needed
magnesium hydroxide	MOM	Saline	Adults: 30-60 ml/day Children: 5-30 ml/day
magnesium sulfate	Epsom Salt	Saline	Adults: 10-15 Gm in glass water Children: 5-10 Gm in glass water
methylcellulose	Citrucel	Bulk-forming	Adults: 5-20 ml liquid 3 × /day or 1 tablespoonful 1-3 × /day (mix w/water, other fluid)
mineral oil	Mineral Oil	Lubricant	Adults: 5-45 ml Children: 5-20 ml
phenolpthalein	Modane	Stimulant	Adults: 60-194 mg at hs
poycarbophil	Mitrolan	Bulk-forming	Adults: 1 Gm 4 × /day; maximum: 6 Gm/day Children 6-12 yrs: 500 mg 1-3 × /day; maximum: 3 Gm/day Children 3-6 yrs: 500 mg 2 × /day; maximum: 2 Gm/day
psyllium	Metamucil	Bulk-forming	Adults: 1 tsp 1-3 × /day (mix w/ water, other fluid)
senna	Senokot	Stimulant	Adults: 2-8 tablets/day Children: 1-4 tablets/day

hs, bedtime.

Castor oil: Acts in small intestine. Reduces absorption of fluid, electrolytes, stimulates intestinal peristalsis. Produces watery stool in 2-6 hrs.

Lactulose: Acts in colon. Similar to saline laxatives. Osmotic action may be enhanced in distal ileum/colon by bacterial metabolism to lactate, other organic acids. This decrease in pH increases motility, secretion. Produces soft stool in 1-3 days.

Saline: Act in small/large intestine, colon (sodium phosphate). Poorly, slowly absorbed, causes hormone cholecystokinin release from duodenum (stimulates fluid secretion, motility), possesses osmotic properties, produces watery stool in 2-6 hrs (low doses produce semifluid stool in 6-12 hrs).

Stimulant: Acts in colon. Enhances accumulation of water/electrolytes in colonic lumen, enhances intestinal motility. May act directly on intestinal mucosa. Produces semifluid stool in 6-12 hrs (NOTE: Bisacodyl suppository acts in 15-60 min).

Surfactants: Act in small and large intestines. Hydrate and soften stools by their surfactant action facilitating penetration of fat and water into stool. Produces soft stool in 1-3 days.

USES

Short-term treatment constipation; evacuate colon before rectal/bowel examination; prevent straining (e.g., after anorectal surgery, myocardial infarction); reduce painful elimination (e.g., episiotomy, hemorrhoids, anorectal lesions); modify effluent from ileostomy, colostomy; prevent fecal impaction; remove ingested poisons.

PRECAUTIONS

CONTRAINDICATIONS: Acute surgical abdomen, abdominal pain, intestinal obstruction or perforation, fecal impaction, undiagnosed rectal bleeding, young children. **CAUTIONS:** Select laxative carefully for diabetics and pts on sodium restricted diet. (No saline laxative.) Avoid overuse/abuse.

INTERACTIONS

Cholinergics increase effects; anticholinergics and CNS depressants decrease effects. Mineral oil impairs absorption of vitamins A, D, E, and K. Antacids decrease laxative action of bisacodyl tablets. Laxative may decrease absorption of other drugs by increasing rate of passage.

SIDE EFFECTS

Cramping, frequent liquid stools, nausea, weakness, perianal irritation.

TOXIC EFFECTS/ADVERSE REACTIONS

Incidence rare. Severe diarrhea may cause dehydration and electrolyte imbalance. Fluid retention with saline laxative may cause edema and electrolyte imbalance. *Bulk-forming laxative:* Allergic reaction, impaction.

NURSING IMPLICATIONS

GENERAL: Give w/at least 8 ounces of water and provide 6-8 glasses of water that day (unless pt on water restriction). Most laxatives should be given on an empty stomach at bedtime to provide morning evacuation. Provide call light and assistance as indicated. **BASELINE ASSESSMENT:** Results of laxative. **PATIENT/FAMILY TEACHING:** Avoid chronic use. Value of high fiber diet, fluid intake, exercise, and regular bowel habits.

neuromuscular blockers

ACTION

Interrupt nerve impulse transmission at skeletal neuromuscular junction and/or autonomic ganglia. (these receptors are called "nicotinic-cholinergic"). Further classified by whether or not they cause depolarization of motor end-plate (nondepolarizing vs. depolarizing). Combine w/nicotinic-cholinergic receptor at postjunctional membrane blocking competitive transmitter action of acetylcholine. When administered, motor weakness gives way to total flaccid paralysis. Cause relaxation of skeletal muscle. Can produce decreased B/P due to release of histamine and to partial ganglionic blockade. Lack CNS effects—does not diminish consciousness or pain perception.

USES

Adjuvant in surgical anesthesia to obtain relaxation of skeletal muscle (esp. abdominal wall) for surgery (allows lighter level of anesthesia, valuable in orthopedic procedures). Neuromuscular blocking agents of short duration often used to facilitate intubation w/endotracheal tube; facilitates laryngoscopy, bronchoscopy and esophagoscopy in combination w/general anesthetics. Provide muscle relaxation in pts undergoing mechanical ventilation, muscle relaxation in diagnosis of myasthenia gravis. Prevent convulsive movements during electroconvulsive therapy.

PRECAUTIONS

CONTRAINDICATIONS: Contraindicated during pregnancy, lactation, hypersensitivity to drug or components, pts who have own or family history of malignant hyperthermia. Use w/extreme caution, if at all, in pts w/myasthenia gravis. **CAUTIONS:** During cesarean delivery (potential respiratory depression in neonate); caution and reduced dosage during delivery when magnesium sulfate has been administered to pregnant woman (potentiates effects). Cautious use in pts w/hepatic, renal, or pulmonary impairment; respiratory depression; geriatric or debilitated pts.

NEUROMUSCULAR BLOCKING AGENTS

Generic Name	Brand Name(s)	Type	Uses
atracurium	Tracrium	Nondepolarizing	Endotracheal intubation Surgery Mechanical ventilation
doxacurium	Nuromax	Nondepolarizing	Endotracheal intubation Surgery
mivacurium	Mivacron	Nondepolarizing	Surgery Mechanical ventilation Endotracheal intubation
pancuronium	Pavulon	Nondepolarizing	Surgery Mechanical ventilation
pipecuronium	Arduan	Nondepolarizing	Endotracheal intubation Surgery
rocuronium	Zemuron	Nondepolarizing	Endotracheal intubation Surgery Mechanical ventilation
succinylcholine	Anectine Quelicin	Depolarizing	Endotracheal intubation Surgery Mechanical ventilation ECT
tubocurarine	Tubocurarine	Nondepolarizing	Surgery Mechanical ventilation ECT Dx: Myasthenia gravis
vecuronium	Norcuron	Nondepolarizing	Endotracheal intubation Surgery Mechanical ventilation

ECT, electroconvulsive therapy; Dx, diagnosis.

INTERACTIONS

General anesthesics, antibiotics (esp. aminoglycosides) may increase effects. Anticholinesterase inhibitors (e.g., neostigmine) may decrease effects.

SIDE EFFECTS

Prolonged apnea, residual muscle weakness, hypersensitivity reactions. Many drugs also cause hypotension, wheezing and bronchospasm, cardiac disturbances, flushing, urticaria, pruritus.

TOXIC EFFECTS/ADVERSE REACTIONS

Malignant hyperthermia is rare, but often fatal (esp. w/halothane or succinylcholine). Severely compromised respiratory function; respiratory paralysis.

NURSING IMPLICATIONS

GENERAL: Have equipment and personnel immediately available to intubate pt and provide mechanical ventilation, including use of positive pressure oxygen. Have anticholinesterase reversal agents immediately available. Drugs do not alter consciousness; pt may be conscious but unable to move, breathe. **INTERVENTION/EVALUATION:** Continuously monitor B/P, pulse, EKG. **PATIENT/FAMILY TEACHING:** Explain to conscious pt, family that muscle tone will return. Provide emotional support and monitor respirations carefully during recovery period.

nitrates

ACTION

Relax most smooth muscles, including arteries and veins. Effect is primarily on veins (decrease left/right ventricular end-diastolic pressure). In angina, nitrates decrease myocardial work and O_2 requirements (decrease preload by venodilation and afterload by arteriodilation). Nitrates also appear to redistribute blood flow to ischemic myocardial areas improving perfusion w/o increase in coronary blood flow.

USES

Sublingual: Acute relief of angina pectoris.

Oral, topical: Long-term prophylactic treatment of angina pectoris.

Intravenous: Adjunctive treatment in CHF associated w/acute myocardial infarction. Produces controlled hypotension during surgical procedures; control B/P in perioperative hypertension, angina unresponsive to organic nitrates or beta-blockers.

PRECAUTIONS

CONTRAINDICATIONS: Hypersensitivity, hypotension, severe anemia, head trauma or cerebral hemorrhage, renal or hepatic dysfunction, closed-angle glaucoma, pregnancy, lactation. **CAUTIONS:** Acute MI, hepatic or renal dysfunction, blood volume decrease from diuretics, systolic B/P below 90 mm Hg. Chronic administration may lead to tolerance.

INTERACTIONS

Alcohol, antihypertensives, vasodilators may increase risk of orthostatic hypotension.

SIDE EFFECTS

Headache, hypotension, dizziness, palpitations, skin or mucous membrane sensitivity to nitrites/nitrates.

TOXIC EFFECTS/ADVERSE REACTIONS

Severe headache, significant hypotension, difficulty breathing, chest pain, hypersensitivity reactions.

NITRATES

Generic Name	Rte Admin	Brand Name(s)	Cardiovascular Effect: Onset	Cardiovascular Effect: Duration	Dosage Range
erythrityl	PO	Cardilate	5-30 min	3-6 hrs	5-10 mg before event, up to 100 mg/day
isosorbide	SL	Isordil Sorbitrate	2-5 min	1-3 hrs	2.5-10 mg q2-3h
	PO	Isordil Sorbitrate	20-40 min	4-6 hrs	10-40 mg q6h
	SR	Dilatrate-SR Isordil Sorbitrate	up to 4 hrs	6-8 hrs	40-80 mg q8-12h
nitroglycerin	SL	Nitrostat	1-3 min	30-60 min	0.3-0.6 mg to 3×/15 min
	SR	Nitrobid Nitroglyn	20-45 min	3-8 hrs	2.5 mg 3-4×/day up to 26 mg 3-4×/day
	Trans	Minitran Nitro-Dur Nitrodisc Transderm-Nitro	30-60 min	Up to 24 hrs	0.2-0.4 mg/hr up to 0.8 mg/hr
	Top	Nitrol	30-60 min	2-12 hrs	1-2 in q8h up to 4-5 in q4h
pentaerythritol	PO	Duotrate Peritrate	PO: 20-60 min	5 hrs	PO: 10-20 mg 3-4×/day up to 40 mg 4×/day
			SR: 30 min	up to 12 hrs	SR: 1 cap/tab q12h

SL, sublingual; SR, sustained release; Trans, trasdermal; Top, topical.

NURSING IMPLICATIONS

GENERAL: IV infusion of nitroglycerin requires special administration set and precise flow rate. **BASELINE ASSESSMENT:** Record onset, type (sharp, dull, squeezing), radiation, location, intensity, and duration of anginal pain and precipitating factors (exertion, emotional stress). Obtain baseline B/P and apical pulse. **INTERVENTION/EVALUATION:** Monitor B/P and apical pulse (withhold and notify physician if systolic B/P below 90 mm Hg). Continuous cardiac monitoring is indicated for unrelieved, acute episodes. Assess for relief of anginal pain. Check for local irritation when given dermally or sublingually. **PATIENT/FAMILY TEACHING:** Avoid high caffeine foods/fluids, such as coffee, colas, chocolate, tea (increase risk of anginal attacks). Do not take alcohol (can cause hypotensive, shocklike state) or other drugs w/o physician approval. Identify precipitating factors. Take sublingual tablets sitting or lying down for anginal relief; may repeat every 5 min, up to 3 tablets in 15 min. If no relief, have ambulance transport to hospital. Do not change brands; discard expired drugs. Notify physician of severe or persistent headache.

nonsteroidal anti-inflammatory drugs (NSAIDs)

ACTION

Exact mechanism for anti-inflammatory, analgesic, antipyretic effects unknown. Inhibition of enzyme cyclooxygenase, the enzyme responsible for prostaglandin synthesis appears to be a major mechanism of action. May inhibit other mediators of inflammation (e.g., leukotrienes). Direct action on hypothalamus heat regulating center may contribute to antipyretic effect.

USES

Provides symptomatic relief from *pain/inflammation* in the treatment of musculoskeletal disorders (e.g., rheumatoid arthritis, osteoarthritis, ankylosing spondylitis); *analgesic* for low to moderate pain; *reduce fever* (many agents not suited for routine/prolonged therapy due to toxicity). By virtue of its action on platelet function, aspirin is used in treatment or prophylaxis of diseases associated w/hypercoagulability (reduce risk of stroke/heart attack).

PRECAUTIONS

CONTRAINDICATIONS: Aspirin sensitivity or allergy to other components; pregnancy; lactation; children <14 yrs of age, gastrointestinal disorders. **CAUTIONS:** Renal or hepatic dysfunctions, cardiac or hypertensive disorders, severe infections, elderly, coagulation defects, otic disease.

INTERACTIONS

Salicylates: Antacids, NSAIDs may increase risk GI effects (e.g., ulceration). Urinary alkalinizers, antacids, increase excretion. Anticoagulants, heparin, thrombolytics increase risk of bleeding. Large doses may increase insulin, oral hypoglycemic effects. Valproic acid, platelet aggregation inhibitors may increase risk of bleeding. May increase toxicity of methotrexate, zidovudine. Ototoxic medications, vancomycin may increase ototoxicity. May decrease effect of probenecid, sulfinpyrazone.

NSAIDs: May increase effects of oral anticoagulants, heparin, thrombolytics. May decrease effect of antihypertensives, diuretics. Salicylates, aspirin may increase risk of GI side effects, bleeding. Bone marrow depressants may increase risk of hematologic reactions. May increase methotrexate toxicity. Probenecid may increase concentration.

NSAIDS

Generic Name	Brand Name(s)	Use: Dosage Range
aspirin	many	Aches/pains: 325-650 mg q4h prn Arthritis: 3.2-6 Gm/day Juvenile rheumatoid arthritis: 60-110 mg/kg/day Acute rheumatic fever: Adults: 5-8 Gm/day Children: 100 mg/kg/day × 14 days; then, 75 mg/kg/day × 4-6 wks Transient ischemic attacks: 1,300 mg/day Myocardial infarction prophylaxis: 300-325 mg/day Analgesic/antipyretic (children): up to 60-80 mg/kg/day or 10-15 mg/kg/dose q4h
choline salicylate	Arthropan	Arthritis/pain/fever: 870 mg (5 ml) q3-4h up to 6×/day
diclofenac	Voltaren	Arthritis: 100-200 mg/day
diflunisal	Dolobid	Arthritis: 0.5-1 Gm/day Pain: 1 Gm, then 0.5 Gm q8-12h
etodolac	Lodine	Arthtitis: 600-800 mg/day Pain: 200-400 mg q6-8h; max: 1200 mg/day
fenoprofen	Nalfon	Arthritis: 300-600 mg 3-4×/day Pain: 200 mg q4-6h prn
flurbiprofen	Ansaid	Arthritis: 200-300 mg/day
ibuprofen	Motrin	Arthritis: 1.2-3.2 Gm/day Pain: 400 mg q4-6h prn Fever: 200 mg q4-6h prn Primary dysmenorrhea: 400 mg q4h prn Juvenile arthritis: 30-40 mg/kg/day
indomethacin	Indocin	Arthritis: 50-200 mg/day Bursitis/tendonitis: 75-150 mg/day Gouty arthritis: 150 mg/day
ketoprofen	Orudis	Arthritis: 150-300 mg/day Pain/primary dysmenorrhea: 25-50 mg q6-8h as needed
ketorolac	Toradol	Pain: PO: 10 mg q4-6h prn; maximum: 40 mg/day IM: Maximum 150 mg/day first day; then max: 120 mg/day
magnesium salicylate	Magan	Arthritis/pain/fever: 3.6-4.8 Gm/day in 3-4 divided doses
meclofenamate	Meclomen	Arthritis: 200-400 mg/day Pain: 50 mg q4-6h prn Primary dysmenorrhea: 100 mg 3×/day
nabumetone	Relafen	Arthritis: 1-2 Gm/day
naproxen	Anaprox	Arthritis: 250-550 mg/day
	Naprosyn	Pain/1° dysmenorrhea/bursitis/tendonitis: 500 mg, then 250 mg q6-8h Juvenile arthritis: 10 mg/kg in 2 divided doses Gouty arthtitis: 750 mg, then 250 mg q8h

1°, primary; prn, according as circumstances may require.

NSAIDS *Continued*

Generic Name	Brand Name(s)	Use: Dosage Range
oxaprozin	Daypro	Arthritis: 600-1800 mg/day
phenylbutazone	Azolid Butazolidin	Arthritis: Initially 300-600 mg; maintenance: 100-400 mg/day Acute gout attack: 400 mg; then 100 mg q4h
piroxicam	Feldene	Arthritis: 20 mg/day
sodium salicylate	Sodium Salicylate	Arthritis/pain/fever: 325-650 mg q4h prn
sulindac	Clinoril	Arthritis: 300 mg/day Acute gouty arthritis/painful shoulder: 400 mg/day
tolmetin	Tolectin	Arthritis: 600-1,800 mg/day Juvenile arthritis: 15-30 mg/kg/day

SIDE EFFECTS

Gastrointestinal upset, dizziness, headache, constipation or diarrhea. *Ophthalmic:* Burning, stinging on instillation, keratitis, elevated intraocular pressure.

TOXIC EFFECTS/ADVERSE REACTIONS

Hypersensitivity reactions, including skin rash or urticaria. Renal or hepatic toxicity, bone marrow suppression, bleeding, esp. of gastrointestinal tract. Tinnitus and hearing disturbances. Reactions vary by individual drug.

NURSING IMPLICATIONS

GENERAL: Check for aspirin sensitivity (cross sensitivity). Administer on schedule to maintain blood levels. Provide rest, positioning, and other comfort measures for pain relief. **BASELINE ASSESSMENT:** Assess pain (type, location, intensity). Check temperature, pulse, respirations. **INTERVENTION/EVALUATION:** Assess pain, therapeutic response (decreased temperature, pain relief, improved mobility). **PATIENT/FAMILY TEACHING:** Take w/meals or on empty stomach, as indicated by individual drug; however, all drugs may be taken w/food, if necessary, to reduce gastrointestinal side effects. Avoid alcohol and consult physician about other medications. Refrain from driving or other activities requiring motor response until certain no dizziness present. Inform other physicians or dentist of drug therapy.

nutrition: enteral

Enteral nutrition (EN), also known as tube feedings, provides food/nutrients via GI tract using special formulas, techniques of delivery, and equipment. All routes of enteral nutrition consist of placement of a tube through which liquid formula is infused.

INDICATIONS

Tube feedings are used in pts w/major trauma, burns, undergoing radiation and/or chemotherapy, w/liver failure, severe renal impairment, w/physical or neurologic impairment, preop and postop to promote anabolism, prevent cachexia, malnutrition.

ROUTES OF ENTERAL NUTRITION DELIVERY

Nasogastric (NG):
INDICATIONS: Most common for short-term feeding in pts unable or unwilling to consume adequate nutrition by mouth. Requires at least partially functioning GI tract. **ADVANTAGES:** Does not require surgical intervention and is fairly easily inserted. Allows full use of digestive tract. Decreases chance hyperosmolar solutions may cause distention, nausea, vomiting. **DISADVANTAGES:** Temporary. May be easily pulled out during routine nursing care. Has potential for pulmonary aspiration of gastric contents, risk of reflux esophagitis, regurgitation.

Nasoduodenal (ND), nasojejunal (NJ):
INDICATIONS: Pts unable or unwilling to consume adequate nutrition by mouth. Requires at least partially functioning GI tract. **ADVANTAGES:** Does not require surgical intervention and is fairly easily inserted. Preferred for pts at risk of aspiration. Valuable for pts w/gastroparesis. **DISADVANTAGES:** Temporary. May be pulled out during routine nursing care. May be dislodged by coughing, vomiting. Small lumen size increases risk of clogging when medication is given through them, more susceptible to rupturing when using infusion device. Must be radiographed for placement, frequently extubated.

Gastrostomy:
INDICATIONS: Pts w/esophageal obstruction or impaired swallowing, pts in whom NG, ND, or NJ not feasible, or when long-term feeding indicated. **ADVANTAGES: Permanent feeding access.** Tubing has larger bore allowing noncontinuous (bolus) feeding (300-400 ml over 30-60 minutes q3-6h). May be inserted endoscopically using local anesthetic (procedure called percutaneous endoscopic gastrostomy [PEG]). **DISADVANTAGES:** Requires surgery, may be inserted in conjunction w/other surgery or endoscopically (see Advantages). Stoma care required. Tube may be inadvertently dislodged. Risk of aspiration, peritonitis, cellulitis, leakage of gastric contents.

ENTERAL FORMULAS

PRODUCT	DESCRIPTION	CAL/ML	OSMOLALITY (MOSM/KG)	PROTEIN GM/L	CHO GM/L	FAT GM/L
Alitrag	Metabolic stress Impaired GI function	1.0	575	52.5	165	15.5
Compleat	Tube feeding	1.1	450	43	130	43
Ensure Plus	Nutrient dense oral supplement	1.5	690	54.9	199	53.2
Glucerna	Glucose intolerance	1.0	375	41.8	93.7	55.7
Isocal HN	Low residue	1.06	—	43.9	122	45.2
Jevity	Tube feeding w/ fiber	1.06	310	44.4	151	36.7
Nepro	Renal dialysis	2.0	635	69.9	212	94.4
Osmolite HN	Low residue	1.06	300	44.4	139	36.7
Pediasure	Children 1-6 yrs	1.0	310	30.0	110	49.9
Perative	Metabolic stress	1.3	425	66.6	176	36.9
Pulmocare	Pulmonary	1.5	465	62.6	106	92
Suplena	Predialysis	2.0	615	30.0	254	95.4
Sustacal	Complete balanced nutrition	1.0	650	61.2	139	23.2
Traumacal	Multiple trauma major burns	1.5	490	82.3	144	68.4
Travasorb HN	Elemental diet	—	560	15.0	58.3	4.5
Twocal HN	Nutrient dense oral supplement	2.0	690	83.7	216	90.3
Vital HN	Elemental diet	1.0	500	41.7	185	10.8

Jejunostomy:
INDICATIONS: Pts w/stomach or duodenal obstruction, impaired gastric motility, pts in whom NG, ND, or NJ not feasible, or when long-term feeding indicated. **ADVANTAGES:** Allows early postop feeding (small bowel function is least affected by surgery). Risk of aspiration reduced. Rarely pulled out inadvertently. **DISADVANTAGES:** Requires surgery (laparotomy). Stoma care required. Risk of intraperitoneal leakage. Can be dislodged easily.

INITIATING ENTERAL NUTRITION

With continuous feeding, initiation of isotonic (about 300 mOsm/L) or moderately hypertonic feeding (up to 495 mOsm/L) can be given full strength usually at a slow rate (30-50 ml/hr) and gradually increased (25 ml/hr q6-24h). Formulas w/osmolality of >500 mOsm/L are generally started at 1/2 strength and gradually increased in rate, then concentration. Tolerance increased if the rate and concentration are not increased simultaneously.

SELECTION OF FORMULAS

Protein: Has many important physiologic roles and is the primary source of nitrogen in the body. Provides 4 kcal/Gm protein. Sources of protein in enteral feedings: sodium caseinate, calcium caseinate, soy protein, dipeptides.

Carbohydrate (CHO): Provides energy for the body and heat to maintain body temperature. Provides 3.4 kcal/Gm carbohydrate. Sources of carbohydrate (CHO) in enteral feedings: corn syrup, cornstarch, maltodextrin, lactose, sucrose, glucose.

Fat: Provides concentrated source of energy. Referred to as "kilocalorie dense" or "protein sparing." Provides 9 kcal/Gm fat. Sources of fat in enteral feedings: corn oil, safflower oil, medium chain triglycerides.

Electrolytes, vitamins, trace elements: Contained in formulas (not found in specialized products for renal and hepatic insufficiency).

All products containing protein, fat, carbohydrate, vitamin, electrolytes, trace elements are nutritionally complete and are designed to be used by pts for long periods.

COMPLICATIONS

MECHANICAL: Usually associated w/some aspect of the feeding tube.

Aspiration pneumonia: Caused by delayed gastric emptying, gastroparesis, gastroesophageal reflux, or decreased gag reflex. May be prevented or treated by reducing infusion rate, using lower fat formula, feeding beyond pylorus, checking residuals, using small bore feeding tubes, elevating head of bed 30-45° during and for 30-60 min after intermittent feeding, and regularly checking tube placement.

Esophageal, mucosal, pharyngeal irritation, otitis: Caused by using large bore NG tube. Prevented by use of small bore whenever possible.

Irritation, leakage at ostomy site: Caused by drainage of digestive juices from site. Prevented by close attention to skin/stoma care.

Tube, lumen obstruction: Caused by thickened formula residue, formation of formula-medication complexes. Prevented by frequently irrigating tube w/clear water (also before and after giving formulas/medication), avoiding instilling medication if possible.

GASTROINTESTINAL: Usually associated w/formula, rate of delivery, unsanitary handling of solutions or delivery system.

Diarrhea: Caused by low-residue formulas, rapid delivery, use of hyperosmolar formula, hypoalbuminemia, malabsorption, microbial contamination or rapid GI transit time. Prevented by using fiber-supplemented formulas, decreasing rate of delivery, using dilute formula and gradually increasing strength.

Cramping, gas, abdominal distention: Caused by nutrient malabsorption, rapid delivery of refrigerated formula. Prevented by delivering formula by continuous methods, giving formulas at room temperature, decreasing rate of delivery.

Nausea, vomiting: Caused by rapid delivery of formula, gastric retention. Prevented by reducing rate of delivery, using dilute formulas, selecting low-fat formulas.

Constipation: Caused by inadequate fluid intake, reduced bulk, inactivity. Prevented by supplementing fluid intake, using fiber-supplemented formula, encouraging ambulation.

METABOLIC: Fluid/electrolyte status should be monitored. Refer to monitoring section below. Additionally, the very young and very old are at greater risk in developing complications such as dehydration or overhydration.

MONITORING

Daily: Estimate nutrient intake, fluid intake/output, weight of pt, clinical observations.

Weekly: Electrolytes (potassium, sodium, magnesium, calcium, phosphorus), blood glucose, BUN, creatinine, liver function tests (e.g., SGOT (AST), alkaline phosphatase), 24 hour urea and creatinine excretion, total iron binding capacity (TIBC) or serum transferrin, triglycerides, cholesterol.

Monthly: Serum ablumin.

Other: Urine glucose, acetone (when blood glucose >250), vital signs (temperature, respirations, pulse, B/P) q8h.

nutrition: parenteral

Parenteral nutrition (PN), also known as total parenteral nutrition (TPN) or hyperalimentation (HAL), provides required nutrients to pts by IV route of administration. The goal of PN is to maintain or restore nutritional status caused by disease, injury, or inability to consume nutrients by other means.

INDICATIONS

Conditions when pt is unable to use alimentary tract via oral, gastrostomy, or jejunostomy routes. Impaired absorption of protein caused by obstruction, inflammation, or antineoplastic therapy. Bowel rest necessary because of GI surgery or ileus, fistulas, or anastomotic leaks. Conditions w/increased metabolic requirements (e.g., burns, infection, trauma). Preserve tissue reserves as in acute renal failure. Inadequate nutrition from tube feeding methods.

COMPONENTS OF PN

In order to meet IV nutritional requirements there are six essential categories in PN needed for tissue synthesis and energy balance.

Protein: In the form of crystalline amino acids (CAA), primarily used for protein synthesis. Several products are designed to meet specific needs for pts w/renal failure (e.g., NephrAmine), liver disease (e.g., HepatAmine), stress/trauma (e.g., Aminosyn HBC), use in neonates and pediatrics (e.g., Aminosyn PF, TrophAmine). Calories: 4 kcal/Gm protein.

Energy: In the form of dextrose, available in concentrations of 5 to 70%. Dextrose <10% may be given peripherally; concentrations >10% must be given centrally. Calories: 3.4 kcal/Gm dextrose.

IV fat emulsion: Available in the form of 10 or 20% concentrations. Provides a concentrated source of energy/calories (9 kcal/Gm fat) and is a source of essential fatty acids. May be administered peripherally or centrally.

Electrolytes: Major electrolytes (calcium, magnesium, potassium, sodium; also acetate, chloride, phosphate). Doses of electrolytes are individualized, based on many factors (e.g., kidney and/or liver function, fluid status).

Vitamins: Essential components in maintaining metabolism and cellular function, vitamins are widely used in PN.

Trace elements: Necessary in long-term PN administration. Trace elements include: zinc, copper, chromium, manganese, selenium, molybdenum, and iodine.

Miscellaneous: Additives include insulin, albumin, heparin and histamine$_2$ blockers (e.g., cimetidine, rantidine, famotidine). Other medication may be included, but compatibility for admixture should be checked on an individual basis.

ROUTE OF ADMINISTRATION

PN is administered via either peripheral or central vein.

Peripheral: Usually involves 2-3 liters/day of 5-10% dextrose w/3-5% amino acid solution along w/IV fat emulsion. Electrolytes, vitamins, trace elements added according to pt needs. Peripheral solutions provide about 2000 kcal/day and 60-90 Gm protein/day. **ADVANTAGES:** Lower risks vs central mode of administration. **DISADVANTAGES:** Peripheral veins may not be suitable (especially in pts w/illness of long duration); more susceptible to phlebitis (due to osmolalities >600 mOsm/L); veins may be viable only 1-2 wks; large volumes of fluid are needed to meet nutritional requirements which may be contraindicated in many pts.

Central: Usually utilizes hypertonic dextrose (concentration range of 15-35%) and amino acid solution of 3-7% w/IV fat emulsion. Electrolytes, vitamins, trace elements added according to pt needs. Central solutions provide 2000-4000 kcal/day. Must be given through large central vein w/high blood flow allowing rapid dilution avoiding phlebitis/thrombosis (usually through percutaneous insertion of catheter into subclavian vein then advancement of catheter to superior vena cava). **ADVANTAGES:** Allows more alternatives/flexibility in establishing regimens; allows ability to provide full nutritional requirements w/o need of daily fat emulsion; useful in pts who are fluid restricted (increased concentration), pts needing large nutritional requirements (e.g., trauma, malignancy), or for whom PN indicated >7-10 days. **DISADVANTAGES:** Risk w/insertion, use, maintenance of central line; increased risk of infection, catheter-induced trauma, and metabolic changes.

MONITORING

May vary slightly from institution to institution.

Baseline: CBC, platelet count, prothrombin time, weight, body length/head circumference (in infants), electrolytes, glucose, BUN, creatinine, uric acid, total protein, cholesterol, triglycerides, bilirubin, alkaline phosphatase, LDH, SGOT (AST), albumin, other tests as needed.

Daily: Weight, vital signs (TPR), nutritional intake (kcal, protein, fat), electrolytes (potassium, sodium, chloride), glucose (serum, urine), acetone, BUN, osmolarity, other tests as needed.

2-3 times/week: CBC, coagulation studies (PT, PTT), creatinine, calcium, magnesium, phosphorus, acid-base status, other tests as needed.

Weekly: Nitrogen balance, total protein, albumin, prealbumin, transferrin, liver function tests (SGOT [AST], SGPT [ALT]), alkaline phosphatase, LDH, bilirubin, Hgb, uric acid, cholesterol, triglycerides, other tests as needed.

COMPLICATIONS

Mechanical: Malfunction in system for IV delivery (e.g., pump failure, problems w/lines, tubing, administration sets, catheter). Pneumothorax, catheter misdirection, arterial puncture, bleeding, hematoma formation may occur w/catheter placement.

Infectious: Infections (pts often more susceptible to infections), catheter sepsis (e.g., fever, shaking chills, glucose intolerance) where no other site of infection identified.

Metabolic: Includes hyperglycemia, elevated cholesterol and triglycerides, abnormal liver function tests.

Fluid, electrolyte, acid-base disturbances: May alter potassium, sodium, phosphate, magnesium levels.

Nutritional: Clinical effects seen may be due to lack of adequate vitamins, trace elements, essential fatty acids.

opioid antagonists

ACTION

Prevents/reverses effects of mu receptor opioid agonists (e.g., increases respiration, reverses sedative effect).

USES

Primarily used to reverse respiratory depression induced by narcotic overdosage. Naloxone is the drug of choice for reversal of respiratory depression.

PRECAUTIONS

CONTRAINDICATIONS: Respiratory depression due to other than narcotic analgesics, hypersensitivity, narcotic dependency, pregnancy, lactation, severe hepatic dysfunction. **CAUTION:** Obstetric and surgical pts should be monitored carefully for bleeding. Care in pts w/cardiac irritability.

INTERACTIONS

Reverses opioid effects. Causes withdrawal symptoms in narcotic-dependent pts.

SIDE EFFECTS

Reduce or eliminate analgesia. Nausea, vomiting, increase in sweating.

TOXIC EFFECTS/ADVERSE REACTIONS

Hypertension, tachycardia. Withdrawal symptoms when administered to pts dependent on narcotics; general achiness, runny nose, restlessness and irritability, insomnia, anorexia, nausea, and vomiting.

NURSING IMPLICATIONS

GENERAL: Have resuscitative equipment immediately available, as well as the antagonist agent. **INTERVENTION/EVALUATION:** Monitor respirations carefully after antagonist is given (naloxone is not as long-acting as some narcotics and dose may have to be repeated). Check B/P and pulse. Be alert to return of pain when narcotic action is reversed. May cause withdrawal symptoms in narcotic-dependent pts.

opioid analgesics

ACTION

Opioids refer to all drugs, natural and synthetic, having actions similar to morphine and to receptors combining w/these agents. Three opioid receptors have been identified: mu, kappa, and delta. Morphine-like opioid agonists act primarily at mu receptors; and opioid w/mixed action are agonists at some receptors, antagonists/weak agonists at other receptors.

Morphine-like: Major effects are on the CNS (produce analgesia, drowsiness, mood changes, mental clouding, analgesia w/o loss of consciousness, nausea and vomiting) and gastrointestinal tract (decrease HCl secretion, diminish biliary, pancreatic, and intestinal secretions; diminish propulsive peristalsis). Also affects respiration (depressed) and cardiovascular system (peripheral vasodilation, decrease peripheral resistance, inhibit baroreceptor reflexes).

Opioids w/mixed action: After binding to receptor, may produce no effect or only limited action. Produce analgesia, euphoria, respiratory

OPIOID ANALGESICS

Generic (Brand) Names	Equianalgesic to 10 mg IM Morphine	Type	Analgesic Effect: Onset	Peak	Duration	Dosage Range
Alfentanil (Alfenta)	—	Agonist	Immediate	—	—	—
Buprenorphine (Buprenex)	IM: 0.3 mg	Mixed	15 min	1 hr	6 hrs	IM, IV: 0.3 mg q6h prn
Butorphanol (Stadol)	IM: 2 mg	Mixed	<10 min	0.5-1 hr	2-4 hrs	IM: 2 mg q3-4h prn IV: 1 mg q3-4h prn
Codeine	PO: 200 mg IM: 120 mg	Agonist	10-30 min	0.5-1 hr	4-6 hrs	PO, SubQ, IM: Adult: 15-60 mg q4-6h prn Children: 0.5 mg/kg q4-6h prn
Dezocine (Dalgan)	IM: 10 mg	Mixed	15-30 min	30-150 min	2-4 hrs	IM: 5-20 mg q3-6h prn IV: 2.5-10 mg q2-4h prn
Fentanyl (Sublimaze)	IM: 0.1 mg	Agonist	7-8 min	—	1-2 hrs	—
Hydrocodone	—	Agonist	—	—	4-8 hrs	—
Hydromorphone (Dilaudid)	PO: 7.5 mg IM: 1.5 mg	Agonist	15-30 min	0.5-1 hr	4-5 hrs	PO: 2 mg q4-6h prn SubQ, IM: 1-2 mg q4-6h prn Rectal: 3 mg q6-8h prn
Levorphanol (Levo-dromoran)	IM: 2 mg	Agonist	0.5-1.5 hr	0.5-1 hr	6-8 hrs	SubQ: 2-3 mg q4h prn
Meperidine (Demerol)	PO: 300 mg IM: 75 mg	Agonist	10-45 min	0.5-1 hr	2-4 hrs	PO, IM, SubQ: Adult: 50-150 mg q3-4h prn Children: 1-1.8 mg/kg q3-4h prn
Methadone (Dolophine)	PO: 20 mg IM: 10 mg	Agonist	30-60 min	0.5-1 hr	4-6 hrs	IM, SubQ, PO: 2.5-10 mg q4h prn
Morphine (Roxanol, MS Contin)	PO: 60 mg	Agonist	15-60 min	0.5-1 hr	3-7 hrs	PO: 10-30 mg q4h prn IM: 5-20 mg q4h prn

OPIOID ANALGESICS *Continued*

Generic (Brand) Names	Equianalgesic to 10 mg IM Morphine	Type	Analgesic Effect Onset	Peak	Duration	Dosage Range
Nalbuphine (Nubain)	IM: 10 mg	Mixed	2-15 min	0.5-1 hr	3-6 hrs	SubQ, IM, IV: 10 mg q3-6h prn
Oxycodone (Roxicodone)	PO: 30 mg	Agonist	15-30 min	1 hr	4-6 hrs	PO: 5 mg or 5 ml q6h prn
Oxymorphone (Numorphan)	IM: 1 mg RTL: 10 mg	Agonist	5-10 min	0.5-1 hr	3-6 hrs	SubQ, IM: 1-1.5 mg q4h prn Rectal: 5 mg q4h prn
Pentazocine (Talwin)	PO: 180 mg IM: 60 mg	Mixed	PO: 15-30 min IM: 15-20 min IV: 2-3 min	1-3 hrs 15-60 min —	3 hrs 3 hrs 3 hrs	PO: 50-100 mg q3-4h prn IM, SubQ, IV: 30 mg q3-4h prn
Propoxyphene (Darvon)	—	Agonist	30-60 min	2-2.5 hrs	4-6 hrs	PO: 100 mg q4h prn
Sufentanil (Sufenta)	IM: 0.02 mg	Agonist	1.3-3 hrs	—	—	IV: 1-2 mcg/kg

and physical depression, have lower abuse potential, may produce withdrawal symptoms in pts w/opioid dependence.

USES

Relief of moderate to severe pain associated w/surgical procedures, myocardial infarction, burns, cancer, or other conditions. May be used as an adjunct to anesthesia, either as a preop medication or intraoperatively as a supplement to anesthesia. Also used for obstetrical analgesia. Codeine and hydrocodone have an antitussive effect. Opium tinctures, such as paregoric, are used for severe diarrhea. Methadone relieves severe pain but is used primarily as part of heroin detoxification.

PRECAUTIONS

CONTRAINDICATIONS: Hypersensitivity, pregnancy or lactation, infants, diarrhea caused by poisoning, respiratory depression, asthma, emphysema, convulsive disorders, severe renal or hepatic dysfunction, prostatic hypertrophy, acute ulcerative colitis, increased intracranial pressure. **CAUTIONS:** Pediatric, geriatric, and debilitated pts may be more susceptible to effects. Caution when using for obstetrical analgesia to prevent respiratory depression in neonate. Respiratory depression is a concern in the severely obese. Care when administered to pts in shock or w/reduced blood volume.

INTERACTIONS

Any of the CNS depressants, including alcohol, potentiate effects. Combination w/MAO inhibitors or administration within 14 days of MAO inhibitors may potentiate effects of either agent. Death has resulted from interactions of the above. There is increased muscle relaxation and respiratory depression w/skeletal muscle relaxants. A few of the narcotics have both agonist and antagonist actions; when administered to pts who have been receiving or abusing narcotics, withdrawal symptoms may develop. Narcotic antagonists are given to reverse respiratory depression of narcotic analgesics.

SIDE EFFECTS

Lightheadedness, dizziness, orthostatic hypotension, drowsiness, constipation.

TOXIC EFFECTS/ADVERSE REACTIONS

Respiratory depression, which can lead to respiratory arrest; bradycardia; hypotension; urinary retention/oliguria; CNS depression w/ slurred speech, dulled mental responses, or stupor. May have converse excitation reaction w/euphoria and tremors. Hypersensitivity may be evidenced by rash, itching, sneezing. Tolerance, physical and/or psychological dependence may develop.

NURSING IMPLICATIONS

GENERAL: When administering intravenously, dilute and give slowly to prevent severe CNS depression and possible cardiac arrest. Give narcotic before pain is intense to break the pain cycle. Maintain appropriate records (most of these are schedule II drugs). **BASELINE ASSESSMENT:** Determine initial B/P, pulse, respirations. Assess pain for type, location, intensity. **INTERVENTION/EVALUATION:** Assess response to pain medication. Monitor B/P, pulse, respirations. Maintain I&O; be alert to decreased urination. Avoid constipation. **PATIENT/FAMILY TEACHING:** Do not smoke (may cause hypoxemia, respiratory depression). Physical and/or mental abilities may be impaired. Do not ambulate w/o assistance; do not drive or engage in activities requiring mental acuity. Refrain from alcohol or other medications. Drug dependence is not likely for short-term medical purposes.

oxytocics

ACTION

Oxytocins (Pitocin, Syntocinon) stimulate frequency/force of contraction of uterine smooth muscle. Responsiveness of uterus increases closer to term. Stimulates breast (contracting of myoepithelial cells surrounding mammary gland) to release milk.

USES

To induce, augment labor when maternal or fetal medical need exists; control of postpartum hemorrhage; cause uterine contraction after cesarean section or during other uterine surgery; induce therapeutic abortion.

PRECAUTIONS

CONTRAINDICATIONS: Hypersensitivity, cephalopelvic disproportions, unfavorable fetal position, fetal distress when delivery is not immediate, prolapsed cord or indication for surgical intervention. Methylergonovine should not be given to hypertensive pts or in toxemia or pregnancy. Ergonovine is used for postpartum hemorrhage and is contraindicated for labor induction. **CAUTIONS:** Pts >35 yrs of age; heart disease, hypertension; renal or hepatic dysfunction; sepsis.

INTERACTIONS

Caudal block anesthetics, vasopressors may increase pressor effects. Other oxytocics may cause uterine hypertonus, uterine rupture or cervical lacerations.

SIDE EFFECTS

Nausea or vomiting.

TOXIC EFFECTS/ADVERSE REACTIONS

Arrhythmias, increased bleeding, uterine hypertonicity, hypotension, water intoxication, anaphylactic reaction. Fetus may develop bradycardia, hypoxia and experience trauma from too rapid birth. Peripheral ischemia, severe hypertension w/ergonovine, methylergonovine.

NURSING IMPLICATIONS

GENERAL: Regulate infusions precisely. **BASELINE ASSESSMENT:** Determine initial maternal B/P, pulse, fetal heart rate. **INTERVENTION/EVALUATION:** Monitor fetal heart rate, maternal B/P and pulse, uterine contractions (duration, strength, frequency) every 15 min. Notify physician of contractions that exceed 1 min; occur more frequently than every 2 min, or stop. Maintain careful I&O; be alert to potential water intoxication. For postpartum hemorrhage: check uterus for firmness, amount of vaginal bleeding, vital signs. Evaluate extremities for warmth, color, movement, pain. **PATIENT/FAMILY TEACHING:** Keep pt, family informed of labor progress. Postpartum: Avoid smoking (added vasoconstriction).

sedative-hypnotics

ACTION

Sedatives decrease activity, moderate excitement, and have calming effects. Hypnotics produce drowsiness, enhance onset/maintenance of sleep (resembling natural sleep). Benzodiazepines are the most widely used agents (largely replace barbiturates): Greater safety, lower incidence of drug dependence. Benzodiazepines potentiate gamma-aminobutyric acid, which inhibits impulse transmission in the CNS reticular formation in brain. Benzodiazepines decrease sleep latency, number of awakenings and time spent in awake stage of sleep; increases total sleep time. Schedule IV drugs. See individual monographs for barbiturates.

USES

Treatment of insomnia, e.g., difficulty falling asleep initially, frequent awakening, awakening too early. For preop sedation.

PRECAUTIONS

CONTRAINDICATIONS: Hypersensitivity. Respiratory depression; respiratory diseases, porphyria, severe renal or hepatic dysfunction, history of alcohol or drug abuse, pregnancy, lactation, children. **CAUTIONS:** Elderly are more sensitive to adverse effects.

INTERACTIONS

Alcohol, narcotic analgesics, and other CNS depressants cause further CNS depressive effects. Combination w/CNS depressants should be avoided when possible.

SIDE EFFECTS

Drowsiness, dizziness, hangover, rebound insomnia due to altered REM, non-REM sleep stages.

TOXIC EFFECTS/ADVERSE REACTIONS

Hypersensitivity reactions: Rash, urticaria. Confusion, extreme drowsiness, diarrhea. Paradoxical excitation may occur, particularly in the elderly. Overdose: Respiratory depression, pulmonary edema, tachycardia and palpitations, marked hypotension, renal and hepatic damage, anoxia, cardiac collapse may proceed to coma and death. Potential for drug abuse and dependence, esp. w/barbiturates.

NURSING IMPLICATIONS

GENERAL: Provide environment conducive to sleep and pain relief. Put side rails up, lower bed, and put call light within reach. Assist in identifying cause of insomnia and encourage pt not to depend on medication. Comply w/federal narcotic laws regarding schedule IV drugs. Consider

HYPNOTICS

Generic Name	Brand Name(s)	Dosage Range
estazolam	ProSom	Adults: 1-2 mg before hs Elderly, Debilitated: 0.5-1 mg at hs
flurazepam	Dalmane	Adults: 15-30 mg before hs Elderly, Debilitated: Initially 15 mg, then based on pt response
quazepam	Doral	Adults: Initially 15 mg, may decrease to 7.5 mg in some pts Elderly, Debilitated: Initially 15 mg, then attempt to decrease dose after 1-2 nights
temazepam	Restoril	Adults: 15-30 mg before hs Elderly, Debilitated: Initially 15 mg, then based on pt response
triazolam	Halcion	Adults: 0.125-0.5 mg before hs Elderly, Debilitated: Initially 0.125 mg until response determined. Range: 0.125-0.25 mg
zolpidem	Ambien	Adults: 10 mg immediately before bedtime Elderly: 5 mg immediately before bedtime

hs, bedtime.

potential for abuse, dependence. Narcotics may need to be reduced when given w/hypnotics. **BASELINE ASSESSMENT:** Determine initial B/P, pulse, respirations, and sleep pattern. **INTERVENTION/EVALUATION:** Assure that pt has swallowed oral medication. Assess response to medication, sleep pattern. Monitor B/P, pulse, and respirations. **PATIENT/FAMILY TEACHING:** Instruct pt not to smoke or get up alone after taking hypnotic. Drowsiness may continue into next day; avoid driving or activities requiring mental acuity until response to drug controlled. Avoid alcohol. Consult physician before taking other medications. Take only as directed; do not increase dosage or abruptly discontinue (possible rebound insomnia).

skeletal muscle relaxants

ACTION

Centrally acting muscle relaxants: Exact mechanism unknown. May act in CNS at various levels to depress polysynaptic reflexes; sedative effect may be responsible for relaxation of muscle spasm.

Baclofen and diazepam: May mimic actions of gamma-aminobutyric acid on spinal neurons; do not directly affect skeletal muscles.

Dantrolene: Acts directly on skeletal muscle relieving spasticity.

SKELETAL MUSCLE RELAXANTS

GENERIC NAME	BRAND NAMES(S)	DOSAGE RANGE
baclofen	Lioresal	Adults: 40-80 mg/kg/day
carisoprodol	Rela Soma	Adults: 350 mg 4 × /day
chlorzoxazone	Parafon Forte DSC	Adults: 250-750 mg 3-4 × /day Children: 125-500 mg 3-4 × /day
cyclobenzaprine	Flexeril	Adults: 10 mg 3 × /day
dantrolene	Dantrium	Adults: 25 mg/day initially, gradually increase to 400 mg/day or less
diazepam	Valium	Adults: 2-10 mg 3-4 × /day Elderly: 2-2.5 mg initially, gradually increase Children: 1-2.5 mg 3-4 × /day
methocarbamol	Robaxin	Adults: 500-1000 mg 4 × /day
orphenadrine	Norflex	Adults: 100 mg morning and evening

USES

Central acting muscle relaxants: Adjunct to rest, physical therapy for relief of discomfort associated w/acute, painful musculoskeletal disorders, i.e., local spasms from muscle injury.

Baclofen, dantrolene, diazepam: Treatment of spasticity characterized by heightened muscle tone, spasm, loss of dexterity caused by multiple sclerosis, cerebral palsy, spinal cord lesions, stroke.

PRECAUTIONS

CONTRAINDICATIONS: Pregnancy, lactation, cross-sensitivity, CNS depression, renal or hepatic dysfunction, children <12 yrs of age. According to specific drug. **CAUTIONS:** Cautious use in pts w/cardiac disease; history of allergy, epilepsy.

INTERACTIONS

Alcohol, narcotic analgesics, sedatives, hynotics, and other CNS depressants may increase CNS effects (e.g., drowsiness, dizziness, fatigue).

SIDE EFFECTS

Drowsiness, orthostatic hypotension, w/dizziness and lightheadedness, nausea or vomiting, stomach cramps, headache, constipation, blurred vision.

TOXIC EFFECTS/ADVERSE REACTIONS

Hypersensitivity reactions. Severe hypotension, tachycardia, blood dyscrasias, GI bleeding, unusual muscle weakness, hepatotoxicity.

NURSING IMPLICATIONS

Provide supportive measures, e.g., bedrest, positioning, exercise, moist heat as indicated. Withdraw drugs slowly. **BASELINE ASSESSMENT:** Determine degree of immobility. Assess pain (type, location, intensity). **INTERVENTION/EVALUATION:** Monitor B/P, pulse, respirations. Assess for therapeutic response (increased mobility and decreased pain). **PATIENT/FAMILY TEACHING:** Administer on schedule to maintain blood levels. Avoid alcohol and consult physician before taking other medications. Do not drive or engage in activities requiring mental acuity (drowsiness, dizziness). Prolonged use may cause dependence.

sympathomimetics

ACTION

Sympathetic nervous system (SNS) is involved in maintaining homeostasis (involved in regulation of heart rate, force of cardiac contractions, B/P, bronchial airway tone, carbohydrate, fatty acid metabolism). The SNS is mediated by neurotransmitters (primarily norepinephrine, epinephrine, and dopamine), which act on adrenergic receptors. These receptors include $beta_1$, $beta_2$, $alpha_1$, $alpha_2$, and dopaminergic. Sympathomimetics differ widely in their actions based on their specificity to affect these receptors. Actions expected by stimulating these receptors include:

$Alpha_1$: Mydriasis, constriction of arterioles, veins.

$Alpha_2$: Inhibits transmitter release.

$Beta_1$: Increases rate, force of contraction, conduction velocity of heart, releases renin from kidney.

$Beta_2$: Dilates arterioles, bronchi, relaxes uterus.

Dopamine: dilates kidney vasculature.

USES

Stimulation of $alpha_1$-receptors: Induces vasoconstriction primarily in skin and mucous membranes; nasal decongestion; combine w/local anesthetics to delay anesthetic absorption; increases B/P in certain hypotensive states; produces mydriasis, facilitating eye exams, ocular surgery.

Stimulation of $alpha_2$-receptors: No therapeutic use.

Stimulation of $beta_1$-receptors: Treatment of cardiac arrest (not primary); treatment of heart failure, shock, AV block (temporary only).

Stimulation of $beta_2$-receptors: Treatment of asthma; delays premature labor.

Stimulation of dopamine receptors: Treatment of shock.

SYMPATHOMIMETICS

Generic Name	Brand Name(s)	Receptor Specificity	Primary Clinical Use
albuterol	Proventil Ventolin	$Beta_2$	Bronchodilator
bitolterol	Tornalate	$Beta_2$	Bronchodilator
dobutamine	Dobutrex	$Beta_1$ $Beta_2$ $Alpha_1$	Inotropic support in pts w/cardiac decompensation
dopamine	Intropin	$Beta_1$ $Alpha_1$ Dopaminergic	Cardiogenic, septic shock Pressor agent
epinephrine	Adrenalin Sus-phrine	$Beta_1$ $Beta_2$ $Alpha_1$	Allergic reaction Bronchodilator Local vasoconstriction (w/anesthetics)
isoetharine	Bronkosol	$Beta_2$	Bronchodilator
isoproterenol	Isuprel	$Beta_1$ $Beta_2$	Heart rate stimulator in bradycardia, heart block Vasopressor in shock Bronchodilator
metaproterenol	Alupent	$Beta_2$	Bronchodilator
metaraminol	Aramine	$Beta_1$ $Alpha_1$	Pressor in acute hypotensive states
norepinephrine	Levophed	$Beta_1$ $Alpha_1$	Pressor in acute hypotensive states
phenylephrine	Neo-synephrine	$Alpha_1$	Arterial vasoconstrictor Nasal decongestant Mydriatic
ritodrine	Yutopar	$Beta_2$	Arrest premature labor
terbutaline	Brethine Bricanyl	$Beta_2$	Bronchodilator

PRECAUTIONS

CONTRAINDICATIONS: Hyperthyroidism, hypertension, cardiovascular disease, narrow-angle glaucoma, Parkinson's disease, psychoneuroses, hypersensitivity. **CAUTIONS:** Diabetes mellitus, urinary tract obstructions, elderly, debilitated, infants and children. See individual monograph for pregnancy, lactation precautions.

INTERACTIONS

Monoamine oxidase (MAO) inhibitors are contraindicated; in combination w/adrenergics, potentiated effects can cause hypertensive crisis, intracranial hemorrhage, and death. Effects of MAO inhibitors may last 3 wks after discontinuation. General anesthetics may increase risk of arrhythmias. Tricyclic antidepressants, maprotiline may increase cardiovascular effects. Norepinephrine may decrease effect of methyldopa.

May have mutually inhibitory effects w/beta-adrenergic blockers. May increase risk of arrhythmias w/digoxin. Ergonovine, oxytocin may increase vasoconstriction. Numerous agents interact with adrenergics and each monograph should be reviewed individually.

SIDE EFFECTS

Palpitations, nervousness, restlessness, sweating, difficulty urinating, headache.

TOXIC EFFECTS/ADVERSE REACTIONS

Nausea and vomiting, tachycardia, pale/cold skin, difficulty breathing, significant increase or decrease in B/P. *Rare:* chest pain and irregular heartbeat.

NURSING IMPLICATIONS

GENERAL: Immediately obtain IV access in cardiac arrest or other emergency. When infusions indicated, pt should be in intensive care unit w/cardiac monitor. Infuse titrate carefully; use infusion pumps for accurate delivery. **INTERVENTION/EVALUATION:** Monitor vital signs frequently, blood gases, electrolytes, renal and hepatic function results. Assess multiorgan response. **PATIENT/FAMILY TEACHING:** Measures to prevent recurrence when given for asthma, COPD such as avoidance of respiratory infection, prevention of allergen exposure, increased hydration.

thyroid

ACTION

Thyroid hormone (T_4 [thyroxine] and T_3 [triiodothyroxine]) are essential for normal growth, development, and energy metabolism. *Promotes growth/development:* Controls DNA transcription and protein synthesis. Necessary in development of nervous system. *Stimulates energy use:* Increases basal metabolic rate (increase O_2 consumption, heat production). *Cardiovascular:* Stimulates heart by increased rate, force of contraction, cardiac output.

USES

Treatment of primary or secondary hypothyroidism, myxedema, cretinism, or simple goiter.

PRECAUTIONS

THYROID

Generic Name	Brand Names(s)	$T_4:T_3$ Ratio	Dosage Equivalent
levothyroxine	Synthroid	T_4 only	50-60 mcg
liothyronine	Cytomel	T_3 only	15-37.7 mcg
liotrix	Thyrolar	4:1	50-60 mcg T_4 12.5-15 mcg T_3
thyroglobulin	Proloid	2.5:1	65 mg
thyroid	Thyroid	2.5:1	65 mg

who have hypertension, cardiac disease, renal insufficiency, diabetes mellitus or are on anticoagulant therapy.

INTERACTIONS

May alter oral anticoagulant effects. Cholestyramine, colestipol may decrease absorption. Sympathomimetics may increase effects, coronary insufficiency.

SIDE EFFECTS

Most reactions are due to excessive dosage w/signs, symptoms of hyperthyroidism: Weight loss, palpitations, increased appetite, tremors, nervousness, tachycardia, increased B/P, headache, insomnia, menstrual irregularities.

TOXIC EFFECTS/ADVERSE REACTIONS

Hypersensitivity reactions; cardiac arrhythmias, possibly death due to cardiac failure.

NURSING IMPLICATIONS

Children need very close monitoring; dosage needs to be higher for growing child. **BASELINE ASSESSMENT:** Check B/P and pulse, weight. **INTERVENTION/EVALUATION:** Monitor pulse for rate, rhythm; notify physician of pulse above 100/min or irregular. Check weight daily; assess food intake. Observe for tremors, nervousness, insomnia. **PATIENT/FAMILY TEACHING:** Do not stop taking medication; generally lifelong therapy. Take medication at the same time each day, preferably in the morning. Teach correct method of taking pulse; check pulse before taking medication, esp. when dosage adjusted. Notify physician of resting pulse that is markedly increased, irregular, 100/min or above. Important to remain under medical supervision, have periodic lab tests. Children may have reversible hair loss, increased aggressiveness during first few months of therapy. Do not take other medications w/o consulting physician. Notify physician promptly of chest pain, weight loss, tremors, insomnia.

Appendix A
COMMONLY USED ABBREVIATIONS

ac—before meals
ACE—angiotensin converting enzyme
ANC—absolute neutrophil count
bid—twice daily
B/P—blood pressure
BSA—body surface area
CBC—complete blood count
Ccr—creatinine clearance
CHF—congestive heart failure
Cl—chloride
CNS—central nervous system
CO—cardiac output
COPD—chronic obstructive pulmonary disease
dL—deciliter
DNA—desoxyribonucleic acid
ECG or EKG—electrocardiogram
EEG—electroencephalogram
esp.—especially
GI—gastrointestinal
Gm—gram
gtt—drop
GU—genitourinary
Hct—hematocrit
h or hr—hour
Hgb—hemoglobin
hs—bedtime
HTN—hypertension
IM—intramuscular
IV—intravenous
K—potassium
kg—kilogram
L—liter
lbs—pounds
LOC—level of consciousness
MAO—monoamine oxidase
m^2—meter squared
mcg—microgram
mEq—milliequivalent
mg—milligram
MI—myocardial infarction
min—minute
ml—milliliter
mo—month
Na—sodium
NaCl—sodium chloride
NSAIDs—nonsteroidal anti-inflammatory drugs
oz—ounce
OD—right eye
OS—left eye
OU—both eyes
pc—after meals
PO—orally, by mouth
prn—as needed
pt—patient
qid—four times daily
qd—daily
qOd—every other day
REM—rapid eye movements
RBC—red blood cell count
RNA—ribonucleic acid
sec—second
SubQ—subcutaneous
SL—sublingual
tid—three times daily
tbs—tablespoon
TPR—temperature, pulse, respirations
tsp—teaspoonful
U—unit
w/—with
w/o—without
WBC—white blood cell count
wk(s)—week, weeks
yr(s)—year, years

Appendix B
BIBLIOGRAPHY

American Hospital Formulary Service Drug Information 94. Bethesda, Md: American Society of Hospital Pharmacists, 1994.

Behrman RE (ed.): *Nelson Textbook of Pediatrics,* 14th ed. Philadelphia: WB Saunders Company, 1992.

Davis J, Sherer K: *Applied Nutrition and Diet Therapy for Nurses.* Philadelphia: WB Saunders Company, 1994.

Drug Facts and Comparisons. St. Louis: JB Lippincott Company, 1995.

Gilman AG, Rall TW, Nies AS, Taylor P (eds.): *Goodman and Gilman's The Pharmacological Basis of Therapeutics,* 8th ed. New York: Pergamon Press, 1990.

Hansten PD, Horn JR: *Drug Interactions,* 7th ed. Philadelphia: Lea & Febiger, 1994.

Johnson GE, Hannah KJ: *Pharmacology and the Nursing Process,* 3rd ed. Philadelphia: WB Saunders Company, 1992.

Lehne RA, Crosby LJ, Hamilton DB, Moore LA (eds.): *Pharmacology for Nursing Care.* Philadelphia: WB Saunders Company, 1994.

Selma TP, Beizer JL, Higbee MD: *Geriatric Dosage Handbook.* Washington, DC: American Pharmaceutical Association, 1993.

United States Pharmacopeia Dispensing Information (USPDI): Drug Information for the Health Care Professional. Rockville, Md: US Pharmacopeial Convention, Inc, 1993, 1994.

Wyngaarden JB, Smith Jr. LD, Bennett JC (eds.): *Cecil Textbook of Medicine,* 19th ed. Philadelphia: WB Saunders Company, 1992.

Appendix C
CALCULATION OF DOSES

Frequently, dosages ordered do not correspond exactly to what is available and must therefore be calculated.

Ratio/proportions: Most important in setting up this calculation is that the units of measure are the same on both sides of the equation.

Problem: Pt A is to receive 65 mg of a medication only available in an 80 mg/2 ml vial. What volume (ml) needs to be administered to the pt?

STEP 1: Set up ratio.

$$\frac{80\text{ mg}}{2\text{ ml}} = \frac{65\text{ mg}}{x(\text{ml})}$$

STEP 2: Cross multiply.

$$(80\text{ mg})(x\text{ ml}) = (65\text{ mg})(2\text{ ml})$$
$$80\,x = 130$$

STEP 3: Divide each side of equation by number with x.

$$\frac{80\,x}{80} = \frac{130}{80}$$

STEP 4: Volume to be administered for correct dose.

$$x = 130/80 \text{ or } 1.625\text{ ml}$$

Calculations in micrograms/kilogram per minute: Frequently, medications given by IV infusion are ordered as micrograms/kilogram per minute.

Problem: 63-year-old pt (weight 165 lbs) is to receive Medication A at a rate of 8 micrograms/kilogram per minute (mcg/kg/min). Given a solution containing Medication A in a concentration of 500 mg/250 ml, at what rate (ml/hr) would you infuse this medication?

STEP 1: Convert to same units. In this problem, the dose is expressed in mcg/kg, therefore convert pt weight to kg (1 kg = 2.2 lbs) and drug concentration to mcg (1 mg = 1,000 mcg).

$$165 \text{ lbs} \times \frac{1 \text{ kg}}{2.2 \text{ lbs}} = \frac{165 \text{ kg}}{2.2} = 75 \text{ kg}$$

$$\frac{500 \text{ mg}}{250 \text{ ml}} \text{ or } \frac{2 \text{ mg}}{\text{ml}} \times \frac{1{,}000 \text{ mcg}}{1 \text{ mg}} = \frac{2{,}000 \text{ mcg}}{1 \text{ ml}} \text{ or } \frac{1 \text{ ml}}{2{,}000 \text{ mcg}}$$

STEP 2: Number of micrograms per minute (mcg/min).

$$\frac{8 \text{ mcg}}{\text{kg}} \times 75 \text{ kg (pt wt)} = \frac{600 \text{ mcg}}{1 \text{ min}} \text{ or } \frac{1 \text{ min}}{600 \text{ mcg}}$$

STEP 3: Number of milliliters per minute (ml/min).

$$\frac{600 \text{ mcg}}{1 \text{ min}} \times \frac{1 \text{ ml}}{2{,}000 \text{ mcg}} = \frac{600 \text{ (ml)}}{2{,}000 \text{ (min)}} = \frac{0.3 \text{ ml}}{\text{min}}$$

STEP 4: Number of milliliters per hour (ml/hr).

$$\frac{0.3 \text{ ml}}{\text{min}} \times \frac{60 \text{ min}}{1 \text{ hr}} = \frac{18 \text{ ml}}{\text{hr}}$$

STEP 5: If the number of drops per minute (gtts/min) were desired, and if the IV set delivered 60 drops per milliliter (gtts/ml) (varies with IV set, information provided by manufacturer), then:

$$\frac{0.3 \text{ ml}}{\text{min}} \times \frac{60 \text{ drops}}{\text{ml}} = \frac{18 \text{ drops}}{\text{min}}$$

Appendix D
CONTROLLED DRUGS

CANADA

Schedule F: Medication requiring a prescription (e.g., antibiotics, antihypertensives)

Schedule G: Medication having mood-modifying effects, may be habit forming; also requires a prescription (e.g., amphetamines).

Narcotics: Have potent psychotropic, addictive properties. Includes derivatives of coca leaves (e.g., cocaine), opiates, and opium derivatives (e.g., morphine).

Schedule H: Substances having no recognized medicinal properties, possess hallucinogenic properties (e.g., LSD).

UNITED STATES

Schedule I: Medication with high abuse potential, no medical use in United States (e.g., heroin, LSD).

Schedule II: Medication with high potential for abuse with currently accepted medical use (e.g., morphine, cocaine).

Schedule III: Medications with accepted medical use and lower potential for abuse than schedule I or II (e.g., nonbarbiturate sedatives).

Schedule IV: Medication with lower abuse potential than schedules I, II, or III with limited physical or psychological dependence (e.g., some sedatives, antianxiety agents).

Schedule V: Lowest abuse potential, primarily small amounts of narcotics (e.g., codeine).

Appendix E
NORMAL LABORATORY VALUES

HEMATOLOGY/COAGULATION

Test	Specimen	Normal Range
Activated partial thromboplastin time (APTT)	Whole blood	25-35 sec
Erythrocyte count (RBC count)	Whole blood	M: 4.3-5.7 million cells/mm^3 F: 3.8-5.1 million cells/mm^3
Hematocrit (HCT, Hct)	Whole blood	M: 39-49% F: 35-45%
Hemoglobin (Hb, Hgb)	Whole blood	M: 13.5-17.5 Gm/dL F: 12.0-16.0 Gm/dL
Leucocyte count (WBC count)	Whole blood	4.5-11.0 thousand cells/mm^3
Leucocyte differential count	Whole blood	
Basophils		0-0.75%
Eosinophils		1-3%
Lymphocytes		23-33%
Monocytes		3-7%
Neutrophils—bands		3-5%
Neutrophils—segmented		54-62%
Mean corpuscular hemoglobin (MCH)	Whole blood	26-34 pg/cell
Mean corpuscular hemoglobin concentration (MCHC)	Whole blood	31-37% Hb/cell
Mean corpuscular volume (MCV)	Whole blood	80-100 fL
Partial thromboplastin time (PTT)	Whole blood	60-85 sec
Platelet count (thrombocyte count)	Whole blood	150-450 thousand/mm^3
Prothrombin time (PT)	Whole blood	11-13.5 sec
RBC count (see Erythrocyte count)		

SERUM/URINE VALUES

Test	Specimen	Normal Range
Alanine aminotransferase (ALT, SGPT)	Serum	0-55 U/L
Albumin	Serum	3.5-5.0 Gm/dL
Alkaline phosphatase	Serum	M: 53-128 U/L F: 42-98 U/L
Anion gap	Plasma or serum	5-14 mEq/L
Aspartate aminotransferase (AST, SGOT)	Serum	0-50 U/L
Bilirubin (total)	Serum	0.2-1.2 mg/dL
Bilirubin (conjugated direct)	Serum	0-0.4 mg/dL
Calcium (total)	Serum	8.4-10.2 mg/dL

Carbon dioxide (CO_2) total	Plasma or serum	20-34 mEq/L
Chloride	Plasma or serum	96-112 mEq/L
Cholesterol (total)	Plasma or serum	<200 mg/dL
C-Reactive protein	Serum	68-8200 ng/mL
Creatine kinase (CK)	Serum	M: 38-174 U/L F: 26-140 U/L
Creatine kinase isoenzymes	Serum	Fraction of total: <0.04-0.06
Creatinine	Plasma or serum	M: 0.7-1.3 mg/dL F: 0.6-1.1 mg/dL
Creatinine clearance	Plasma or serum and urine	M: 90-139 mL/min/1.73m^2 F: 80-125 mL/min/1.73m^2
Free thyroxine index (FTI)	Serum	1.1-4.8
Glucose	Serum	Adults: 70-105 mg/dL >60 yrs: 80-115 mg/dL
Hemoglobin A_{1c}	Whole blood	5.6-7.5% of total Hgb
Homovanillic acid (HVA)	Urine, 24 hr	1.4-8.8 mg/day
17-Hydroxycorticosteroids (17-OHCS)	Urine, 24 hr	M: 3.0-10.0 mg/day F: 2.0-8.0 mg/day
Iron	Serum	M: 65-175 mcg/dL F: 50-170 mcg/dL
Iron binding capacity, total (TIBC)	Serum	250-450 mcg/dL
Lactate dehydrogenase (LDH)	Serum	0-250 U/L
Magnesium	Serum	1.3-2.3 mg/dL
Oxygen (Po_2)	Whole blood, arterial	83-100 mm Hg
Oxygen saturation	Whole blood, arterial	95-98%
pH	Whole blood, arterial	7.35-7.45
Phosphorus, inorganic	Serum	2.7-4.5 mg/dL
Potassium	Serum	3.5-5.1 mEq/L
Protein (total)	Serum	6.0-8.5 Gm/dL
Sodium	Plasma or serum	136-146 mEq/L
Specific gravity	Urine	1.002-1.030
Thyrotropin (hTSH)	Plasma or serum	2-10 μU/mL
Thyroxine (T_4) total	Serum	5-12 mcg/dL
Triglycerides (TG)	Serum, after 12 hr fast	20-190 mg/dL
Triiodothyronine resin uptake test (T_3RU)	Serum	22-37%
Urea nitrogen	Plasma or serum	7-25 mg/dL
Urea nitrogen/creatinine ratio	Serum	12/1-20/1
Uric acid	Serum	M: 3.5-7.2 mg/dL F: 2.6-6.0 mg/dL
Vanillylmandelic acid (VMA)	Urine, 24 hr	2-7 mg/day

Appendix F
FDA PREGNANCY CATEGORIES

A: No demonstrated risk to the fetus in any trimester of pregnancy.

B: No demonstrated risk to the fetus in animal studies, no human studies available in pregnant women.

OR

Animal studies have shown adverse effects but human studies with pregnant women have not demonstrated risk to the fetus in any trimester of pregnancy.

C: Animal studies show adverse effect on fetus but no adequate studies in humans; benefits from drug during pregnancy may outweigh risks.

OR

No animal reproduction studies and no adequate human studies.

D: Definite human fetal risks but benefits of use in pregnant women may be acceptable despite risks.

X: Animal and human studies show fetal abnormalities or adverse reaction indicating risk to fetus. Risk of use in pregnant women clearly outweighs benefits.

Appendix G

SIGNS AND SYMPTOMS OF TOXIC EFFECTS/ ADVERSE REACTIONS

HYPOGLYCEMIA (excessive insulin):
Tremulousness, cold/clammy skin, mental confusion, rapid/shallow respirations, unusual fatigue, hunger, drowsiness, anxiety, headache, muscular incoordination, paresthesia of tongue/mouth/lips, hallucinations, increased pulse/blood pressure, tachycardia, seizures, coma.

HYPERGLYCEMIA (insufficient insulin):
Hot/flushed/dry skin, fruity breath odor, excessive urination (polyuria), excessive thirst (polydipsia), acute fatigue, air hunger, deep/labored respirations, mental changes, restlessness, nausea, polyphagia (excessive appetite).

HYPOKALEMIA (serum potassium level <3.5 mEq/L):
Weakness/paresthesia of extremities, muscle cramps, nausea, vomiting, diarrhea, hypoactive bowel sounds, absent bowel sounds (paralytic ileus), abdominal distention, weak/irregular pulse, postural hypotension, difficulty breathing, disorientation, irritability.

HYPERKALEMIA (serum potassium level >5.0 mEq/L):
Diarrhea, muscle weakness, heaviness of legs, paresthesia of tongue/hands/feet, slow/irregular pulse, decreased blood pressure, abdominal cramps, oliguria/anuria, respiratory difficulty, cardiac abnormalities.

HYPONATREMIA (plasma Na level <130 mEq/L):
Abdominal cramping, nausea, vomiting, diarrhea, cold/clammy skin, poor skin turgor, tremulousness, muscle weakness, leg cramps, increased pulse rate, irritability, apprehension, hypotension, headache.

HYPERNATREMIA (plasma Na level >150 mEq/L):
Hot/flushed/dry skin, dry mucous membranes, fever, extreme thirst, dry/rough/red tongue, edema, restlessness, postural hypotension, oliguria.

DEHYDRATION:
Poor skin turgor, dry mucous membranes, thirst, flushed/dry skin, sunken eye sockets/darkening of skin under eyes (adults), sunken fontanelle (infants) rapid respirations, increased pulse rate, longitudinal furrows in tongue, decreased blood pressure, postural hypotension, oliguria/anuria, urine specific gravity greater than 1.030.

SUPERINFECTION:
Fever, diarrhea, ulceration (white patches) on mucous membranes of

mouth, inflammation of tongue (glossitis), black furry tongue, anogenital itching, vaginal itching/discharge.

STOMATITIS:
Redness/burning of oral mucous membranes, inflammation of gums (gingivitis), inflammation of tongue (glossitis), difficulty swallowing, ulceration of oral mucosa.

CONGESTIVE HEART FAILURE:
Dyspnea, cough, distended neck veins, fatigue with exertion, orthopnea, cool extremities, nail bed cyanosis, peripheral edema, weight gain, rales at base of lungs, wheezing, rust-colored/brown-tinged sputum.

BONE MARROW DEPRESSION (IMMUNOSUPPRESSION):
Fever, chills, sore throat, increased pulse rate, cloudy/foul smelling urine, urgency/burning/increased frequency of urination, white blood cells/bacteria in urine, redness/irritation of oral mucous membranes, redness/swelling/draining at injection sites/cuts, easy bruising/bleeding, perineal/rectal pain, vaginal/rectal discharge.

Appendix H

RATES OF INTERMITTENT IV (PIGGYBACK) ADMINISTRATION

Generic Name	Brand Name(s)	Compatibility 0.9% NaCl	Compatibility 5% Dextrose	Usual Infusion Time
acyclovir	Zovirax	YES	YES	At least 1 hr
amikacin	Amkin	YES	YES	Adults, children: 30-60 min Infants: 1-2 hrs
amphotericin	Fungizone	NO	YES	2-6 hrs
ampicillin	Polycillin	YES	YES	15-30 min
ampicillin/ sulbactam	Unasyn	YES	YES	15-30 min
aztreonam	Azactam	YES	YES	20-60 min
cefamandole	Mandol	YES	YES	15-30 min
cefazolin	Ancef Kefzol	YES	YES	15-30 min
cefmetrazole	Zefazone	YES		10-60 min
cefonicid	Monocid	YES	YES	20-30 min
cefoperazone	Cefobid	YES	YES	15-30 min
cefotaxime	Claforan	YES	YES	20-30 min
cefotetan	Cefotan	YES	YES	20-30 min
cefoxitin	Mefoxin	YES	YES	15-30 min
ceftazidime	Fortaz Tazidime	YES	YES	15-30 min
ceftizoxime	Cefizox	YES	YES	15-30 min
ceftriaxone	Rocephin	YES	YES	Adults: 15-30 min Children: 10-30 min
cefuroxime	Zinacef	YES	YES	15-60 min
cephalothin	Keflin	YES	YES	15-30 min
cephapirin	Cefadyl	YES	YES	15-30 min
cephradine	Velosef	YES	YES	15-30 min
chloramphenicol	Chloromycetin	YES	YES	15-30 min
cimetidine	Tagamet	YES	YES	15-20 min
ciprofloxacin	Cipro	YES	YES	60 min
clindamycin	Cleocin	YES	YES	300-600 mg: 10-20 min 900 mg-1.2 Gm: 30-40 min
doxycycline	Vibramycin	YES	YES	1-4 hrs
erythromycin	Erythrocin	YES	YES	20-60 min
famotidine	Pepcid	YES	YES	15-30 min
fluconazole	Diflucan	—	YES	200 mg/hr
glanciclovir	Cytovene	YES	YES	1 hour
gentamicin	Garamycin	YES	YES	30-120 min
granisetron	Kytril	YES	YES	5 min
hydrocortisone	Solu-Cortef	YES	YES	15-30 min

imipenem cilastatin	Primaxin	YES	YES	250-500 mg: 20-30 min 1 Gm: 40-60 min
methicillin	Staphcillin	YES	YES	30-120 min
methyl-prednisolone	Solu-Medrol	YES	YES	15-30 min
metoclopramide	Reglan	YES	YES	15-30 min
metronidazole	Flagyl	YES	YES	30 min
mezlocillin	Mezlin	YES	YES	30 min
miconazole	Monistat IV	YES	YES	30-60 min
minocycline	Minocin	YES	YES	6 hours
nafcillin	Nafcil Unipen	YES	YES	30-60 min
netilmicin	Netromycin	YES	YES	30-120 min
ofloxacin	Floxin	YES	YES	60 min
ondansetron	Zofran	YES	YES	15 min
penicillin G	Pfizerpen	YES	YES	Adults: 1-2 hrs Children: 15-30 minutes
pentamidine	Pent AM 300	YES	YES	At least 1 hour
piperacillin	Pipracil	YES	YES	30 min
piperacillin/ tazobactam	Zosyn	YES	YES	30 min
ranitidine	Zantac	YES	YES	15-20 min
rifampin	Rifadin	YES	YES	100 mg/30 min 500 mg/3 hrs
ticarcillin	Ticar	YES	YES	Adults: 30-120 min Neonates: 10-20 min
ticarcillin/ clavulanate	Timentin	YES	YES	30 min
tobramycin	Nebcin	YES	YES	20-60 min
trimethoprim/ sulfamethoxazole	Bactrim, Septra	NO	YES	60-90 min
vancomycin	Vancocin	YES	YES	At least 1 hour
vidarabine	Vira-A	YES	YES	12-24 hrs
zidovudine	Retrovir	—	YES	Over 60 min

NOTE: Compatibility information of medications to large volume parenterals or admixture with other medications is beyond the scope of this chart. Refer inquiries to the Pharmacy Department or Drug Information Centers.

INDEX

INDEX

Generic drugs appear in boldface type; U.S. trade names are in regular type, Canadian trade names appear in small caps, and classifications are in lower case italics. Italicized page numbers indicate the page in the classification section on which the drug is listed.

Generic drugs appear in boldface type; U.S. trade names are in regular type, Canadian trade names appear in small caps, and classifications are in lower case italics. Italicized page numbers indicate the page in the classification section on which the drug is listed.

Generic drugs appear in boldface type; U.S. trade names are in regular type, Canadian trade names appear in small caps, and classifications are in lower case italics. Italicized page numbers indicate the page in the classification section on which the drug is listed.

Generic drugs appear in boldface type; U.S. trade names are in regular type, Canadian trade names appear in small caps, and classifications are in lower case italics. Italicized page numbers indicate the page in the classification section on which the drug is listed.

Generic drugs appear in boldface type; U.S. trade names are in regular type, Canadian trade names appear in small caps, and classifications are in lower case italics. Italicized page numbers indicate the page in the classification section on which the drug is listed.

Generic drugs appear in boldface type; U.S. trade names are in regular type, Canadian trade names appear in small caps, and classifications are in lower case italics. Italicized page numbers indicate the page in the classification section on which the drug is listed.

Generic drugs appear in boldface type; U.S. trade names are in regular type, Canadian trade names appear in small caps, and classifications are in lower case italics. Italicized page numbers indicate the page in the classification section on which the drug is listed.

Generic drugs appear in boldface type; U.S. trade names are in regular type, Canadian trade names appear in small caps, and classifications are in lower case italics. Italicized page numbers indicate the page in the classification section on which the drug is listed.

Generic drugs appear in boldface type; U.S. trade names are in regular type, Canadian trade names appear in small caps, and classifications are in lower case italics. Italicized page numbers indicate the page in the classification section on which the drug is listed.

Generic drugs appear in boldface type; U.S. trade names are in regular type, Canadian trade names appear in small caps, and classifications are in lower case italics. Italicized page numbers indicate the page in the classification section on which the drug is listed.

Generic drugs appear in boldface type; U.S. trade names are in regular type, Canadian trade names appear in small caps, and classifications are in lower case italics. Italicized page numbers indicate the page in the classification section on which the drug is listed.

Generic drugs appear in boldface type; U.S. trade names are in regular type, Canadian trade names appear in small caps, and classifications are in lower case italics. Italicized page numbers indicate the page in the classification section on which the drug is listed.

Generic drugs appear in boldface type; U.S. trade names are in regular type, Canadian trade names appear in small caps, and classifications are in lower case italics. Italicized page numbers indicate the page in the classification section on which the drug is listed.

Generic drugs appear in boldface type; U.S. trade names are in regular type, Canadian trade names appear in small caps, and classifications are in lower case italics. Italicized page numbers indicate the page in the classification section on which the drug is listed.

Generic drugs appear in boldface type; U.S. trade names are in regular type, Canadian trade names appear in small caps, and classifications are in lower case italics. Italicized page numbers indicate the page in the classification section on which the drug is listed.

Generic drugs appear in boldface type; U.S. trade names are in regular type, Canadian trade names appear in small caps, and classifications are in lower case italics. Italicized page numbers indicate the page in the classification section on which the drug is listed.

Generic drugs appear in boldface type; U.S. trade names are in regular type, Canadian trade names appear in small caps, and classifications are in lower case italics. Italicized page numbers indicate the page in the classification section on which the drug is listed.

LATEST DRUG SUPPLEMENT

ACITRETIN
ALENDRONATE
APROTININ
BUDESONIDE
CALCIPOTRIENE
CELIPROLOL
CETIRIZINE
CILAZAPRIL
CYSTEAMINE
BITRATRATE
DALTEPARIN
DORZOLAMIDE
FAMCICLOVIR
FENOFIBRATE
FLEROXACIN
FLUTICASONE
FLUVOXAMINE
IMIGLUCERASE
LAMOTRIGINE
LANSOPRAZOLE
LOSARTAN
METFORMIN
NALTREXONE
NEFAZODONE
PEGASPARGASE
(PEG-L ASPARAGINASE)
PERINDOPRIL
PREDNICARBATE
RIMEXOLONE
SPIRAPRIL
STAVUDINE (d4T)
TACROLIMUS
TEICOPLANIN
TIRILAZAD
TRAMADOL
TRIMETREXATE
VALACYCLOVIR
VIGABATRIN
VINORELBINE

acitretin

ah-sa-tree'tin
(Soriatane)

CLASSIFICATION

Antipsoriatic

ACTION

Exact mechanism unknown. Possesses immunomodulating and anti-inflammatory effects. May inhibit polymorphonuclear accumulation in stratum corneum, inhibit lymphocytic blastogenesis, and stimulate T-cell–mediated cytotoxicity.

USES

Treatment of psoriasis (reduces severity of scaling, erythema, and epidural induration and percent of body surface involvement).

INDICATIONS/DOSAGE/ROUTES

Psoriasis:
PO: Adults, elderly: 30-50 mg/day. **Range:** 10-75 mg/day.

SIDE EFFECTS

FREQUENT: Drying of eyes/nose/lips, cheilitis, desquamation of palms/soles. Alopecia, nail abnormalities, pruritus, fatigue. **OCCASIONAL:** Nausea, headache, sweating, chills, sensation of cold.

alendronate

ah-len'droo-nate
(Fosamax)

CLASSIFICATION

Bone resorption inhibitor, calcium regulator

ACTION

Binds to hydroxyapatite crystals, inhibiting their formation/dissolution (prevents soft tissue calcification, may inhibit normal calcification). Primary effect is inhibition of bone resorption at doses without retarding mineralization (corrects hypercalcemia / hypercalciuria, decreases pain/occurrences of fractures).

USES

Treatment of hypercalcemia of malignancy, Paget's disease, hypertrophic ossification; prevention of osteoporosis in postmenopausal women.

INDICATIONS/DOSAGE/ROUTES

Postmenopausal (osteoporosis):
PO: Adults, elderly: 5 mg/day.

Malignant hypercalcemia:
IV: Adults, elderly: 10 mg as single dose infused over 2-24 hrs.

Paget's disease:
IV: Adults, elderly: 10 mg daily for 5 days, infused over 1 hr.

SIDE EFFECTS

OCCASIONAL: *IV:* Mild fever, transient lymphopenia, serum transaminase elevation.

aprotinin

ah-pro'teh-nin
(Trasylol)

CLASSIFICATION

Hemostatic

ACTION

Inhibits fibrinolysis, turnover of coagulation factors and decreases bleeding. A protease inhibitor, inhibits plasmin and kallikrein (inhibiting fibrinolysis), inhibits contact phase activation of coagulation, preserves adhesive glycoproteins in platelet membrane (resistant to damage from increased plasmin levels, mechanical injury).

USES

Reduce blood loss and need for blood transfusions in pts undergoing cardiopulmonary bypass in repeat coronary artery bypass graft (CABG) surgery and in primary CABG surgery in pts w/high risk of bleeding (e.g., impaired hemostasis) or where access to blood is unavailable or unacceptable.

INDICATIONS/DOSAGE/ROUTES

Hemostatic
IV: Adults, elderly: 1-2 million kIU, then 1-2 million kIU into pump prime volume, then IV infusion of 250,000-500,000 kIU/hr of operation.

SIDE EFFECTS

NOTE: Side effects reported are seen in open heart surgery and not necessarily due to aprotinin.
FREQUENT: Atrial fibrillation, myocardial infarction, heart failure, atrial flutter. **OCCASIONAL:** Ventricular tachycardia, supraventricular tachycardia, hypotension, pneumonia, respiratory disorder, kidney failure, sepsis, apnea, confusion.

budesonide

bew-deh'sew-nide
(Rhinocort)

CLASSIFICATION

Corticosteroid

ACTION

Exact mechanism unknown. Decreases immediate and late-phase allergic reactions. Reduces influx of inflammatory cells.

USES

Relief of symptoms of seasonal/perennial allergic rhinitis (adults, children) and nonallergic perennial rhinitis (adults only).

INDICATIONS/DOSAGE/ROUTES

NOTE: Each spray = 32 mcg budesonide.

Seasonal/perennial allergic rhinitis:
INTRANASAL: Adults, elderly, children >6 yrs: Initially, two sprays in each nostril in morning and evening or four sprays each nostril in morning. After desired clinical effect is obtained, decrease dose gradually q2-4wks to lowest effective dose.

Nonallergic perennial rhinitis:
INTRANASAL: Adults, elderly: Same as above.

SIDE EFFECTS

FREQUENT: Mild nasopharyngeal irritation, pharyngitis, increased cough, burning, stinging, headache, dryness. **OCCASIONAL:** Dry mouth, dyspepsia.

calcipotriene

cal-sip'oh-try-ene
(Dovonex)

CLASSIFICATION

Antipsoriatic

ACTION

Synthetic vitamin D_3 analog regulates skin cell production/development. (Scaly red patches of psoriasis caused by abnormal growth/production of skin cells known as keratinocytes.)

USES

Treatment of moderate plaque psoriasis.

INDICATIONS/DOSAGE/ROUTES

Psoriasis:
TOPICAL: Adults, elderly: Apply thin layer two times/day to affected areas (rub in gently, completely).

SIDE EFFECTS

FREQUENT: Burning, itching, skin irritation. **OCCASIONAL:** Dermatitis, dry skin, erythema, peeling, rash, worsening of psoriasis.

celiprolol

cell-ih-pro'loll
(Selecor)

CLASSIFICATION

Beta-adrenergic blocker

ACTION

Selectively blocks $beta_1$-adrenergic receptors, slowing sinus heart rate, decreasing cardiac output, decreasing B/P. Decreases myocardial ischemia severity by decreasing oxygen requirements. Possesses some $beta_2$ activity (vasodilation/bronchodilation) and intrinsic sympathomimetic activity.

USES

Management of hypertension alone or in combination w/other medication. Management of chronic stable angina.

INDICATIONS/DOSAGE/ROUTES

Hypertension:
PO: Adults, elderly: 200-500 mg/day as single dose.

Angina:
PO: Adults, elderly: 300-600 mg/day.

SIDE EFFECTS

FREQUENT: Nausea, diarrhea, abdominal discomfort, headache, fatigue, dizziness. **OCCASIONAL:** Insomnia, Raynaud's phenomena, orthostatic hypotension, bronchial obstruction, tremor, rash, muscle cramps, impotence.

cetirizine

seh-tear'ih-zeen
(Reactine)

CLASSIFICATION

Antihistamine

ACTION

Inhibits histamine release and eosinophil chemotaxis during secondary phase of allergic response, reduces inflammatory cell infiltration in late phase allergic response, inhibits release of cytotoxic mediators of inflammatory response from platelets.

USES

Treatment of seasonal and perennial allergic rhinitis and chronic idiopathic urticaria.

INDICATIONS/DOSAGE/ROUTES

Allergic rhinitis, urticaria:
PO: Adults, elderly: 5-10 mg/day. May increase up to 20 mg/day.

SIDE EFFECTS

FREQUENT: Somnolence, sedation, headache, dry mouth, fatigue. **OCCASIONAL:** Nausea, vomiting.

cilazapril

sigh-lay'zah-prill
(Inhibace)

CLASSIFICATION

Angiotensin converting enzyme (ACE) inhibitor

ACTION

Suppresses renin-angiotensin-aldosterone system (prevents conversion of angiotensin I to angiotensin II, a potent vasoconstrictor; may inhibit angiotensin II at local vascular, renal sites). Decreases plasma angiotensin II; increases plasma renin activity; decreases aldosterone secretion. In hypertension, reduces peripheral arterial resistance. In CHF, increases cardiac output and decreases peripheral vascular resistance, B/P, pulmonary capillary wedge pressure, pulmonary vascular resistance.

USES

Treatment of hypertension alone or in combination w/other antihypertensives. Adjunctive therapy for management of CHF.

INDICATIONS/DOSAGE/ROUTES

Hypertension:
PO: Adults, elderly: 2.5-5 mg/day as single dose.

Heart failure:
PO: Adults, elderly: 10 mg/day as single dose.

SIDE EFFECTS

FREQUENT: Headache, dizziness, fatigue, cough. **OCCASIONAL:** Chest pain, skin rash, somnolence, taste disturbances.

cysteamine bitartrate

sis-tea'ah-mean
(Cystagon)

CLASSIFICATION

Urinary tract: Cystine depletor

ACTION

Cystine-depleting agent, lowering cystine content of cells in pts w/cystinosis (an autosomal recessive inborn error of metabolism: abnormal transport of cystine out of lysosomes). Nephropathic form (accumulation of cystine, crystal formation) may lead to organ damage (esp. kidney, producing end-stage renal failure).

USES

Management of nephropathic cystinosis in adults and children.

INDICATIONS/DOSAGE/ROUTES

Nephropathic cystinosis:
PO: Adults, elderly, children: Initially, ¼-⅙ maintenance dose gradually increased over 4-6 wks. **Maintenance:** *Adults, children*

>12 yrs, >49.5 kg: 2 Gm/day in 4 divided doses. *Children (up to 12 yrs):* 1.3 Gm/m^2/day given in 4 divided doses. **NOTE:** Do not give intact capsule to children 6 yrs or less. Sprinkle capsule over food.

SIDE EFFECTS

FREQUENT: Vomiting, anorexia, fever, diarrhea, lethargy, rash. **OCCASIONAL:** Nausea, abdominal pain, dyspepsia, ataxia, confusion, dizziness, nervousness.

dalteparin

dall-teh-pear'inn
(Fragmin)

CLASSIFICATION

Anticoagulant

ACTION

Contains antithrombin III. Also binds antithrombin III, accelerating natural function of antithrombin III (inhibition of factor Xa and thrombin).

USES

Prevention of postop deep vein thrombosis (DVT).

INDICATIONS/DOSAGE/ROUTES

Prevention of DVT:
SubQ: Adults, elderly: 200 IU/kg once daily or 100 IU/kg q12h.

SIDE EFFECTS

OCCASIONAL: Mild, local skin irritation, pain, erythema at injection site. **RARE:** Skin necrosis, increased liver enzymes.

dorzolamide

door-zoll'ah-mide
(TruSopt)

CLASSIFICATION

Carbonic anhydrase inhibitor

ACTION

Reduces intraocular pressure (IOP) by inhibiting carbonic anhydrase in ciliary processes of eye, decreasing secretion of aqueous humor. Exact mechanism unknown. May slow formation of bicarbonate ions, reducing sodium and fluid transport.

USES

Treatment of psoriasis (reduces severity of scaling, erythema, and epidural induration and percent of body surface involvement).

INDICATIONS/DOSAGE/ROUTES

Reduction of IOP:
OPHTHALMIC: Adults, elderly: 1 drop in affected eye 3 times/day.

SIDE EFFECTS

FREQUENT: Ocular burning, stinging, discomfort immediately after administration; bitter taste; superficial punctate keratitis; ocular allergic reactions. **OCCASIONAL:** Blurred vision, tearing, dryness, photophobia, headache, nausea, asthenia/fatigue.

famciclovir

fam-sigh'klo-veer
(Famvir)

CLASSIFICATION

Antiviral

ACTION

Converted to active compound penciclovir, a selective antiherpesvirus agent. Intracellularly, inhibits viral DNA polymerases and viral DNA synthesis.

USES

Management of acute herpes zoster (shingles).

INDICATIONS/DOSAGE/ROUTES

Acute herpes zoster (shingles):
PO: Adults, elderly: 500 mg q8h for 7 days.

Dosage in renal impairment:
Dosage is based on creatinine clearance.

CREATININE CLEARANCE (ML/MIN)	DOSAGE
≥60	500 mg q8h
40-59	500 mg q12h
20-39	500 mg q24h

SIDE EFFECTS

FREQUENT: Fatigue, nausea, diarrhea, headache. **OCCASIONAL:** Fever, vomiting, constipation, dizziness, pruritus.

fenofibrate

feen-oh-fi'brate
(Lipidil)

CLASSIFICATION

Antihyperlipoproteinemic

ACTION

Reduces plasma triglycerides (VLDL) concentration, increases HDL, may increase LDL. Exact mechanism unknown. May inhibit lipolysis of fat in adipose tissue, reduce liver extraction of free fatty acids reducing triglyceride production, or inhibit synthesis and clearance of VLDL carrier apolipoprotein B reducing VLDL production.

USES

Adjunct to diet in pts w/severe hypertriglyceridemia (types IV and V) at risk of pancreatitis and not responding to diet alone.

INDICATIONS/DOSAGE/ROUTES

Hypertriglyceridemia:
PO: Adults, elderly: Initially 100 mg/day w/meals. May increase up to 300 mg/day.

SIDE EFFECTS

FREQUENT: Upper gastrointestinal symptoms (e.g., dyspepsia, abdominal pain, nausea), cholesterol gallstones, muscular pain, painful extremities, myositis, myalgia, arthralgia.

fleroxacin

fleur-ox'ah-sin
(Megalone)

CLASSIFICATION

Anti-infective: quinolone

ACTION

Inhibits DNA gyrase in susceptible microorganisms, interfering w/bacterial DNA replication and repair. Bactericidal.

USES

Treatment of infections of urinary tract, skin and soft tissue, bone and joint, gastrointestinal tract and sexually transmitted diseases.

INDICATIONS/DOSAGE/ROUTES

Usual anti-infective dosage:
PO: Adults, elderly: 200-400 mg/day as single dose.

SIDE EFFECTS

FREQUENT: Nausea, vomiting, insomnia. **OCCASIONAL:** Diarrhea, constipation, headache, dizziness, fatigue, photosensitivity.

fluticasone

flew-tih-kay'sown
(Flonase)

CLASSIFICATION

Corticosteroid

ACTION

Exact mechanism unknown. May inhibit influx/activation of inflammatory cells, release of inflammatory mediators. Primarily has effect on late-phase allergic reactions.

USES

Management of seasonal and perennial allergic rhinitis in pts 12 yrs and older.

INDICATIONS/DOSAGE/ROUTES

Allergic rhinitis:
INTRANASAL: Adults, elderly: Initially, 200 mcg (2 sprays each nostril once daily or 1 spray each nostril q12h). **Maintenance:** 1 spray each nostril once daily. **Maximum:** 200 mcg/day. **Children, 12 yrs or older:** Initially, 100 mcg (1 spray each nostril once daily). **Maximum:** 200 mcg/day.

SIDE EFFECTS

FREQUENT: Mild nasopharyngeal irritation, burning, stinging, dryness, headache. **OCCASIONAL:** Rebound congestion, bronchial asthma, rhinorrhea, loss of sense of taste.

fluvoxamine

flu-vocks'ah-meen
(Luvox)

CLASSIFICATION

Antidepressant

ACTION

Selectively inhibits serotonin (5-HT) uptake in CNS enhancing serotonergic function.

USES

Treatment of depression, obsessive compulsive disorder (OCD).

INDICATIONS/DOSAGE/ROUTES

Depression, OCD:
PO: Adults, elderly: Initially, 50-100 mg/day (50 mg may decrease incidence of nausea). **Maintenance:** 100-300 mg/day.

SIDE EFFECTS

FREQUENT: Nausea, somnolence, asthenia, headache, dry mouth, insomnia. **OCCASIONAL:** Abdominal pain, dizziness, nervousness, tremor, vomiting, dyspepsia.

imiglucerase

im-ih-gloo'sir-ace
(Cerezyme)

CLASSIFICATION

Enzyme

ACTION

Analogue of enzyme β-glucocerebrosidase, which catalyzes hydrolysis of glycolipid glucocerebroside to glucose and ceramide.

USES

Treatment of Gaucher's disease (characterized by deficiency of β-glucocerebrosidase activity) results in accumulation of glucocerebrosidase in tissue macrophages becoming engorged. Secondary hematologic sequelae include severe anemia, thrombocytopenia, progressive hepatosplenomegaly, skeletal complications.

INDICATIONS/DOSAGE/ROUTES

Gaucher's disease:
IV INFUSION (over 1-2 hrs): Adults, elderly, children: Initially, 2.5 U/kg 3 times/wk up to 60 U/kg/wk. **Maintenance:** Progressive reduction in dosage while monitoring pt response.

SIDE EFFECTS

FREQUENT: Headache. **OCCASIONAL:** Nausea, abdominal discomfort, dizziness, pruritus, rash, small decrease in B/P or urinary frequency.

lamotrigine

lah-moe'tri-gene
(Lamictal)

CLASSIFICATION

Anticonvulsant

ACTION

Stabilizes neuronal membrane by blocking voltage-dependent sodium channels (prevents release of excitatory neurotransmitters).

USES

Add-on therapy for treatment of refractory partial seizures in adults.

INDICATIONS/DOSAGE/ROUTES

NOTE: Initiate therapy slowly (avoid rash).

Partial seizures:
PO: Adults, elderly: *(w/valproic acid only):* Initially, 50 mg/day, may increase by 50 mg q2wks. **Maintenance:** 100-200 mg/day as single dose. *W/only enzyme-inducing drugs (e.g., phenytoin, carbamazepine):* Initially, 25-50 mg 2 times/day, may increase by 100 mg every week. **Maintenance:** 400-500 mg/day in 2 divided doses. *W/both valproic acid and enzyme-inducing drugs:* Initially, 50 mg/day; may increase by 50 mg q2wks. **Maintenance:** 100-200 mg/day in 2 divided doses.

SIDE EFFECTS

FREQUENT: Dizziness, diplopia, ataxia, asthenia, somnolence, headache. **OCCASIONAL:** Nausea, vomiting, nystagmus, tremor, rash, abdominal pain, nervousness, irritability, confusion.

lansoprazole

lan-sew-prey'zoll
(Prevacid)

CLASSIFICATION

Gastric acid pump inhibitor

ACTION

Irreversibly binds to H^+/K^+ ATPase (an enzyme on surface of parietal cells). Inhibits H^+ transport into gastric lumen. Inhibits basal, stimulated gastric acid secretion regardless of stimulus.

USES

Short-term treatment of duodenal ulcers; treatment and maintenance treatment of reflux esophagitis; long-term treatment of hypersecretory conditions (e.g., Zollinger-Ellison syndrome).

INDICATIONS/DOSAGE/ROUTES

Duodenal ulcer:
PO: Adults, elderly: 30 mg/day up to 4 wks.

Reflux esophagitis:
PO: Adults, elderly: 30 mg/day.

Hypersecretory conditions:
PO: Adults, elderly: 60-120 mg/day as single dose or 2 divided doses.

SIDE EFFECTS

FREQUENT: Diarrhea, headache, nausea, abdominal pain, pharyngitis. **OCCASIONAL:** Anorexia, constipation, dizziness, tiredness.

losartan

low-sar'tan
(Cozaar)

CLASSIFICATION

Angiotensin II inhibitor

ACTION

Selectively inhibits angiotensin receptor subtype I (responsible for hypertensive, increased inotropic, sodium-retaining properties of angiotensin II).

USES

Treatment of hypertension either alone or in combination w/ other antihypertensives.

INDICATIONS/DOSAGE/ROUTES

Hypertension:
PO: Adults, elderly: Initially, 12.5 mg/day. Increase gradually over 2-4 wks. **Range:** 50-150 mg/day.

SIDE EFFECTS

OCCASIONAL: Hypotension.

metformin

met-fore'man
(Glucophage)

CLASSIFICATION

Hypoglycemic: Oral

ACTION

Exact mechanism unknown. May decrease gastrointestinal absorption of glucose, increase glucose uptake by muscle/adipose tissue, decrease hepatic glucose production, increase insulin production/action, increase peripheral utilization of glucose.

USES

Adjunct to diet/exercise in management of non–insulin-dependent diabetes mellitus (type II). May be used as monotherapy or in combination w/oral hypoglycemics or insulin.

INDICATIONS/DOSAGE/ROUTES

Diabetes mellitus:
PO: Adults, elderly: Initially, 500 mg/day. **Maintenance:** 500 mg 3 times/day or 850 mg 2 times/day. **Maximum:** 3000 mg/day in divided doses.

SIDE EFFECTS

FREQUENT: Anorexia, nausea, abdominal discomfort, diarrhea. **RARE:** Lactic acidosis (more common w/higher doses and in pts w/ kidney or liver disease, the elderly, alcoholics, or pts w/cardiorespiratory insufficiency.

naltrexone

nal-trecks'own
(Revia)

CLASSIFICATION

Opioid antagonist, alcohol deterrent

ACTION

Opioid antagonist: Blocks effects of opioids by competitively binding to opioid receptors. *Alcohol deterrent:* Exact mechanism unknown. Decreases craving, drinking days, relapse rate.

USES

Adjunct to maintenance opioid-free state in detoxified, formerly opioid-dependent individuals. Adjunct to treatment following alcohol detoxification in alcohol-dependent pts, esp. to prevent alcohol relapse.

INDICATIONS/DOSAGE/ROUTES

Opioid-free state:
PO: Adults, elderly: Initially, 25 mg; then 50 mg/day (may be given as 100 mg every other day or 150 mg q3day).

Adjunct in treatment of alcohol dependence:
PO: Adults, elderly: 50 mg/day.

SIDE EFFECTS

FREQUENT: Difficulty sleeping, anxiety, nervousness, headache, low energy, nausea, vomiting, joint/muscle pain, abdominal pain/ cramps. **OCCASIONAL:** Irritability, dizziness, loss of appetite, diarrhea, constipation, skin rash, chills, increased thirst.

nefazodone

neh-fay'zo-done
(Serzone)

CLASSIFICATION

Antidepressant

ACTION

Inhibits 5-HT (serotonin) re-uptake (increasing brain levels of serotonin), blocks a specific serotonin receptor in brain. Possesses minimal antihistaminic, anticholinergic, alpha-adrenergic, and sedative activity.

USES

Treatment of depression often w/psychotherapy.

INDICATIONS/DOSAGE/ROUTES

Depression:
PO: Adults, elderly: Initially, 200 mg/day in 2 divided doses. May increase after 1 wk based on clinical response.

SIDE EFFECTS

FREQUENT: Nausea, headache, drowsiness, asthenia, dizziness. **OCCASIONAL:** Insomnia, sexual dysfunction.

pegaspargase (PEG-L asparaginase)

peg-ah-spar'gase
(Oncaspar)

CLASSIFICATION

Antineoplastic

ACTION

Breaks down asparagine (required for cell survival [certain malignant cells are not able to synthesize, but normal cells can synthesize asparagine]). Interferes w/ protein synthesis, DNA, RNA synthesis. Cell-cycle specific for G_1 phase of cell division.

USES

Treatment of acute lymphoblastic leukemia (ALL) in combination w/other chemotherapeutic agents for pts requiring L-asparaginase but who have developed hypersensitivity to native forms of L-asparaginase.

INDICATIONS/DOSAGE/ROUTES

ALL:
IV/IM: Adults, elderly, children ≥0.6 m²: 2500 IU/m² q14days. **Children <0.6 m²:** 82.5 IU/kg q14 days.

SIDE EFFECTS

FREQUENT: Decrease in blood clotting factors, hepatotoxicity, pancreatitis, allergic reactions (trouble breathing, rash, itching, joint pain), nausea, vomiting, decreased weight, anorexia. **OCCASIONAL:** Confusion, drowsiness, unusual tiredness, swelling of feet, lower legs, stomatitis, lower back pain.

perindopril

pare-inn'doe-prill
(Aceon)

CLASSIFICATION

Angiotensin converting enzyme (ACE) inhibitor

ACTION

Suppresses renin-angiotensin-aldosterone system (prevents conversion of angiotensin I to angiotensin II, a potent vasoconstrictor). Lowers peripheral arterial resistance, mean diastolic/systolic B/P. Systolic B/P decrease results from reduction of total peripheral resistance. Reduces secretion of aldosterone.

USES

Treatment of essential hypertension alone or in combination w/ other antihypertensives, particularly thiazide diuretics.

INDICATIONS/DOSAGE/ROUTES

Hypertension:
PO: Adults, elderly: Initially, 2-4 mg/day. **Maintenance:** 2-8 mg/day as single or two divided doses. **Maximum:** 16 mg/day.

Dosage in renal impairment:
Dosage based on creatinine clearance.

Creatinine Clearance (mL/min)	Dosage
>60	4 mg/day
30-60	2 mg/day
15-30	2 mg every other day
<15	2 mg on day of dialysis

SIDE EFFECTS

FREQUENT: Cough (dry). **OC-**

CASIONAL: Dizziness, lightheadedness, rash, fever, joint pain, headache, diarrhea, loss of taste, unusual tiredness, upset stomach.

prednicarbate

pred-nih-car'bate
(Dermatop)

CLASSIFICATION

Corticosteroid: Topical

ACTION

Diffuses across cell membranes forming complexes w/cytoplasm. Complexes stimulate protein synthesis of inhibitory enzymes responsible for anti-inflammatory effects (e.g., inhibits edema, erythema, pruritus, capillary dilation, phagocytic activity).

USES

Provide relief of inflammation/pruritus associated w/corticosteroid responsive disorders.

INDICATIONS/DOSAGE/ROUTES

Usual topical dosage:
TOPICAL: Adults, elderly: Apply sparingly 2-4 times/day.

SIDE EFFECTS

FREQUENT: Contact dermatitis (burning/itching of skin), painful, red, itchy, pus-containing blisters, thinning of skin w/easy bruising, dryness, irritation, skin redness or scaling of skin lesions, skin rash.

rimexolone

rye-mecks'oh-loan
(Vexol)

CLASSIFICATION

Corticosteroid: Ophthalmic

ACTION

Exact mechanism unknown. May produce anti-inflammatory effect by potentiating epinephrine vasoconstriction, stabilize lysosomal membrane, retard macrophage movement, inhibit function of lymphocytes/neutrophils, inhibit prostaglandin synthesis.

USES

Symptomatic relief of inflammatory conditions of the conjunctiva, cornea, lid, anterior segment of the globe. Adjunct to prevent fibrosis, scarring, potential visual impairment from chemical, radiation, or thermal burns or penetration of foreign bodies.

INDICATIONS/DOSAGE/ROUTES

Usual ophthalmic dosage:
OPHTHALMIC: Adults, elderly: Instill 1-2 drops into conjunctival sac every hour during day and q2h at night. May decrease to 1 drop 3-4 times/day after 24-48 hrs of favorable response.

SIDE EFFECTS

FREQUENT: Temporary mild blurred vision, burning, stinging, redness, or watering of eyes.

spirapril

spy'rah-prill
(Renormax)

CLASSIFICATION

Angiotensin converting enzyme (ACE) inhibitor

ACTION

Suppresses renin-angiotensin-aldosterone system (prevents conversion of angiotensin I to angiotensin II, a potent vasoconstrictor; may inhibit angiotensin II at local vascular, renal sites). Decreases plasma angiotensin II, increases plasma renin activity, decreases aldosterone secretion. Reduces peripheral arterial resistance.

USES

Treatment of hypertension alone or in combination w/other antihypertensives.

INDICATIONS/DOSAGE/ROUTES

Hypertension:
PO: Adults, elderly: 6-24 mg/day as single dose.

SIDE EFFECTS

FREQUENT: Headache, dizziness, fatigue. **OCCASIONAL:** Rash, diarrhea, nausea, cough, loss of taste perception.

stavudine (d4T)

stay'view-deen
(Zerit)

CLASSIFICATION

Antiviral

ACTION

Inhibits viral reverse transcriptase interfering w/retrovirus replication.

USES

Management of HIV infection w/evidence of impaired immunity (decreased CD4 cell count).

INDICATIONS/DOSAGE/ROUTES

HIV infection:
PO: Adults 60 kg or greater: 20-40 mg 2 times/day. **Adults 40 to <60 kg:** 15-30 mg 2 times/day. **Adults <40 kg:** 10-20 mg 2 times/day.

SIDE EFFECTS

FREQUENT: Peripheral neuropathy (pain, burning, aching, weakness or pins and needles of extremities). **OCCASIONAL:** Fever, headache, infection, asthenia, Kaposi's sarcoma, lymphoma, increased CPK, confusion, pneumonia, dyspnea.

tacrolimus

tah-crow-lie'mus
(Prograf)

CLASSIFICATION

Immunosuppressant

ACTION

Inhibits T-lymphocyte activation. Binds to protein intracellularly forming a complex preventing generation of nuclear factor of activated T-cells.

USES

Prophylaxis of organ rejection in pts receiving allogenic liver transplants. Use concomitantly w/adrenal corticosteroids.

INDICATIONS/DOSAGE/ROUTES

Organ rejection prophylaxis:
IV INFUSION: Adults, children: 0.05-0.1 mg/kg/day beginning no sooner than 6 hrs after transplantation. Continue only until oral therapy tolerated.

PO: Adults, children: 0.15-0.3 mg/kg/day in two divided doses q12h. Give initial dose no sooner than 6 hrs after transplantation or 8-12 hrs after discontinuing the IV infusion.

SIDE EFFECTS

FREQUENT: Tremor, headache, diarrhea, hypertension, nausea, renal impairment, abdominal pain, fever, insomnia. **OCCASIONAL:** Paresthesia, constipation, vomiting, pruritus, back pain, peripheral edema.

teicoplanin

ty-co-plan'inn
(Targocid)

CLASSIFICATION

Antibiotic

ACTION

Bactericidal. Inhibits bacterial cell wall synthesis by binding to cell wall. May alter cell wall permeability, inhibit RNA synthesis.

USES

Treatment of infections caused by gram-positive organisms. Treatment of skin/soft tissue, septicemia, bone/joint, endocarditis, respiratory infections.

INDICATIONS/DOSAGE/ROUTES

NOTE: Reduce dosage in pts w/ renal impairment.

Infections:
IM/IV: Adults, elderly: Initially, 6 mg/kg q12h for 3 doses, then 6 mg/kg daily. **Children:** Initially, 10 mg/kg q12h for 3 doses, then 6-10 mg/kg daily.

SIDE EFFECTS

FREQUENT: Fatigue, headache, diarrhea, pain, redness, phlebitis, hypersensitivity, skin reactions, urticaria, pruritus, eosinophilia, neutropenia, increased platelet counts. **OCCASIONAL:** Nephrotoxicity, high-frequency hearing loss, bronchospasm.

tirilazad

tie-ril'ah-zad
(Freedox)

CLASSIFICATION

Antioxidant

ACTION

Blocks lipid peroxidation. Cytoprotective agent oxidizes peroxyl radicals and stabilizes cell membranes. Preserves membrane content of vitamin E (an antioxidant). Promotes tissue survival in vicinity of CNS injury.

USES

Prevention of progressive neuronal degeneration and associated complications after brain/spinal injury, subarachnoid hemorrhage, stroke.

INDICATIONS/DOSAGE/ROUTES

Prevention of neuronal degeneration:
IV INFUSION: Adults, elderly: Up to 6 mg/kg/day for 3 days.

SIDE EFFECTS

FREQUENT: Mild to moderate pain at injection site.

tramadol

tram-ah-dole′
(Ultram)

CLASSIFICATION

Opioid analgesic

ACTION

Alters processes affecting pain perception, emotional response to pain. Appears to primarily involve serotonergic and noradrenergic mechanisms. Potentiates activity of serotonin by competitive inhibition of neuronal serotonin uptake and stimulation of serotonin release. Also binds w/opioid receptors within CNS (low affinity).

USES

Relief of moderate pain (e.g., cancer, sports injuries, obstetrics).

INDICATIONS/DOSAGE/ROUTES

Analgesic:
IV/IM/SubQ/PO: Adults, elderly: 100 mg 4 times/day. Increased dosage intervals in pts w/renal or hepatic impairment.

SIDE EFFECTS

FREQUENT: Nausea, dizziness. **OCCASIONAL:** Constipation, dry mouth, sweating, respiratory depression.

trimetrexate

try-meh-trecks′ate
(Neutrexin)

CLASSIFICATION

Anti-infective

ACTION

Folate antagonist, inhibits enzyme dihydrofolate reductase (DHFR). Disrupts DNA, RNA, protein synthesis causing cell death. Given w/leucovoran. Leucovoran is transported into mammalian cells providing a source of reduced folates needed for normal cellular biosynthesis (leucovoran is prevented from entering *Pneumocystic carinii* organism allowing for cytotoxicity of trimetrexate).

USES

Treatment of moderate-to-severe *Pneumocystis carinii* pneumonia (PCP) in immunocompromised pts (given w/leucovoran).

INDICATIONS/DOSAGE/ROUTES

PCP:
IV INFUSION: Adults: 45 mg/m^2 over 60-90 min daily for 21 days. Dosage modified in pts w/hematologic toxicity.

SIDE EFFECTS

FREQUENT: Fever, rash/pruritus, neutropenia, thrombocytopenia, anemia, increased SGOT (AST), SGPT (ALT), hyponatremia. **OCCASIONAL:** Nausea, vomiting, confusion, fatigue, increased alkaline phosphatase.

valacyclovir

val-ah-sigh′klo-veer
(Valtrex)

CLASSIFICATION

Antiviral

ACTION

Prodrug of acyclovir. Converted

to acyclovir triphosphate, becoming part of DNA chain, interfering w/DNA synthesis and viral replication. Virustatic.

USES

Treatment of shingles and herpes.

INDICATIONS/DOSAGE/ROUTES

Antiviral:
PO: Adults: 1000 mg 2-3 times/day.

SIDE EFFECTS

FREQUENT: Nausea, vomiting. **OCCASIONAL:** Headache, diarrhea, stomach pain, rash.

vigabatrin

vig-ah-bay'trin
(Sabril)

CLASSIFICATION

Anticonvulsant

ACTION

Appears to increase brain GABA levels by inhibiting GABA metabolism. May also decrease excitation-related amino acids, aspartate, glutamate, and glutamine concentrations in brain.

USES

Treatment of complex partial seizures. Less effective against primary generalized seizures.

INDICATIONS/DOSAGE/ROUTES

Anticonvulsant:
PO: Adults, elderly: 1-4 Gm/day in divided doses. **Children:** 50-150 mg/kg/day in divided doses.

SIDE EFFECTS

FREQUENT: Adults: Somnolence, fatigue, irritability, dizziness, headache, depression, confusion, lack of concentration, abdominal pain, anorexia. **Children:** Insomnia, agitation.

vinorelbine

vin-oh-rell'bean
(Navelbine)

CLASSIFICATION

Antineoplastic

ACTION

Cell cycle–specific antimitotic agent. Disrupts mitotic microtubules. Inhibits cell division.

USES

Treatment of metastatic breast cancer, non-small cell lung cancer, ovarian cancer, Hodgkin's disease.

INDICATIONS/DOSAGE/ROUTES

NOTE: Dosage individualized based on clinical response, tolerance to adverse effects. When used in combination therapy, consult specific protocols for optimum dosage, sequence of drug administration.

Antineoplastic:
IV: Adults, elderly: 30 mg/m^2 weekly.

SIDE EFFECTS

FREQUENT: Myelosuppression, peripheral neurotoxicity, constipation, loss of deep tendon reflexes, diarrhea, stomatitis, injection site reactions, nausea, vomiting, alopecia.